# Reproduction in Farm Animals

## 7th Edition

# Reproduction in Farm Animals
# 7th Edition

Edited by
**B. Hafez/E.S.E. Hafez**
*Co-Directors*
*Reproductive Health Center*
*IVF/Andrology International*
*Kiawah Island, South Carolina, USA*

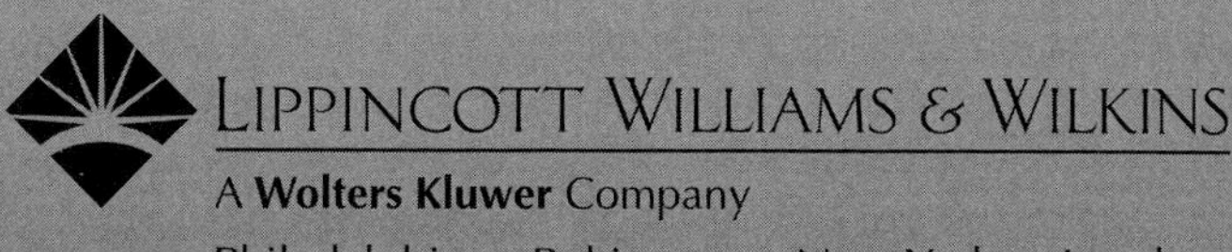


Philadelphia • Baltimore • New York • London
Buenos Aires • Hong Kong • Sydney • Tokyo

*Editor:* Donna Balado
*Managing Editor:* Karen Gulliver
*Marketing Manager:* Annie Smith
*Production Editor:* Paula C. Williams



351 West Camden Street
Baltimore, Maryland 21201-2436 USA

530 Walnut Street
Philadelphia, Pennsylvania 19106-3621 USA



*Printed in the United States of America*

First Edition, 1962
Japanese translation, 1965
Spanish translation, 1967
Second Edition, 1968
Japanese translation, 1971
Third Edition, 1974
Fourth Edition, 1980
Reprinted, 1982
Portuguese translation, 1982
Italian translation, 1985
Fifth Edition, 1987
Japanese translation, 1992
Spanish translation, 1992
Sixth Edition, 1993

**Library of Congress Cataloging-in-Publication Data**

Reproduction in farm animals / edited by B. Hafez, E.S.E. Hafez.—7th ed.
p. cm.
Includes bibliographical references.
ISBN 0-683-30577-8
1. Livestock—Reproduction. 2. Veterinary physiology. I. Hafez, B. II. Hafez, E. S. E. (Elsayed Saad Eldin), 1922–

SF871.R47 2000
636.089'26—dc21 99-053783

*The publishers have made every effort to trace the copyright holders for borrowed material. If they have inadvertently overlooked any, they will be pleased to make the necessary arrangements at the first opportunity.*

To purchase additional copies of this book, call our customer service department at **(800) 638-3030** or fax orders to **(301) 824-7390.** International customers should call **(301) 714-2324.**

04 05 06 07
2 3 4 5 6 7 8 9 10

# PREFACE

The first edition, published in 1962, covered the basic and comparative aspects of reproductive physiology in a simplified manner to meet the needs of students in reproductive biology, veterinary medicine, and animal sciences. This objective is maintained in the seventh edition, which represents a condensed, concise treatise on the physiology and biochemistry of reproduction of farm animals. The book is divided into major sections and these, in turn, are loosely arrayed into two domains, the components of the reproductive system and the regulation of the reproductive process, from the control of ovulation to the initiation of parturition. The reader will note the profound differences among the various animal species. To address this issue we provided separate coverage of the major species, where this seemed appropriate, so that the student of reproduction could ascertain the similarities and differences among them.

During the past decade there were significant advances in the main concepts of animal reproduction as a result of modern biotechnology, such as the use of gonadotropin releasing hormones and their analogs, assisted reproductive technology/andrology (ARTA), genetics, molecular biology, immunology, toxicology, and pharmacology. Five new chapters have been added to the 7th edition:

1. Reproduction in Llamas and Alpacas
2. Genetic Engineering
3. Pharmacotoxologic Factors and Reproduction
4. Immunology of Reproduction
5. Molecular Biology of Reproduction

Modern techniques of bioengineering of farm animals involve microinsemination, recombination of DNA, and *in vitro* manipulation, transfer, and expression of genes. These techniques were greatly improved with the use of computers, microcomputers, and commercially available diagnostic and analytical kits. A wide variety of techniques have been employed for the evaluation of semen, such as: evaluation of sperm fertilizability using zona-free hamster egg (fresh or frozen); motility pattern as viewed by videotape microscopy; *in vitro* penetrability of sperm in bovine cervical mucus; and cryopreservation of embryos and semen using computerized freezers. Most of the investigations reviewed in this edition are based more on holistic research than on research at the submicroscopic or molecular level. However, the excitement generated by recent advances in molecular biology and development tend to downgrade the value of whole-animal research. No attempt was made to provide a detailed bibliography, but a selected number of classic papers and review articles are listed at the end of each chapter.

This edition could not have been revised without the cooperation of the contributing authors and their willingness to follow the editorial guidelines. The chapters have been concisely edited, and the major concepts have been summarized in tables supplemented by line drawings and scanning electron micrographs. All chapters have been completely revised and condensed. There have been numerous deletions from the sixth edition, as well as integration of new and modern concepts such as "growth factors," molecular biology, genetics, and *in vitro* micromanipulation of gametes and embryos.

Some tabulated appendices include: chromosome numbers and reproductive ability of bovine, caprinae, and equine species and some of their hybrids; preparation of physiologic solutions, sperm stains, tissue culture media, and cryoprotectants. These appendices proved to be helpful for staging demonstrations, laboratory exercises, and training workshops for teachers, laboratory technicians, and students. It is hoped that the seventh edition will be of some help to undergraduate students in animal sciences and veterinary medicine.

B. Hafez/E.S.E. Hafez
Kiawah Island, South Carolina USA
March, 2000

# Acknowledgments

Included in the seventh edition, the contributions and the valuable information were provided by: S.E. Abdelgadir, L.L. Anderson, A.E. Archibong, R.L. Ax, M. Dally, B.A. Didion, D.P. Froman, D.L. Garner, R.D. Geisett, P.J. Hansen, J.D. Kirby, S.S. Koide, R.W. Lenz, C.C. Love, J.R. Malayer, J.A. Proudman, J. Sumar, D.D. Varner, H. Wahid, and Professor M.R. Jainudeen, my friend and long-time associate, who has contributed greatly to the improvement of the table of contents and detailed structure of several chapters. Sincere thanks are due to Ms. Donna Balado and Crystal Taylor of Lippincott Williams & Wilkins for their meticulous and painstaking efforts during the preparation of the book. Special thanks are also due to Vice President Timothy Satterfield for his excellent cooperation and continued interest in the development of animal and veterinary sciences.

# Contributors

***S.E. Abdelgadir***
Asst. Professor of Reproduction Endocrinology/Infertility
Director of Andrology/Embryology
Department of OB/GYN
University of Nevada School of Medicine
Las Vegas, Nevada 89102 USA

***L.L. Anderson***
Department of Animal Science
Iowa State University
11 Kildee Hall
Ames, Iowa 50011 USA

***A.E. Archibong***
Director of Andrology/Research
Department of OB/GYN and
Asst. Professor
Department of Anatomy/Physiology
Meharry Medical College
Nashville, Tennessee 37208 USA
615-327-6284 (Tel) 615-327-6296 (Fax)

**R.L. *Ax*, Ph.D.**
Professor and Head Department of Animal Science
Adjunct Professor
Department of OB/GYN
University of Arizona
Tucson, Arizona 85721-00038 USA
520-621-7623 (Tel) 520-621-9435 (Fax)

**M.R. *Dally*, Ph.D.**
Professor of Animal Science
Hopland Research and Extension Center
University of California
Hopland, California 95449 USA

**B.A. *Didion*, Ph.D.**
Dekalb Swine Breeders, Inc.
3100 Sycamore Road
Dekalb, Illinois 60115 USA

***D.P. Froman***
Department of Animal Sciences
Oregon State University
112 Withycombe Hall
Corvallis, Oregon 97331-6702 USA
541-737-5060 (Tel) 541-737-4174 (Fax)

***D.L. Garner***
Department of Animal Science
School of Veterinary Medicine
University of Nevada
Mail Stop 202, Reno, Nevada 89557-0104 USA
702-784-6135 (Tel) 702-784-1375 (Fax)

***R.D. Geisert***
Division of Agricultural Sciences and Natural Resources
Department of Animal Sciences
114 Animal Science
Oklahoma State University
Stillwater, Oklahoma 74078-6051 USA
405-744-6077 (Tel) 405-744-7390 (Fax)

***B. Hafez***
Reproductive Health Center
78 Surfsong Road
Kiawah Island, South Carolina 29455 USA
843-768-5556 (Tel) 843-768-6494 (Fax)

***E.S.E. Hafez***
Reproductive Health Center
IVF Andrology Laboratory
78 Surfsong Road
Kiawah Island, South Carolina 29455 USA
843-768-5556 (Tel) 843-768-6494 (Fax)
Ivfreprod@aol.com (e-mail)

***P.J. Hansen***
Department of Dairy/Poultry Sciences
Institute of Food and Agricultural Sciences
University of Florida
Bldg. 499, Shealy Drive
PO Box 110920
Gainesville, Florida 32611-0920 USA
352-393-5590 (Tel) 352-392-5595 (Fax)

***M.R. Jainudeen***
University Business Centre
University Administration Building
43400 UPM
Serdang, Selangor, Malaysia
603-948-5649 (Tel/Fax)
(Home Address)
60 Jalan SS 19/5B
47500 Subang Jaya, Selangor, Malaysia
603-734-5694 (Tel/Fax)
jain@pop.jaring (e-mail)

***R. Juneja***
8402 Timberline Court
Monmouth Junction, New Jersey 08852 USA
732-422-8895 (Tel) 732-940-5711 (Fax)
ARJuneja@aol.com (e-mail)

***J.D. Kirby***
Dept. of Animal Sciences
Oregon State University
112 Withycombe Hall
Corvallis, Oregon 97331-6702 USA
541-737-5060 (Tel) 541-737-4174 (Fax)

***S.S. Koide***
Population Council
1230 York Avenue
New York, New York 10021 USA
212-327-8731 (Tel) 212-327-7678 (Fax)

***R.W. Lenz, Ph.D.***
Sire Power, Inc.
R.R.2
Tunkhannock, Pennsylvania 18657 USA

***C.C. Love, D.V.M., Ph.D.***
Diplomate
American College of Theriogenology
Department of Large Animal Medicine & Surgery
College of Veterinary Medicine
Texas A&M University
College Station, Texas 77843-4475 USA

***J.R. Malayer***
Division of Agricultural Sciences and Natural Resources
Department of Animal Science
114 Animal Science
Oklahoma State University
Stillwater, Oklahoma 74078-6051 USA
405-744-6077 (Tel) 405-744-7390 (Fax)

***C.A. Pinkert***
The University of Alabama at Birmingham
Department of Comparative Medicine
227 Volker Hall
1670 University Boulevard
Birmingham, Alabama 35294-0019 USA
205-934-9574 (Tel) 205-975-4390 (Fax)
Pinkert@uab.edu (e-mail)

***J.A. Proudman***
Research Physiologist
Germplasm and Gamete Physiology Laboratory
Livestock and Poultry Sciences Institute
BARC-East
Building 262
Beltsville, Maryland 20705 USA
301-504-8094 (Tel) 301-504-8546 (Fax)
JohnP@lpsi.barc.usda.gov (e-mail)

***J.B. Sumar***
Avenida De Los Incas 1412
Wanchaq, Cusco, Peru
51 (84) 224 614 (Tel) 51 (84) 221 632 (Fax)

***D.D. Varner, D.V.M., M.S.***
Diplomate
American College of Theriogenology
Department of Large Animal Medicine & Surgery
College of Veterinary Medicine
Texas A&M University
College Station, Texas 77843-4475 USA

***H. Wahid***
Department of Veterinary Science
Clinical Studies
University Putra
Malaysia, 43400
Serdang, Selangor, Malaysia
603-948-6101 X1829 (Tel) 603-948-6317 (Fax)
wahid@vet.upm.edu.my (e-mail)

# Contents

# Part I

# *Functional Anatomy of Reproduction*

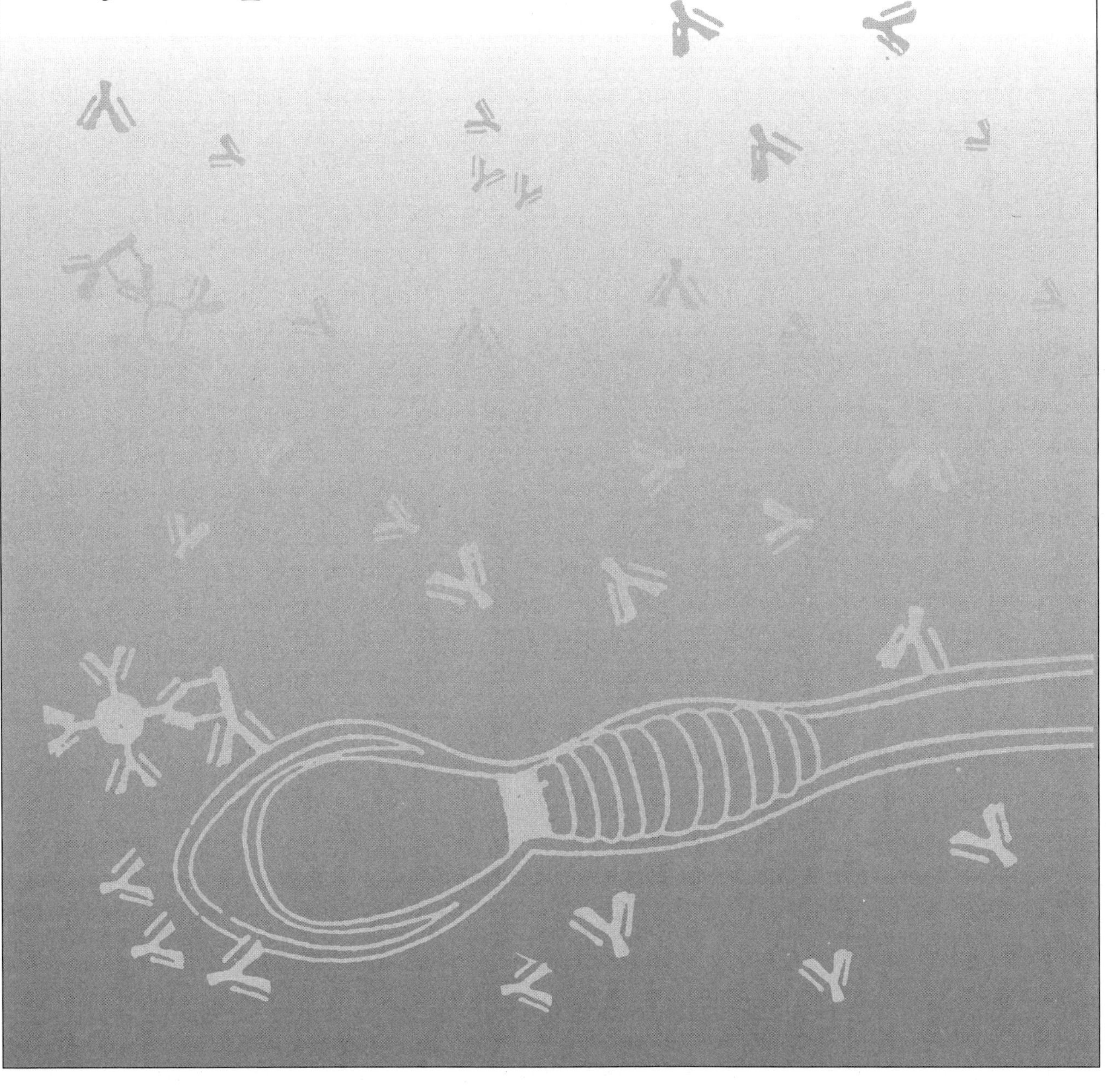

CHAPTER 1

# Anatomy of Male Reproduction

E.S.E. HAFEZ

The male gonads, the testes, lie outside the abdomen within the scrotum, which is a purselike structure derived from the skin and fascia of the abdominal wall. Each testis lies within the vaginal process, a separate extension of the peritoneum, which passes through the abdominal wall at the inguinal canal. The deep and superficial inguinal rings are the deep and superficial openings of the inguinal canal. Blood vessels and nerves reach the testis in the spermatic cord, which lies within the vaginal process; the *ductus deferens* accompanies the vessels but leaves them at the orifice of the vaginal process to join the urethra. Besides permitting the passage of the vaginal process and its contents, the inguinal canal also gives passage to vessels and nerves supplying the external genitalia.

The spermatozoa leave the testis by efferent ductules that lead into the coiled duct of the epididymis, which continues as the straight ductus deferens. Accessory glands discharge their contents into the ductus deferens or into the pelvic portion of the urethra.

The urethra originates at the neck of the bladder. Throughout its length it is surrounded by cavernous vascular tissue. Its pelvic portion, which is enclosed by striated urethral muscle and receives secretions from various glands, leads into a second penile portion at the pelvic outlet. Here it is joined by two more cavernous bodies to make up the body of the penis, which lies beneath the skin of the body wall. A number of muscles grouped around the pelvic outlet contribute to the root of the penis. The apex or free part of the penis is covered by modified skin—the penile integument; in the resting condition it is enclosed within the prepuce. The topographic features of the organs of the important farm species are shown in Figure 1-1.

The testis and epididymis are supplied with blood from the testicular artery, which originates from the dorsal aorta near the embryonic site of the testes. The internal pudendal artery supplies the pelvic genitalia and its branches leave the pelvis at the ischial arch to supply the penis. The external pudendal artery leaves the abdominal cavity via the inguinal canal to supply the penis, scrotum, and prepuce. Lymph from the testis and epididymis passes to the lumbar aortic lymph nodes. Lymph from the accessory glands, urethra, and penis passes to the sacral and medial iliac nodes. Lymph from the scrotum, prepuce, and peripenile tissues drains to the superficial inguinal lymph nodes.

Afferent and efferent (sympathetic) nerves accompany the testicular artery to the testis. The pelvic plexus supplies autonomic (sympathetic and parasympathetic) fibers to the pelvic genitalia and to the smooth muscles of the penis. Sacral nerves supply motor fibers to the striated muscles of the penis and sensory fibers to the free part of the penis. Afferent fibers from the scrotum and prepuce travel mainly in the genitofemoral nerve.

## DEVELOPMENT

### *Prenatal Development*

The testes develop in the abdomen, medial to the embryonic kidney (mesonephros). The plexus of ducts within the testis becomes connected to mesonephric tubules and so to the mesonephric duct, to form the epididymis, ductus deferens, and vesicular gland. The prostate and bulbourethral glands form from the embryonic urogenital sinus and the penis forms by tubulation and elongation of a tubercle that develops at the orifice of the urogenital sinus.

Two agents produced by the fetal testis are responsible for this differentiation and development (1). Fetal androgen causes development of the male reproductive tract. "Müllerian inhibiting substance," a glycoprotein, is responsible for suppression of the paramesonephric (Müllerian) ducts from which the uterus and vagina develop (2). Abnormalities in differentiation and development of gonads and ducts can result in varying degrees of intersexuality (3).

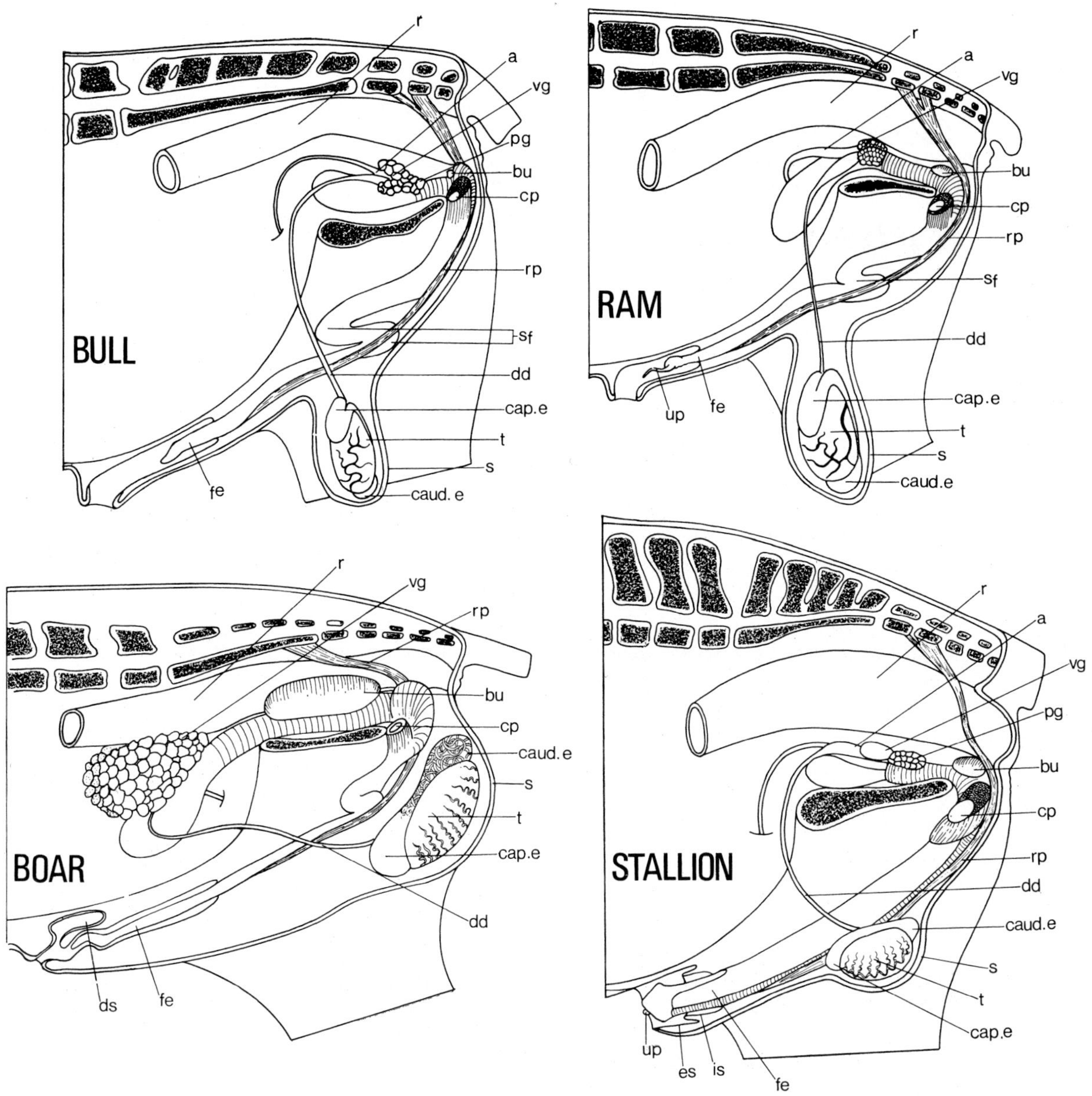


FIGURE 1-1. Diagram of the male reproductive tracts as seen in left lateral dissections. *a*, Ampulla; *bu*, bulbourethral gland; *cap. e*, caput epididymidis, *caud. e*, cauda epididymidis; *cp*, left crus of penis, severed from the left ischium; *dd*, ductus deferens; *ds*, dorsal diverticulum of prepuce; *es*, prepenile prepuce; *fe*, free part of the penis; *is*, preputial fold; *pg*, prostate gland; *r*, rectum; *rp*, retractor penis muscle; *s*, scrotum; *sf*, sigmoid flexure; *t*, testis; *up*, urethral process; *vg*, vesicular gland. (Adapted from Popesko, Atlas der topographischen anatomie der Haustiere. Vol. 3, Jena: Fischer, 1968.)

## *Descent of the Testis*

During testicular descent (4), the gonad migrates caudally within the abdomen to the deep inguinal ring. It then traverses the abdominal wall to emerge at the superficial inguinal ring, which is, in fact, the much-enlarged foramen of the genitofemoral nerve (L3, L4). The testis completes its migration by passing fully into the scrotum. Descent is preceded by the formation of the vaginal process, a peritoneal sac extending through the abdominal wall and enclosing the inguinal ligament of the testis. The inguinal ligament of the gonad is often called the *gubernaculum testis*, and it terminates in the region of the scrotal rudiments. Descent follows the line of the *gubernaculum testis*. The time of descent varies (Table 1-1). In the horse, the epididymis commonly enters the inguinal canal before the testis, and that part of the inguinal ligament connecting testis and epididymis (proper ligament of testis) remains extensive until after birth.

TABLE 1-1. *Development of the Male Reproductive Tract in Farm Animals (weeks)*

| | BULL | RAM | BOAR | STALLION |
|---|---|---|---|---|
| Primary spermatocytes | | | | |
| In seminiferous tubules | 24 | 12 | 10 | Variable throughout seminiferous tubules of each testis |
| Sperm in seminiferous tubules | 32 | 16 | 20 | 56 |
| Sperm in cauda epididymidis | 40 | 16 | 20 | 60 |
| Sperm in ejaculate | 42 | 18 | 22 | 64–96 |
| Completion of separation between penis and penile part of prepuce | 32 | >10 | 20 | 4 |
| Age at which animal can be considered sexually "mature" | 150 | >24 | 30 | 90–150 (variable) |

Testicular descent enters scrotum half-way through fetal life (bull, ram), last quarter of fetal life (boar), or just before/after birth (stallion).

Sometimes the testis fails to enter the scrotum. In this condition (cryptorchidism), the special thermal needs of testis and epididymis are not met, although the endocrine function of the testis is unimpaired. Bilaterally cryptorchid males therefore show more or less normal sexual desire but are sterile. Occasionally some of the abdominal viscera pass through the orifice of the vaginal process and enter the scrotum; scrotal hernia is particularly common in pigs.

### *Postnatal Development*

Each component of the reproductive tracts of all farm animals grows in size relative to overall body size and undergoes histologic differentiation. Functional competence is not achieved simultaneously in all components of the reproductive system. Thus, in the bull, the capacity for erection of the penis precedes the appearance of sperm in the ejaculate by several months. In rams, the terminal segment of the epididymis is morphologically "adult" at 6 weeks, but the initial segment is not so until 18 weeks (5). At puberty all the components of the male reproductive system have reached a sufficiently advanced stage of development for the system as a whole to be functional. The period of rapid development that precedes puberty is known as the prepubertal period, although this period is itself sometimes referred to as "puberty." During the postpubertal period, development continues and the reproductive tract reaches full sexual maturity months or even years after the age of puberty. In horses, significant increases in testicular weight, daily sperm production, and epididymal sperm reserves occur at 15 years of age. Some important anatomic changes that occur during postnatal development are summarized in Table 1-1.

## TESTIS AND SCROTUM

The testis is secured to the wall of the vaginal process along the line of its epididymal attachment. The position in the scrotum and the orientation of the long axis of the testis differ with the species (Fig. 1-1). The arrangement of tubules and ducts within the testis in the bull is shown in Figure 1-2. The histologic and cytologic characteristics of the cellular components of the seminiferous tubules are summarized in Table 1-2. The rete testis is lined by a nonsecretory cuboidal epithelium.

Testicular size varies throughout the year in seasonal breeders (ram, stallion, camel). Removal of one testis results in considerable enlargement of the remaining gonad (up to 80% increase in weight). In the unilateral cryptorchid, removal of the descended testis may be followed by descent of the abdominal testis as it enlarges.

The interstitial (Leydig) cells, which lie between the seminiferous tubules, secrete male hormones into the testicular veins and lymphatic vessels. The spermatogenic cells of the tubule divide and differentiate to form spermatozoa. Just before puberty, the sustentacular (Sertoli) cells of the tubule form a barrier (6), which isolates the differentiating germ cells from the general circulation. These sustentacular cells contribute to fluid production by the tubule and may

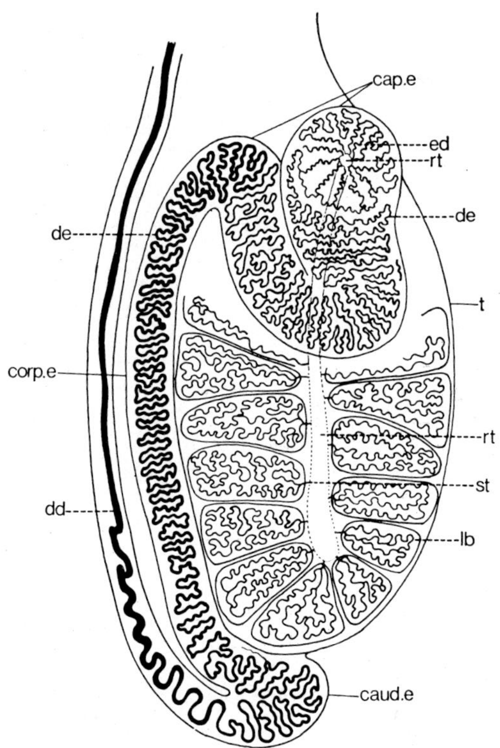


FIGURE 1-2. Schematic drawing of the tubular system of the testis and epididymis in the bull (for clarity the duct system of the rete testis is omitted). *cap. e*, Caput epididymidis; *caud. e*, cauda epididymidis; *corp. e*, corpus epididymidis; *dd*, ductus deferens; *de*, duct of the epididymis; *ed.*, efferent ductule; *lb*, lobule with seminiferous tubules; *rt*, rete testis; *st*, straight tubule; *t*, testis. (Simplified from Blom and Christensen. Nord Vet Med 1968;12:453.)

produce the Müllerian-inhibiting factor found in the rete fluid of adult males (2). The sustentacular cells do not increase in numbers after puberty is attained. This may limit spermiogenesis. Sperm production increases with age in the postpubertal period and is subject to seasonal changes in many species. Castration of prepubertal males suppresses sexual development. Regressive changes in behavior and structure take place following castration of adult males. Castration is a standard procedure in animal husbandry to modify aggressive male behavior and to eliminate undesirable carcass qualities, e.g., boar taint.

Spermatogenesis disorders are monitored by changes in sperm parameters in the ejaculate or by infertility. Turner et al, (7) conducted extensive studies to identify the proteins which play major roles in spermatogenesis and are subsequently transported into the blood stream.

Autonomic innervation of the testis plays a major role in regulating the functions of the male genitourinary tract. Adrenergic, cholinergic, and nonadrenergic noncholinergic (NANC) mechanisms operate in a highly orchestrated fashion to ensure reliable storage and release of urine from the bladder to regulate the transport and storage of sperm in

TABLE 1-2. ***Functional Histology of the Mammalian Testis***

| SEGMENT | HISTOLOGIC CHARACTERISTICS |
|---|---|
| Tunica albuginea | A thick, white capsule of connective tissue surrounding the testis; made primarily of interlacing series of collagenous fiber. |
| Seminiferous tubules | Appear as large isolated structures, round or oblong in outline; varying appearance due to the complex coiling of the tubules at many different angles and levels. Between the tubules are masses of interstitial (Leydig) cells, which produce the male sex hormones. |
| Spermatogonia | Lie in the outermost region of the tubule; round nuclei appear as an irregular layer within surrounding connective tissue. Nuclei are small size and dark stain due to presence of large numbers of chromatin granules. |
| Primary spermatocytes | Located just inside an irregular layer of spermatogonia and Sertoli cells; nuclei are larger than those of the spermatogonia and stain lighter. |
| Secondary spermatocytes | Maturation divisions and secondary spermatocytes are not seen in the average tubule owing to the short duration of these stages. |
| Spermatids | Located internally to primary spermatocytes. Layer of spermatids may be several cells in thickness. Sperm lie along the border of the lumen. The sperm heads are lodged in deep indentations of the surface of the Sertoli cell. |
| Sertoli cells | Large and relatively clear except for the prominent, dark-staining nucleolus. Cytoplasm is diffuse, and its limits are indefinite. |

the reproductive tract and coordinate the emission/ejaculation of the sex accessory glands (8).

The adrenergic innervation may play a role in mediating epididymal function. The sympathetic innervation within the epididymis is necessary for neuromuscular events required for the transport of sperm. The neuronal input may play an important role in the maintenance of epididymal function (8).

### *Thermoregulation of the Testis*

For effective functioning, the mammalian testes must be maintained at a temperature lower than that of the body. Anatomic features of the testis and scrotum permit the regulation of testicular temperature. Temperature receptors in the scrotal skin can elicit responses that tend to lower *whole* body temperature and provoke panting and sweating (9). The scrotal skin is richly endowed with large adrenergic sweat glands, and its muscular (dartos) component enables it to alter the thickness and surface area of the scrotum and vary the closeness of the contact of the testes with the body wall. In the horse, this action may be supported by the smooth muscle within the spermatic cord and tunica albuginea, which can lower or raise the testis. In cold conditions, these smooth muscles contract, elevating the testes and wrinkling and thickening the scrotal wall. In hot conditions the muscles relax, lowering the testes within the thin-walled pendulous scrotum. The advantages offered by these mechanisms are enhanced by the special relationship of the veins and arteries.

In all farm animals, the testicular artery is a convoluted structure in the form of a cone, the base of which rests on the cranial or dorsal pole of the testis. These arterial coils are intimately enmeshed by the so-called pampiniform plexus of testicular veins (10). In this countercurrent mechanism, arterial blood entering the testis is cooled by the venous blood leaving the testis. In the ram, blood in the testicular artery falls 4 °C in its course from the superficial inguinal ring to the surface of the testis; the blood in the veins is warmed to a similar degree between the testis and the superficial ring. The position of the arteries and veins close to the surface of the testis tends to increase direct loss of heat from the testis. In the boar, the scrotum is less pendulous (Fig. 1-1) and sweating is less efficient. This may explain the smaller difference between scrotal and rectal temperatures (3.2 °C) (11).

## EPIDIDYMIS AND DUCTUS DEFERENS

Three anatomic parts of the epididymis are recognized (Fig. 1-2). The caput epididymidis (head), in which a variable number of efferent ductules (13 to 20) (12) join the duct of the epididymis. It forms a flattened structure applied to one pole of the testis. The narrow corpus epididymidis (body) terminates at the opposite pole in the expanded cauda epididymidis (tail). The middle region of each efferent duct shows marked secretory activity (13). The convoluted duct of the epididymis is very long (bull, 36 m; boar, 54 m). The wall of the duct of the epididymis has a prominent layer of circular muscle fibers and a pseudostratified epithelium of columnar cells. Three segments of the duct of the epididymis can be distinguished histologically; these do not coincide with the gross anatomic regions (14).

There is a progressive decrease in the height of the epithelium and stereocilia and a widening of the lumen throughout the three segments. The first two segments are concerned with sperm maturation, whereas the terminal segment is for sperm storage.

The lumen of the epididymal tubules is lined with epithelium made of a basal layer of small cells and a surface layer of tall columnar ciliated cells.

The mucosa of the ductus deferens is thrown into longitudinal folds. Near the epididymal end, the epithelium resembles that of the epididymis: the nonciliated cells have little secretory activity. The lumen is lined with pseudostratified epithelium. The ampulla of the ductus deferens is furnished with branched tubular glands, which, in the stallion, are highly developed and contribute ergothioneine to the ejaculate. The ejaculatory duct enters the urethra. Fluid uptake and spermiophagy take place in the epithelium of the ejaculatory duct (15). Scanning electron microscopy has been used to evaluate functional ultrastructure of male reproductive organs with emphasis on spermatogenesis (Fig. 1-3). Large volumes of fluid (up to 60 ml in the ram) leave the testis daily, and most of this is absorbed in the caput epididymidis by the initial segment of the duct of the epididymis. Transport of sperm through the epididymis takes about 9 to 13 days. Maturation of sperm occurs during transmit through the epididymis; motility increases as sperm enter the corpus epididymidis. The environment of the sperm in the cauda epididymidis provides factors that enhance fertilizing ability. Sperm from this region give higher fertility than those from the corpus epididymidis (14).

Spermatozoa stored in the epididymis retain fertilizing capacity for several weeks; the cauda epididymidis is the principal storage organ, and it contains about 75% of the total epididymal spermatozoa. The special ability of the cauda epididymidis to store sperm depends on low scrotal temperatures and on the action of male sex hormone (16). Sperm stored in the ampullae constitute only a small part of the total extra-gonadal sperm reserves. Small numbers of nonmotile sperm appear in ejaculates collected weeks or even months after castration.

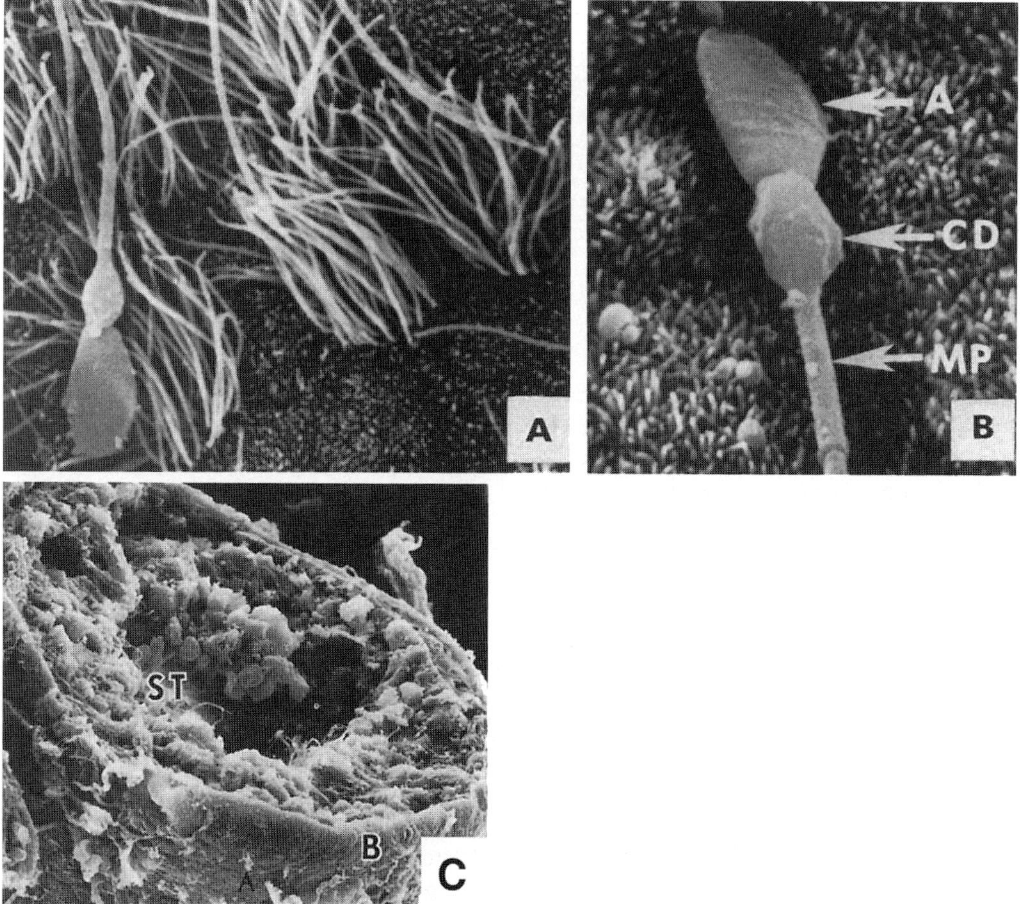


FIGURE 1-3. Scanning electron micrographs (SEM) (**A**) Luminal surface of an efferent duct with ciliated and nonciliated cells and a sperm. (**B**) Short microvilli on the luminal surface of nonciliated cells in the efferent ducts. The spermatozoal cytoplasmic droplet (*CD*), acrosome (*A*), and middle piece (*MP*) are distinguishable (×6,500). (**C**) Cross section of a seminiferous tubule (*ST*). Note several "stages" of spermatogenesis, encased in a muscular boundry tissue. (**A** and **B** from Connell CJ. Spermatogenesis. In: Hafez ESE, ed. Scanning Electron Microscopy of Human Reproduction. Ann Arbor, MI: Ann Arbor Science Pubs, 1978. **C** courtesy of Dr. Larry Johnson, from Johnson L, et al. Am J Vet Res 1978.)

## ACCESSORY GLANDS

The prostate and bulbourethral glands pour their secretions into the urethra, where at the time of ejaculation, they are mixed with the fluid suspension of sperm and ampullary secretions from the ductus deferens. Weber et al (17) have demonstrated volumetric changes in the accessory glands of the stallion resulting from sexual stimulation (increased volume) and ejaculation (reduced volume).

### *Comparative Anatomy*

THE SEMINAL VESICLES. These lie laterally to the terminal parts of each ductus deferens. In ruminants, they are compact lobulated glands. In the boar, they are large and less compact. In the stallion, they are large pyriform glandular sacs. The duct of the seminal vesicles and the ductus deferens may share a common ejaculatory duct that opens into the urethra.

THE PROSTATE GLAND. A distinct lobulated external part of body lies outside the thick urethral muscle, and a second internal or disseminated part surrounds the pelvic urethra. The disseminate prostate extends caudally as far as the ducts of the bulbourethral glands. The body of the prostate is small in the bull and large in the boar. In the stallion, the prostate gland is wholly external.

THE BULBOURETHRAL GLANDS. These are dorsal to the urethra near the termination of its pelvic portion. In the bull they are almost hidden by the bulbospongiosus muscle. They are large in the boar and contribute the gel-like component of boar semen. In ruminants and the boar, the ducts of the bulbourethral glands open into urethral recesses (18).

**THE URETHRAL GLANDS.** The bull lacks urethral glands comparable with those found in man (19). Glands of this name in the horse have been considered comparable to the disseminate prostate of ruminants.

### *Function*

Apart from providing liquid vehicle for the transport of sperm, the function of the accessory glands is obscure although much is known about the specific chemical agents contributed by the glands to the ejaculate (20, 21). Fructose and citric acid are important components of seminal vesicle secretions of domestic ruminants. Citric acid alone is found in stallion seminal vesicle; boar seminal vesicle also contain little fructose and are characterized by a high content of ergothioneine and inositol.

Spermatozoa from the cauda epididymidis are capable of fertilization when inseminated without the addition of

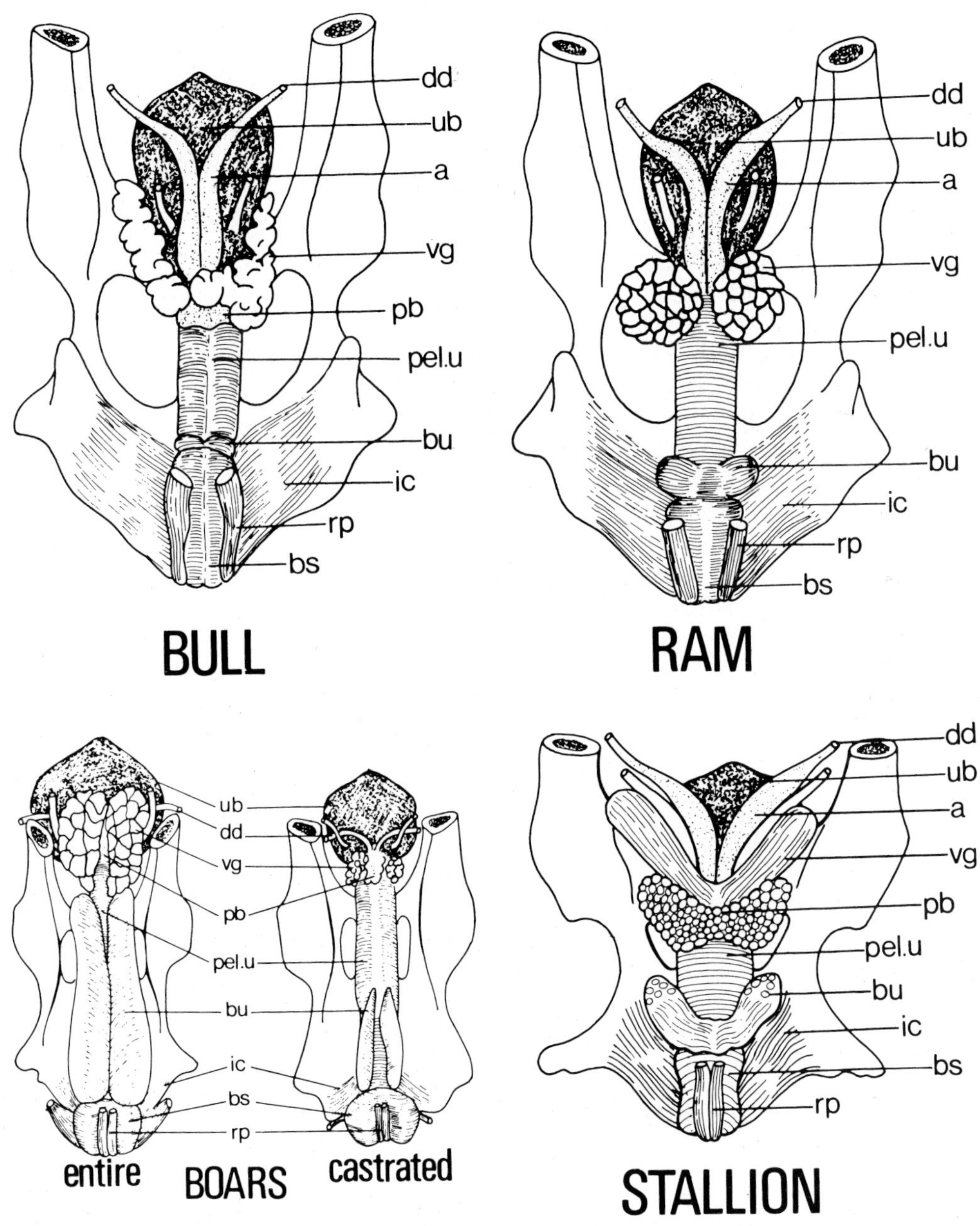


FIGURE 1-4. The pelvic genitalia, within the pelvic bones, as seen from a dorsal view. *a*, ampulla; *bs*, bulbospongiosus muscle; *bu*, bulbourethral gland; *dd*, ductus deferens; *ic*, ischiocavernosus muscle; *pb*, body of prostate gland; *pel. u*, pelvic urethra; *rp*, retractor penis muscle; *ub*, urinary bladder; *vg*, vesicular gland. (Diagrams of bull, boar and stallion redrawn from Nickel R. Tierarztl Umschau 1954;9:386.)

accessory gland secretions. The gel-like fraction of the boar ejaculate forms a plug in the vagina of mated females. In commercial insemination practice, this fraction is removed from the semen by filtration.

In large animals, rectal palpation of some of the accessory glands is possible. The positions of these glands relative to the bony pelvis are shown in Figure 1-4.

In the pig, the size of the bulbourethral glands can be used to differentiate the cryptorchid from the castrated state. After prepubertal castration, the bulbourethral glands are small. In boars with retained testes, the glands are of normal size (22). These differences can easily be felt, ventral to the rectum, with a finger inserted through the anus.

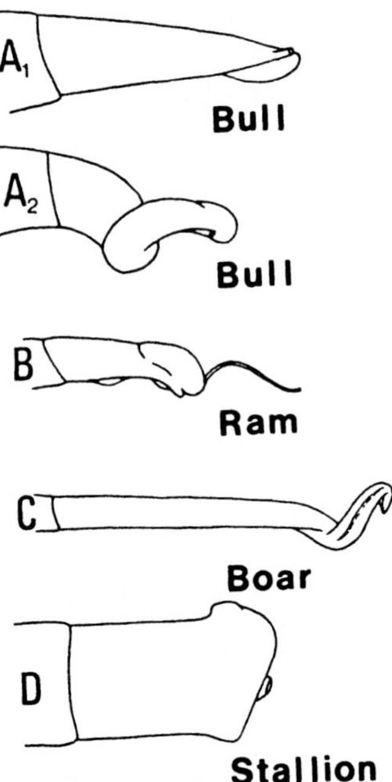


FIGURE 1-5. Diagrams to show the shape of the free end of the penis. (A1) The shape of the penis just before intromission. (A2) The shape after intromission when spiral deviation has occurred. (B) The shape of the penis during natural service. (C) Does not show the full degree of spiralling that occurs during service. (D) Drawn after injection and shows enlargement of the erectile bodies. (A1, A2, and B from photographs. C and D from fixed specimens. Not drawn to scale.)

## PENIS AND PREPUCE

### *Structure*

In the mammalian penis, three cavernous bodies are aggregated around the penile urethra. The *corpus spongiosum penis*—which surrounds the urethra—is enlarged. This bulb is covered by the striated bulbospongiosus muscle. The corpus cavernosum penis arises as a pair of crura from the ischial arch, which are covered by ischiocavernosus muscles. A thick covering (tunica albuginea) encloses the cavernous bodies. The retractor penis muscles in ruminants and swine control the effective length of the penis by their action on the sigmoid flexure.

In the stallion, the cavernous bodies contain large cavernous spaces; during erection, considerable increases in size result from accumulation of blood in these spaces. In bull, ram, and boar the cavernous spaces of the corpus cavernosum penis is small, except in the crura and at the distal bend of the sigmoid flexure.

In ruminants and swine, the orifice of the prepuce is controlled by the cranial muscle of the prepuce; a caudal muscle may also be present. In the boar there is a large dorsal diverticulum in which urine and epithelial debris accumulate.

### *Erection and Protrusion*

Sexual stimulation produces dilatation of the arteries supplying the cavernous bodies of the penis (especially the crura). Stiffening and straightening of the penis in ruminants is caused by the ischiocavernosus muscle, which pumps blood from the cavernous spaces of the crura into the rest of the corpus cavernosum penis.

Erection failures (impotence) arise from structural defects rather than from psychological causes (23). Rising pressure in the corpus cavernosum penis produces considerable elongation of the ruminant and porcine penis with little dilation (24). When the penis of the bull is protruded, the prepuce is everted and stretched over the protruded organ.

In normal service, this occurs after intromission. If it occurs before the penis enters the vestibule, intromission cannot be achieved.

Intromission in the bull lasts for about 2 seconds, and straightening of the penis after withdrawal often occurs abruptly as the dorsal apical ligament reasserts its action in keeping the penis straight. Withdrawal into the prepuce follows as the pressure in the cavernous spaces subsides. The fibrous architecture of the corpus cavernosum penis in the region of the sigmoid flexure tends to reform the flexure; this is assisted by shortening of the retractor penis muscle. The terminal 5 cm or so of the boar penis are spiraled (Fig. 1-5), and during erection the whole visible length of the free end of the penis becomes spiraled (24). Intromission lasts for up to 7 minutes, during which time a large volume of semen is ejaculated. Spiral deviation does not occur in the ram or goat, and intromission is of short duration. In the horse intromission lasts for several minutes.

### *Emission and Ejaculation*

Emission consists of movement of the spermatic fluid along the ductus deferens to the pelvic urethra, where it is mixed

TABLE 1-3. *Age and Weight of First Breeding and Semen Characteristics*

| | Beginning of Breeding Life | | | Volume of Ejaculate | | Sperm Concentration $10^8$ per ml |
|---|---|---|---|---|---|---|
| Species | *Age (months)* | *Body Weight* | *Range* | *Mean* | *Range* | *Mean* |
| Cat | 9 | 3.5 kg | 0.01–0.3 | 0.04 | 1.5–28 | 14 |
| Dog | 10–12 | varies | 2–25 | 9.0 | 0.6–5.4 | 1.3 |
| Guinea pig | 3–5 | 450 gm | 0.4–0.8 | 0.6 | 0.05–0.2 | 0.1 |
| Rabbit | 4–12 | varies | 0.4–6 | 1.0 | 0.5–3.5 | 1.5 |

From Hamner CE. The semen. In: Hafez ESE, ed. Reproduction and Breeding Techniques for Laboratory Animals. Philadelphia: Lea & Febiger, 1970.

with secretions from the accessory glands. Ejaculation is the passage of the resultant semen along the penile urethra. Emission is brought about by smooth muscles, under the control of the autonomic nervous system. Electrical stimulation of ejaculation in farm animals is a crude imitation of the complex natural mechanisms. During natural service, the sensory nerve endings in the penile integument and the deeper penile tissues are essential to the process of ejaculation.

Passage of semen along the ductus deferens is continual during sexual inactivity. Prinz and Zaneveld (25) suggest that during sexual rest a complex random or cyclic process of sperm removal from the cauda epididymidis may aid the regulation of sperm reserves. Sexual excitement and ejaculation are accompanied by contractions of the cauda epididymidis and ductus deferens, which increase the rate of flow. Overall, the number of sperm passing through the ductus deferens is not increased by sexual activity.

Muscular contraction of the wall of the duct is controlled by sympathetic autonomic nerves of the pelvic plexus derived from the hypogastric nerves. In normal stallions, $\alpha$-receptor stimulation and $\beta$-receptor blockade increase the sperm concentration in the ejaculate (26).

During ejaculation the bulbospongiosus muscle compresses the penile bulb and so pumps blood from the penile bulb into the remainder of the corpus spongiosum penis. Unlike the corpus cavernosum penis, this cavernous body is normally drained by distal veins; peak pressures recorded during ejaculation are much lower than those in the corpus cavernosum penis (27). The waves of pressure passing down the penile urethra may help to transport the ejaculate. Pressure changes in the corpus spongiosum penis during ejaculation are transmitted to the corpus spongiosum glandis; the glans penis enlarges in the ram, goat, and stallion but not in the bull.

## LABORATORY ANIMALS

Species differences in the male reproductive organs are shown in Figure 1-1. These organs can move from a wholly scrotal to a wholly abdominal position. Differences in relative size of the accessory glands are reflected in the semen characteristics (Table 1-3).

## REFERENCES


1. Gondos B. Development and differentiation of the testis and male reproductive tract. In: Steinberger A, Steinberger E, eds. Testicular Development: Structure and Function. New York: Raven Press, 1980.
2. Vigier B, Tran D, duMesuil du Brusson F, Heyman Y, Josso N. Use of monoclonal antibody techniques to study the ontogeny of bovine anti-Müllerian hormone. J Reprod Fertil 1983;69:207.
3. Hare WCD, Singh E. Cytogenetics in animal reproduction. Farnham: Royal Commonwealth Agricultural Bureau, 1979.
4. Wensing CJG. Testicular descent in the rat and a comparison of this process in the rat with that in the pig. Anat Rec 1986;214:154.
5. Nilnophakoon N. Histological studies on the regional postnatal differentiation of the epididymis in the ram. Anat Histol Embryol 1978;7:253.
6. Vazama F, Nishida T, Kurohmara M, Hayashi Y. The fine structure of the blood-testis barrier in the boar. Jap J Vet Sci 1988;50:1259.
7. Turner KJ, McKinnell C, McLaren TT, Qureshi SJ, Saunders TK, Foster MD, Sharpe RM. Detection of germ cell-derived proteins in potential for monitoring spermatogenesis in vivo. J Androl 1996;17:127–136.

8. Ricker D, Chamness SL, Hinton BT, Chang TK. Changes in luminal fluid protein composition in the rat cauda epididymidis following partial sympathetic denervation. 1996;17: 117–126.
9. Robertshaw D, Vercoe JE. Scrotal thermoregulation of the bull. (Bos sp). Aust J Agric Res 1980;31:401.
10. Hees H, Kohler T, Leiser R, Hees I, Lips T. Gefäss-Morphologie des Rinderhodens Licht-und rasterelektron-mikroskopische Studien. Anat Anz 1990;170:119.
11. Stone BA. Thermal characteristics of the testis and epididymis of the boar. J Reprod Fertil 1981;63:551.
12. Hemeida NA, Sack WO, McEntee K. Ductuli efferentes in the epididymis of boar, goat, ram, bull and stallion. Am J Vet Res 1978;39:1892.
13. Goyal HO, Eljack A, Mobini C. Regional differences in the morphology of the ductuli efferentes of the goat. Anat Histol Embryol 1988;17:369.
14. Amann RP. Function of the epididymis in bulls and rams. J Reprod Fertil Suppl 1987;34:115.
15. Abou-Elmagd A, Wrobel KH. The epithelial lining of the bovine ejaculatory, duct. Acta Anat 1990;139:60.
16. Foldesey RG, Bedford JM. Biology of the scrotum (1): Temperature and androgen as determinants of the sperm storage capacity of the rat cauda epididymidis. Biol Reprod 1982; 26:673.
17. Weber JA, Geary RT, Woods GL. Changes in accessory sex glands of stallions after sexual preparation and ejaculation. J Am Vet Med Assoc 1990;196:1084.
18. Garrett PD. Urethral recess in male goats, sheep, cattle and swine. J Am Vet Med Assoc 1987;191:689.
19. Kainer RA, Faulkner LC, Abdel-Raouf M. Glands associated with the urethra of the bull. Am J Vet Res 1969;30:963.
20. Spring-Mills E, Hafez ESE, eds. Accessory glands of the male reproductive tract. Ann Arbor: Ann Arbor Science Pubs, 1979.
21. Spring-Mills E, Hafez ESE, eds. Male accessory organs. New York: Elsevier, 1980.
22. Lauwers J, Nicaise M, Simoens O, de Vos NR. Morphology of the vesicular and bulbourethral glands in barrows and the changes induced by diethyl stilboestrol. Anat Histol Embryol 1984;13:50.
23. Glossop CE, Ashdown RR. Cavernosography and differential diagnosis of impotence in the bull. Vet Rec 1986;118:357.
24. Ashdown RR, Barnett SW, Ardalani G. Impotence in the boar. (1): Angioarchitecture and venous drainage of the penis in normal boars. Vet Rec 1981;109:375.
25. Prinz GS, Zaneveld LJD. Radiographic study of fluid transport in the rabbit vas deferens during sexual rest and after sexual activity. J Reprod Fertil 1980;58:311.
26. Klug E, Deegen E, Lazarz B, Rojem I, Merkt M. Effect of adrenergic neurotransmitters upon the ejaculatory process in the stallion. J Reprod Fertil Suppl 1982;32:31.
27. Beckett SD. Circulation to male reproductive organs. In: Shepherd ST, Aboud FM, eds. Handbook of Physiology—The Cardiovascular System III. Washington, D.C., American Physiological Society, 1983.


## SUGGESTED READING


Ardalani G, Ashdown RR. Venous drainage of the bovine corpus cavernosum penis in relationship to penile dimensions and age. Res Vet Sci 1988;45:174.

Ashdown RR, Barnett SW, Ardalani G. Impotence in the bull. (2): Occlusion of the longitudinal canals of the corpus cavernosum penis. Vet Rec 1979;104:598.

Ashdown RR, Smith JA. The anatomy of the corpus cavernosum penis of the bull and its relationship to spiral deviation of the penis. J Anat 1969;104:153.

Dixson AF, Kendrick KH, Blank MA, Bloom SR. Effects of tactile and electrical stimuli upon release of vasoactive intestinal polypeptide in the mammalian penis. J Endocrinol 1984; 100:249.

Domer FR, Wessler G, Brown RL, Charles HC. Involvement of the sympathetic nervous system in the urinary bladder internal sphincter and in penile erection in the anaesthetized cat. Invest Urol 1978;15:404.

Goyal HO, Williams CS. The rete testis of the goat, a morphological study. Acta Anat 1987;130:151.

Hafez ESE. Scanning electron microscopic atlas of mammalian reproduction. New York: Springer, 1975.

Hochereau-de-Reviers MT, Monet-Kunz C, Courot M. Spermatogenesis and Sertoli cell numbers and function in rams and bulls. J Reprod Fertil 1987;34(Suppl):101.

Hoffer AP, Hinton BT. Morphological evidence for a blood-epididymis barrier and the effects of gossypol on its integrity. Biol Reprod 1984;30:991.

Johnson L, Tatum ME. Temporal appearance of seasonal changes in numbers of Sertoli cells, Leydig cells and germ cells in stallions. Biol Reprod 1989;40:994.

McKenzie FF, Miller JC, Baugess LC. The reproductive organs and semen of the boar. Res Bull Mo Agric Exp Sta 1938; 279.

Nickel R, Schummer A, Seiferle E. The viscera of the domestic mammals. Sack WO, trans. and ed. Berlin: Parey, 1973.

Seidel GE Jr, Foote RH. Motion picture analysis of ejaculation in the bull. J Reprod Fertil 1969;20:313.

CHAPTER 2

# Anatomy of Female Reproduction

B. HAFEZ AND E.S.E. HAFEZ

The female reproductive organs are composed of ovaries, oviducts, uterus, cervix, uteri, vagina, and external genitalia. The internal genital organs (the first of four components) are supported by the broad ligament. This ligament consists of the mesovarium, which supports the ovary; the mesosalpinx, which supports the oviduct; and the mesometrium, which supports the uterus. In cattle and sheep, the attachment of the broad ligament is dorsolateral in the region of the ileum, so that the uterus is arranged like a ram's horns, with the convexity dorsal and the ovaries located near the pelvis.

## EMBRYOLOGY

The fetal reproductive system consists of two sexually nondifferentiated gonads, two pairs of ducts, a urogenital sinus, a genital tubercle, and vestibular folds (Fig. 2-1). This system arises primarily from two germinal ridges on the dorsal side of the abdominal cavity, and it can differentiate into a male or a female system.

The sex of the fetus depends on inherited genes, gonadogenesis, and the formation and maturation of accessory reproductive organs.

Wolffian and Müllerian ducts are both present in the sexually undifferentiated embryo. In the female, the Müllerian ducts develop into a gonaductal system and the Wolffian ducts atrophy. The opposite is true in the male. The female Müllerian ducts fuse caudally to form a uterus, a cervix, and the anterior part of a vagina.

In the male fetus, testicular androgen plays a role in the persistence and development of the Wolffian ducts and the atrophy of the Müllerian ducts.

## THE OVARY

The ovary, unlike the testis, remains in the abdominal cavity. It performs both exocrine (egg release) and endocrine (steroidogenesis) functions. The predominate tissue of the ovary is the cortex. The primordial germ cells arise extragonadally and migrate through the yolk sac mesentery to the genital ridges. During fetal development, the oogonia are produced by mitotic multiplication. This is followed by the first meiotic division to form several million oocytes, a process that is arrested in the prophase. Subsequent atresia reduces the number of oocytes at the time of birth, a further reduction occurs at puberty, and only a few hundred are present during reproductive senescence.

At birth, a layer of follicular cells surrounds the primary oocytes in the ovary to form the primordial follicles. The shape and size of the ovary vary both with the species and the stage of the estrous cycle (Fig. 2-2). In cattle and sheep, the ovary is almond-shaped, whereas in the horse it is bean-shaped owing to the presence of a definite ovulation fossa, and indentation in the attached border of the ovary. The porcine ovary resembles a cluster of grapes because the protruding follicles and corpora lutea obscure the underlying ovarian tissue.

The part of the ovary that is not attached to the mesovarium is exposed and bulges into the abdominal cavity. The ovary, composed of the medulla and cortex, is surrounded by the superficial epithelium, commonly known as germinal epithelium. The ovarian medulla consists of irregularly arranged fibroelastic connective tissue and extensive nervous and vascular systems that reach the ovary through the hilus. The arteries are arranged in a definite spiral shape. The ovarian cortex contains ovarian follicles and/or corpora lutea at various stages of development of regression (Table 2-1).

The vascular pattern of the ovary changes with different hormonal states. Variations in the architecture of the vessels allow adaptation of the blood supply to the needs of the organ. The intraovarian distribution of blood undergoes remarkable changes during the preovulatory period.

Arterial blood flow to the ovary varies in proportion to luteal activity. Hemodynamic changes seem to be impor-

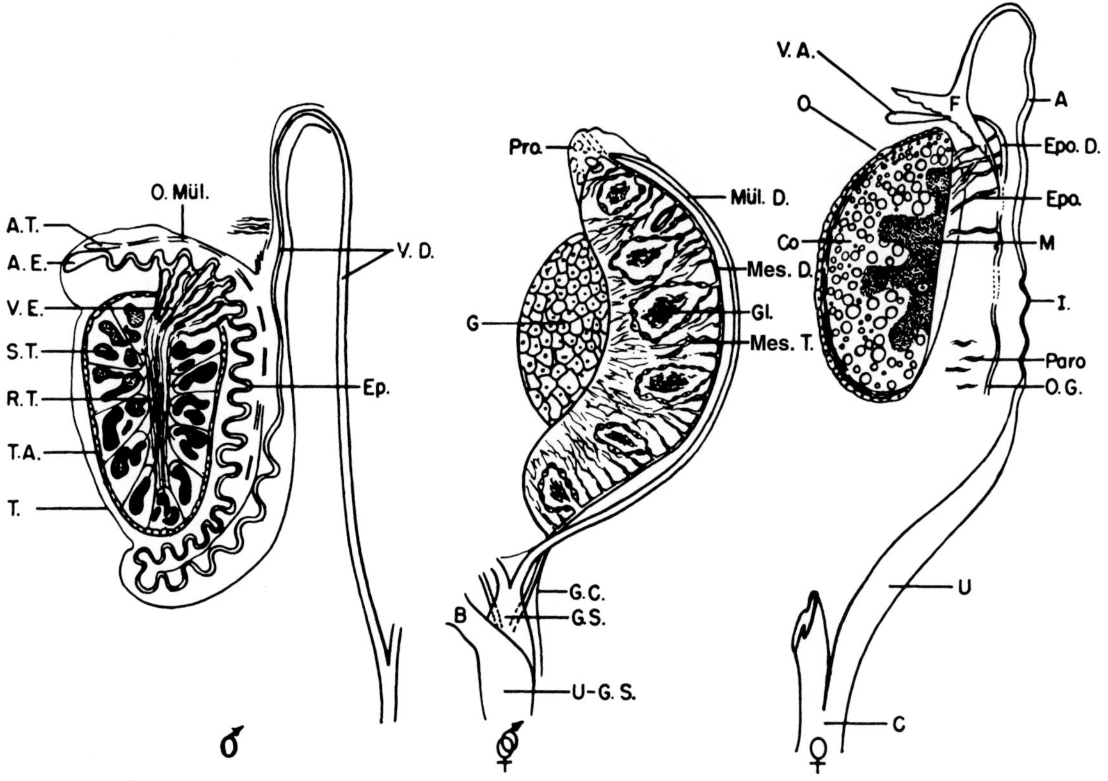


FIGURE 2-1. Simplified scheme of embryonic differentiation of male and female genital systems. (**Center**) The undifferentiated system with its large mesonephros, mesonephric duct, Müllerian duct and undifferentiated gonad. Note that the Müllerian and Mesonephric ducts cross before they enter the genital cords. (**Right**) The female system, in which the ovary and Müllerian ducts differentiate while the remnants of the Mesonephros and Mesonephric ducts atrophy into the epoophoron, paroophoron, and Gartner's duct. (**Left**) The male system in which the testes and Mesonephric (Wolffian) ducts differentiate; the sole remnants of the Müllerian ducts are the testicular appendix and prostatic utricle (vagina masculinus). *A*, Ampulla; *B*, Bladder; *C*, Cervix; *Co*, Ovarian cortex; *Ep*, Epididymis; *Mul.D.*, Müllerian duct; *O*, Ovary; *S.T.*, Seminiferous tubules; *T*, Testis; *U*, Uterus; *U-G.S.*, Urogenital sinus; *V.D.*, Vas deferens.

tant in regulating corpus luteum (CL) function and lifespan. Thus, changes in blood flow precede the decline in progesterone secretion, whereas restriction of ovarian blood flow causes premature CL regression. At the time of luteolysis in ewes, there is a reduction in ovarian blood flow (1).

Blood flow to the bovine ovary is highest during the luteal phase, decreases with luteal regression, and reaches a nadir just before ovulation. Ovarian blood flow increases with the newly developing CL. The decline in blood flow seems to follow the abrupt decline at the time of regression of the CL (2).

### *Corpus Luteum*

The CL develops after the collapse of the follicle at ovulation. The inner wall of the follicle develops into macroscopic

FIGURE 2-2. The ovarian/oviductal anatomy of farm animals. (**A**) Changes in estrus cycle of bovine ovary: *1*, ripe follicle; *2*, collapsed follicle surface, wrinkled/walls bloodstained; *9*, corpus albicans (Arthur 1964). (**B**) Organization of cells in estrous ovine corpus luteum: *a*, corpus haemorrhagicum; *b*, corpus luteum of the second day following estrus; *c*, corpus luteum, day 4 after estrus. (**C**) Graffian follicle: *Co*, cumulus oophorus; *Ge*, germinal epithelium; *Lf*, liquor folliculi; Mg, membrana granulosa. (**D**) Structure of wall of graafian follicle showing how the granulosa cells are deprived of a blood supply by basement membrane (Baird 1972). (**E**) Fully formed zona pellucida (*ZP*) around an oocyte in a graafian follicle. Microvilli arising from oocyte inter-digitate with processes from granulosa cells (**G**). These processes penetrate into cytoplasm of oocyte (**C**) provide nutrients/maternal protein (*N*) oocuyte nucleus (Baker 1972). (**F**) Anatomy of the bovine ovarian vasculature (J.H. Wise et al, 1982). (**G**)Anatomy of ovine ovary/oviduct. A, ampulla; F, fimbriae; *In*, infundibulum; *Is*, isthmus; M.*o*., mesovarium; O, ovary; O.*a*, ovarian artery; O.*b*, ovarian bursa; *U*, uterus. Note the suspended loop to which the ovarian bursa is attached. The oviduct in the ewe is pigmented. (**H**) Major segments of the oviduct. (**I**) Cross and longitudinal sections of different segments of the oviduct; *1* represents the isthmus; *8* represents the infundibulum. Note the variability in the degree of complexity of the mucosal folds.

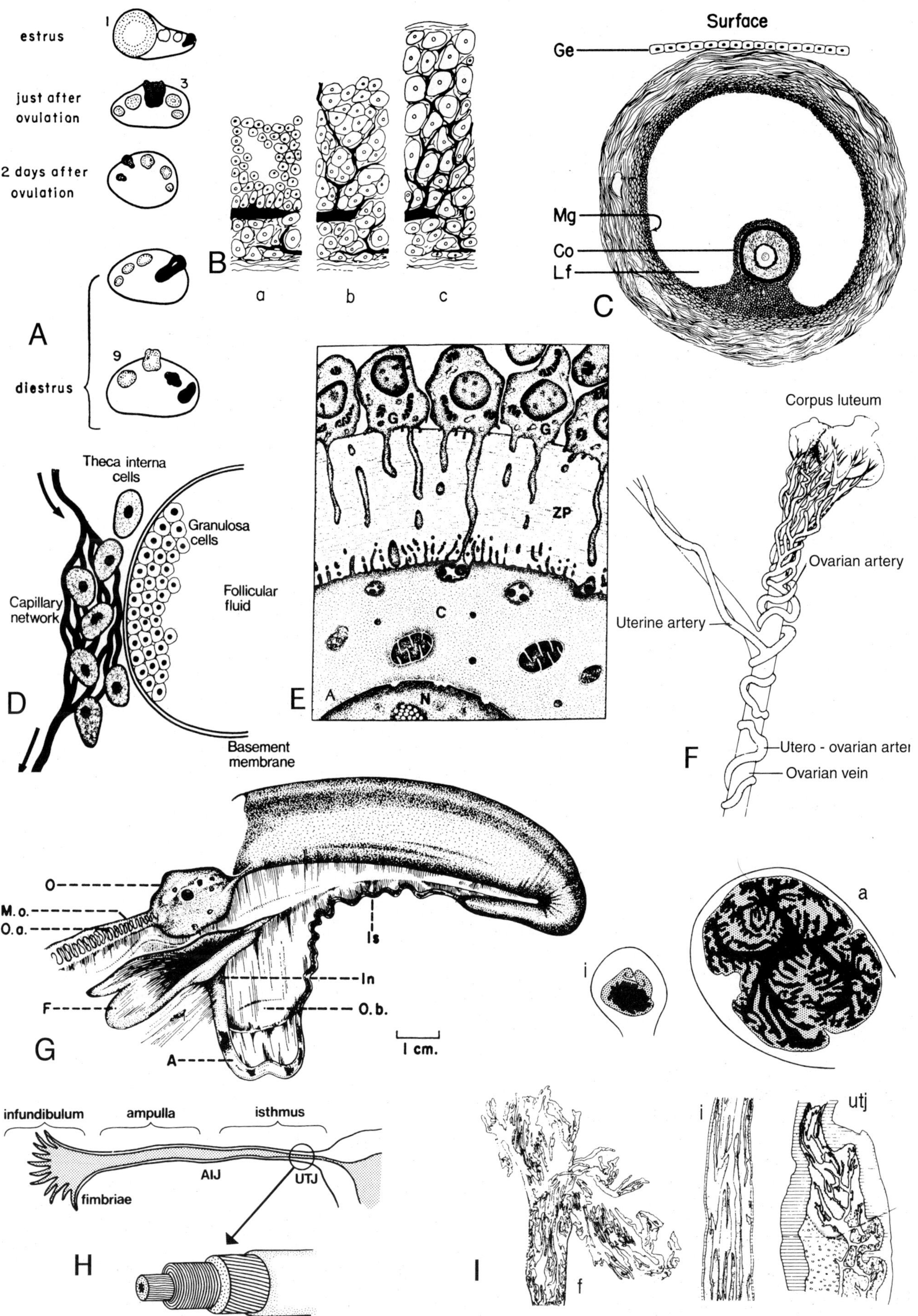
estrus
1
just after ovulation
3
2 days after ovulation
A
9
diestrus
B
a
b
c
Surface
Ge
Mg
Co
Lf
C
Theca interna cells
Granulosa cells
Capillary network
Follicular fluid
Basement membrane
D
G
ZP
C
A
N
E
Corpus luteum
Ovarian artery
Uterine artery
Utero - ovarian arter
Ovarian vein
F
O
M.o.
O.a.
Is
In
F
O.b.
A
G
1 cm.
a
i
infundibulum
ampulla
isthmus
AIJ
UTJ
fimbriae
H
I
f
i
utj

TABLE 2-1. ***Functional Histology of the Mammalian Ovary/Ovarian Follicle***

| ANATOMIC FUNCTIONAL UNIT | HISTOLOGIC CHARACTERISTICS |
|---|---|
| Superficial epithelium | Surface layer of flattened epithelium (commonly incorrectly known as germinal epithelium). |
| Tunica albuginea | Dense, fibrous connective tissue covering the whole ovary just beneath the superficial epithelium. |
| Ovarian cortex | Contains several primary follicles (with oocytes in a quiescent state) and a few large follicles. During each estrous cycle, variable numbers of follicles undergo rapid growth and development, culminating in ovulation. |
| Ovarian medulla | Loose connective tissue contains nerves, lymphatics, and tortuous thin-walled blood vessels, collagen and elastic fibers, fibroblasts. |
| Ovarian stroma | Poorly differentiated, embryonal-mesenchymal-like cells capable of undergoing complex morphologic alterations during the reproductive life; stromal cells can give rise to theca interna cells. |
| Smooth muscle | Smooth muscle cells throughout the ovary, especially in the cortical stroma. Ovarian myoid cells are similar to smooth muscle cells of other tissues. Large numbers of microfilaments arranged in characteristic bundles.<br>Smooth muscle cells and neural elements directly involved in ovulation. Smooth muscle cells, especially in the perifollicular regions, involved in "squeezing the follicle" during ovulation. |
| OVARIAN FOLLICLES | |
| Primary follicle | Oocyte enclosed by a single layer of flattened or cuboidal follicular cells. |
| Growing follicle | Oocyte with increased diameter/increased number of layers of follicular cells; zona pellucida is present around oocyte. |
| Secondary follicle | Flattened granulosa cells of the primordial or unilaminar follicle proliferate. |
| Tertiary (vesicular) follicle | Under the influence of pituitary gonadotrophins, the granulosa cells of multilayered follicles secrete a fluid, liquor folliculi, which accumulates in the intercellular spaces.<br>Continued secretion/accumulation of liquor folliculi result in dissociation of granulosa cells causing formation of a large, fluid-filled cavity—the antrum.<br>Zona pellucida is surrounded by a solid mass of radiating follicular cells, forming the corona radiata. |
| Graafian follicle | Follicular cells increase in size; antrum filled with follicular fluid. Oocyte pressed to one side, surrounded by accumulation of follicular cells (cumulus oophorus); elsewhere in the follicular cavity an epithelium of fairly uniform thickness called the membrana granulosa has formed. |
| Preovulatory follicle | Blister-like structure protruding from ovarian surface due to rapid accumulation of follicular fluid/thinning of the granulosa layer. The viscous liquor folliculi is formed from the secretions of granulosa cells and plasma proteins transported into the follicle by transudation.<br>Dramatic changes at subcellular level, particularly in the golgi complex, involved in formation of the zona pellucida.<br>Oocyte, in the prophase of meiosis, resumes several hours before ovulation.<br>First meiotic (maturational) division associated with extrusion of first polar body. |

and microscopic folds that penetrate the central cavity. These folds consist of a central core of stromal tissue and large blood vessels, which become distended. The cells develop a few days before ovulation. They regress quickly, and within 24 hours after ovulation all remaining thecal cells are in an advanced stage of degeneration. Hypertrophy and luteinization of the granulosa cells commence after ovulation.

Progesterone is secreted by the luteal cells as granules. In the ewe, this process appears to be maximal at day 10 of the cycle and begins to taper off noticeably at day 12. The secretory activity declines gradually until day 14.

In aged animals, the functions of the CL decline as a result of an inability of follicular cells (granulosa and theca interna) to respond fully to hormonal stimuli, changes in the quantity and/or quality of hormone secretion, and a reduced stimulus for hormone secretion.

DEVELOPMENT. The increase in the weight of the CL is initially rapid. In general, the period of growth is slightly longer than half the estrous cycle. In the cow, the weight and progesterone content of the CL increase rapidly between days 3 and 12 of the cycle and remain relatively constant until day 16, when regression begins. In the ewe and sow, corpora lutea increase rapidly in weight and progesterone content from day 2 to day 8, and remain relatively constant until day 15, when regression begins (3). The diameter of the mature CL is larger than that of a mature graafian follicle except in the mare, in which it is smaller.

REGRESSION. If fertilization does not occur, the CL regresses, allowing other larger ovarian follicles to mature. As these cells degenerate, the whole organ decreases in size, becomes white or pale brown, and is known as the *corpus albicans*. After two or three cycles, a barely visible scar of connective tissue remains. Remnants of the bovine corpus albicans persist during several successive cycles. The bovine CL of the estrous cycle begins to regress 14 to 15 days after estrus, and its size may decrease by half within 36 hours.

LUTEOLYSIS. Estrogen-induced luteolysis, probably mediated through stimulation of uterine prostaglandin during the estrous cycle of the ewe, is responsible for the normal regression of the CL. An embryo must be in the uterus of ewes on days 12 and 13 after mating in order for the CL to be maintained. This time represents the state at which the uterus initiates steps leading to luteolysis.

The main uterine vein and the ovarian artery are the proximal and distal components of a local venoarterial pathway involved in the luteolytic and antiluteolytic effects. Hysterectomy abolishes the luteolytic effect and causes persistence of the CL. Luteolysis in the pig is associated with increased plasma prostaglandin PGF in the uteroovarian vein (4).

The changes in blood flow to the luteal tissue can be attributed to changes in flow to the CL, which receives most of the blood supply. Blood flow to the CL plays a role in the regulation of this gland and in regulating the activity of gonadotropins at the luteal cell level.

CORPUS LUTEUM AND PREGNANCY. Progestogens are necessary for the maintenance of pregnancy. Some progestogens serve as immediate precursors to other steroids that are also necessary during pregnancy. Except in the mare, there is an obligatory requirement for continued secretory activity of the CL throughout pregnancy because the placenta does not secrete progesterone in these species. Overiectomy of the gilt at any time during pregnancy results in abortion within 2 to 3 days. After removing one ovary or the corpora lutea from each ovary on day 40 of gestation, a minimum of five corpora lutea is needed to maintain gestation.

MATERNAL RECOGNITION OF PREGNANCY. Blastocytes must be present by day 12 after ovulation in ewes and day 13 in gilts to extend the lifespan of the CL. Maternal recognition of pregnancy in cattle occurs between day 15 and 17 of gestation. Plasma concentrations of progesterone are higher in pregnant than in nonpregnant cows within 8 days after breeding.

The CL of pregnancy is known as the *corpus luteum vernum* and may be larger than the *corpus luteum spurium* (false yellow body) of the estrous cycle. In cattle it increases in size for 2 to 3 months of gestation, then regresses for 4 to 6 months. Thereafter it remains relatively constant until calving, when it degenerates within 1 week postpartum.

## THE OVIDUCT

There is an intimate anatomic relationship between the ovary and the oviduct. In farm mammals, the ovary lies in an open ovarian bursa, in contrast to some species in which it lies in a closed sac (e.g., rat, mouse). This bursa in farm animals is a pouch consisting of a thin peritoneal fold of mesosalpinx, which is attached to a suspended loop at the upper portion of the oviduct. In cattle and sheep, the ovarian bursa is wide and open. In swine it is well-developed, and although open, it largely encloses the ovary. In horses it is narrow and cleft-like and encloses only the ovulation fossa.

### Anatomy

The length and degree of coiling of the oviduct vary in farm mammals. The oviduct may be divided into four functional segments: the fringe-like *fimbriae*; the funnel-shaped abdominal opening near the ovary—the *infundibulum*; the more distal dilated *ampulla*; and, the narrow proximal portion of the oviduct connecting the oviduct with the uterine lumen—the *isthmus* (Fig. 2-3). The fimbriae are unattached except for one point at the upper pole of the ovary. This ensures close approximation of the fimbriae and the ovarian surface. In vivo and in vitro techniques used to study the functions of the oviduct are summarized in Table 2-2.

The ampulla, accounting for about half of the oviductal length, merges with the constricted section known as the *isthmus*. The isthmus is connected directly to the uterus; it enters the horn in the form of a small papilla in the mare. In the sow, however, this junction is guarded by long finger-like mucosal processes. In the cow and ewe, there is a flexure at the uterotubal junction, especially during estrus. The thickness of the musculature increases from the ovarian to the uterine end of the oviduct.

### Oviductal Mucosa

The oviductal mucosa is made of primary, secondary, and tertiary folds. The mucosa in the ampulla is thrown into high, branched folds that decrease in height toward the isthmus and become low ridges in the uterotubal junction.

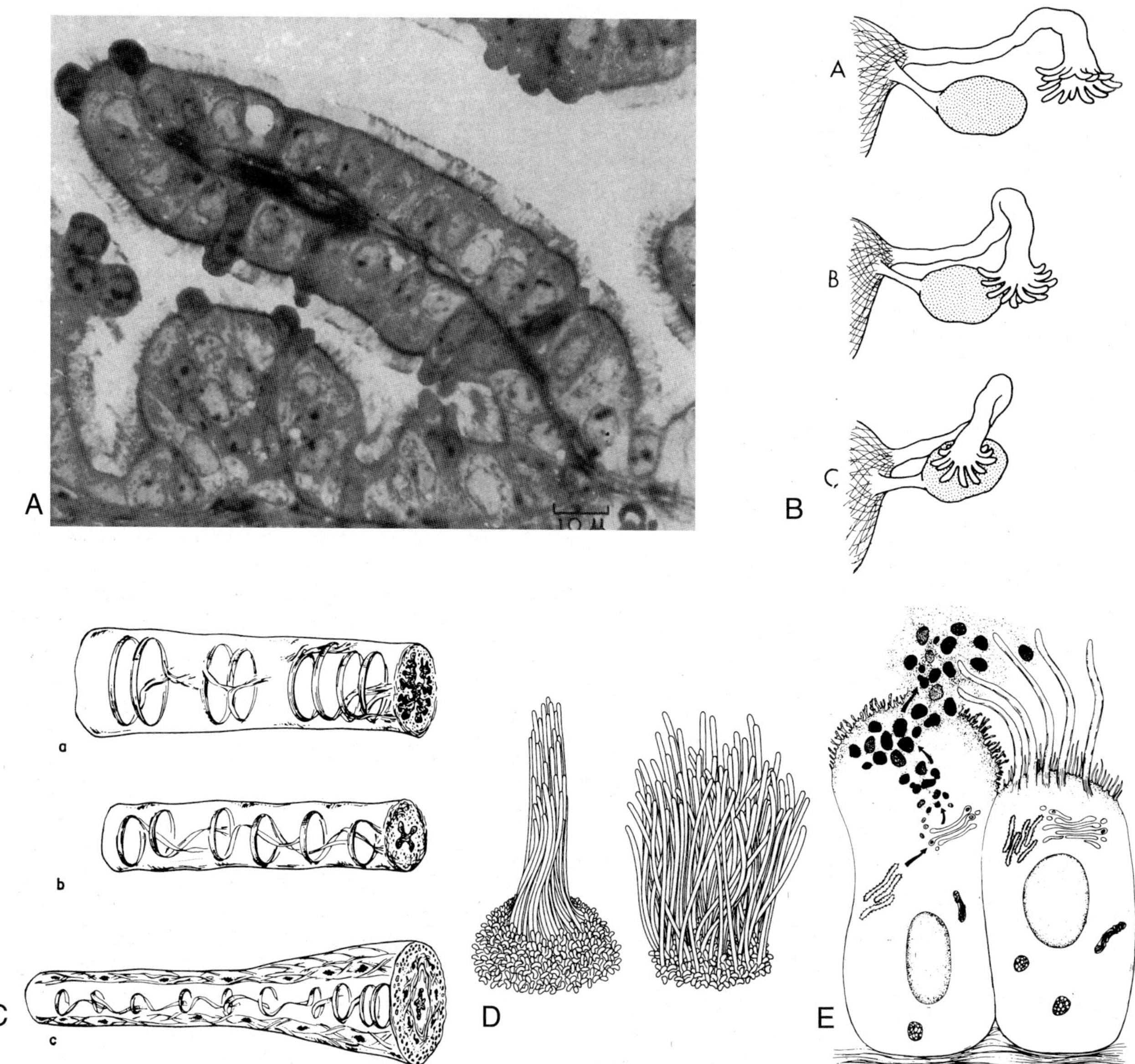


FIGURE 2-3. Physiology, histology, and cytology of the oviduct. (**A**) Oviductal epithelium. *A*, secretory cells with bulging secretory material/ciliated cells with kinocilia (Photo by Professor S. Reinius). (**B**) Contraction of fimbria in relation to ovarian surface, a mechanism by which eggs are picked up into the infundibulum. (**C**) The musculature in the oviduct of ungulates. *A*, ampulla: the musculature consists of spiral fibers arranged almost circularly; *B*, isthmus: note difference in morphology of muscle fibers; *C*, uterotubal junction: note the longitudinal muscle coat of uterine origin, as well as peritoneal fibers (Schilling. Zentralbl Veterinaermed 1962;9:805). (**D**) Ciliated cells from the oviduct (*right*) and uterus (*left*). Note the presence of microvilli on the apical surface of the cell. (**E**) Secretory cells showing the biosynthesis, packaging, storage, release, and distribution of secretory material, which is the main component of the luminal fluid in the oviduct and uterus. The action of kinocilia facilitates the release of secretory granules from the surface cells.

The complex arrangement of these mucosal folds in the ampulla almost completely fills the lumen so that there is only a potential space. Fluid is at a minimum; thus, the cumulus mass is the intimate contact with the ciliated mucosa (Fig. 2-4). The mucosa consists of one layer of columnar epithelial cells. The epithelium contains ciliated and nonciliated cells.

CILIATED CELLS. The ciliated cells of the oviductal mucosa have a slender motile cilia (kinocilia) that extend

TABLE 2-2. *In Vivo and In Vitro Techniques Used to Study Functions of the Oviduct*

| FUNCTION UNDER STUDY | TECHNIQUES |
|---|---|
| Structure and ultrastructure of epithelium, secretory activity, and cilia | Scanning and transmission electron microscopy<br>Culture of fragments of oviductal mucosa<br>Histochemical observations of frozen section |
| Identification of adrenergic or cholinergic receptors | Fluorescence histochemical technique<br>Physiopharmacology of oviductal contractility (e.g., response to drugs) |
| Contractility of oviductal musculature | Visual observation of oviduct through abdominal wall or abdominal window |
| Biochemical composition of oviductal fluid | Extra-abdominal or intra-abdominal device to collect fluid |
| Detection of protein uptake in oviductal epithelium | Immunofluorescence<br>Pharmacology/neuropharmacology |
| Egg transport in oviduct | Effects of prostaglandins, steroid hormones<br>Segmental flushing of oviduct<br>Use of surrogate eggs<br>Recovery of eggs from uterus in vivo |
| Sperm transport in oviduct | Segmental flushing of oviduct at intervals following artificial insemination<br>Flushing of oviduct from fimbriae, by laparoscopy, at intervals following breeding or A.I. |
| Kinetics of cilia beat | High-speed cinematography |

into the lumen. The rate of beat of cilia is affected by the levels of ovarian hormones, activity being maximal at ovulation or shortly afterward when the stroke of the cilia in the fimbriated portion of the oviducts is closely synchronized and directed toward the ostium. The action of ciliary beat seems to enable the egg within the surrounding cumulus cells to be stripped from the surface of the collapsing follicles toward the ostium of the oviduct. The percentage of ciliated cells decreases gradually in the ampulla toward the isthmus and reaches a maximum in the fimbriae and infundibulum. Ciliated cells are noted in large numbers at the apices of the mucosal folds. Variations in the percentage of ciliated and secretory cells along the length of the oviduct have some function significance. Ciliated cells are most abundant where the egg is picked up from the ovarian surface, whereas secretory cells are abundant where luminal fluids are needed as a medium for the interaction of eggs and sperm.

The cilia beat toward the uterus. Their activity, coupled with oviductal contractions, keeps oviductal eggs in constant rotation, which is essential to bring egg and sperm together (fertilization) and preventing oviductal implantation. Ciliation of the oviduct is hormonally controlled in the rhesus monkey: cilia disappear almost completely after hypophysectomy and develop in response to administration of exogenous estrogens. The oviducts atrophy and deciliate during anestrus, hypertrophy and become reciliated during proestrus and estrus, and atrophy and deciliate during pregnancy.

Infections of the female reproductive tract are associated with dramatic changes in cell morphology. Infection is usually associated with the loss of ciliated cells. A decrease in the number of cilia may lead to the accumulation of tubal fluid and inflammatory exudate, which contributes to the agglutination of tubal plicae and subsequent development of salpingitis.

NONCILIATED CELLS. The secretory cells of the oviductal mucosa are nonciliated and characteristically contain secretory granules, the size and number of which vary widely among species and during different phases of the estrous cycle. The apical surface of the nonciliated cells is covered with numerous microvilli. Secretory granules accumulated in epithelial cells during the follicular phase of the cycle are released into the lumen after ovulation, causing a reduction in epithelial height.

The oviductal fluid has several functions, including sperm capacitation, sperm hyperactivation, fertilization, and early preimplantation development. The oviductal fluid is composed of a selective transudate of serum and secretory products of the granules from the secretory cells of the oviductal epithelium (5). Oviductal secretions are regulated by steroid hormones.

Several protein components are common to oviductal fluid and serum. Some of these, however, are present in different proportions in these two body fluids; for example, the quantity of a transferrin and prealbumin in oviductal fluid is far greater relative to albumin than is the quantity of these proteins in the serum. Many serum proteins have

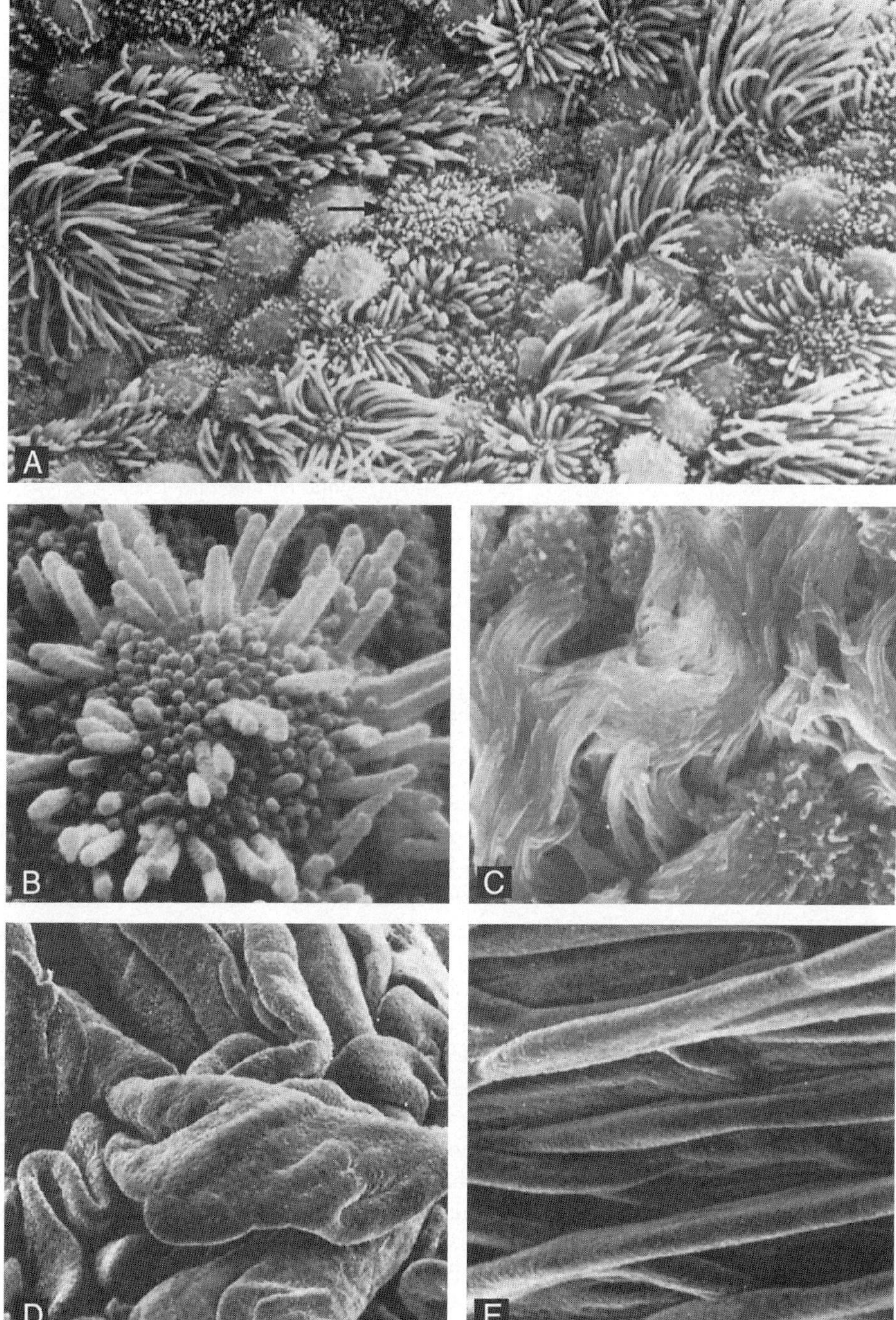


FIGURE 2-4. Scanning electron micrographs of the oviduct. (**A**) The oviductal epithelium showing secretory (*arrow*) cells heavily coated with microvilli and ciliated cells. Note that some cells are fully ciliated while others have cilia on the periphery. (**B**) Rosette-like structure of a ciliated cell ciliogenesis, a process that occurs at random, culminating in complete ciliation as shown in here. (**C**) Fully ciliated cells in the fimbriae that assist in the pick-up of ova after its release from the Graafian follicle. (**D**) *E*, oviductal epithelium. Mucosal folds which protrude in the lumen of ampulla (37™). (**E**) Mucosal folds that protrude in the lumen of the isthmus (40™).

no counterparts in oviductal fluid and conversely, several proteins are unique to oviductal fluid.

### *Oviductal Musculature and Related Ligaments*

Oviductal contractions facilitate mixing of oviductal contents, help to denude the ova, promote fertilization by increasing egg-sperm contact, and partly regulate egg transport. Unlike intestinal peristalsis, oviductal peristalsis tends to delay slightly the progression of the ovum instead of transporting it.

PATTERNS OF OVIDUCTAL CONTRACTIONS. The oviductal musculature undergoes various types of complex contractions: localized peristalsis-like contractions originating in isolated segments or loops and traveling only a short distance; segmental contractions; and worm-like writhings of the entire oviduct. Contractions in an abovarian direction are more common than those in an adovarian direction. In general the ampulla is less active than the isthmus. Additional complicating factors are the contractile activities of the mesosalpinx, the myometrium and the supporting ligaments, and ciliary movement.

Oviductal muscular contractions are stimulated by contractions of two major membranes that contain smooth musculature and are attached to the fimbriae, ampulla, and ovary: the mesosalpinx and the mesotubarium superius. The frequency and amplitude of spontaneous contractions vary with the phase of the estrous cycle. Before ovulation, contractions are gentle with some individual variations in the rate and pattern of contractility. At ovulation, contractions become most vigorous. At ovulation, the fringe-like folds contract rhythmically and "massage" the ovarian surface.

The pattern and amplitude of contraction vary in different segments of the oviduct. In the isthmus, peristaltic and antiperistaltic contractions are segmental, vigorous, and almost continuous. In the ampulla, strong peristaltic waves move in a segmented fashion toward the midportion of the oviduct.

Utero-Ovarian and Related Ligaments. The utero-ovarian ligament contains smooth muscle cells arranged primarily in longitudinal bundles, which continue into the myometrium but not into the ovarian stroma. The smooth muscles in the mesovaria and the various ligaments of the mesenteries attached to the ovaries and the fimbriae contract intermittently. These rhythmic muscular contractions ensure that the fimbriae remain in a constant position relative to the surface of the ovaries.

## The Uterus

The uterus consists of two uterine horns (cornua), a body, and a cervic (neck) (Fig. 2-5). The relative proportions of each, as well as the shape and arrangement of the horns, vary according to species. In swine, the uterus is of the bicornuate type (uterus bicornis). The horns are folded or convoluted and may be as long as 4 to 5 feet, while the body of the uterus is short (Fig 2-6). This length is an anatomic adaptation for successful litter bearing. In cattle, sheep, and horses, the uterus is of the bipartite type (uterus bipartitus). These animals have a septum that separates the two horns and a prominent uterine body (the horse has the largest). In ruminants the uterine epithelium has several caruncles. Both sides of the uterus are attached to the pelvic and abdominal walls by the broad ligament.

### *Endometrial Glands and Uterine Fluid*

The endometrial glands are branched, coiled, tubular structures lined with columnar epithelium. They open onto the endometrial surface, except in the caruncular areas (in ruminants). The glands are relatively straight at the time of estrus; they grow, secrete, and become more coiled and complex as the level of progesterone produced by the developing CL rises. They begin to regress when the first signs of luteal regression are also noted. The endometrial epithelial cells are relatively tall during estrus; following a period of active secretion during estrus, they become low and cuboidal at 2 days postestrus.

The volume and biochemical composition of the uterine fluid show consistent variation during the estrus cycle. In sheep the volume of the fluid in the uterus exceeds that of the oviduct during estrus, whereas during the luteal phase, the reverse is true.

Uterine Proteins. The endometrial fluid contains mainly serum proteins and small amounts of uterine-specific proteins. The ratio and amounts of these proteins vary according to the reproductive cycle. Differences in concentration as well as distribution of components in the uterine fluids compared to the blood serum provide evidence that secretion as well as transudation occurs. In the rabbit, a protein named *blastokinin* (uteroglobulin) can influence blastocyst formation from morulae. The uterine fluid in the mouse contains a factor that initiates implantation. Uterine secretions provide an optimal environment for the survival and capacitation of spermatozoa and the cleavage of the early blastocyst before implantation.

Specific proteins of uterine and/or conceptus origin have been characterized during early pregnancy in the ewe. One of the proteins, a purple-colored, iron-containing glycoprotein named *uteroferin* has been purified (6). Uterine secretions play a part in the control of embryonic growth and the implantation.

Uterine Contraction. The contraction of the uterus is coordinated with the rhythmic movements of the oviduct and ovary. There is considerable variation in the origin, direction, amplitude degree, and frequency of contractions in the reproductive tract.

During the estrous cycle the frequency of myometrial contractions is maximal at and immediately after estrus. At estrus, uterine contractions originate in the posterior part of the reproductive tract and more predominantly toward the oviduct. During the luteal phase, the frequency of contractions is reduced and only a small percentage moves toward the oviducts. Estradiol increases the frequency of uterine contractions in ovariectomized ewes, where the progesterone reduces the frequency. High levels of progesterone are noted when contractile activity is relatively quiescent.

### *Uterine Metabolism*

The endometrium metabolizes carbohydrates, lipids, and proteins to supply the necessary requirements for cell nutri-

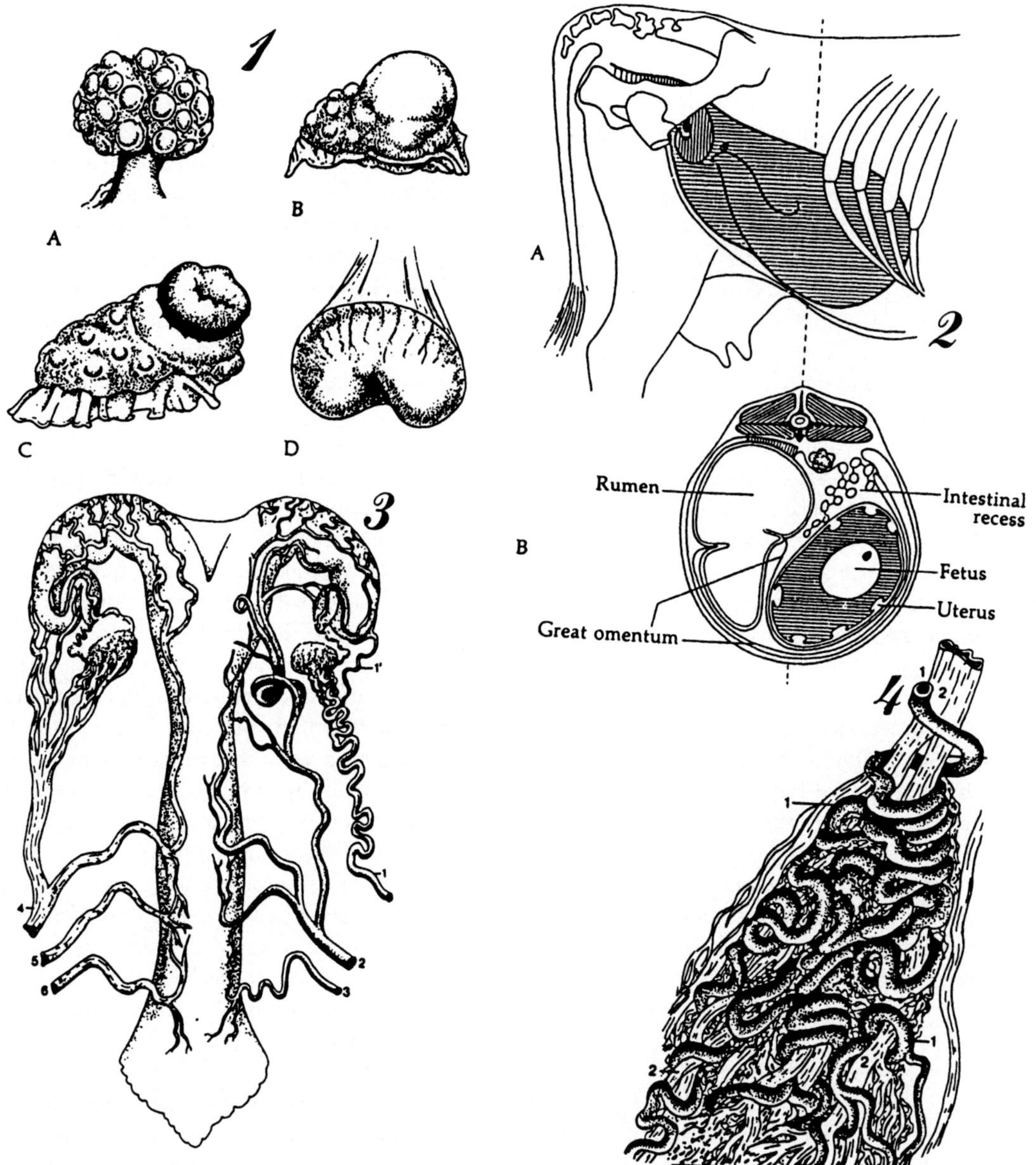


FIGURE 2-5. Comparative parameters of female reproductive anatomy. (**1**) Ovarian differences resulting from species morphology and functional changes. *A*, sow ovary (berry-shaped); *B*, cow ovary (almond-shaped) with ripening follicle; *C*, cow ovary with fully developed corpus luteum; *D*, mare ovary (kidney-shaped) with ovulation fossa (identation) (Dyce KM, Sack WO, Wensing CJG. Textbook of veterinary anatomy. Philadelphia: W.B. Saunders, 1987). (**2**) Position of the cow's uterus at the third and sixth months of pregnancy. *A*, superimposed uterus and ovary (*left*) (vertical striping, uterus; blackened circle, ovary) represents the uterus at the third month of pregnancy; *B*, cross section of uterus at sixth month of pregnancy with its contained fetus relative to adjoining abdominal viscera (rumen on left/uterus on right side of abdomen) (Dyce KM, Wensing CJG. Essentials of bovine anatomy. Philadelphia: Lea & Febiger, 1971). (**3**) Blood supply to the reproductive tract of the cow. The arteries are shown on the right side and the veins on the left. *1*, ovarian artery; *1'*, uterine branch; *2*, uterine artery; *3*, vaginal artery; *4*, ovarian vein; *5*, uterine vein; *6*, vaginal vein (Dyce KM, Sack WO, Wensing CJG. Textbook of veterinary anatomy. Philadelphia: W.B. Saunders, 1987). (**4**) Relationship of the ovarian artery of a ruminant and its branches; *1*, to those of the uterine vein; *2*, the intertwining ensures a large area of contact (Dyce KM, Sack WO, Wensing CJG. Textbook of veterinary anatomy. Philadelphia: W.B. Saunders, 1987).

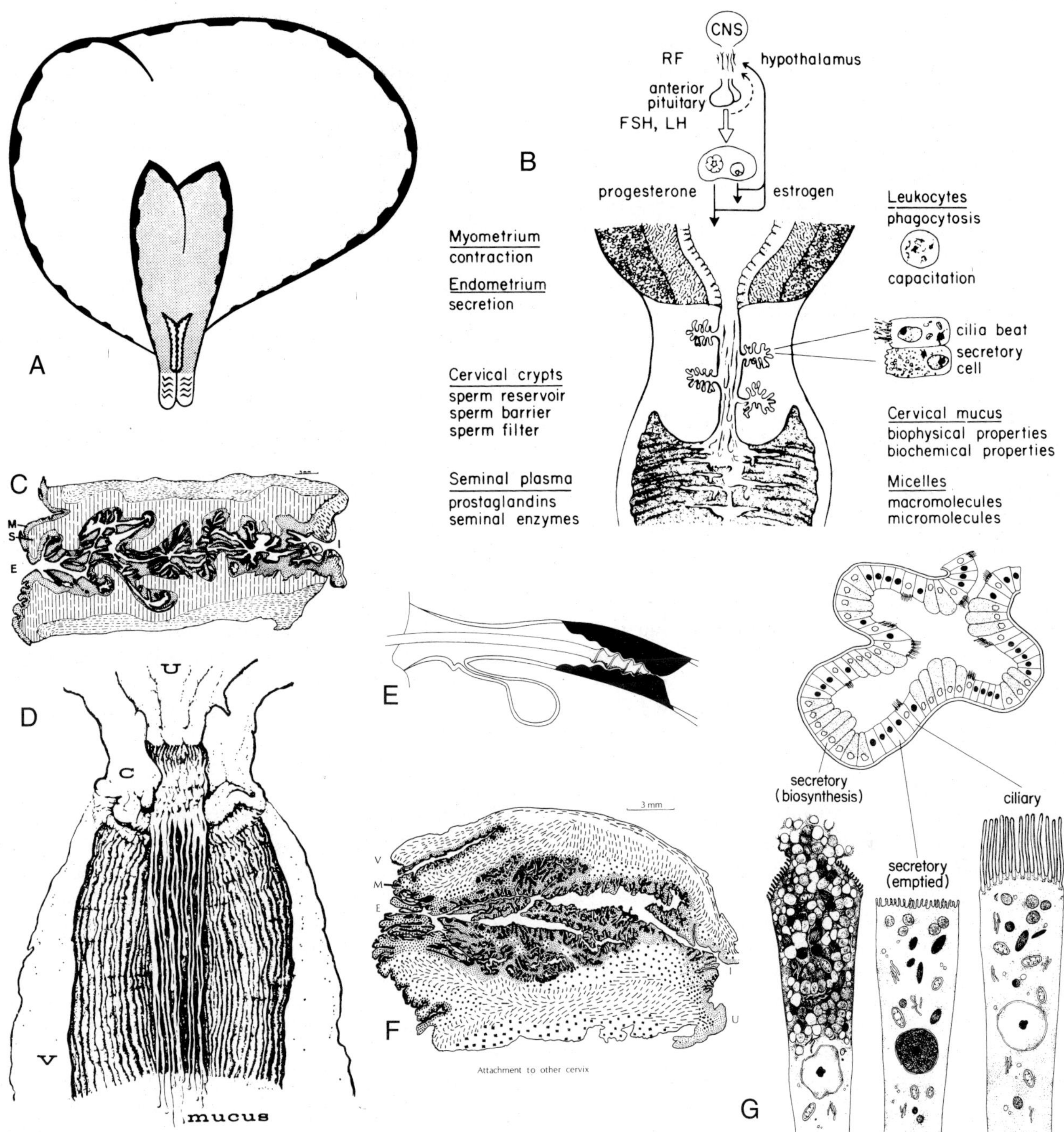


FIGURE 2-6. Functional anatomy of the uterus and cervix. (**A**) Changes taking place in size and shape of the ruminant uterus during pregnancy. Three uteri are shown in the diagram; the inner one represents a nonpregnant uterus; the outer one represents a gravid uterus prior to delivery, and the middle one represents a uterus after delivery in the process of involution. (**B**) Comparative anatomy and physiology of the cervix. (**C**) Tracing of a longitudinal section of the bovine cervix showing the complexity of the cervical crypts which attract massive numbers of spermatozoa. *E*, external, or *I*, internal, or *M*, mucus-secreting mucosa; *S*, cervical stroma. (**D**) The strands of cervical mucus flow from the crypts of the cervix (*C*) to the epithelium of the vagina (*V*). The biophysical characteristics of cervical mucus and arrangement of the macromolecules of mucus facilitate sperm transport from the vagina to the uterus (*U*). (**E**) Corkscrew structure of the cervical canal to accommodate similar structure of the penis (Hunter, 1983). (**F**) Cervix of the rabbit. Note the complexity of cervical canal of the double cervix. (**G**) Cervical crypt (*top*) and secretory cells before and after secretion of mucus (*bottom*).

tion, rapid proliferation of the uterine tissue, and development of the conceptus. These reactions depend on four phenomena: (a) the enzymatic reactions involved in glucose metabolism; (b) the increase in circulation through the spiral arterioles; (c) the morphologic changes that occur in the endometrium and myometrium; and (d) the stimulating action of the ovarian and other hormones.

Ovarian hormones play a substantial role in regulating uterine metabolism. Growth of the uterus (both protein synthesis and cell division) is induced by estrogen. A rapid change occurs in the metabolism of the endometrium about the time the egg passes through the uterotubal junction.

### *Function of the Uterus*

The uterus serves a number of functions. The endometrium and its fluids play a major role in the reproductive process: (a) sperm transport from the site of ejaculation to the site of fertilization in the oviduct; (b) regulation of the function of the CL; and (c) initiation of implantation, pregnancy and parturition.

SPERM TRANSPORT. At mating, the contraction of the myometrium is essential for the transport of sperm from the site of ejaculation to the site of fertilization. Large numbers of sperm aggregate in the endometrial glands. As sperm are transported through the uterine lumen to the oviducts, they undergo "capacitation" in endometrial secretions.

LUTEOLYTIC MECHANISMS. There is a local utero-ovarian cycle whereby the CL stimulates the uterus to produce a substance that in turn destroys the CL. The uterus plays an important role in regulating the function of the CL. Corpora lutea are maintained in a functional state for long periods following hysterectomy of cattle, sheep, and swine. If small amounts of uterine tissue remain in situ, luteal regression occurs and cycles are resumed after variable periods. Following unilateral hysterectomy, corpora lutea adjacent to the excised uterine horn are usually better maintained than those adjacent to the remaining horn.

Intramuscular or intrauterine administration of prostaglandin causes complete luteal regression in the cow and ewe. The gravid uterine horn exerts an antiluteolytic effect at the level of the adjacent ovary. This effect is exerted through a local utero-ovarian venoarterial pathway.

IMPLANTATION AND GESTATION. The uterus is a highly specialized organ that is adapted to accept and nourish the products of conception from the time of implantation until parturition. Uterine "differentiation" is governed by the ovarian steroid hormones. This process must evolve to some critical stage when the uterus is prepared to selectively accept the blastocyst. Unless such differentiation occurs, the uterus is unsuited to permit implantation.

After implantation, the embryo depends on an adequate vascular supply within the endometrium for its development. Throughout gestation, the physiologic properties of the endometrium and its blood supply are important for the survival and development of the fetus. The uterus is capable of undergoing tremendous changes in size, structure, and position to accommodate the needs of the growing conceptus.

PARTURITION AND POSTPARTUM INVOLUTION. The contractile response of the uterus remains dormant until the time of parturition, when it plays the major role in fetal expulsion. Following parturition, the uterus almost regains its former size and condition by a process called *involution*. In the sow, the uterus continuously declines in both weight and length for 28 days after parturition; thereafter it remains relatively unchanged during the lactation period. However, immediately after the young are weaned, the uterus increases in both weight and length for 4 days.

During the postpartum interval, the destruction of endometrial tissue is accompanied by the presence of large numbers of leukocytes and the reduction of the endometrial vascular bed. The cells of the myometrium are reduced in number and size. These rapid and disproportional changes in the uterine tissue are a possible cause of low postpartum conception rate. Neither the presence of suckling calves nor anemia delays uterine involution. Caruncular tissues are sloughed off and expelled from the uterus 12 days after calving.

EFFECTS OF FOREIGN BODIES AND IUDs. The stimulation of the uterus during the early stages of the estrous cycle hastens regression of the CL and causes precocious estrus. Uterine stimulation can be initiated by placing a small foreign body in the lumen. The subsequent estrous cycle will be either shortened or prolonged, depending on when the foreign body was inserted and on the nature and size of the material introduced. The fact that the estrous cycle is unaffected when the uterine segment containing the foreign body is denervated implies that the nervous system is responsible for this effect.

Although intrauterine devices (IUDs) have an antifertility effect in several domestic animals, their apparent mode of action varies widely. The major antifertility effect of IUDs seems to be exerted between the time the embryo enters the uterus and the time of implantation. The insertion of large-diameter IUDs in sheep and cattle alter the estrous cycle by shortening the functional lifespan of the CL. In sheep, large-diameter IUDs inhibit sperm transport and fertilization.

## CERVIX UTERI

The cervix is a sphincter-like structure that projects caudally into the vagina (Fig. 2-7). The cervix is a fibrous organ

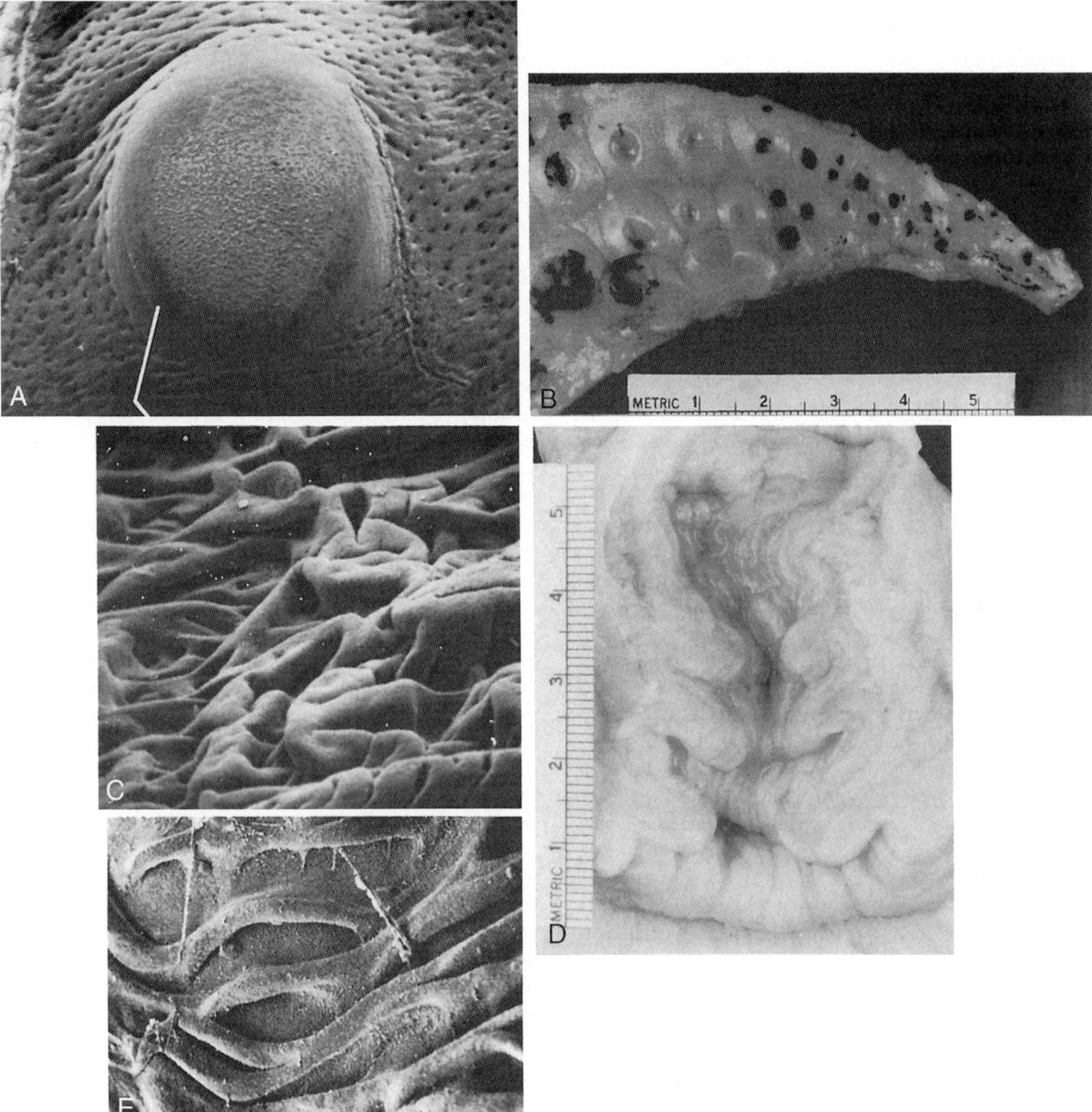


FIGURE 2-7. Scanning electron micrographs (SEM) of female reproductive organs. (**A**) Ovine endometrium: caruncle surrounded by openings of endometrial glands. (**B**) Mucosa of uterine horn of the nonpregnant ewe. Note caruncles and pigmentation of the endometrium. (**C**) Rabbit vagina showing the rugae of the vaginal epithelium for expansion during copulation and parturition. (**D**) Morphology and histology of the cervix (cut open) of a heifer four days after estrus. Note the annual rings around the cervical canal. (**E**) Bovine cervix showing complexity of cervical crypts (59™).

composed predominantly of connective tissue with only small amounts of smooth muscle tissue present. The cervix is characterized by a thick wall and constricted lumen. Although the structure of the cervix differs in detail among farm mammals, the cervical canal has various prominences. In ruminants these are in the form of transverse or spirally interlocking ridges known as *annular rings*, which develop to varying degrees in the different species. They are especially prominent in the cow (usually four rings) and in the ewe, where they fit into each other to close the cervix securely. In the sow, the rings are in a corkscrew arrangement that is adapted to the spiral twisting of the tip of the boar's penis. Distinguishing features of the mare's cervix are the conspicuous folds in the mucosa and the projecting folds into the vagina.

The cervix is tightly closed except during estrus, when it relaxes slightly, permitting sperm to enter the uterus. Mucus discharged from the cervix is expelled from the vulva.

### *Cervical Stroma and Physiologic Changes*

The connective tissue of the cervical stroma is made of ground substance, fibrous constituents, and cellular elements. The ground substance contains proteoglycan, and hyaluronic acid, chondroitin-4,6-sulfate, dermatan sulfate, heparan sulfate, and keratan sulfate associated with proteins. The fibrous constituents include collagen, elastin, and reticulin. Cellular elements comprise mast cells, fibroblasts, and wandering cells. Collagen is made of chains of several amino acids such as glycine, proline, hydroxyproline, lysine, or hydroxylysine. The patterns of reticulin, elastin, and interfibrous ground substances facilitate the dilation of the cervix at delivery. The dissociation of the collagen fibers, which become widely separated from one another, causes the loosening of cervical tissues and increases clear spaces between collagen bundles.

Gross changes in the biochemical composition of the cervix during pregnancy indicate that the cervix during pregnancy is preparing for a change in its functional properties by alterations in the parameters that regulate the physical properties of connective tissue matrices. Morphologically, these pregnancy-related changes do not become apparent until quite late during gestation, when tissue breakdown and destruction of the collagen network become apparent.

During the course of pregnancy, the cervix may show as much as eightfold increase in mass. The enhanced growth and the decreased concentrations of the matrix components may be a consequence of several factors, including increased vascularization and increased concentrations of glycoproteins.

Cervical softening and ripening are not due exclusively to enzymatic activity involving only matrix degradation. The dynamic nature of the cervix at the time of parturition may provide an anabolic basis by which a new matrix with altered physical properties is produced. The major characteristics of the parturient cervix include (a) increased rates of proteoglycan and hyaluronate synthesis with a concomitant decrease in hexuronate concentration, (b) the appearance of a new type of proteoglycan, and (c) a breakdown in the structure and organization of the collagen network.

### *Cervical Mucus*

Cervical mucus consists of macromolecules of mucin of epithelial origin which are composed of glycoproteins (particularly of the sialomucinous type) that contain about 25% amino acids and 75% carbohydrates. The mucin is composed of a long, continuous polypeptide chain with numerous oligosaccharide side chains. The carbohydrate portion is made of glactose, glucosamine, fucose, and silic acid. The proteins of cervical mucus include prealbumin, lipoprotein, albumin, $\beta$-globulins, and $\gamma$-globulins. The cervical mucus contains several enzymes, including glucuronidase, amylase, phosphorylase, esterase, and phosphatases.

Owing to its unique biophysical characteristics, the cervical mucus has several rheologic properties such as ferning, elasticity, viscosity, thixotrophy, and tack (stickiness). The cervical mucus during estrus shows a fern pattern of crystallization on drying on a glass slide. This fern pattern, associated with the high chloride content of the mucus, does not occur with drying of mucus obtained at stages of the cycle when progesterone levels are high or during pregnancy. The phenomenon may have some value, when combined with other observations, for early pregnancy diagnosis. The secretion of cervical mucus is stimulated by ovarian estrogen and inhibited by progesterone.

Cyclic qualitative changes in the cervical mucus throughout the estrous cycle and cyclic variations in the arrangement and viscosity of these macromolecules cause periodic changes in the penetrability of spermatozoa in the cervical canal. Optimal changes of cervical mucus properties—such as an increase in quantity, viscosity, ferning, and pH, and decrease in viscosity and cell content—occur during estrus and ovulation, and these are reversed during the luteal phase when sperm penetration in the cervix is inhibited. Under the influence of estrogens, the macromolecules of glycoprotein of the mucus are oriented so that the spaces between them measure 2 to 5$\mu$m. In the luteal phase, the spaces of the meshwork of macromolecules become increasingly smaller. Thus, at the time of estrus and ovulation, the larger size of the meshes allows the transport of sperm through the meshwork of filaments and through the cervical canal.

### *Functions*

The cervix plays several roles in the reproductive process: (a) it facilitates sperm transport through the cervical mucus to the uterine lumen; (b) it acts as sperm reservoir; and (c) it may play a role in the selection of viable sperm, thus preventing the transport of nonviable and defective sperm.

SPERM TRANSPORT. Upon ejaculation, sperm are oriented toward the internal os. As the flagellum beats and vibrates, the sperm head is propelled forward in the channels of least resistance. The macrorheologic and microrheologic properties of cervical mucus play a major role in sperm migration. Sperm penetrability increases with the cleanliness of mucus, since cellular debris and leukocytes delay sperm migration. The aqueous spaces between the micelles permit the passage of sperm as well as diffusion of soluble substances. Proteolytic enzymes may hydrolyze the backbone protein or some of the crosslinkages of the mucin and reduce the network to a less resistant mesh with more open channels for the migration of sperm. When cervical mucus and semen are placed in apposition *in vitro*, phase lines immediately occur between the two fluids. Sperm phalanges soon appear and develop high degrees of arborization, the terminal aspects of which consist of channels through which one or two sperm can pass.

After mating or artificial insemination, massive numbers of sperm are lodged in the complicated cervical crypts. The cervix might act as a reservoir for sperm, thus providing the upper reproductive tract with subsequent releases of sperm. It is also possible that sperm that are trapped in the cervical crypts are never released, thus preventing excessive numbers of sperm from reaching the site of fertilization.

In ruminants prolonged survival of sperm in the cervix relative to other parts of the reproductive tract suggest that the cervix acts as a sperm reservoir. In the cervices of cattle and goats, most sperm are not randomly distributed but are located between cervical crypts. Penetration of sperm to these sites in the cervix depends on sperm viability and on the structure and, consequently, the rheologic properties of the cervical mucus.

The Cervix During Pregnancy. During pregnancy, a highly viscid, nonferning, thick, and turbid mucus occludes the cervical canal, acting as an effective barrier against sperm transport and invasion of bacteria in the uterine lumen, thus preventing uterine infections. The only other time the cervix is open is before parturition. At this time the cervical plug liquefies and the cervix dilates to permit the expulsion of the fetus and fetal membranes.

## The Vagina

The vaginal wall consists of surface epithelium, muscular coat, and serosa. The muscular coat of the vagina is not as well developed as the outer parts of the uterus. It consists of a thick inner circular layer and a thin outer longitudinal layer; the latter continues for some distance into the uterus. The muscularis is well supplied with blood vessels, nerve bundles, groups of nerve cells, and loose and dense connective tissue. The cow is unique in possessing an anterior sphincter muscle in addition to the posterior sphincter found in the other farm mammals.

There are species differences in vaginal changes during the estrous cycle. These differences probably reflect different secretion rates for estrogen and progesterone and ultimately for the gonadotrophins. Vaginal smears, however, are not useful in diagnosing the stage of the cycle or hormonal abnormalities.

The surface of the vaginal cells is made of numerous microridges that run longitudinally or in circles. In this multilayered stratified epithelium, the cells are wedged on each other by interlocking opposed microridges, thus forming a firm surface. The morphology and pattern of these microridges, which affect the firmness of the epithelium, vary throughout the reproductive cycle.

### *Physiologic Responses*

Vaginal Contractions. Vaginal contractility plays a major role in psychosexual responses and possibly sperm transport. The contraction of the vagina, uterus, and oviducts is activated by fluid secreted into the vagina during precoital stimulation.

Immunologic Responses. The vagina appears to be one of the major sites for sperm antigen-antibody reaction since the vagina is more exposed to sperm antigen than are the uterus and oviduct. Local production of antibodies to sperm antigens may occur within the vaginal tissue.

Immature and mature plasma cells, located beneath the epithelium, seem to be under endocrine control since these cells increase in number during the luteal phase, following ovariectomy and during the postmenopausal stage. These plasma cells seem to be involved in the secretion of immunoglobulins A and G, which seem to prevent bacterial infection and produce antibodies against spermatozoa.

Vaginal Fluid. The vaginal fluid is composed primarily of transudate through the vaginal wall, mixed with vulvar secretions from sebaceous glands and sweat glands and contaminated with cervical mucus, endometrial, and oviductal fluids and exfoliated cells of the vaginal epithelium. As estrus approaches, the vascularity of the vaginal wall increases and the vaginal fluid becomes thinner.

A specific and distinct odor is present in the urogenital tract of cows during estrus. This odor apparently disappears or is greatly attenuated during diestrus. Dogs can be trained to detect and respond to the odors associated with estrus in cattle (7).

Microbiologic Flora. The vaginal flora is made of a dynamic mixture of aerobic, facultatively anaerobic, and strictly anaerobic microorganisms with new strains constantly being introduced. The flora of microorganisms varies throughout the life cycle. The various populations of microorganisms are equipped enzymatically to survive and replicate under a given vaginal environment. During periods of high glycogen content, acidophilic organisms predominate, but other organisms are present among the heterogeneous group making up the normal flora.

### *Functions of the Vagina*

The vagina has multiple functions in reproduction. It is a copulatory organ in which semen is deposited and coagulated until sperm are transported through the macromolecules of the cervical mucus column. The dilated bulbous vagina provides a postcoital semen pool to supply sperm for cervical reservoirs. The rugae vaginales and the fence-like, rhomboidshaped arrangement of the musculature allow distention of the vagina during mating and parturition. Although the vagina contains no glands, its walls are moistened by transudates through the vaginal epithelium (incorrectly called *mucosa*), by cervical mucus, and by endometrial secretions.

Following ejaculation, the seminal plasma is not transported into the uterus; most of it is expelled or absorbed through the vaginal walls. Some of the biochemical components of the seminal plasma, when absorbed in the vagina, exert physiologic responses in other parts of the female reproductive tract.

The pH of the vaginal secretion is unfavorable to sperm. A complex interaction of the cervical mucus, vaginal secretion, and seminal plasma induces a buffering system that protects sperm until they are transported through the micelles of cervical mucus. Pathologic conditions resulting in insufficient buffering of the seminal pool (e.g., low volume of ejaculate, scanty amounts of thick cervical mucus, and leakage of semen) may cause rapid immobilization of spermatozoa. The vagina serves as an excretory duct for secretions of the cervix, endometrium, and oviduct; it also serves as the birth canal during parturition. These functions are accomplished through various physiologic characteristics, namely, contraction, expansion, involution, secretion, and absorption.

## EXTERNAL GENITALIA

The vestibule, the labia majora, the labia minora, the clitoris, and the vestibular glands compose the external genitalia.

### *Vestibule*

The junction of the vagina and vestibule is marked by the external urethral orifice and frequently by a ridge (the vestigial hymen). In some cattle, the hymen may be so prominent that it interferes with copulation.

The vestibule of the cow extends inward for approximately 10 cm, where the external urethral orifice opens into its ventral surface. Gartner tubes (remnants of the Wolffian ducts) open into the vestibule posteriorly and laterally to Gartner's ducts. The glands of Bartholin, which secrete a viscid fluid, most actively at estrus, have a tuboalveolar structure similar to the bulbourethral glands in the male.

### *Labia Majora and Labia Minora*

The integument of the labia majora is richly endowed with sebaceous and tubular glands. It contains fat deposits, elastic tissue, and a thin layer of smooth muscle. It has the same outer surface structure as the external skin. The labia minora have a core of spongy connective tissue.

### *Clitoris*

The ventral commissure of the vestibule conceals the clitoris, which has the same embryonic origin as the male penis. It is composed of erectile tissue covered by stratified squamous epithelium, and it is well-supplied with sensor nerve endings. In the cow, the greater part of the clitoris is buried in the mucosa of the vestibule. In the mare, however, it is well developed, and in the sow it is long and sinuous, terminating in a small point or cone.

Extensive investigations have been conducted on comparative anatomy of female reproductive organs of farm mammals (8–12).

## REFERENCES

1. Niswender GD, Reimers TJ, Diekman MA, Nett TM. Blood flow: a mediator of ovarian function. Biol Reprod 1976;13:381.
2. Wise TH, Caton D, Thatcher WW, Barron DH, Fields MJ. Ovarian function during the estrous cycle of the cow: ovarian blood flow and progesterone release rate. J Anim Sci 1982;55:627–637.
3. Erb RE, Randel RD, Callahan CJ. Female sex steroid changes during the reproductive cycle. J Anim Sci 1971;32(Suppl 1):80.
4. Guthrie HD, Rexroad CE Jr. Endometrial prostaglandin F release in vitro and plasma 13,14-Dihydro-15-KETO Prostaglandin $F_2$ in pigs with luteolysis blocked by pregnancy estradiol bensoate or human chorionic gonadotrophin. J Anim Sci 1981;52:330–339.
5. Oliphant G, Reynolds AB, Smith PF, Ross PR, Marta JS. Immunocytochemical localization and determination of hormone-induced synthesis of the sulfated oviductal glycoproteins. Biol Reprod 1984;31:165–174.
6. Basha S, Bazer FW, Geiser RD, Roberts RM. Progesterone-induced uterine secretions in pigs. Recovery from pseudopregnant and unilaterally pregnant gilts. J Anim Sci 1980; 50:113–123.
7. Kiddy CA, Mitchell DS, Bolt DJ, Hawk HW. Detection of estrus-related odors in cows by trained dogs. Biol Reprod 1978;19:389.
8. Curry TE Jr, Lawrence IE Jr, Burden HW. Effect of ovarian sympathectomy on follicular development during compensatory ovarian hypertrophy in the guinea pig. J Reprod Fertil 1984;71:39–44.
9. Garris DR, Ingenito AJ, McConnaughey MM, Dar MS. Regu-

lation of estrogen-induced uterine hyperemia and contractility in guinea pig: cholinergic modulation of an alpha-adrenergic response. Biol Reprod 1984;30:863–868.

10. Moor RM, Hay MR, Seamark RF. The sheep ovary: regulation of steroidogenic, haemodynamic and structural changes in the largest follicle and adjacent tissue before ovulation. J Reprod Fertil 1975;45:595.

11. Oliphant G, Cabot C, Ross P, Marta J. Control of the humoral immune system within the rabbit oviduct. Biol Reprod 1984;31:205–212.

12. Silvia WJ, Fitz TA, Mayan MH, Niswender GD. Cellular and molecular mechanisms involved in luteolysis and maternal recognition of pregnancy in the ewe. Anim Reprod Sci 1984;7:57–74.

# PART II

# *Physiology of Reproduction*

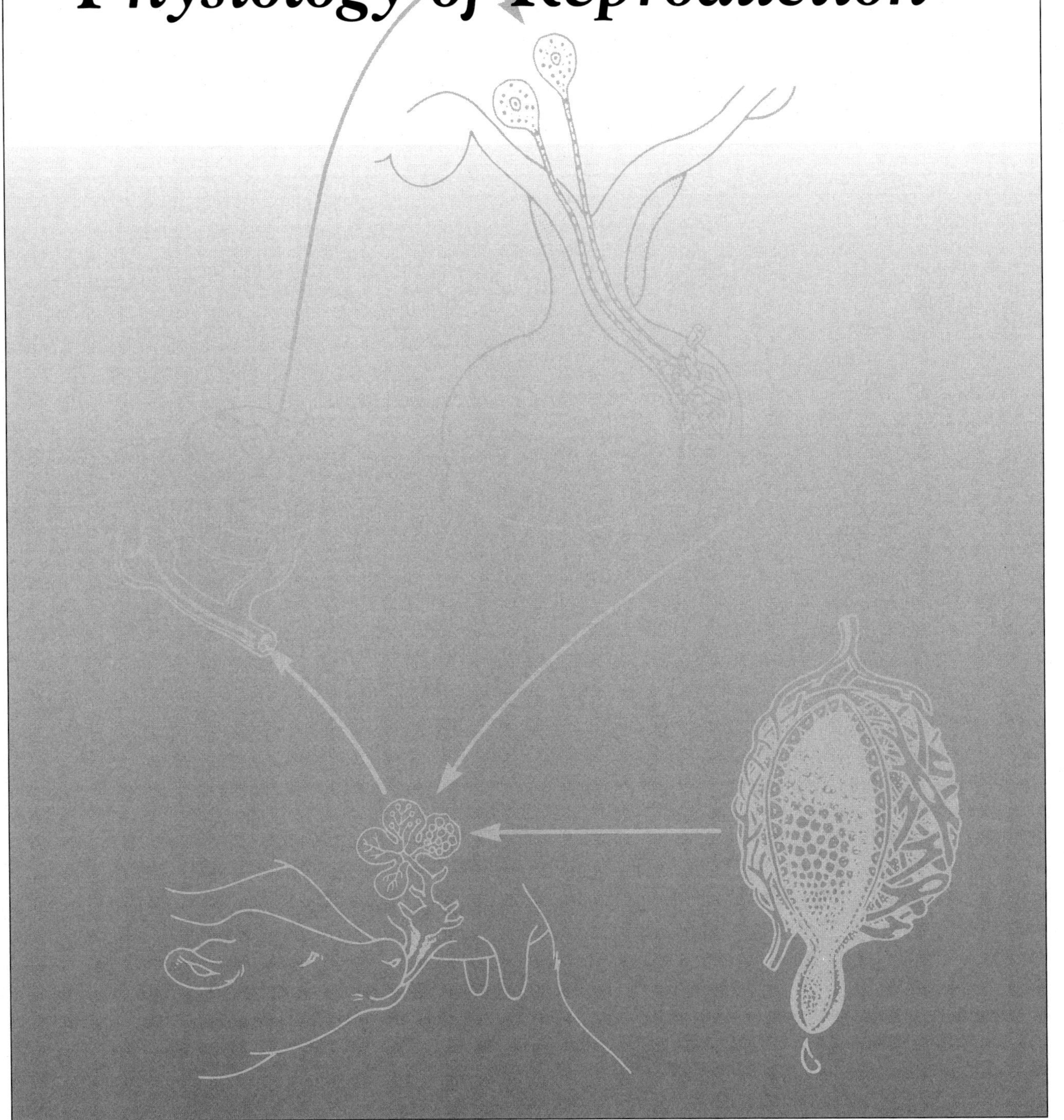

# CHAPTER 3

# *Hormones, Growth Factors, and Reproduction*

E.S.E. HAFEZ, M.R. JAINUDEEN, AND Y. ROSNINA

Over the passage of time, the control of mammalian reproduction has shifted from the central nervous system (CNS) to regulation by two separate systems, the CNS and the endocrine systems (Fig. 3-1). Then followed the discovery that the hypothalamus linked the two systems through the hypothalamo-hypophyseal portal system to coordinate the functions of the gonads. However, many phenomena could not be explained solely on neuroendocrine control. Therefore, the past decade has witnessed the discovery of chemical messengers (growth factors) and the presence of regulatory autocrine/paracrine systems within the gonads. These advances have helped to unravel phenomena that hitherto could not be explained solely on neuroendocrine control.

Both the endocrine and nervous systems function to initiate, coordinate, or regulate the functions of the reproductive system. Unlike the nervous system, which controls body function through rapid, electric nerve impulses e.g., musculoskeletal system, the endocrine system uses chemical messengers or hormones to regulate slow body processes, e.g., growth and reproduction.

The classic definition of a hormone is a physiologic, organic, chemical substance synthesized and secreted by a ductless endocrine gland, which passes into the circulatory system for transport. Hormones inhibit, stimulate, or regulate the functional activity of the target organ or tissue. However, organs like the uterus and the hypothalamus produce hormones, which do not meet the classic definition of a hormone.

Besides hormones from the endocrine glands, extensive investigations during the last decade have revealed the role of peptide growth factors, commonly known as "Growth Factors" in reproduction. Growth factors are hormone-related substances controlling the growth and development of several organs, tissues, and cultured cells. Unlike hormones, growth factors are produced and secreted by cells from different tissues to diffuse into target cells.

This chapter is presented in two sections. The first deals with the biochemical structure, modes of communication, and function feedback mechanisms of the major reproductive hormones in farm animals. The second section reviews Growth Factors, their mode of communication and roles in the reproductive process in farm animals. More details are found in later chapters.

## ENDOCRINE GLANDS

Before discussing the hormones of reproduction, it is worthwhile to review briefly the functional anatomy of the hypothalamus, the pituitary, and the gonads.

### *Hypothalamus*

The hypothalamus occupies only a very small portion of the brain. It consists of the region of the third ventricle, extending from the optic chiasma to the mammillary bodies (Fig. 3-2). There are neural connections between the hypothalamus and the posterior lobe through the hypothalamic-hypophyseal tract and vascular connections between the hypothalamus and the anterior pituitary lobe (Fig. 3-3). Arterial blood enters the pituitary by way of the superior hypophyseal artery and inferior hypophyseal artery. The superior hypophyseal artery forms capillary loops at the median eminence and pars nervosa. From these capillaries, blood flows into the hypothalamo-hypophyseal portal system, which begins and ends in capillaries without going through the heart. Part of the venous out flow from the anterior pituitary is by way of a retrograde back flow, which exposes the hypothalamus to high concentrations of anterior pituitary hormones. This blood flow provides the pituitary gland the negative feedback mechanism of regulating the functions of the hypothalamus. This type of feedback has been termed the short-loop feedback.

### *Pituitary Gland*

The pituitary gland is located in the sella turcica, a bony depression at the base of the brain. The gland is subdivided

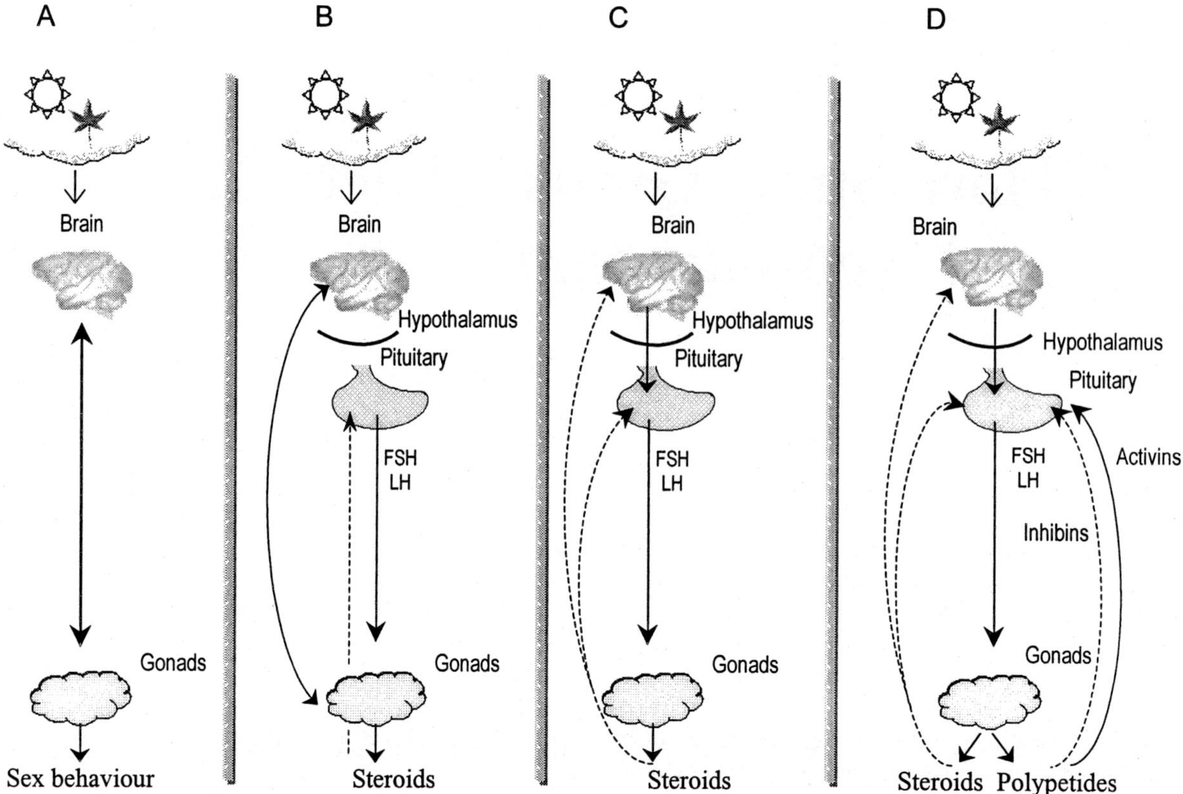


FIGURE 3-1. Chronology of the changing concepts on regulation of mammalian reproduction. (**A**) Central nervous system acts via nerve pathways (neural control). (**B**) The discovery of the endocrine system (ES) shifted the emphasis from the CNS to ES (endocrine control). The gonadotropic hormones from the anterior pituitary controlled gonadal hormone secretion (steroids). The steroids through a negative feedback mechanism decreased/increased hormone output from the anterior pituitary gland. (**C**) Later, the recognition of the hypothalamus-hypophyseal portal system provided the route for hypothalamic hormones to control the anterior pituitary gland (neuroendocrine control). (**D**) The intragonadal regulators or "growth factors" acting via autocrine/paracrine mechanisms modulate the secretion of pituitary gonadotropic hormones.

into three distinct anatomic parts: anterior, intermediate, and posterior lobes. There are remarkable species variations in the anatomy of the pituitary gland. For example, the pars intermedia is well developed in the hypophysis of cattle and horses.

The cell types in the anterior pituitary have traditionally been classified on their staining characteristics into agranular and granular chromophils. The chromophils are divided into acidophils and basophils. This classification has been revised with the advent of immunochemistry and electron microscopy. The anterior pituitary has five different cell types secreting six hormones. By cell type, the somatotropes secrete growth hormone, corticotropes secrete adenocorticotropic hormone (ACTH), mammotropes secrete prolactin, thyrotropes secrete thyroid stimulating hormone (TSH), and gonadotropes which secrete follicle stimulating hormone (FSH) and luteinizing hormone (LH).

### *Gonads*

In both sexes, the gonads play a dual role: the production of germ cells (gametogenesis) and the secretion of gonadal hormones. The interstitial cells that are located among the seminiferous tubules are named the Cells of Leydig. The Leydig cells secrete testosterone in the male whereas the theca interna cells of the Graafian follicle are the primary source of circulating estrogens. Following rupture of the follicle (ovulation), the granulosa and thecal cells are replaced with the corpus luteum (CL) that secretes progesterone.

### *Pineal Gland*

The pineal gland (epiphysis) originates as a neuroepithelial evagination from the roof of the third ventricle under the posterior end of the corpus callosum. The pineal gland of

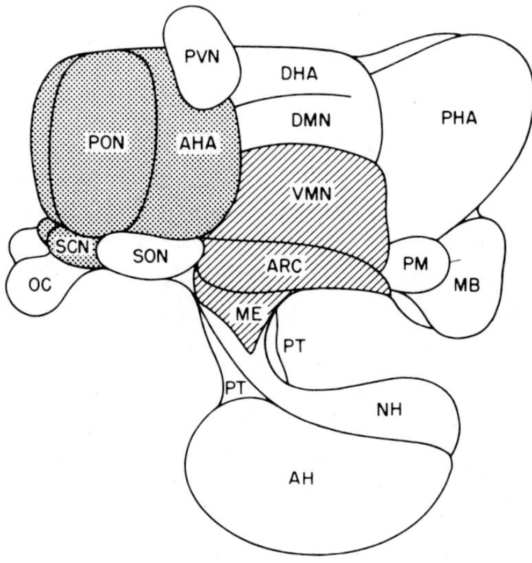


FIGURE 3-2. Schematic drawing of hypothalamic nuclei and pituitary. *AH*, adenohypophysis; *ARC*, arcuate nucleus; *AHA*, anterior hypothalamic area; *DHA*, dorsal hypothalamic area; *DMN*, dorsal medial nucleus; *ME*, median eminence; *NH*, neurohypophysis; *MB*, mammillary body; *PM*, premammillary nucleus; *OC*, optic chasm; *PVN*, paraventricular nuclei; *PON*, preoptic nuclei; *PHA*, posterior hypothalamic area; *PT*, pars tuberalis; *SCN*, suprachiasmatic nucleus; *SON*, supraoptic nuclei; *VMN*, ventromedial nucleus.

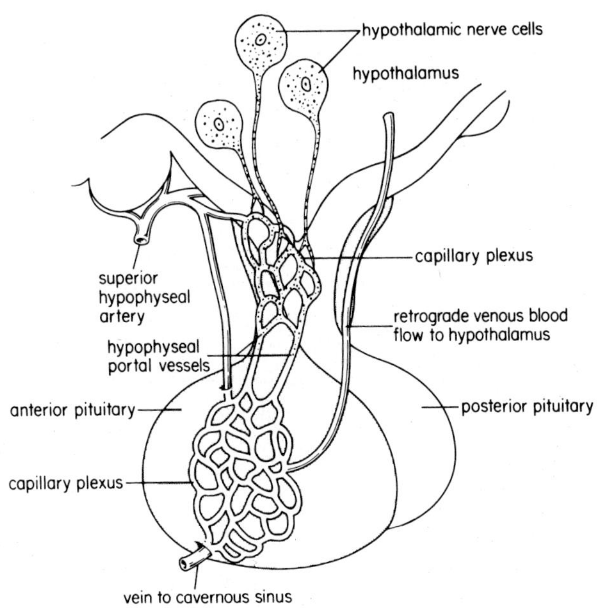


FIGURE 3-3. Hypothalamus-pituitary-gonadal complex. Hypothalamic nerve cells releasing neurohormones into the portal vessels for transport to the anterior pituitary via the hypothalamopypophyseal vessels. Solid particles in nerve cells represent neurohormones. Blood is transported by the retrograde venous system back to the hypothalamus.

the amphibian is a photoreceptor that sends information to the brain, whereas the mammalian pineal is an endocrine gland.

The hormonal activity of the pineal gland is influenced by both the dark-light cycle and the seasonal cycle, causing it to play an important role in the neuroendocrine control of reproduction. The gland converts neural information from the eyes about daylight length into an endocrine output of melatonin, which is secreted into the blood stream and cerebrospinal fluid.

## Hormones

Hormones may be classified according to either their biochemical structure or mode of action. The biochemical structure of hormones includes glycoproteins, polypeptides, steroids, fatty acids, and amines.

### *Structure of Hormones*

According to their chemical structure, the hormones of reproduction are divided into four groups:

Proteins: These are polypeptide hormones ranging from a molecular weight of 300 up to 70,000 daltons, e.g., oxytocin, FSH, and LH.

Steroids: These are derived from cholesterol and have a molecular weight of 300 to 400 daltons, e.g., testosterone.

Fatty acids: These are derived from arachidonic acid and have a molecular weight of about 400 daltons.

Amines: These compounds are derived from tyrosine or tryptophan, e.g., melatonin.

### *Modes of Intercellular Communication*

The CNS was considered to be the coordinator of all body systems until the discovery of endocrine glands. Then the view became that regulation of reproduction was shared by two separate systems with the hypothalamus as the interface between the two systems. Currently, chemical messengers that do not fit either system—Growth Factors—are being discovered that play a role in the control of reproduction.

Cells communicate with each other via chemical messengers such as amines, amino acids, steroids, and polypeptides. Thus, there are four modes of intercellular communications:

Neural communication, in which neurotransmitters are released at synaptic junctions from nerve cells and act across narrow synaptic clefts between as neurotransmitters.

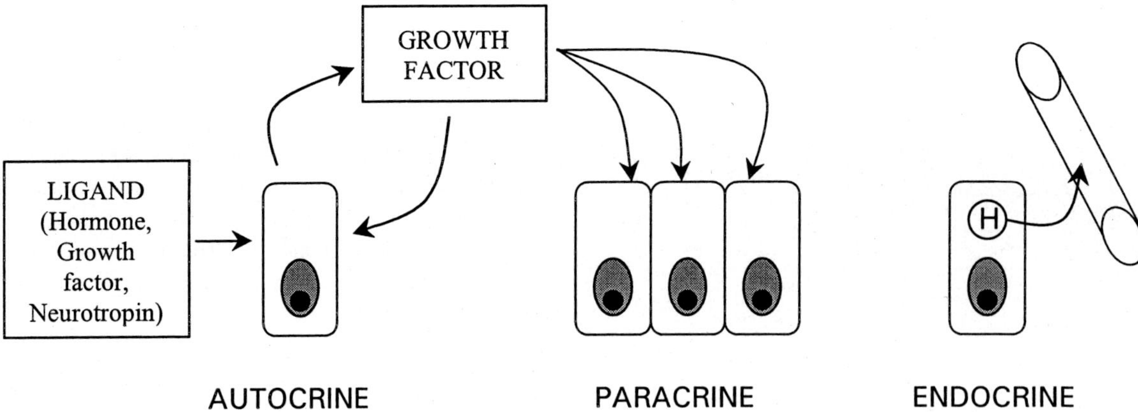


FIGURE 3-4. Modes of intercellular communication. Locally produced growth factors acting in an autocrine/paracrine manner mediate endocrine action in target cells.

Endocrine communication, in which hormones transported through blood circulation, typical of most hormones.

Paracrine communication, in which the products of the cells diffuse through extracellular fluid to affect neighboring cells that are at a distance., e.g., prostaglandins.

Autocrine communication, in which cells secrete chemical messengers that bind to receptors on the same cell that secreted the messenger (Fig. 3-4).

## Regulation of Hormone Secretion

The nervous system plays an essential role in the regulation of gonadal activity by means of endocrine feedback mechanism, neural pathways, and immunoendocrine control.

### ENDOCRINE FEEDBACK

***Gonad.*** A target gland hormone (e.g., estrogen) can influence the secretion of the tropic stimuli that caused its own release (e.g., FSH). The feedback control occurs at the level of the hypothalamus and the pituitary gland (Fig. 3-3). Depending on their concentration in the blood, steroid hormones may exert a stimulatory (positive) or an inhibitory (negative) feedback.

***Inhibitory or negative feedback.*** This system involves reciprocal interrelationships between two or more glands and target organs. For example, as stimulation of the ovary increases estrogen secretion, FSH levels decline. Similarly, when pituitary hormones reach a certain level, some hypothalamic nuclei respond by decreasing the production of their particular releasing hormone, a decline in secretion of pituitary tropic hormone, and a lower level of target gland function.

***Stimulatory or positive feedback.*** In this system, an increasing level of hormone(s) causes subsequent increase of another hormone. For example, increasing levels of estrogen during the preovulatory phase trigger an abrupt release of pituitary LH. These two events are precisely synchronized, because a LH surge is necessary for the rupture of ovarian follicle.

***Hypothalamic hormones.*** Both pituitary and steroid hormones regulate the synthesis, storage, and release of hypothalamic hormones through two feedback mechanisms: a long and a short loop. Long feedback involves interaction among the gonad, pituitary, and hypothalamus while the short feedback system permits pituitary gonadotropins to influence the secretory activity of the releasing hormones without mediation of the gonads (see Hypothalamus—retrograde back flow in the hypothalamus).

NEUROENDOCRINE REFLEX. Apart from the feedback mechanisms mentioned above, the nervous system may control release of hormones through neural pathways, e.g., oxytocin in milk-let down and LH release following copulation, as will be pointed out later.

IMMUNOENDOCRINE CONTROL. The endocrine and immune systems interact extensively to regulate each other. Several endocrine organs are involved in some aspect of this regulatory process: hypothalamus, pituitary, gonads, adrenals, pineal, thyroid, and thymus. Many of these organs are themselves affected by immune function.

## Hormone Receptors

Each hormone has a selective effect on one or more target organs. This effect is achieved through two mechanisms:

Each target organ has a specific method of binding that hormone not found in other tissue.

The target organs have certain metabolic pathways capable of responding to the hormone-metabolic pathways not shared by nontarget tissue.

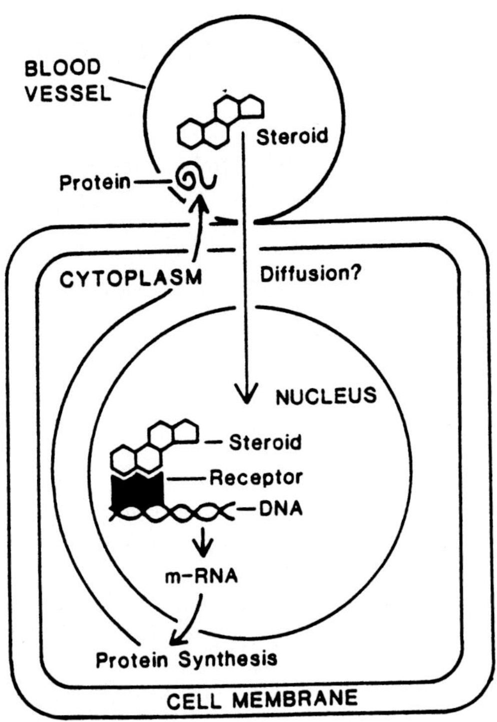


Figure 3-5. Schematic mechanism of action of steroid hormones. The steroid passes through the cell membrane and into the nucleus to bind to its receptor.

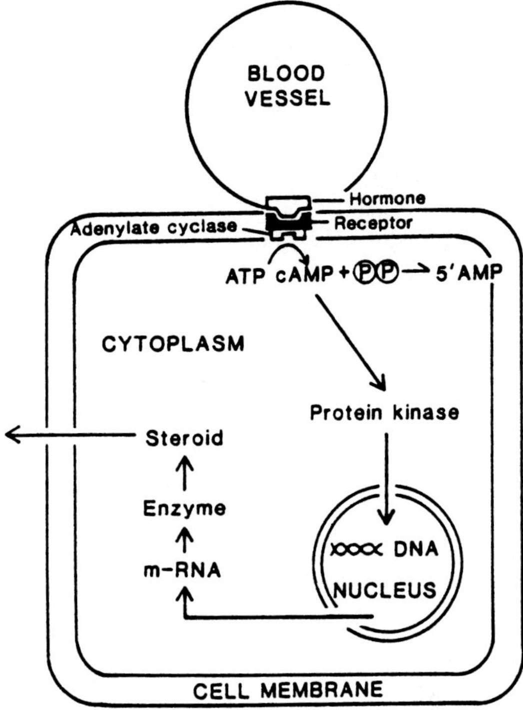


Figure 3-6. Schematic mechanism of action of protein hormones. The sequence of cellular events that occur following binding of a protein hormone to a receptor in the membrane of a target cell is shown.

Specific binding is the usual mechanism. For example, all target tissues that respond to steroid hormones contain a receptor protein within the cell, which specifically binds the activating hormone. Within the target cell, the steroid hormone is found in the cytoplasm, bound to a relatively large protein (molecular weight, 200,000 daltons). Binding results in transformation or activation of the steroid protein complex, allowing it to move (translocate) into the cell nucleus. At the nuclear site the steroid complex binds to specific receptor and causes a sequence of physiologic responses specific for that cell (Fig. 3-5).

The target cells of the anterior pituitary possess cell membrane receptors that recognize and selectively bind the protein hormones, including gonadotropins (Fig. 3-6). The binding phenomenon triggers the synthesis and secretion of the pituitary hormone via the cyclic AMP-protein kinase system of the cell. Estrogen levels, in turn, influence the gonadotropin receptors (1).

### *Hormone Assays*

Several techniques are used to study endocrinology: ablation of a gland, organ replacement therapy, and isolation of hormones. Quantitative at measurements of hormones are based on bioassays, immunologic assays, and radioimmunoassays (RIAs).

Biologic assays have been used to measure activity of all hormones. The hormone is administered to the animal to induce a measurable biologic response. The RIA, one of the major advances in analytic endocrinology, allows rapid measurement of large numbers of samples containing low concentrations of hormones. The principle of the RIA is based on the theory that in the absence of unlabeled antigen or hormone (H), the labeled radioactive hormone (H*) has maximal opportunity to react with a limited number of antibody-binding sites (Ab).

## Primary Hormones of Reproduction

Primary hormones regulate the various reproductive processes, whereas secondary or metabolic hormones indirectly influence reproduction. The latter hormones are not discussed in this chapter. The primary hormones are involved in many aspects of reproductive processes—spermatogenesis, ovulation, sexual behavior, fertilization, implantation, maintenance of gestation, parturition, lactation, and maternal behavior.

Reproductive hormones are derived primarily from four major systems or organs: various areas of the hypothalamus, anterior and posterior lobes of the pituitary gland, gonads (testis and ovary including their interstitial tissues and corpus luteum), and the uterus and placenta.

TABLE 3-1. *Summary of Origin and Function of Neurohormones Regulating Reproduction*

| HORMONES | ORIGIN | NEURAL PATHWAYS | PRINCIPAL FUNCTIONS |
|---|---|---|---|
| Prolactin-inhibiting hormone (PIH)<br>Prolactin-releasing hormone (PRH) | Hypothalamus | Neurons containing dopamine in the arcuate nucleus | Inhibits prolactin release<br>Stimulates prolactin release |
| Gonadotropin releasing hormone (GnRH) | Ventromedial nucleus<br>Arcuate nucleus<br>Median eminence | Negative feedback from gonads | Stimulates tonic release of FSH and LH |
| Gonadotropin releasing hormone (GnRH) | Anterior hypothalamic area<br>Preoptic nuclei<br>Suprachiasmatic nucleus | Hypothalamic cells sensitive to estrogen, touch receptors in skin and genitalia of reflex ovulating species | Stimulates preovulatory surge of FSH and LH |
| Oxytocin | Paraventricular nuclei<br>Supraoptic nuclei | Tactile sensations from the mammary gland, uterus, and cervix | Induces uterine contractions, milk letdown, and facilitates gamete transport |
| Melatonin | Pineal | Retina via retinohypothalamic fibres | Inhibits gonadotropic activity in long-day breeders, e.g., hamster<br>Stimulates the onset of the breeding season in short-day breeders, e.g., sheep |

### *Hypothalamic Releasing/Inhibiting Hormones*

The hormones of the hypothalamus that regulate reproduction are gonadotropin-releasing hormone (GnRH or LH-RH), ACTH, and prolactin-inhibiting factor (PIF). The hypothalamus is also the source of oxytocin and vasopressin, which are stored in the neurohypophysis (posterior lobe of the pituitary gland). The neuroendocrine control of hypothalamic hormones, sensory pathways, and integrating areas are summarized in Table 3-1.

In 1977, two American scientists, Schally and Guillemin, shared the Nobel prize for their independent research on determining the chemical structures of hormones of the hypothalamus that control pituitary function. GnRH is a decapeptide (10 amino acids) with a molecular weight of 1183 daltons. It is synthesized and then stored in the medial basal hypothalamus. GnRH provides a humoral link between the neural and endocrine systems. In response to neural signals, pulses of GnRH are released into the hypophyseal portal system for the release of LH and FSH from the anterior pituitary.

### *Adenohypophyseal Hormones*

The anterior pituitary gland secretes three gonadotropic hormones: FSH, LH, and prolactin (Table 3-2) (see cell types under Pituitary Gland). LH and FSH are glycoprotein hormones with a molecular weight of about 32,000 daltons. Gonadotropes in the anterior pituitary secrete both hormones. Each hormone consists of two dissimilar subunits termed the alpha and beta subunits. The alpha subunit is common to both FSH and LH within species, whereas the beta subunit is distinct and confers specificity of each gonadotropin. The alpha and beta subunits of any of these hormones by themselves have no biologic activity. Prolactin is not a glycoprotein.

As stated above GnRH and the gonadal steroids regulate secretion of gonadotropins. Additionally, gonadal peptides regulate FSH secretion. These either stimulate (activins) or inhibit (inhibins, follistatin) FSH secretion as will be discussed later in this chapter.

FOLLICLE STIMULATING HORMONE. Follicle stimulating hormone stimulates the growth and maturation of the ovarian follicle or the Graafian follicle. FSH does not cause secretion of estrogen from the ovary by itself; instead, it needs the presence of LH to stimulate estrogen production. In the male, FSH acts on the germinal cells in the seminiferous tubules of the testis and is responsible for spermatogenesis up to the secondary spermatocyte stage; later androgens from the testis support the final stages of spermatogenesis.

LUTEINIZING HORMONE. Luteinizing hormone is a glycoprotein composed of an alpha and a beta subunit with a molecular weight of 30,000 daltons and a biologic half-life of 30 minutes. Tonic or basal levels of LH act in conjunction with FSH to induce estrogen secretion from the large ovar-

**TABLE 3-2. *Summary of Reproductive Hormones Secreted by the Pituitary Gland***

| HORMONE | STRUCTURE AND SOURCE | PRINCIPAL FUNCTIONS |
|---|---|---|
| Follicle-stimulating hormone (FSH) | Glycoprotein, Gonadotropes in anterior lobe | Stimulates follicular growth in female and spermatogenesis in male secretion |
| Luteinizing hormone (LH) | Glycoprotein, Gonadotropes in anterior lobe | Stimulates ovulation and luteinization of ovarian follicles (corpus luteum) in female and testosterone secretion in male |
| Prolactin (PRL) | Protein, Mammatropes in anterior lobe | Promotes lactation and maternal behavior |
| Oxytocin | Protein, Stored in posterior lobe pituitary | Stimulates contractions of pregnant uterus, causes milk ejection |

ian follicle. The preovulatory surge of LH is responsible for rupture of the follicle wall and ovulation. LH stimulates the interstitial cells of both the ovary and testis. In the male, the interstitial cells (Leydig cells) produce androgens after LH stimulation.

**PROLACTIN.** Prolactin is a polypeptide hormone secreted by the adenohypophysis. As stated earlier, it is not a glycoprotein like other gonadotropins. Ovine prolactin is a 198 amino acid protein with a molecular weight of 24,000 daltons. Prolactin molecules are similar in structure to growth hormones, and in some species, these hormones have similar biologic properties.

An inhibiting hormone termed prolactin inhibiting factor (PIF) regulates secretion of prolactin. PIF is probably the catecholamine, dopamine, that is an amine of low molecular weight synthesized from L-tyrosine. It is secreted from nerve terminals mostly in the arcuate nucleus located in the median eminence and transported through the hypophyseal portal system to the adenohypophysis.

Prolactin initiates and maintains lactation. It is regarded as a gonadotropic hormone because of its luteotropic properties (maintenance of corpus luteum) in rodents. However, in domestic animals, LH is the main luteotropic hormone, with prolactin being of less importance in the luteotropic complex. Prolactin may mediate the seasonal and lactational effects on reproduction in farm animals.

### *Neurohypophyseal Hormones*

The hormones of the posterior pituitary (neurohypophysis) differ from the other pituitary hormones in that they do not originate from the pituitary, but are only stored there until needed. The two hormones, oxytocin (milk letdown hormone) and vasopressin (antidiuretic hormone or ADH) are actually produced in the hypothalamus. These hormones are transferred from the hypothalamus to the posterior pituitary not through the vascular system, but along the axons of the nervous system.

**OXYTOCIN.** Oxytocin is synthesized in the supraoptic nucleus of the hypothalamus and is transported in small vesicles enclosed by a membrane down the hypothalamic-hypophyseal nerve axons. They are stored at the nerve endings next to the capillary beds in the neurohypophysis until their release into the circulation (Fig. 3-3). As stated earlier, oxytocin is also produced in the corpus luteum. Thus, oxytocin has two sites of origin, the ovary and the hypothalamus.

Oxytocin also plays an important part in reproductive processes. During the follicular phase of the estrous cycle and during the late stages of gestation, oxytocin stimulates uterine contractions, which facilitate sperm transport to the oviduct at estrus.

The stretching of the cervix at parturition caused by the passage of the fetus stimulates a reflex release of oxytocin (Ferguson's reflex). However, the best known action of oxytocin is the reflex release of milk. In the lactating female, visual and tactile stimuli associated with suckling or milking induce the release of oxytocin into the circulation. Oxytocin causes contraction of myoepithelial cells (smooth muscle cells) that surround the alveoli in the mammary gland, resulting in milk letdown (Fig. 3-7).

Ovarian oxytocin is involved in luteal function. It acts on endometrium to induce prostaglandin $F_{2\alpha}$ ($PGF_{2\alpha}$) release, which has a luteolytic action (regression of the corpus luteum).

**MELATONIN.** Melatonin (N-acetyl-5-methoxytrptamine) is synthesized in the pineal gland. Pineal parenchymal cells take up the amino acid, tryptophan, from the circulation and convert it to serotonin (2). Two steps in the metabolism of serotonin are under neural control. The first is the conversion of serotonin to N-acetylserotonin, which is followed by the conversion N-acetylserotonin to melatonin. The second step involves the melatonin-forming enzyme, hydroxyindole-O-methyl-transferase (HIOMT) (Fig. 3-8).

Synthesis and secretion of melatonin is greatly elevated during darkness. Long daily periods of elevated secretion of melatonin are probably responsible for the induction of ovarian cycles in ewes and the inhibition of cyclicity in mares.

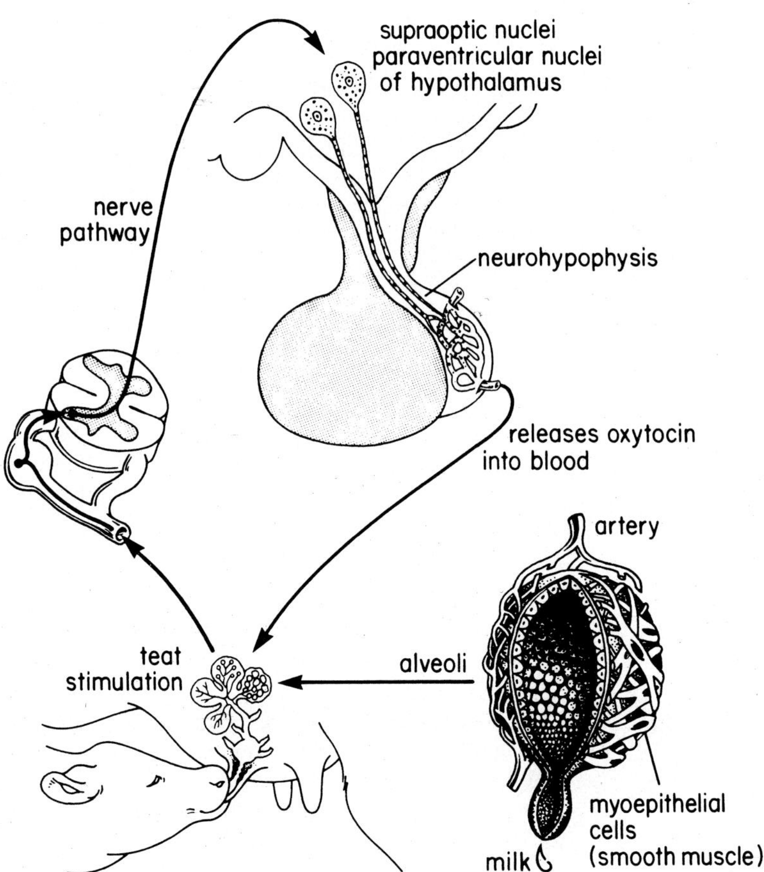


FIGURE 3-7. Milk letdown may be considered a neuroendocrine reflex. The stimulation of the teat induced a neural signal to the hypothalamus to release oxytocin from the neurohypophysis, which stimulates the myoepithelial cells to constrict the alveoli, resulting in milk secretion.

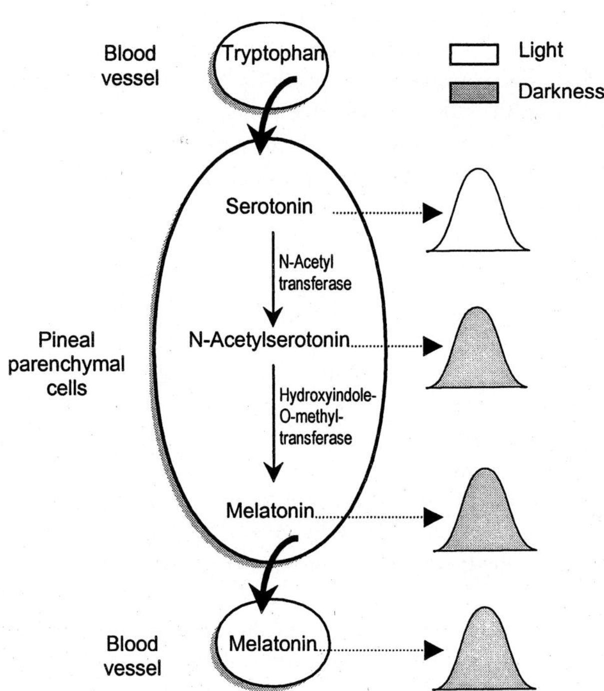


FIGURE 3-8. Formation of melatonin and diurnal rhythms in the pineal and melatonin in blood.

Species differences exist in the effects of exogenou melatonin on the gonads and on the timing of the treatmen Exogenous melatonin regulates ovine gonadal activity; con tinuous melatonin administration effectively induces breec ing activity in acyclic ewes around midsummer.

## *Gonadal Steroid Hormones*

The ovaries and testes primarily secrete gonadal steroi hormones. Nongonadal organs such as the adrenals and th placenta also secrete steroid hormones to some extent. The are of four types: androgens, estrogens, progestins, and re laxin. The first three types are steroids while the fourth i a protein. The ovaries produce two steroid hormones, estra diol and progesterone, and a protein hormone, relaxin; th testis secretes a single hormone testosterone (Table 3-3).

Steroid hormones secreted by the ovary, testes, placenta, and adrenal cortex have a basic or common nucleus called the cyclopentanoperhydrophenanthrene nucleus. It consists of three, six-member fully hydrogenated (perhydro) phenanthrene rings designated A, B, and C, and one five-member cyclopentane ring designated D (Fig. 3-9). An 18-carbon steroid has estrogen activity, a 19-carbon steroid has androgen activity, and a 21-carbon steroid has progestogen properties. Cholesterol, a 27-carbon steroid, becomes

**TABLE 3-3. *Summary of Hormones Secreted by Reproductive Organs***

| HORMONE | STRUCTURE AND SOURCE | PRINCIPAL FUNCTIONS |
|---|---|---|
| Estrogen | 18-carbon steroid, Secreted by the theca interna of the ovarian follicle | Promotes sexual behavior; stimulates development of secondary sex characteristics, anabolic effects |
| Progesterone | 21-carbon steroid, Secreted by the corpus luteum | Acts synergistically with estrogen in promoting estrous behavior and preparing reproductive tract for implantation |
| Testosterone | 19-carbon steroid, Secreted by Leydig cells in the testis | Develops and maintains accessory sex glands; stimulates secondary sexual characteristics, sexual behavior, and spermatogenesis; possesses anabolic effects |
| Relaxin | Polypeptide hormone with $\alpha$ and $\beta$ subunits, Secreted by the corpus luteum | Dilates cervix; causes uterine contractions |
| Prostaglandin $F_{2\alpha}$ | 20-carbon unsaturated fatty acid, Secreted by almost all body tissues | Causes uterine contractions assisting in sperm transport in the female tract and parturition<br>Causes regression of the corpus luteum (luteolytic) |
| Activins | Protein, Found in follicular fluid in female and rete testis fluid in male | Stimulates FSH secretion |
| Inhibins | Protein, Found in Sertoli cells in male and the granulosa cells in female | Inhibits release of FSH to a level, which maintains species specific number of ovulations |
| Follistatin | Protein, Found in ovarian follicular fluid in the female | Modulates the secretion of FSH |

pregnenolone (20-carbon) when its side chain is cleaved. Pregnenolone is subsequently converted to progesterone, which is in turn converted to an androgen and on to estrogens (Fig. 3-10).

The biosynthetic pathways in all endocrine organs that produce steroid hormones are similar, the organs differing only in the enzyme systems they contain. The testis primarily synthesizes androgens, whereas the ovaries synthesize two major types of steroids: 18-carbon estrogens and the 21-carbon progestins.

In blood plasma, steroid hormone is mostly bound to albumin, a plasma protein with low affinity and high capacity for steroids. Another portion of the steroid hormone is bound to one or more specific proteins with high affinity.

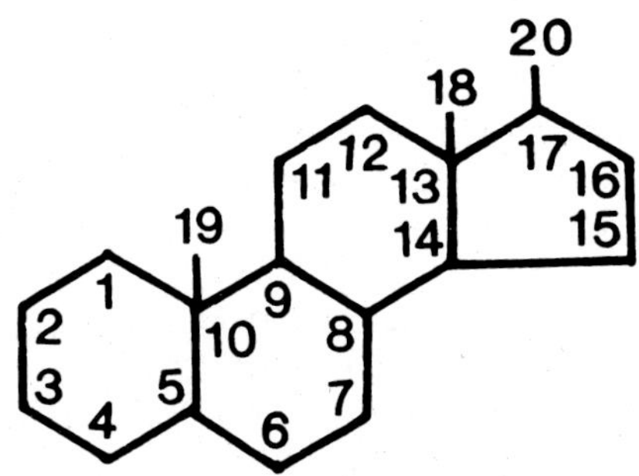


FIGURE 3-9. International Union of Pure and Applied Chemistry (IUPAC) nomenclature of the steroid nucleus. Letters designate ring and numbers designate carbon.

The half-life of naturally occurring steroids in the body is very short. Therefore, several steroids with modified biochemical structure have been synthesized for clinical use.

The secretory activity of steroid hormones by the gonads is under endocrine control of the anterior pituitary. Hypophysectomy or removal of the hypophysis before or after puberty causes atrophy of the gonads, whereas injection of pituitary preparation or implantation of pituitary tissue restores the secretory activity.

ESTROGENS. Estradiol is the primary estrogen (Fig. 3-10), with estrone and estriol representing other metabolically active estrogens (Table 3-3). Several substances of estrogenic activity are found in both the animal and plant kingdom.

Estradiol is the biologically active estrogen produced by the ovary with smaller quantities of estrone. Except for the possible secretion of small amounts of estriol in the luteal phase of the cycle, most estriol and related urinary estrogens are metabolic breakdown products of secreted estradiol/estrone. All ovarian estrogens are produced from androgenic precursors.

Plant estrogens (isoflavons) are found primarily in legumes such as subterranean clover and alfalfa. Two of these compounds, genistein and coumestrol cause infertility in females and, less frequently, in males. Zeronal (Ralgro) is a compound with estrogenic activity produced by a mold. As an ear implant, it promotes growth of feedlot animals.

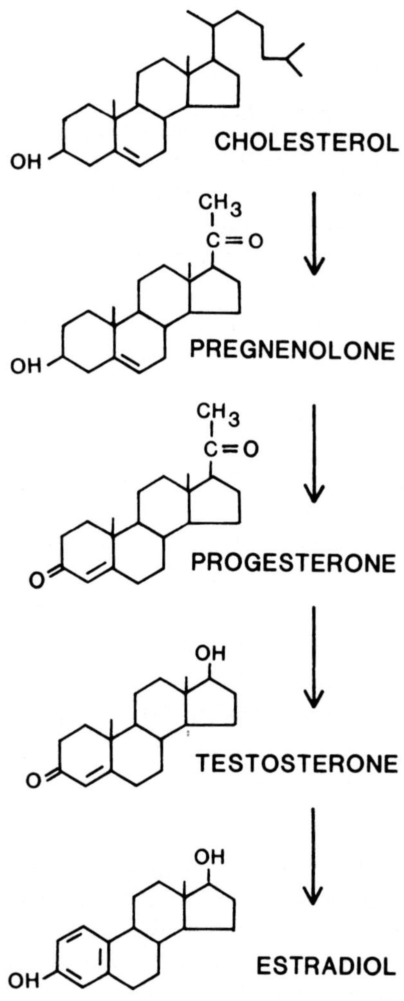

CHOLESTEROL

PREGNENOLONE

PROGESTERONE

TESTOSTERONE

ESTRADIOL

FIGURE 3-10. The biosynthesis of steroid hormones from cholesterol. This scheme provides a simplistic view of a highly organized and complicated process that requires multiple enzyme systems.

These compounds act like estrogens but do not have the 18-carbon steroid nucleus.

Binding proteins in the circulation carry estrogens. Of all the steroids, estrogens have the widest range of physiologic functions. Some of these functions are:

Act on the CNS to induce behavioral estrus in the female; however, small amounts of progesterone with estrogen are needed to induce estrus in some species such as the ewe and cow.

Act on the uterus to increase both amplitude and frequency of contractions by potentiating the effects of oxytocin and $PGF_{2\alpha}$.

Physical development of female secondary sexual characteristics.

Stimulate duct growth and cause the development of the mammary gland.

Exert both negative and positive feedback controls on LH and FSH release through the hypothalamus. The negative effect is on the tonic center in the hypothalamus, and the positive effect is on the preovulatory center.

In ruminants, estrogens also have a protein anabolic effect to increase body weight gain and growth. The possible mechanism for increased growth may be due to the ability of estrogens to stimulate the pituitary to release more growth hormone.

Diethylstibesterol (DES), a synthetic nonsteroidal estrogen, was formerly used for growth promotion in cattle and sheep. DES binds to estrogen receptor, and acts with the same potency as 17$\beta$-estradiol. Because of its carcinogenic effects, it has been replaced by other estrogenic implants.

Estrogens have been used to abort cows and sheep because of their luteolytic properties (regression of CL) whereas in the sow, estrogens have a luteotrophic action (helps to maintain CL).

PROGESTOGENS. Progesterone (Fig. 3-10) is the most prevalent, naturally occurring progestogen and is secreted by luteal cells of the corpus luteum (Table 3-3), the placenta, and adrenal gland. Progesterone is transported in blood by a binding globulin as for androgens and estrogens. LH primarily stimulates progesterone secretion.

Progesterone performs the following functions:

Prepares the endometrium for implantation and maintenance of pregnancy by increasing activity of secretory glands in the endometrium and by inhibiting the motility of the myometrium.

Acts synergistically with estrogens to induce behavioral estrus.

Develops the secretory tissue (alveoli) of the mammary glands.

Inhibits estrus and the ovulatory surge of LH at high levels. Thus, progesterone is important in the hormonal regulation of the estrous cycle.

Inhibits uterine motility.

Synthetic progestogens are available to synchronize the estrous cycles of ruminants. The progestogens act by inhibiting LH secretion from the pituitary. The hormone is either fed or inserted into the vagina as an intravaginal device for a period of one estrous cycle length. On cessation of the treatment, animals will display estrus and ovulate 48 to 72 hours later.

ANDROGENS. Androgens are 19-carbon steroids with a hydroxyl or oxygen at positions 3 and 17 and a double bond at position 4. The androgens are called 17-ketosteroids when oxygen is found at position 17 (Fig. 3-10). Testosterone is an androgen produced by the interstitial cells (Leydig cells) of the testes (Table 3-3), with a limited amount produced by the adrenal cortex.

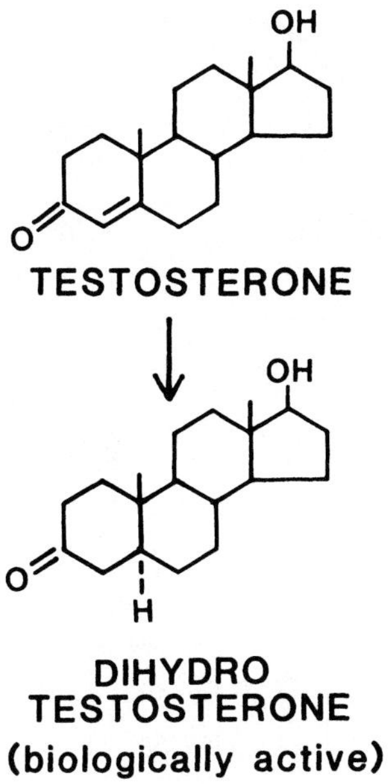

OH

O

TESTOSTERONE

OH

O

H

DIHYDRO TESTOSTERONE (biologically active)

FIGURE 3-11. Testosterone is not the biologically active form, but it is converted to dihydrotestosterone, which binds to the nuclear receptor.

Testosterone (Fig. 3-11) is transported in the blood by a $\alpha$-globulin designated steroid-binding globulin. Some 98% of circulating testosterone is bound. The remaining testosterone is free to enter the target where an enzyme in the cytoplasm converts testosterone to dihydrotesterone, which can act on the nuclear receptor.

The horse is a unique species because the seminiferous tubules and epididymis also produce high levels of testosterone. Horsemen have known for centuries that if part of the epididymis is left attached to the vas deferens during castration, the gelding will look and behave like a stallion. This is because androgens are produced by the remaining epididymis. Allowing part of the epididymis to remain is termed "cutting a horse proud." This high level of androgen prolongs the life of epididymal sperm in the stallion rather than acting on the secondary sex characteristics.

The functions of testosterone are:

Stimulate late stages of spermatogenesis and prolong the life span of epididymal sperm.

Promote growth, development, and secretory activity of the accessory sex organs of the male.

Maintain secondary sex characteristics and sexual behavior or libido of the male

The synthetic androgens, testosterone propionate and androstenedione, are often used to prepare teasers for the detection of estrus. These androgenized cows and ewes have the advantage of not transmitting venereal diseases.

### *Relaxin*

Relaxin is a polypeptide hormone consisting of alpha and beta subunits that are connected by two disulfide bonds. It has a molecular weight of 5700 daltons. Inhibins and insulin are structurally similar, but their biologic actions are different. Relaxin is secreted primarily by the corpus luteum during pregnancy (Table 3-3). In some species, the placenta and uterus also secrete relaxin. The main biologic action of relaxin is dilation of the cervix and vagina before parturition. It also inhibits uterine contractions and causes increased growth of the mammary gland if given in conjunction with estradiol. In the guinea pig, relaxin causes separation of the pubic symphysis bone within 6 hours after injection. Separation of the pubic symphysis normally occurs during parturition in this species.

### *Inhibins and Activins*

Inhibins and activins were isolated from gonadal fluids because of their effects on the production of FSH (Table 3-3). Inhibins and activins are paracrine regulators whereby they modulate the endocrine LH signal.

INHIBINS. The gonads are the main source of inhibin and related proteins, which contribute to the endocrine regulation of the reproductive system. Sertoli cells in the male and the granulosa cells in the female produce inhibins. Inhibins are not steroids but proteins comprising two disulfide bridged subunits called $\alpha$ and $\beta$. In the male, inhibins are secreted via the lymph and not by venous blood as in the female (3).

Inhibins play an important role in the hormonal regulation of ovarian folliculogenesis during the estrous cycle. Inhibins act as chemical signals to the pituitary gland on the number of growing follicles in the ovary. Inhibins reduce the secretion of FSH to a level, which maintains the species-specific number of ovulation in both single and litter bearing species (4). By inhibiting FSH release without altering LH release, inhibins may be partly responsible for the differential release of LH and FSH from the pituitary.

Besides the regulation of pituitary FSH, inhibin related proteins regulate Leydig cell function (5).

ACTIVINS. Follicular fluid contains a fraction that stimulates rather than inhibits the secretion of FSH (6). The proteins responsible for this activity were characterized as activins (Fig. 3-12). Activins are potent FSH-releasing dimers (dimers of inhibin-subunits, $\beta$) and are present in gonadal fluids, e.g., follicular fluid and rete testis fluid. These heterodimeric hormones are composed of a $\alpha$-subunit and one of two $\beta$-subunits ($\beta$A or, $\beta$B). Activin is a fully functional member of the growth factors (6).

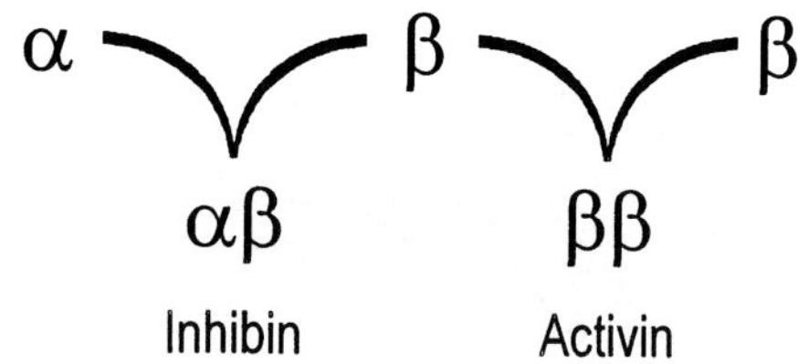


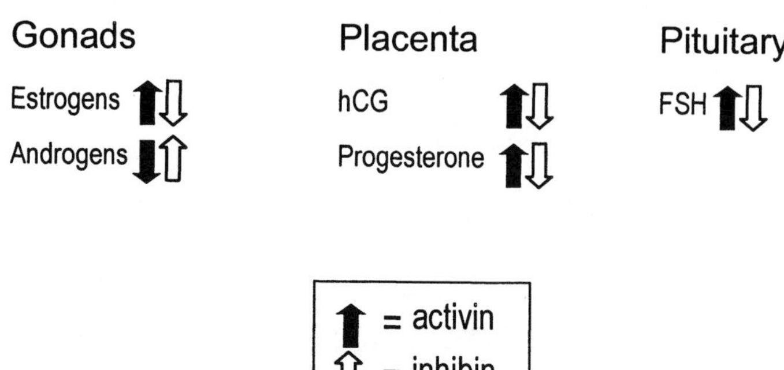


FIGURE 3-12. Summary of the physiological actions of inhibins and activins (adapted from Vale W, Bilezikjian LM, River C. Reproductive and other roles of inhibins and activins. In: Knobil E, Neill JD, eds. Reproductive Physiology, Vol 1, 2nd Ed. New York: Raven Press, 1994;34).

FOLLISTATIN. Follistatin is another protein isolated from follicular fluid. Follistatin not only inhibits the secretion of FSH similar to that of inhibins but also binds activin and neutralizes its biological activity. Thus, it modulates the secretion of FSH.

### *Placental Hormones*

The placenta secretes several hormones either identical to, or with biologic activity similar to, hormones of mammalian reproduction: equine chorionic gonadotropin (eCG), human chorionic gonadotropin (hCG), placental lactogen (PL), and protein B (Table 3-4).

EQUINE CHORIONIC GONADOTROPIN. The hormone eCG (PMSG) was discovered when blood from pregnant mares produced sexual maturity in immature rat. eCG is a glycoprotein with $\alpha$ and $\beta$ subunits similar to LH and FSH but with a higher carbohydrate content, especially sialic acid. The higher sialic acid content appears to account for the long half-life of several days for eCG. Thus, a single injection of eCG has biologic effects on the target gland for more than a week.

The equine uterus secretes this placental gonadotropin. The endometrial cups are the source for the eCG. The cups that are formed at about day 40 of pregnancy persist until day 85 of pregnancy. eCG has both FSH and LH biologic actions, with the FSH actions being dominant. eCG circulates in the blood of pregnant mares and is not excreted in urine. The secretion of eCG stimulates development of ovarian follicles (Table 3-4). Some follicles ovulate, but most become luteinized follicles, due to the LH like action of the eCG. These accessory corpora lutea produce progestogens, which maintain pregnancy in the mare. eCG was one of the first commercially available gonadotropins used to induce superovulation in farm animals.

HUMAN CHORIONIC GONADOTROPIN. The glycoprotein hCG consists of $\alpha$ and $\beta$ subunits with a molecular weight of 40,000 daltons. The $\alpha$ subunit has 92 amino acids and two carbohydrate chains. The $\alpha$ subunit of hCG is similar to the $\alpha$ subunits of human, porcine, ovine, and bovine LH. The $\beta$ subunit has 145 amino acids and five carbohydrate chains. hCG is primarily luteinizing and luteotropic and has little FSH activity. The syncytiotrophoblastic cells in the primate placenta synthesize hCG of the placenta of primates; hCG is found in both blood and urine (Table 3-4). Its presence in the urine in early pregnancy is the basis of the various laboratory tests for human pregnancy. It is detected in the urine 8 days after conception by sensitive immunoassays.

PLACENTAL LACTOGEN. Placental lactogen is a protein with chemical properties similar to prolactin and growth hormone. Its molecular weight is 22,000 to 23,000 daltons in the ovine with 192 amino acids. Placental lactogen is isolated from placental tissue but cannot be detected in the serum of the pregnant animal until the last trimester of pregnancy (Table 3-4). Placental lactogen is more important for its growth hormone properties than its prolactin properties. It is important in regulating maternal nutrients to the fetus and possibly is important for fetal growth. Placental lactogen may play a role in milk production because the level is higher in dairy cows (high milk producers) than in beef cows (low milk producers).

TABLE 3-4. *Summary of Hormones Secreted by the Placenta*

| HORMONE | SPECIES | STRUCTURE AND SITE | BODY FLUIDS WHERE PRESENT | PRINCIPAL FUNCTIONS |
|---|---|---|---|---|
| Human chorionic gonadotropin (primates only) (hCG) | Human, monkey | Glycoprotein, Syncytiotrophoblastic cells | Blood, urine | LH activity, maintains corpus luteum of pregnancy in primates |
| Equine chorionic gonadotropin (eCG/PMSG) | Horse | Glycoprotein, Endometrial cups of fetal origin | Blood | FSH activity, stimulates formation of accessory corpora lutea in mare |
| Estrogens | Sheep, cattle | Steroid, Fetoplacental unit | Blood | |
| Progesterone | Sheep, cattle | Steroid, Fetoplacental unit | Blood | Maintenance of pregnancy |
| Placental lactogen | Sheep, cattle | Protein, Placental tissue | Blood | Regulates transport of nutrients from dam to fetus, but not fully elucidated |
| Pregnancy protein B | Sheep, cattle | Protein, from conceptus | Blood | Maternal recognition of pregnancy |

PROTEIN B. The bovine conceptus produces numerous signals during early pregnancy. Currently only one protein from placental tissue has been partially purified–pregnancy-specific protein B (bPSPB) (7). The physiologic action of protein B may be involved in preventing destruction of the corpus luteum in early pregnancy of the cow or ewe (Table 3-4). This placental hormone has the potential to be the first reliable hormonal pregnancy test for cattle.

## *Prostaglandins*

Prostaglandins, first isolated from accessory sex gland fluids, were termed prostaglandins because of their association with the prostate gland. Almost all body tissues secrete them. All prostaglandins are 20-carbon unsaturated hydroxy fatty acids with a cyclopentene ring. Arachidonic acid, an essential fatty acid, is the precursor for prostaglandins most closely associated with reproduction, mainly $PGF_{2\alpha}$ and prostaglandin $E_2$ ($PGE_2$) (Fig. 3-13).

Most prostaglandins act locally at the site of their production on a cell-to-cell interaction and therefore do not conform exactly to the classic definition of a hormone. Unlike other humoral agents, prostaglandins are not localized in any particular tissue. They are transported in the blood to act on a target tissue away from the site of production. Some forms never appear in the blood, whereas others are degraded after they circulate throughout the liver and lungs. $PGF_{2\alpha}$ is the natural luteolytic agent that ends the luteal phase (corpus luteum) of the estrous cycle and allows for the initiation of a new estrous cycle in the absence of fertilization. It is particularly potent in ending early pregnancy.

Prostaglandins may be considered hormones, which regulate several physiologic and pharmacologic phenomena, such as contraction of smooth muscles in the reproductive and gastrointestinal tracts, erection, ejaculation, sperm transport, ovulation, formation of the corpus luteum, partu-

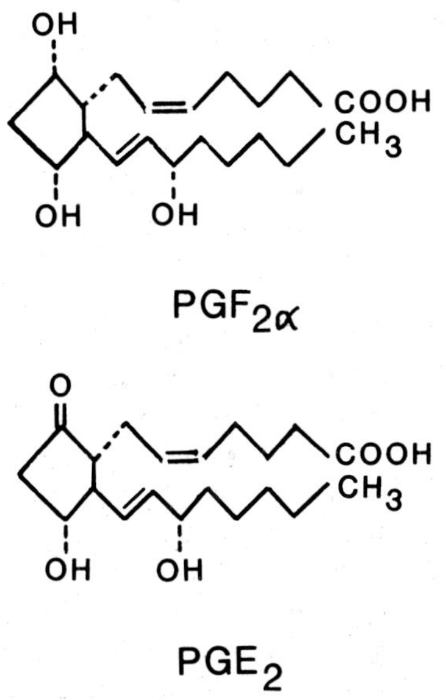

FIGURE 3-13. Chemical structure of $PGF_{2\alpha}$ and $PGE_2$.

rition, and milk ejection. Prostaglandins are involved in ovulation (8). For example, in the ewe and cow, ovulation is blocked by the administration of indomethacin, an inhibitor of prostaglandin synthesis (9). Since LH release is unaffected in these animals, the action at the level of the ovarian follicle involves either or both $PGF_{2\alpha}$, and $PGE_2$.

An increase in estrogen, which promotes myometrium growth in the uterus, stimulates $PGF_{2\alpha}$ synthesis and release. In pregnant animals, the developing embryo sends a signal to the uterus (maternal recognition of pregnancy), preventing luteolytic effects of $PGF_{2\alpha}$ (see Chapter 10 Immunolgy of Reproduction).

The capacity of $PGF_{2\alpha}$ to induce luteolysis has been exploited for manipulating the estrous cycle and the induction of parturition.

## CLINICAL USES OF HORMONES

Almost all the hormones discussed above are used in improving reproductive efficiency in farm animals. The reader is referred to several chapters in this book for a plethora of hormonal applications in animal production and veterinary medicine.

## HORMONAL REGULATION OF REPRODUCTION

The hypothalamus functions as an interface between the nervous and endocrine systems and plays an important role in the hormonal regulation of reproduction. Edqvist has reviewed the endogenous control of reproductive processes in domestic animals (10). As stated earlier, the gonadal hormones inhibit the release of LH and FSH in both sexes (negative feedback) whereas they enhance the release of LH and FSH only in the female (positive feedback).

### *Endocrine Mechanisms*

The endocrine mechanisms to be discussed here include puberty, estrous cycle, pregnancy and parturition, testicular function, Sertoli cells, and activins and inhibins.

PUBERTY. By definition, a male or female has reached puberty when it is able to release gametes and exhibit sexual behavior. The onset of puberty is regulated by the maturity of the hypothalamic-adenohypophyseal axis rather than by the inability of the pituitary to produce gonadotropins or by an ovarian insensitivity to their effects. It is well known that the prepubertal calf, pig, and lamb will ovulate following exogenous gonadotropins.

The prepubertal female responds to the pulsatile secretion of gonadotropin by gradually secreting estrogen. In ewes and heifers, the frequency of LH-peaks increases followed by a transient rise in the preovulatory surge of LH. This is associated with behavioral estrus during this pubertal period.

Prepubertal males in response to gonadotropin stimulation, secrete testosterone progressively. Every pulse of LH is followed at a one-hour interval by a transitory rise in testosterone secretion. As puberty progresses the increase of testosterone in blood causes a decrease in gonadotropin secretion via a negative feedback effect.

ESTROUS CYCLE. During the estrous cycle, LH and FSH are released in a tonic manner or as a surge. Neural pathways are also associated with the timing of ovulation (Fig. 3-14).

***Tonic LH and FSH Release.*** Tonic levels of LH and FSH are controlled by negative feedback from the gonads. The tonic level of LH is not stationary but shows oscillations about every hour. Tonic serum LH levels are elevated after gonadectomy in both males and females. The increased levels of LH and FSH after gonadectomy are due to the

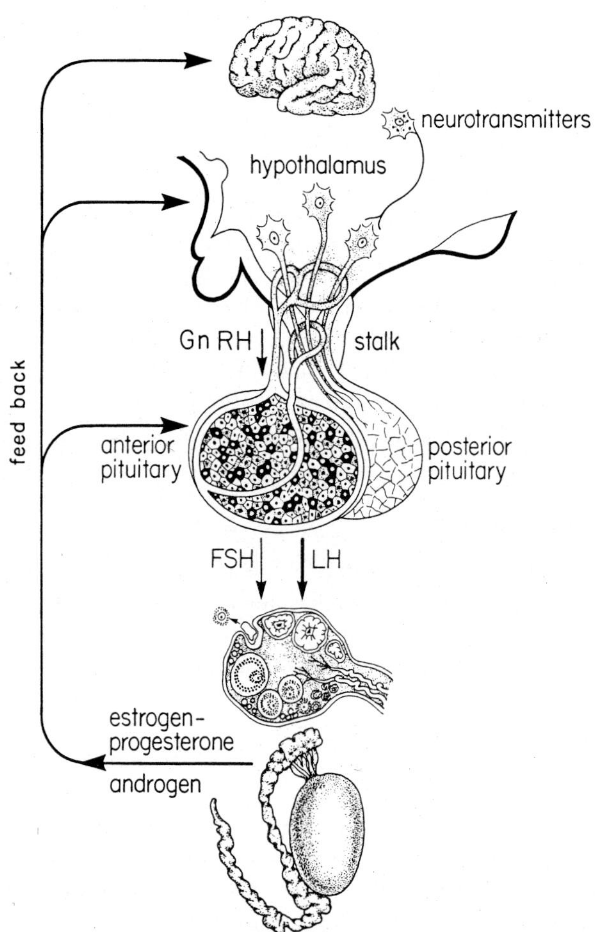


FIGURE 3-14. Endocrine-neuroendocrine relationship among hypothalamus, pituitary gland, and gonad (ovary-testis). Hypothalamic neurosecretory materials (GnRH) are transported by the portal blood capillaries to the cells of the anterior pituitary. FSH and LH stimulate the gonads. Estrogens and androgens secreted by the gonads exert a feedback.

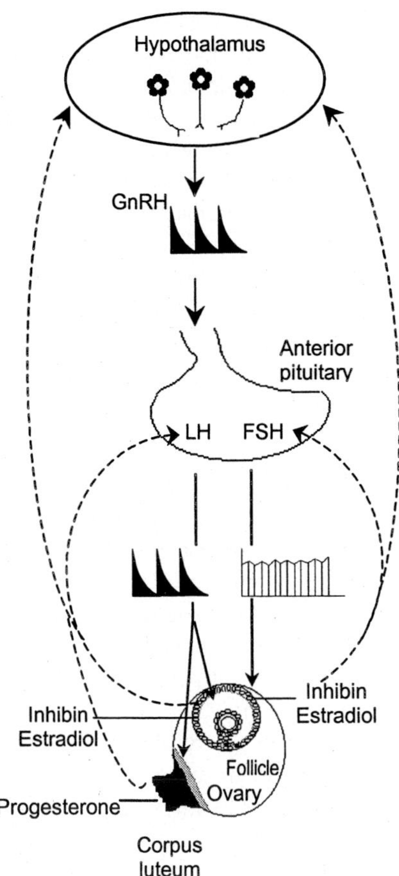


FIGURE 3-15. Hypothalamus, anterior pituitary, and ovary interrelationships. Solid arrows indicate stimulatory effects, dashed arrows indicate inhibitory effects.

lack of a negative feedback from the gonadal steroids on the tonic LH control center in the hypothalamus (Fig. 3-15).

The LH and FSH surges also induce the final stages of oocyte maturation, just before ovulation, to metaphase II.

***Preovulatory LH and FSH Release.*** A second type of LH and FSH release, called the preovulatory surge of LH and FSH, is evident in the female before ovulation. An increase in the circulating estrogen concentration has a positive feedback effect on the hypothalamus, inducing a sudden surge of GnRH release, which is accompanied, by the preovulatory surge of LH and FSH. The preovulatory surges of LH and FSH lasts 6 to 12 hours, are responsible for ovulation.

The levels of estradiol decline after the LH and FSH surges, and the psychical manifestations of estrus abate. The animal will ovulate 24 to 30 hours after the initial maximal gonadotropin surge.

NEURAL PATHWAYS. Various neural pathways exist between the reproductive system and hypothalamic-pituitary axis. Mating can modulate the preovulatory surge of LH by prolonging the duration of LH release rather than by increasing plasma concentrations.

Mating affects the time of ovulation in spontaneously ovulating species such as sheep. In beef cattle, clitoral stimulation hastens the onset of ovulation, and stimulation of the cervix reduces the time from the beginning of estrus to the occurrence of LH surge. In sows, natural mating affects ovulation by shortening the interval from onset of estrus to ovulation and by reducing the interval from the first to last ovulation. Naturally mated sows have higher concentrations of plasma LH immediately after mating.

PREGNANCY AND PARTURITION. Both the maintenance of pregnancy and the initiation of parturition are under endocrine control. Progesterone is the important hormone required for continuation of pregnancy. In all farm animals, progesterone secreted by the corpus luteum is essential for maintenance of early pregnancy. However in the horse, the placenta takes over the function of progesterone secretion (see Chapter 9 Pregnancy). As parturition approaches, the declining progesterone levels trigger a complex interaction involving the fetus and the mother. $PGF_{2\alpha}$, estrogens, oxytocin and fetal cortisol are some of the hormones associated with parturition.

TESTICULAR FUNCTION. The neuroendocrine control of testicular function is similar to those as in the female. The endocrine control of male reproduction has been reviewed (3). Both FSH and androgens maintain the gametogenic function, whereas LH controls the secretion of testosterone from the Leydig cells. Unlike in the female, there is no positive feedback system. Thus, after castration, both concentration and pulse frequency of LH and FSH are retained.

Testosterone secretion is regulated by long, short, and ultrashort loops. The long loop involves FSH, inhibin, and LH-testosterone interactions (Fig. 3-16). The short loop between the interstitial and seminiferous epithelium involves growth factors and hormones. The ultrashort loop regulates Sertoli cell-germ cell-myoid cell interactions. In the bull, each pulse of LH results in a peak of testosterone about 30 to 45 minutes later.

Stallions produce and excrete large quantities of estrogens compared to those produced by males of most other mammalian species. The testes produce the estrogens. Concentrations of 17$\beta$-estradiol (estradiol) are seasonal in stallions and are parallel to the concentrations of LH and testosterone

SERTOLI CELLS. Sertoli cells and germ cells reciprocally regulate each other's cyclic secretion of proteins along the length of the seminiferous tubule. Myoid cells amplify this process through transforming growth factors, humoral modulators, and extracellular matrix. Sertoli cells are provided with low-resistance pathways for intercellular transport of cell metabolites, which coordinate the activity of the seminiferous epithelium.

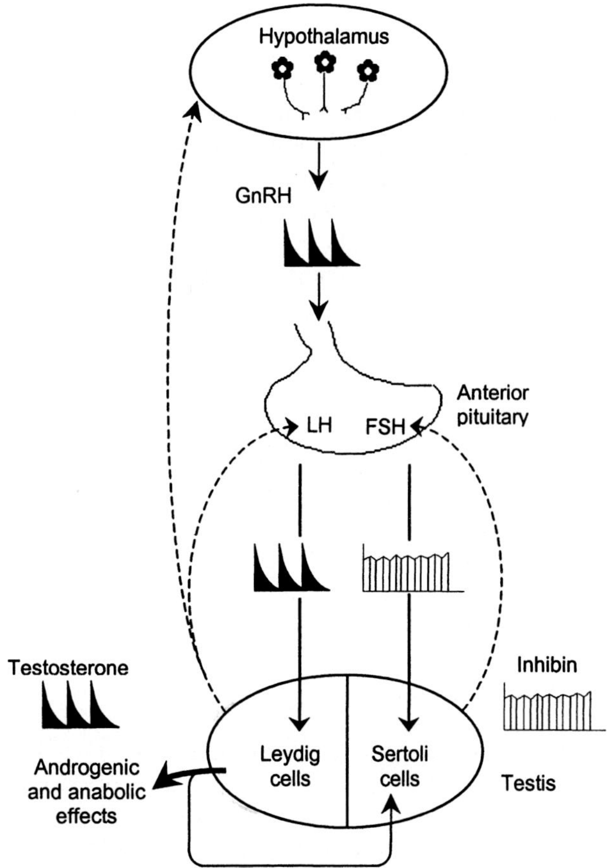


Figure 3-16. Hypothalamus, anterior pituitary, and testis interrelationships. Solid arrows indicate stimulatory effects, dashed arrows indicate inhibitory effects.

Several circulating proteins are internalized through the basal compartment into Sertoli cells by endocrine mechanisms: transferrin, androgen bound protein (ABP), insulin-like growth factors (IGF), and related growth factors. Proteins secreted by Sertoli cells in the adluminal compartment are internalized by a paracrine mechanism in germ cells. Spermatocytes and early spermatids are preferential targets of Sertoli cell proteins in the testis.

Activins and Inhibins. Activins and inhibins act within the gonads and placenta as autocrine and paracrine modulators of the production of steroids and other hormones, and growth factors. As previously mentioned, inhibins and activins are produced by the Sertoli cells. These regulate FSH secretion but have minimal effect on LH secretion. For a detailed discussion of the reproductive and other roles of activins and inhibins, the reader should refer elsewhere (6).

### *Sexual Behavior*

Male Sexual Behavior. Castration of males is a routine procedure in a reproductive management program in farm animals. The depressing action of castration varies with the species, the individual, and the physiologic and behavioral status of the animal at the time of operation.

Some mounting activity is retained after prepubertal castration in bulls and rams, but the underdevelopment of the genital tract resulting from the lack of androgen during ontogeny drastically inhibits mating.

Two parameters of normal sexual behavior seem to be somewhat independent: the animal's desire to mount and thrust and the ability to ejaculate. After castration, the desire to mount is retained for a longer period than the ability to ejaculate. The attainment of an erection is the last aspect of normal sexual behavior to disappear after castration.

Female Sexual Behavior. Female sexual behavior depends on an appropriate endocrine balance resulting in the development of the ovarian follicles. Ovariectomy inhibits sexual behavior, but in the cow and sow, sexual behavior is restored in ovariectomized females after the injection of a minimal dose of estrogen following 8 to 12 days of progesterone pretreatment. In the sow and ewe, there is a linear dose-response relationship between the duration of estrus and the logarithm of the dose of estrogen. There is also a relationship between duration of natural estrus and the number of ovulations in the sow and ewe.

Sex Specificity. The sex specificity of steroid hormones—androgens for males, estrogens and progestogens for females—raises the possibility of a direct influence of the hormone on the behavioral response. The rhythm of secretion, however, differs between the sexes, and a possible sexualization of the brain may influence the reaction. The treatment of gonadectomized animals with the hormone of the opposite sex shows that the sex specificity of the hormone is limited as far as the behavioral responses are concerned. Daily injections of estrogen allow a complete recovery of male activity in castrated rams, whereas a single treatment with testosterone induces a normal female receptivity in the ovariectomized female.

Neural Mechanisms. The physiologic signal that initiates sexual motivation is the secretion of steroid hormones. Once released in the bloodstream, hormones are rapidly bound to receptor sites in the CNS. Maximal estrogen levels in the blood of the ewe and sow occur about 24 hours before onset of estrus. When the animal is sexually motivated, behavioral events are initiated. Specific or unspecific sensory stimuli acting on the sense organs, through innate or acquired mechanisms, are integrated in the brain to elicit appropriate motor reactions.

## Growth Factors

Growth factors have become increasingly important in many areas of reproductive physiology. Growth factors are hormone-like polypeptides and proteins, which are predominantly paracrine and autocrine in promoting mitogenic activity in local tissue proliferation and remodeling, e.g., transformation of the ovarian follicle into a corpus luteum. Much of the research on growth factors is focused on their growth promoting actions.

Growth factors may be divided into three classes:

Agents that promote the multiplication and/or development of various types of cells—nerve growth factor, insulin-like growth factor I (IGF-1), activins and inhibins, and epidermal growth factors (EGF).

Cytokines, produced by macrophages and lymphocytes, are important in the regulation of the immune system.

Colony stimulating factors (CSF) that regulate proliferation and maturation of red and white bloods.

### Methods of Study

Growth factors are usually defined by their ability to induce stimulation of target cell multiplication, and their activity is measured by assays where either the increase of cell populations or the incorporation of labeled thymidine into DNA is determined. During the past few years, several studies have been conducted on growth factors related to male and female reproduction in both man and animal.

### Mechanism of Action

Growth factors elicit cellular responses by binding to specific cell, surface receptors in their target tissues. Polypeptide growth factors regulate the proliferation on many cell types and regulate growth of the reproductive tract. These factors have a wide range of cell types that express the appropriate growth factor receptors (11).

### Growth Factors

The discussion of growth factors in this chapter will be restricted to ovarian and testicular physiology. Table 3-5 lists some growth factors related to reproduction in farm animals. Table 3-6 presents recent studies on the regulation of ovarian function (12–31).

Descriptions of the growth factors relevant to this chapter were gleaned from several sources (2, 6, 32–34).

**Cytokines.** Cytokines are hormone-like chemical messengers secreted by lymphocytes and macrophages that affect the immune system. Once the amino acid sequence of a factor is established, the name changes to interleukin, e.g., interleukin-1 (IL-1) or interleukin-2 (IL-2). IL-2 is a growth factor produced by T4 cells that increases the synthesis of T8 and $\beta$B cells.

**Epidermal Growth Factor (EGF).** EGF is a polypeptide with potent mitogenic activity in several types of cells in vivo and in vitro. The factor was originally isolated from the submaxillary glands of mice, human urine, and other sources.

**Fibroblast Growth Factor (FGF).** FGF, originally isolated from bovine pituitary, is a polypeptide. It is angiogenic (i.e., it stimulates the growth of blood vessels) as well as mitogenic. The synthesis of FGF in the ovary stimulates bovine luteal cells but delays the differentiation of bovine granulosa cells in culture.

**Inhibins and Activins.** Inhibins and activins are important paracrine/autocrine regulators of FSH and LH. Their structure, sources, and actions were discussed earlier.

**Insulin and Insulin-Like Growth Factors (IGFs).** IGFs or somatomedins are polypeptide growth factors secreted by the liver and several tissues in response to stimulation by growth hormone. They mediate most of the growth-promoting actions of growth hormone. The insulin-like growth factors (IGF-I and IGF-II) are single-chain polypeptides with structural homology to proinsulin. They regulate proliferation and differentiation of several cell types and exert insulin-like metabolic effects. Unlike insulin, most tissues produce them. IGFs have the capacity to act via endocrine as well as autocrine and/or paracrine mechanisms.

**Interferons (IFNs).** Interferons (IFNs) are a group of proteins which were initially identified by their ability to protect cells against viral infections. There are at least three classes: $\alpha$, $\beta$, and $\gamma$. Both $\alpha$ and $\beta$ IFNs are synthesized in response to viral infection, whereas an IFN-$\gamma$ is produced in T lymphocyte following mitogenic or antigenic stimulation.

**Nerve Growth Factor (NGF).** NGF is a protein growth factor required for the growth and maintenance of sympathetic neurons.

**Platelet-Activating Factor.** Platelet-activating factor (PAF) is a potent phospholipid mediator produced by several cell types: neutrophils, macrophages, endothelial cells, and preimplantation embryos. PAF induces a wide range of physiologic and pharmacologic responses involving reproductive processes (35), platelet aggregation, anaphylaxis, and vascular permeability. PAF, produced by sperm, enhances sperm motility and in vitro fertilization during coincubation of sperm and egg.

**Platelet-Derived Growth Factor (PDGF).** PDFG is a polypeptide produced by platelets, macrophages, and endothelial cells. It is a potent mitogen for vascular smooth

TABLE 3-5. ***Putative Autocrine/Paracrine Regulators and Reproductive Function in Farm Animals (Compiled from the Literature)***

| PUTATIVE REGULATOR | PRINCIPAL FUNCTIONS |
|---|---|
| EGF (epidermal growth factor) | May stimulate regrowth of epithelium following disruption of ovarian surface at ovulation |
| ECG-I like (ECG-I like peptides) | Growth and development of neonatal uterus; relation of these peptides with estrogen action unknown |
| FGF (fibroblast growth factor) | 18,000-Dalton protein stimulates proliferation of various cell types required with blastocyst implantation and embryonic development |
| GHRH (Growth Hormone Releasing Hormone) | Modulatory action of GHRH on gonadal function is FSH dependent<br>Locally formed GFR exerts synergistic action during ovarian follicle maturation |
| GM-CSF (granulocyte-macrophage colony-stimulating factor) | Secreted by placental cells, autocrine within certain cells of fetal placenta<br>An important cytokine that serves as a basis for interaction between maternal immune system and reproductive tissues during mammalian pregnancy |
| IFN (Interferon) | Cytokines with complex effects on cells of immune system in ovine and bovine<br>Conceptus produce IFN as their major secretory factor before implantation |
| IGF (insulin growth factor) | Plays a role in early pregnancy in ruminants<br>Endometrium synthesizes and secretes four IGF<br>Testicular EGF plays a role in regulation of spermatogonial division and testicular IGF-I production stimulated by retinol without cyclic changes in testicular IGF-I concentrations |
| Intrafollicular growth factor | Regulates steroidogenesis in granulosa cells in large ovarian follicles via aromatase activity |
| PAF (platelet-activating factor) | Phospholipid secreted by human blastocyst, an autocrine growth factor, needed for implantation<br>PAF performs antiluteolytic and luteotropic function during pregnancy |
| PDGF (platelet-derived growth factor) | Promotes hatching and blastocyst outgrowth after in vitro microinjection of anti-PDGF antibodies into uterine lumen |
| Relaxin | Polypeptide, closely related structure to insulin and insulin-like growth factors, synthesized and secreted by corpus luteum |
| TNF (tumor necrosis factor) | Immunohistochemically localized in ovary: granulosa cells of antral follicle<br>Increases thecal progesterone production and inhibits basal and FSH-stimulated progesterone in granulosa cells<br>TNF and hCG increase progesterone secretion above maximal dose of hCG |

muscle, and fosters wound healing. PDFG also increases FSH-stimulated progestin production.

**RELAXIN-LIKE FACTOR (RLF).** RLF is a new member of the insulin/insulin-like growth factor family, which appears to be predominantly expressed in the Leydig cells of the testis. In addition, it is produced in the ovary of a number of species in both follicular theca cells and in the corpus luteum of the cycle and pregnancy (36). RLF might functionally substitute for relaxin in the cow (37).

**TRANSFORMING GROWTH FACTOR (TGF).** Transforming growth factor $\alpha$ (TGF$\alpha$), closely related to EGF, binds to EGF receptors and exerts similar effects. TGF$\beta$ is produced in the granulosa and theca cells and the oocyte.

**TUMOR NECROSIS FACTOR (TNF).** Tumor necrosis factor-$\alpha$ (TNF$\alpha$) has traditionally been associated with inflammation, but several reports describe a potential function for TNF in the female tract. TNF is involved in gamete development, cyclic changes in uterus, cancers of the female reproductive tract, placental maturation, and embryonic development (38).

**VASCULAR ENDOTHELIA GROWTH FACTOR (VEGF).** The female reproductive organs exhibit marked, periodic growth and regression, accompanied by equally striking changes in their rates of blood flow. These are some of the few adult tissues in which angiogenesis occurs as a normal process. Ovarian follicles and corpora lutea produce angiogenic factors. These angiogenic factors appear to be heparin-binding and belong to the fibroblast growth factor (FGF) and vascular endothelial growth factor (VEGF) families of proteins. VEGF was first demonstrated in bovine corpus luteum and later in ovine corpus luteum. The cyclic changes associated with the formation and regression of the corpus

**TABLE 3-6. *Recent Advances in Putative Autocrine/Paracrine Regulators and Ovarian Function in Farm Animals***

| PUTATIVE REGULATOR | EXPERIMENTAL DESIGNS/ HYPOTHESIS | RESULTS/FINDINGS/CONCLUSIONS | REFERENCES |
|---|---|---|---|
| ECF | Bovine/Oocyte maturation or embryo culture in defined medium | The maturation-promoting effect was evident for denuded oocytes | Lonergan et al (12) |
| ECF + IGF-I | Bovine oocytes in vitro | Stimulate cumulus expansion, nuclear maturation, and cleavage after fertilization of bovine oocytes in vitro | Rieger et al (13) |
| EGF + IGF-I | Bovine oocytes matured in vitro in serum-free media | Both growth factors, acting alone or together, stimulate cumulus expansion, enhance nuclear maturation in oocytes surrounded by compact cumulus cells | Lorenzo et al (14) |
| EGF, TGF | Bovine cumulus cell-enclosed oocytes | Increases the number of fertilized ova that developed to the blastocyst stage | Kobayashi et al (15) |
| PDGF | In vitro-matured and in vitro-fertilized bovine embryos by platelets | Stimulatory effects of PDGF on bovine embryo development may be derived from both the oviductal epithelium and platelets | Thibodeaux et al (16, 17) |
| EGF, IGF | Intraovarian regulation in the pig ovary | At least four EGF-related peptides are expressed in pig ovaries, but difficult to predict their physiological regulation | Hammond et al (18) |
| VEGF | Luteal tissues from ewes at different stages of the oestrous cycle | VEGF is expressed in luteal tissue throughout the ovine oestrous cycle and that expression of mRNA encoding VEGF is up-regulated during rapid luteal development | Redmer et al (19) |
| TGF-$\alpha$ | Secretory function of bovine corpus luteum during the oestrous cycle and pregnancy in vitro | TGF-$\alpha$ and PDGF stimulate P4 release particularly during late pregnancy | Liebermann et al (20) |
| GM-CSF | Stimulates development of bovine embryos | Useful molecule for increasing blastocyst production rates in serum-free culture systems | De Moraes and Hansen (21) |
| IGF-I | Blastocyst development of bovine embryos produced in vitro | Culture media containing high concentrations of IGF-I combined with oestrous cow serum and granulosa cells improves the development of embryos produced in vitro | Palma et al (22) |
| IGF-I, Insulin | Bovine, one-cell embryos cultured in a chemically defined, protein-free medium | Insulin and IGF-I improve the in vitro development of bovine embryos | Matsui et al (23) |
| Bovine interferon $\tau$ ($IFN_{\tau}$) | Secretion of $PGF_{2\alpha}$ and $PGF_2$ by epithelial and stromal cells in endometrium | $bIFN_{\tau}$ suppresses prostaglandin secretion in epithelial cells of endometrium which is suggestive an antiluteolytic role | Danet-Denoyers et al (24) |
| Inhibins, activins, IGF-I | Alterations in intrafollicular amounts during selection of the first-wave dominant follicle (DFI) | Decline in serum follicle-stimulating hormone concentrations alters key intrafollicular growth factors involved in selection of the dominant follicle in heifers | Mihn et al (25) |

*continued*

TABLE 3-6. **(Continued)**

| PUTATIVE REGULATOR | EXPERIMENTAL DESIGNS/ HYPOTHESIS | RESULTS/FINDINGS/CONCLUSIONS | REFERENCES |
|---|---|---|---|
| IGF-I + IGFBPs | Changes associated with the steroidogenic capacity that occur in follicle | The absence of IGFBPs, other than IGFBP-3, in bovine preovulatory follicles may allow for increased availability of IGF-I, which is important for oocyte maturation and ovulation | Funston et al (26) |
| IGF-I + IGFBPs | Change during growth of the dominant follicle in lactating Holstein cows | Low amounts of IGFBP-2 and increased thecal binding sites for hCG/LH are related to establishment of the dominant follicle during the first follicular wave in cattle | Stewart et al (27) |
| IGF-I | Progesterone and androstenedione production by bovine thecal cells | Significant role in thecal cell mitogenesis and LH-induced thecal cell steroidogenesis during follicular development in cattle | Stewart et al (28) |
| IGF-I | Granulosa and thecal cells from dominant preovulatory (DO) and nonovulatory (DNO) bovine follicles | Proliferation potential appeared to be switched off during the late stages of maturation of DNO follicles and switched on after induced luteal regression and rescue of DO follicles | Bao et al (29) |
| IGF-I | Ovarian follicular steroidogenesis during the follicular phase of the bovine estrous cycle | A possible regulatory role for IGFBPs in follicular maturation and on aromatase activity | Echternkamp et al (30) |
| IGF-I | The influence of body energy reserves on postpartum anestrous beef cows after early weaning | The number of LH pulses at weaning, serum IGF-I, and the interval to the onset of ovarian activity after early weaning of anestrous beef cows influenced by BCS | Bishop et al (31) |

luteum is associated with the formation of new blood vessels—angiogenesis (19).

### *Growth Factors and Reproduction*

It is widely held that FSH and LH regulate both ovarian and testicular functions. However, it is difficult to explain reproductive processes such as folliculogenesis, selection of ovulatory and atretic follicles, and oocyte maturation solely by changes in gonadotropin levels. During the past decade, attention has been directed on locally produced factors acting by autocrine or paracrine mechanisms that are able to modulate the target cells' responsiveness to FSH and LH. These autocrine or paracrine agents may serve to alter the sensitivity or responsiveness of FSH or LH in either a stimulatory or an inhibitory manner.

INTRAOVARIAN REGULATORS. The ovarian follicle undergoes rapid cell proliferation during its early growth, which apparently is independent of circulating gonadotropins. Perhaps ovarian autocrine and paracrine agents regulate the initiation of follicular growth.

Many growth factors and cytokines alter the responsiveness of theca cells to LH and the granulosa cells to LH and FSH in vitro (39). These include activins, inhibins, IGF-1, EGF, FGF, TGF-$\alpha$ and TGF-$\beta$, TNF$\alpha$, interleukin-1, interferon-$\gamma$ and endothelin. However, the actions of only a few of these factors have been demonstrated in vivo.

In 1995 Campbell tested growth factors in vivo by intra-arterial infusion in ewes with ovarian transplants (40). They found that EGF, TGF$\alpha$, basic FGF, inhibin, and steroid free bovine follicular fluid inhibited ovarian function, whereas IGF-1 stimulated hormone secretion.

Apparently, control of development and selection of the ovulatory follicle occurs at three levels (21):

gonadotropins initiate follicle development;

ovulatory follicle produces growth factors that suppress development of other follicles through gonadotropin-dependent mechanisms; and

factors within the ovulatory follicle, which modulate the actions of gonadotropins.

In this respect, the inhibins and activins are potential intraovarian regulatory systems. The biochemistry of activins and inhibins has been dealt with earlier. Each is composed of two of three peptide units. In the ovary, the expression of subunit peptides inhibins and activins appears to be developmentally regulated.

**IMPLANTATION AND GESTATION.** Growth factors mediate cell proliferation, differentiation, migration, and invasion during preimplantation development, implantation, and subsequent stages of gestation. In the ewe, the major product of preimplantation blastocyst is ovine trophoblast protein-1 (oTP-1) which is now classified as an $\vartheta$-interferon (IFN). A similar trophoblast interferon (IFN), bovine trophoblast protein-1 (bTP-1) or IFN$\tau$, is a secretory product of the bovine conceptus. In vivo, these interferons prolong the length of the estrous cycle via an antiluteolytic effect on uterine production of $PGF_{2\alpha}$ (24).

**EARLY EMBRYO.** Several growth factors are involved in implantation of the blastocyst. PDGF, a glycoprotein (molecular weight, 30,000 daltons) supports the growth of serum-dependent cells (Table 3-6). PDGF is normally confined to paracrine and autocrine actions. PDGF is secreted by some human blastocysts and is present in human uterine secretions. Growth factors in the zygote, morula and blastocysts include transforming growth factor (TGFB1), transforming growth factor-$\alpha$ (TGFF-$\alpha$), IGF (IGFII), PDGF, and interleukin-6 (IL-6).

Other growth factors and related isoforms that are not transcribed by the morula and blastocyst include IGF-I, epidermal growth factor (EGF), and nerve growth factor.

**UTERINE CONTRACTIONS.** Platelet-derived growth factor (PDGF) and insulin receptors have profound effects on endometrial and myometrial cells by stimulation of their proliferation. PDGF releases arachidonic acid and subsequent conversion to prostaglandins, $PGF_{2\alpha}$ stimulates uterine contractions.

**LEYDIG CELL FUNCTION.** The role of inhibins and related proteins is not confined to the regulation of pituitary FSH. These proteins are now recognized as growth and differentiation factors and in the testis they regulate both epithelial and interstitial cell functions. In species such as rodents and pigs, inhibins and activins are paracrine regulators of steroidogenesis whereby they modulate the endocrine LH signal. Activins have a significant role in Leydig cell development in the fetal testis and at puberty, i.e., activins (like TGF$\beta$) hold Leydig cell growth in abeyance until differentiation or puberty (5).

Endogenous opioid peptides (EOP) seem to have an autocrine and paracrine regulation on Leydig cell steroidogenesis and participate in the intratesticular control of vascular permeability. $\beta$Endorphin is present in the testicular interstitial fluid (TIF), in a concentration many fold higher than that found in plasma.

## REFERENCES


1. Capen CC, Martin SL. The pituitary gland. In: McDonald LE, Pineda MH, eds. Veterinary Endocrinology and Reproduction. Philadelphia: Lea & Febiger, 1989.
2. Ganong WF. Review of Medical Physiology. 17th ed. Connecticut: Appleton & Lange.
3. Setchell BP. Male Reproduction. In: Reproduction in Domestic Animals. King GJ, ed. New York: Elsevier Science Publishers BV, 1993.
4. Taya K, Kaneko H, Takedomi T, Kishi H, Watanabe G. Role of inhibin in the regulation of FSH secretion and folliculogenesis in cow. Anim Reprod Sci 1996;42:563–570.
5. Risbridger GP. Regulation of Leydig cell function by inhibins and activins. Anim Reprod Sci 1996;42:343–349.
6. Vale W, Bilezikjian LM, River C. Reproductive and other roles of inhibins and activins. In: Knobil E, Neill JD, eds. Reproductive Physiology, Vol 1, 2nd ed. New York: Raven Press, 1994;34.
7. Sasser RG, Ruder CA, Ivani KA, Butler JE, Hamilton WC. Detection of pregnancy by radioimmunoassay of a novel pregnancy-specific protein in serum of cows and a profile of serum concentrations during gestation. Biol Reprod 1986;35: 936–942.
8. DeSilva M, Reeves JJ. Ovulation blockage by intrafollicular injection of indomethacin in the cow. J Anim Sci 1985; 75:547.
9. Murdock WJ, Dunn TG. Luteal function after ovulation blockage by intra-follicular injections of indomethacin in the ewe. J Reprod Fert 1983;69:671.
10. Edqvist LE, Stabenfeldt GH. The Endogenous Control of Reproductive Processes. In: King GJ, ed. Reproduction in Domestic Animals. New York: Elsevier Science Publishers BV, 1993.
11. Earp S. The epidermal growth factor receptor: control of synthesis and signaling function. In: Schomberg DE, ed. Serono Symposium. New York: Springer-Verlag, 1991.
12. Lonergan P, Khatir H, Carolan C, Mermillod P. Bovine blastocyst production in vitro after inhibition of oocyte meiotic resumption for 24 h. J Reprod Fertil 1997;109:355–365.
13. Rieger D, Luciano AM, Modina S, Pocar P, Lauria A, Gandolfi F. The effects of epidermal growth factor and insulin-like growth factor I on the metabolic activity, nuclear maturation and subsequent development of cattle oocytes. J Reprod Fertil 1998;112:123–130.
14. Lorenzo PL, Illera MJ, Illera JC, Illera MJ. Enhancement of cumulus expansion and nuclear maturation during bovine oocyte maturation in vitro by the addition of epidermal growth factor and insulin-like growth factor I. J Reprod Fertil 1994; 10:697–701.
15. Kobayashi K, Yamashita S, Hoshi H. Influence of epidermal growth factor and transforming growth factor-alpha on in vitro maturation of cumulus cell-enclosed bovine oocytes in a defined medium. J Reprod Fertil 1994;100:439–446.
16. Thibodeaux JK, Del Vecchio RP, Hansel W. Role of platelet-derived growth factor in development of in vitro matured and

in vitro fertilized bovine embryos. J Reprod Fertil 1993;98: 61–66.

17. Thibodeaux JK, Del Vecchio RP, Broussard JR, Dickey JF, Hansel W J. Stimulation of development of in vitro-matured and in vitro-fertilized bovine embryos by platelets. J Anim Sci 1993;71:1910–1916.
18. Hammond JM, Samaras SE, Grimes R, Leighton J, Barber J, Canning SF, Guthrie HD. The role of insulin-like growth factors and epidermal growth factor-related peptides in intraovarian regulation in the pig ovary. J Reprod Fertil 1993;48(Suppl):117–125.
19. Redmer DA, Dai Y, Li J, Charnock-Jones DS, Smith SK, Reynolds LP, Moor RM. Characterization and expression of vascular endothelial growth factor (VEGF) in the ovine corpus luteum. J Reprod Fertil 1996;108:157–165.
20. Liebermann J, Schams D, Miyamoto A. Effects of local growth factors on the secretory function of bovine corpus luteum during the oestrous cycle and pregnancy in vitro. Reprod Fertil Dev 1996;8:1003–1011.
21. de Moraes AA, Hansen PJ. Granulocyte-macrophage colony-stimulating factor promotes development of in vitro produced bovine embryos. Biol Reprod 1997;57:1060–1065.
22. Palma GA, Muller M, Brem G. Effect of insulin-like growth factor I (IGF-I) at high concentrations on blastocyst development of bovine embryos produced in vitro. Fertil 1997; 110:347–353.
23. Matsui M, Takahashi Y, Hishinuma M, Kanagawa H. Insulin and insulin-like growth factor-I (IGF-I) stimulate the development of bovine embryos fertilized in vitro. J Vet Med Sci 1995;57:1109–1111.
24. Danet-Desnoyers G, Wetzels C, Thatcher WW. Natural and recombinant Interferon $\tau$ regulate basal and oxytocin induced secretion of prostaglandins $F_{2\alpha}$ and $E_2$ by epithelial cells and stromal cells in the endometrium. Reprod Fertil Dev 1994;6:193–202.
25. Mihm M, Good TE, Ireland JL, Ireland JJ, Knight PG, Roche JF. Decline in serum follicle-stimulating hormone concentrations alters key intrafollicular growth factors involved in selection of the dominant follicle in heifers. Biol Reprod 1997;57:1328–1337.
26. Funston RN, Moss GE, Roberts AJ. Insulin-like growth factor-I (IGF-I) and IGF-binding proteins in bovine sera and pituitaries at different stages of the estrous cycle. Endocrinology 1995;136:62–68.
27. Stewart RE, Spicer LJ, Hamilton TD, Keefer BE, Dawson LJ, Morgan GL, Echternkamp SE. Levels of insulin-like growth factor (IGF) binding proteins, luteinizing hormone and IGF-I receptors, and steroids in dominant follicles during the first follicular wave in cattle exhibiting regular estrous cycles. Endocrinology 1996;137:2842–2850.
28. Stewart RE, Spicer LJ, Hamilton TD, Keefer BE. Effects of insulin-like growth factor I and insulin on proliferation and on basal and luteinizing hormone-induced steroidogenesis of bovine thecal cells: involvement of glucose and receptors for insulin-like growth factor I and luteinizing hormone. J Anim Sci 1995;73:3719–3731.
29. Bao B, Thomas MG, Griffith MK, Burghardt RC, Williams GL. Steroidogenic activity, insulin-like growth factor-I production, and proliferation of granulosa and theca cells obtained from dominant preovulatory and nonovulatory follicles during the bovine estrous cycle: effects of low-density and high-density lipoproteins. Biol Reprod 1995;53:1271–1279.
30. Echternkamp SE, Howard HJ, Roberts AJ, Grizzle J, Wise T. Relationships among concentrations of steroids, insulin-like growth factor-I, and insulin-like growth factor binding proteins in ovarian follicular fluid of beef cattle. Biol Reprod 1994;51:971–981.
31. Bishop DK, Wettemann RP, Spicer LJ. Body energy reserves influence the onset of luteal activity after early weaning of beef cows. J Anim Sci 1994;72:2703–2708.
32. Pimental E. Hormones, Growth Factors, and Oncogenes. Florida: CRC Press, 1987.
33. Schomberg DW, ed. Growth Factors in Reproduction. New York: Springer-Verlag, 1990.
34. Tsafriri A, Adashi EY. Local nonsteroidal regulators of ovarian function. In: Knobil E, Neill JD, eds. Reproductive Physiology, Vol 1, 2nd Ed. New York: Raven Press, 1994;15.
35. Harper MJK. Platelet-activating factor: a paracrine factor in preimplantation stages of reproduction. Biol Reprod 1989; 40:907–913.
36. Ivell R. Biology of the relaxin-like factor (RLF). Rev Reprod 1997;2:133–138.
37. Bathgate R, Balvers M, Hunt N, Ivell R. Relaxin-like factor gene is highly expressed in the bovine ovary of the cycle and pregnancy: sequence and messenger ribonucleic acid analysis. Biol Reprod 1996;55:1452–1457.
38. Hunt JS. Expression and regulation of the tumour necrosis-$\alpha$ gene in the female reproductive tract. Reprod Fertil Dev 1993;5:141–153.
39. Findlay JK, Drummond AE, Fry RC. Intragonadal regulation of follicular development and ovulation. Anim Reprod Sci 1986;42:321–331.
40. Campbell BK, Scaramuzzi RJ, Webb R. Control of antral follicle development and selection in sheep and cattle. J Reprod Fertil 1995;49(Suppl):334–350.

CHAPTER 4

# Reproductive Cycles

E.S.E. HAFEZ AND B. HAFEZ

| Term | Definition |
|---|---|
| Corona cells | radiant, slightly expanded, compact or absent, even or clumped |
| Expanded cumulus mass | present in thin matrix of acid mucopholysacchardide, dense matrix or absent, even distribution or clumped |
| Follicular membrana granulosa cells | amount of cytoplasm, loose aggregation or compact appearance, pale color, or dark and clumped |

The reproductive cycle relates to various phenomena: puberty and sexual maturity, the breeding season, the estrous cycle, postpartum sexual activity, and aging. These components are regulated by environmental, genetic, physiologic, hormonal, behavioral, and psychosocial factors. The level of fertility initiated at the time of puberty is maintained for a few years before it begins to gradually decline due to aging. Farm animals, however, are slaughtered well before the decrease in fertility levels.

## PRENATAL AND NEONATAL PHYSIOLOGY

### Gonadotropins

Secretion of the gonadotropins FSH and LH and their hypothalamic-releasing factor, hormone LHRH, begins during fetal life. In the ewe and cow it starts early, shortly after sex differentiation (month 1 or 2 of pregnancy) and in the sow only toward the end of fetal life (about 1.5 months after gonadal sex differentiation). This secretion temporarily regresses; it is slightly reduced 2 months before birth in cattle, near term in sheep, and 1 month after birth in pigs. Gonadotropin levels remain low up to the onset of puberty. The duration of this "infancy" is highly variable. It lasts a few days in the rat, 1 month in sheep and pig, 3 months in cattle, and 6 to 7 years in humans.

At the onset of the pubertal period, gonadotropin secretion rises. This process occurs in normal animals as well as in animals that had been castrated early in which the process is clearer, owing to the absence of negative feedback from the gonadal steroid. Gonadotropin rise results in the removal of the inhibitory control of the central nervous system when the body's development progressively attains a level compatible with reproduction (Fig 4-1).

### The Gonads

During prenatal and neonatal life, gametogenesis and steroidogenesis seem independent, while at the onset of puberty they become closely related (Table 4-1).

THE TESTIS. Leydig cells are gonadotropin sensitive and their continued steroidogenic activity closely depends on gonadotropic secretion. In swine, a transitory testosterone secretion occurs about day 55 when the Leydig cells differentiate; this secretion then drops until the fetus begins to secrete LH shortly before birth. At the onset of puberty, gonadotropin secretion resumes and Leydig cells are reactivated. In swine the Leydig cells, which were active during fetal and neonatal life, occupy large areas between the tubules, while after puberty the peritubular cells are more active.

THE OVARY. Initial ovarian structure is not fundamentally different from that of the testis. The appearance of meiotic prophase early in life is one of the main differences between ovarian and testicular germ cell evolution. Moreover, as oogonia completely disappear, the oocytes formed during the fetal and neonatal period are the only source of oocytes available during the entire sexual life.

## PUBERTY

From a practical point of view, a male or female animal has reached puberty when it is able to release gametes and to manifest complete sexual behavior sequences. Puberty is basically the result of a gradual adjustment between increas-

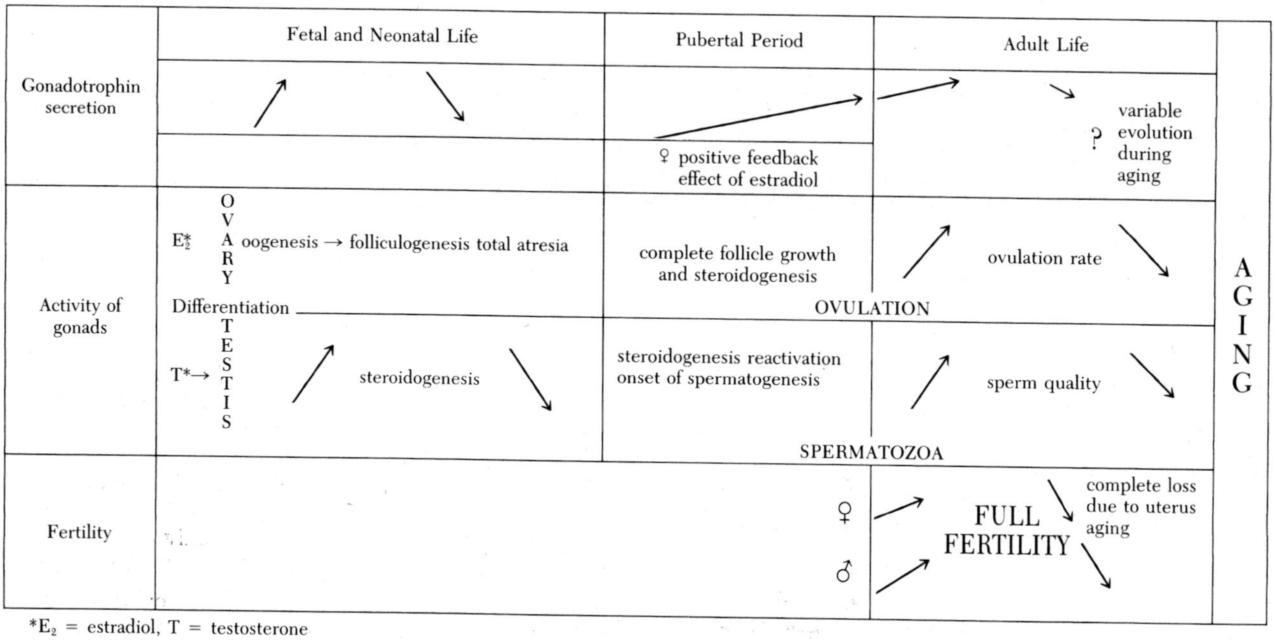

| | Fetal and Neonatal Life | Pubertal Period | Adult Life | |
|---|---|---|---|---|
| Gonadotrophin secretion | ↗ ↘ | ↗<br>♀ positive feedback effect of estradiol | ↗ ↘ ? variable evolution during aging | AGING |
| Activity of gonads | OVARY: $E_2^*$ → oogenesis → folliculogenesis total atresia | complete follicle growth and steroidogenesis | ↗ ovulation rate ↘ | |
| | Differentiation | OVULATION | | |
| | TESTIS: $T^*$ → ↗ steroidogenesis ↘ | steroidogenesis reactivation onset of spermatogenesis | ↗ sperm quality ↘ | |
| | | SPERMATOZOA | | |
| Fertility | | ♀ ↗<br>♂ ↗ | FULL FERTILITY ↘ complete loss due to uterus aging ↘ | |

$^*E_2$ = estradiol, T = testosterone

Figure 4-1. Neonatal, pubertal, and maturity stages.

## Table 4-1. *Comparative Physiology of Pubertal Events in the Two Sexes*

| | Male | Female |
|---|---|---|
| Gonads | Basic structure of testis (seminiferous cords/interstitial tissue) remains unchanged from gonadal sex differentiation at beginning of fetal life to onset of puberty.<br>Interstitial tissue fills space between sex cords, composed of elongated cells/steroidogenic cells. Leydig cells secrete androgens as soon as the testis differentiates/before gonadotropic function is triggered. | Initial ovarian structure is similar to that of testis.<br>Sex cords, formed by somatic and germ cells, are present at the beginning of ovarian/testicular differentiation; these structures remain basically unchanged.<br>Oocytes are wrapped by a few somatic cells to form primordial follicles within a framework of interstitial tissue.<br>As soon as primordial follicle reserve is constituted, it rapidly diminishes by atresia. A cow fetus that has 2,700,000 oocytes at day 110 of gestation has only 70,000 oocytes at birth. |
| Endocrine Control of Puberty | In response to gonadotropin secretion, testosterone rises from very low to adult levels.<br>Extent of testosterone secretion increases as puberty advances, finally testosterone level remains definitively high. Increase of blood testosterone level eventually causes a decrease in gonadotropin secretion by a negative feedback effect. | Estrogen secretion increases in response to pubertal gonadotropin rise as long as antral follicle formation has begun (in the ewe/cow). Estrogen level only rises in gilts toward week 11 after birth, when first antral follicles appear.<br>Pubertal gonadotropic secretion begins 3 weeks earlier at 8 weeks of age. |
| Gametogenesis | At puberty gonocytes migrate to periphery of tubules/differentiate into spermatogonia; supporting cells produce Sertoli cells.<br>These changes occur at the elevation of prepubertal gonadotropins.<br>Sertoli cells remain present during whole sexual life; their number is limiting factor in sperm production. | First antral follicles appear during prepubertal period (sow, rabbit) or even earlier (cow, ewe).<br>Complete follicular development, resumption of oocytes meiosis/ovulation occur only when FSH/LH reach adult profile. |

ing—gonadotropic activity and the ability of the gonads to simultaneously assume steroidogenesis and gametogenesis.

### *Endocrine Mechanisms of Puberty*

At the onset of puberty, the circulating concentrations of gonadotropins increase, which is due to the rise of both the amplitude and the frequency of the periodic impulses of gonadotropins. This results from sex steroids and possibly from an increase in responsiveness of the hormone GnRH, secreted from the hypothalamus to regulate gonadotropins. In 2 to 8 week old lambs, pulse frequencies increase from 1 to 5 in a 6-hour period (Fig. 4-2).

### *Gametogenesis*

Manipulation of certain factors during the prepubertal period may reduce the onset of puberty further or increase testicular growth rate. Gonocytes develop at random through the testis into definitive A-spermatogonia. This, together with the formation of Sertoli cells, marks the end of the prepubertal period and the onset of spermatogenesis (1). The concentration of the sperm's progressive motility, the seminal protein concentration, and the percentage of sperm with a normal head, tail, and acrosomal morphology increases from puberty through 16 weeks after puberty. Rapid increases in the percentage of sperm exhibiting normal head morphology (excluding acrosomes) and motility are associated with rapid decreases in percentage of sperm with proximal cytoplasmic droplets (2). The first antral follicles appear during the prepubertal period (sow, rabbit) or even earlier (cow, ewe). However, complete follicular development, resumption of oocyte meiosis, and ovulation are observed only when FSH and LH have reached adult profiles (Figs. 4-2–4-4).

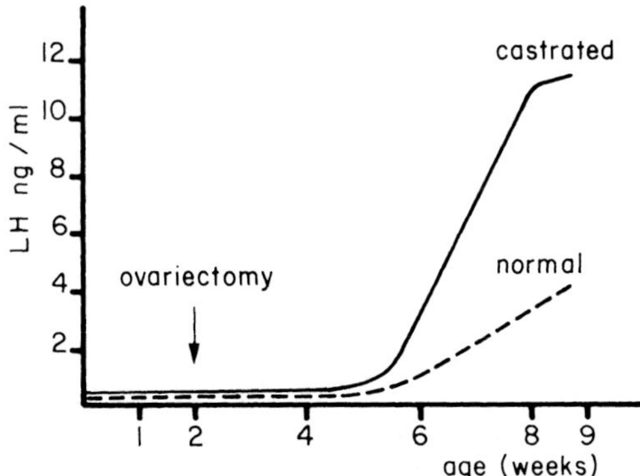


FIGURE 4-2. Comparative evolution of plasma LH levels in normal and castrated ewe lambs. The pubertal rise occurs at the same age in both animals, but the increase is more pronounced in the castrated. (From Foster DL, Lemons JA, Jaffe RB, Niswender GD. Sequential patterns of circulating luteinizing hormone and follicle-stimulating hormone in female sheep from early postnatal life through the first estrous cycles. Endocrinology 1975;97:985.)

### *Age at Puberty*

In normal breeding conditions puberty occurs at about 3 to 4 months of age in rabbits; 6 to 7 months in sheep, goats, and swine; 12 months in cattle; and 15 to 18 months in horses.

The age of puberty is influenced by physical environment, photoperiod, age and breed of dam, breed of sire, and sires within breed, heterosis, environmental temperature, body weight as affected by nutrition, and growth rates before and after weaning. The onset of puberty is more closely related to body weight than to age. Dairy cattle reach puberty when the body weight is 30 to 40% that of the adult weight, whereas in beef cattle this percentage is higher (45 to 55% that of adult body weight) (3). The same difference occurs in sheep (Romney ewes: 40%; Suffolk: 50%; Scottish Blackface: 63% of adult body weight) (4). Nutritional levels modulate age at puberty. If growth is accelerated by overfeeding, the animal reaches puberty at a younger age. On the other hand, if growth is slowed down by underfeeding, puberty is delayed.

Puberty and regularity of estrous cycles in gilts is affected by the breed, type of housing, and season of the year during sexual maturation. Both gilts reared in confinement and gilts not reared in confinement that were exposed to a boar reached puberty at an earlier age than gilts reared without exposure. In seasonal breeders, the age of puberty depends on the birth season. Ewes born in January attain puberty 8 months later, whereas those born in April become pubertal when 6 months old (during full adult breeding season in both cases). Puberty occurs earlier in gilts bred in a group than those bred alone. The presence of an adult boar hastens puberty in both situations (5). Full reproductive efficiency is not attained in any species at the first estrus or ejaculation. There is a period of "adolescent sterility." This period is remarkably short (some weeks) in domestic animals as compared with humans (1 year or more).

PRACTICAL APPLICATIONS FOR AGE OF PUBERTY. The age of sexual maturity in ewes is related to adequate energy intake and the attainment of sufficient body weight. Early onset of sexual maturity provides economic advantages through increased lifetime reproductive rate. Thus, it is advantageous to maximize growth rates in ewe lambs being added to the breeding flock. The application of multiple lambing systems permits the rearing of lambs throughout various seasons of the year.

The genetic improvement achieved by artificial insemination and embryo transfer of dairy cattle has resulted from the use of proven-tested sires. Obtaining semen at the earliest possible age from bulls being proven-tested is desirable to hasten identification of superior sires. Ultimately, the genetic impact of a superior sire is limited by the number of sperm produced, which is a direct function of testicular size.

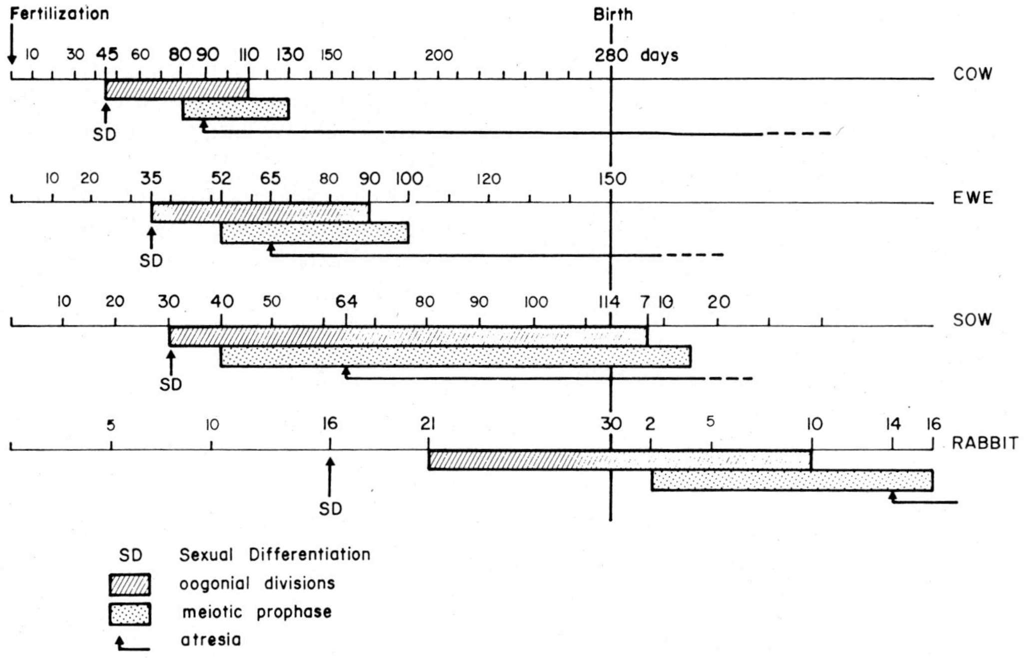


FIGURE 4-3. Species differences in patterns of oogenesis in some mammals.

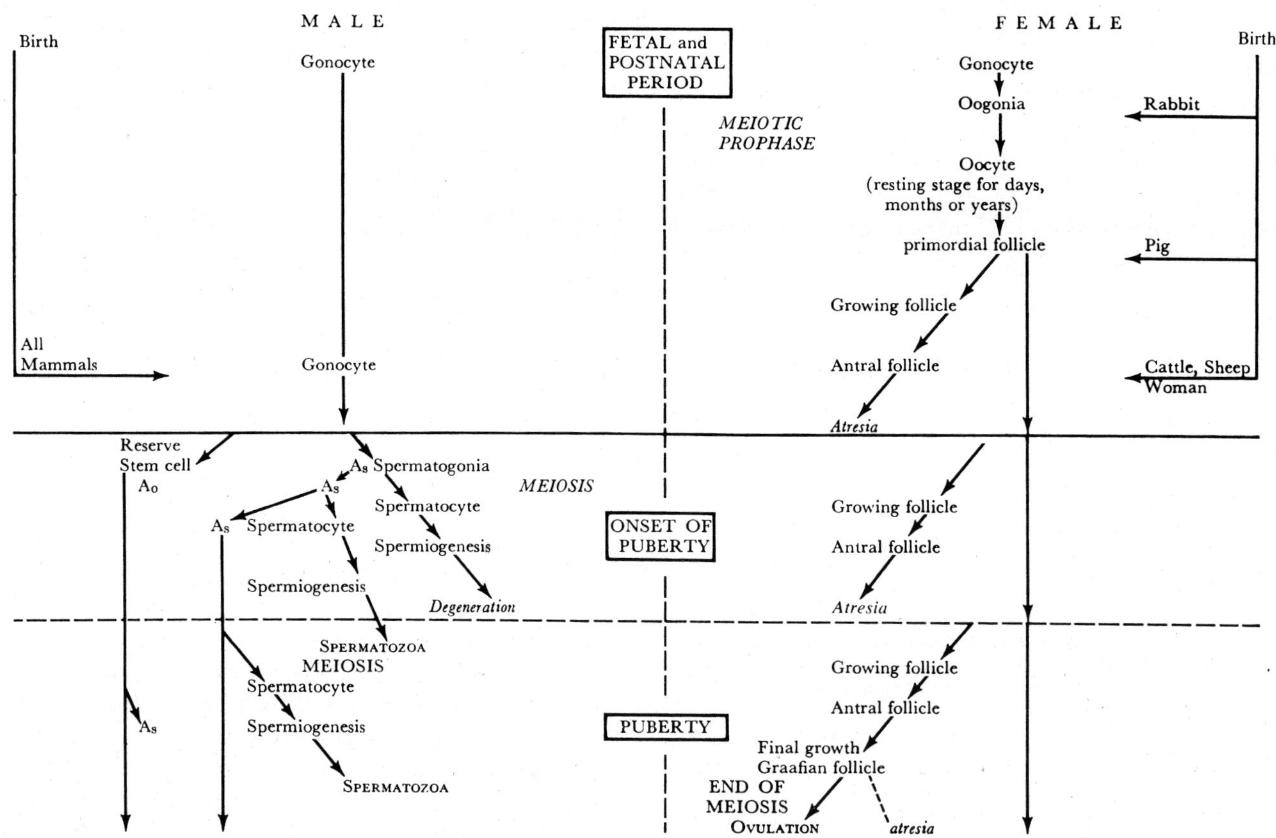


FIGURE 4-4. Comparison of gametogenesis in male and female mammals from fetal life to active sexual life. $A_o$, reserve stem cells; $A_s$, stem cell spermatogonia.

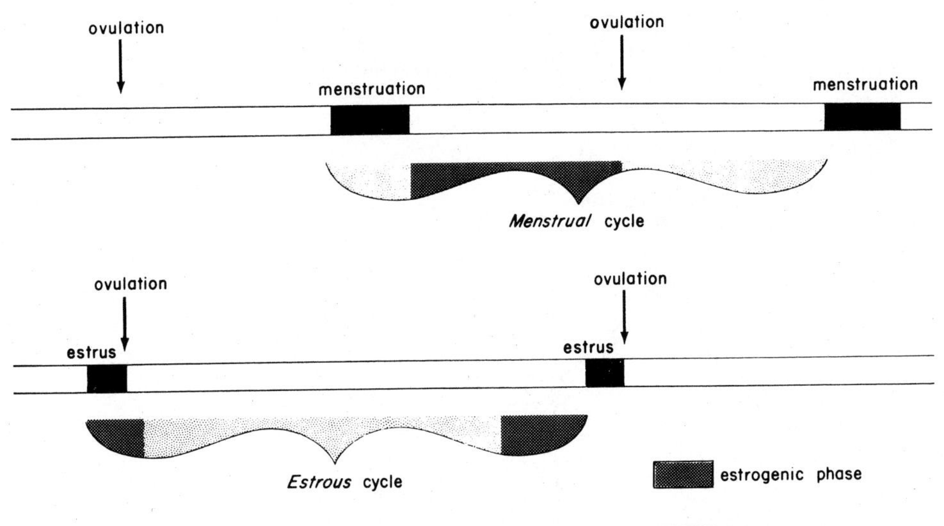


FIGURE 4-5. Comparative diagram to show differences in the patterns and stages of the estrous cycle in farm animals as compared to the menstrual cycle in women. Note the incidence of ovulation in relation to estrus and menstruation. (Adapted from an illustration by Professor C. Thibault.)

## Estrous Cycles

Mating is limited during estrus, coinciding with the time of ovulation. In humans and other primates, mating is not restricted at any time of the menstrual cycle, and ovulation occurs during midcycle (Fig. 4-5). The length of the estrous cycle in different species is: ewe, 16 to 17 days; cow, sow, goat, 20 to 21 days; mare, 20 to 24 days. The duration of estrus is species dependent and varies slightly from one female to another within the same species. This is also true in respect to the time of ovulation, which occurs 24 to 30 hours after the onset of estrus in most ewes and cows, 35 to 45 hours in sows, and 4 to 6 days in mares (Table 4-2).

TABLE 4-2. ***Estrous Cycle, Estrus, and Ovulation in Farm Animals***

| | Length of Estrous Cycle (Days) | Duration of Estrus (Hours) | Time of Ovulation |
|---|---|---|---|
| Ewe | 16–17 | 24–36<br>32–40 | 30–36 hours from beginning of estrus |
| Goat | 21 (also short cycles) | 20–35 | Unavailable |
| Sow | 19–20 | 48–72 | 35–45 hours from beginning of estrus |
| Cow | 21–22 | 18–19 | 10–11 hours after end of estrus |
| Mare | 19–25 | 4–8 days | 1–2 days before end of estrus |

The cervical mucus undergoes remarkable ultrastructural changes throughout the cycle.

The length of estrus and the time of ovulation also vary in relation to internal and external factors. In ewes the interval between the onset of estrus and LH ovulatory surge (and therefore the interval between estrus and ovulation) lengthens as the number of ovulations increases.

### *Endocrine Regulation of Estrous Cycles (Figs. 4-6 to 4-9)*

The estrous cycle is regulated by endocrine and neuroendocrine mechanisms, namely the hypothalamic hormones, the gonadotropins, and the steroids secreted by the testis and ovary. Regulation of gonadotropin secretion during the es-

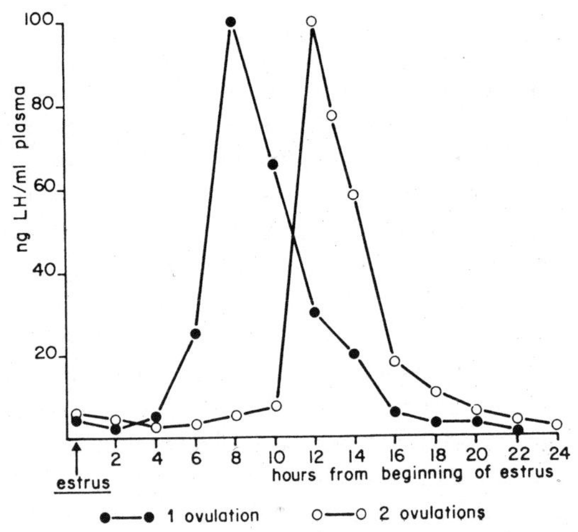


FIGURE 4-6. Timing of LH surge in ewe according to number of ovulations (Ile-de-France breed). (From Thimonier, Pelletier. Ann Biol Anim Biochim Biophys 1971;11:559.)

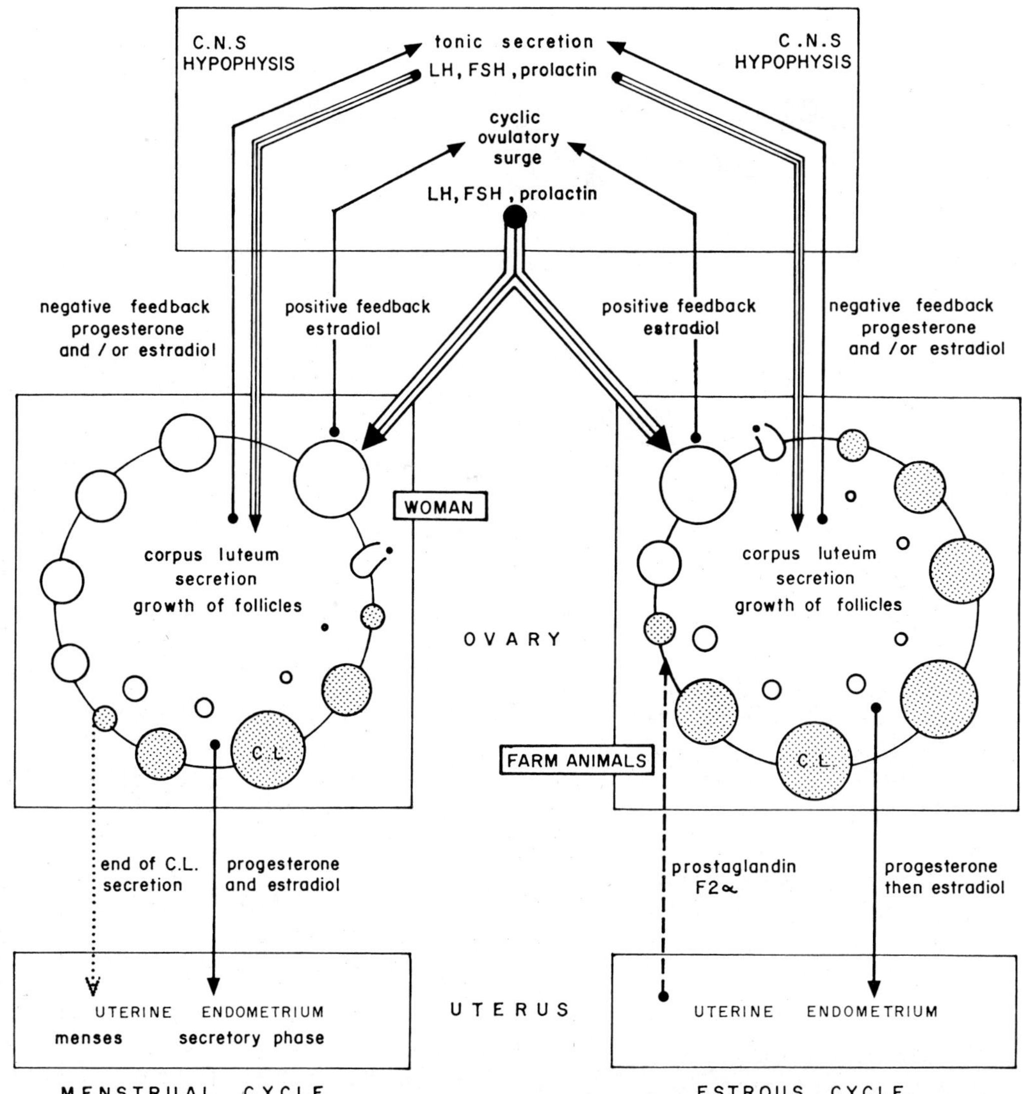


FIGURE 4-7. Interrelationship between ovary and hypothalamohypophysis and between ovary and uterus.

trous cycle requires a delicate balance among complex hormonal interactions. One component known to be an important influence is gonadotropic hormone-releasing hormone (GnRH). Changes in the rates of GnRH synthesis and release, as well as the rate of degradation of this hormone, are additional factors that modify its role in influencing gonadotropin release (6). At the ovarian level, the estrous period is characterized by high estrogen secretion from preovulatory Graafian follicles. Estrogens stimulate uterine growth by a mechanism that involves interaction of the hormone with receptors and the increase in synthetic processes within cells. Estrogens also stimulate the production of prostaglandins by the uterus.

At the end of estrus, ovulation occurs followed by corpus luteum formation resulting in progesterone secretion. The corpus luteum is made of two distinct steroidogenic cell types, both of which contribute significantly to the total progesterone secreted during the luteal phase of the estrous cycle. The small luteal cells secrete little progesterone unless stimulated by LH, while large luteal cells spontaneously secrete progesterone at a high rate. The corpus luteum of pregnancy is resistant to the luteolytic effect of $PGF_{2\alpha}$. The corpus luteum is the main source of progesterone and relaxin in pregnant swine where relaxin may play a role in parturition and the onset of lactation. The ovary is the primary source of relaxin in several species that require this organ throughout gestation, that is, pigs and rodents. Relaxin is distributed uniformly throughout ovarian tissue and is not confined to corpora lutea.

Prostaglandin $F_{2\alpha}$ ($PGF_{2\alpha}$) is the uterine luteolytic hormone in several mammalian species. Uterine $PGF_{2\alpha}$ controls the life span of the corpus luteum, which in turn regulates the length of the cycle. If pregnancy occurs, the luteolytic influence of the uterus has to be negated since progesterone

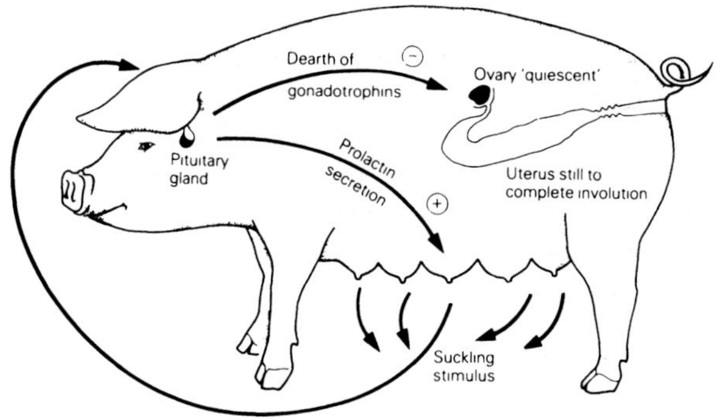


FIGURE 4-8. Endocrine relationships in the post-partum sow showing the active secretion of prolactin early in the suckling period and the relative dearth of gonadotrophin secretion associated with lactational anestrus and incomplete involution anestrus and incomplete involution of the uterus. A change in the relative secretion of gonadotropins and prolactin occurs as the incidence of suckling decreases with the interval after birth. (Hunter RHF. Reproduction of Farm Animals. New York: Longman, 1982.)

secreted by the corpus luteum is necessary for the maintenance of pregnancy. The period of corpus luteum activity is called the *luteal phase*; it lasts 14 to 15 days in ewes and 16 to 17 days in cows and sows. The follicular phase, from the regression of the corpus luteum to ovulation, is relatively short: 2 to 3 days in ewes and goats and 3 to 6 days in cows and sows. This short follicular phase does not reflect the true duration of Graafian follicle growth. Thus, estrous cycle length is closely related to the duration of the luteal phase. Corpus luteum regression is not caused by a decreased secretion of pituitary luteotrophic hormones (LH and prolactin) but by the action of a luteolytic factor, $PGF_{2\alpha}$.

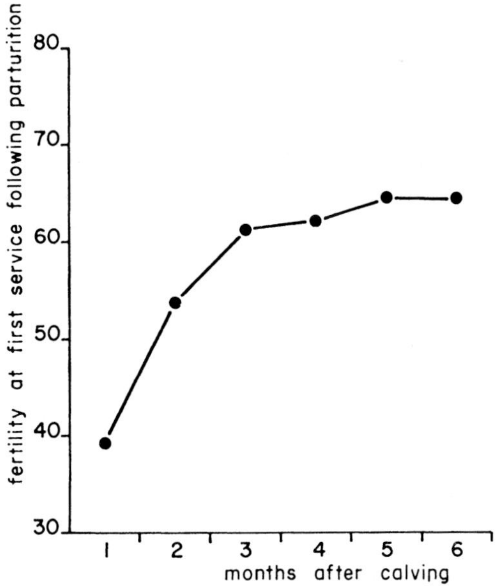


FIGURE 4-9. Fertility of dairy cattle at first service following parturition. (From Casida. Wisc Expt Sta Research Bull No. 270. 1968.)

## *Postpartum Estrus and Ovulation*

The duration of postpartum anestrus is affected by several environmental, genetic, physiologic, and metabolic factors including breed, strain, nutritional level, suckling, milk production, frequency of milking, and level of and genetic potential for milk yield. The duration of postpartum anestrus is also affected by the rate of uterine involution, the rate of development of ovarian follicles, pituitary and peripheral concentrations of gonadotropins, peripheral levels of estrogens and progesterone, onset of episodic secretion, and changes in body weight and energy intake (7). In cattle energy balance during the first 20 days of lactation is important in determining the onset of postpartum ovarian activity (8). The time required for postpartum uterine involution varies from 4 to 6 weeks.

In modern swine production systems, it is important that sows return to estrus rapidly following weaning. Several factors influence the weaning to estrus interval such as type of feed and feed intake during gestation, lysine intake during lactation, protein intake during gestation and lactation, postweaning feed intake, lactation length, and altered suckling stimulus (9). Altering the nursing pattern of pigs may be effective in either inducing estrus in the dam before weaning or decreasing the interval to remating after weaning. In general sows exhibiting prolonged weaning to estrus intervals are thin. Energy intake during lactation is inversely related to sow weight loss during lactation, thus low energy intake during the lactation may cause delayed estrus following weaning (Fig. 4-8).

ENDOCRINE FACTORS. A relatively high level of progesterone is absolutely necessary throughout gestation. Progesterone is secreted by the corpus luteum and in some species (cow, ewe) mainly by the placenta. The continuous progesterone secretion suppresses estrus and, in most mammals, ovulation.

Following parturition, progesterone drops to undetectable levels and estrus and ovulation can resume. The sow exhibits estrus within 48 hours after parturition, but there is no ovulation. The high plasma estrogen rise after farrowing (10) may explain the estrous behavior. In mares there is a fertile estrus 1 to 3 weeks after parturition. In cows, ewes, and goats silent ovulations can occur 2 to 3 weeks following parturition; however, fertile estrous cycles return later (11–13). Postpartum anestrous females have short estrous cycles in response to weaning. Approximately 80% of the postpartum anestrous cows that exhibited estrus within 10 days after weaning their calves have estrous cycles of 7 to 12 days in length with a short serum progesterone rise after the first estrus. The early decline of progesterone after the first estrus is not due to lack of LH in serum. However, lower levels of FSH before this first ovulation may be due to the reduced life span of the subsequent corpus luteum (Tables 4-1, 4-2) (14).

It would appear that the corpora lutea associated with the short cycles in cattle have a short life span as a result of (a) lack of luteotrophic support; (b) failure of the luteal tissue to recognize a luteotropin; and/or (c) enhanced secretion of a luteolytic agent.

**SUCKLING, NURSING, AND LACTATION.** The extent of postpartum anestrus depends on the degree of mammary stimulation the dam receives and on the nutritional status of the dam during late gestation and early lactation. During this period of frequent nursing, serum concentrations of prolactin are elevated and are inversely related to the concentrations of circulating FSH and LH (15). In dairy cattle the interval from parturition to first ovulation is related to the level of milk production and is longer in cows with a higher genetic potential for milk yield. Because high-producing cows cannot maintain a positive energy balance during the early lactation and must mobilize body reserves, the postpartum ovarian activity is more closely associated with milk production than with total digestible nutrient intake (8).

The inhibitory relationship between the mammary gland and reproductive function may be due to neural stimulation, secretion of an inhibitory substance, or the hormonal milieu. The level of nutrition also influences postpartum reproduction, although the effect of suckling is not related to the nutritional effect. The interval from parturition to uterine involution may be shortened by nursing. Nursing cows exhibit shorter intervals to uterine involution.

The interval from parturition to first ovulation is shortened in unilateral ovariectomized cattle when surgery is performed 5 days postpartum. There is also a significant interaction between the effect of suckling and unilateral ovariectomy. Unilateral ovariectomy shortens the interval to the first postpartum estrus, and compensatory ovarian hypertrophy occurs in suckled animals. In nonsuckled animals, unilateral ovariectomy does not further shorten the already short interval (16).

In nursing beef cattle, the interval from parturition to first estrus varies from 60 to 100 days. Several attempts were made to initiate ovarian cycles in anestrous-suckled beef cows through early weaning, limited nursing, gonadotropin-releasing hormone treatment, and treatment with a combination of sex steroids. Early weaning, limited nursing, GnRH, and steroids all induce ovulation in anestrous beef cows. However, the luteal phase of the first postpartum estrous cycle and the first estrous cycle following early weaning limited nursing, and GnRH treatment is shorter than in normal estrous cycles.

The importance of suckling on the duration of postpartum anestrus is demonstrated in sheep by experimentally induced pregnancy during seasonal anestrus so that lambing occurs during the breeding season. Dried off ewes usually return to estrus after about 1 month, while nursing ewes present the first estrus some weeks later. In sheep and cattle, the duration of postpartum anestrus varies with the breed and seems to be constant for the same female during successive pregnancies.

Fertility is low during the first estrus, particularly when the female nurses. Maximal fertility in the cow occurs 60 to 90 days after calving. In sows fertility is nil during weaning; a highly fertile estrus occurs a few days after weaning.

The sequence of uterine involution are as follows:

Parturition

a) preliminary shrinkage of endometrium
b) necrosis of caruncles
c) sloughing/discharge of tissue
d) regeneration/renovation of endometrium
e) new epithelial lining fully restored
f) delayed renovation during non-breeding season

There are remarkable species differences in the mechanisms of sloughing/renovation/regeneration of the mammalian endometrium. In ruminants the caruncles are sloughed off and discharged within 4 to 6 weeks. In pigs, there is slight fluid discharges for up to one week postpartum; this followed by regeneration of the columnar epithelium and full restoration of the endometrium within 3 to 4 weeks.

## BREEDING SEASON

In wild animals, there is a well-defined breeding season when both sexes have sexual activity. The Barbary sheep, a wild breed, exhibit two sexual seasons, one in October through January and the other in April through June. In domestic mammals, the nature and extent of the breeding season is variable. Cattle and swine exhibit no seasonality of breeding, whereas sheep, goats, and horses have a breeding season that also varies in duration.

**NATURE OF BREEDING SEASON.** In sheep and goats there are important breed differences in the duration of the sexual season. Préalpes and Mérino sheep are long-season breeders, whereas Blackface and Southdown are short-season breeders. The length of the sexual season in these breeds is 260, 200, 139, and 120 days, respectively. A long sexual season is a dominant genetic character. All Mérino crosses exhibit a long sexual season like the Mérino. A cross of Dorset Horn and Persian ewe has produced a breed—the Dorper—which has only a 1-month anestrus (Fig. 4-10).

Silent ovulatory cycles always occur at the beginning and end of the sexual season. These ovarian cycles continue during the anestrous period in a variable number of ewes. In Ile-de-France Préalpes ewes, the frequency of silent cycles rises temporarily in spring. If a ram is present, behavioral estrus appears, thus permitting a second annual sexual season in these breeds. In goats the sexual season is well defined in temperate climates. The ovaries in the Alpine goat are slightly active from February to March and quiescent from

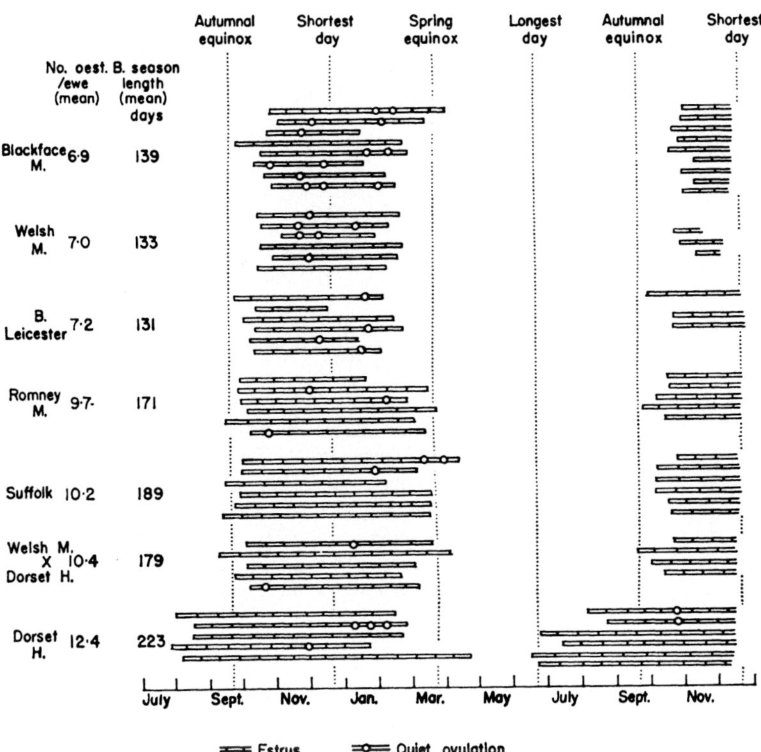


FIGURE 4-10. Breed differences in the duration of the sexual season and nonsexual season in adult ewes in Great Britain. Some breeds such as the Dorset Horn had a prolonged sexual season, whereas those such as the Welsh Mountain had a restricted sexual season. In nearly all cases, the sexual season was within the period from the autumnal equinox and the spring equinox, and the middle of the season corresponded rather closely to the shortest day of the year, or December 21. This illustrates the close relationship between the sexual season and length of day. Note that some estrous cycles double or triple the usual length occurred, which is due to quiet ovulations or to the failure to detect heat in the nonpregnant females observed. (After Hafez ESE. J Agric Sci 1952;42:305.)

April to July; activity is abruptly resumed in all goats in September. Quiet ovulations are less frequent than in ewes. As in sheep in tropical climates, Creole goats exhibit continuous sexual activity.

Although rams can mate throughout the year, testis weight, testosterone, and gonadotropin levels are minimal from January to May during female anestrus (Fig. 4-11). Similarly, in the billy goat the plasma testosterone level remains low from January to August, when it rises suddenly at the beginning of the breeding season. An annual reproductive cycle in horses is well documented from both hemispheres. In northern temperate countries, ovarian silence in mares and low plasma testosterone and LH levels in stallions are observed from October to February.

In cattle and pigs estrus occurs regularly throughout the year, and seasonality is discrete. Local breeding conditions often mask its expression. In cattle a seasonal variation of fertility in temperate climates only becomes evident after studying a large number of herds over a period of several years (Fig. 4-12). Minimal fertility occurs in June and maximal fertility in November. This variation may be related to photoperiodism rather than to temperature and breeding, which can fluctuate from year to year. Cows are mainly responsible for the seasonal variation of fertility, as shown by nonreturn rates after insemination in spring and fall with frozen semen collected in fall or spring. Fertility in the sow is lower in the summer than in other seasons, and the litter size is also smaller then (Fig. 4-13).

**ROLE OF PHOTOPERIODISM AND TEMPERATURE.** Photoperiods and environmental temperature affect the annual sexual cycles; the former is the most efficient factor.

The most conclusive experience showing the control of reproduction by photoperiodism has been conducted in sheep. Using two photoperiodic cycles per year, ewes experience two annual breeding seasons (Fig. 4-14). When the ewe is allowed to mate regularly, lambing occurs every 6 1/2 months, since the 5-month gestation is followed by a lactational anestrus of 1 1/2 months. The mare is a long-day seasonal breeder with reproductive cyclicity occurring from early May to October in northern latitudes. The arbitrary assignment of January 1st as the birth date for all foals born in a given year has created a demand in the equine industry for the administration of hormones to advance the onset of the natural breeding season in mares by 3 to 4 months. Thus foals would be born nearer to the first of the year.

In the northern hemisphere, increasing the daylight ratio up to 16 hours in November and December advances the beginning of the sexual season in the mare; first ovulation occurs up to 3 months earlier than under natural photoperiod. Induced cycles are endocrinologically normal and fertile (17). Several hormonal treatments were used with varying success, such as pregnant mare serum gonadotropin (PMSG), human chorionic gonadotropin (hCG), gonadotropin-releasing hormone (GnRH), progesterone, and equine pituitary extracts (18). Similar manipulations are

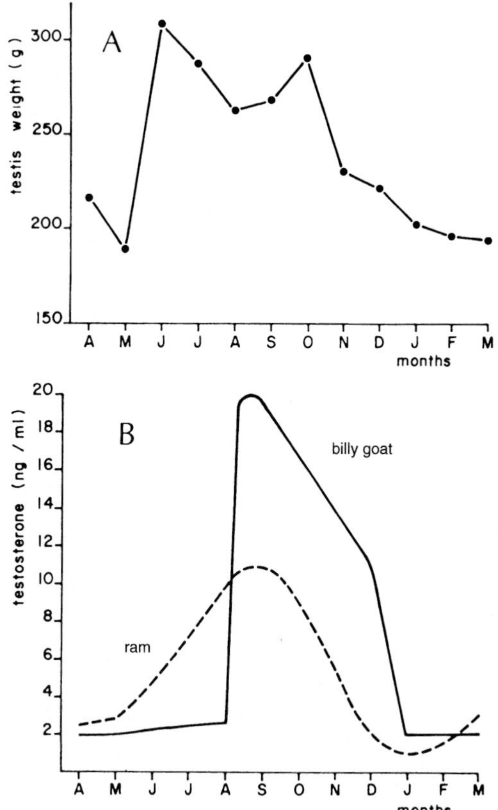


FIGURE 4-11. (A) Seasonal variation of testis weight in Ile-de-France ram (testis weight is adjusted to body weight) (47° N). (From Pelletier. PhD Thesis. University of Paris, 1971.) (B) Seasonal variations of testosterone plasma levels in Ile-de-France ram and Alpine billy goat. (ram: from Attal. PhD Thesis, University of Paris, 1970; billy goat: from Saumande, Rouger. C R Acad Sci Paris D 1972;274:89.)

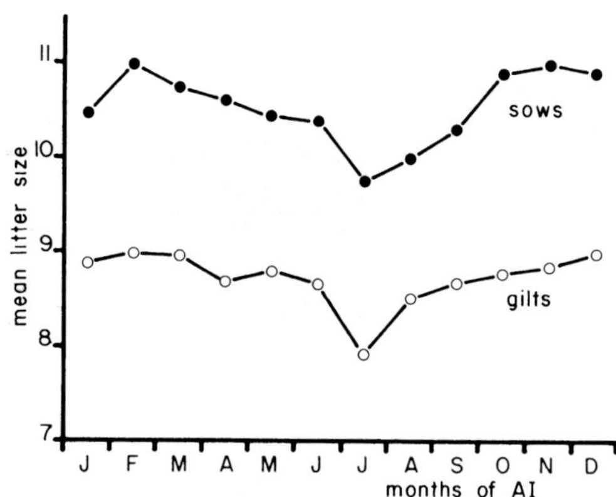


FIGURE 4-13. Evolution of litter size in artificially inseminated sows and gilts in the west of France (46° N). This study includes 4,510 gilts and 13,324 sows and covers three consecutive years. (From Courot, Bariteau. Personal communication, 1978.) Pig fertility is minimal under conditions of long days and high temperatures, as evidenced in sows and gilts by the smaller litter size in July. Note that adult sows have 1.5 piglets more per litter than gilts all the year round.

also effective with rams. Using two photoperiodic cycles per year, the ram exhibits two periods of decreasing spermatogenetic activity coinciding with the two periods of increasing day length (19). Photoperiodism is basically a synchronizer of sexual activity. When ewes are placed under 12 hours of daylight every day or under constant illumination for many years, a breeding season is maintained for 1 or 2 years, then estrus becomes more random throughout the year.

Seasonal variation of temperature plays a major role in the regulation of sexual function in lower vertebrates, particularly in reptiles. In mammals, when environmental temperatures remain within the limit compatible with thermoregulatory mechanisms, seasonal temperature variation effect on fertility is rarely reported (20). Nevertheless, the postfertilization period appears to be a critical one in domestic females. Cow, ewe, and sow embryos are susceptible to damage during the first 10 days of development (21). In swine, photoperiodism and temperature interact unfavorably on fertility. Sperm output, sperm motility, and farrowing rate are severely lowered when boars are submitted to summer temperatures (35°C) under long days (16 hours).

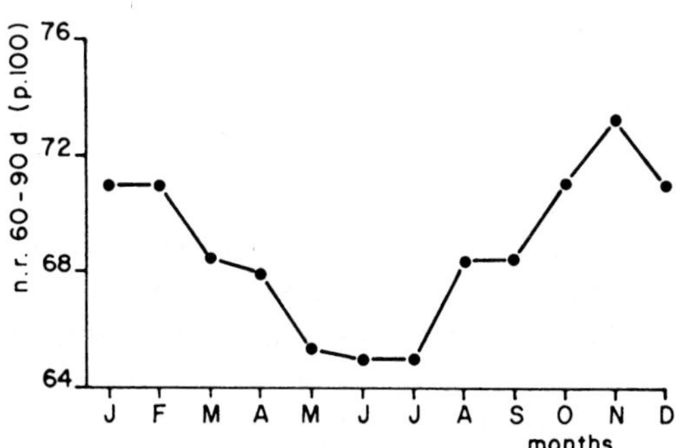


FIGURE 4-12. Seasonal variation of fertility in cattle from 320,000 artificial inseminations over seven years (Montbéliard breed in French Jura, 47° N). The nonreturn rate is lower in spring and higher in autumn. (From Courot et al. Ann Biol Anim Biochim Biophys 1968;8:209.)

### *Breeding Season in Males*

The duration of the breeding season of males is longer than in the females of the species. Although rams can mate throughout the year, testis weight, testosterone, and gonadotropin levels are minimal from January to May during female anestrus (Fig. 4-11). Similarly, in the billy-goat, the plasma testosterone level remains low from January to August, when it rises suddenly at the beginning of the breeding season. An annual reproductive cycle in stallions is also well documented from both hemispheres. In northern temperate countries, low plasma testosterone and LH levels in stallions are observed from October to February. Breed differences exist in mature rams with regard to secretory patterns of hormones. Breed differences in serum gonadotropin and testosterone are apparent only during the short days of the year when the hypothalamo-pituitary-testicular axis is considered most active. Likewise, breed differences in prolactin are noted only during the long days, when secretion of this

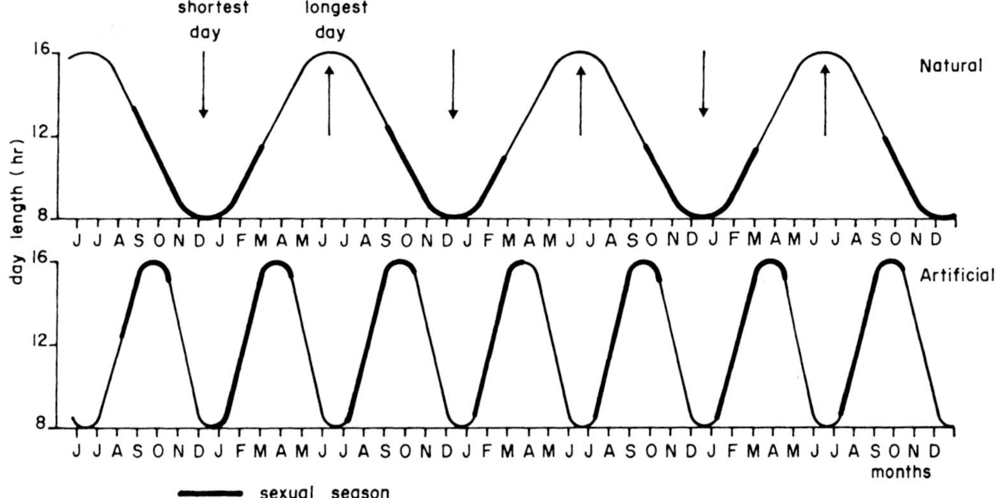


FIGURE 4-14. Periods of sexual activity in Limousine ewes. **Top:** Under natural photoperiodicity, estrus normally occurs during decreasing daylight period. **Bottom:** Under 6-month photoperiodic cycles, estrus occurs during the increasing daylight period. (From Mauleon, Rougeot. Ann Anim Biochim Biophys 1962;2:209.)

hormone is enhanced. Breed differences in LH, FSH, and testosterone secretion in rams during short days might be related to seasonality of mating and/or fecundity or breed types (22).

There are distinct breed differences in hormone secretion in rams. These differences seem to be related to both seasonality of mating and fecundity of breed types and thus may provide important insight into the neuroendocrine mechanisms underlying seasonal variations in reproduction of this species. The between animal variability in gonadotropin secretion, noticeable particularly in Dorsets and Rambouillets, may similarly prove useful in identifying the most prolific individuals within a breed (22).

FACTORS REGULATING BREEDING SEASON. Environmental, physiologic, and social factors regulate the onset and maintenance of the breeding season. The patterns of photoperiod, rainfall, and temperature are considered environmental cues that either entrain an endogenous rhythm or directly trigger the physiologic changes of the breeding season (23). These are mediated by endocrine and neuroendocrine mechanisms.

Among the domesticated bovine species, the Zebu cattle exhibits the most distinct seasonality in reproductive efficiency. For example, the frequency of estrus and ovulation, as well as conception rate in Zebu cattle is higher during the summer than during the winter in Kenya (24). Temperature may modify the seasonal effect of photoperiod on reproductive function.

### *Endocrine and Neuroendocrine Mechanisms*

Photoperiodicity effect involves at least two separate mechanisms. First, there is a direct action on the hypothalamic pituitary axis. In the castrated ram and spayed mare, in which negative feedback from sexual steroids does not occur, gonadotropin levels reach a maximum during the normal breeding season and decrease during the nonbreeding season. Secondly, there is a simultaneous change in the sensitivity of the central nervous system to negative feedback from steroids.

The photosensitive period is short in birds (about 1 hour) and remarkably broad in the ram (7 hours). In rams submitted to 8 hours of light per day given in two parts (7 hours plus 1 hour given at various intervals in the night), LH level was higher when the one-hour flash was given 11 to 20 hours after the beginning of the 7-hour light period (Fig. 4-15). Under natural condition, LH levels are higher in the summer than in the winter months.

Prolactin and thyroxine secretion are also modulated photoperiodically. Under the same photoperiod of 8 hours of light given in a 7-hour period plus a 1-hour period, maximal prolactin secretion was obtained in the ram when the 1-hour flash was given 17 hours after light on. Moreover, a photoperiod enhancing either gonadotropin and prolactin secretion or maximal testis enlargement is never followed by sustained pituitary and gonadal responses.

## AGING AND FERTILITY

Herd fertility is evaluated by the percentage of pregnant females and the litter size. These parameters increase for a few years after puberty, reach a maximum, and then decrease slowly. The maximal pregnancy rate is reached around 3 to 4 years in sows, 4 to 6 years in ewes, and 5 to 7 years in cows. Maximal litter size occurs in third, fourth, and fifth pregnancies in the sow. Maximal frequency of two pregnan-

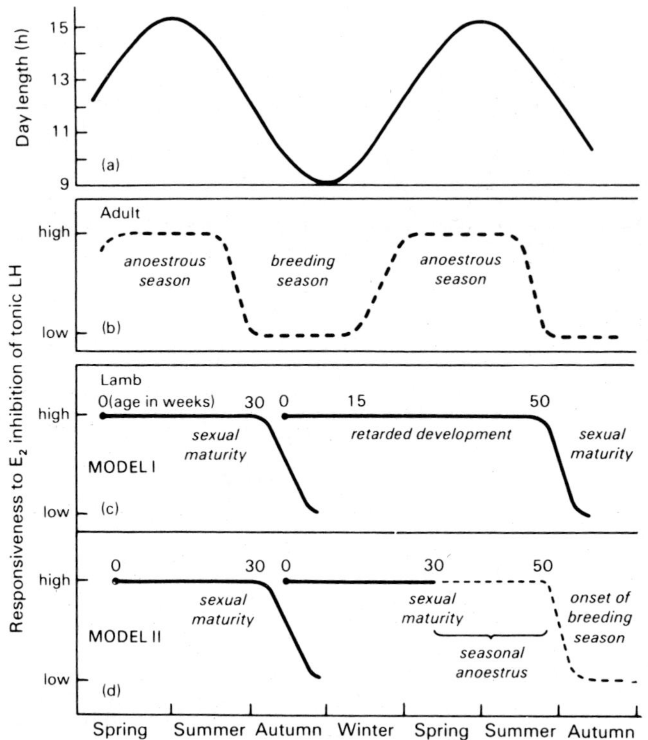


FIGURE 4-15. Alternative models for the influence of photoperiod on the decrease in responsiveness to estradiol inhibition of tonic LH secretion in the lamb. Models I and II are based on the age and season of the decrease in responsiveness to estradiol feedback and initiation of ovulation in lambs born in the spring and autumn in relation to (a) natural photoperiod and (b) annual changes in responsiveness and ovarian cyclicity in the adult. Responsiveness is schematically illustrated as the inverse of circulating LH concentrations in chronically estradiol treated ovariectomized females. Responsiveness is considered to be high when LH secretion is suppressed and is low when LH secretion is not suppressed; intact females are acyclic during periods of high responsiveness and are cyclic during periods of low responsiveness. (Foster DL. Mechanism for delay of first ovulation in lambs born in the wrong season. Biol Reprod 1981;25:85–92.)

TABLE 4-3. *Twinning Frequencies in the Cow According to Age (Gestation Number)*

| GESTATION NUMBER | TWIN PREGNANCIES (%) MONOZYGOTIC | TWIN PREGNANCIES (%) DIZYGOTIC |
|---|---|---|
| 1 | 0.15 | 0.33 |
| 2 | 0.17 | 1.36 |
| 3 | 0.14 | 1.96 |
| 4 | 0.24 | 2.30 |
| 5 | 0.17 | 2.54 |

Swedish breed, from Johansson I, Lindhe B, Pirchner F. Hereditas 1974;78:201.

cies appears from the fifth pregnancy onward in cows (Table 4-3). In ewes the rate of twins increases up to 6 to 7 years and then decreases slowly (Fig. 4-16).

As in other mammals, ovulation and fertilization rates decrease only slightly in aged domestic females, but embryonic mortality, stillbirth, and postpartum losses increase. Early embryonic mortality may result from poor egg quality in aging female, as shown in the rabbit by the relatively unsuccessful development of blastocysts transferred from old donors to young foster mothers (25). However, high rates of embryonic and perinatal loss mainly result from the fact that the aging uterus reacts too slowly to the demands of the rapidly growing fetus and to the stimulus initiating parturition. Increased sperm production continues during aging, but at a slower rate. Apart from pathologic disturbances, male fertility, sperm production, and semen quality decrease slowly during aging. In bulls, the daily sperm output falls from $6 \times 10^9$ at 3 to 4 years to $4 \times 10^9$ between 6 and 13 years. Fertility decreases in the same proportion from 65% of nonreturn at 3 to 4 years to 54% at 12 years (26).

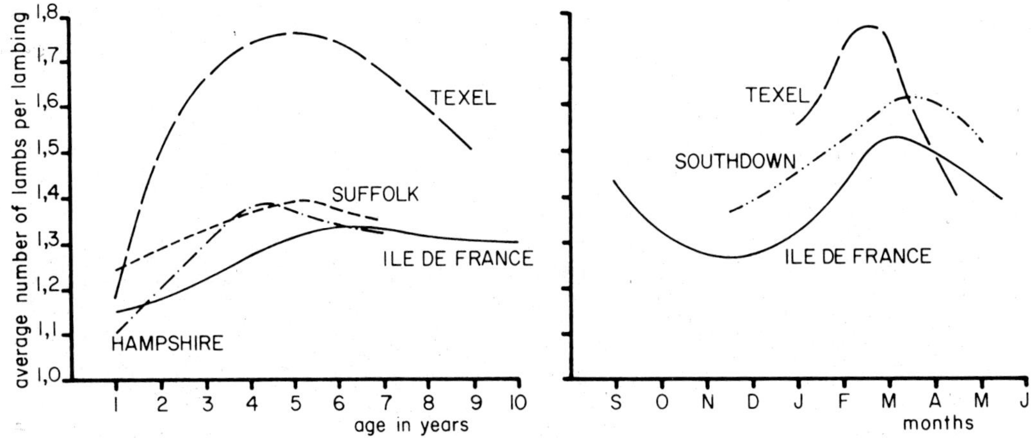


FIGURE 4-16. Effect of age on lambs per lambing and of season on lambing rate. (Institut technique de l'Elevage ovin et caprin. Paris, France, 1972.)

The remarkable decline in the reproductive parameters may be due to endocrine factors that affect body growth, sexual development, metabolism, and homeostasis. Endocrine failure may represent either a reduction in hormone secretion or a reduction in the response of target cells to hormonal stimulation (27).

## REFERENCES


1. Curtis SK, Amann RP. Testicular development and establishment of spermatogenesis in Holstein bulls. J Anim Sci 1981;53:1645–1659.
2. Lunstra DD, Echternkamp SE. Puberty in beef bulls: acrosome morphology and semen quality in bulls of different breeds. J Anim Sci 1982;55:638–648.
3. Roy JHB, Gillies CM, Shotton SM. Factors affecting the first oestrous in cattle and their effect on early breeding. In: Taylor JC, ed. The Early Calving of Heifers and its Impact on Beef Production. Brussels: European Economic Communities, 1975.
4. Hafez ESE. Studies on the breeding season and reproduction of the ewe. J Agric Sci 1952;42:189.
5. Mavrogenis AP, Robinson OW. Factors affecting puberty in swine. J Anim Sci 1976;42:1251.
6. O'Conner JL, Lapp CA, Mahesh VB. Peptidase activity in the hypothalamus and pituitary of the rat: fluctuations and possible regulatory role of luteinizing hormone releasing hormone-degrading activity during the estrous cycle. Biol Reprod 1984;36:855–862.
7. Stevenson JS, Britt JH. Models for prediction of days to first ovulation based on changes in endocrine. J Anim Sci 1980; 50:103–112.
8. Butler WR, Everett RW, Coppick CE. The relationships between energy balance, milk production and ovulation in postpartum Holstein cows. J Anim Sci 1981;53:742–749.
9. Reese DE, Moser BD, Peo ER Jr, Lewis AJ, Zimmerman DR, Kinder JE, Stroup WW. Influence of energy intake during lactation on the interval from weaning to first estrus in sows. J Anim Sci 1982;55:590–598.
10. Shearer IJ, Purvis K, Jenkin G, Haynes NB. Peripheral plasma progesterone and oestradiol 17$\beta$ levels before and after puberty in gilts. J Reprod Fertil 1972;30:347.
11. Casida LE. Studies on the postpartum cow. Wisc Exp Station Res Bull No 270, 1968.
12. Hunter GL. Increasing frequency of pregnancy in sheep. Anim Breed Abstr 1968;36:347.
13. Hunter GL. Increasing frequency of pregnancy in sheep. Anim Breed Abstr 1968;36:533.
14. Ramirez-Godinez JA, Kiracofe GH, Schalles RR, Niswender GD. Endocrine patterns in the postpartum beef cow associated with weaning: a comparison of the short and subsequent normal cycles. J Anim Sci 1982;55:153–158.
15. Moss GE, Adams TE, Niswender GD, Nett TM. Effects of parturition and suckling on concentrations of pituitary gonadotropins, hypothalamic GnRH and pituitary responsiveness to GnRH in ewes. J Anim Sci 1980;50:496.
16. Grass J, Hauser ER. The influence of early age mastectomy and unilateral ovariectomy on reproductive performance of the bovine. J Anim Sci 1981;53:171–176.
17. Oxender WD, Noden PA, Hafs HD. Estrus, ovulation and serum progesterone, estradiol and LH concentrations in mares after an increased photoperiod during winter. Am J Vet Res 1977;38:203.
18. Hart et al., 1984.
19. Ortavant R, Thibault C. Influence de la durée d'éclairement sur les productions spermatiques du Bélier. C R Soc Biol 1956;150:358.
20. Hafez ESE. Environmental Effect on Animal Productivity. In: Hafez ESE, ed. Adaptation of Domestic Animals. Philadelphia: Lea & Febiger, 1968.
21. Ortavant R, Loir M. The environment as a factor in reproduction in farm animals. World Congr Anim Prod: Buenos Aires, 1978.
22. D'Occhio MJ, Schanbacher BD, Kinder JE. Profiles of luteinizing hormone, follicle-stimulation hormone, testosterone and prolactin in rams of diverse breeds: effects of contrasting short (8L:16D) and long (16L:8D) photoperiods. Biol Reprod 1984;30:1039–1054.
23. Ruiz de Elvira MC, Herndon JG, Wilson ME. Influence of estrogen-treated females on sexual behavior and male testosterone levels of a social group of Rhesus monkeys during the nonbreeding season. Biol Reprod 1982;26:825–834.
24. Rhodes RC III, Randel RD, Long CR. Corpus luteum function in the bovine: in vivo and in vitro evidence for both a seasonal and breed type effect. J Anim Sci 1982;55:159–168.
25. Adams CE. Ageing and reproduction in the female mammal with particular reference to the rabbit. J Reprod Fertil 1970; 12(Suppl):1.
26. Bishop MWH. Ageing and reproduction in the male. J Reprod Fertil 1970;12(Suppl):65.
27. Morrison MW, Davis SL, Spicer LJ. Age-associated changes in secretory patterns of growth hormone, prolactin, and thyrotropin and the hormonal responses to thyrotropin-releasing hormone in rams. J Anim Sci 1981;53:160–170.


## SUGGESTED READING


Foster DL, Lemons JA, Jaffe RB, Niswender GD. Sequential patterns of circulating luteinizing hormone and follicle-stimulating hormone in female sheep from early postnatal life through the first estrous cycles. Endocrinology 1975;97:985.

Hunter RHF. Reproduction of Farm Animals. London: Longman, 1982.

Reardon TF, Robinson TJ. Seasonal variation in the reactivity to oestrogen of the ovariectomized ewe. Aust J Agric Res 1961;12:320.

CHAPTER 5

# Folliculogenesis, Egg Maturation, and Ovulation

E.S.E. HAFEZ AND B. HAFEZ

The ovary performs two major functions. One is the cyclic production of fertilizable ova. The second is the production of a balanced ratio of steroid hormones that maintain the development of the genital tract, facilitate the migration of the early embryo, and secure its successful implantation and development in the uterus. The follicle is the ovarian compartment that enables the ovary to fulfill its dual function of gametogenesis and steroidogenesis.

## FOLLICULOGENESIS

In the primordial follicle reserve, formed during fetal life or soon after birth, some primordial follicles begin to grow continuously throughout life or at least until the reserve is exhausted. When any follicle is released from this reserve, it continues to grow until ovulation or until the follicle degenerates, which is the case with the majority of follicles (Table 5-1). The largest follicle is responsible for most estrogen secretion by the ovary at estrus. Estrogen secretion by the largest follicle decreases rapidly at the time of the LH peak.

Cattle ovulate a single follicle that can be identified by its size about 3 days before onset of estrus, when there are one or two large follicles on ovaries. In sheep, one or two large follicles secrete more estrogens and bind more gonadotropins to granulosa cells than smaller follicles. In sows, recruitment of the ovulatory follicles into the ovulatory population continues during the follicular phase. Thus, the development of smaller follicles may be promoted rather than inhibited by larger "dominant" follicles.

The final follicular growth in ewes, cows, and sows ranges between 12 and 34 days; the total duration of follicular growth is longer than 20 days and presumably about six months. The growth of the follicle up to the stage of antrum formation is not strictly gonadotropin dependent. In hypophysectomized females the formation of preantral follicles continues at a more or less normal rate. On the other hand, antrum formation and final growth are entirely FSH/LH dependent (Figures 5-1 and 5-2).

### Follicle Growth

Follicular growth and maturation represent a series of sequential subcellular and molecular transformations of various components of the follicle: the oocyte, granulosa, and theca (1). These are governed by several intraovarian factors, intrafollicular factors, and hormonal signals, which lead to the secretion of androgens and estrogens (mainly estradiol).

Follicle growth involves hormonally induced proliferation and differentiation of both theca and granulosa cells, leading ultimately to the increased ability of follicles to produce estradiol and to respond to gonadotropins. Production of estradiol determines which follicle will gain the LH receptors necessary for ovulation and luteinization. Disturbances in the responsiveness of the granulosa and theca to the gonadotropin signals, lead to cessation of follicle growth and initiation of follicle atresia.

### Recruitment and Selection of Ovarian Follicles

The ovarian follicle is a balanced physiologic unit whose structure/function depend on extracellular factors such as gonadotropins and complex system of intrafollicular relationships. In sheep, all healthy follicles 2 mm in diameter are recruited, and once selection has occurred, recruitment is blocked. Booroolas sheep differ from Merinos because of the extended time during which recruitment takes place, the low incidence of selection, and the ability of fully grown follicles to wait for the LH peak. In contrast, Romanov sheep differ from Ile-de-France ewes because of a higher number of follicles recruited between days 13 and 15 (2).

TABLE 5-1. *Some Morphologic, Physiologic, and Biochemical Aspects of Ovarian Follicles*

| COMPONENTS | MORPHOLOGIC/PHYSIOLOGIC CHARACTERISTICS |
|---|---|
| Thecal cells | Produce androgens in response to increasing basal LH.<br>After ovulation, theca develop in theca lutein cells. |
| Follicular wall | Made of granulosa/theca, separated by basement lamina, undergo developmental changes related to organogenesis of an endocrine/exocrine gland. |
| Granulosa cells | In preovulatory follicles, granulosa cell projections connect through ruptured basal lamina.<br>After ovulation, granulosa layer is invaded by vessels/connective material. |
| Corona radiata | Before ovulation, the egg lies at one side of the ovarian follicle.<br>Embedded in a solid mass of follicular cells, cumulus oophorus. |
| Primordial follicle | Follicles with centrally located oocytes/single layer of granulosa cells.<br>Differentiate from primordial germ cells (oogonia) and remain in an arrested meiotic prophase until they resume maturation/ovulation atresia.<br>Follicle growth, proliferation of granulosa cells, zona pellucida formation, theca cell differentiation. |
| Secondary follicle | Increase in number of granulosa cells by mitosis, cells become cuboidal. |
| Vesicular follicle | Follicles with accumulation of follicular fluid in antrum within epithelial cells. |
| Follicular fluid (in antrum) | Some components are physiologically active: oocyte maturation inhibitor, LH-binding inhibitor, inhibin, and various enzymes and chondroitin sulphuric acid.<br>Contains only in large follicles, high percentage of estradiol-17$\beta$ in follicular phase/progesterone at ovulation.<br>High concentration of progesterone after LH surge inhibits aromatoze activity locally in ovary. |
| Follicular fluid (between granulosa cells) | Viscous/rich in hyaluronic acid.<br>Fluid accumulates as ovulation approaches.<br>Many old oocytes remain on the follicular surface after ovulation until removed by fimbria.<br>Lutein cells develop after ovulation are major source of progesterone in corpus luteum. |

### *Follicular Fluid*

Follicular fluid originates mainly from the peripheral plasma by transudation across the follicle basement lamina and accumulates in the antrum.

BIOCHEMICAL COMPOSITION OF FOLLICULAR FLUID. Follicular fluid, a serum transudate modified by follicular metabolic activities, contains specific constituents such as steroids and glycoproteins synthesized by the cells of the follicle wall. During follicular growth, an equilibrium is established between serum and follicular fluid. The metabolite concentrations in the two compartments are similar. These concentrations are similar to those in oviductal secretions. The fluid contains several compounds of major physiologic significance, and most of them are concentrations similar to blood serum (Table 5-2).

In large antral follicles (but not in small follicles), the follicular fluid contains remarkably high levels of 17$\beta$-estradiol in the follicular phase and progesterone as ovulation approaches. Polycystic ovaries, however, have high levels of androstenedione.

Viable ovarian follicles also accumulate and secrete several physiologically active nonsteroids:

- oocyte maturation inhibitor (OMI), a polypeptide weighing about 1,500 daltons
- luteinization inhibitor, a complex protein
- inhibitory protein, a protein of about 1,400 daltons
- relaxin, polypeptide of about 9,000 daltons
- inhibin (FSH-suppressing activity), a protein of high molecular weight (Table 5-3).

FUNCTIONS OF FOLLICULAR FLUID. The follicular fluids play a major role in the physiologic biochemical and metabolic aspects of the nuclear and cytoplasmic maturation of the oocyte. The follicular fluid undergoes remarkable changes throughout the estrous cycle and performs several functions including the following:

a) regulation of the functions of the granulosa cells, initiation of follicular growth, and steroidogenesis
b) oocyte maturation, ovulation, and egg transport to the oviduct
c) preparation of the follicle for the formation of the subsequent corpus luteum
d) the stimulatory and inhibitory factors in the fluid regulate the follicle cycle
e) the volume of fluid released at ovulation is also impor-

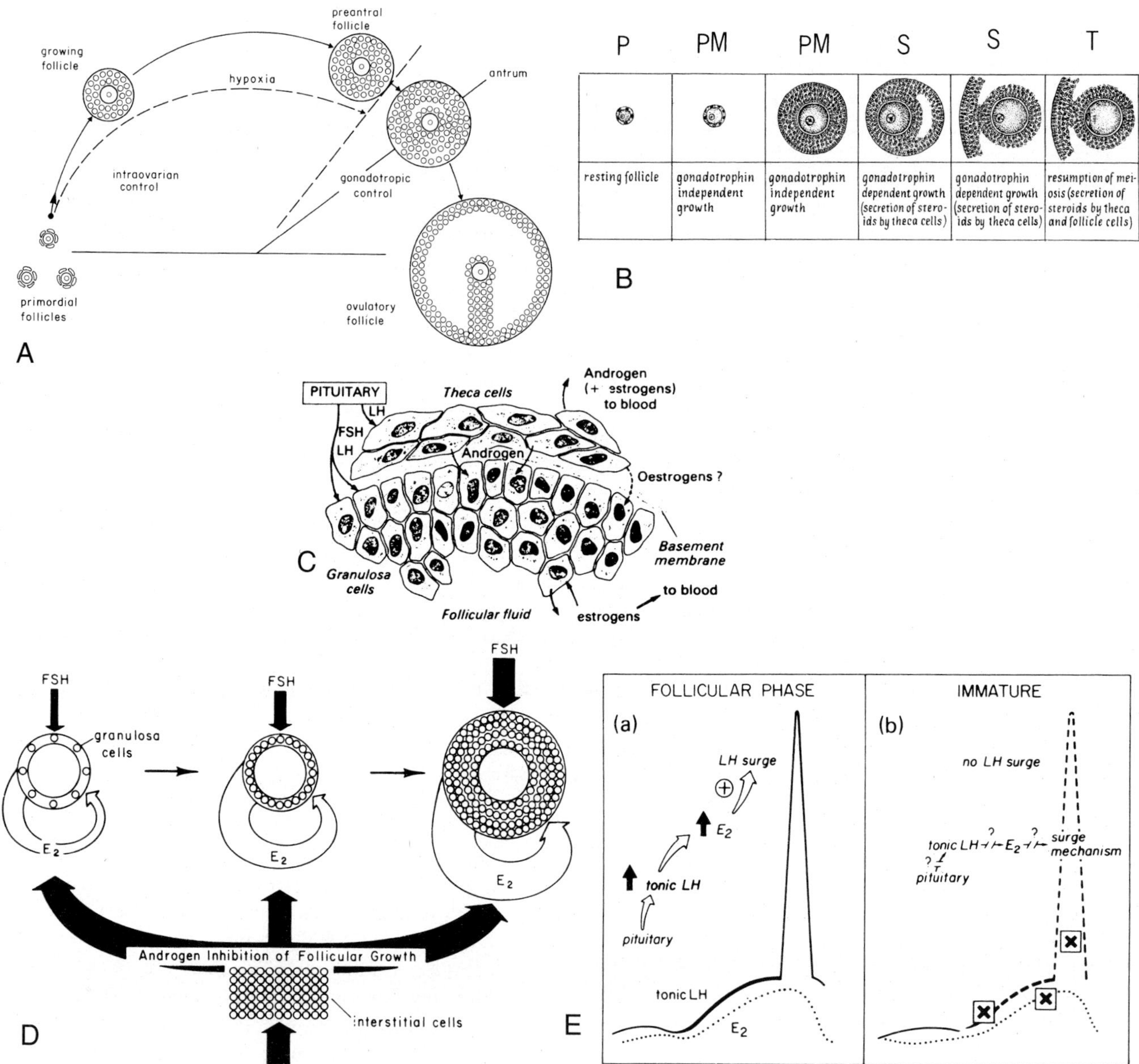


FIGURE 5-1. (A) Some follicles begin to grow every day. The number of primordial follicles beginning growth every day is controlled by intraovarian factor. Antrum formation and final follicle growth up to the ovulatory size is gonadotropin dependent. (Thibault C, Levasseur MC. La fonction ovarienne chez les Mammiferes. Paris: Masson, 1978.) (B) Physiologic and morphologic classification of ovarian follicles: *P*, primordial follicle; *PM*, primary follicle; *S*, secondary follicle; and *T*, tertiary follicle. (Dvorak M, Tersarik J. Ultrastructure of human ovarian follicles. In: Motta PO, Hafez ESE, eds. Biology of the Ovary. London: Martinus Nijhoff, 1980.) (C) Part of follicle showing sites of action of gonadotropins/production/action of steroids. (Peters H, McNatty KP. The development of the ovary in the embryo. In: The Ovary. Berkeley: University of California Press, 1980.) (D) Relationship between pituitary hormones and ovarian steroids in growing preantral follicles. (Peters H, McNatty KP. The development of the ovary in the embryo. In: The Ovary. Berkeley: University of California Press, 1980.) (E) *a*. Follicular phase: relationships between LH/estradiol during follicular phase of estrous cycle of the ewe. *b*. Immature phase: three possible endocrine events that may fail in immature female. (Foster DL, Ryan KD. Endocrine mechanisms governing transition into adulthood in female sheep. In: Scaramuzzi RJ, Lincoln DW, Weir BJ, eds. Reproductive Endocrinology of Domestic Ruminants. J Reprod Fertil 1981;30(Suppl):75–90).

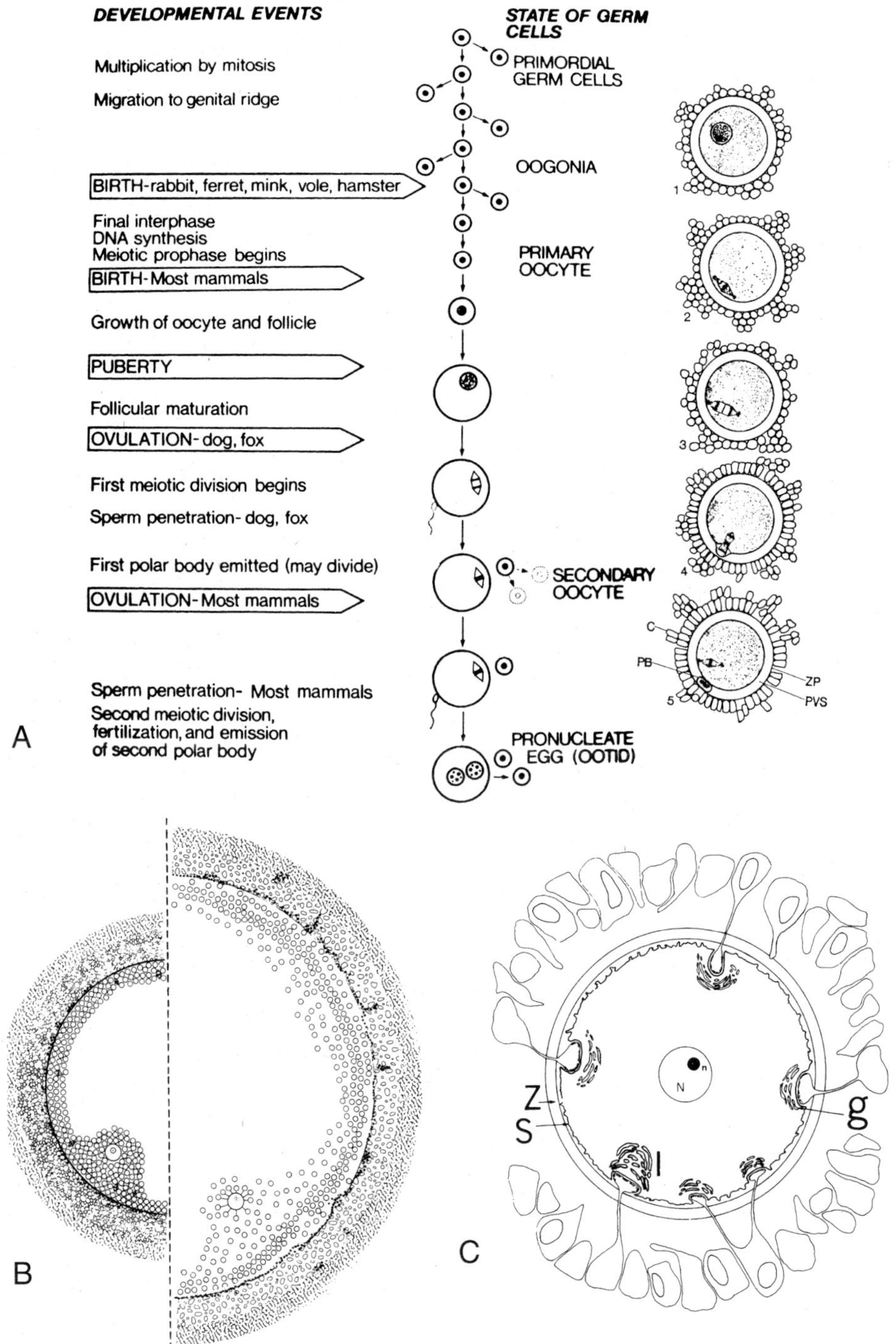


Figure 5-2. (**A**) Developmental events of animals. (Baker TG. Oogenesis and ovulation. In: Austin CR, Short RW, eds. Reproduction in Mammals. Cambridge: Univesity Press, 1972.) (**B**) Bovine ovarian follicle (*after*) and 24 hours (*before*) shows ovulation edema of the theca with dissociation of the round cells of the theca interna. (Thibault C, Levasseur MC. La Fonction Ovarienne chez les Mammiferes. Paris: Masson, 1979.) (**C**) Anatomic and physiologic relationships between the egg and the surrounding follicular cells: g, Golgi body; S, perivitelline space; Z, zona pellucida. (Thibault C, Levasseur MC. La Fonction Ovarienne chez les Mammiferes. Paris: Masson, 1979.)

**TABLE 5-2. *Some Components and Metabolites of the Follicular Fluid That Exhibit Physiologic Functions***

| BIOCHEMICAL COMPONENTS | COMPOUNDS |
|---|---|
| Proteins | Albumins, globulins, IgA, IgM, fibrinogen, lipoproteins, peptides |
| Amino acids | Asp, Thr, Glu, Gln, Ala, Gly, Asn |
| Enzymes | Intracellular/extracellular |
| Carbohydrates | Glucose, fructose, fucose, galactose, mannose |
| Glycoproteins | Glucosamine, galactosamine, hyaluronic acid, heparin, plasminogen |
| Gonadotropins | FSH, LH/prolactin |
| Steroids | Cholesterol, androgens, progestins, estrogens |
| Prostaglandins | PGE, $PGF_{2\alpha}$ |
| Elements/salts | Sodium, potassium, magnesium, zinc, copper, calcium, sulphur, chloride, inorganic phosphate, phosphorus |
| Immunoglobulins | IgG is predominant immunoglobulin<br>IgA is present in amounts second to IgG<br>Concentration of IgG is fluid increases as the follicles enlarge to preovulatory size |

Large healthy follicles are characterized by a high estradiol content and relatively low testosterone value. When large follicles are atretic, estradiol level is lower than that of testosterone. The same low estradiol:testosterone ratio is observed in small healthy follicles; however, their progesterone content is lower than that of large follicles, whether they are atretic or not. Intrafollicular steroid content reflects the steroidogenic potency of these follicles.

tant, along with the oviductal secretions, of the environment in which sperm metabolism, capacitation, and early embryonic development take place.

## ENDOCRINOLOGY OF FOLLICULAR GROWTH AND OVULATION

Growth, maturation, ovulation, and luteinization of the Graafian follicle depend on appropriate patterns of secretion, sufficient concentrations, and adequate ratios of FSH and LH in the serum. These hormones include steroids, prostaglandins, and glycoproteins (combinations of sialic acid and bichained polypeptide).

FSH plays a major role in the initiation of antrum formation. This gonadotropin stimulates granulosa cell mitosis and follicular fluid formation. Moreover, FSH induces granulosa cell sensitivity to LH by increasing the number of LH receptors. In sows, LH receptors increase from 300 in small follicles to 10,000 large preovulatory follicles. The LH-receptor increment prepares the luteinization of granulosa cells in response to LH ovulatory surge.

### *Steroidogenesis*

Steroidogenic activity of the follicle also depends on FSH and LH acting on granulosa and theca cells, respectively. The androgen-estrogen ratio in the follicular fluid reflects

**TABLE 5-3. *Regulatory Function of Follicular Fluid with Inhibitory or Stimulatory Responses***

| SUBSTANCES | PHYSIOLOGIC RESPONSE |
|---|---|
| **INHIBITORS:** | |
| Oocyte maturation inhibitor (OMI) | Inhibits completion of oocyte meiosis |
| Luteinization inhibitor | Prevents or inhibits luteinization of granulosa cells |
| FSH receptor-binding inhibitor | Depresses binding of FSH to granulosa cells |
| Inhibin (FSH suppressing substance) | Depresses secretion of FSH |
| Other factors | Promote capacitation/acrosome reaction of sperm |
| **STIMULATOR:** | |
| Luteinization stimulator | Stimulates luteinization of granulosa cells |

the physiologic integrity and viability of the follicle. In the ewe, granulosa cells secrete only estradiol when testosterone is present in the culture medium; secretion is higher if FSH is added. On the other hand, theca cells from large follicles of cattle and sheep synthesize testosterone. Because FSH mainly stimulates granulosa cells, testosterone production, the FSH-LH ratio is an important endocrine parameter to evaluate ovarian steroid production.

### *Follicular Growth During "Follicular" and "Luteal" Phases*

Active corpora lutea are present in the ovaries during a large part of the estrous cycle called the luteal phase. The follicular phase, the period from corpus luteum regression to the following ovulation, is apparently short (2 days in ewes and 4 to 5 days in cows and sows). However, the presence of antral follicles through the luteal phase suggests that the real duration of the follicle phase is longer than 2 to 5 days, if "follicular phase" refers to the period from antral follicle formation to ovulation. Therefore, the luteal phase in domestic mammals would partially overlap the true follicular phase, obscuring the relationship between basal plasma FSH and LH levels and follicular growth.

There are certain species differences regarding these phases:

a) animal species with no luteal phase, such as rodents with 4-day estrous cycles
b) primates with quite distinct follicular and luteal phases
c) domestic mammals with overlapping "follicular" and "luteal" phases

In domestic mammals, there is also a second rise of FSH 20 to 30 hours after the preovulatory surge of LH and FSH. This postovulatory FSH rise triggers antrum formation in the follicle population that includes candidates for ovulation 1 or 2 cycles later. In ewes the second peak of FSH is significantly larger in those animals with a higher ovulation rate, and the magnitude of this peak is highly correlated with the number of antral follicles present in the ovary 17 days later. Only a few of these differentiated antral follicles grow to ovulation; the others become atretic and degenerate.

The relatively long duration of the follicular phase in domestic mammals as compared to rodents probably results from the slowing down of follicular growth by progesterone from the corpus luteum. When fully functional corpora lutea are induced in rodents by cervical stimulation, the duration of the estrous cycle and of follicular growth increases several days. On the other hand, reduction of the progesterone level during the luteal phase in cows and ewes by corpus luteum enucleation or prostaglandin luteolysis is followed by shortening of the cycle; ovulation occurs within 3 days showing an immediate acceleration of follicular growth. This is the physiologic basis of the well-known practice of estrus synchronization in cattle after prostaglandin luteolytic treatment or in sheep after withdrawal of exogenous progestogens (vaginal sponge).

## EGG MATURATION

The maturation of oocytes comprises two stages:

a) a period of growth
b) a period of final nuclear and cytoplasmic preparation prerequisite to fertilization and normal development.

### *Oocyte Growth*

When a primordial follicle is released from the reserve, the oocyte and its follicle begin to grow. Oocyte growth is almost complete at the time of antrum formation. Through cellular processes, the inner cumulus cells actively cooperate to achieve oocyte growth, as they establish close contact with the oocyte cell membrane. During the formation of the external membrane of the oocyte (zona pellucida), the cumulus cell processes are strengthened. The cytologic, morphologic, metabolic, chromosomal, physiologic, biochemical, and hormonal aspects of oocyte growth are summarized in Tables 5-4 and 5-5.

The maturation of oocytes is independent of:

a) the nature of follicular stimulation
b) the diameter of the follicle from which oocytes have been removed
c) the source of the follicular fluid or its filtrate from diverse follicles and different females.

In gilts, the removal of one ovary results in compensatory growth of the other ovary as measured by the increased number of growth follicles in an increased volume of follicular fluid (3). Thus, the removal of one ovary from a sow results in nearly the same litter size per farrowing as in an intact sow. However, the lifetime production of piglets by a sow with a unilateral ovariectomy appears to be reduced.

### *Oocyte Preparation for Fertilization*

From oogenesis onward, the diplotene nucleus of the oocyte remains in the resting stage called the *dictyate nucleus*. Meiosis never resumes normally before gonadotropin ovulatory surge (Figures 5-3 and 5-4). The gonadotropin ovulatory discharge suppresses production of the granulosa cell meiotic-inhibiting factor. The gonadotropin surge is followed by metabolic modification of that follicular layer (Figure 5-5). Meiotic resumption (nuclear maturation) is only one aspect of egg maturation; cytoplasmic maturation must also occur.

TABLE 5-4. ***Major Physiologic, Biochemical, Biophysical, and Neuroendocrine Characteristics of Follicular Growth and Maturation***

| PARAMETERS | PHYSIOLOGIC MECHANISMS |
|---|---|
| Recruitment and selection of follicles to ovulate | Throughout the estrous cycle, each ovary has numerous antral follicles on its surface. Two processes lead to development of preovulatory follicles.<br>Recruitment process establishes a group of follicles capable of ovulating.<br>Individual follicles are selected to continue development to ovulation from a cohort of grossly similar follicles that degenerate. |
| Development of follicles | Follicles classified according to:<br>size of follicle<br>number of layers of granulosa cells<br>development of theca layers<br>position of oocyte within its surrounding cumulus oophorus<br>presence of an antrum (fluid-filled space). |
| Number of follicles that develop | Number of follicles that develop per estrous cycle depends on hereditary/environmental factors.<br>In cattle/horses, one follicle usually develops more rapidly than others, so that at each estrus only one egg is released; remaining follicles regress/become atrophied.<br>In swine, 10–25 follicles ripen at each estrus.<br>In sheep, one to three follicles may reach maturity depending on breed, age/stage of sexual season. |
| Nuclear maturation | Resting or immature oocytes have a large nucleus germinal vesicle.<br>Meiosis progresses from germinal vesicle (prophase of the first reduction division) to metaphase of second reduction division where it stops once again.<br>First polar body is extruded into perivitelline space. |
| Cytoplasmic maturation | Resumption of meiosis results from release of an inhibitory effect exerted by follicular cells on oocyte.<br>Inhibition release coincides with loosening of granulosa/other cells around the oocyte. |
| Ovum maturation | Upon appropriate stimulation from circulating FSH/LH.<br>Final maturation of the oocyte within the mature, preovulatory follicle(s). |
| Stigma formation | A thin area of follicular apex, the whole apical wall becomes thin; prior to ovulation, inner layers of the follicular wall protrude through a gap to form a papilla.<br>Stigma thins out, bulges on ovarian surface/becomes completely avascular.<br>At ovulation the bulging stigma ruptures at the apex, releasing some of follicular fluid. |
| Release of eggs | Cumulus-oocyte complex oozes out in viscous follicular fluid.<br>Gelatinous mass comprising contents of follicle is gradually extruded until it is released to be picked up by cilia heat of fimbria. |

# OVULATION

Preovulatory follicles undergo three major changes during the ovulatory process:

a) cytoplasmic and nuclear maturation of the oocyte
b) disruption of cumulus cell cohesiveness among the cells of the granulosa layer
c) thinning and rupture of the external follicular wall

After the ovulatory surge of gonadotropins, blood flow increases to all classes of follicles. The follicle destined to ovulate, however, receives the largest volume of blood in absolute terms (as measured in ml/min).

### *Follicular Atresia*

The ovarian follicles undergo degenerative changes during which the follicles lose their integrity. Most oocytes are lost at variable stages of their growth, as well as during all stages of the ovarian cycle. This loss occurs more frequently in the advanced stages of follicular growth.

Atresia is associated with several morphologic, bio-

**TABLE 5-5. *Physiological Mechanisms of Steroidogenesis: Anomalies of Follicular Growth/Ovulation and Association of Ovarian Follicles/Corpus Luteum***

| PARAMETERS | PHYSIOLOGIC MECHANISMS |
|---|---|
| Steroidogenesis | All cell types of the ovary, particularly granulosa cells and theca cells, have the capacity to make steroids.<br>Steroid hormones secreted by a particular cell type are determined by stage of estrous cycle.<br>Following ovulation, the luteinized granulosa cells become vascularized and secrete increased amounts of progesterone in ovarian vein. |
| Anomalies of follicular growth and ovulation | Various anomalies occur in follicular growth, ovulation, and luteinization of the ruptured follicle. Growth can be arrested at specific stages, leading to conditions in which the follicles release androgens and other steroids, as in the development of cystic ovaries.<br>Abnormal follicle growth may arise through deficiencies in the hypothalamic-pituitary axis.<br>Luteinized unruptured follicle: luteinization of a follicle without the release of the egg; luteinization of follicles proceeds normally in the absence of follicle rupture. This condition is due to subtle defects in the endocrine profile or in follicular maturation that may accelerate, delay, or even prevent rupture of follicle release of ova. |
| Association of follicle/corpus luteum | Physiologic association between follicles/functional corpora lutea exists because follicular development is enhanced in ovary containing a corpus luteum.<br>Progesterone may act both systemically and locally to alter time-dependent changes in follicle size, thus making it possible for some follicles to grow while others undergo atresia.<br>Estrogens affect follicles directly, both preventing atresia and stimulating growth. |

Data from: diZerega GS, Hodgen GD. Folliculogenesis in the primate ovarian cycle. Endocr Rev 1981;2:27–49.
Draincourt MA, Cahill LP. Preovulatory follicular events in sheep. J Reprod Fertil 1984;71:205–211.
Sluss PM, Reichert LE Jr. Porcine follicular fluid contains several low molecular weight inhibitors of follicle-stimulating hormone binding to receptor. Biol Reprod 1984;30:1091.

chemical, and histologic changes that vary greatly with the stage of follicle growth, as well as with the animal species. They may be related to an altered role of granulosa cells and also to an altered passage of nutritive substances from the plasma in the follicles. Degeneration is accompanied by loss of the oocyte, granulosa cells, and receptors for various hormones.

FACTORS AFFECTING ATRESIA. Several factors regulate follicular atresia: age, the stage of the reproductive cycle, pregnancy, lactation, the balance between estrogen and androgen of extraovarian or intraovarian sources, a genetic "program," nutrition, and ischemia. There may be several processes and mechanisms of atresia depending on the stage of follicular growth. Different hormonal treatments influence the rate at which the follicles become atretic. The ability of a developing follicle to release high concentrations of estrogens, which stimulate growth and cell differentiation of granulosa, is central to selection of a given follicle for maturation and ovulation. Interruption of estrogen production at any step results in atresia of follicles.

The effect of the corpus luteum on the ovarian follicle is determined by the type of follicle and the stage of pregnancy. The reduction in the diameter of the largest follicle and the accumulation of the medium-sized follicles is due to the effect of the corpus luteum on reducing the rate of growth and atresia of the follicle.

### *Site of Ovulation*

The mammalian ovary is normally arranged so that ovulation can occur at any point on its surface, except at the hilus. However, ovulation in mares always occurs in a limited ovarian area called the *ovulation fossa.* The ovary of horses begins its development in the usual way, and the germinal epithelium covers the whole ovary.

In cattle, sheep, and horses ovulation occurs at random with respect to which ovary contains the previous corpus luteum. However, in some mammals ovulation consistently alternates between the ovaries. In the ewe, the site of ovulation is independent of the location of the corpus luteum of the previous ovarian cycle, and the duration of the estrous cycle is unaffected by the relative locations of the corpus luteum.

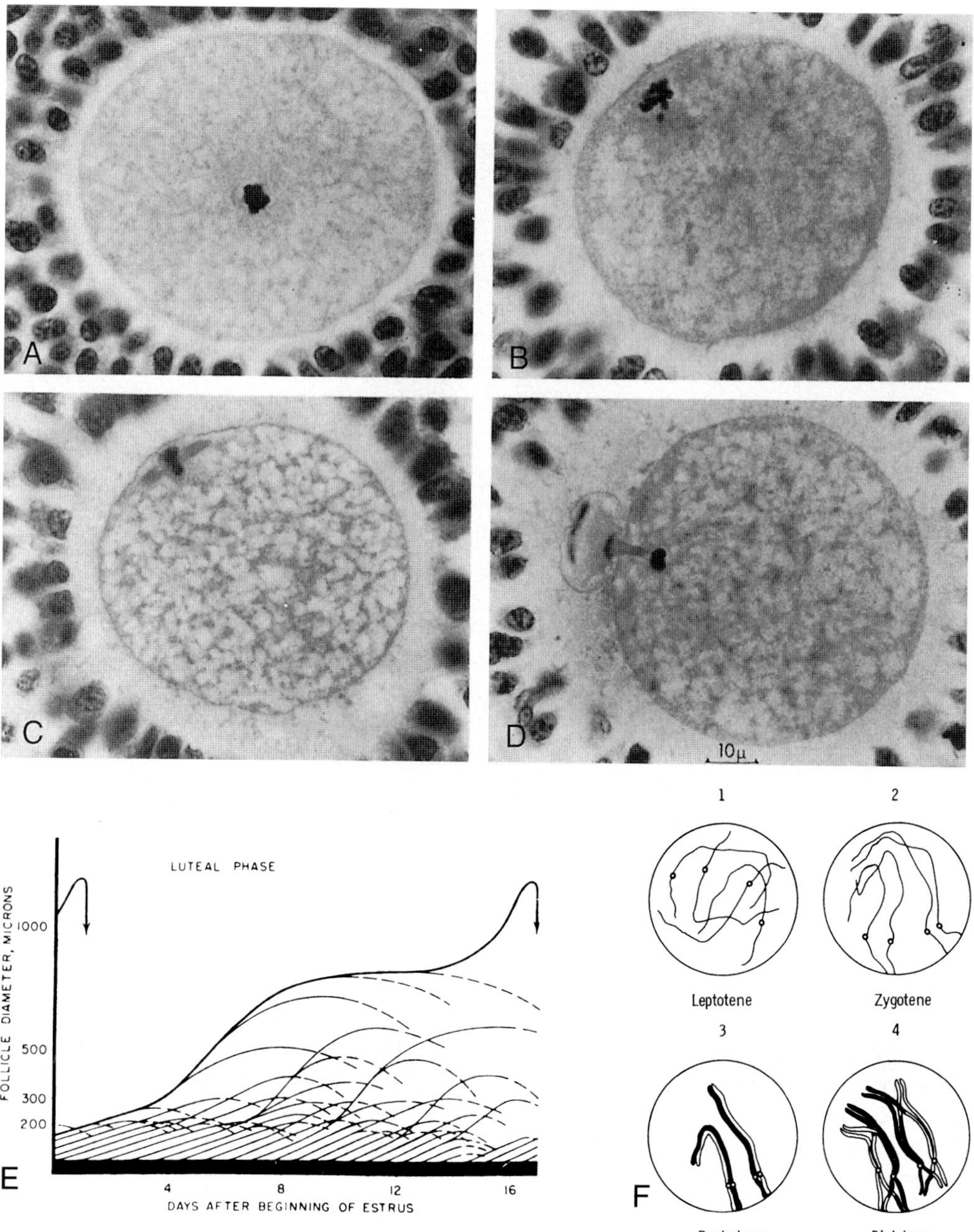


**FIGURE 5-3.** Mammalian oocytes showing typical maturation changes. (**A**) Dense chromatin mass in late germinal vesicle; cells of cumulus surround oocyte. (**B**) Diakinesis; nucleus has migrated to the periphery, and its envelope is about to break down; corona radiata forms around oocyte. (**C**) First metaphase; spindle axis is parallel to surface of oocyte. (**D**) Late first telephase; spindle is perpendicular to oocyte surface, and polar body is almost separated. (Hill R, Franchi LL, Baker TG. Oogenesis and follicular growth. In: Hafez ESE, Evans TN, eds. Human Reproduction: Conception and Contraception. 2nd ed. Hagerstown, MD: Harper & Row, 1980.) (**E**) Follicular cycle in the guinea pig. The heavy solid line indicates the average diameter of the largest follicles. Ovulation occurs at the arrow. The other solid and broken lines represent the concomitant growth and atresia, respectively. (**F**) Cytogenetic changes in mammalian oocytes showing typical chromosomal events during meiosis. For simplicity, only two pairs of homologues are shown. (Franchi LL, Baker TG. Oogenesis and follicular growth. In: Hafez ESE, Evans TN, eds. Human Reproduction: Conception and Contraception. Hagerstown, MD: Harper & Row, 1973.)

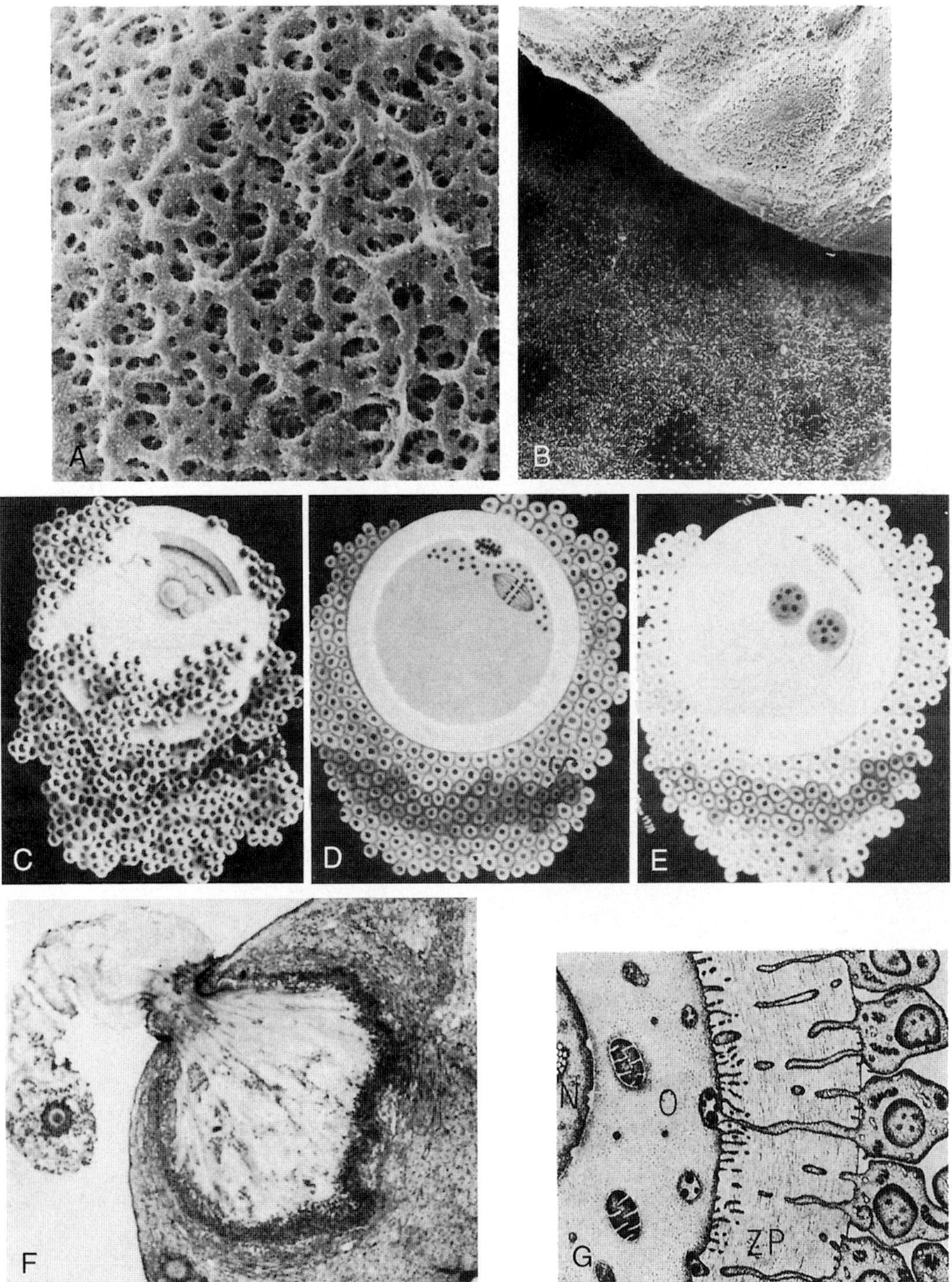


FIGURE 5-4. Scanning electron micrographs of the oocyte/zona pellucida. (**A**) Zona pellucida as shown from the outside surface and inside surface. (**B**) Characteristic mesh of the zona through which sperm penetrate. Spongy appearance of inner surface of the zona (*ZZ*) as it is peeled off the trophoblastic layer of blastocyst. Trophoblastic cells (*TT*) are characterized by microvilli. Species differences in thickness of zona pellucide: opossum, 1 μm; mouse, 5 μm; hamster, 8 μm; human, 13 μm; sheep, 15 μm; pig, 16 μm; cow, 27 μm. (**C–E**) Arrangements and cytologic connections between granulosa and the zona pellucida of the oocyte. Note some cytologic differences in distinct layers (*SS*) of the granulosa cells. (**F**) Section through follicle of rabbit immediately after ovulation protrusion of cumulus/matrix through the stigma and its adherence to ovarian surface (54™). (Blandau RJ. Gamete transport: comparative aspects. In: Hafez ESE, Blandau RJ, eds. The Mammalian Oviduct. Chicago: University of Chicago Press, 1996.) (**G**) Zona pellucida (*ZP*) around an oocyte in Graafian follicle. Microvilli arising from oocyte interdigitate with processes from granulosa cells (*G*). These processes penetrate into cytoplasm of oocyte (O) and may provide nutrients and maternal protein. (*N*), oocyte nucleus. (Baker TG. Oogenesis and ovulation. In: Austin CR, Short RW, eds. Reproduction in Mammals. Cambridge: Univesity Press, 1972.)

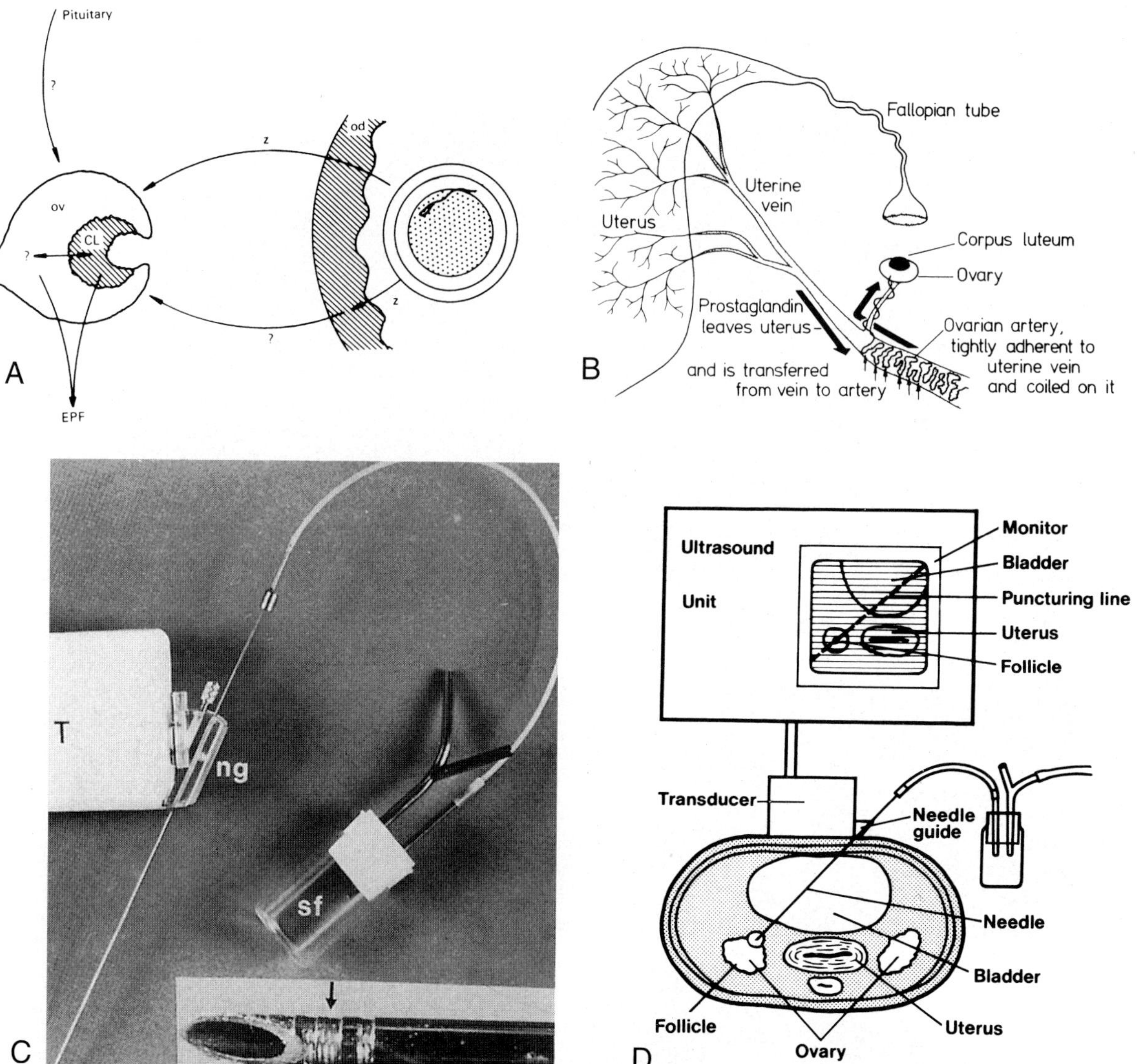


FIGURE 5-5. (A) Production of early pregnancy factor (EPF). *CL*, corpus luteum; *od*, oviduct; *ov*, ovary; *z*, zygotin. (Nancarrow. The early pregnancy factor of sheep and cattle. In: Scaramuzzi RJ, Lincoln DW, Weir BJ, eds. Reproductive Endocrinology of Domestic Ruminants. J Reprod Fertil 1982:30[Suppl].) (B) Utero-ovarian vasculature in the sheep and of the route that $PGF_{2\alpha}$ travels from the uterus to the ovary. (Peters H, McNatty KP. The development of the ovary in the embryo. In: The Ovary. Berkeley: University of California Press, 1980.) (C) Aspiration equipment for ultrasonically guided percutaneous follicle puncture: *T*, transducer; *ng*, needle guide; *sf*, sampling flask. (D) Needle tip with the shallow tracks (*arrow*) in the needle tip. Schematic illustration of the ultrasonically guided puncture technique. (Wickland M, Nilsson L, Hansson R, Hamberger ML, Janson P. Collection of human oocytes by the use of sonography. Fertil Steril 1983;39:603.)

There is no difference between left and right ovaries in size or occurrence of ovulation in horses. The frequency of multiple ovulations for ponies is about 10%. The ovulatory season appears to be shorter, with ponies ovulating during the fall in the younger age groups (under 5 years) less than in the older groups, indicating a shorter breeding season for young mares. Ovarian activity appears to decrease after 15 years. The onset of puberty occurs at 12 to 15 months of age (4). In ponies there is a decrease in the number of large follicles during late estrus.

### *Cellular Events*

Several tissue layers separate the oocyte from the outside of the follicle. These are the surface epithelium, the collagen-rich tunica albuginea, the theca externa, the thin basement lumina separating the capillary network from the membrana granulosa, and the membrana granulosa itself. Before ovulation, all tissue layers are broken down. Moreover, the necessary increase in follicular elasticity during preovulatory growth is associated with changes in granulosa and theca cell relationships. Such changes are also prerequisite to further corpus luteum organization.

As the enlarging follicle begins to protrude from the surface of the ovary, the vascularity of the follicular surface increases except at its center, which seems devoid of blood vessels. This avascular area is the future point of rupture.

OOCYTE. Only the cumulus cells anchored in the zona pellucida remain, surrounding the oocyte and forming the corona radiata. Cumulus cell dissociation frees the oocyte from the granulosa layer, and meiosis resumes about 3 hours after the gonadotropin surge.

Cumulus cells actively secrete glycoproteins, which form a viscous mass enclosing the oocyte and its corona. After follicular rupture the viscous mass spreads at the ovarian surface to facilitate the "pick up" of the oocytes by the fimbriae. Ultrasonography is used extensively to recover preovulatory eggs from the ovarian follicle to be used *in vitro* fertilization (IVF).

GRANULOSA CELLS. The granulosa layer is completely dissociated only at the follicular apex and finally disappears. About 2 hours before ovulation, granulosa cell growth processes penetrate through the lamina basalis, preparing the invasion of theca cells and blood vessels into the granulosa after ovulation in the developing corpus luteum. This process is associated with the production of the early pregnancy factor (EPF).

THECA CELLS. The follicular volume rapidly increases in the few hours preceding ovulation without any increment of follicular fluid pressure, owing to the increased elasticity of the follicle. This results from a looser cohesion of the theca externa cells owing to the invasive edema of this layer and to collagen fiber dissociation, which begins 4 hours after coitus.

APEX CHANGES. The rupture of the follicle involves interaction between the ovarian epithelium and the underlying follicular wall. The wall of the follicle apex becomes exceedingly thin in an area called the "stigma." The stigma thins out, bulges on the surface of the ovary, and becomes completely avascular. At ovulation the bulging stigma ruptures at the apex, releasing some of the follicular fluid and the viscous glycoprotein mass embedding the oocyte.

### Mechanisms of Ovulation

Ovulation occurs in response to several physiologic, biochemical, and biophysical mechanisms (Fig. 5-4):

a) neuroendocrine/endocrine mechanisms, GnRH steroids, and prostaglandins
b) neurobiochemical/pharmacologic mechanisms
c) neuromuscular and neurovascular mechanisms, and enzymatic interactions (Table 5-6).

Prostaglandins may stimulate ovarian contractions and activate thecal fibroblasts to proliferate and release proteolytic enzymes that digest the follicle wall and basement lamina. Steroids, especially progesterone, may also be involved.

### Biochemical Mechanisms of Ovulation

The gonadotropin preovulatory surge first induces an immediate and temporary rise in steroid levels due to an increased secretion of progesterone and related progestins. Later, estradiol and $PGF_2$ secretion are also augmented. Inhibition of either prostaglandin or steroid secretion prevents ovulation.

CHANGES IN STEROID SECRETION. The enhancement of steroid secretion and the switch of the estradiol-progesterone ratio that follow the gonadotropin surge are easily detectable in the follicular fluid. Inhibition of progesterone synthesis prevents ovulation. The role of progesterone is to stimulate collagenase activity in the follicular wall.

PROSTAGLANDINS. The increase of $PGF_{2\alpha}$ and $PGE_2$ levels in follicular fluid does not immediately follow the gonadotropin surge, as the steroid elevations do. In sows an increase of prostaglandins begins only 30 hours after ovulatory discharge, and the maximal level occurs about 40 hours later as ovulation approaches. When prostaglandin synthesis is inhibited, the oocyte remains inside the luteinizing follicle or may be "ovulated" inside the ovary. $PGF_{2\alpha}$ is involved in follicular rupture; and $PGE_2$ in the remodeling of the follicular layers, terminating in corpus luteum formation.

### Neuromuscular Mechanisms

The ovarian stroma and the concentric layers of the theca externa of preovulatory follicles contain smooth muscle cells that are richly innervated by autonomic nerve terminals. Ovarian contractions facilitate follicular rupture after the follicular apex has been thinned. Before rupture, the follicle itself does not contract spontaneously. After follicular rupture, the thecal neuromuscular system, stimulated by $PGF_{2\alpha}$ contributes to the extrusion of the oocyte.

### Neuroendocrine Control of Ovulatory Gonadotropic Discharge

A preovulatory gonadotropin surge occurs at the beginning of estrus when progesterone has fallen to its minimal blood levels and when estradiol reaches its highest cyclic values.

Estradiol acts at two levels: the pituitary and the hypo-

TABLE 5-6. *Some Neuroendocrine and Endocrine Mechanisms of Ovulation*

| PARAMETERS | PHYSIOLOGIC AND BIOCHEMICAL MECHANISMS |
|---|---|
| Neuroendocrine | Gonadotropins secreted in a pulsatile fashion in response to similar pulsatile release from GnRH from neurosecretory neurons in hypothalamus. |
| | Gonadal steroids exert feedback effects both directly on the pituitary and through modulation of pulsatile pattern of GnRH secretion. |
| | Dopamine inhibits prolactin release. |
| | Endorphins are endogenous apiate peptides through modulation of neurotransmitter mechanisms, endorphins affect prolactin/gonadotropin secretion. |
| Endocrine | LH is at a steady level during early follicular phase/rises slightly before ovulation. |
| | Remarkable surge of LH occurs prior to ovulation; LH levels return to low level during luteal phase. |
| | Number of ovarian follicles that develop/proportion that subsequently degenerate are regulated by FSH/LH ratio. |
| | Cyclic changes in estradiol/FSH levels stimulate one or two waves of follicular growth and regulate ovulation rates. |
| | Granulosa cells secrete progesterone into follicular fluid/act as precursor for estrogen synthesis in surrounding theca interna cells. |
| | LH reaches critical concentrations in plasma, it exerts a negative feedback within the CNS. |
| | Several follicles grow during first stages of the estrous cycle, but few reach preovulatory maturity. |
| | Less FSH may be required to initiate growth of small follicles than to maintain larger follicles and bring them to ovulatory size. |
| Prostaglandins | Theca is the predominant site of prostaglandin production, and the capacity of both granulosa/theca cells increases with the stage of follicular developments; rupture of follicles is associated with follicular synthesis of prostaglandin. |
| | Concentration of prostaglandins E and F in follicular fluid of preovulatory follicles increases as time of ovulation approaches; indomethacin blocks follicular rupture by inhibiting prostaglandin production. |
| | Exogenous LH increases prostaglandin E and prostaglandin F within the whole ovaries, Graafian follicles, and follicular fluid. |

thalamus. Estradiol increases the sensitivity of pituitary gonadotropin-producing cells to the competent hypothalamic hormone GnRH. During post partum anestrus in lactating females, estradiol positive feedback may be prevented by high prolactin levels related to the suckling stimulus.

### *Egg "Pick-Up"*

The ovary, attached to the back of the broad ligament, lies free in the peritoneal cavity. The oviduct curls over the ovary to facilitate egg "pick-up" by the mucosal folds of the fimbriae. At the time of ovulation, the ovum, together with the surrounding cells in the gelatinous mass, protrudes at the ovarian surface and is swept into the ostium of the oviduct by the action of the motile kinocilia of the fimbriae.

### *In Vitro Ovulation*

Several culture media are used to induce ovulation *in vitro* with or without ovarian perfusion. The selection of quality follicles is favored by the choice of season for the experiments and also by the absence of any ovarian stimulation when the follicle ovulates; thus, the granulosa cell mass will be well preserved. The same culture system is used for *in vitro* fertilization of oocytes matured in their follicles *in vitro*. The proportion of follicles ovulating, particularly after addition of progesterone to the medium, is appreciably higher than that previously obtained after the culture of whole ovaries.

### *Anomalies of Ovulation and Reproductive Failure*

The absence of ovulation and the subsequent formation of follicular cysts are the main causes of reproductive failure in cows and aged sows. An efficient treatment for preventing cyst formation, which reduces fertility in cystic cows, is the stimulation of gonadotropin release by GnRH or the direct stimulation of the ovary with hCG. It is probable that the presence of cystic follicles reflects a disorder in gonadotrophic function at the hypothalamic level.

## REFERENCES

1. Testart J, Thebault A, Frydman R, Papiernik E. Oocyte and cumulus oophorus changes inside the human follicle cultured

with gonadotrophins. In: Hafez ESE, Semm K, eds. In-vitro Fertilization and Embryo Transfer. Lancaster, England: MTP Press, 1982.
2. Draincourt MA, Cahill LP. Preovulatory follicular events in sheep. J Reprod Fertil 1984;71:205–211.
3. Redmer DA, Christenson RK, Ford JS, Day BN. Effect of unilateral ovariectomy on compensatory ovarian hypertrophy, peripheral concentrations of follicle-stimulating hormone and luteinizing hormone, and ovarian venous concentrations of estradiol-17$\beta$ in pre-puberal gilts. Biol Reprod 1984;31:59–66.
4. Wesson JA, Ginther OJ. Influence of season and age on reproductive activity in pony mares on the basis of a slaughterhouse survey. J Anim Sci 1981;52:119–129.

## Suggested Reading

Blandau RJ. Gamete transport: comparative aspects. In: Hafez ESE, Blandau RJ, eds.The Mammalian Oviduct. Chicago: University of Chicago Press, 1969.

diZerega GS, Hodgen GD. Folliculogenesis in the primate ovarian cycle. Endocr. Rev. 1981;2:27–49.

Dvorak M, Tesarik J. Ultrastructure of human ovarian follicles. In: Motta PP, Hafez ESE, eds. Biology of the Ovary. London: Martinus Nijhoff, 1980.

Foster DS, Ryan KD. Endocrine mechanisms governing transition into adulthood in female sheep. In: Scaramuzzi RJ, Lincoln DW, Weir BJ, eds. Reproductive Endocrinology of Domestic Ruminants. J Reprod Fertil 1981;30(Suppl):75–90.

Franchi LL, Baker TG. Oogenesis and follicular growth. In: Hafez ESE, Evans TN, eds. Human Reproduction: Conception and Contraception. Hagerstown, MD: Harper & Row, 1973.

Guraya SS. Recent advances in the cellular and molecular biology of ovarian follicles. In: Puett D, ed. Human Fertility, Health and Food: Impact of Molecular Biology and Biotechnology. New York: United Nations Fund for Population Activities, 1984.

Hafez ESE, Levasseur MC, Thibault C. Folliculogenesis, egg maturation and ovulation. In: Hafez ESE, ed. Reproduction in Farm Animals. 4th ed. Philadelphia, Lea & Febiger, 1980.

Hunter RHF. Reproduction of Farm Animals. London: Longman's, 1982.

Peters H, McNatty KP. Morphology of the ovary. In: Peters H, McNatty KP, eds. The Ovary. Berkeley: University of California Press, 1980a.

Peters H, McNatty KP. Corpus luteum function. In: Peters H, McNatty KP, eds. The Ovary. Berkeley: University of California Press, 1980b.

Sluss PM, Reichert LE Jr. Porcine follicular fluid contains several low molecular weight inhibitors of follicle-stimulating hormone binding to receptor. Biol Reprod 1984;30:1091.

Thibault C, Levasseur MC. La Fonction Ovarienne chez les Mammiferes. Paris: Masson, 1979.

Wickland M, Nilsson L, Hansson R, Hamberger ML, Janson P. Collection of human oocytes by the use of sonography. Fertil Steril 1983;39:603.

CHAPTER 6

# Transport and Survival of Gametes

E.S.E. HAFEZ AND B. HAFEZ

The sperm-egg complex undergoes various maturational changes in preparation for fertilization (Table 6-1). While the female sheds 1 or 2 ova (or 10 to 15 ova in the case of swine), each estrous cycle, the male discharges massive numbers of sperm at copulation. Since the survival time of ova and sperm is relatively short (20 to 48 hours), fertilizations depends primarily on the synchronous transport of the gametes in the female reproductive tract. Gamete transport is the result of the inherent contractility of the female tract as modified by central nervous system reflexes and hormonal activity. Pharmacologically active substances in the semen stimulate and modulate the contractility of the female reproductive tract. The oviductal cilia and fluids, cervix, uterotubal junction, and ampullary-isthmic junction play roles in gamete transport.

## SPERM TRANSPORT IN THE FEMALE TRACT

Species differences exist in the sites at which the ejaculate is deposited in the female reproductive tract during copulation (Table 6-2). In cattle and sheep, the small volume of semen is ejaculated into the cranial end of the vagina and onto the cervix (Fig. 6-1). In horses and swine, the voluminous ejaculate is deposited through the relaxed cervical canal into the uterus. The sperm are unique because they are transported through various luminal fluids of completely different physiologic and biochemical characteristics, such as testicular fluid, epididymal fluid, seminal plasma, vaginal fluid, cervical mucus, uterine fluid, oviductal fluid, and peritoneal fluid (Fig. 6-1).

Physiochemical and immunologic factors in the vagina and cervix at the time of insemination play an important role in sperm survival and transport into the uterus and oviduct (Table 6-2 and Figs. 6-2 and 6-3). The vaginal secretions immobilize sperm within 1 to 2 hours of insemination. The rapid elimination and immobilization of sperm in the vagina make the rapid transport of sperm to a more favorable environment essential.

Seminal plasma plays a major role in the transport and physiology of sperm. However, sperm removed from the vas deferens and epididymis are successfully used in artificial insemination, and the removal of various accessory organs of the male tract rarely decreases fertility so long as ejaculation still results in the release of a few million sperm.

Unlike the vagina, the epithelial lining of the cervix, uterus, and oviduct is composed of nonciliated secretory cells and kinociliated cells. In general, secretory cells have a dome-shaped surface covered with numerous microvilli, and their cytoplasm contains numerous secretory granules. The percentage of kinociliated cells in the epithelium, which varies in different parts of the reproductive tract, is maximal in the fimbriae and oviductal ampulla and minimal in the uterus and uterine cervix. The ciliated cells are covered with kinocilia that beat rhythmically toward the vagina (Fig. 6-3).

### *Sperm Distribution in the Female Reproductive Tract*

Three stages are recognized in sperm transport in the female reproductive tract: short, rapid sperm transport; colonization of reservoirs; and slow, prolonged release.

RAPID TRANSPORT. Immediately after insemination, sperm penetrate the micelles of the cervical mucus where some are quickly transported through the cervical canal. This phase takes 2 to 10 minutes and may be facilitated by sperm motility as well as increased contractile activity of the myometrium and mesosalpinx during courtship and coitus. Some sperm reach the internal os of the cervix within 1.5 to 3 minutes after insemination. Thus, some sperm can reach the site of fertilization rapidly. Whether the first sperm

TABLE 6-1. ***Sperm and Egg Physiology Related to Fertilization***

| PARAMETERS | OOGENESIS AND CHARACTERISTICS OF OVA | SPERMATOGENESIS AND CHARACTERISTICS OF SPERM |
|---|---|---|
| First maturational division in gamete | First maturational division is completed in preovulatory follicle | First meiotic division results in two cells of equal size |
| Second maturational division | Second maturational division is completed only when egg is penetrated by sperm | Not comparable |
| Number of gametes produced during reproductive life | Thousands of oogonia are found in neonate ovary | Millions of sperm are produced in each ejaculate from puberty, with reduced numbers during senility |
| Sex chromosome in gamete | X | X or Y |
| Amount of cytoplasm in gamete | As oocyte matures, the amount of its cytoplasm increases | As spermatid develops into sperm, the amount of cytoplasm decreases, acrosome and tail develop in late spermatid |
| Motility of gamete | Oocytes, surrounded by follicular cells, are immotile | Sperm motility develops gradually in various parts of epididymis and increases at ejaculation |
| Plasma membrane at fertilization | Egg acquires plasma membranes from sperm | Sperm loses its plasma membranes to egg |
| Survival in female reproductive tract | 12–24 hours after ovulation | Fertilizability is maintained 24 hours after ejaculation |

TABLE 6-2. ***Species Differences in the Site of Ejaculation and Semen Characteristics in Mammals***

| SITE OF EJACULATION | SEMEN CHARACTERISTICS | SPECIES |
|---|---|---|
| VAGINA | | |
| Incipient plug | Slight coagulation of ejaculate | Human; Rabbit |
| Incipient plug | Instant coagulation of ejaculate | Monkey |
| Little accessory fluid | Semen with high sperm concentration | Cattle; Sheep |
| UTERUS | | |
| Voluminous | Distention of cervix | Horse |
| Voluminous | Retention of penis during copulation | Dog; Pig |
| Vaginal plug | Spasmodic contraction of vagina | Rodents |

entering the oviduct participate in fertilization of the ovum is not known; it has been proposed that fertilization occurs only when a minimal number of sperm reach the site of fertilization.

COLONIZATION OF SPERM RESERVOIRS. Massive numbers of sperm are trapped in the complex mucosal folds of the cervical crypts. This process is facilitated by the fact that the micelles of the cervical mucus direct sperm to the cervical crypts where the reservoir is formed. Fewer leukocytes are found in the cervical secretions compared with those of the vagina or uterus; this suggests that less phagocytosis of sperm takes place in the cervix. Concentration gradients of sperm in different segments of the reproductive tract are important for fertility. The more sperm that enter the cervical reservoir, the more that will reach the oviduct, thus increasing the chance of fertilization. In addition, the larger the reservoir, the longer an adequate population of sperm will be maintained in the oviduct.

In species in which ejaculation occurs in the uterine horns, sperm reservoirs are localized in the uterotubal junction, as in the pig, or in the endometrial glands, as in the dog. No evidence indicates that sperm are released after their entry into the endometrial glands of any species. Sperm transport is affected by prostaglandins (Figs. 6-3 and 6-4) in the semen of some species.

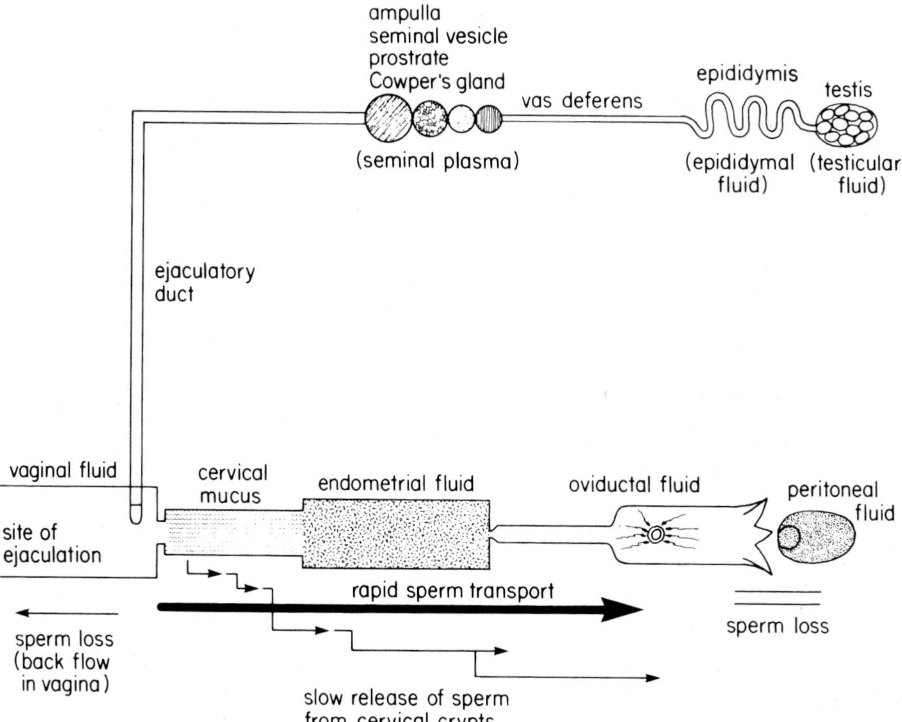


FIGURE 6-1. The various luminal fluids in which sperm are suspended from the time of sperm production in the seminiferous tubules to the time of fertilization in the oviduct.

SLOW RELEASE AND TRANSPORT. After adequate sperm reservoirs have been established within the reproductive tract, the sperm are released sequentially for a prolonged period. This slow release, which involves the innate motility of sperm and the conctractile activity of the myometrium and mesosalpinx, ensures the continued availability of sperm for entry to the oviduct to effect fertilization of the egg. However, various anatomic and physiologic barriers prevent massive numbers of sperm in the ejaculate from reaching the site of fertilization presumably to avoid polyspermy, which is lethal to the fertilized egg.

## *Sperm Transport in the Cervix*

The endocervical mucosa is an intricate system of clefts, grooves, and crypts grouped together. Several functions have been ascribed to the cervix and its secretion:

a) it is receptive to sperm penetration at or near ovulation and inhibits migration at other phases of the cycle;
b) it acts as a sperm reservoir;
c) it protects sperm from the hostile environment of the vagina and from phagocytosis;
d) it provides sperm with energy requirements;
e) it filters defective and immobile sperm, and
f) it possibly participates in the capacitation of sperm.

CERVICAL MUCUS. Cervical mucus that accumulates in the vaginal pool may contain endometrial, oviductal, follicular, and peritoneal fluids as well as leukocytes and cellular debris from uterine, cervical, and vaginal epithelia. The cervical mucus is a hydrogel, which consists of water and a solid component composed of three or more units forming a three-dimensional network. The secretions are heterogeneous in composition, due to the presence of two types of low-viscosity and high-viscosity components. Cervical mucus has rheologic properties such as viscosity, flow elasticity, spinnbarkeit, thixotropy, and tack (stickiness). Low-molecular-weight organic components include free simple sugars (glucose, maltose, and mannose) and amino acids. The mucus also contains proteins, trace elements, and enzymes.

A physiologic balance of ovarian steroids is necessary for the initiation and maintenance of a cervical population of sperm following artificial insemination, particularly after estrus synchronization.

SPERM PENETRATION IN CERVICAL MUCUS. Ejaculated sperm rapidly penetrate watery cervical mucus during mid-cycle, aided principally by sperm motility as well as the microrheologic and macrorheologic properties of mucus. The rate of sperm penetration in the mucus varies throughout the estrous cycle.

Sperm are mechanically oriented toward the cervical internal os. As the flagellum beats and vibrates, the sperm head is propelled forward in the channels of least resistance. The tail frequency sets up a mechanical resonance between itself and the oscillation frequency of the molecular lattice. Hydrodynamic principles seem to apply to sperm motility;

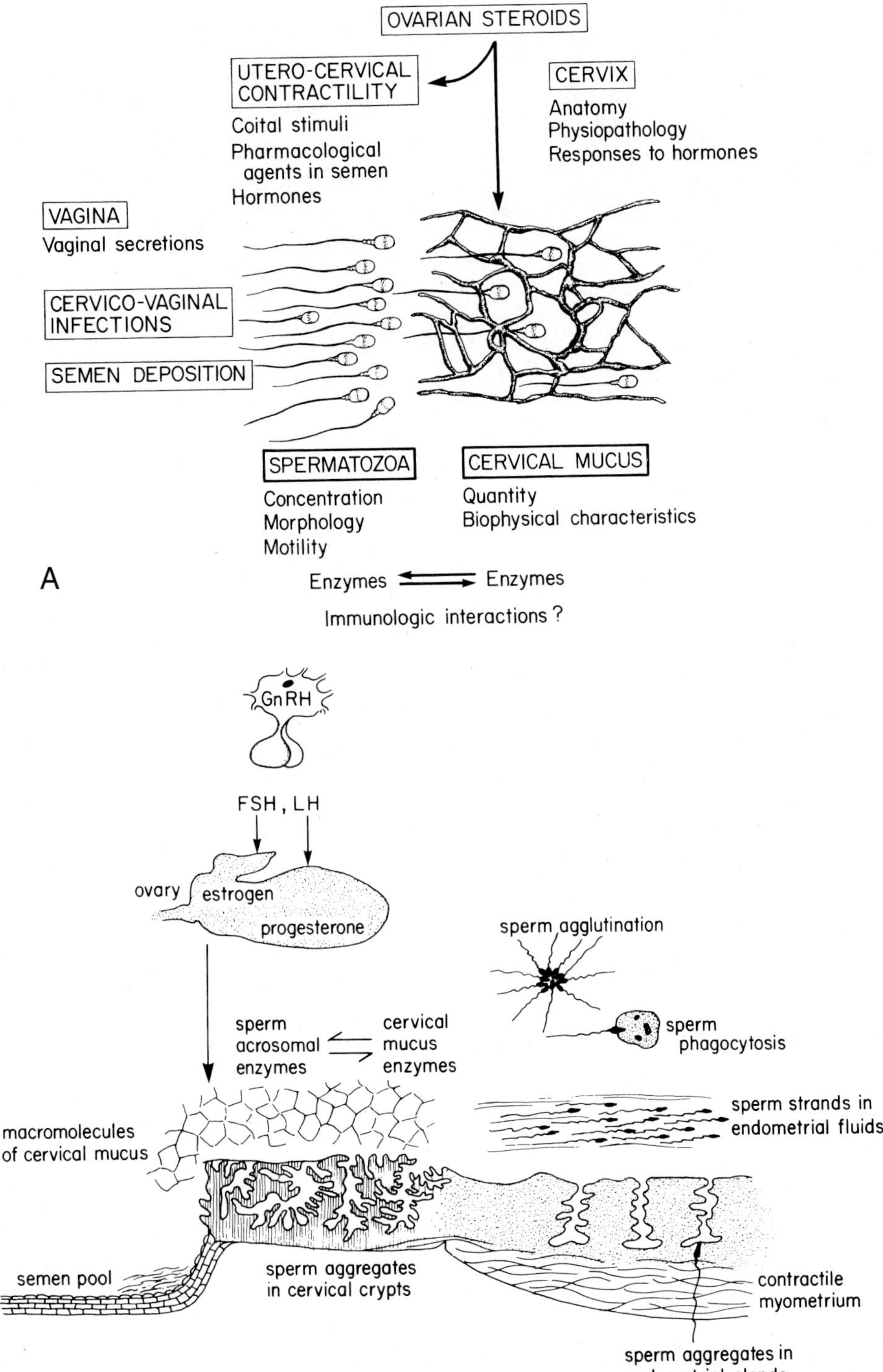


FIGURE 6-2. (A) The biophysical, physiologic, biochemical and immunologic interaction among sperm, cervical mucus, and various segments of the female reproductive tract. (B) Sperm transport through the cervix to the uterine lumen involves biochemical mechanisms as well as biophysical/physiologic changes in cervical mucus, which in turn are controlled by endocrine factors.

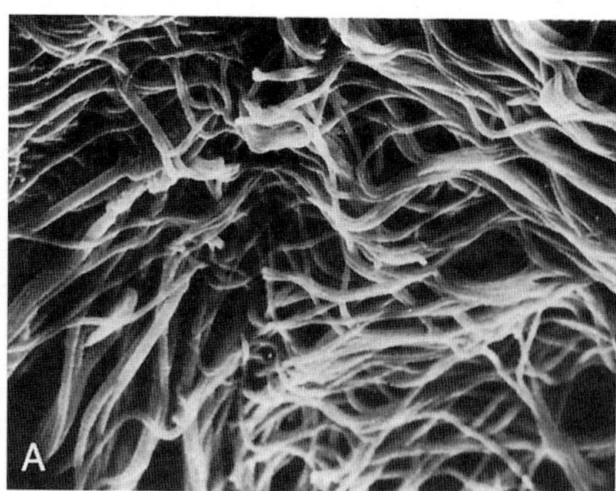


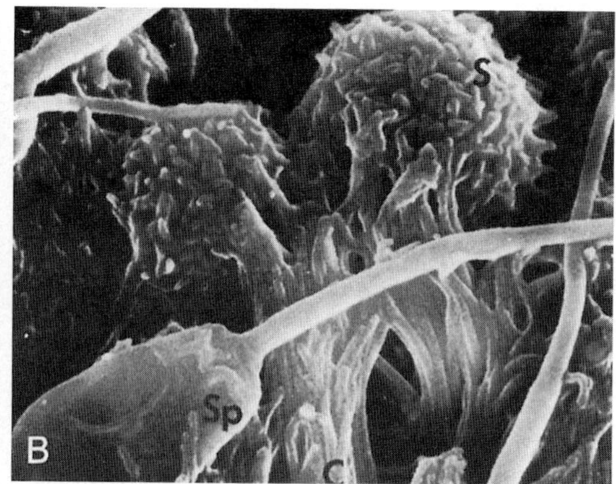


FIGURE 6-3. Scanning electron micrographs showing the relationship between sperm ultrastructure of cervical mucus. (**A**) Sperm on the cervical epithelium one hour postcoital. Note the arrangement of sperm tail in a parallel formation (From Hafez ESE. J Reprod Fertil 1973;73:217.) (**B**) Cervical epithelium showing nonciliated secretory cells (S) with microvilli and ciliated cells.

thus, motile sperm are in dynamic equilibrium with the viscous force of the medium rather than being affected by the inertial force that influences large moving objects.

Dead pig sperm inseminated in pigs were transported to the oviduct less efficiently than live sperm. It appears that sperm mobility facilitates penetrability but is not absolutely necessary.

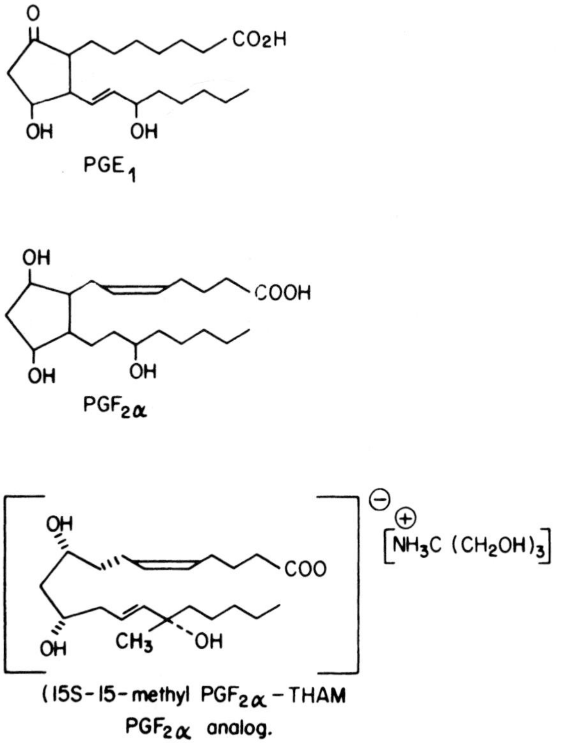

Although sperm appear to move at random in the cervical secretion, they probably follow the path of least resistance along strands of cervical mucus. When migration of a sperm in mucus is impeded, the sperm usually resumes its forward course with a sudden deflection into an adjacent parallel path. When semen is mixed with cervical mucus *in vitro*, a sharp boundary occurs between the two fluids and the cervical mucus is penetrated by fingerlike phalanges. Phalange formation may function to increase the surface area between semen and cervical mucus, provide pockets of semen within the mucus to protect sperm from the hostile vaginal environment, or facilitate sperm migration into the uterine cavity.

PGE$_1$

PGF$_{2\alpha}$

(15S-15-methyl PGF$_{2\alpha}$-THAM
PGF$_{2\alpha}$ analog.

FIGURE 6-4. Chemical formula of various types of prostaglandins found in the semen. On ejaculation in the vagina, some of these prostaglandins cause an increase in the tone and patterns of contractility of the musculature of the uterus and/or the oviduct. These responses affect the quantitative and qualitative components of sperm transport.

## *Sperm Transport in the Uterus*

The contractile activity of the vagina and myometrium plays a major role in the transport of sperm into and through the uterus. Massive numbers of sperm invade the endometrial glands. It is believed that the presence of sperm in the uterus induces endometrial leukocytic response, which enhances phagocytosis of excessive numbers of living and probably dead sperm.

SPERMOPHAGY. The uptake of sperm by phagocytes is of special physiologic significance because infiltration of leukocytes into the uterine lumen, and their activation to ingest sperm following mating seems to be a major mechanism for the removal of these cells from the female reproductive tract (1). Sperm in the uterus are taken into phagocytic vacuoles and digested by the macrophages (Fig. 6-5). Phagocytotic sperm may not have been initially damaged or necrotic.

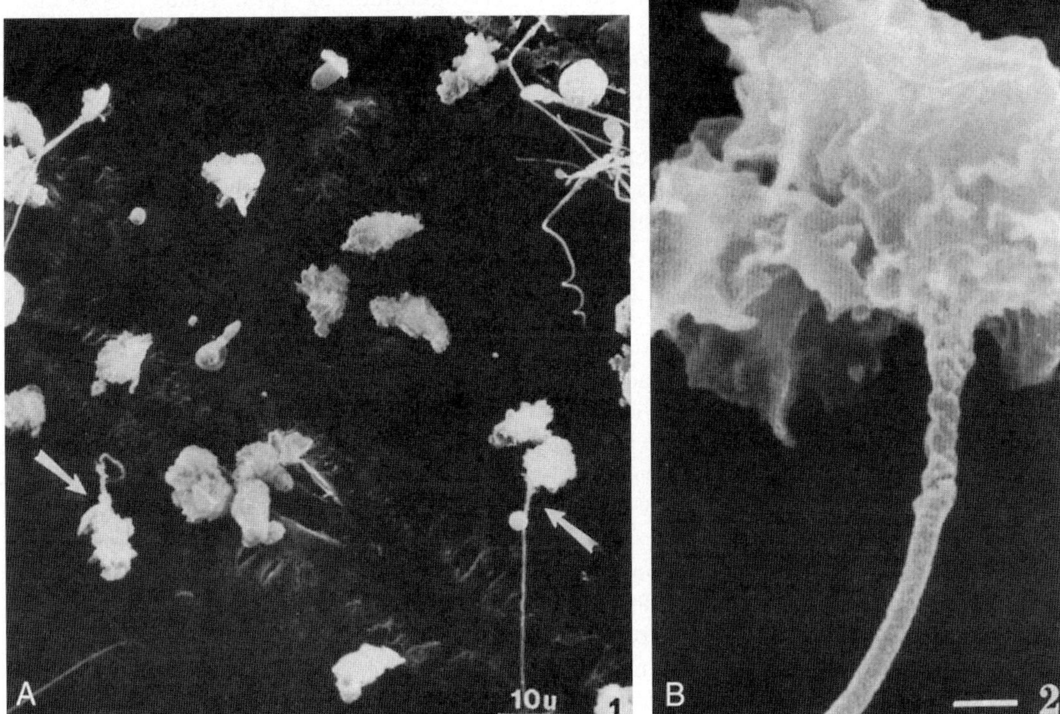


FIGURE 6-5. Scanning electron micrographs of human sperm. (A) Human ejaculate from a patient with unexplained infertility showing massive infiltration of leukocytes. Few "free" sperm are present; most associated with the ruffled white cells. The smooth contoured cells may be immature forms of early spermatid (13,000™). (B) Ruffled leukocyte with a sperm during spermaphagy. (From Koehler JK, et al. Spermaphagy. In: Hafez ESE, Kenemans P, eds. Atlas of Human Reproduction Scanning Electron Microscopy. Lancaster, England: MTP Press, 1982.)

## *Transport in the Oviduct*

The oviduct has the unique function of conveying sperm and eggs in opposite directions almost simultaneously. The pattern and rate of sperm transport through the oviduct are controlled by several mechanisms, such as peristalsis and antiperistalsis of oviductal musculature, complex contractions of the oviductal mucosal folds and the mesosalpinx, fluid currents and countercurrents created by ciliary action, and possibly the opening and closing of the intramural portion. The relative importance of these mechanisms in sperm transport through the oviduct is unknown. Oviductal contractions alter the configuration of the oviductal compartments momentarily, so that fluids and suspended sperm may be transported toward the fimbriae from one compartment to the next. In the oviducts of the pigeon and the tortoise, there are two systems of kinocilia: one beats toward the ovary and the other toward the cloaca. These two ciliary systems are capable of moving particles in opposite directions.

The rate and pattern of sperm transport through the oviduct are attributed to peristalsis and antiperistalsis of musculature and contractions of the mucosal folds and mesosalpinx. The frequency and amplitude of contractions of oviductal circular and longitudinal musculature, mesosalpinx, and mesotubarium are controlled by ovarian hormones, adrenergic and nonadrenergic activity, and such components of seminal plasma as prostaglandin.

The pattern and amplitude of contractions vary in different segments of the oviduct. In the isthmus, peristaltic and antiperistaltic contractions are segmental, vigorous, and almost continuous. In the ampulla, strong peristaltic waves move in a segmental fashion toward the midportion of the oviduct.

## *Endocrine Control of Sperm Transport*

Ovarian hormones affect:

a) the structure, ultrastructure, and secretory activity of the cervical, uterine, and oviductal epithelia;
b) the contractile activity of the uterotubal musculature; and
c) the quantitative and qualitative characteristics of cervical mucus and uterine and oviductal secretions.

Changes are noted in the protein content, enzyme activity, electrolyte composition, surface tension, and conductivity of these fluids. Increasing the amount of endogenous estrogen during the preovulatory phase of the cycle or administering synthetic estrogens produces copious amounts of thin, watery, cervical secretions. Endogenous progesterone during the luteal phase of the cycle or in pregnancy produces scanty, viscous, cellular cervical mucus with low spinnbarkeit and ferning properties. The penetrability of sperm is inhibited greatly in progestational cervical mucus. It is possible that the cycle changes that occur in cervical mucus are mechanisms to protect the female from unnecessary exposure to the foreign proteins of semen (Table 6-3).

### *Hyperactivation of Sperm Motility*

Cumulus cells, by using substances in the culture medium, can provide the ovum with intermediary metabolites for maturation and/or zygote cleavage. Cumulus cells also act as a sperm "reservoir," maintaining many sperm within a close cellular matrix immediately apposing the zona pellucida.

The velocity of sperm and the pattern of sperm motility are altered as the sperm are transported through different segments of the female reproductive tract. Sperm hyperactivation occurs primarily in the oviduct near the time of ovulation and may be instrumental in the final sperm transport, the completion of sperm capacitation, and the acrosome reaction. Sperm are normally retained in the isthmus portion of the oviduct. Biophysical and biochemical properties of the isthmus may impede the upward migration of sperm and facilitate sperm storage. Physical characteristics of the isthmus include narros isthmic lumen, a viscous isthmic mucus, reduced local temperatures, prouterine ciliary beat, and oviductal muscular contractions, which are directed primarily towards the uterus. Physiologic interaction between the sperm and the isthmic environment involves the modulation of sperm motility (Table 6-3).

Active swimming of sperm is readily induced by dilution of the isthmic contents with ampullary fluid or an artificial media. When pyruvate is present in the medium, hyperactivated flagellar bending is stimulated, whereas these movements are virtually absent when glucose alone is present. Alterations in the concentrations of both $K^+$ and pyruvate may have a role in regulating the motility of sperm in the oviductal isthmus, $K^+$ being inhibitory and pyruvate stimulatory (2). When *in vitro* fertilization media are used, immediate vigorous sperm motility is noted and many of the isthmic sperm display hyperactivation. The depression of isthmic sperm motility may be accomplished by the presence of one or more motility inhibitors in the isthmic environment. A similar suppression of sperm movement occurs in the epididymal lumen (2).

The pH of the female reproductive tract fluids varies considerably. The vagina is acidic, around pH 4.0; cervical mucus is basic, pH 8.4, and the uterus is intermediate, pH 7.8. The pH of oviductal fluid is around 7.1 to 7.3 in the follicular phase and 7.5 to 7.8 in the luteal phase. Thus it is important that sperm maintain good motility over a relatively wide range of extracellular pH values.

### *Sperm Transport and Fertility*

The continuous flow of sperm from the cervix is associated with phagocytosis of sperm within the uterus and sperm loss into the peritoneal cavity. Thus, a population of fertile sperm is maintained at the site of fertilization near the ampullary-isthmic junction of the oviduct. The percentage of morphologically normal sperm is higher in the oviducts and uterus than in the ejaculate. Some morphologically abnormal sperm may reach the oviduct, although to a lesser extent than normal sperm. The filtering of dead, abnormal, and incompetent sperm during their passage through the reproductive tract ensures the greatest viability of the zygote.

Head-to-head and tail-to-tail sperm agglutination may occur, causing inhibition in sperm transport (Fig. 6-6). The immunologic significance of sperm agglutination in relation to infertility is not known.

Effect of Estrous Synchronization on Sperm Transport. The survival and transport of sperm in the female reproductive tract generally decrease after any alteration of the estrous cycle. The number of sperm in the oviduct is reduced after regulation of estrus by the administration of progestogen and prostaglandin $F_2$ (Fig. 6-4), which cause regression of the corpora lutea. Regulation of estrus with progestogen or prostaglandin allows only limited numbers of sperm to reach the oviducts, thus causing lowered ovum fertilization rates and low fertility.

Uterine contractions, observed *in vivo* or measured *in vitro*, differ between control ewes and ewes in regulated estrus. Three compounds, when added to semen used for

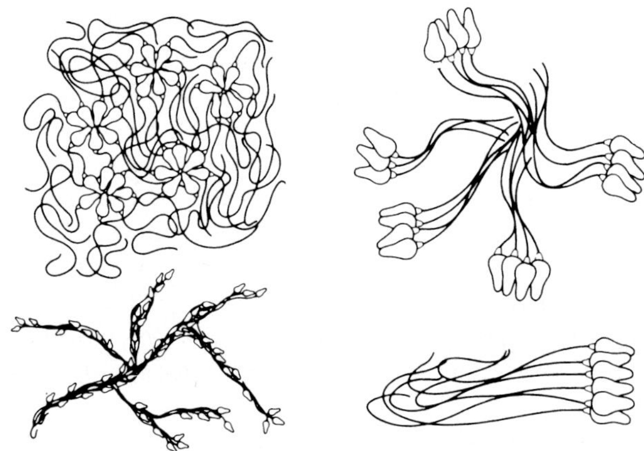

Figure 6-6. Different patterns of head-to-head and tail-to-tail sperm agglutination, a phenomenon that interferes with sperm transport. Little is known about the immunologic significance of sperm agglutination in relation to infertility in farm animals.

TABLE 6-3. ***Sequence of Major Physiologic Phenomena Associated with Sperm Transport in the Male and Female Reproductive Tract***

| | PHYSIOLOGIC PHENOMENA | MECHANISMS INVOLVED |
|---|---|---|
| Reproductive tract | Sperm stored in cauda epididymidis undergo maturation. | Neuromuscular |
| | At ejaculation, sperm released from epididymis mixed with male accessory secretions. | Metabolic |
| Vagina | Semen deposited in several ejaculatory pulsations. | Copulatory motor activities |
| | Semen mixed with vaginal and cervical secretions. | Copulatory motor activities |
| Cervix | Sperm migrate through micelles of cervical mucus. | Biophysical |
| | Cervical crypts establish "sperm reservoir" or rid excessive sperm causing massive reduction in sperm number. | Mechanical (kinocilia of epithelium) |
| Uterus | Sperm separated from seminal plasma transported to oviduct. | Myometrial contraction |
| | Surface plasma of sperm removed. | Agglutination of sperm |
| | Metabolic changes and capacitation of sperm. | Phagocytosis of sperm by leukocytes |
| Uterotubal junction | Quantitative selection of sperm. | Mechanical |
| Isthmus | Sperm numbers reduced. | |
| Ampullary-isthmic junction | Control of egg transport in oviduct. | Neural |
| | Sperm plasma membrane changes (acrosome reaction), sperm capacitation. | Biochemical |
| Ampulla | Sperm motility increases in oviductal fluid to be able to penetrate corona radiata and zona pellucida. | Mechanical |
| | Acrosomal proteinases released. | Enzymatic |
| Fimbriae | Excessive sperm lost into peritoneal cavity. | Sperm motility |

insemination or injected into females near the time of insemination, increase the number of sperm in the oviducts. These compounds include a combination of prostaglandins $E_1$ and $F_2$ for sheep, and estradiol-17$\beta$ for rabbits and sheep (3).

A positive relationship exists between the number of sperm in the oviduct around the time of ovulation and the number of accessory sperm per ovum and the resulting percentage of ova fertilized. The increased fertilization rate is associated with increased numbers of accessory sperm per ovum. Moreover, the number of sperm in the oviduct around the time of ovulation is reduced in hormone-treated ewes when compared with untreated ewes.

### *Survival of Sperm*

Once ejaculation has occurred, sperm have a finite life span. Certain components of the seminal plasma stimulate sperm motility, whereas others inhibit motility. Much information is known about the duration of sperm motility, but little is known about the duration of fertilizing capacity, which is lost long before motility. A relationship exists between the pH of the intravaginal seminal pool and the motility of the sperm.

When migrating into the genital tract, sperm are separated rapidly from the seminal plasma and resuspended in the female genital fluid. In the oviduct, sperm are greatly diluted. Since only a few sperm appear in the oviduct, their survival time is difficult to estimate, and if they remain motile, they migrate into the peritoneal cavity.

During transport to the site of fertilization, sperm are significantly diluted with luminal secretions from the female reproductive trace and are susceptible to changes in the pH of luminal fluids. Acidity or excessive alkalinity of the mucus immobilizes sperm, whereas moderately alkaline mucus enhances their motility.

The cervical mucus secreted at the time of ovulation

provides an environment suited to the maintenance of metabolic activity of sperm. This mucus undergoes biochemical changes, such as a decrease in albumin, alkaline phosphatase, peptidase, antitrypsin, esterase, and sialic acid, as well as an increase in mucins and sodium chloride.

Transport of sperm into the uterus may influence capacitation because the sperm are separated from an excess of "decapacitation factor" and from other enzyme inhibitors in the seminal plasma.

### *Loss of Sperm*

Although millions of sperm are deposited into the reproductive tract of the female, few ever reach the egg at the site of fertilization. Most sperm perish at the selective barriers: uterine cervix, uterotubal junction, and oviductal isthmus. In the uterine cavity, sperm undergo phagocytosis by leukocytes (Fig. 6-5). A continual loss of sperm also occurs in the vaginal and peritoneal cavities.

The introduction of semen into the uterine cavity initiates the leukocytic response: the appearance of polymorphonuclear leukocytes. The biologic relationship between leukocytes and sperm with respect to capacitation and/or sperm survival is not known. In the bovine cervix, the majority of leukocytes occur in the central mass of the mucin, a fact indicating that most of them have invaded the cervix from the uterus. Most viable sperm, lodging in the cervical crypts, escape the leukocytes, so an adequate population of sperm would survive.

Damaged sperm are carried passively back through the ectocervix with the help of ciliated cells beating toward the vagina. Such sperm, advancing only a short distance into the cervical mucus core, do not reach the cervical crypts and greatly decrease in number within a few hours after coitus. Since sperm that become immotile elsewhere are not rapidly eliminated, the ratio of immotile sperm that are being eliminated is higher in the cervix than in other segments of the female reproductive tract. Large amounts of cervical mucus are produced, and numerous sperm are expelled with the mucus through the vulva in cattle. Sperm that reach the fimbriae may be released into the peritoneal cavity.

## RECEPTION OF EGGS (OVA PICKUP)

The viscid mass of cumulus oophorus that contains oocyte and corona cells adheres to the stigma and remains attached to it unless it is removed by the action of the kinocilia of the fimbriae. Ovum transport through the ostium itself and the first few millimeters of the ampulla is effected by the action of the cilia.

The physiologic mechanism by which freshly ovulated eggs are picked up into the oviducts depends on four main factors:

1. The structural characteristics of the fimbriae of the infundibulum and its relationship to the surface of the ovary at the time of ovulation.
2. The pattern of release of the cumulus oophorus and its contained egg from the follicle at the time of ovulation.
3. The biophysical properties of the follicular fluids and the fluids that comprise the matrix of the cumulus oophorus.
4. The coordinated contraction of the fimbriae and the utero-ovarian ligaments.

At the time of ovulation, the fimbriae are engorged with blood and are brought into close contact with the surface of the ovary by the muscular activity of the mesotubarium. The ovary is moved slowly to and from and around its longitudinal axis by contractions of the ligamentum ovarii proprium.

The ovary is located inside the ovarian bursa to which the ampulla of the oviduct and part of the fimbriae are attached. The ovary can move readily from this location to the surface of the fimbriae, which is positioned at the open portion of the ovarian bursa. This movement is controlled by both the *ligamentum ovarii proprium* and the mesovarium, which hold the ovary and oviduct in position.

The contractile activities of the fimbriae, oviduct, and ligaments are partly coordinated by hormonal mechanisms involving the estrogen/progesterone ration. Egg reception is most efficient about the time of estrus, but it occurs to some degree throughout the cycle.

## EGG TRANSPORT IN THE OVIDUCT

The transport time of ova in the oviduct varies with the species (Tables 6-4 and 6-5). In cattle, sheep, and swine, the transport time ranges from 72 to 90 hours (Fig. 6-7). Unfertilized ova are retained in the oviduct of the mare for several months. It is critical that fertilized eggs reach the uterus at an appropriate progestational stage of the estrous cycle.

The rate of egg transport is faster from the infundibulum to the ampullary-isthmic junction than through the isthmic portion. This delay in ovum transport appears to be required for subsequent implantation of the embryo. The time of entry of the ovum into the uterus is relatively precise compared with the movement of the ovum past the ampullary-isthmic junction into the isthmus.

The transport of the egg through the oviduct is regulated by four primary forces:

**TABLE 6-4. *Transport Time of Ova in the Oviduct of Farm Animals Compared with Some Other Mammals***

| SPECIES | TIME IN OVIDUCT (HOURS) |
|---|---|
| Cattle | 90 |
| Sheep | 72 |
| Horse | 98 |
| Pig | 50 |
| Cat | 148 |
| Dog | 168 |
| Monkey, rhesus | 96 |
| Opossum | 24 |
| Woman | 48–72 |

1. The frequency, force, and programming of contraction of oviductal musculature and related ligaments, as influenced by endocrine, pharmacologic, and neural mechanisms.
2. The direction and rate of currents and countercurrents of luminal fluids as affected by the rate and direction of the beat of kinocilia lining the mucosal folds
3. The secretory activity of nonciliated cells in the oviductal epithelium as influenced by the estrogen progesterone ratio
4. The hydrodynamics and rheologic properties of luminal fluids at the critical times that ova are being transported (Fig. 6-8).

**TABLE 6-5. *Patterns of Egg Transport in the Oviduct as Affected by Type of Oviductal Contractility***

| TYPE OF OVIDUCTAL CONTRACTILITY | PATTERN OF EGG TRANSPORT |
|---|---|
| Peristaltic contractions from ampulla to ampullary-isthmic junction | Fast progress of egg |
| Peristaltic contraction from uterotubal junction to ampullary-isthmic junction | Obstruction of egg transport |
| Segmental contraction | Forward/backward shuttling of egg |
| Outbursts of spastic contraction of circular musculature | Complete obstruction of egg transport at a sphincter |
| Contraction of related ligaments causing bending of oviduct | Regulation of rate of egg transport |

### *Oviductal Contraction*

The various patterns of oviductal contraction regulate to some extent the rate of egg transport (Table 6-5). After follicular rupture, the ovum is picked up by the oviductal fimbriated end, which is brought in contact with the ovary by means of myometrium contraction, the smooth muscle of the mesosalpinx, as well as the tubo-ovarian ligaments. After a fast passage of the ovum through the distal ampulla, which takes place in a pattern of to-and-fro movement, the ovum is retained in the proximal part of the ampullary region, near the ampullary-isthmic junction, allowing fertilization to take place (4).

### *"Locking" and "Unlocking" of Ova in Oviduct*

Various mechanisms cause the slow transport of the ova through the isthmus: tubal peristalsis, ciliary activity, and fluid currents and countercurrents within the lumen. The physiologic and pharmacologic mechanisms that regulate oviductal locking/unlocking of ova follow:

1. Mechanical blocking (e.g., edema).
2. Myogenic blocking from
   a) sustained contraction of circular musculature of the isthmus;
   b) contractions regulated by myogenic pacemakers, which are somehow coupled in time and space so that they do not force ova transport prematurely to the uterus;
   c) local or general relaxation of muscle.
3. Neurogenic blocking controls one of the myogenic mechanisms.

### *Gamete Transport and Conception Rate*

The rapid transport of live or dead sperm to the upper oviduct within a matter of minutes infers the importance of smooth muscle contractions in this situation. In natural breeding, sperm are deposited during estrus at least 10 to 12 hours before ovulation, and the rate of sperm transport is unlikely to become a critical factor determining conception. In the case of artificial insemination, particularly when this forms part of an estrous synchronization and/or gonadotropin treatment program, the rate and efficiency of sperm transport to the site of fertilization are of fundamental importance.

The condition of the cervical mucus is critical for successful colonization of the cervix, the latter region providing the principal postcoital reservoir of sperm in ruminants, at

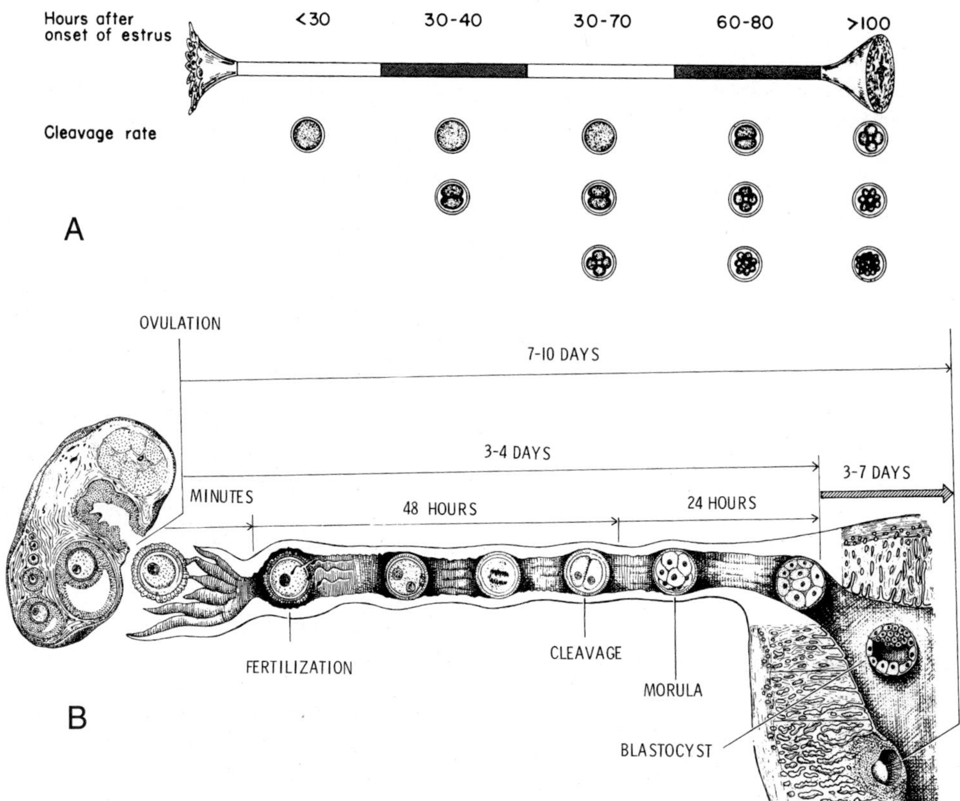


FIGURE 6-7. (A) Rate of transport and cleavage of eggs in swine. Eggs pass through the first half of the oviduct rapidly, and they remain the third quarter, which contains the ampullary-isthmic junction, until 60 to 75 hours after onset of estrus. The eggs enter the uterus between 66 and 90 hours after onset of estrus. (Data from Oxenreider, et al. Anim Sci 1965;24:413.) (B) Temporal relationships of the major reproductive events that take place in the oviduct such as ova pick-up by the fimbriae and fertilization, cleavage and formation of the blastocyst in the uterus.

least during the first 24 hours. Sperm are stored for 2 to 3 days in the endometrial glands and in the folds of the lower isthmus and region of the uterotubal junction. Thus, sperm may be protected from phagocytosis.

Significant numbers of sperm enter the oviducts of estrous cows within 2 hours of mating, although they are found in the ampulla by 8 hours. Only a small fraction of the ejaculate reaches the upper tube. This phenomenon is important to avoid the pathologic condition of polyspermic fertilization.

Thus, the probability of postovulatory aging of the egg before sperm penetration is extremely low under conditions of natural mating. However, if artificial insemination is employed or under systems of controlled breeding, the eggs may deteriorate before sperm reach the ampulla, even though the fertilizable life of the egg is 20 to 24 hours.

An accelerated descent of eggs through the oviduct occurs after superovulation treatment in cattle, although experiments with pregnant mare serum gonadotropin (PMSG) have not produced this particular response. The disturbance of egg transport in laboratory animals under steroid hormone treatment is well-known, so excessive progesterone production or progestogenic treatments shortly after ovulation may produce a similar result in farm animals, leading to temporary infertility.

## FERTILIZABLE LIFE AND AGING OF EGGS

The fertilizable life of the egg is the maximal period during which it remains capable of fertilization and normal development. In most species, the egg is capable of being fertilized for some 12 to 24 hours (Table 6-6). It rapidly loses its fertilizability upon reaching the isthmus and is completely nonfertilizable after reaching the uterus.

The egg may be fertilized near the end of its fertilizable life as a result of delayed breeding. Such eggs may or may not implant and, if so, they produce mostly nonviable embryos. Guinea pigs show a high percentage of abnormal pregnancies and decrease in litter size as the age of the egg increases prior to fertilization (Fig. 6-9). Fertilization of aged eggs in swine is associated with polyspermy and hence abnormal embryonic development. In single-bearing animals, aging

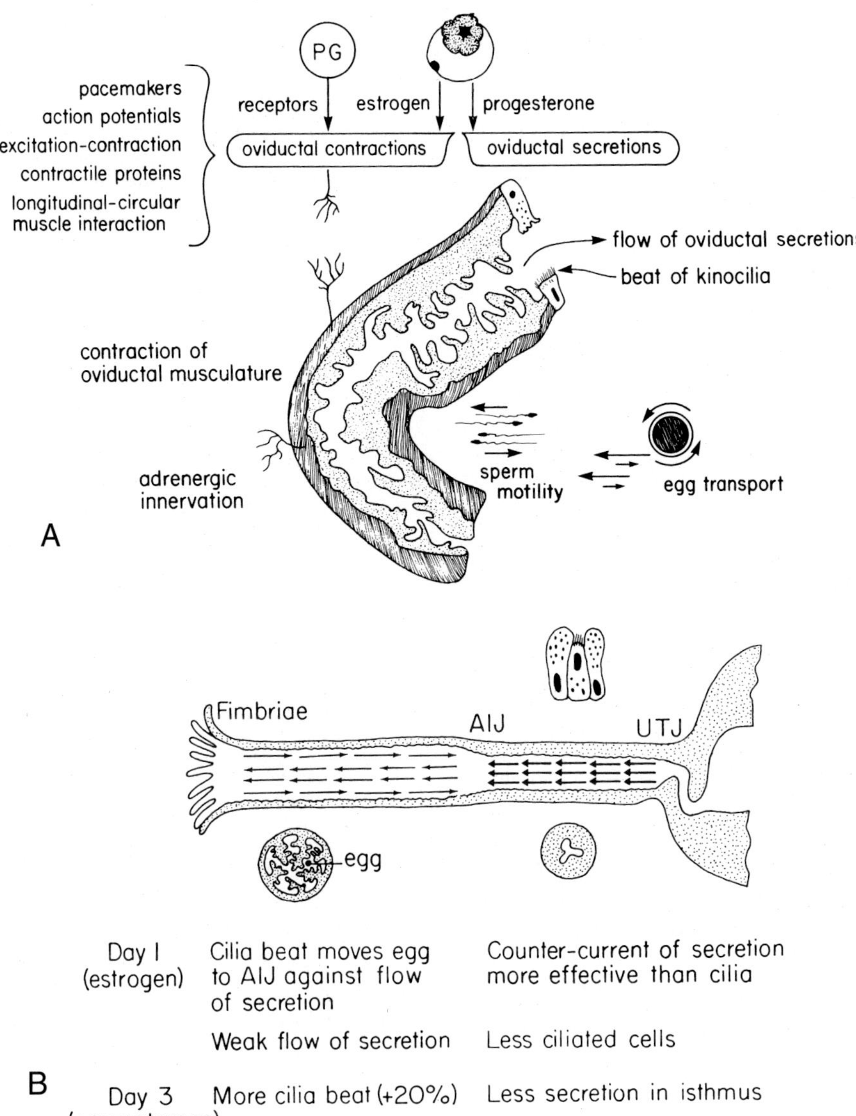


FIGURE 6-8. (**A**) Anatomic and physiologic mechanisms that regulate egg and sperm transport in the oviduct. (**B**) The effect of estrogen and progesterone in the flow of oviductal secretions in the ampulla and isthmus (shown by *arrows* toward the fimbriae), the flow of oviductal cilia (shown by *arrows* toward the uterotubal junction [*UTJ*]), and egg transport in the oviduct. *AIJ*, ampullary-isthmic junction.

of the egg may cause abortion, embryonic resorption, or abnormal development of the embryo. Similar abnormalities may result from aged sperm.

In general, fertilization of aged gametes involves one of the following possibilities:

a) aged egg and aged sperm
b) aged egg and freshly ejaculated sperm
c) freshly ovulated egg and aged sperm

Nonviable embryos resulting from any of the foregoing combinations may cause low conception rates in certain herds and flocks. Fertilization with aged sperm increases subsequent embryonic mortality in swine and poultry. At present there is insufficient evidence in farm mammals concerning the relative deleterious effects of gamete aging in fertilization, implantation, and prenatal development. It is possible that some of the congenital abnormalities in postnatal life are a consequence of aged gametes (Fig. 6-9).

## TRANSUTERINE MIGRATION AND LOSS OF EGGS

Transuterine migration of the egg through the common body of the uterus is common in ungulates. For example, when one of the ovaries is removed from a sow, approximately half of the embryos develop in each uterine horn, irrespective of which ovary was removed. There is also a tendency in the normal sow for the number of embryos to be equalized between the two horns. Transuterine migration is more common in swine and horses than in cattle and sheep. Nonetheless, cattle and sheep that have double ovu-

TABLE 6-6. ***Estimates of the Fertile Life of Sperm and Ova, and the Tempo of Embryonic Development***

| | FERTILE LIFE[a] (HOURS) | | DAYS AFTER OVULATION[b] | | |
|---|---|---|---|---|---|
| SPECIES | *Sperm* | *Ovum* | *8-Cell* | *Into Uterus* | *Blastocyst* |
| Cattle | 30–48 | 20–24 | 3 | 3–3 1/2 | 7–8 |
| Horse | 72–120 | 6–8 | 3 | 4–5 | 6 |
| Human | 28–48 | 6–24 | 2 1/2 | 2–3 | 4 |
| Rabbit | 30–36 | 6–8 | 2 1/2 | 3 | 4 |
| Sheep | 30–48 | 16–24 | 2 1/2 | 3 | 6–7 |
| Swine | 24–72 | 8–10 | 2 1/2 | 2 | 5–6 |

[a]*Fertile life* is a relative concept since fertility declines progressively over a period of hours. For sperm, only the period in the female genital tract is included. The life of ova is timed from ovulation. For both, longevity probably depends on a variety of factors, including the hormonal state of the female.
[b]*These estimates are only approximate since developmental rate is subject to considerable variation both among individuals and among breeds*. In addition, accurate information on the time of ovulation is lacking in several species.

lations from one ovary usually have one embryo in each uterine horn. The physiologic mechanisms that govern the movement of eggs, both within the individual horns and between horns, is unknown.

Transperitoneal migration of eggs can be accomplished by experimental conditions, for example, removal of one ovary leaving the fimbriae and oviduct intact and ligation of the other oviduct. In this case, the remaining oviduct has the ability to pick up the ovum released by the contralateral ovary and a normal pregnancy may follow. Transperitoneal migration may be avoided by currents and surface tension of the peritoneal fluid.

The egg may never reach the infundibulum as a result of many causes. For example, eggs entrapped in the ruptured follicles can be found in the developing corpora lutea. The egg may also be lost into the peritoneal cavity; such an egg usually degenerates but in rare cases may result in ectopic pregnancy (pregnancy located outside the uterus). Egg loss in the peritoneal cavity may be caused by the immobilization of the oviduct as a result of faulty rectal palpation of the ovaries, postpartum or postabortium infections, emdometritis, or nonspecific abdominal infections.

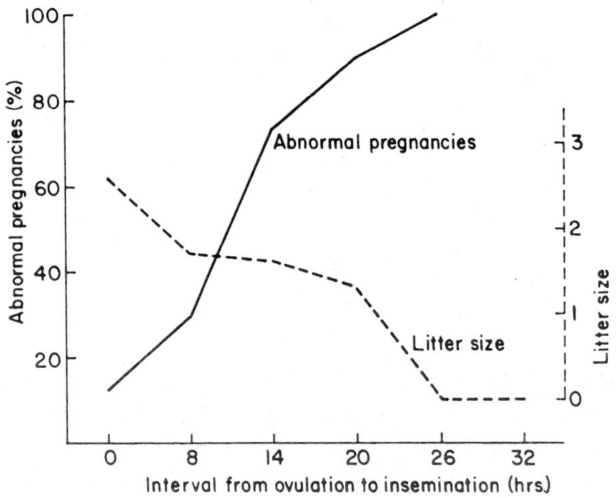


FIGURE 6-9. The effect of aging on ova (delayed insemination) on percentage of abnormal pregnancies and litter size in guinea pigs. The ova were fertilized and implanted when the animals were inseminated at 26 hours after ovulation, yet the embryos did not continue development. (Data from Blandau RJ, et al. Am J Anat 1939;64:303.)

# EMBRYONIC DEVELOPMENT IN OVIDUCT

The oviduct takes an active part in maintaining and preparing the eggs for fertilization and subsequent cleavage. The oviductal fluid is rich in substrates and cofactors involved in ovum development, such as pyruvate and bicarbonate, free amino acids, oxygen, $CO_2$, and carbohydrates, perhaps lipids, nucleosides, steroids, and other compounds. These substances are contributed by the cells of the oviductal mucosa to the luminal fluid milieu.

Endocrine factors are important in the early development of embryos in the oviduct. Eggs at early cleavage stages require specific substances provided by the oviduct for their development. Thus, premature entry of morulae into the uterus will cause their degeneration. After a certain time, the blastocysts need to enter the uterus for final development and implantation.

## REFERENCES


1. Koehler JK, Berger RE, Smith D, Karp L. Spermophagy. In: Hafez ESE, Kenemans P, eds. Atlas of Human Reproduction Scanning Electron Microscopy. Lancaster, England, MTP Press, 1982.
2. Burkham LJ, Overstreet JW, Katz DF. A possible role for potassium and pyruvate in the modulation of sperm motility in the rabbit oviductal isthmus. U Reprod Fertil 1984;71:367–376.
3. Hawk HW, Cooper BS, Conley HH. Increased numbers of sperm in the oviducts and improved fertilization rates in rabbits after administration of phenylephrine or ergonovine near the time of insemination. J Anim Sci 1982;55: 878–890.
4. Aref I, Hafez ESE (1973). Oviductal contractility in relation to egg transport in the rabbit. Obstet Gynecol 1973;42:165.


## SUGGESTED READING


Blandau RJ, Verdugo P. An overview of gamete transport-comparative aspects. In: Harper MJK, Pauerstein CJ, Adams CE, Coutinho EM, Croxatto HB, Paton DM, eds. Ovum Transport and Fertility Regulation. Copenhagen, Scriptor, 1976.

Daunter B, Lutjen, P. Cervical mucus. In: Hafez ESE, Kenemans P, eds. Atlas of Human Reproduction by Scanning Electron Microscopy. Lancaster, England: MTP Press, 1982.

Hawk HW, Cooper BS. Sperm transport in the cervix of the ewe after regulation of estrous prostaglandin or progestogen. J Anim Sci 1977;44:63.

McLaren A. Fertilization and Implantation. In: Hafez ESE, ed. Reproduction of Farm Animals. 4th ed. Philadelphia: Lea & Febiger, 1980.

Pedersen H, Fawcett DW. Functional anatomy of the human spermatozoon. In: Hafez ESE, ed. Human Semen and Fertility Regulation in Men. St. Louis, MO: C.V. Mosby, 1976.

CHAPTER 7

# Spermatozoa and Seminal Plasma

D.L. GARNER AND E.S.E. HAFEZ

## SEMEN

Semen is the liquid cellular suspension containing spermatozoa, the male gametes, and secretions from the accessory organs of the male reproductive tract. The fluid portion of this suspension, which is formed at ejaculation, is known as seminal plasma. A comparison of the seminal characteristics of some farm animals appears in Table 7-1.

## SPERM CELLS

Spermatozoa are formed in the *seminiferous tubules* of the testes. These tubules contain a complex series of developing germ cells that ultimately form the male gametes. Fully-formed spermatozoa are elongated cells consisting of a flattened head containing the nucleus and a tail containing the apparatus necessary for cell motility (Fig. 7-1). The entire spermatozoan is covered by the plasmalemma or plasma membrane. The acrosome or acrosomal cap is a double-walled structure situated between the plasma membrane and the anterior portion of the sperm head. A neck connects the sperm head with its tail (flagellum), which is subdivided into the middle, principal, and end pieces (Fig. 7-1).

### Sperm Morphology

SPERM HEAD. The major feature of the head is the oval, flattened nucleus containing highly compact chromatin (Fig. 7-2). The condensed chromatin is comprised of deoxyribonucleic acid (DNA) complexed to a special class of basic proteins known as sperm *protamines*. The chromosome number and hence the DNA content of the sperm nucleus is haploid or half the DNA of somatic cells of the same species. The haploid sperm cell results from the meiotic cell divisions that occur during sperm formation.

ACROSOME. The anterior end of the sperm nucleus is covered by the acrosome, a thin, double-layered membranous sac that is layered over the nucleus during the last stages of sperm formation (Figs. 7-2 and 7-3). This cap-like structure, which contains acrosin, hyaluronidase, and other hydrololytic enzymes, is involved in the fertilization process. The equatorial segment of the acrosome is important because it is this part of the spermatozoon, along with the anterior portion of the postacrosomal region, which initially fuses with the oocyte membrane during fertilization.

SPERM TAIL. The tail of the male gamete is composed of the neck, middle, principal, and end pieces (Fig. 7-1). The neck or connecting piece forms a basal plate that fits into a depression in the posterior aspect of the nucleus. The basal plate of the neck is continuous posteriorly, with nine outer coarse fibers that project posteriorly throughout most of the tail.

The region of the tail between the neck and the annulus is the middle piece. The central core of the middle piece together with the entire length of the tail comprises the axoneme. The axoneme itself is composed of nine pairs of microtubules that are arranged radially around two central filaments. In the middle piece this 9 + 2 arrangement of microtubules is surrounded by the nine outer coarse or dense fibers that appear to be associated with the nine doublets of the axoneme (Fig. 7-2). The axoneme and associated dense fibers of the middle piece are covered peripherally by numerous mitochondria (Fig. 7-2). The mitochondria are arranged in a helical pattern around the longitudinal fibers of the tail (Fig. 7-2), and are the source of energy needed for sperm motility.

The principal piece, which continues posteriorly from the annulus and extends to near the end of the tail, is

TABLE 7-1. *Characteristics and Chemical Components of Semen from Farm Animals*

| CHARACTERISTIC OF COMPONENT | BULL | RAM | BOAR | STALLION | COCK[a] |
|---|---|---|---|---|---|
| Ejaculate volume (ml) | 5–8 | 0.8–1.2 | 150–200 | 60–100 | 0.2–0.5 |
| Sperm concentration (million/ml) | 800–2000 | 2000–3000 | 200–300 | 150–300 | 3000–7000 |
| Sperm/ejaculate (billion) | 5–15 | 1.6–3.6 | 30–60 | 5–15 | 0.06–3.5 |
| Motile sperm (%) | 40–75 | 60–80 | 50–80 | 40–75 | 60–80 |
| Morphologically normal sperm (%) | 65–95 | 80–95 | 70–90 | 60–90 | 85–90 |
| Protein (g/100 ml) | 6.8 | 5.0 | 3.7 | 1.0 | 1.8–2.8 |
| pH | 6.4–7.8 | 5.9–7.3 | 7.3–7.8 | 7.2–7.8 | 7.2–7.6 |
| Fructose | 460–600 | 250 | 9 | 2 | 4 |
| Sorbitol | 10–140 | 26–170 | 6–18 | 20–60 | 0–10 |
| Citric acid | 620–806 | 110–260 | 173 | 8–53 | nil |
| Inositol | 25–46 | 7–14 | 380–630 | 20–47 | 16–20 |
| Glyceryl phosphoryl choline (GPC) | 100–500 | 1100–2100 | 110–240 | 40–100 | 0–40 |
| Ergothioneine | 0 | 0 | 17 | 40–110 | 0–2 |
| Sodium | 225 ± 13 | 178 ± 11 | 587 | 257 | 352 |
| Potassium | 155 ± 6 | 89 ± 4 | 197 | 103 | 61 |
| Calcium | 40 ± 2 | 6 ± 2 | 6 | 26 | 10 |
| Magnesium | 8 ± 0.3 | 6 ± 0.8 | 5–14 | 9 | 14 |
| Chloride | 174–320 | 86 | 260–430 | 448 | 147 |

Adapted from Lake. In: Bell, Freeman, eds. Physiology and Biochemistry of the Domestic Fowl. New York: Academic Press, 1971; and from Foote, Gilbert, White. In: Hafez ESE, ed. Reproduction in Farm Animals. 4th ed. Philadelphia: Lea & Febiger, 1980.

[a]Mean values of chemical components (mg/100 ml ± S.E.) unless otherwise indicated.

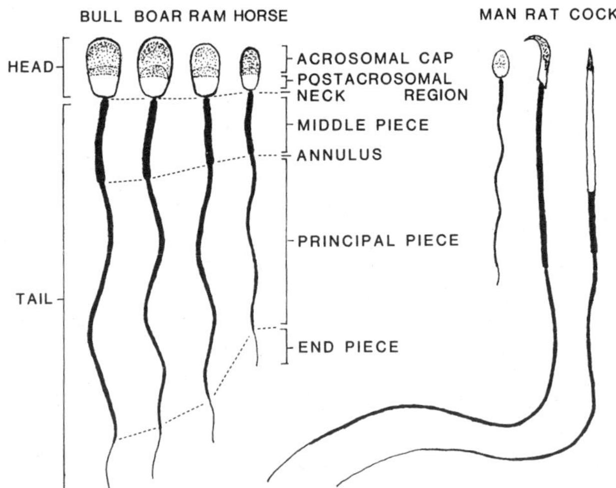


FIGURE 7-1. Comparison of the spermatozoa of farm animals and other vertebrates. The major structural features are given. Note the differences in the relative size and shape.

composed centrally of the axoneme and its associated coarse fibers. A fibrous sheath provides stability for the contractile elements of the tail.

The end piece, which is posterior to the termination of the fibrous sheath, contains only the central axoneme covered by the plasma membrane. The axoneme is responsible for sperm motility. The outer pairs of microtubules of the 9 + 2 pattern generate the bending waves of the tail by a sliding movement between adjacent pairs.

The protoplasmic or cytoplasmic droplet, which is usually detached from ejaculated spermatozoa, is composed of residual cytoplasm. Although considered abnormal for ejaculated spermatozoa from most species, the droplet may be retained either in the neck region, where it is known as a proximal droplet, or near the annulus, where it is called a distal droplet.

## *Chemical Composition of Spermatozoa*

The principal chemical components of spermatozoa are nucleic acids, proteins, and lipids. Nearly one-third of the dry

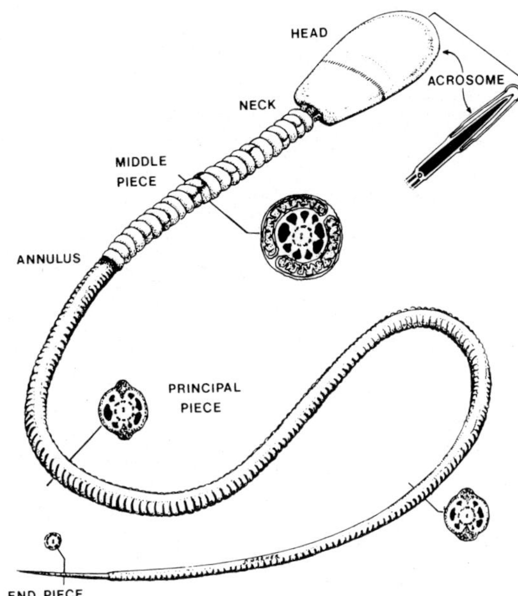


FIGURE 7-2. Features of a bovine spermatozoon without the overlying plasma membrane. The head with its acrosomal cap and the tail with its four anatomical divisions are shown. Cross sections of the middle piece, principal piece (2) and tail piece show the central axonemal core of 9 + 2 microtubules, the nine-coarse outer fibers, the mitochondrial sheath, the dorsal and ventral longitudinal columns, and the circumferential ribs.

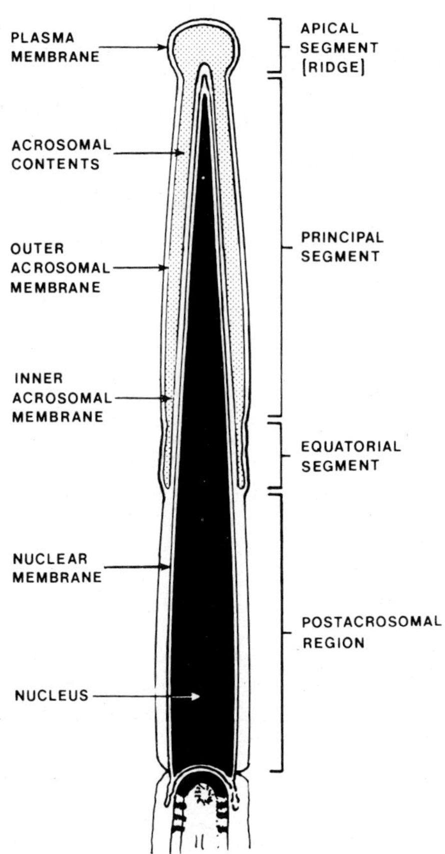


FIGURE 7-3. A sagittal section of a bovine sperm head showing the various anatomical subdivisions. The acrosome includes the apical (apical ridge), the principal, and the equatorial segments. The outer membranes of the apical and principal segments make up what is called the *acrosomal cap*. The relationship of the acrosome, with its inner and outer membranes, to the nuclear and plasma membranes is also shown.

weight of a single sperm cell is contributed by the nucleus. The nuclear chromatin is composed of approximately half DNA and half protein. The acrosomal cap contains a variety of enzymes. Many structural proteins, enzymes, and lipids are found in the tail.

### Inorganic Constituents of Spermatozoa

Spermatozoa are high in phosphorus, nitrogen, and sulfur. Most of the phosphorus is associated with DNA, whereas the sulfur is derived from both basic nuclear proteins and the keratinoid components of the tail.

### Biochemical Components of Spermatozoa

The spermatozoal nucleus is composed of condensed chromatin in which the DNA is stabilized by protamines. Sperm nuclei from most species contain only protamines, whereas spermatozoa from some species contain varying amounts of the larger arginine-rich histones. These basic nuclear proteins, which are important for condensation and stabilization of the DNA, are held together by sulfhydryl bonds. The sulfhydryl bonding increases as the cells pass through the epididymis.

During fertilization the spermatozoon undergoes an acrosome reaction in which most of the contents of the acrosome are released or exposed by openings created by fusion of the plasma and outer acrosomal membranes (Fig. 7-3). The released hyaluronidase disperses the cumulus cells that surround newly ovulated ova. Procrosin is the precursor for the proteolytic enzyme, acrosin, which is thought to assist the penetrating spermatozoon in digesting a pathway through the zona pellucida. The equatorial segment differs from the acrosomal cap in that its contents are not released during the initial acrosome reaction but are exposed when the spermatozoon penetrates the zona pellucida. The spermatozoa, however, may be capable of mechanically penetrating the zona pellucida by means of their own motility.

The mitochondrial sheath of spermatozoa, which is rich in phospholipid, varies greatly among species in the number of mitochondria and in the chemical makeup. Spermatozoa contain enzymes of the cytochrome-cytochrome oxidase respiratory system and the glycolytic pathway. Other metabolic enzymes, including the sperm-specific lactate dehydrogenase known as LDH-X, are also present. The energy-rich adenine and guanine nucleotides are important components in sperm energetics as are the axonemal proteins, tubulin and dynein. Sperm dynein, which is the principal protein in the arms of the axonemal microtubules, has been shown to be a divalent cation-activated ATPase.

### *Sex Chromosomes: X and Y Spermatozoa*

The process of sperm formation in most mammals results in two types of spermatozoa relative to sex chromatin. Mammalian males are *heterogametic* in that one-half of the spermatozoa contain an X-chromosome and the other half a Y-chromosome. Of the two types of gametes produced by mammalian males, spermatozoa carrying the X-chromosome produce female embryos upon fertilization of an oocyte, whereas spermatozoa carrying the Y-chromosome produce male embryos. The males of avian species, however, are *homogametic* in that they produce spermatozoa with only one kind of sex chromosome. Sex determination in birds occurs with the egg.

Although the difference in DNA content between X-chromosome-bearing and Y-chromosome-bearing spermatozoa in domestic livestock is only about 3 to 4%, this small difference can be resolved using fluorescent staining and flow cytometric analyses. Furthermore, flow cytometers have been modified so that they can sort viable mammalian spermatozoa into relatively pure X and Y sperm populations. When these sorted sperm were inseminated into females the sex ratio of the progeny was nearly identical to that predicted by the ratio of X-spermatozoa to Y-spermatozoa in the flow-sorted inseminate. Considerable effort is being focused on developing this approach as a practical means of predetermining the sex of domestic livestock.

## SEMINIFEROUS EPITHELIUM

### *Spermatogenesis: Spermatogonia, Spermatocytes, and Spermatids*

The seminiferous epithelium, lining the seminiferous tubules, is composed of two basic cell types: the Sertoli cells and the developing germ cells. The germ cells undergo a continuous series of cellular divisions and developmental changes, beginning at the periphery and progressing towards the lumen of the tubule (Fig. 7-4). The stem cells, called spermatogonia, divide several times before forming spermatocytes. The spermatocytes then undergo meiosis, thereby reducing the DNA content of the cells to one-half that of somatic cells. This series of cellular divisions, including the proliferation of the spermatogonia and the meiotic divisions, is known as *spermatocytogenesis*. The haploid cells resulting from this process are called spermatids. The spermatids then undergo a progressive series of structural and developmental changes to form spermatozoa. These metamorphic changes are known as *spermiogenesis*. The developing germinal cells are closely associated with the much larger Sertoli cells that surround them during development (Fig. 7-4).

### *Spermatocytogenesis*

During embryonic development, special primordial germ cells migrate from the yolk sac region of the embryo into the undifferentiated gonads. After reaching the fetal gonad, these primordial cells divide several times forming cells called gonocytes. In the male, these gonocytes seem to undergo differentiation before puberty to form the type AO spermatogonia from which the other germ cells originate. The type A1 spermatogonia divide progressively to form type A2, type A3, and type A4 spermatogonia (Fig. 7-5). The type A4 divide again to form intermediate spermatogonia (type In) and then again to form type B spermatogonia. These various types of spermatogonia, which can be identified in histologic sections of the seminiferous epithelium, are the basis for proliferation of the germ cell line.

Some variation exists regarding how spermatogonia are classified, and in certain species, only three rather than four type A spermatogonia are evident. The type A2 cells divide not only to produce the many germinal cells that eventually form sperm, but also a specific division is thought to be used to replace the stem cell population of type A1 spermatogonia. Special reserve stem cells, type AO spermatogonia, replace the stem cell population.

The type B spermatogonia divide at least once and probably twice to form the primary spermatocytes. The primary spermatocytes duplicate their DNA and undergo progressive nuclear changes of meiotic prophase known as preleptotene, leptotene, zygotene, pachytene, and diplotene before dividing to form secondary spermatocyte. Without further DNA synthesis, the resultant secondary spermatocytes divide again to form the haploid cells known as spermatids. The entire divisional process of spermatocytogenesis, from spermatogonia to spermatid, takes approximately 45 days in the bull. These divisions are, however, incomplete in that small cytoplasmic or intercellular bridges are retained between a series or "clone" of developing germ cells. These bridges are thought to be important in coordinating simultaneous development of germ cells as a group.

### *Spermiogenesis*

The round spermatids are transformed into spermatozoa by a series of progressive morphologic changes collectively known as spermiogenesis. These changes include condensation of the nuclear chromatin, formation of the sperm tail or flagellar apparatus, and development of the acrosomal cap (Fig. 7-5). The various developmental stages of spermatid transformation are divided into four phases: the Golgi, cap, acrosomal, and maturation phases.

GOLGI PHASE. The Golgi phase of spermiogenesis is characterized by formation of proacrosomal granules within the Golgi apparatus, the coalescence of the granules into a single acrosomal granule, the adherence of the resultant

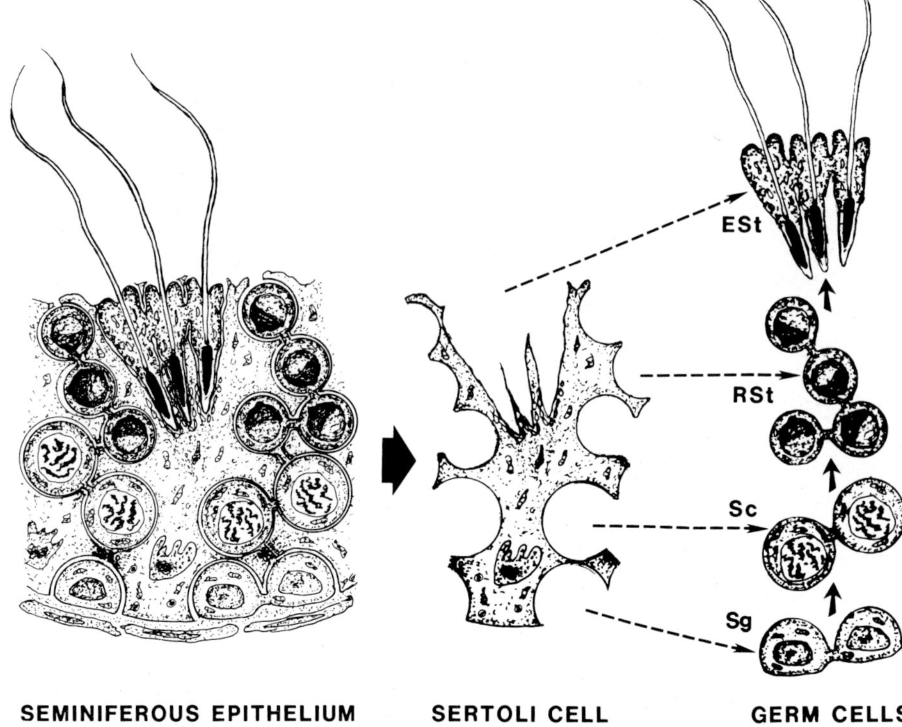


FIGURE 7-4. The seminiferous epithelium showing the complex nature of the association between Sertoli cells and the developing germ cells along with an illustration depicting dissociation of this cellular complex. The developing germ cells occupy intracellular spaces between adjacent Sertoli cells and move from the basement membrane toward the lumen during spermatogenic process. The germ cells begin their developmental process as spermatogonia (*Sg*), become spermatocytes (*Sc*), then round spermatids (*RSt*) and finally elongated spermatids (*ESt*). Schematic dissociation of the seminiferous epithelium shows how the germ cells occupy the expanded intercellular spaces between adjacent Sertoli cells. (Adapted from Fawcett DW. In: Mancini RE, Martini L, eds. Male Fertility and Sterility. New York: Academic Press, 1974.)

acrosomal granule to the nuclear envelope, and the early stages of tail development at the pole opposite that of the adherence of the acrosomal granule (Fig. 7-5, steps 1–3). The proximal centriole migrates closest to the nucleus where it is thought to form a basis for attachment of the tail to the head.

CAP PHASE. The cap phase is characterized by a spreading of the adherent acrosomal granule over the surface of the spermatid nucleus (Fig. 7-5, steps 4–7). This process continues until nearly two-thirds of the anterior portion of each spermatid nucleus is covered by a thin, double-layered membranous sac that closely adheres to the nuclear envelope. During this cap phase, the developing axonemal components of the tail, which are formed from elements of the distal centriole, elongate well beyond the periphery of the cellular cytoplasm. During the early development, the axoneme closely resembles the structure of a cilium in that it consists of two central tubules surrounded peripherally by nine pairs of tubules.

ACROSOMAL PHASE. The acrosomal phase of spermiogenesis is characterized by major changes in the nuclei, the acrosomes, and the tails of the developing spermatids. The developmental changes are facilitated by rotation of each spermatid so that the acrosome is directed toward the basement or outer wall of the seminiferous tubule and the tail toward the lumen (Fig. 7-5, steps 8–12). The nuclear changes include condensation of the chromatin into dense granules and reshaping of the spheroidal nucleus into an elongated, flattened structure. At this point in development, the nuclear histones are progressively replaced by transitional proteins. The acrosome, which is closely adherent to the nucleus, also condenses and elongates to correspond to the shape of the nucleus. These modifications in nuclear and acrosomal shape appear to be "molded" by the surrounding Sertoli cells. The morphologic changes are slightly different for each species and thus result in elongated spermatids and resultant spermatozoa that are characteristic for each species.

The changes in nuclear morphology are accompanied by displacement of the cytoplasm to the caudal aspect of the nucleus where it surrounds the proximal portion of the developing tail. Within this cytoplasm, microtubules associate to form a temporary cylindrical sheath called the manchette, which projects posteriorly from the caudal border of the acrosome where it loosely surrounds the axoneme. Within the cylindrical manchette, a specialized cytoplasmic structure called the chromatoid body condenses around the axoneme to form the ring-like structure known as the annulus. The annulus first forms near the proximal centriole and then during subsequent development migrates posteriorly along the tail. The mitochondria, which were previously distributed throughout the cytoplasm of the spermatid, begin to concentrate close to the axoneme where they form the sheath that characterizes the middle piece of the tail.

MATURATION PHASE. The maturation phase of spermiogenesis involves final transformation of the elongated

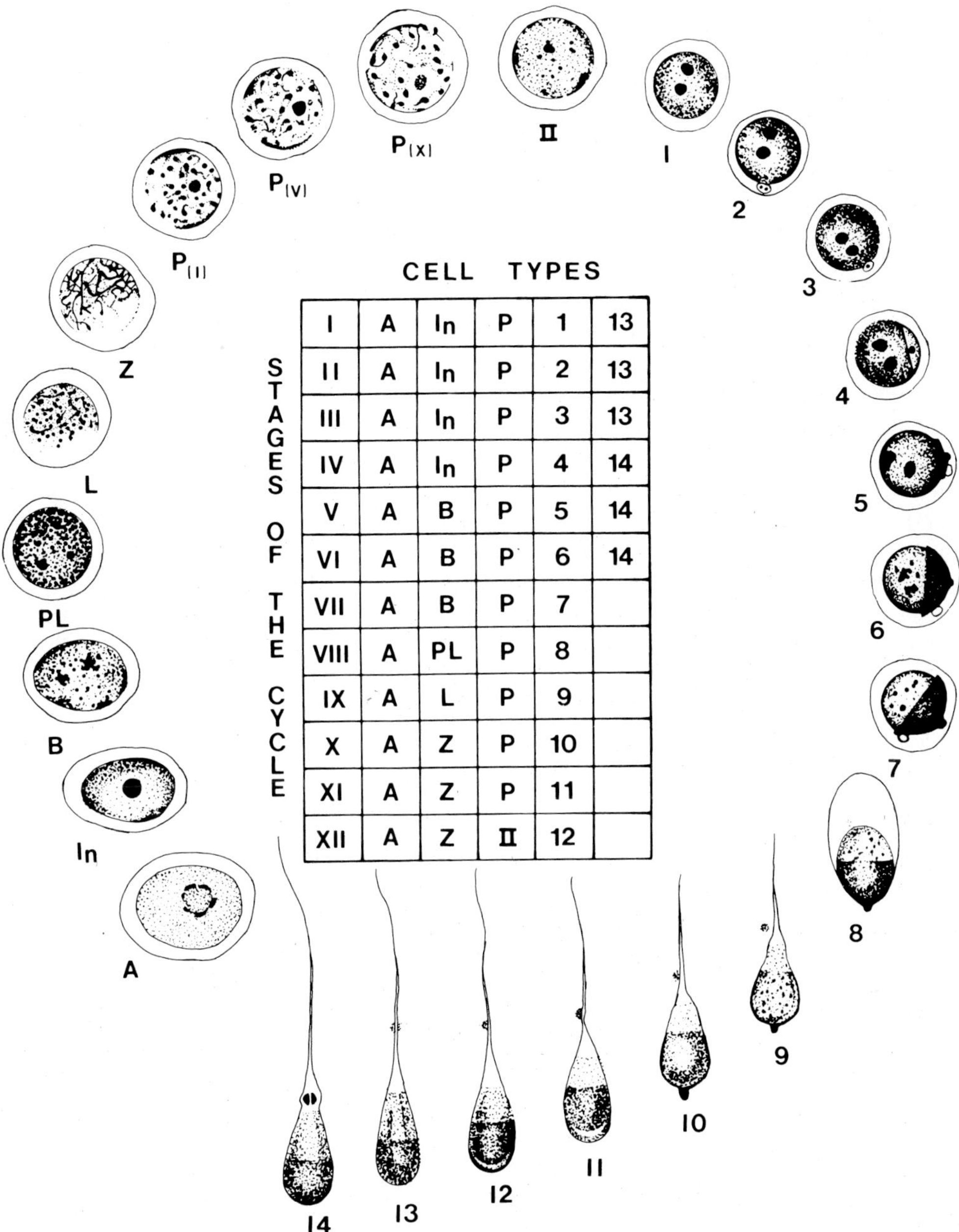

| STAGES OF THE CYCLE | CELL TYPES | | | | |
|---|---|---|---|---|---|
| I | A | In | P | 1 | 13 |
| II | A | In | P | 2 | 13 |
| III | A | In | P | 3 | 13 |
| IV | A | In | P | 4 | 14 |
| V | A | B | P | 5 | 14 |
| VI | A | B | P | 6 | 14 |
| VII | A | B | P | 7 | |
| VIII | A | PL | P | 8 | |
| IX | A | L | P | 9 | |
| X | A | Z | P | 10 | |
| XI | A | Z | P | 11 | |
| XII | A | Z | II | 12 | |



FIGURE 7-5. The various steps in spermatogenesis in the bull beginning with a type A spermatogonium. The table in the center indicates the particular cellular association of the 12 stages of the cycle of the seminiferous epithelium. The various cell types are: A, *I*, *B*, successive stages of spermatogonia, *PL*, preleptotene spermatocyte; *L*, leptotene spermatocyte; *Z*, zygotene spermatocyte; *P*, pachytene spermatocytes from stages I, V, and X; *II*, secondary spermatocyte; 1 through 14 are steps of spermiogenesis showing the Golgi phase (steps 1 to 3), the cap phase (steps 4 to 7), the acrosome phase (steps 8 to 12) and the maturation phase (steps 13 and 14). (Adapted from Berndtson WE, Desjardins C. Am J Anat 1974;140:167–180.)

spermatids into cells to be released into the lumen of the seminiferous tubule. The reshaping of the nucleus and acrosome of each spermatid, initiated during the previous phase, produces spermatozoa characteristic for each species. Within the nucleus, the chromatin granules undergo progressive condensation as the transitional proteins are replaced by protamines as they form a fine homogeneous material that uniformly fills the entire sperm nucleus (Fig. 7-5, steps 13–14).

During the maturation phase a fibrous sheath and the underlying nine coarse fibers are formed around the axoneme. The coarse fibers appear to be associated individually with the nine pairs of microtubules of the axoneme and are continuous with columns in the neck of the connecting piece of the spermatid. The fibrous sheath covers the axoneme from the neck to the beginning of the end piece. The annulus migrates distally from its position adjacent to the nucleus along the tail to a point where it will subsequently separate the middle piece from the principal piece of the tail. The mitochondria become tightly packed into a continuous sheath extending from the neck to the annulus.

During the later stages of spermiogenesis, the manchette disappears and the Sertoli cell then shapes the cytoplasm remaining after elongation of the spermatid into a spheroidal lobule called the residual body. This lobule of cytoplasm, which remains connected to the elongated spermatid by a slender thread of cytoplasm, is also interconnected with other residual bodies by intercellular bridges that resulted from the incomplete division of the germ cells during spermatocytogenesis (Fig. 7-5). Formation of the residual body completes the final maturation, and the elongated spermatids are ready for release as spermatozoa.

### *Spermiation*

The release of formed germ cells into the lumen of the seminiferous tubules is known as spermiation. The elongated spermatids, which are oriented perpendicularly to the tubular wall, are gradually extruded into the lumen of the tubule. The lobules of residual cytoplasm through which groups of spermatids are connected by intercellular bridges remain embedded in the epithelium. Extrusion of the spermatozoal components continues until only a slender stalk of cytoplasm connects the neck of the spermatid to the residual body. Breakage of the stalk results in formation of the cytoplasmic droplet in the neck region of the released spermatozoa (proximal droplet) and retention of the interconnected residual bodies. Following release of the spermatozoa, the residual bodies are phagocytized by the Sertoli cells to recycle the protoplasmic components. Not only do the Sertoli cells phagocytize the residual bodies remaining from the spermatogenic process, but these cells must also remove considerable numbers of degeneration germ cells. Because the spermatogenic process is relatively inefficient, large numbers of potential sperm degenerate before becoming spermatozoa.

### *Duration of Spermatogenesis*

The various cell types within any cross section of the seminiferous epithelium form well-defined cellular associations that undergo cyclic changes. As many as 14 distinct cellular associations or stages are identifiable in some species, whereas only 6 stages are identifiable in man. In the bull, as many as 12 stages of this cycle have been described (Fig. 7-5). A complete, time-dependent cycle of the stages known as the cycle of the seminiferous epithelium is defined as "a series of changes in a given area of seminiferous epithelium between two appearances of the cellular association or developmental stages." The steps in spermiogenesis are used to classify the various stages of the cycle. The time necessary to complete a cycle of the seminiferous epithelium varies among domestic species. Duration of the cycle is about 9 days in the boar, 10 days in the ram, 12 days in the horse, and 14 days in the bull. Depending on the species, four to nearly five epithelial cycles are required before the type A spermatogonia from the first cycle have completed the metamorphosis of spermiogenesis. Each epithelial cycle is analogous to a student attending college (e.g., freshman, sophomore, junior, or senior) in that it takes four or more cycles or "years" before a spermatogonial stem cell or "incoming freshman" has completed the process of spermatogenesis or "finished the senior year" (Fig. 7-6). Spermiation, which can be thought of as "graduation," occurs for the three previous cycles or classes before the stem cell completes the developmental process to become spermatozoa or "the incoming freshman completes the four-year curriculum." The relative time that it takes each cell to go through a particular phase of the spermatogenic cycle differs greatly. Although differences in the rate of spermatogenesis exist among mammalian species, the process is uniform within a species.

### *Spermatogenic Wave*

The stages of the cycle of the seminiferous epithelium change not only with time, but also along the length of the tubular loop (Fig. 7-7). A portion of tubule at one stage is usually adjacent to portions of tubule in stages just preceding or following it in time (Fig. 7-8). This sequential change in stage of cycle along the length of the tubule is known as the wave of the seminiferous epithelium. Examination of a loop of seminiferous tubule along its length also reveals that the wave involves a sequence of stages beginning with the less advanced stages in the middle of the loop to progressively more advanced stages nearer the rete testis. Certain irregularities or breaks in the sequential order are noted. Such breaks in sequence, called modulations, occur occasionally but involve relatively short lengths of tubule.

## BLOOD-TESTIS BARRIER

### *Cellular Junctions*

The seminiferous tubules are not penetrated by blood or lymph vessels. In addition, the developing germ cells within the tubules are protected from chemical changes in the blood by a specialized permeability barrier. This blood-testis barrier has two principal components: (a) the incomplete or partial barrier of the myoid cells that surround the tubule and (b) the unique junctions between adjacent Sertoli cells.

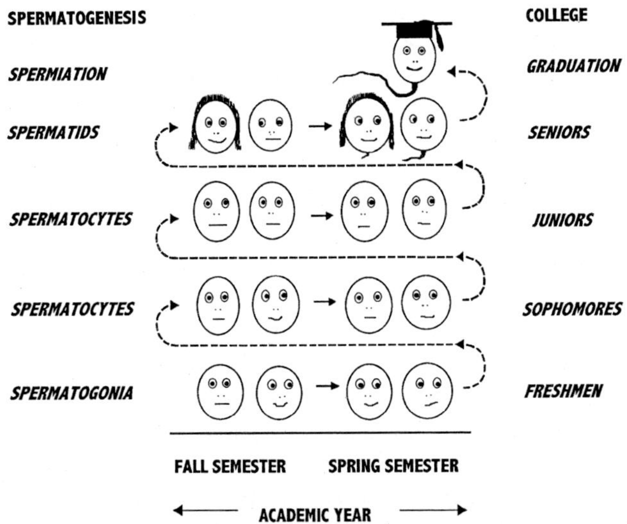


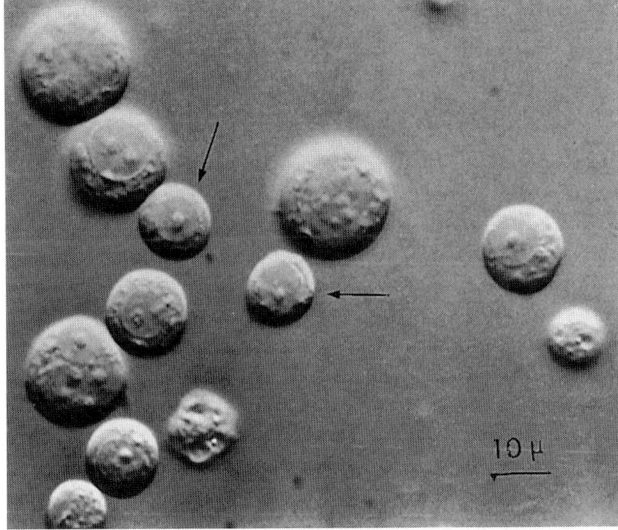


Figure 7-6. (*Top*) The journey of spermatogonial stem cells through the process of forming spermatozoa within the seminiferous tubule is analogous to students attending college (e.g., freshman, sophomore, junior, or senior). This illustration shows that it takes four or more cycles, or "years," before a spermatogonial stem cell, or "incoming freshman," has completed the process of spermatogenesis, or "finished the senior year." The release of spermatozoa from the Sertoli cells, which is termed spermiation, can be thought of as "graduation." This process occurs sequentially for the three previous cycles or classes before the stem cell completes the developmental process to become a spermatozoon, or "the incoming freshman student completes the four-year curriculum as a college graduate." The analogy breaks down by the fact that the stem cells divide many times during the spermatogonial and primary spermatocyte stages resulting in more than a hundred fully-formed sperm or graduating seniors. (Adapted from Johnson L. In: Cupps PT, ed. Reproduction in Domestic Animals. 4th ed. San Diego: Academic Press, 1991.) (*Bottom*) Isolated spermatogonial cells.

Myoid Layer. The basement membrane or tunica propria that surrounds the seminiferous tubules contains a layer of contractile myoid cells (Fig. 7-9). In some species a majority of the cell junctions of this layer are sealed by tight

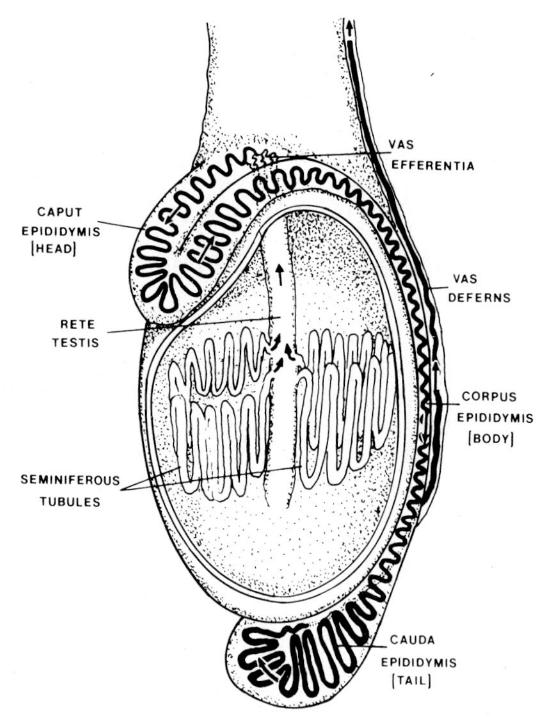


Figure 7-7. Loops of the seminiferous tubules, the rete testis, and the excurrent duct system of the ram. The pathway by which spermatozoa are transported to the exterior is indicated by arrows. (Modified from Setchell BP. In: Cole HH, Cupps PT, eds. Reproduction in Domestic Animals. New York: Academic Press, 1977.)

apposition of the adjacent cell membranes. This barrier, however, is not well developed in the bull, ram, or boar and may be a relatively unimportant permeability barrier in the testis of farm animals.

Sertoli Cell Junctions. The principal permeability barrier between the blood and testis is thought to be the complexes at junctions between adjacent Sertoli cells. These Sertoli-Sertoli junctions, which are situated near the cellular base, contain multiple zones of adhesion (tight junctions) where the opposing membranes are fused. The occluding junctions divide the seminiferous tubules into two distinct compartments: (1) a basal compartment containing spermatogonia and preleptotene spermatocytes and (2) an adluminal compartment, containing the more advanced stages of spermatocytes and spermatids, which freely communicates with the lumen of the tubule.

The basal compartment is freely accessible to components that have previously penetrated the myoid layer. The second barrier, composed of the occluding junctions between Sertoli cells, demonstrates a wide range of permeability from complete exclusion of some substances to nearly free transfer of others. This differential permeability appears to be important in maintaining an environment suitable for the spermatogenic function of the tubules. The blood-testis barrier not only excludes entry of certain substances

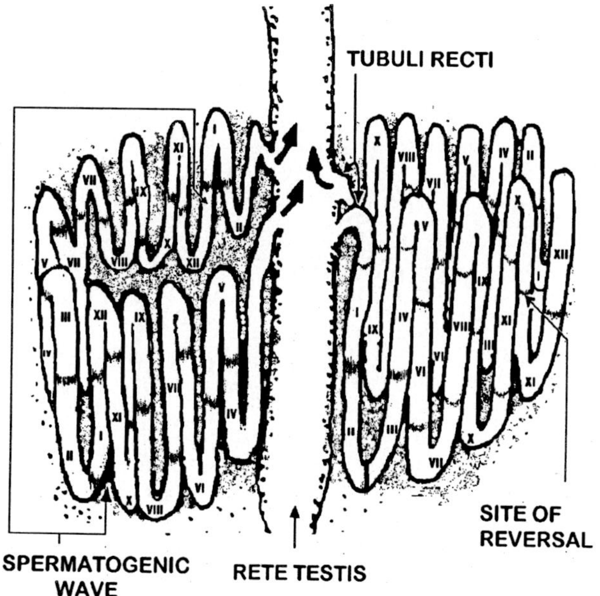


Figure 7-8. A seminiferous tubule in which the wave of the seminiferous epithelium is schematically represented along the length of the tubule. The succession of stages I to XII, the site of reversal in the middle of the tubule and the relationship of the wave to the rete testis are shown. The more advanced stages of each wave are located nearer the rete testis. An actual seminiferous tubule may contain 15 or more complete spermatogenic waves. (Adapted from Perey B, Clermont Y, Leblond CP. The wave of the seminiferous epithelium in the rat. Am J Anat 1961;108:47–77.)

but also appears to function in retaining specific levels of other substances, such as androgen-binding protein (ABP), inhibin, and enzyme inhibitors, within the luminal compartments of the tubules.

### *Fluid Secretions*

The spermatids produced during the final phase of spermiogenesis are released during spermiation into the lumen of the seminiferous tubules as immature spermatozoa. These sperm cells, which are immotile, are swept from the tubules by fluid secretions originating from the Sertoli cells. Transit into the epididymis is aided by secretions from the rete testis, by the contractile elements of the testis (e.g., myoid cells and testicular capsule), and by the cilia lining the efferent ducts.

Testicular fluid is a composite secretion of both the Sertoli cells and the epithelial cells lining the rete testis (Fig. 7-9). The Sertoli cells, however, are thought to be the predominant source of fluid leaving the testis. Fluid secretion from Sertoli cells is thought to occur because active transport processes push solutes into the adluminal compartment, thereby forming an osmotic gradient. This fluid contains several unique proteins including ABP, which is secreted into the lumen of the seminiferous tubule by the Sertoli cells. The ABP forms a complex with the androgens produced by the Leydig cells. The resultant complex assists transit of androgen into the caput epididymis.

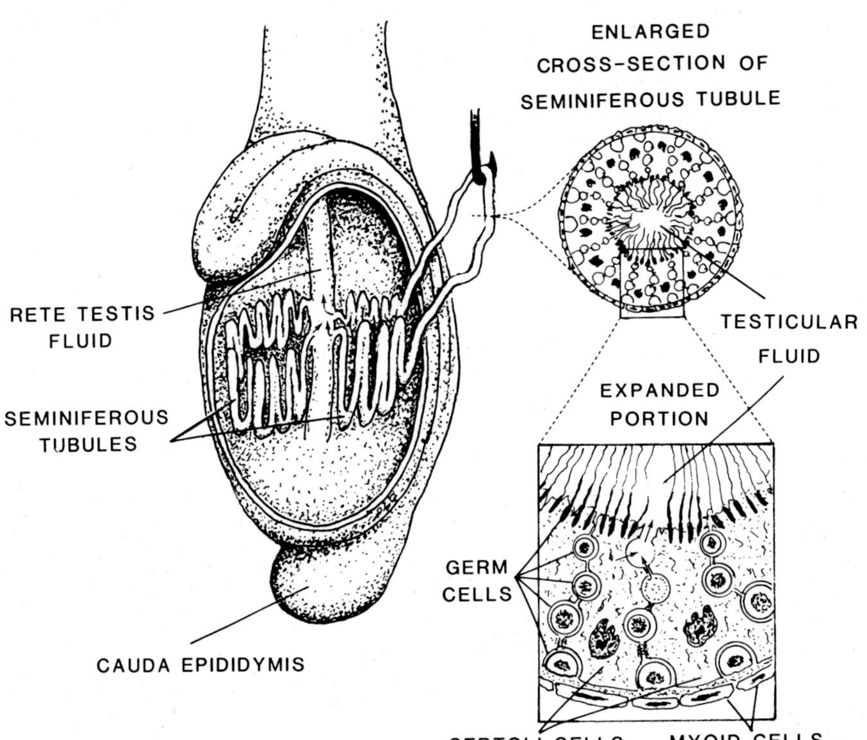


Figure 7-9. Source of testicular and rete testis fluid. These fluids become mixed in the rete testis and are excreted into the excurrent duct system of the male. Testicular fluid is secreted by the Sertoli cells into the lumen of the tubule. One seminiferous tubule has been pulled from the testis and enlarged and expanded in cross section to show the microanatomy of the seminiferous epithelium.

## *Endocrine Control of Spermatogenesis*

Normal testicular function requires hormonal stimulation by pituitary *gonadotrophins*, which are in turn controlled by pulsatile secretion gonadotrophin-releasing hormone (GnRH) from the hypothalamus (Fig. 7-10). Restoration of spermatogenesis can be achieved in the hypophysectomized rat by treatment with both FSH and LH or with FSH and testosterone, indicating that pituitary support is essential because hypophysectomy, surgical removal of the pituitary, results in cessation of spermatogenesis. High doses of testosterone alone, however, will maintain spermatogenesis in hypophysectomized rats, provided treatment begins immediately after removal of the pituitary. Other species, however, require FSH in addition to the steroid for maintenance of spermatogenesis. Other pituitary hormones (e.g., prolactin, growth hormone, and thyroid-stimulating hormone) may have secondary roles in support of testicular function.

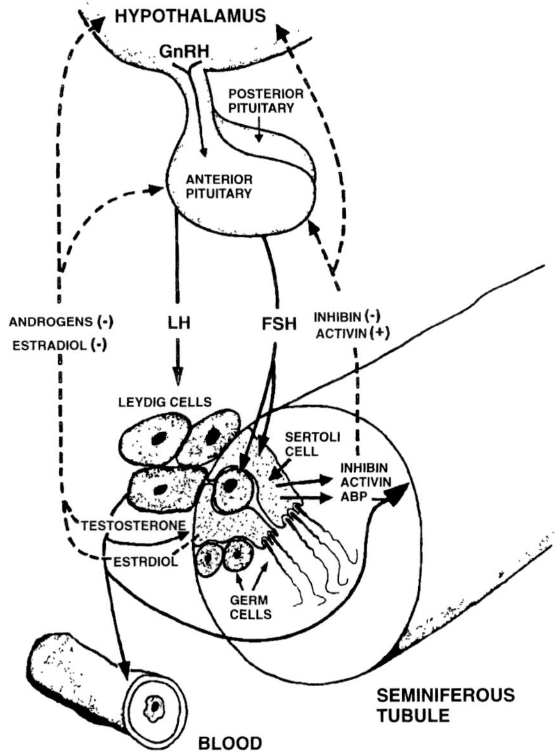


FIGURE 7-10. The endocrine control of testicular function in mammals. The hypothalamus secretes gonadotropin, a hormone-releasing hormone (GnRH), that stimulates the secretion of LH and FSH from the anterior pituitary. The LH stimulates the interstitial cells of Leydig to produce androgens, mainly testosterone. The androgens are secreted into the bloodstream where they cause the development of secondary sex characteristics of the male and development and maintenance of the male reproductive tract. The androgens suppress GnRH, LH, and FSH secretion by negative feedback on the pituitary and hypothalamus. Testosterone is also secreted into the seminiferous tubule where it is necessary for maintenance of spermatogenesis. The FSH interacts with receptors on the Sertoli cells to cause production of androgen-binding protein (ABP), conversion of testosterone to dihydrotestosterone and estrogen, stimulation of the spermatocytogenesis, completion of sperm release (spermiation) and secretion of inhibin. The inhibin secreted into the bloodstream has a negative feedback effect on FSH but not on LH secretion. (From Kaltenback CC, Dunn TG. Endocrinology of reproduction. In: Hafez ESE. Reproduction in Farm Animals. 4th ed. Philadelphia: Lea & Febiger, 1980.)

The testes not only produce the major *androgen*, testosterone, but also a series of related steroid hormones. The major action of androgens is on the Sertoli cells rather than directly on the germ cells. The myoid cells also appear to be androgen dependent. This steroid dependency is met by pulsatile production of androgens by the interstitial Leydig cells, which are adjacent to the seminiferous tubules (Fig. 7-10). The Leydig cells are stimulated to secrete androgens by pulses of pituitary LH. The androgens produced by the Leydig cells not only diffuse into the adjacent Sertoli cells but are secreted into the blood where they feed back both at the hypothalamus and the pituitary to block release of additional LH (Fig. 7-10). The other principal gonadotrophin, FSH, stimulates production of ABP and inhibin by the Sertoli cells. ABP forms a complex with androgen and is carried along with the spermatozoa into the epididymis. The epithelial cells of the epididymis require relatively high levels of androgen for normal function. Inhibin has a negative feedback effect on FSH secretion but not on LH. Although much of the testosterone secreted into the seminiferous tubules is converted into *dihydrotestosterone* (DHT) by the enzyme, 5$\alpha$-steroid reductase, some of the testosterone is converted to estrogens by the enzyme *aromatase*. A relatively high level of testosterone is required for spermatid maturation.

Sertoli and germ cells reciprocally regulate each other's cyclic secretion of proteins along the length of the seminiferous tubles. This process is amplified by the myoid cells through transforming growth factors, humoral modulators, and extracellular matrix modification. *Activin* and *inhibin*, which are secreted by the Sertoli cells, have remarkable characteristics to generate a diverse series of signals. Activins, potent FSH-releasing dimers (dimers of inhibin $\beta$-subunits), have paracrine (inhibiting growth hormone and adrenocorticotropin secretion), and autocrine (stimulating FSH secretion) mechanisms. Activin and inhibin also act within the gonads as autocrine and paracrine modulators of the production of steroids, other hormones, and growth factors. Transforming growth factor (TGF), a multifunctional peptide induced in response to steroids, may be involved with regulation of testicular function. Two groups of compounds are involved with regulation of the hypothalamo-pituitary-gonadal axis. These include (a) neurotransmitters, dopamine, serotonin, and norepinephrine and (b) brain opioids and other peptides. Other physiological modulators of cell proliferation such as chalones influence the cell cycle of the seminiferous epithelium.

## EPIDIDYMAL TRANSIT, SPERM MATURATION AND STORAGE

Testicular spermatozoa are transported from the testis through a highly convoluted duct known as the *epididymis* (Fig. 7-7). The epididymis not only transports spermatozoa distally from the testis into the vas deferens but during this transit the spermatozoa also undergo a maturation process in which they gain the potential ability to fertilize ova. This maturation involves several functional changes, including development of the *potential* for sustained motility, progressive loss of water and distal migration, and eventual loss of the cytoplasmic droplet. The functional capabilities of the various epithelial cells lining the epididymis, and, hence, their influence on the sperm maturation process, are maintained by testicular androgens.

### *Transport Mechanisms*

The passage of spermatozoa through the epididymis depends on localized contractions of the duct wall at a frequency of about three per minute. Spermatozoa are transported through the epididymis in about 7 days in the bull, 12 days in the boar and 16 days in the ram. The transit time may be reduced by 10 to 20% by an increased frequency of ejaculation. The contractile elements of the epididymal wall show regional differences in that the content of smooth muscle cells increases progressively from the tail of the epididymis to the vas deferens.

### *Maturation and Storage of Spermatozoa*

The functional changes occurring during epididymal transit of spermatozoa involve maturation of cell organelles. For instance, the development of the capacity for sperm motility reflects both qualitative and quantitative changes in the metabolic patterns of the flagellar apparatus. Although mature epididymal spermatozoa are relatively quiescent within the epididymis, they rapidly demonstrate motility upon removal and examination. The maturation process in which epididymal spermatozoa attain the capacity for progressive motility involves progressive changes in the flexibility and patterns of movement of their flagella. Rapid forward progression appears first in the middle of the corpus epididymis in a few spermatozoa and becomes the predominating motility pattern in spermatozoa from the cauda and vas deferens.

Secretory components of epithelial cells lining the epididymis, such as "immobilin" in some laboratory animals and "quiescence factor" in the bull, probably prolong sperm survival by preventing unnecessary metabolism. Forward motility protein appears to be important to the attainment of progressive motility in bovine epididymal spermatozoa.

Transit through the epididymis is associated with significant changes within the chromatin of the sperm nucleus. This DNA-protein complex, which was once thought to be relatively inert following its condensation during the latter phases of spermiogenesis, undergoes an additional compaction during the epididymal transit.

During epididymal transit, the droplet migrates from the neck region to a position near the annulus. Presence of the droplet on a significant number of ejaculated spermatozoa is a sign of immaturity. Also, changes associated with maturation of the acrosome have been noted in most species during epididymal passage. Although marked changes occur in some species, those occurring in farm animals are limited to a rather subtle reduction in the dimensions of the acrosome.

### *Development of Fertilizing Potential in the Epididymis*

Spermatozoa develop their initial ability to fertilize ova during their transport through the epididymis. Their fertilizing capacity is considered potential since they must undergo capacitation before they can penetrate ova. Testicular spermatozoa are infertile even when inseminated in relatively large numbers. The lack of fertility of caput epididymal spermatozoa may be related to motility. Spermatozoa from the caput epididymis possess active circular swimming movement, but yet are incapable of the vigorous unidirectional movement of spermatozoa possessing the ability to undergo longitudinal rotation. Changes occurring during epididymal transport such as droplet movement and loss, and the increase in specific gravity are difficult to interpret from a functional standpoint. The development of fertilizing ability is associated with changes in several aspects of the functional integrity of the spermatozoa: (a) development of the potential for sustained progressive motility, (b) alteration of the metabolic patterns and the structural state of specific tail organelles, (c) changes in nuclear chromatin, (d) changes in nature of the surface of the plasma membrane, (e) movement and loss of the protoplasmic droplet, and (f) modification, at least in some species, of the form of the acrosome.

### *Storage of Spermatozoa*

The major site of sperm storage within the male reproductive tract is the caudal portion or tail of the epididymis. The tail of the epididymis contains 70% of the total number of spermatozoa in the excurrent ducts, whereas the vas deferens contains only 2%. The spermatozoa contained within the epididymal duct from the head to the tail are termed the extragonadal reserves even though only those in the distal section of the tail can be ejaculated. Although the environment is favorable to their survival, spermatozoa are not preserved indefinitely.

### *Disposal of Unejaculated Spermatozoa*

Most unejaculated spermatozoa are gradually eliminated by excretion into the urine. Those spermatozoa that are not eliminated in the urine undergo a gradual senescence. They first lose their fertilizing ability, then their motility, and finally they disintegrate. Ejaculates collected after prolonged sexual rest usually contain a high percentage of degenerating or "stale" spermatozoa.

## Seminal Plasma

The functional significance of seminal plasma is questionable in that pregnancy can be induced in some species by insemination with epididymal spermatozoa. It, however, appears to be an essential component in natural mating because it serves as a carrier and protector of the spermatozoa. The importance of this role varies because spermatozoa are ejaculated directly into the uterus in some species (e.g., sow and mare). Seminal plasma appears to be more important in natural mating of the ewe and cow where the ejaculate is deposited in the vagina.

## Accessory Glands

The source of the constituents of seminal plasma varies with the species as does the number and size of the accessory organs. It is a composite secretion arising from a number of sources including the testes, epididymides, and accessory glands of the male (Fig. 7-11). The only accessory gland common to all mammals is the prostate. The epididymis or its functional analogue and the vas deferens are the only accessory organs present in male birds and reptiles.

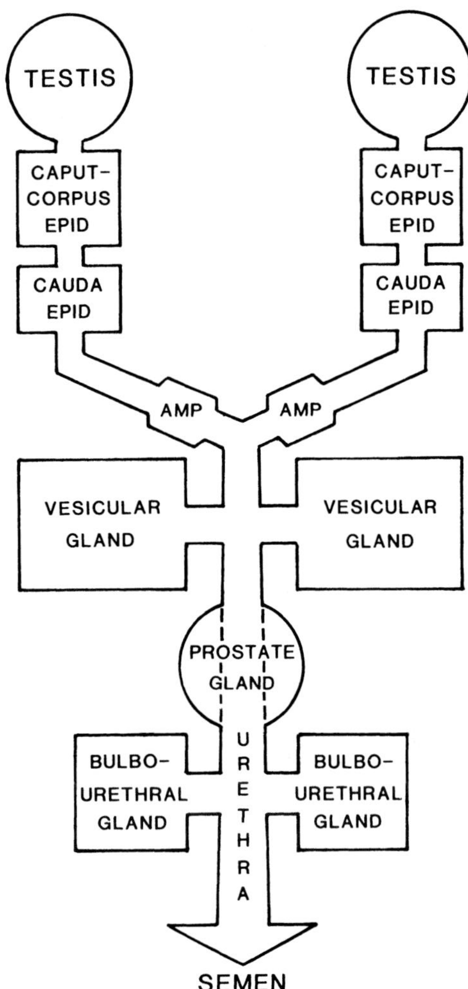


Figure 7-11. Ejaculated semen of most farm animals is composed of, in addition to a small amount of testicular fluid, contributions from several accessory organs including the epididymis (*CAPUT-CORPUS EPID* and *CAUDA EPID*), ampullary glands (*AMP*), vesicular glands, prostate gland, and bulbourethral glands. The relative contribution of the glands vary not only among species, but also among individuals within a species and among ejaculates from the same animal.

### *Biochemical Constituents of Seminal Plasma*

Seminal plasma contains unusually high levels of citric acid, ergothioneine, fructose, glycerylphosphorylcholine, and sorbitol (Table 7-1). Appreciable quantities of ascorbic acid, amino acids, peptides, proteins, lipids, fatty acids, and numerous enzymes are also present. Antimicrobial constituents including immunoglobulins of the IgA class are constituents of seminal plasma. In addition, a variety of hormonal substances including androgens, estrogens, prostaglandins, FSH, LH, chorionic gonadotrophin-like material, growth hormone, insulin, glucagon, prolactin, relaxin, thyroid releasing hormone, and enkephalins have been detected in seminal plasma.

## Spermatozoal Metabolism

The motile character of spermatozoa provides an easily discernible means of assessing their physiologic status. But motility, by itself, is not an accurate predictor of potential fertilizing capacity. The energy required for motility is apparently derived from intracellular stores of ATP (adenosine triphosphate). The utilization of ATP appears to be regulated by the endogenous level of cAMP. The cAMP not only regulates ATP breakdown, but also has a direct effect on sperm motility.

Although spermatozoa lack many of the organelles associated with metabolic processes, they are metabolically active because they possess the enzymes necessary to carry out the biochemical reactions of glycolysis (Embden-Meyerhof pathway), the tricarboxylic acid cycle, fatty acid oxidation, electron transport, and possibly the hexose monophosphate shunt.

### *Glycolysis*

Under anaerobic conditions, that is in the absence of oxygen, spermatozoa break down glucose, fructose, or mannose

TABLE 7-2. **Age, Weight, and Semen Characteristics at First Breeding**

| SPECIES | BEGINNING OF BREEDING LIFE *Months* | *Body Weight (kg)* | VOLUME OF EJACULATE (ml) | SPERM CONCENTRATION ($10^8$ PER ml) |
|---|---|---|---|---|
| Boar | 5–8 | 250 | 100–150 | 0.1–0.2 |
| Bull | 12–14 | 500 | 3–5 | 0.8–1.2 |
| Ram | 6–8 | varies | 0.3–1.0 | 1.2–2.0 |
| Stallion | 20–24 | 500 | 50–100 | 0.1–1.5 |
| Cock | 4–6 | varies | 0.10–0.3 | 50–90 |
| Cat | 9 | 3.5 | 0.01–0.3 | 1.5–28 |
| Dog | 10–12 | varies | 2–25 | 0.6–5.4 |
| Guinea pig | 3–5 | 0.450 | 0.4–0.8 | 0.05–0.2 |
| Rabbit | 4–12 | varies | 0.4–0.6 | 0.5–3.5 |

Adapted from Foote, In: Hafez ESE, ed. Reproduction in Farm Animals. 4th ed. Philadelphia: Lea & Febiger, 1980. Garner, Hafez. In: Hafez ESE, ed. Reproduction in Farm Animals. 6th ed. Philadelphia: Lea & Febiger, 1986.

to lactic acid. This glycolytic activity, or more correctly fructolytic activity because fructose is the principal seminal sugar, allows spermatozoa to survive under the anaerobic conditions. This characteristic is important during storage of spermatozoa for use in artificial insemination.

### *Respiration*

Spermatozoa use a variety of substrates in the presence of oxygen. Their respiratory activity provides the means of using the lactate or pyruvate resulting from the breakdown of fructose to yield carbon dioxide and water. This oxidative pathway, which is located in the mitochondria, is considerably more efficient in the production of energy than fructolysis. Using these catabolic processes, the spermatozoa convert most of the energy into ATP. Although much of the ATP is used for the energy-consuming process of motility, some is used to maintain the integrity of the active transport processes of spermatozoal membranes. These active transport processes prevent loss of vital ionic components from

TABLE 7-3. *In Vitro* Manipulation of Sperm

| TECHNIQUE | PROCEDURE | RATIONALE |
|---|---|---|
| Sperm washing | Percoll®, Sperm ISolate®, Modified Ham's F-10 medium, Tyrodes salt solution, or other isotonic media, prewarmed and filtered before use | Retrograde ejaculation<br>Cryopreserved semen<br>Oligozoospermia, low sperm motility<br>Eliminate antisperm antibodies<br>Intrauterine insemination preparation |
| Sperm swim up | Selection of sperm<br>Increase sperm quality | Decreased motility, eliminate potential pathogens, eliminate leukocytes |
| Swim down | Increase sperm quality | Oligospermia |
| Semen manipulation for IVF[a] | Swim up and swim down<br>*In vitro* capacitation | Eliminate cryopreservation media constituents |
| Semen and oocyte manipulation for enhancing fertilization | Microfertilization | Sperm transfer using zona drilling to enhance sperm access to the oocyte |
| Micromanipulation of sperm | Intracytoplasmic sperm insertion (ICSI) | Micromanipulators used to introduce one sperm into a matured oocyte |
| Semen sexing | Flow cytometric sorting | Live sorting of X and Y sperm |

[a]IVF = in vitro fertilization.

the sperm cell. In the absence of exogenous substrates, spermatozoa use their intracellular stores of plasmalogen to provide energy on a short term basis.

## IMMUNOLOGIC ASPECTS OF SPERMATOZOA

### *Antigenicity of Spermatozoa*

An important function of the blood-testis barrier is the immunologic isolation of developing gametes. Its importance is that the spermatocytes, spermatids, and spermatozoa are readily recognized as foreign cells by the immune system of the adult male. Thus, sequestering of the developing germ cells behind an immunologic barrier prevents an adult male from developing antibodies against his own sperm.

### *Autoimmunity*

Immunization of a male against spermatozoa or isolated spermatozoal antigens results in varying degrees of autoimmune orchitis (inflammation of the testis) and, in some cases, cessation of spermatogenesis. As a result of autoimmunity, the concentration of antispermatozoal antibodies can be high in the seminal fluid. Such spermatozoal-specific antibodies can interfere with spermatozoal functioning thereby reducing male fertility. In more severe cases, damage to the blood-testis barrier or the epididymal portion of the excurrent duct system through traumatic injury or infection often results in autoimmune orchitis affecting both testes. Vasectomy, the transectioning and ligation of the vas deferens, also results in varying degrees of testicular inflammation. The severity of the orchitis depends on the species and the postoperative time. The autoimmune response of vasectomized males is thought to occur because intermittent distention and rupture of the ligated duct results in release of spermatozoa into the peritoneal cavity.

## *IN VITRO* EVALUATION OF SEMEN

Males should be evaluated for seminal quality before use as breeding animals (Table 7-2). Once the semen has been collected from the male, several approaches may be used to assess the quality of the sample. Classic semen evaluation techniques, as well as new automated semen assessment technologies, yield only estimates of potential fertilizing capacity of spermatozoa.

## ASSISTED REPRODUCTIVE TECHNOLOGIES

Various techniques for micromanipulation of spermatozoa (Table 7-3) can be used to enhance the reproductive potential of genetically superior sires. *In vitro* fertilization (IVF) procedures can be used if sperm numbers are insufficient for fertilization to take place within the female tract. Another technique is to physically insert a single spermatozoon into an appropriately matured oocyte using micromanipulation. This procedure, which is called intracytoplasmic sperm injection (ICSI), can overcome a variety of male infertility problems. The application of this method remains controversial in that the actual fertilizing sperm is selected bypassing the screening systems inherent to the female reproductive tract that prevent defective spermatozoa from fertilizing oocytes. Considerable laboratory skill is required when manipulating the gametes *in vitro*.

## SUGGESTED READING


What is semen? How does semen analysis assist in understanding the reproductive status of the male? In: Robaire B, Pryor JL, Trasler JM. eds. Handbook of Andrology. Am Soc Andrology.

Amman RP, Hammerstedt RH. *In vitro* evaluation of sperm quality: An opinion. J Androl 1993;14:397–406.

Dadoune JP, Demoulin A. Structure and functions of the testis. In: Thibault C, Levasseur MC, Hunter RHF, eds. Reproduction in Mammals and Man. Paris: Ellipses, 1993.

Garner DL. Ancillary tests of bull sperm semen quality. In: Van Camp SD, ed. Veterinary Clinics of North America: Food Animal Practice. 1997;13:313–330.

Garner DL. Artificial Insemination. In: Cupps PT, ed. Reproduction in Domestic Animals. 4th ed. San Diego, CA: Academic Press, 1991.

Johnson L. Spermatogenesis. In: Cupps PT, ed. Reproduction in Domestic Animals. 4th ed. San Diego, CA: Academic Press, 1991.

Lamming GE. Marshall's Physiology of Reproduction: Vol. 2, Reproduction in the Male. New York: Churchill Livingstone, 1990.

Mann T, Lutwak-Mann C. Male Reproductive Function and Semen. New York: Springer-Verlag, 1981.

Ott RS. Breeding soundness of bulls. In: Current Therapy in Theriogenology: Diagnosis, Treatment and Prevention of Reproductive Diseases in Small and Large Animals. Philadelphia: WB Saunders, 1986:125–136.

Senger PL. Pathways to Pregnancy and Parturition. Pullman, WA: Current Conceptions, 1997.

# CHAPTER 8

# *Fertilization and Cleavage*

E.S.E. HAFEZ AND B. HAFEZ

During the course of mammalian evolution there have been dramatic changes leading to biosexual reproduction and internal fertilization and cleavage of the gametes. These adaptive mechanisms in evolution were associated with various parameters to avoid irreversible accumulation of detrimental mutations in the face of a competitive and constantly changing environment. Sperm and eggs are equal from the standpoint of their genome but their life history and behavior before and during fertilization are quite different. The sperm have remarkable motility patterns which change constantly in order to fuse with and activate the egg. When activated by the fertilizing sperm, the egg, with a dual complement of the female and male genomes, eliminates all or almost all of the nonnuclear elements of the sperm.

Extensive investigations have been conducted on several parameters of fertilization and related phenomena in domestic and laboratory mammals: structure and ulstructure of sperm (1, 2); maturation of epididymal sperm (3–7); capacitation (8–13); acrosome reaction (14, 15); gamete binding (16–21); and gamete interaction (22–29).

The sequence of events of sperm capacitation/penetration of zona pellucida, block of polysperm/cotical granules reaction, and development of male and female pronuclei/fusion/cleavage are summarized in Tables 8-1 through 8-6, and illustrated in Figures 8-1 through 8-7.

## FERTILIZATION

### *Ovum Maturation*

The ovum resumes meiosis from prophase I of the first meiotic division as it begins to mature during folliculogenesis. The ovum is in metaphase 11 of the second meiotic division when ovulated. However, ova of the horse, dog, and fox are only in their first meiotic division at the time of ovulation. Ovum maturation and meiosis are not completed until fertilization is completed, when the ovum becomes a zygot.

### *Sperm Maturation*

Sperm require maturational changes that occur during a ten to fifteen day transport through the epididymis, after which fertilization is possible. Sperm maturational changes depend on epididymal secretions and transport time, which are essential for sperm to fertilize the ovum. To achieve their fertilizability and gamete fusion sperm undergo several known and unknown sequestial maturational changes including "capacitation" and acrosome reactions.

CAPACITATION. Chang and Austin noted that sperm must reside in the female reproductive tract before becoming capable of attaching to and penetrating the ovum. This process was termed sperm capacitation, which seems to take place in the uterus, specifically, the isthmic region of the oviduct. Sperm surface components are *modified* or *removed* by genital tract secretions causing the phospholipid bilayer to become destabilized, permitting acrosomal activation. Such changes may include depletion of sperm cholesterol at the sperm surface, alteration in glycosaminoglycans, and changes in ions as sperm traverse the genital tract. Capacitation leads to acrosomal changes needed for sperm penetration of the ovum investments. Therefore, capacitation functions to prevent premature acrosome activation until the sperm reach the site of fertilization and come in contact with the ovum. The true acrosome reaction involves fusion of the sperm plasma membrane with the outer acrosomal membrane (Fig. 8-1) followed by extensive vesiculation over the anterior segment of the acrosome. This differs from the "false" acrosome reaction that occurs during senescence or degeneration of sperm. Fusion and vesiculation of the acrosome release hydrolytic enzymes, for example, hyaluronidase and acrosin, which are implicated in penetration of the ovum.

### *Interaction of Sperm and Ovum*

The fertile lifespans of sperm and ovum (Table 8-2) dictate synchronous insemination and ovulation to achieve high

TABLE 8-1. ***Epididymal Sperm Maturation, Capacitation, and Acrosome Reaction in Farm Animals***

| | EPIDIDYMAL MATURATION OF SPERM |
|---|---|
| Site Sperm Acquire Fertilizing | a. Ability of testicular sperm to move is due to immaturity of plasma membrane |
| Development of Sperm's Motility | b. Transfer of substances: glycerol-3-phosphorylcholine a forward motility protein from the epididymal fluid |
| Maturation Sperm Plasma | c. Sperm unable to move progressively or interact with and fertilize eggs |
| Membrane | d. Sperm attain motility in caput epididymis or in corpus epididymis according to species |
| Maturational Sperm Structures | e. Sperm do not gain fertilizability simultaneously in same region |
| | f. Most sperm attain full fertilizability in cauda, major sperm storage site |
| Deposit, Storage, Ascent in Female Tract | g. Sperm fertilizability is evaluated: i) sperm's ability to fertilize zona-free hamster eggs, ii) motility patterns, iii) surface characteristics, and iv) structural stability of head/tail |
| | h. Epididymis/vas deferens secrete specific components necessary for functional maturation |

conception rate. Females ovulate at various times after onset of estrus. Sperm longevity in the female reproductive tract appears related to the length of estrus. For example, swine and horse sperm have greater longevity than do that of sheep and cattle. Longevity of sperm in the pig and horse increases the probability of viable sperm being present at ovulation when insemination occurs well in advance of ovulation. Regardless of the timing of ovulation, high conception rates result if sperm are present in the oviduct shortly before ovulation. Insemination too early reduces conception rates, which results from loss of sperm viability and the number of sperm at the site of fertilization, whereas loss of ovum viability can result from insemination after ovulation even though fertilization occurs.

TABLE 8-2. ***Time of Events in Early Embryonic Development***

| | SPECIES | | | |
|---|---|---|---|---|
| PARAMETER | *Cattle* | *Horse* | *Sheep* | *Swine* |
| Gamete Longevity (hours) | | | | |
| Sperm | 30–48 | 72–120 | 30–48 | 34–72 |
| Ovum | 20–24 | 6–8 | 16–24 | 8–10 |
| Embryonic Development (days)[a] | | | | |
| 2-cell | 1 | 1 | 1 | 0.6–0.8 |
| 4-cell | 1.5 | 1.5 | 1.3 | 1 |
| 8-cell | 3 | 3 | 1.5 | 2.5 |
| Blastocyst | 7–8 | 6 | 6–7 | 5–6 |
| Hatching | 9–11 | 8 | 7–8 | 6 |
| Blastocyst Transport to Uterus | | | | |
| Hours | 72–84 | 140–144[b] | 66–72 | 46–48 |
| Cell Stage | 8–16 | Blastocyst | 8–16 | 4 |
| Blastocyst Elongation (days) | 13–21 | NE[c] | 11–16 | 11–15 |
| Initial Placentation (days) | 22 | 37 | 15 | 13 |
| Birth (days) | 278–290 | 335–345 | 145–155 | 112–115 |

[a]Days after ovulation.
[b]Unfertilized ova remain in the oviduct.
[c]No elongation occurs to form filamentous blastocysts.

TABLE 8-3. ***Capacitation: Factors Controlling/Affecting Capacitation Events During Capacitation***

a. Sperm acquire fertilizability after residing in the female tract for some time.
b. Capacitation involves removal or alteration of a stabilizer or protective coat from sperm plasma membrane; this is under autonomic nerve and hormonal controls.
c. Sperm are found in close contact with epithelial cells of the isthmus and the uterotubal junction.
d. Most of capacitance occurs in lower segment of isthmus where fertilizing sperm are stored, capacitation within the isthmus progresses faster when females mate after ovulation than when they mate before ovulation.
e. Capacitation is facilitated by "rubbing off" sperm surface-adsorbed materials (including seminal plasma proteins) against cervical mucus.
f. Specificity/speciality of female tract: sperm fully capacitated in uterus without ascending to oviduct. Women have successful pregnancy following gamete intra fallopian transfer (GIFT) or direct intra-peritoneal insemination (DIPI); capacitation is possible in peritoneal cavity and/or ampulla. Capacitation is not strictly organ specific. Sperm adhering to epithelium of isthmus undergo capacitation slowly.
g. *In vitro* sperm capacitation (IVC) and *in vitro* fertilization (IVF) are routinely applied using several commercially available tissue culture media or in modified Tryode's/Krebs-Ringer's solutions supplemented with energy sources (e.g., glucose, lactate, and pyruvate) and albumin, (e.g., Ham F10) supplemented with blood serum. Serum are also commonly used, particularly for human IVF.
h. Sperm maintain ionic gradients across plasma membrane; the concentration of $K^+$ inside cell is higher than outside; reverse is true for $Na^+$.
i. IVC of bovine sperm facilitated by heparin which assists removal of seminal plasma component from sperm surface. Because plasma membrane is directly exposed to capacitating environment, significant changes occur in this membrane during capacitation. The removal or alteration of coating material from sperm surface constitutes an important part of capacitation. The coating materials removed or altered during capacitation include decapacitation factors.

Although the male ejaculates billions of sperm into the female reproductive tract, approximately 1,000 to 10,000 spermatozoa are present in the isthmus and only 10 to 100 sperm may be in the ampulla after 4 to 12 hours. Low numbers of sperm in the oviduct do not result from slow sperm transport but rather from their controlled movement into the ampulla by the uterotubal junction and lower isthmus (in the pig), as well as from their movement from the vagina and cervix into the uterus (in ruminants). This relationship regulates the number of sperm at the fertilization site (preventing polyspermy), while providing a sperm reservoir to ensure that capacitated sperm are present until ovulation.

The ability of sperm to adhere to and release from the epithelial lining of the ampulla may assist in maintaining adequate numbers of sperm at the site of fertilization (30). When present in the ampulla, sperm become hyperactivated, which increases the probability that they will make contact with the ovum. Although the complete roles of the oviduct and its lumenal contents in ensuring fertilization are not understood, the process is efficient because fertilization rates in all domestic species exceed 90%.

SPERM-OOCYTE ENCOUNTER. Fertilization in mammals requires three critical events: (a) sperm migration between cumulus cells (if present); (b) sperm attachment and migration through the zona pellucida; and (c) fusion of sperm and ovum plasma membranes.

A substance produced by the cumulus oophorus of rabbit ova may stimulate sperm motility. This factor may play a secondary role in the sperm-ovum encounter since peristaltic contractions of the ampulla increase the chance of ovum-sperm contact (28).

### *Sperm Attachment*

Attachment of the sperm head to the zona pellucida is regulated by receptor sites on the zona surface. Treatment of ova with antizona antibodies or the proteolytic enzyme trypsin blocks sperm attachment. Binding to the zona pellucida can also be inhibited by pretreatment of sperm with antisperm antibodies or glycoproteins extracted from the zona pellucida (Fig. 8-2). Antibodies to sperm or zona pellucida, therefore, block or mask sperm receptor sites on sperm and zona surfaces. The presence of glycosyl transferase, proteinases, and glycosi-

**Table 8-4. *Acrosome/Acrosome Reaction***

| | |
|---|---|
| | a. Acrosome consists of anteriorly located acrosomal cap and posteriorly located equatorial segment, relative size, topographical relationship between two segments of acrosome in seven acrosomal cap is located with hydrolyzing enzymes, the equatorial segment enzymatically "empty." Hyaluronidase/acrosin are acrosomal enzymes extensively studied/characterized. |
| Acrosome Enzymes | b. The acrosome contains several powerful hydrolyzing enzymes. Structural proteins maintain acrosome shape/positioning of different functional components within acrosomal matrix, acrosome organization is required to insure release of acrosome components in precise order so sperm traverse the egg vestments. |
| Functional Significance | c. To fertilize eggs, sperm must be highly motile as well as capable of undergoing acrosome reaction (AR) penetrating through egg investments/fusing with egg. |
| Morphology, Detection, Kinetics of | d. Acrosome reaction (AR) as indicator of completed capacitation. Because sperm do not undergo AR either spontaneously or mediated by ligands (e.g., zona pellucida), unless they become capacitated. |
| Acrosome Reaction *In Vivo*<br>Zona-Mediated Acrosome Reaction vs. Spontaneous<br>Acrosome Reaction | e. Massive influx of $Ca^{2+}$ occurs during AR. Concentration of intracellular $Ca^{2+}$ in sperm is low, in both head and tail regions, because of presence of ATPase-mediated $Ca^{2+}$ antiporter, and a $Ca^{2+}/H^{+}$ exchange system in plasma membrane. |
| Mechanism of Reaction | f. Carbohydrate is distinct component of acrosomal matrix. Glycoprotein layer covering inner surface of outer acrosomal membrane holds vesiculated (fenestrated) plasma/outer acrosomal membranes together during acrosome reaction. |
| | g. Form of acrosome does not change during capacitation, enzymatically inactive proacrosin in sperm acrosome is converted to enzymatically active acrosin by glycosaminoglycans in uterine fluid. |
| | h. Function of AR: eggs are surrounded by glycoprotein coats through which sperm must pass before reaching egg plasma membrane. Acrosome-reacted sperm dissolve coat locally to produce a "hole" through which the sperm swim. Outer acrosomal membrane overlying plasma membrane destroyed (partially or totally) or become detached from main body of sperm. |

dases on the plasma membrane covering the sperm head could result in binding to ZP3 through a lock/key mechanism such as that for an enzyme and its substrate (16).

### *Sperm Penetration*

Penetration of the zona by sperm occurs within 5 to 15 minutes after sperm attachment. The acrosome reaction may occur before or after attachment of the sperm head to the glycoprotein receptors on the zona, but an acrosome-intact sperm is essential for attachment. Binding of the sperm head to ZP3 allows interactions with other zona components that stimulate acrosome activation.

Acrosin was long considered the essential zona lysin for sperm penetration, but the number of enzymes present in or attached to the acrosomal membranes suggests that a combination of enzymes acts synergistically during penetration. This is consistent with the heterogenous glycoprotein structure of the zona pellucida. Enzymes exposed during the acrosome reaction are needed for the passage of sperm through the zona, but sperm motility is also required (28). As acrosomal reacted sperm initiate zona pellucida penetration, the glycoprotein ZP2 may serve as a secondary sperm receptor to maintain sperm attachment during passage through the zona.

Gamete Fusion. The vitelline membrane may have less specificity than the zona pellucida in binding foreign sperm; however, some degree of selectivity is apparent since the plasma membrane of the ovum will competitively bind more homologous sperm.

The acrosome reaction is a prerequisite for fusion between ova and spermatozoa plasma membranes, and zona free ova cannot undergo fusion with nonacrosomal activated sperm even though attachment to the membrane surface occurs (Fig. 8-3).

TABLE 8-5. ***Sperm/Zona Attachment and Interaction During Fertilization***

| | | |
|---|---|---|
| Sperm Attachment to Zona | | a. Specific sperm receptor in the zona pellucida is one of three major glycoproteins that form extracellular matrix of zona pellucida.<br>b. Three glycoproteins, ZP1, ZP2, and ZP3, are synthesized by maturing oocytes. These are present in all mammals but with variations in these proteins.<br>c. ZP3 functions as sperm receptor to which only sperm with an intact acrosome can bind.<br>d. Binding of sperm to sperm receptors occurs through an interaction with O-linked oligosaccharides on ZP3. |
| Cumulus and Sperm Attachment | | a. Role of cumulus cells in sperm attachment cells in sperm attachment is debated in domestic animals (especially the cow), since they are usually absent 3 to 4 hours after ovulation.<br>b. Hyaluronidase in bull acrosome allows penetration of cumulus oophorus.<br>c. Arylsulfatase from boar acrosome causes cells of the cumulus oophorus to disperse. Enzymes necessary for cumulus penetration or dispersion are present in these species. |
| Sperm Interaction/ Cumulus Oophorus | Properties of Cumulus Oophorus<br>Sperm Entry into Cumulus<br>Inhibition of Sperm Penetration in Cumulus<br>Role of Cumulus<br>Acrosome Hyaluronidase | a. Acrosome reaction allows release of zona lysin by which sperm digest a path through the zona pellucida to vitelline membrane.<br>b. Acrosome contains several enzymes: hyaluronidase, acrosin, proacrosin (inactive form of acrosin), esterase, phospholipase $A_2$, acid phosphatases, aryl sulphatase, $\beta$-N-acetyl glucosaminidase, aryl amidase, and nonspecific acid proteinases; with quantitative/qualitative species differences. |
| Sperm Zona Pellucida Interaction | Function of Zona<br>Properties of Zona<br>Sperm Binding/Penetration through Zona | a. Acrosome is activated by the time of sperm attachment and penetration of zona. Once sperm has traversed the zona pellucida, the head moves into vitelline space/contacts vitelline membrane.<br>b. Sperm tail propels sperm into vitelline space, rotating the vitelline membrane within zona pellucida. |

The vitelline membrane is covered by dense microvilli, except for an elevated area adjacent to the surface where the second polar body will be extruded after fertilization. Sperm attachment is seldom observed in this area of the vitelline membrane. Attachment of sperm occurs initially at the equatorial segment of the sperm head with either the microvilli or the intervillous area of the vitelline membrane. Fusion of sperm and egg does not involve the plasma membrane over the equatorial segment and postacrosomal region of the sperm head. Subsequently, the surface of the equatorial region of the sperm is incorporated into the plasma membrane of the ovum. The equatorial region of the sperm plasma membrane becomes intermixed with the ovum plasma membrane and can be identified in the egg membrane as late as the eight-cell stage.

### *Block to Polyspermy*

Immediately following fertilization, the ovum surface changes to prevent fusion of additional spermatozoa. When this mechanism fails, polyspermic fertilization can result with formation of polyploid embryos that undergo embryonic death or abnormal development.

Although physiologic polyspermy is common in birds and reptiles, the incidence of polyspermy in most mammalian species is only 1 or 2% (31). The pig appears most susceptible to polyspermy, expecially as a result of delayed mating or insemination when up to 15% of the eggs are penetrated by more than one spermatozona. In sheep, Killeen and Moore (32) found that late insemination, that is 36 to 48 hours after onset of estrus, was associated with abnormal fertilized eggs in which 39% were polyspermic or contained multinucleated blastomeres.

### *Development of Pronuclei and Syngamy*

On penetration of the vitelline membrane by the spermatozona, the activated ovum completes meiosis and expels the first and/or second polar body into the perivitelline space

TABLE 8-6. ***Sperm/Egg Fusion, Cortical Reaction, Polyspermy Block, Sperm Decondensation, and Pronuclei Development***

| | | |
|---|---|---|
| SPERM-EGG FUSION | Sperm Become Capable of Fusing with Eggs<br>Fusion of Subnormal/Abnormal Sperm/Oolemma<br>Fusion Competence of Oolemma<br>Detection of Sperm-Egg Fusion<br>Control of Sperm-Egg Fusion | a. Sperm/egg fusion does not involve inner acrosomal membrane of anterior region, involves the plasma membrane over equatorial segment/postacrosomal region of sperm head.<br>b. Surface of equatorial region of sperm is incorporated into plasma membrane of ovum.<br>c. Equatorial region of sperm plasma membrane is intermixed with ovum plasma membrane/is identified in egg membrane as late as eight-cell stage. |
| CORTICAL REACTION<br>POLYSPERMY BLOCK | Cortical Granules/Cortical Reaction<br>Block to Polyspermy | a. Block to polyspermy is at zona pellucida in most mammals (e.g., sheep, swine) with a secondary physiologic block at vitelline membrane in rabbits.<br>b. Initiation of block is at sperm penetration of ovum when cortical granules are released into perivitelline space.<br>c. Release of content of these granules cause extensive reorganization of zona pellucida and/or vitelline surface the "cortical reaction." Cortical reaction results in release of enzymes that cause hardening of zona pellucida/inactivation of sperm receptors (ZP3).<br>d. Enzymatic digestion of O-linked oligosaccharides on ZP3 would remove specific carbohydrates involved in zona binding of sperm.<br>e. Proteolysis of ZP2 may also alter physical characteristics of the zona to prevent further penetration of unwanted accessory sperm. |
| DECONDENSATION OF SPERM NUCLEUS IN OOPLASM | Sperm Nucleus<br>Sperm Nucleus Decondensation | a. After fusion with egg plasma membrane, sperm nuclear envelope disintegrates, released chromatin material undergoes decondensation.<br>b. Sperm nuclear envelope is rapidly replaced by a new envelope within the ovum cytoplasm, forming male pronucleus. Decondensation of sperm nuclear envelope requires specific components in cytoplasm of ovum.<br>c. Immature cow oocytes are unable to decondense sperm nuclei even when matured *in vitro*. Factor necessary for decondensation is termed *male pronucleus growth factor*. |
| COMPLETION OF MEIOSIS, PRONUCLEI DEVELOPMENT | Completion of Pronuclei Development Syngamy | a. Once the male/female pronuclei are in close proximity, the nuclear envelopes disperse, allowing intermixing of chromosomes.<br>b. Associated with these events is the initiation of DNA synthesis from cytoplasmic precursors.<br>c. The chromosomes then aggregate in prophase of first cleavage division, resulting in formating of a zygot/restoration of diploid state.<br>d. Process of fertilization allows combining of maternal and paternal hereditary elements.<br>e. During fusion of sperm/egg, sperm constituents from cell membranes/sperm head are released into ooplasm. |

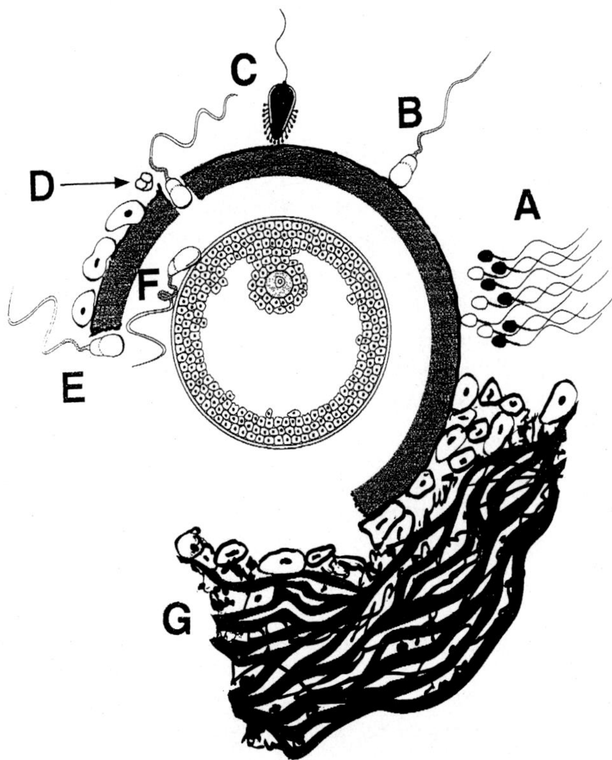


FIGURE 8-1. Sequence of events during sperm hyperactivation, capacitation, acrosome reaction, and fertilization: (A) Sperm subsets (capacitated active, capacitation latent, non-capacitated, and dysfunctional) penetrate cumulus cells. (B) Initial binding of sperm with zona glycoprotein ZP2. (C) Acrosome reaction follows sperm/egg recognition. (D) Acrosomal cap discarded as sperm penetrates zona pellucida. (E) Acrosin exposed on inner acrosomal membrane; may mediate secondary binding to ZP3. (F) Fusion between plasma membranes of sperm; oocyte/sperm membranes fuse. (G) Cumulus matrix.

(Fig. 8-4). The remaining matemal haploid chromosomes are then enclosed by a pronucleus. Male and female pronuclei migrate to the ovum center, for rearrangements in the cytoskeletal framework of the ovum after activation.

Although possible in theory, attempts to produce homozygous diploid (two male or female pronuclei) mice have failed (33). Contributions from both the male and female pronuclei appear necessary for normal embryonic development.

INTERSPECIES FERTILIZATION. Interspecies fertilization has been demonstrated only between the snowshoe hare and rabbit, mink, and ferret; sheep and goat; and horse and donkey. In addition, *Bos laurus* and *Bos incficus*, European and Asian domestic cattle, will readily produce fertile hybrids that demonstrate a greater disease resistance and heat tolerance than *Bos laurus* cattle. Domestic cattle and American bison (*Bison bison*) have also been crossed successfully to produce a hybrid that may have superior cold resistance and forage use capability. Failure in the hybridization process can occur during fertilization and/or cleavage so that successful interspecies fertilization is rare. Development of semen and egg collection methods *followed by* successful *in vitro* fertilization techniques allow this problem to be addressed. Results using these techniques indicate that from the time of the early cleavage divisions to blastocyst formation the mammalian ovum is tolerant of a foreign environment. After this time, hybrids succumb, which indicates their dependence on highly specific conditions during the postblastocyst period.

When successful hybridization has been demonstrated, there are marked differences in the success of reciprocal crosses such that a high rate of fertilization is possible in one direction but not in the other; that is, a male snowshoe hare and female rabbit is successful, but a female snowshoe hare and male rabbit is much less so. Fertilization failure between different species is not primarily a result of differences in genetic constitution of sperm or egg but is attributed to genetically determined differences in the physiologic constitution of these gametes in the genital tract.

The importance of the trophoblast in the maintenance of pregnancy has been demonstrated in studies involving interspecies pregnancy, and immunologic involvement has been implicated in the failure of a portion of such pregnancies. This problem has been circumvented using the techniques of embryo micromanipulation. Blastomeres from early (four-cell to eight-cell) sheep and goat embryos were used to construct chimeric embryos. Blastomeres were positioned so that the outside cells were from the species into which the embryos would be transferred. Trophoblast components, which originate from the outer cell layer, were able to protect cells from the foreign species positioned on the inner cell layer, which gives rise to the embryonic tissue proper. Thus, maternal immune rejection of cells from the "foreign" species could be prevented and the pregnancy maintained.

## CLEAVAGE

After the zygote stage, embryos enter into several mitotic divisions. The zygote, or one-cell stage, is quite large, having a low nuclear to cytoplasmic ratio. To attain a ratio similar to somatic cells, cell divisions occur without an increase in cell mass. This process is referred to as cleavage. Growth during this period may be considered negative since cellular mass decreases from 20% in the cow to 40% in sheep, however, nuclei do increase in size, and the proper amount of nucleic acid is maintained in the chromosomes (31). Since cells of mammalian embryos contain little yolk (except for swine and horses), they rely on the mother for much of their metabolic support during early pregnancy. This is provided by oviductal and uterine secretions (histotroph). During early cleavage there is little increase in meta-

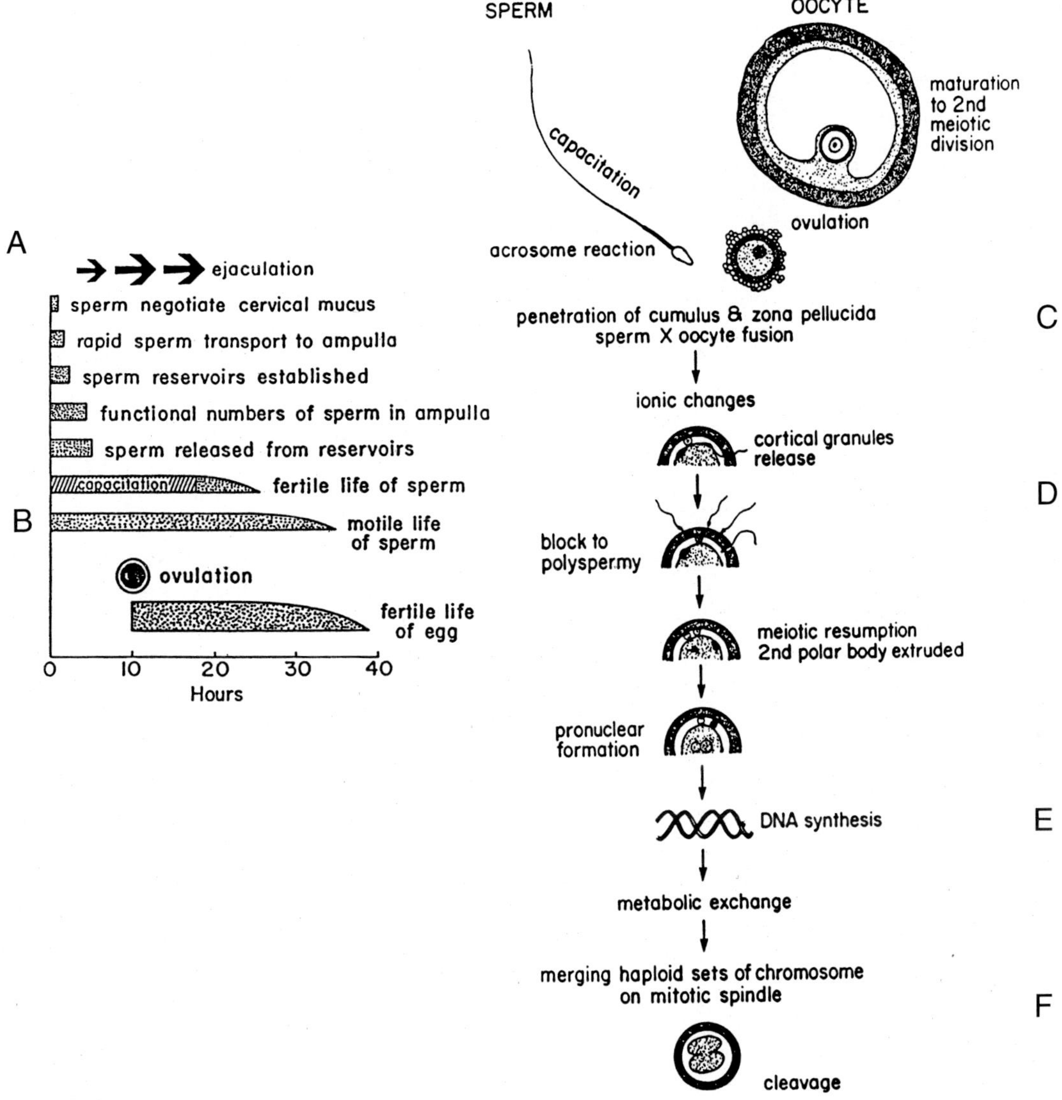


FIGURE 8-2. Diagrammatic illustration of the sequence of events of sperm/oocyte interaction: (A) ejaculation, (B) sperm migration, (C) sperm release from reservoirs, (D) penetration of zona pellucida, (E) fertilization, (F) cleavage.

bolic rate, but a sharp rise occurs between the morula and blastocyst stage.

### Normal Time Course

Cleavage of the zygote is by vertical division through the main axis of the egg from animal (site of polar body extrusion) to vegetal (area of yolk reserve) pole. The cleavage furrow often goes through the area where the pronuclei resided at the initiation of syngamy. The resulting daughter cells are called *blastomeres*. The plane of the second division is also vertical and passes through the main axis but at a right angle to the initial plane of cleavage, producing four blastomeres. The third cleavage division occurs approximately at a right angle to the second, producing eight blastomeres. This doubling sequence is carried on through the remainder of early cleavage. The initial cleavage divisions usually occur simultaneously in all the blastomeres, but the synchronization is inevitably lost and blastomeres start dividing independently of each other.

Cleavage divisions are always mitotic with each daughter cell (blastomere) receiving the full assortment of chromosomes. Blastomeres from the two-cell to eight-cell stage in the rabbit are totipotent, that is, fully capable of giving rise to an intact embryo. Totipotency of sheep blastomeres is maintained up to the eight-cell stage (34). In four-cell embryos no more than three of four blastomeres are totipotent and in eight-cell embryos no more than one of eight

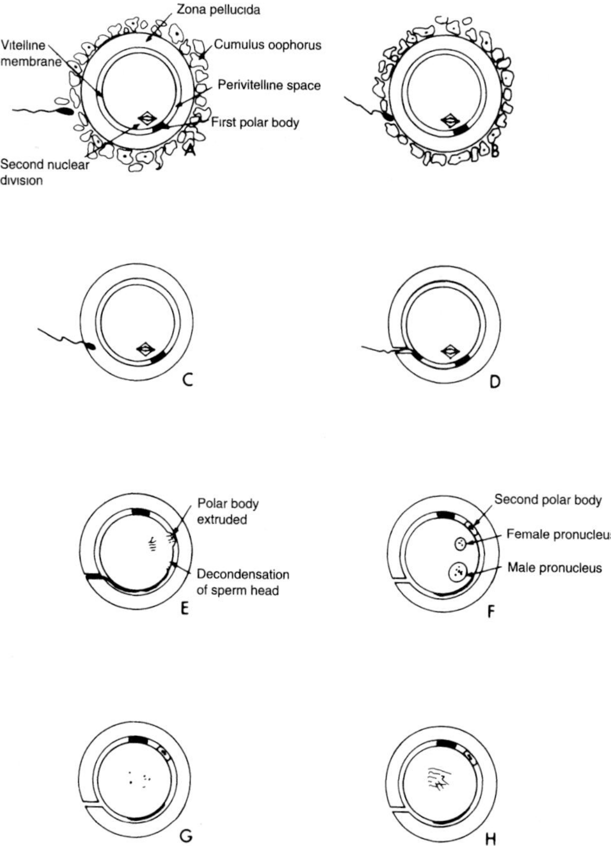


FIGURE 8-3. Steps during fertilization. (A) Spermatozoon first encounters and penetrates the cumulus oophorus. First polar body is present in the perivitelline space with the metaphase spindle of the secondary oocyte present in the cytoplasm. (B) A spermatozoon having undergone acrosomal activation. (C) The inner acrosomal membrane of a spermatozoon contacts the zona pellucida. (D) Enzymes exposed on the membrane surface allow penetration into the perivitelline space. (E) The equatorial region of the sperm head attaches and fuses with the vitelline membrane stimulating completion of the second meiotic division. (F) The large male pronucleus and smaller female pronucleus form following extrusion of the second polar body. (G) The pronuclei migrate to the oocyte center, where the nuclear envelopes disperse. (H) The prophase of the first mitosis division begins. (From McLaren A. In: Hafez ESE, ed. Reproduction in Farm Animals. 4th ed. Philadelphia: Lea & Febiger, 1980;229.)

blastomeres is totipotent. After this time, however, the blastomeres appear to differentiate according to their position in the morula.

While blastomeres are encased within the zona pellucida, they must accommodate themselves to this limited area. Once the embryo has formed 9 to 16 blastomeres, but in some cases more, it is referred to as a *morula,* because of its resemblance to a mulberry. Segregation of the inner and outer cells of the 16-cell mouse embryo (or morula) may be initiated by morphogenic changes occurring at the 8-cell stage. At this time, blastomeres flatten on each other to form a rounded embryo and internal cellular components, and surface microvilli become asymmetrically positioned in a process termed polarization. The combined processes of flattening of the blastomeres and polarization are referred to as "compaction." Before the 16-cell stage, there is variability in the rate of compaction among embryos as well as in the time of its onset (35).

The polarization hypothesis states that the asymmetry between the apical and basal aspects of the blastomeres at the 8-cell stage provides the basis for the differences between the inner and outer cells of the morula. The way in which the plane of division occurs during the fourth cleavage division, that is, 8-cell to 16-cell stage, could segregate the structurally different regions of the 8-cell blastomeres into heterogenous populations. In this situation, division planes that occurred parallel to the blastomere surface or across the axis of polarity would split the blastomere into two daughter cells having different morphologic and behavioral characteristics. Sutherland et al. (35) demonstrated that during the fourth cleavage division in mice there were three major division plane orientations; anticlinal (perpendicular to the outer surface of the blastomere); perioclinal (parallel to the outer surface of the blastomere); and oblique (at an angle between the other two) (Fig. 8-4).

The relative number of inner and outer cells in the 16-cell morula would, therefore, depend on the proportion of the types of division during the fourth cleavage. By tracing the lineages of four-cell and eight-cell blastomers, Sutherland et al. (35) found that the division order of the blastomers during third or fourth cleavage was associated with the division order of the parent blastomeres during the previous cleavage. Some preimplantation pig embryos have inner cells by the 12-cell to 16-cell stage (34). The proportion of inner cells was low in morula but increased during differentiation of the ICM and trophectoderm in early blastocysts. The proportion of ICM cells then decreased as blastocysts expanded and hatched.

Tight junctions form within the trophoblast layer of 8-cell to 16-cell mouse embryos (36) when the blastomeres are in close apposition during the process of compaction (Fig. 8-5). The formation of tight junctions provides a permeability seal that allows fluid to move from the outside to the inside of the blastocyst without substantial leakage, and form the blastocoele. The formation of gap and tight junctions between presumptive trophoblast cells also plays an important role in separating cells from contact with the maternal environment, thereby allowing the blastocyst to positionally differentiate into two populations of cells. One population forms the inner cell mass and gives rise to the embryo proper, and the other gives rise to the trophectoderm or trophoblast, which forms the chorion.

### Cleavage Rates and Variation

The lower region of the ampulla is the site of fertilization in most mammalian species. When the embryo has developed to the 8-cell to 16-cell stage (4-cell stage in the pig), it is transported into the uterus, where it continues to prolif-

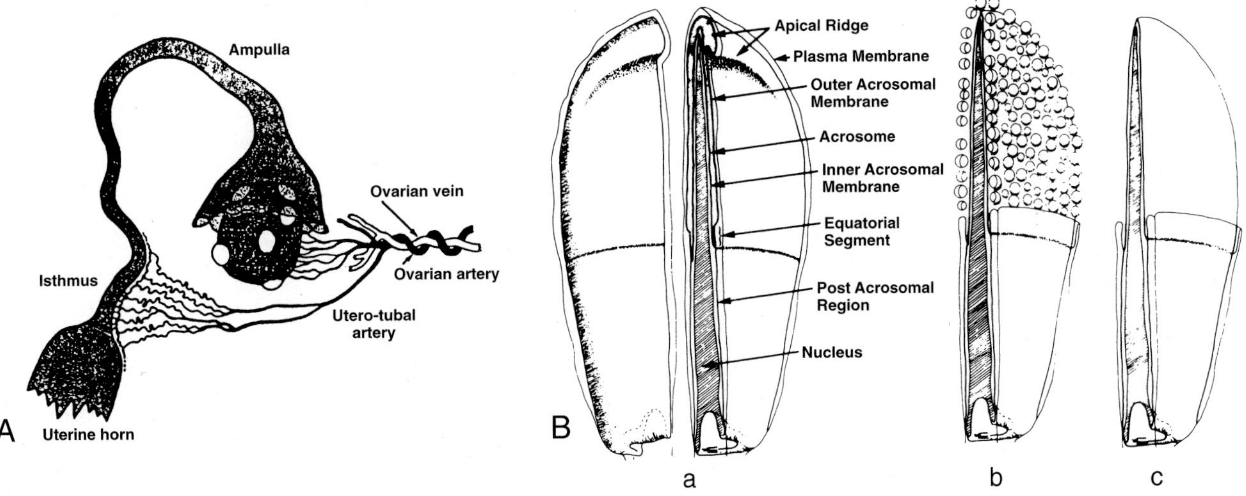


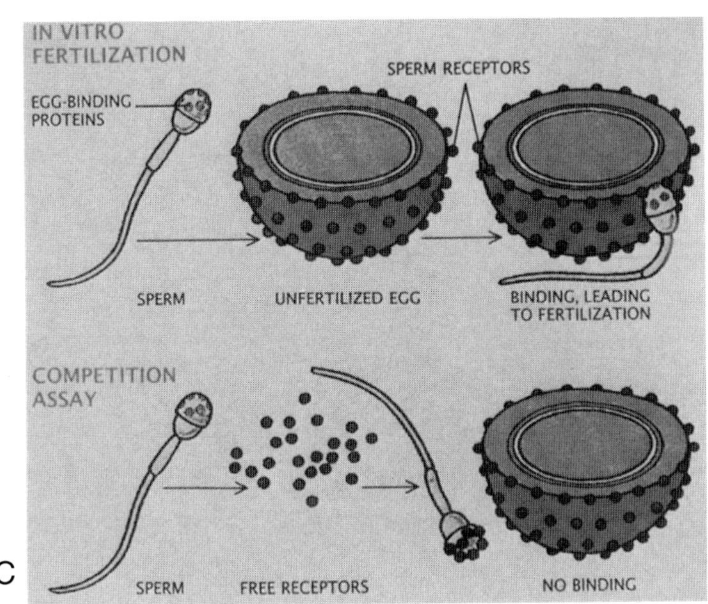


FIGURE 8-4. (**A**) Representation of the arterial blood supply to the ovary and isthmus of the pig oviduct. (From the literature.) (**B**) The sequence of events during acrosome reaction in mammalian spermatozoa. (*a*) Intact plasma and acrosomal membrane of an unreacted spermatozoon. (*b*) Initiation of the acrosome reaction showing multiple fusion points between the plasma membrane and outer acrosomal membrane. Fusion leaves the appearance of numerous vesicles over the cell surface. Note that fusion is absent in the equatorial and postacrosomal regions. Acrosomal enzymes involved with ovum penetration are released and exposed on the inner acrosomal membrane. (*c*) The acrosome swells and is eventually lost during penetration of the zona pellucida, leaving only the inner acrosomal membrane exposed on the upper portion of the sperm head. (Adapted from R.G. Saacke and J.M. White, [1972] Proc. 4th Tech. Conf. A.I. and Reprod., Trinto, Italy pp. 22–27.) (**C**) The protein ZP3 in the zona pellucida is the sperm receptor. Exposure of sperm to unfertilized ova results in sperm binding to ZP3 (top). In the competition assay (bottom), sperm are incubated with ZP3 first and then exposed to ova; however, the sperm are unable to bind to the ZP3 proteins on the zona pellucida because their ZP3 binding proteins are already occupied (blocked) by the free ZP3 to which the sperm were introduced before introduction of ova. (Reproduced from Paul M. Wassarman [1988]. Scientific American December, p. 83.)

erate. The time embryos spend in the oviduct allows the uterus to prepare for the nutritive role that it must provide once the embryo comes into residence (Table 8-2).

The rate at which the developing embryo moves through the oviduct and into the uterus is thought to be entirely a maternal function controlled by factors that affect the muscular function of the isthmus, such as the local adrenergic system, which can be modified by estrogen/progesterone. Prostaglandins of the F series, acting locally, appear to impede transport of the embryo into the uterus,

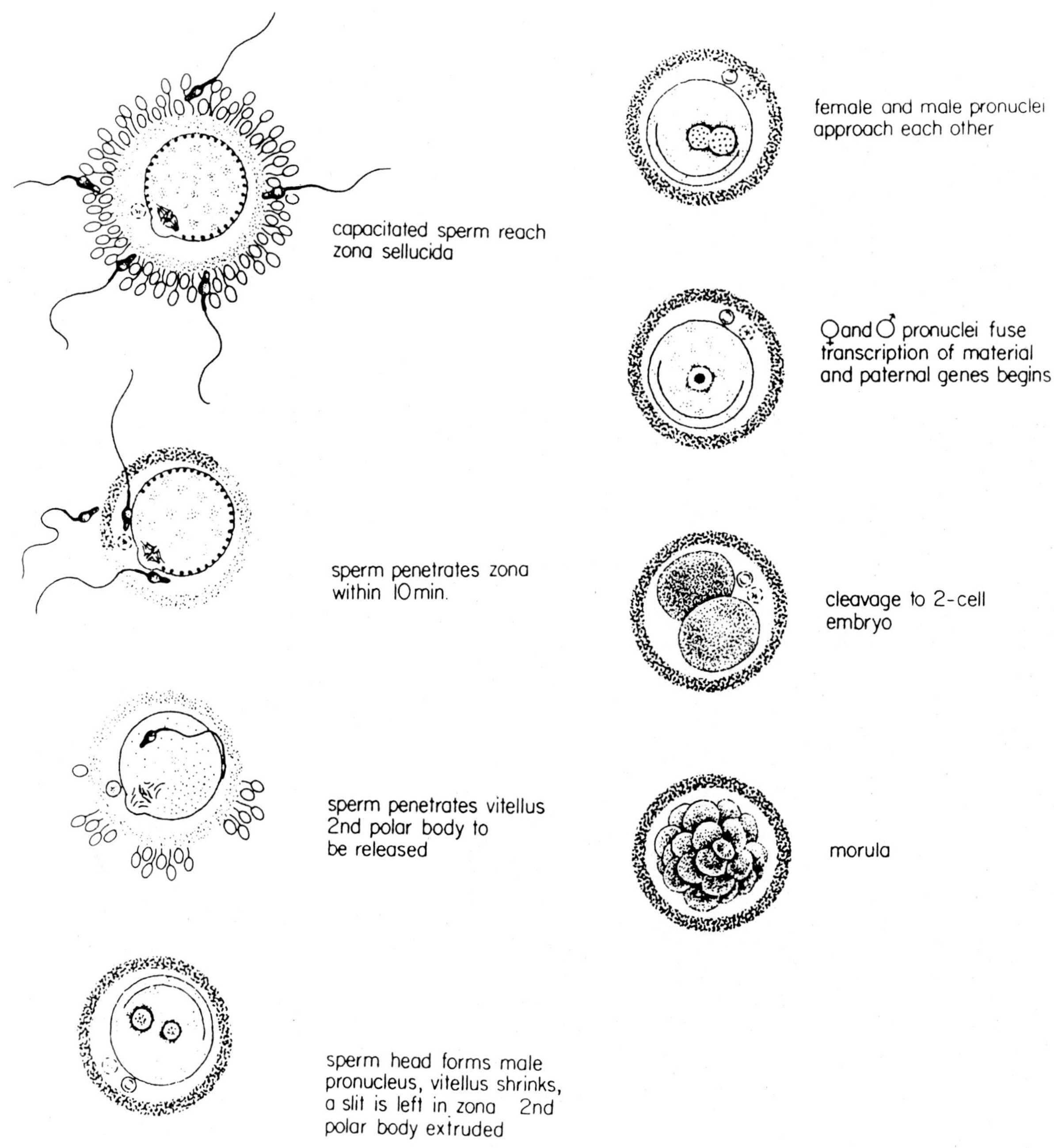


FIGURE 8-5. Sequence of events of fertilization/cleavage to the 2-cell blastomere, morula, and early blastocyst.

whereas prostaglandins of the E series appear to accelerate their delivery to the uterus.

Eggs are transported from the oviduct into the uterus whether or not fertilization has taken place, the horse being an exception. In the mare, unfertilized eggs remain within the isthmus and slowly degenerate over several months, while developing embryos pass by them and enter the uterus (37). The rate at which cleavage divisions progress is impacted by environmental and genetic influences. Warner et al. (38) described a gene in preimplantation mouse embryos which is associated with the murine histocompatibility complex which influences rate of cleavage of mouse embryos.

### *Expression of Genome*

At ovulation, eggs contain rRNA, mRNA, tRNA, and ribosomes and are fully equipped to synthesize proteins. An ordered set of changes in the synthesis and modification of proteins occurs during oocyte maturation, fertilization, and

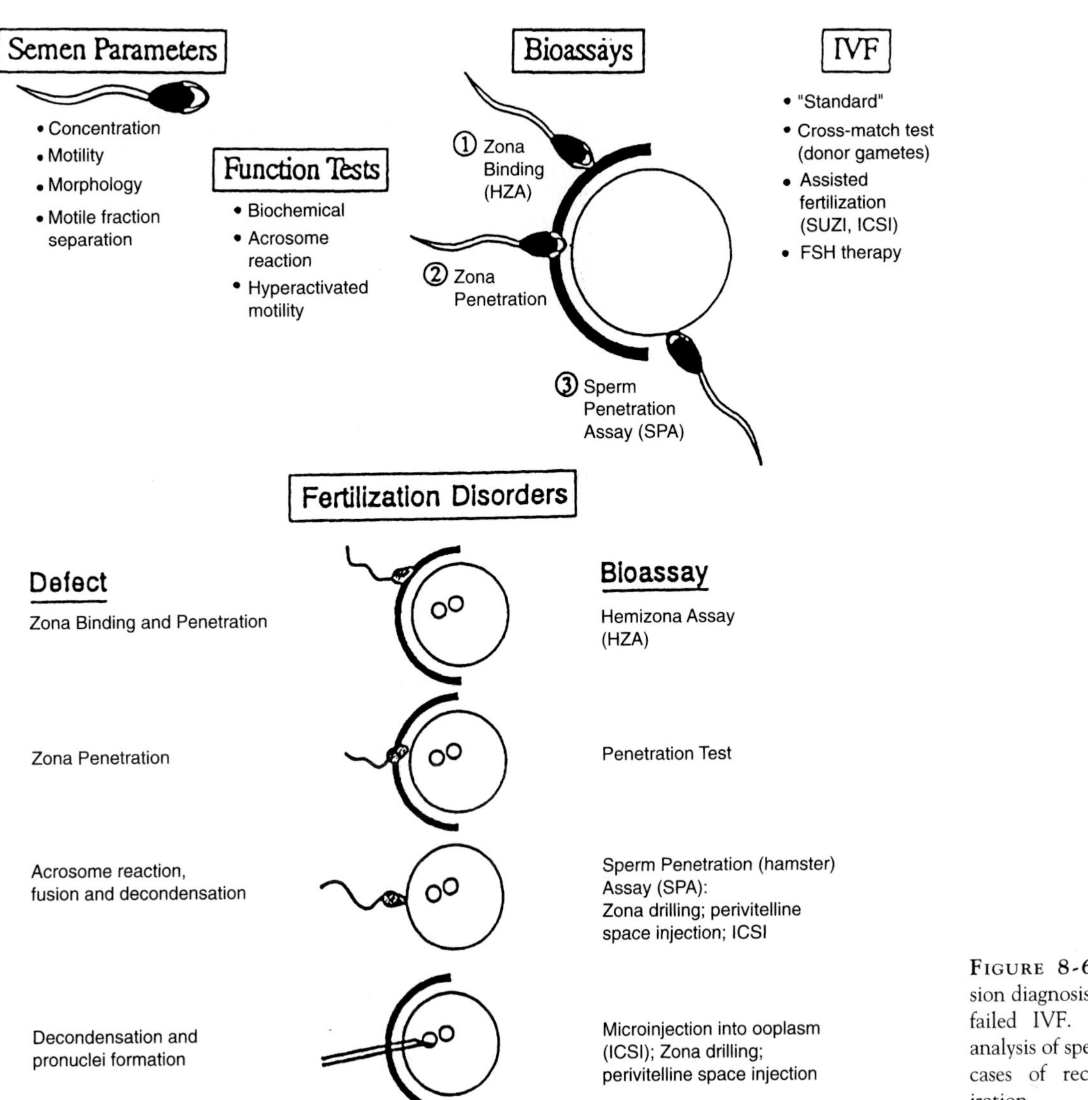


FIGURE 8-6. Stepwise progression diagnosis in cases of recurrent failed IVF. (*Bottom*) Sequential analysis of specific sperm defects in cases of recurrent failed fertilization.

development until the two-cell stage. Embryos proceed in their development from the first cleavage division to the blastocyst stage, where there is an active transcription and accumulation of new mRNA from the zygote genome (39). The embryo becomes dependent on transcription just after the first cleavage division with a concomitant increase in synthesized protein occurring by the two-cell stage (40). In sheep, total protein synthesis is high during the first two cleavage divisions, decreases by 95% by the third cleavage division, remains low in the fourth cleavage division (8 to 16 cells) and increases again in the fifth cleavage division (16 to 32 cells) (41). Full activation of transcription in sheep embryos occurs in the fourth cleavage division. Similar findings are reported for cow embryos (42). Shortly after initiation of embryogenesis, synthesis of all commonly identified classes of RNA is initiated.

Embryonic gene products such as specific enzymes or antigens can be produced in different ways. For instance, these proteins could be produced at all stages in most, or all, embryonic cells. Proteins in this category include enzymes essential for normal metabolic activity as well as ubiquitous structural proteins such as actin, tubulin, and spectrin. In contrast, other proteins during development are referred to as temporal gene products. For example, the serine protease plasminogen activator is present in trophoblast and primitive endoderm cells. This protease is a temporal product of swine, cow, and sheep (43) embryos during peri-implantation development.

Studies concerning mechanisms for controlling expression of development gene products in domestic species are few. Simmen and Simmen (44) suggest that peptide growth factors and their associated proteins may play an important role in critical aspects of conceptus growth and uterineconceptus interactions during the peri-implantation period.

### *Parthenogenesis*

Parthenogenesis, the development of an egg without intervention of the sperm, occurs in many invertebrate species and in some vertebrate species. Early stages of parthenogenesis can be induced or may occur spontaneously; however, the activated eggs do not usually cleave more than twice before dying.

Mammalian oocytes and eggs do on occasion start developing into embryos in the absence of any detected stimulus. In such cases female germ cells may possess an inherent tendency to divide and differentiate, which is enhanced by fertilization or inducers of the parthenogenic response.

Generation of one-cell embryos using nuclear transfer with two male pronuclei to form "androgenones" or with two female pronuclei to form "gynogenones" can be accomplished experimentally, but both fail to develop to term (33). Paternal and maternal contributions to the diploid genome of embryonic cells are necessary because they play complementary roles in the development process. Surani et al. (33) demonstrated that the parental origin of chromosomes determines their influence during embryogenesis, and therefore contributions from parental genomes are not functionally equivalent during conceptus development. Parthenogenic and normal embryonic cells can be combined to form "chimeras" that can survive to term. Renard et al. (45) used embryo reconstruction techniques with mouse embryos to produce gynogenetic and androgenetic haploid embryos from which blastomeres were obtained at the four-cell stage. Single blastomeres from the androgenones and gynogenones were then fused and allowed to form diploid doublets. Two or three of these doublets were then transferred to a foster mother and some developed to term.

### *Twinning and Embryo Manipulation*

Twinning in monotocous domestic species is most frequently of the dyzygotic type in which more than one egg is ovulated and the eggs are fertilized by different sperm, resulting in offspring no more identical than other full siblings. The twinning rate in domestic animals is affected by breed, age, and environment.

Among cattle, dairy breeds have twinning rates of about 3.5%, whereas in beef breeds the average is less than 1.0%. Twin pregnancies, one conceptus per uterine horn, have no detrimental effect on calf viability; therefore, in cattle the major factor limiting increased multiple births appears to be ovulation rate. With twin pregnancy in cattle, fusion of the chorioallantois of adjacent conceptuses results in a common blood circulation. Therefore, 91% of heifers born co-twin with a male are sterile freemartins. Although rare, similar conditions have been reported in sheep, goats, and pigs.

Highly prolific ewes such as Finnsheep and Booroola Merino often produce two or more offspring per lambing. These ewes have a high ovulation rate which, in the Booroola Merino ewe, has been linked to a major F (fecundity) gene (46). This gene may be responsible for elevated levels of FSH in both ewe lambs and adult ewes, an observation also reported for other prolific breeds of sheep.

The incidence of dizygotic twins is 1 to 2% in thoroughbred mares and near 3% in draft-type mares. Double ovulations are fairly common in mares, but one or both embryos usually die early in development, while those that continue to develop are prone to abortion, mummification or, if born alive, neonatal death. Fetal death among twins in utero is often attributed to placental insufficiency or inadequate uterine capacity since total placental surface area of twins is only slightly greater than that of a single fetus. Twins occurring naturally reflect differences in ovulation rate as well as the ability of the female to maintain a twin pregnancy.

A major factor regulating the number of twin pregnancies is the number of eggs ovulated. Ovulation rate can be increased by exogenous gonadotropin (usually equine chorionic gonadotropin, ECG) administration in cattle and sheep; however, ovarian response is variable and not conducive to twinning. When two ovulations occur unilaterally, the twin pregnancy rate is low, whereas when a single ovulation occurs on each ovary, the incidence of twinning is higher. This difference has been attributed to competition between embryos since transfer of two embryos to the same uterine horn leads to reduced numbers of cotyledonary attachments compared to results when one embryo was transferred to each uterine horn. A twinning rate of about 60% can be achieved using bilateral embryo transfer.

Immunization against ovarian steroids, particularly androstenedione or estrone, leads to a dramatic increase in the ovulation rate in ewes and to a lesser degree in cows. In ewes, the mean ovulation rate was increased by 0.6 ovulations per ewe, which resulted in an increase in the number of lambs reared. This process, however, results in increased embryonic deaths in sheep. Immunization against recombinant $\alpha$-subunit of bovine inhibin results in a three-fold to four-fold increase in ovulation rate in sheep and a 35% increase in ovulation rate in pigs (47).

Twins can also be monozygotic, in which case a single fertilized egg gives rise to two identical offspring. The incidence of naturally occurring monozygotic twins is rare with only a few species such as humans and cattle having well-documented occurences. In cattle, monozygotic twins represent 10% or less of twins born. Monozygotic twins usually originate after implantation when the inner cell mass differentiates into two primitive streaks, giving rise to two identical offspring.

Nuclear transplantation involves the transfer of individual nuclei from preimplantation embryos to unfertilized mature oocytes and has been used successfully in the "cloning" of sheep, cow, and rabbit embryos, which has resulted in birth of viable offspring. Offspring produced by nuclear transfer may not be true clones, because most of the mitochondrial genome originates from the cytoplasm of the recipient oocyte. The principle behind this procedure is that nuclei from embryos contain all of the genetic information necessary to give rise to a complete individual having the same genetic makeup. As embryonic development proceeds, the genetic potential of nuclei become increasingly restricted as a result of differentiation, and they are no longer "totipotent" and can give rise only to specific tissues within the embryo. Nuclei can be transplanted to the cytoplasm of a mature oocyte. Factors within the cytoplasm of the mature oocyte "reprogram" the transplanted nucleus to allow it to give rise to a new embryo. Cytoplasm from pronuclear or two-cell embryos is not able to "reprogram" the transplanted nucleus. Initial results of cloning in rabbits and cows indicated that fewer than 4% and 1%, respectively, of the embryos developed to term. Willadsen et al. (48), working with cattle, and Collas and Robl (49), working with rabbits, have increased those percentages to 33% and 21%, respectively.

Production of monzygotic twins can also be achieved by microsurgical separation of blastomeres of two-cell embryos. The technical details of this are discussed in a later chapter.

## EARLY EMBRYONIC DEVELOPMENT

### *Blastocyst Formation*

Development of tight intercellular junctions of the morula during compaction is followed by accumulation of fluid within the central cavity forming the blastocoele. Differentiation of two distinct cell populations occurs after blastocyst formation. The majority of cells form the outside peripheral cuboidal layer, termed *trophoblast* or *trophectoderm*, which is covered by dense microvilli and functions in selective nutrient uptake. Later in development, the trophoblast will form the chorion. A second group of cells residing at one pole beneath the trophoblast form the embryoblast (inner cell mass), which develops into three primary germ layers of the embryo (ectoderm, mesoderm, and endoderm) during the process of gastrulation.

### *Zona Hatching*

Release (hatching) of the blastocyst from the zona pellucida (Fig. 8-6) occurs in the uterus 4 to 8 days postovulation (Table 8-2). Changes in zona integrity that are due to enzymatic factors produced by the uterus or embryo have been implicated in hatching of pig blastocysts. Exposure to the estrogen-stimulated uterine environment may cause a softening of the zona pellucida and allow the blastocyst to expand and rupture the zona layer. Expansion and contraction of the cow blastocyst appears to play the major role in hatching as the zona becomes torn by distension of the blastocyst, although enzymes involved with zona weakening may also play a role. The zona ruptures on the equatorial plane, allowing the blastocyst to squeeze between the two edges of the opening.

Prostaglandins (especially of the E series) are involved with the hatching process since prostaglanding antagonists prevent both blastocyst expansion and hatching. Thus expansion of the blastocyst appears to be a vital process for zona hatching with production of uterine or blastocyst enzymatic factors playing a supporting role. On day 11 postestrus in the sheep and pig, and day 13 in the cow, the blastocyst undergoes a logarithmic elongation phase. The cow blastocyst transforms from a 3 mm spherical shape on approximately day 13 to a 25 cm filamentous threadlike form on day 17. By day 18 of gestation, the blastocyst has extended into the contralateral horn. This rapid lateral conceptus elongation in sheep and cattle occurs through continual hyperplasia of trophectoderm and extraembryonic endoderm.

Rapid growth of cow and sheep blastocysts occurs over several days, but the rate of elongation of the pig blastocyst is unsurpassed. Pig blastocysts develop from 2 mm spheres on approximately day 10 of pregnancy to 10 mm tubular blastocysts on day 11 to 12. The tubular blastocysts transform (at a rate of 30 to 40 mm/hr) into a thin filamentous form that measures approximately 20 cm in length. This occurs by cellular reorganization rather than cellular-hyperplasia. After this initial elongation phase, the pig blastocyst continues to increase in length and diameter as a result of cellular hyperplasia and reaches lengths of 800 to 1000 mm by day 16.

Rapid blastocyst elongation in pigs is unique to each blastocyst within the litter. Those that reach the tubular stage earliest may have a competitive edge for survival over slower developing blastocysts by obtaining sufficient uterine surface area necessary to support continued development.

Horse blastocysts do not change from a spherical to a filamentous morphology during early development. The embryonic vesicle diameter increases at 2 to 3 mm per day and retains its spherical form until days 17 to 19, when it conforms to the shape of the uterine lumen.

### *Intrauterine Migration and Spacing*

Intrauterine migration and equidistant spacing between embryos is essential to embryonic survival in polytocous species. Pig embryos are found near the tip of the uterine horn 5 to 6 days after initiation of estrus and then migrate toward the uterine body, with embryos entering and mixing with embryos in the opposite uterine horn as early as day 9. Migration and spacing of the embryos is terminated on approximately day 12, when rapid blastocyst elongation occurs.

Transuterine migration is rare in mono-ovulatory ewes and cows. However, intrauterine migration will occur in sheep but not cows when multiple ovulations occur on the same ovary. This is a major problem when superovulation is used to increase the twinning rate in cattle.

Using ultrasound to monitor embryonic movement in mares, transuterine migrations occurred approximately 13 times per day between days 10 to 16 of gestation (50). Fixation of the embryo within the uterine lumen occurs on day 16, although migration is possible as late as days 25 to 30 gestation.

## REFERENCES


1. Eddy EM. The spermatozoa. In: Knobil E, Neil J, eds. The physiology of reproduction. New York: Raven Press, 1988;27–68.
2. Bellve AR, O'Brien R. The mammalian spermatozoa: structure and temporal assembly. In: Harrman IF, ed. Mechanism and Control of Animal Fertilization. New York: Academic Press, 1983;55–137.
3. Flechon JE. Ultrastructural and cytochemical analysis of the mammalian sperm plasma membrane during epididymal maturation. Prog Reprod Biol 1981;8:90–99.
4. Eddy EM, Vernon RB, Muller CH, Hahnel AC, Fenderson BA. Immunodissection of sperm surface modifications during epididymal maturation. Am J Anat 1985;174:225–237.
5. Hirayania T, Quinn P, Marrs R. Fertilizing ability of mouse spermatozoa from different regions of the epididymis microsurgically injected into the perivitelline space of oocytes. Fertil Steril 1991; (Suppl):S-II.
6. Olson GE, Orgebin-Crist MC. Sperm surface changes during epididymal maturation. Ann NY Acad Sci 1982;383: 372–391.
7. Courot M. Transport and maturation of spermatozoa. Prog Reprod Biol 1981;8:67–79.
8. Storey BT. Sperm capacitation and the acrosome reaction. Ann NY Acad Sci 1991;637:457–473.
9. Fraser LR, Ahuja KK. Metabolic and surface events in fertilization. Gamete Res 1988;20;491–519.
10. Fraser LR. Sperm capacitation and its modulation. In: Bavister BD, et al., ed. Mammalian Fertilization. Norwell, Massachusetts: Serono Symposia, USA, 1990;141–153.
11. O'Rand MG. Modification of the sperm membrane during capacitation Ann NY Acad Sci 1982;383:392–404.
12. Holt WV. Membrane heterogeneity in the mammalian spermatozoa. Int Rev Cytol 1984;81:159–194.
13. Clegg EC. Mechanisms of mammalian sperm capacitation. In: Hartmann JF, ed. Mechanism and Control of Animal Fertilization. New York: Academic Press, 1983;177–212.
14. Fraser LR. Mechanisms controlling mammalian fertilization In: Finn CA, ed. Oxford Review of Reproductive Biology. Oxford: Clarendon Press, 1984;6:174–225.
15. Hirst PJ, DeMayo FJ, Dukelow WR. Xenogenous fertilization of laboratory and domestic animals in the oviduct of the pseudopregnant rabbit. Theriogenology 1981;15:67–75.
16. Wassarman PM. Profile of a mammalian sperm receptor. Development 1990;108:1–17.
17. Schatten H, Schatten G, eds. The Molecular Biology of Fertilization. New York: Academic Press, 1989.
18. Michod RF, Levin BR, eds. The Evolution of Sex. Saunderland, Massachusetts: Sinauer Associates, 1987.
19. Metz CB, Monroy A, eds. Biology of Fertilization. New York: Academic Press, 1985;1:111.
20. Koehler J, Nudelman ED, Hakomori S. A collagen-binding protein of the surface of ejaculated rabbit spermatozoa. J Cell Biol 1980;86:529–536.
21. Bedford JM, Cooper GW. Membrane fusion events in fertilization of vertebrate eggs. In: Poste G, Nicolson GL, eds. Membrane Surface Reviews (Membrane Fusion). Amsterdam: North Holland, 1978;5:65–125.
22. Saling PM. Mammalian sperm interaction with extracellular matrices of the egg. In: Milligan SR, ed. Oxford Review of Reproductive Biology. Oxford: Oxford University Press, 1989;11:339–388.
23. Rankin TL, Tsuruta KJ, Holland MY, Griswold MD, Orgebin-Crist MC. Isolation, immunolocalization and sperm-association of three proteins of 18, 25 and 29 killodaltons secreted by the mouse epididymis. Biol Reprod 1992;46:747–766.
24. Koehler JK ed. Gamete Surfaces and Their Interactions. New York: Alan R Liss, 1985.
25. Longo FJ. Fertilization. New York: Chapman & Hall, 1987.
26. Hartmann JF, ed. Mechanism and Control of Animal Fertilization. New York: Academic Press, 1983.
27. Dunbar BS, O'Rand MG, eds. A comparative overview of mammalian fertilization. New York: Plenum Press, 1991.
28. Yanagimachi R. Mechanisms of fertilization in mammals. In: Fertilization and Embryonic Development *in Vitro*. New York: Plenum Press, 1981;81–187.
29. Moore HDM, Bedford JM. The interaction of mammalian gametes in the female. In: Hartmann JF, ed. Mechanism and Control of Animal Fertilization. New York: Academic Press, 1983;453–497.
30. Suarez SS, Drost M, Redfern, Gottibe W. Sperm motility in oviduct. In: Bavister BB, Cummins J, eds. Fertilization in Mammals, 1990.
31. McLaren A. Fertilization, cleavage and implantation. In: Hafez ESE, ed. Reproduction in Farm Animals. Philadelphia: Lea & Febiger, 1974.
32. Killeen ID, Moore NW. Fertilization and survival of fertilized eggs in the ewe following surgical insemination at various times after the onset of oestrus. Aust J Biol Sci 1970;23:1279–1287.
33. Surani MAH, Barton SC. Development of gynogenetic eggs in the mouse: implications for parthenogenic embryos. Science 1983;22:1034.
34. Papaioannou VE, Ebert KM. Comparative aspects of embryo manipulation in mammals. In: Rossant J, Pedersen RA, eds. Experimental Approaches to Mammalian Embryonic Development. New York: Cambridge University Press, 1986.
35. Sutherland AE, Speed TP, Calarco PG. Inner cell allocation in the mouse morula: the role for oriented division during fourth cleavage. Dev Biol 1990;137:13–25.
36. Ducibelle T. Surface changes in the developing trophoblast

cell. In: Johnson MH, ed. Development in Mammals. North Holland: Amsterdam, 1977;1:5–30.

37. Van Neikerk CH, Gerneke WH. Pesistence, and parthenogenetic cleavage of tubal ova in the mare. Onderstepoort J Vet Res 1966;33:195–232.
38. Warner CA, Gollnick SO, Goldbard SB. Linkage of the preimplantation-embryo development (ped) gene to the mouse major histocompatability complex (MHC). Biol Reprod 1987;36:606–610.
39. Schultz GA. Utilization of genetic information in the preimplantation mouse embryo. In: Rossant J, Pederson RA, eds. Experimental Approaches to Mammalian Embryonic Development. New York: Cambridge University Press, 1986.
40. Bolton VN, Oades PJ, Johnson ME. The relationship between cleavage, DNA replication and gene expression in the 2-cell mouse embryo. J Embryol Exp Morph 1984;79:139–163.
41. Crosby IM, Gandolfi F, Moor RM. Control of protein synthesis during early cleavage of sheep embryos. J Reprod Fertil 1988;82:769–775.
42. King WA, Niar A, Chartrain I, Betterridge KJ, Quay P. Nucleolus organizer regions and nucleoli in preattachment bovine embryos. J Reprod Fertil 1988;82:87–95.
43. Menino AR, Dyk AR, Gardiner CS, Gorbner MA, Kaaekuahiwi MA, Williams JS. The effects of plaminogen on *in vitro* ovine embryo development. Biol Reprod 1989;41:899–905.
44. Simmen FA, Simmen RCM. Peptide growth factors and protooncogenes in mammalian conceptus development. Biol Reprod 1991;44:1–5.
45. Renard JP, Babinet B, Barra J. Participation of the paternal genome is not required before the eight-cell stage for full-term development of mouse embryos. Dev Biol 1991;143:199–202.
46. Bindon BM, Piper LR. Endocrine differences in ovine prolificacy. Proc Int Cong Animal Reprod Artif Insem. 1984; 4;17–26.
47. Brown RW, Hungerford JW, Greenwood PE, Bloor RJ, Evans DF, Tsonis CG, Forage RG. Immunization against recombinant bovine inhibin a subunit causes increased ovulation rates in gilts. J Reprod Fertil 1990;90:199–205.
48. Willadsen SM, Janzen RE, McAlister JJ, Shea BF, Hamilton G, McDermand D. The viability of late morula and blastocysts produced by nuclear transplantation in cattle. Theriogenology 1991;35:161–170.
49. Collas P, Robl JM. Factors affecting the efficiency of nuclear transplantation in the rabbit embryo. Biol Reprod 1990; 43:877–884.
50. Leith GS, Ginther OJ. Intrauterine mobility of the early equine conceptus. Proc 10th Int Congress on Animal Reprod and Artif Insem. 1984;11;118.

CHAPTER 9

# Implantation

R.D. GEISERT AND J.R. MALAYER

## EARLY EMBRYONIC DEVELOPMENT

### *Blastocyst Formation*

Development of tight intercellular junctions of the morula during compaction is followed by the accumulation of fluid with the central cavity forming the blastocoele. Fluid accumulation within the blastocoele results from the movement of water, a result of mitochondrial metabolism, following the localization of active $Na^+/K^+$ pumps on the basal membrane of the trophectoderm. Because of the placement of the $Na^+/K^+$ pumps for active ion transport, a solute gradient is established which induces fluid movement into the blastocoele forming the blastocyst.

Expansion of the blastocoele positions cells of the tight morula to be either on the outside or inside of the fluid filled vesicle. This positioning leads to the formation of the trophoblast (outside cell layer) and the inner cell mass (embryoblast) which resides at one pole beneath the trophoblast (Fig. 9-1). Differentiation of these two specific cell layers provides the initial cells that eventually contribute to formation of the placenta and embryo. The inner cell mass develops three primary germ layers of the embryo (ectoderm, mesoderm, and endoderm) during the process called gastrulation. These primary germ layers differentiate into the skin, hair, muscle, nervous system, skeleton, and organs that form the embryo. Outside the trophoblast is covered by dense microvilli that function to contact and adhere to the maternal uterine epithelium for placental attachment and nutrient uptake. Following hatching from the zona pellucida, trophectoderm of the trophoblast will become lined with mesoderm which expands out from the inner cell mass to form the outer membrane of the placenta called the chorion (Fig. 9-2).

### *Zona Hatching*

Blastocyst hatching or escape from the zona pellucida occurs within the uterine lumen between 4 to 8 days post-ovulation (Fig. 9-1). Blastocyst hatching occurs through the combined physical and enzymatic actions of the expanding vesicle. During hatching, rhythmic expansion and contraction of the blastocyst will stretch the zona. Expansion of the blastocyst involves both cellular hyperplasia and increased fluid accumulation in the blastocoele. Fluid movement within the blastocyst and hatching appears to involve blastocyst prostaglandin synthesis (especially prostaglandin E) as prostaglandin antagonists can prevent blastocyst expansion and hatching. Activation of enzymes such as plasmin and trypsin by the blastocyst and/or uterus causes softening of the zona matrix allowing the blastocyst to expand and rupture the zona along its equatorial plane. Rupture of the zona permits the blastocyst to squeeze between the two edges of the opening (Fig. 9-1).

### *Intrauterine Migration and Spacing*

Blastocyst escape from the zona pellucida provides the first cell to cell contact between the conceptus (embryo and its extraembryonic membranes) and maternal uterine epithelium. Cellular contact is essential for nutrient exchange and placental attachment. In addition, initially the conceptus of domestic farm species must physically cover a large portion of the maternal endometrium to regulate release of prostaglandin $F_{2\alpha}$ to prevent luteolysis.

Intrauterine migration and equidistant spacing between embryos is essential to embryonic survival in polytocous species. Porcine embryos are found near the tip of the uterine horns 5 to 6 days after initiation of estrus and then migrate toward the uterine body, mixing with embryos in the opposite uterine horn as early as day 9. Migration and equal spacing continue until approximately day 12, when conceptuses undergo a rapid process of trophoblast elongation (Fig. 9-3). Intrauterine migration and spacing appear to be modulated through peristaltic contractions of the myometrium stimulated by the developing conceptus. Conceptus production of histamine, estrogen, and prostaglandins all serve a role in stimulating local myometrial activity to move the conceptus (1). Intrauterine migration in the pig is essential

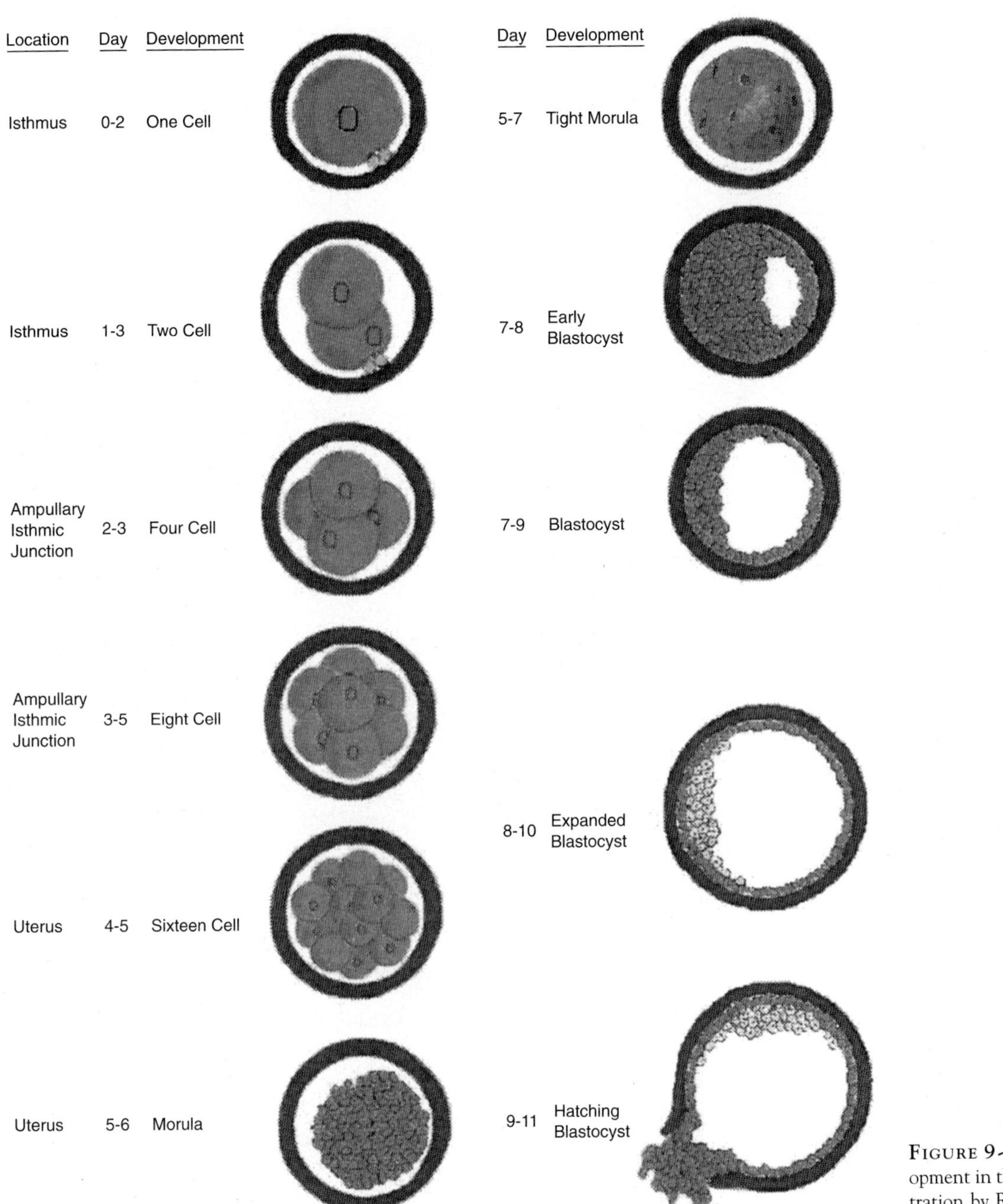


FIGURE 9-1. Stages of early development in the bovine embryo. (Illustration by Randy G. Bradley.)

to not only cover the uterine surface, as maintenance of pregnancy requires the presence of at least two embryos in each uterine horn, but provide space for placental development of the littermate embryos.

Transuterine migration is rare in monovulatory ewes and cows. However, intrauterine migration will occur in sheep when multiple ovulations occur on the same ovary. Migration appears to be stimulated by conceptus estrogen and prostaglandin release.

The conceptus of the mare probably demonstrates the most spectacular form of intrauterine migration of any species. Following hatching from its zona pellucida, the equine conceptus is surrounded by an acellular capsule that forms between the trophoblast and zona when the embryo enters the uterus on day 5. The origin of the capsule appears to be from uterine secretions (2). The capsule will remain for several weeks and may play a role in conceptus migration and protection. Transuterine migration (Fig. 9-4A) can occur from 10 to 13 times per day between days 10 to 16 of gestation (2). Migration of the vesicle back and forth between the uterine horns is essential to inhibit luteolysis in the mare. Conceptus production of prostaglandin E is

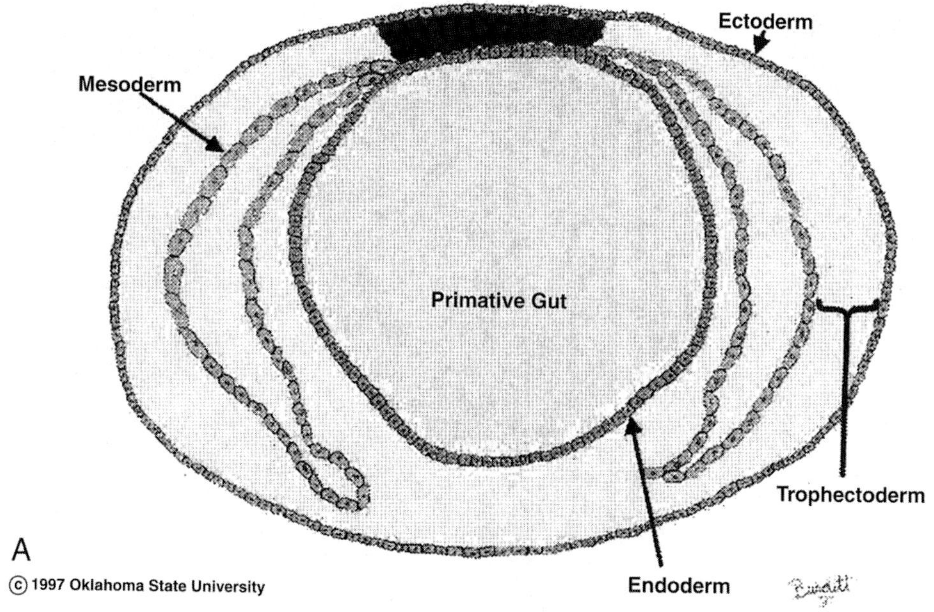


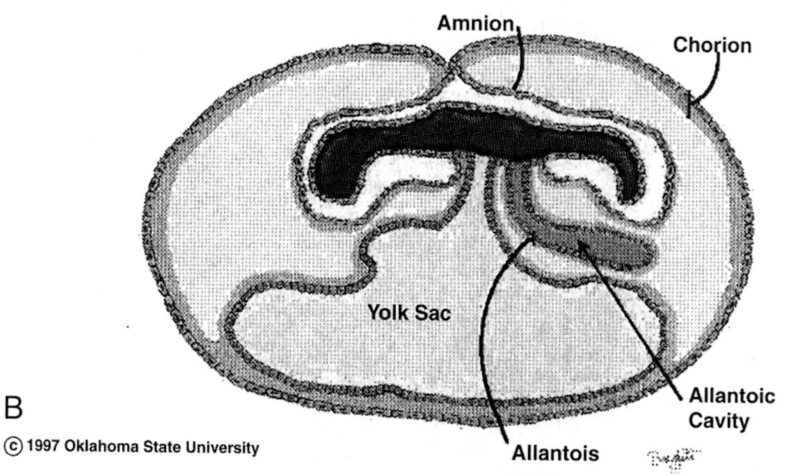


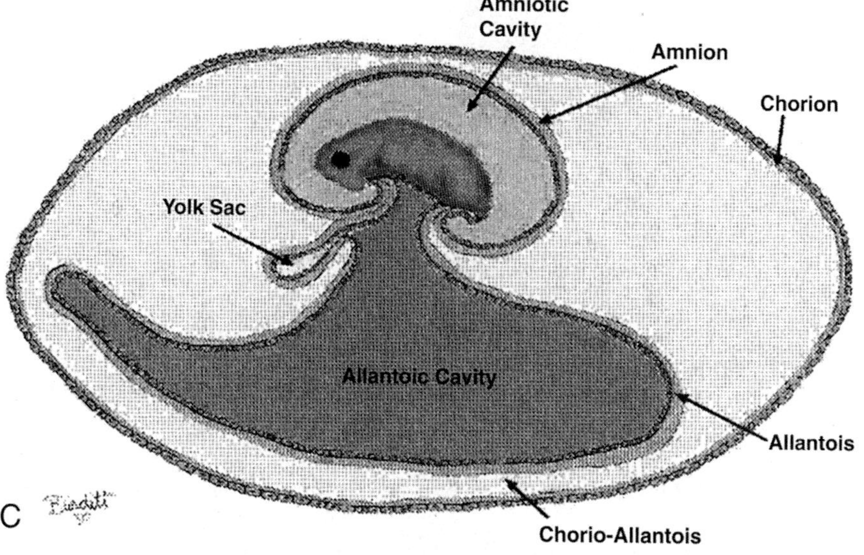


FIGURE 9-2. (**A**) Development of the primary layers for the extraembryonic membranes in the pig on day 13. (**B**) Formation of the yolk sac, amnion, and outgrowth of the allantoic sac on day 16 of gestation. (**C**) Regression of the yolk sac and continued expansion of the allantois from the hindgut which fuses with the chorion to form the chorioallantois. (Illustration by Larry G. Burditt.)

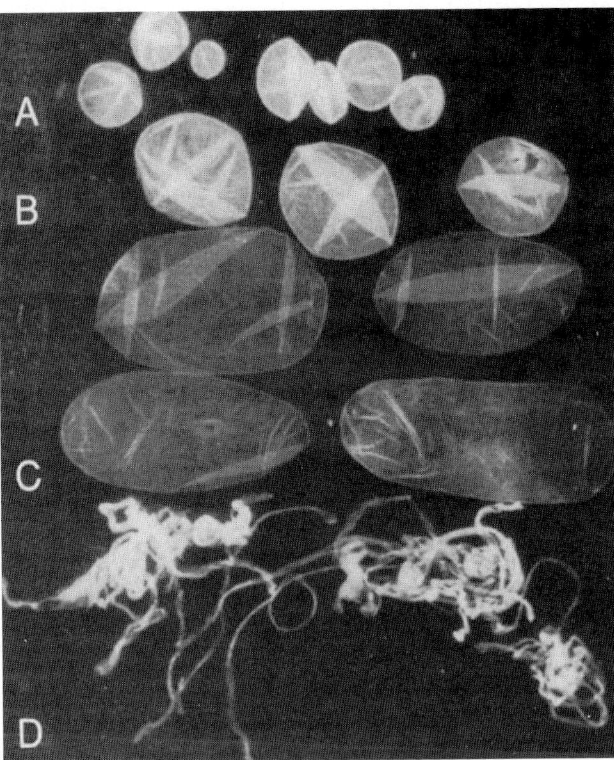


**FIGURE 9-3.** Collage showing rapid development of pig conceptuses through early spherical (**A**, Day 10.5), late spherical (**B**, Day 11), tubular (**C**, Day 11.5), and early filamentous (**D**, Day 12) forms. Pig conceptuses rapidly elongate to block release of $PGF_{2\alpha}$ into the vascular system and gain surface area in the uterus for placental development. (From Rodney Geisert and Fuller Bazer.)

involved with stimulating myometrial contractility to propel the vesicle through the uterine horns. Increase in vesicle diameter, uterine tone, and thickening of the uterine wall induced by conceptus production of estrogen causes fixation of vesicle within the uterine lumen on day 16 of gestation. However, suboptimal concentrations of serum progesterone and/or small vesicle diameter can lead to continued vesicle mobility and possible embryonic loss following day 16. When the embryonic vesicle can no longer migrate and is fixed within the uterine horn, myometrial contractions continue causing the vesicle to rotate so the embryo is oriented to the ventral region of the vesicle (Fig. 9-4**A**). Proper orientation of the embryo results from regional differences in the chorion thickness as mesodermal layer migrates down between the trophectoderm and endoderm.

### *Conceptus Expansion*

Shortly following hatching the blastocyst enters into a phase of rapid growth and development. During this phase, an inner layer of extraembryonic endodermal cells originating from the embryoblast encloses the blastocoele, forming a bilaminar blastocyst. The extraembryonic endoderm cells develop into a continuous membrane that will become a constituent of the yolk sac (Fig. 9-2**B**). Embryoblast (inner cell mass) is visible on the outside of the blastocyst as the layer of trophectoderm covering it (called Rauber cells) has degenerated exposing the embryoblast to the maternal environment. On day 11 postestrus in the ewe and sow, and day 14 or 15 in the cow, the conceptus undergoes a logarithmic growth and elongation phase. The bovine conceptus transforms from a 3 mm spherical shape on approximately day 13, to a 25 cm filamentous form on day 17. By day 18 of gestation, the conceptus has extended into the contralateral (opposite to CL) horn (Fig. 9-4**B**). This rapid lateral conceptus elongation in the ewe and cow occurs through continual hyperplasia of trophoblast. The developing embryoblast that will form the embryo remains in the horn ipsilateral to corpus luteum. Expansion of the trophoblast permits the conceptus to extend its placental membranes throughout the uterus and block the epsilateral horn synthesis of $PGF_{2\alpha}$ to prevent luteolysis.

Rapid growth and expansion of the cow and ewe conceptus throughout the uterus occurs over several days, but the rate of conceptus elongation in the sow is unsurpassed. Porcine conceptuses develop from 2 mm spheres on approximately day 10 of gestation to 10 mm tubular shapes on day 11 or 12 (Fig. 9-3). Tubular conceptuses rapidly (within 2 to 3 hr) elongate (30 to 40 mm/hr) into a thin filamentous thread-like form measuring 20 cm in length (3). Conceptus elongation occurs by cellular reorganization and remodeling rather than cellular hyperplasia as occurs in the ewe and cow. The rapid expansion of each conceptus provides a mechanism for the early embryo to cover the vast uterine surface in the sow (Fig. 9-4**C**). After this initial elongation phase, the conceptus will continue to increase in length and diameter as a result of cellular hyperplasia, reaching lengths of 80 to 100 cm by day 16. Rapid elongation coincides with conceptus estrogen synthesis, which stimulates uterine secretion and is involved with maintenance of the corpora lutea during early pregnancy.

The signal for the rapid transformation of the porcine conceptus on day 12 has not been established. Timing of conceptus elongation in the pig may involve uterine secretions, which includes movement of retinol and appearance of retinoic acid receptors in the conceptus during early development (4). Retinoic acid is known to alter embryonic development, influence extracellular matrix and cell surface adhesive molecules, and induce expression of several peptide growth factors. Rapid elongation of the pig conceptus occurs through trophoblast and endodermal remodeling and movement. This change in morphology would involve changes in the cellular matrix, which is made of collagen and laminin, and cell adhesion through the interaction of integrins (cell adhesion factors). Through its receptor in the conceptus, retinoic acid can stimulate a cascade of cellular remodeling steps possibly by inducing cell production of transforming growth factor-$\beta$, a major modifier of extracellular matrix. Transforming growth factor-$\beta$ activation of proteo-

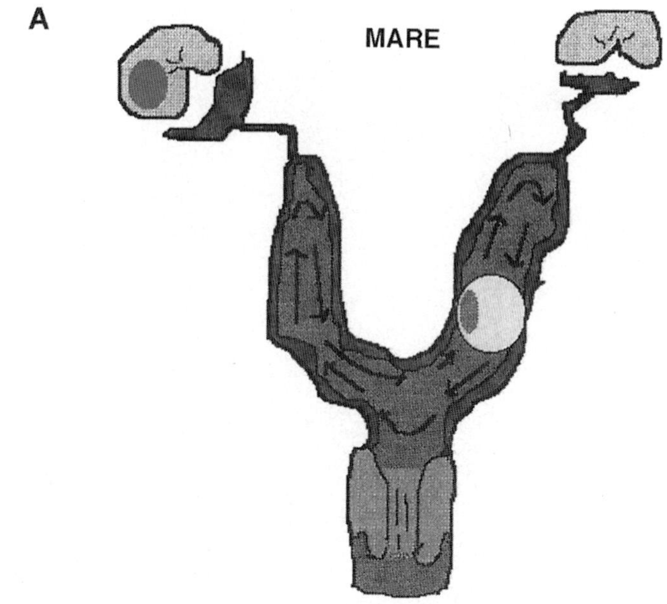


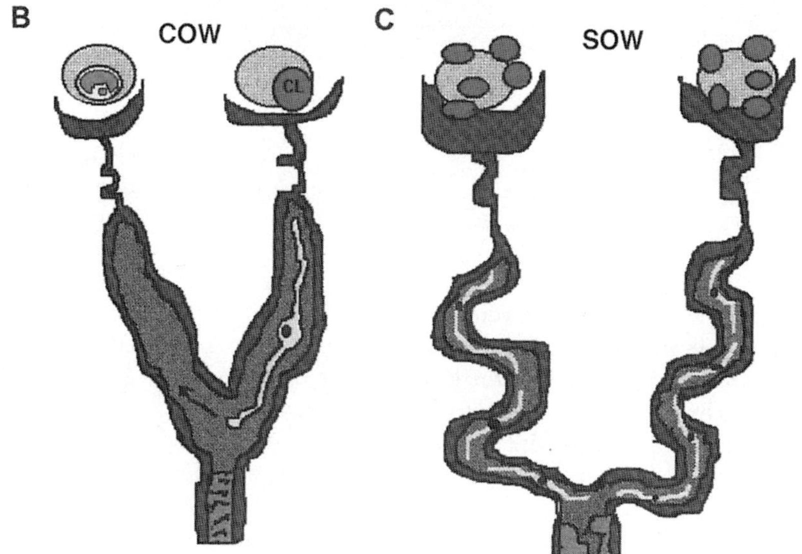


FIGURE 9-4. Methods cover the uterus for inhibition of luteolysis in domestic farm animals. (A) The horse conceptus will migrate between the uterine horns 10 to 13 times per day between day 10 and 16 of gestation. On day 16 the conceptus will become fixed in the uterine lumen of the horn and orient itself so that the embryo is ventral to the vesicle. (B) The bovine conceptus will elongate throughout the ipsilateral horn on day 15 to 17 of gestation, reaching into the contralateral by day 18. (C) Porcine conceptuses rapidly elongate throughout the uterus on day 12 of gestation. Each conceptus can develop a placenta that is close to a meter in length by day 16.

lytic enzymes such as plasminogen activator and metalloproteases may induce breakdown of the extracellular matrix and remodeling of the cells during the rapid morphological change in shape.

Although the majority of littermate conceptuses in the sow are at a similar morphological stages of development and elongation occurs simultaneously, elongation is initiated through gene activation within each conceptus. Spherical conceptuses within a litter can range in diameter, which if the difference is large can lead to a difference of 4 to 24 h in the time of elongation on day 12. These conceptuses most likely represent embryos that are behind in development and could run the highest risk of being lost if uterine space is limited. Because elongation is so rapid and there is a minimum placental surface necessary for survival to term, conceptuses that reach the tubular stage earliest may have a competitive edge for survival over less developed littermates by obtaining sufficient uterine surface area necessary to support continued development.

The conceptus of the mare does not undergo a transformation from spherical to a filamentous morphology during early development. The embryonic vesicle diameter increases at 2 to 3 mm per day until it becomes fixed in the uterine horn on day 16 as described earlier. Embryonic vesicle retains its spherical shape even up to day 50 of gestation. Following continued growth and expansion of the allantochorion, the shape of the placenta will conform to shape of the uterus.

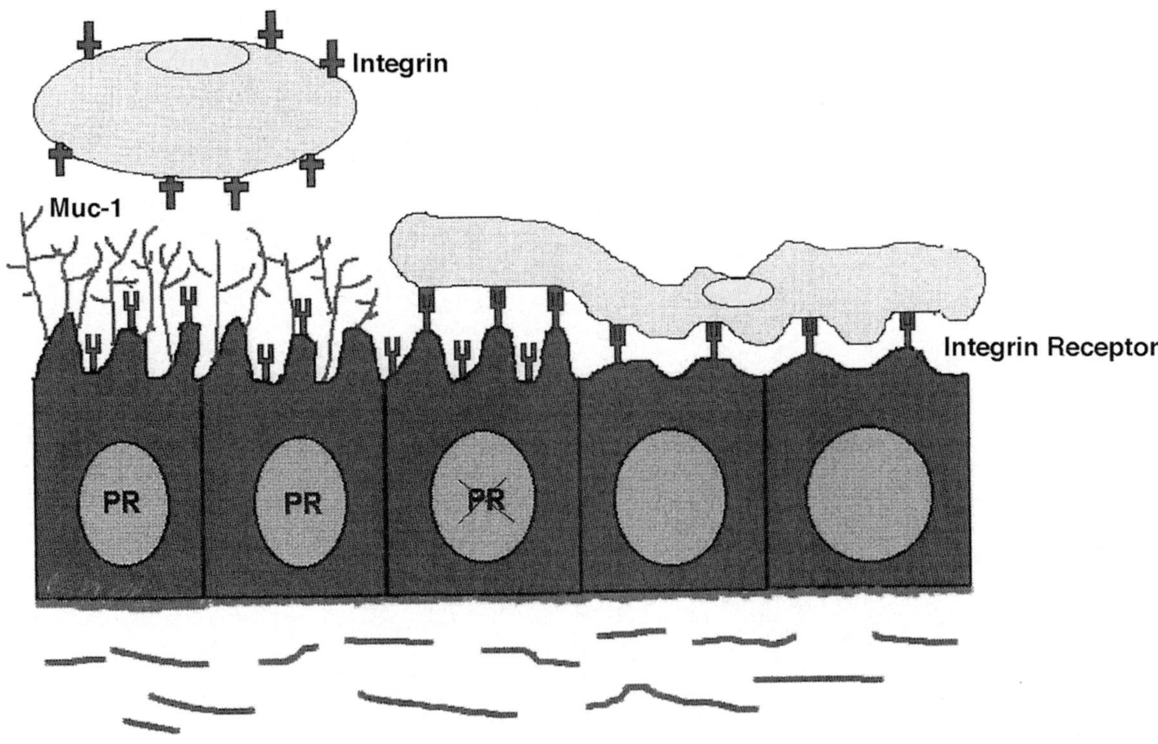


FIGURE 9-5. Implantation of the conceptus in domestic farm species is noninvasive. The conceptus cannot attach to the uterine epithelial surface until the large glycoprotein called Muc-1 has been removed. Muc-1 is stimulated by progesterone which loses its effect on the epithelium when progesterone receptor (PR) down-regulates. The loss of Muc-1 from the epithelial surface permits the contact of integrins with their receptors bringing the conceptus in close contact with the uterine surface and forming epitheliochorial type of placentation. (Illustration by Randy G. Bradley.)

### *Implantation*

What regulates the time in which uterus becomes receptive to attachment by the blastocyst? The apical surface of the uterine epithelium is initially covered by a thick glycocalyx that diminishes as the time for conceptus attachment approaches. One transmembrane glycoprotein, termed Muc-1, is abundant during the nonreceptive phase of pregnancy and could serve as an antiadhesion factor (5). The presence of Muc-1 is greatly reduced, if not absent, during the period of conceptus attachment to the uterine surface. Timing of implantation, or in the case of domestic farm species placental attachment, may be regulated by length of time the uterine endometrium is exposed to progesterone stimulation. Serum concentrations of progesterone rapidly rise following formation of the corpus luteum. Over an 8 to 10 day exposure to progesterone, nuclear progesterone receptors in the uterine epithelium down-regulate leading to a loss of the direct effect of progesterone on this cell type. Since epithelial synthesis of Muc-1 is stimulated by progesterone, loss of progesterone receptor from the uterine epithelium would reduce Muc-1 production and open a receptive state for conceptus attachment (Fig. 9-5).

Rodents and primates have blastocysts that penetrate into the uterine mucosa (6) by phagocytizing and digesting through the uterine luminal epithelium as they migrate into the uterine stroma. These embryos are thus encapsulated beneath the uterine luminal surface. Transformation and proliferation of the uterine stromal cells (referred to as decidualization) accompany this invasive process in the vicinity of the developing blastocyst. The implantation in the mouse and rat is triggered by estrogen release from ovarian follicles on day 4 of pregnancy. Inhibition of follicle estrogen production prevents implantation and induces a state of delayed blastocyst development until estrogen is administered.

In contrast to rodents and primates, implantation in large domestic farm species is superficial and noninvasive (7), and involves phases of trophoblast-uterine epithelial cell apposition and adhesion. The porcine trophoblast, however, does exhibit invasive properties when placed in an ectopic site, such as the kidney capsule. This invasive property results from conceptus production of proteolytic enzymes such as plasminogen activator and other proteases. Invasive implantation like that seen in rodents does not occur in the pig since the conceptus proteases are regulated by uterine secretion of protease inhibitors to plasmin, trypsin, and many serine proteases.

Porcine conceptuses begin to attach to uterine surface on day 13, with attachment completed across the trophoblastic surface between days 18 to 24. Attachment is through interdigitation of uterine and trophoblastic microvilli cov-

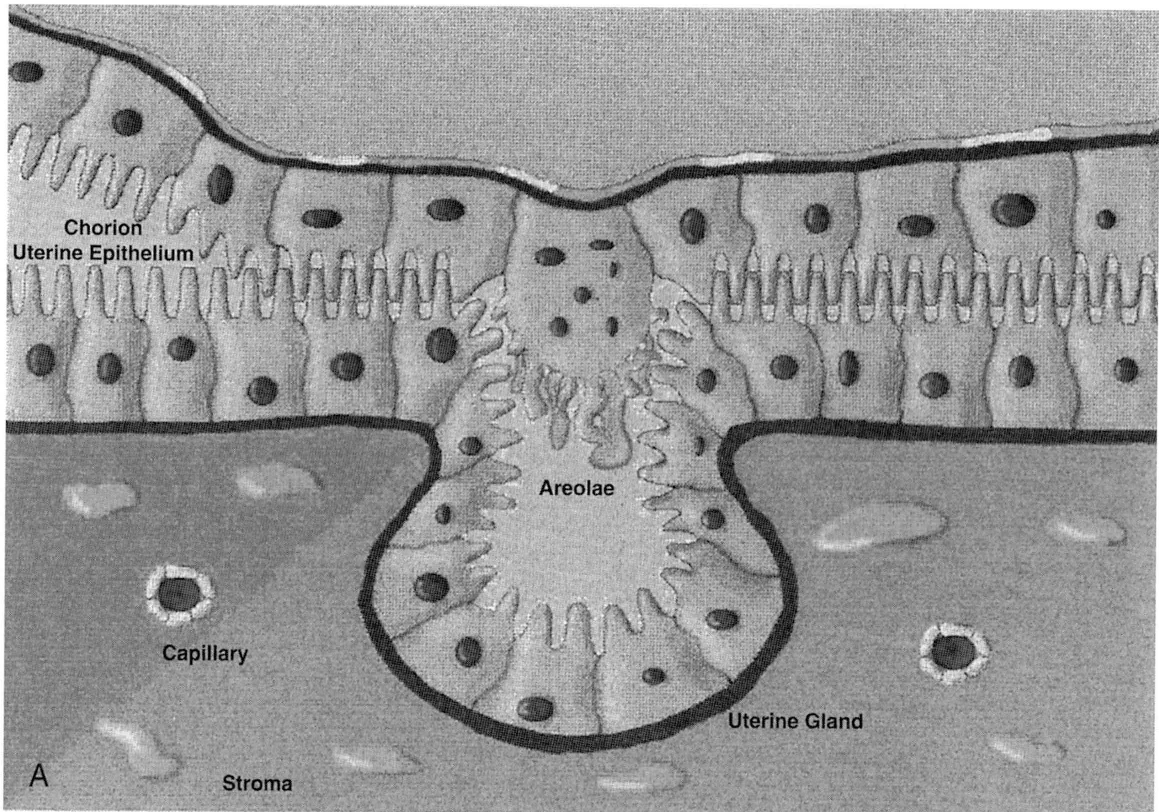


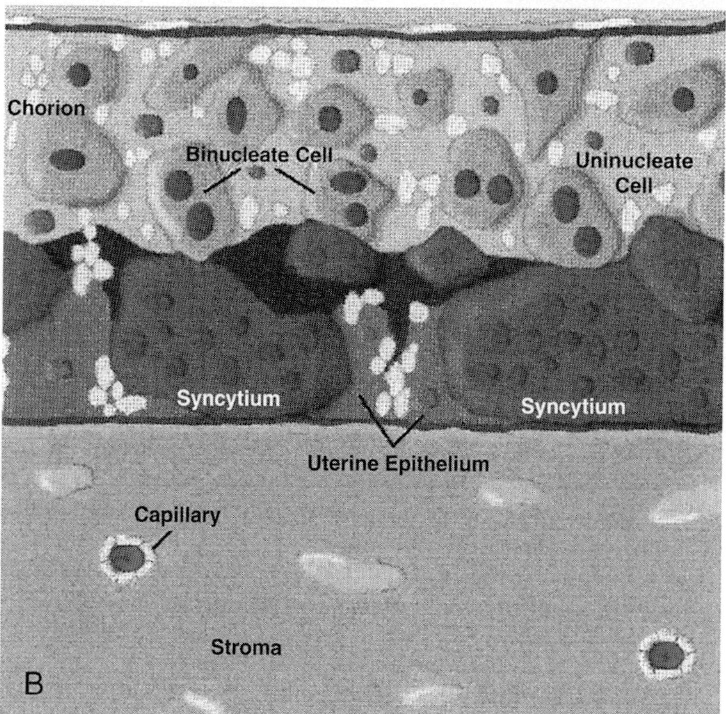


Figure 9-6. Placental attachment. (**A**) Formation of the epitheliochorial type of placental attachment in the pig. Microvilli of the chorion and uterine lumenal epithelium interconnects through a sticky glycocalyx that holds the layers together throughout gestation. Areolae form over the mouths of the uterine glands serving to absorb nutrients for fetal development throughout gestation. (**B**) Initially the chorion forms a epitheliochorial type of attachment similar to the pig. On day 17 some of mononucleate cells of the chorion form into binucleate cells which migrate into the uterine lumenal epithelium. The binucleate cells will fuse with the uterine epithelial cells forming a multinucleated syncytium. Formation of a syncytium may play an immunoprotective role for the developing fetus and also allow the transport of placental lactogen into the maternal vascular to control nutrient movement and mammary gland development. (Illustration by Randy G. Bradley.)

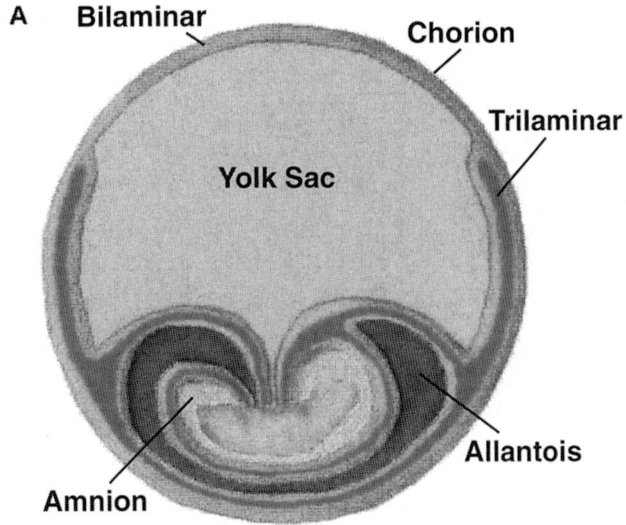


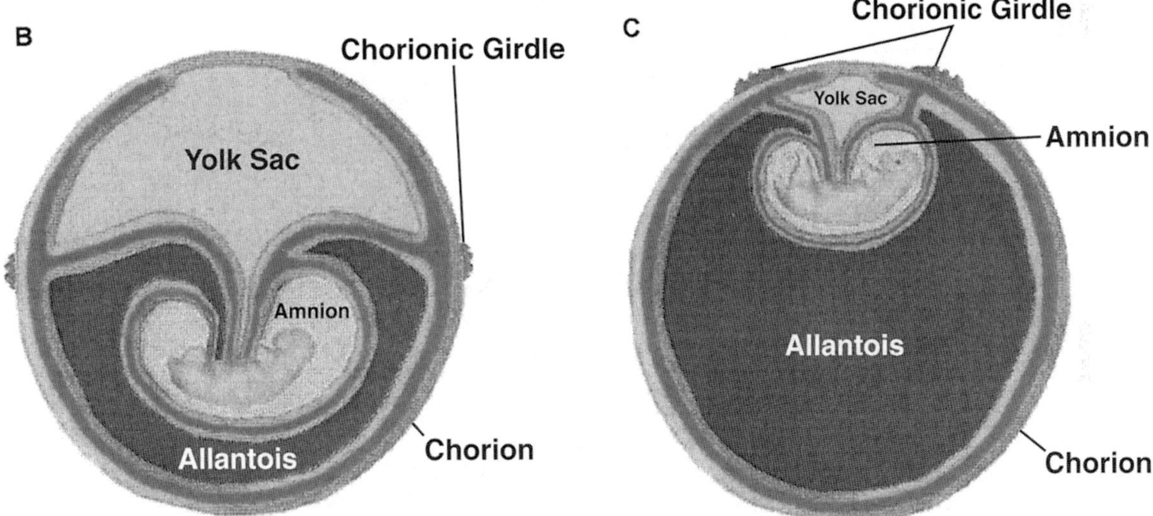


FIGURE 9-7. Placental development in the horse. (**A**) On day 24 the horse conceptus is spherical with placental absorption occurring through the yolk sac which is connected to the chorion. The allantois is beginning to expand from the hindgut. The embryo is ventral to the vesicle when in the uterine lumen at this time. (**B**) The allantois continues to expand as the yolk sac regresses on day 30. Chorionic girdle develops in the region between the allantois and yolk sac. (**C**) The yolk sac is almost completely regressed by day 40 and the allantois has expanded to fill the space within the chorion. With expansion of the allantois, the embryo is now positioned on the dorsal side of the vesicle. The chorionic girdle has descended with the expansion of the allantois and will invade into the endometrium to form endometrial cups shortly. (Illustration by Randy G. Bradley.)

ering the complete interface between the two layers, except where the trophoblast overlies the openings of uterine glands (Fig. 9-6**A**). The trophoblastic surface in these areas becomes modified to form specialized absorptive structures, called areolae, that allow nutrient uptake by the developing conceptus. Loss of Muc-1 allows adhesion between the trophoblast and uterine epithelium of many species including the pig. Removal of the large glycoprotein may permit interaction between adhesive factors such as the integrins (5) and their receptors (Fig. 9-5).

Conceptus attachment in ruminant species involves both caruncular and intercaruncular areas of the uterine endometrium. A transitory attachment first occurs as the bovine and ovine conceptus develop finger-like villi (papil-

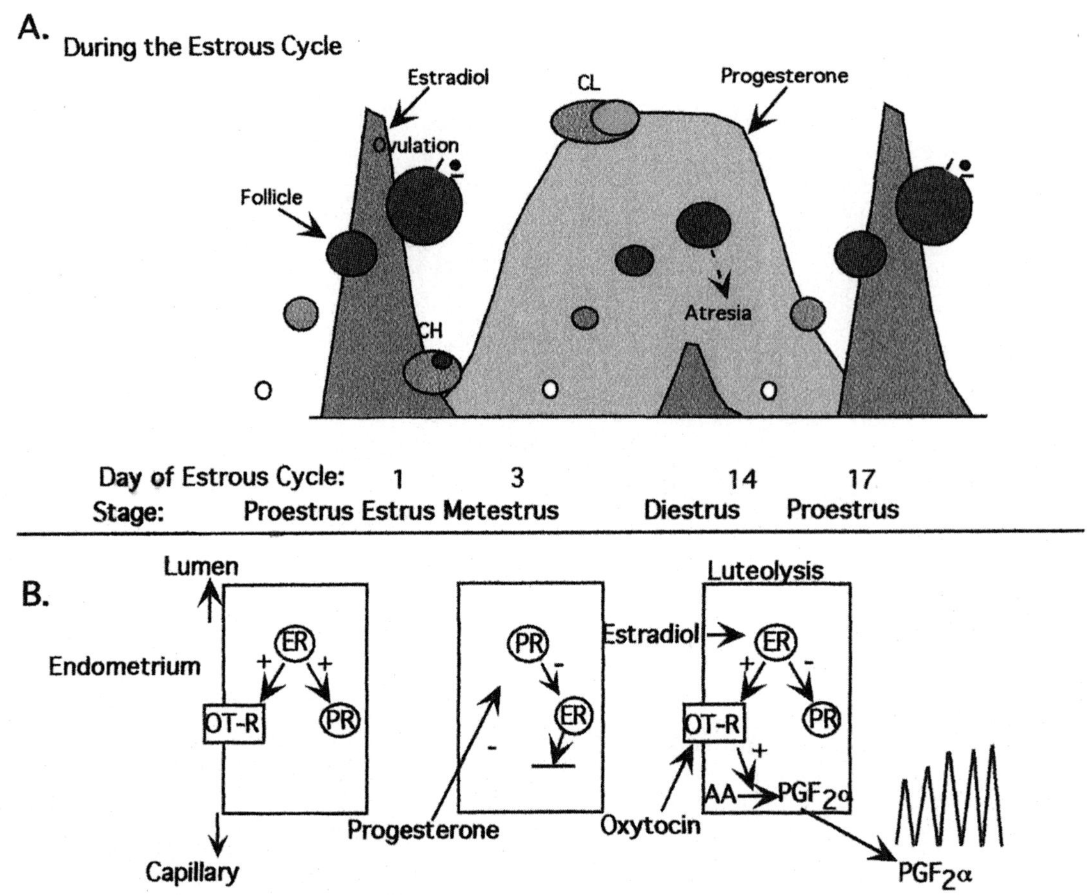


FIGURE 9-8. (A) Relative changes in circulating hormone levels and ovarian changes during the estrous cycle in the sheep. Estrus is characterized by elevated levels of circulating estrogens resulting in sexual receptivity and elevation in endometrial expression of estrogen receptor (*ER*) and progesterone receptor (*PR*). Following ovulation, the ovulatory follicle is transformed into the corpus hemorrhagicum (*CH*) and subsequently into the corpus luteum (*CL*). During metestrus and diestrus, from 3 to 14 days, the CL is producing progesterone at maximum capacity. Additional waves of developing preovulatory follicles produce estrogen before undergoing a programmed regression termed "atresia." (**B**) Changes in endometrial hormone response during the estrous cycle. In cyclic ewes, numbers of endometrial estrogen and progesterone receptors are high between estrus and day 12 of the cycle. Under the influence of progesterone, the uterine endometrium releases very little $PGF_2\alpha$ and appears insensitive to estrogen or oxytocin stimulation, the "progesterone block." By day 14, prolonged exposure to progesterone results in down-regulation of the progesterone receptor, resulting in elevation of estrogen receptor expression and "estrogen dominance." This allows endometrial synthesis of oxytocin receptors to increase, resulting in the endometrium becoming sensitive to oxytocin. Oxytocin stimulation mediated through endometrial oxytocin receptors increases conversion of arachidonic acid to prostaglandins and results in episodic release of $PGF_2\alpha$ and luteolysis.

lae) that project into the lumen of the uterine glands. These papillae provide a temporary anchor and absorptive structure for the conceptus as more complete attachment progresses. Loss or reduction in the height of trophoblastic surface microvilli permits close surface contact with the uterine epithelial microvilli. The uterine epithelium presses into the trophoblastic surface, interlocking with the cytoplasmic projections on the trophoblast surface until the trophoblast microvilli redevelop, forming a more complex attachment.

Placental attachment in ruminants is characterized by the appearance of binucleate cells arising from uninucleate cells of the trophoblast. Binucleate cells first appear on day 17 and are present throughout gestation (Fig. 9-6**B**). These cells migrate and fuse with the underlying uterine surface epithelium to form multinucleate cells or a syncytium. The syncytium may be involved in immunologic protection of the conceptus and the transfer of placental lactogen synthesized by the binucleate cells into the maternal vascular circulation.

Placental attachment does not occur until days 24 to 40 in the mare. Early attachment is through interdigitation between surface epithelium of the embryonic vesicle and uterine lining. On day 25 of gestation, a specialized band of cells called the chorionic girdle forms between the yolk

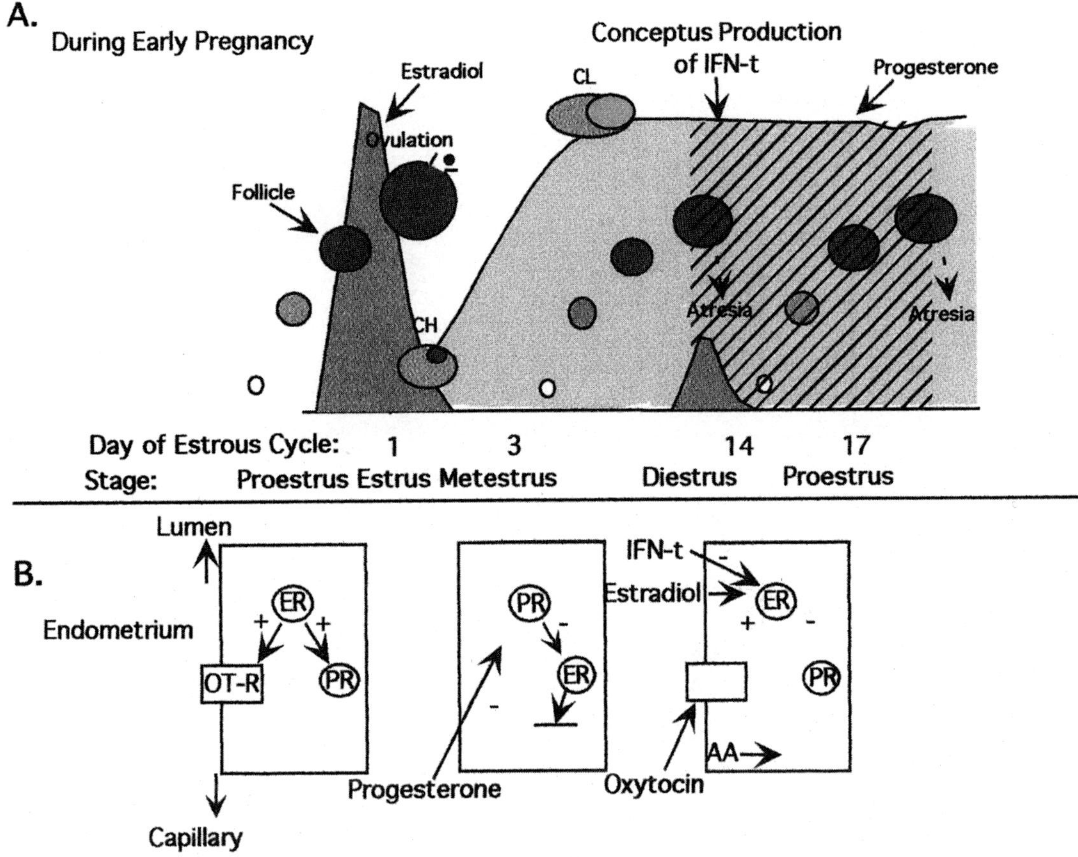


FIGURE 9-9. (A) Relative changes in circulating hormone levels and ovarian changes during early pregnancy in the sheep. Circulating hormone levels and ovarian structures are identical through the first 12 days to the nonpregnant animal. In pregnant ewes, however, conceptus IFN-$\tau$ produced between days 12 and 21 is responsible for maintenance of the CL and progesterone production through suppression of endometrial $PGF_{2\alpha}$ release. (B) Changes in endometrial hormone response during early pregnancy. In pregnant as well as cyclic ewes, numbers of endometrial estrogen and progesterone receptors are high between estrus and day 12 of the cycle. Following the loss of the "progesterone block," conceptus IFN-$\tau$ produced between days 12 and 21 acts on the endometrium to suppress expression of the estrogen receptor. This results in lack of up-regulation of oxytocin receptor numbers and insensitivity to luteal oxytocin release and serves to dampen the pulsatile release of $PGF_{2\alpha}$ to a level below the critical threshold of five pulses per 24 hours.

sac and the expanding allantois (Fig. 9-7). This band of cells, which surround the conceptus, moves with the expansion of the allantois and regression of the yolk sac. Chorionic girdle cells detach from the chorion on day 38 and invade into the uterine stroma to form endometrial cups that produce equine chorionic gonadotropin (eCG). Endometrial cup formation may protect the placenta from maternal immune attack. With continued expansion of the placenta throughout the uterus, microvillous attachment between the chorion and uterine epithelium becomes more complex to give rise to thousands of microcotyledonary structures that hold the placenta firmly in place.

### Placentation

During and following implantation in domestic farm animals, an outgrowth of extraembryonic mesoderm originates from the embryoblast and migrates between the trophectoderm and endoderm (Fig. 9-2**A**). This mesodermal layer will split and combine with the trophectoderm to form the yolk sac (Fig. 9-2**B**). The mesoderm will also contribute to formation of the amnion and the allantois, which is formed from an outgrowth of the embryo hindgut. Amnion forms over the embryo as it drops down into the vesicle and the chorion folds and fuses over the top. The yolk sac regresses during the second to third week of pregnancy as the allantois expands to fuse with the chorion (Fig. 9-2**C**). However, the yolk sac function is extended in the spherical mare placenta as the allantois gradually expands to replace it on day 30 of gestation (Fig. 9-7).

### Maternal Recognition of Pregnancy

The farm animal species are spontaneous ovulators and exhibit uterine-dependent estrous cycles. A close coordination between dynamic processes in the uterine endometrium

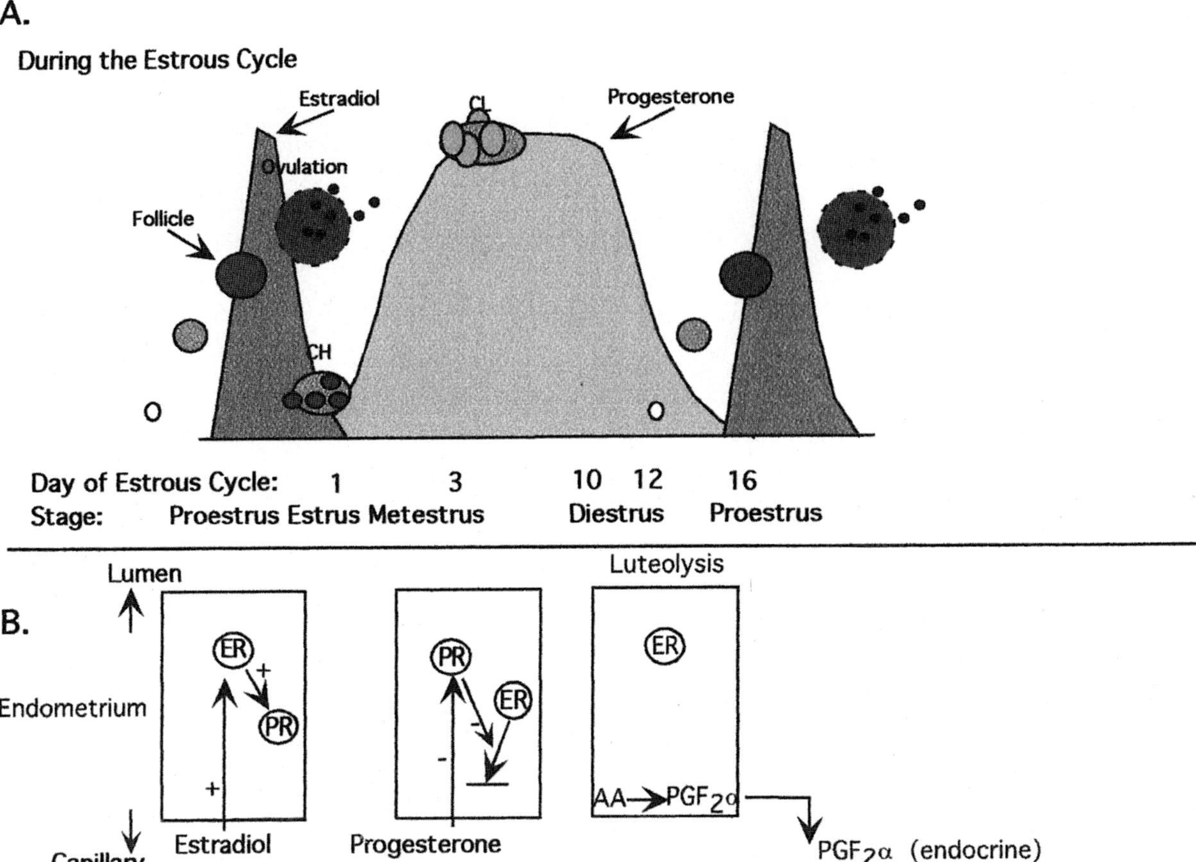


FIGURE 9-10. (A) Relative changes in circulating hormone levels and ovarian changes during the estrous cycle in the pig. Estrus is characterized by elevated levels of circulating estrogens resulting in sexual receptivity, and elevation in endometrial expression of estrogen receptor (ER) and progesterone receptor (PR). Following ovulation, the multiple ovulatory follicles are transformed into the corpora hemorrhagica (CH) and subsequently into the corpora lutea (CL). During metestrus and diestrus, from 3 to 10 days, the CL is producing progesterone at maximum capacity; progesterone production then drops dramatically as luteolysis occurs in response to endometrial release of $PGF_{2\alpha}$. (B) Changes in endometrial hormone response during the estrous cycle. The uterine endometrium is not responsive to estrogen until day 10 of the cycle. Estrogen receptor numbers increase from estrus threough day 5, remain steady through day 12, and then decline after day 15. Ongoing synthesis and release of $PGF_{2\alpha}$ into the uterine-ovarian venous blood following loss of the "progesterone block" at day 10 results in luetolysis.

and the ovary is critical to the establishment of an appropriate uterine environment for pregnancy coincident with the timing of sexual receptivity and ovulation. Following successful mating and fertilization, the conceptus must signal its presence to the maternal system and block the regression of the corpus luteum (CL), a process termed luteolysis, in order to maintain luteal progesterone production. Maintenance of CL is essential for the establishment of pregnancy in all farm animals. The conceptus synthesizes and secretes steroids and/or proteins in order to signal its presence to the maternal system. These molecules serve to modulate synthesis and/or release of luteolytic prostaglandin $F_{2\alpha}$ ($PGF_{2\alpha}$) from the uterus and prevent CL regression. During the critical period of uterine $PGF_{2\alpha}$ release, the conceptus must cover a large portion of the maternal endometrium to regulate the production of $PGF_{2\alpha}$. In the pig, this is accomplished by multiple conceptuses; in the horse, by conceptus migration. The critical period for signaling by the conceptus to block luteolysis and allow pregnancy to be established is called "maternal recognition of pregnancy."

In the absence of successful mating and fertilization, the uterus synthesizes and releases luteolytic $PGF_{2\alpha}$ to initiate morphological regression of the CL and the cessation of progesterone production. This process serves to initiate a new cycle of sexual receptivity (return to estrus) in preparation for mating and fertilization in another attempt to establish pregnancy.

SHEEP AND COW. In the ewe, proteins secreted by the conceptus between days 12 and 21 of pregnancy inhibit

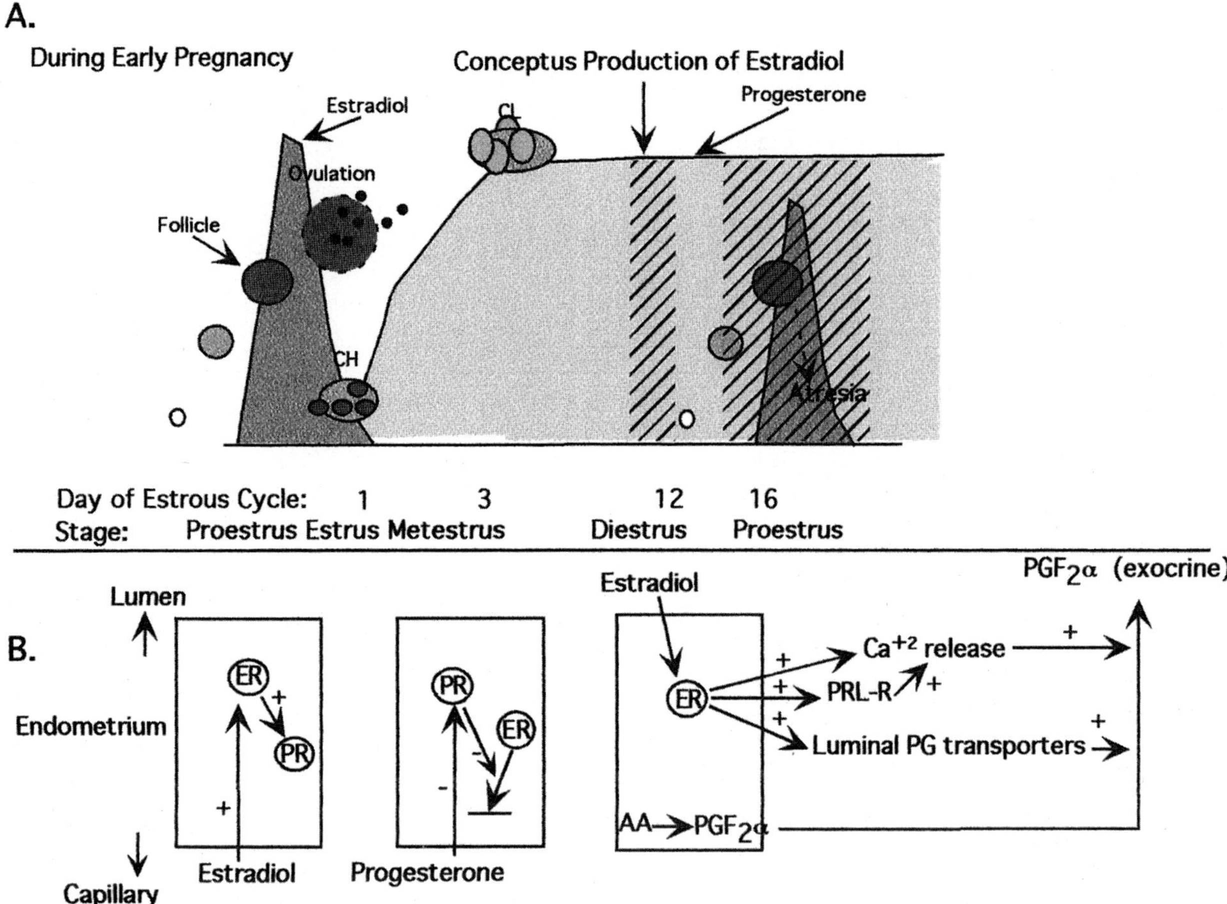


FIGURE 9-11. (A) Relative changes in circulating hormone levels and ovarian changes during early pregnancy in the pig. Circulating hormone levels and ovarian structures are identical through the first 10 days to the nonpregnant animal. During pregnancy, however, conceptus estrogens produced between days 11 to 12 and 14 to 30 are responsible for maintenance of the CL and progesterone production through redirection of endometrial $PGF_{2\alpha}$ release. (B) Changes in endometrial hormone response during early pregnancy in the pig. Estrogen receptor numbers in pregnant gilts increase from estrus through day 5, remain steady through day 12, and then decline after day 15. Estrogen receptor expression then increases at day 18. Loss of the "progesterone block" after day 10 allows estrogen receptors to mediate the action of conceptus estrogens. Actions of conceptus estrogens include stimulation of endometrial protein synthesis and secretion, release of histamine, release of calcium, and the critical alteration of $PGF_{2\alpha}$ release. Mechanisms involved in directional $PGF_{2\alpha}$ release may include: 1) redistribution of prostaglandin transporters within the endometrial cells; 2) stimulation of $Ca^{+2}$ release from intracellular stores, which is associated with $PGF_{2\alpha}$ release; 3) causing an increase in numbers of endometrial prolactin receptors, also associated with increased calcium cycling across the endometrial epithelium and further facilitation of directional release of $PGF_{2\alpha}$; and, 4) conceptus proteins may enhance release of $PGF_{2\alpha}$ toward the uterine lumen.

$PGF_{2\alpha}$ production by the uterine endometrium. Luteolysis in the ewe (Fig. 9-8) involves episodic release of $PGF_{2\alpha}$ between days 14 and 16 of the estrous cycle. These pulses increase in frequency until five pulses are released within a 24-hour period, resulting in luteal regression (8). In pregnant ewes, episodic $PGF_{2\alpha}$ release average 1.3 pulses between days 14 and 15 of pregnancy versus an average of 7.6 pulses in nonpregnant ewes during the same period. Oxytocin released from the CL and/or posterior pituitary stimulates this episodic $PGF_{2\alpha}$ release. Expression of receptors for oxytocin in the uterine endometrium is stimulated by estrogen produced by preovulatory follicles on the ovary.

Conceptus proteins have no effect on the CL lifespan when injected into the utero-ovarian circulation or systemic blood circulation and must be infused into the uterine lumen; thus their action is local to the uterine endometrium and not a systemic effect. The antiluteolytic product in the homogenates is a low molecular weight, acidic protein produced by the sheep conceptus between days 12 and 21 of pregnancy, first termed ovine trophoblast protein 1 (oTP-1). This protein has high amino acid sequence homology to a class of proteins called interferons and is now classified as a unique interferon type called ovine interferon-tau (oIFN-$\tau$) (9).

In cyclic ewes, numbers of endometrial estrogen and progesterone receptors are high between estrus and day 12 of the cycle. Under the influence of progesterone, the uterine endometrium releases very little $PGF_{2\alpha}$ and appears insensitive to estrogen or oxytocin stimulation. This period is referred to as the "progesterone block" (8). Prolonged exposure to progesterone eventually results in down-regulation of the progesterone receptor however, and reduced progesterone influence results in elevation of estrogen receptor expression. Reduced endometrial progesterone receptor numbers and increased numbers of estrogen receptors allows endometrial synthesis of oxytocin receptors to increase, resulting in the endometrium becoming sensitive to oxytocin release from the CL and/or posterior pituitary. Oxytocin stimulation, mediated through endometrial oxytocin receptors and activation of the protein kinase C second messenger system, increases conversion of arachidonic acid to prostaglandins and results in episodic release of $PGF_{2\alpha}$ and luteolysis as described above. In pregnant ewes (Fig. 9-9) conceptus IFN-$\tau$ produced between days 12 and 21 suppresses expression of estrogen receptors resulting in lack of upregulation of oxytocin receptor numbers and insensitivity to luteal oxytocin release (10). This serves to dampen the pulsatile release of $PGF_{2\alpha}$ to a level below the critical threshold of five pulses per 24 hours.

In the cow, maternal recognition of pregnancy occurs between days 16 and 19 of pregnancy (11). The model for maternal recognition of pregnancy in the cow is very similar to that for the sheep, although it is less clear that a direct relationship exists between oxytocin stimulation and release of $PGF_{2\alpha}$ in the cow. The bovine conceptus produces a number of low molecular-weight acidic proteins which include bovine trophoblast protein-1 (bTP-1). Like oTP-1, this protein is classified as an IFN-$\tau$ and called bovine IFN-$\tau$ (bIFN-$\tau$).

Endometrium of pregnant cows produces an endometrial prostaglandin synthesis inhibitor (EPSI) which specifically depresses synthesis of $PGF_{2\alpha}$ (12, 13). This inhibitor appears to be linoleic acid. The ratio of linoleic acid to arachidonic acid (the precursor of $PGF_{2\alpha}$) is much higher in pregnant cows than nonpregnant cows suggesting a critical role for alterations in lipid composition of the uterine tissue in maternal recognition of pregnancy in the cow (14). There is no evidence for an EPSI in the ewe.

**PIG.** Production of estrogens by the developing conceptuses is the signal for maternal recognition of pregnancy in the pig (15). Periods of estrogen production between days 11 and 12 and days 14 to 30 of pregnancy allows for maintenance of the corpora lutea. Both periods of estrogen stimulation of the uterine endometrium appear to be critical since estrogen stimulation in both phases is required to extend the lifespan of the CL. Injection of exogenous estrogens (estradiol benzoate) on days 11 and 14 of the estrous cycle results in extended CL lifespan. Injection of pharmacologic doses of estradiol valerate on days 11 through 15 of the estrous cycle results in maintenance of the corpora lutea for a period equivalent or slightly longer than normal 114 day gestation (16). This is referred to as pseudopregnancy. Pig conceptuses secrete an array of proteins, including interferons, but these do not affect the lifespan of the CL.

The uterine endometrium is not responsive to estrogen until day 10 of the cycle or early pregnancy. Estrogen receptor numbers in both cyclic and pregnant gilts increase from estrus through day 5, remain steady through day 12, and then decline after day 15 (Fig. 9-10). Lack of estrogen responsiveness in the tissue in spite of receptor expression is likely a result of the action of progesterone. Loss of the "progesterone block" after day 10 allows estrogen receptors to mediate the action of conceptus estrogens. Actions of conceptus estrogens include stimulation of endometrial protein synthesis and secretion, release of histamine, release of calcium, and alteration of prostaglandin release.

Utero-ovarian plasma concentrations of $PGF_{2\alpha}$ are elevated between days 12 and 16 of the estrous cycle (Fig. 9-10). Concentrations of $PGF_{2\alpha}$ are significantly lower in utero-ovarian venous plasma between days 12 and 16 in pregnant and pseudopregnant gilts. On the other hand, $PGF_{2\alpha}$ concentrations are significantly higher in uterine flushings from pregnant and pseudopregnant gilts. Thus, estrogens do not appear to inhibit uterine production of $PGF_{2\alpha}$ but instead cause $PGF_{2\alpha}$ to be sequestered in the uterine lumen. Secretion of luteolytic $PGF_{2\alpha}$ into the uterine lumen, termed exocrine secretion, results in $PGF_{2\alpha}$ being unavailable to cause luteolysis (Fig. 9-11). This effect of conceptus estrogens, modification of the direction of $PGF_{2\alpha}$ release away from the bloodstream (endocrine release), is called the endocrine-exocrine model of maternal recognition of pregnancy in the pig (17).

Conceptuses must be present in both uterine horns for pregnancy to be established, and at least two conceptuses must be present in each horn for a sufficient area of the uterine endometrium to be covered and $PGF_{2\alpha}$ release altered. Pigs generally cannot maintain unilateral pregnancy because $PGF_{2\alpha}$ released from one uterine horn may cause luteolysis and CL regression on both ovaries; this also suggests that conceptus factors associated with maternal recognition of pregnancy act locally on the uterine endometrium, not systemically. A second type of prostaglandin ($PGE_2$) is produced by the pregnant endometrium, continues to be released to the utero-ovarian venous blood, and may provide stimulation to the CL for progesterone synthesis and also provide protection from luteolytic effects of $PGF_{2\alpha}$ (18).

**HORSE.** In the cycling mare, $PGF_{2\alpha}$ in uterine venous plasma and in uterine flushings increases from day 8 to day

16 when CL regression occurs and progesterone production ceases. Synthesis of $PGF_{2\alpha}$ is reduced in the presence of the conceptus. Pregnant mares have only very low levels of $PGF_{2\alpha}$ in uterine venous plasma and in uterine flushings, and PGFM in peripheral blood plasma shows no episodic pattern of release (19). Endometrium from both pregnant and nonpregnant mares synthesizes considerable quantities of $PGF_{2\alpha}$ in the absence of a conceptus and the CL of both pregnant and nonpregnant mares is sensitive to $PGF_{2\alpha}$.

The conceptus migrates within the uterine lumen from one horn to the other 10 to 13 times per day between days 10 and 16 of pregnancy, likely in an effort to inhibit or modify endometrial $PGF_{2\alpha}$ production. It remains unclear what product of the conceptus is responsible for modulating endometrial $PGF_{2\alpha}$ production. Between day 8 and 20 of pregnancy, the equine conceptus produces and secretes estrogens, including estradiol and estrone. The conceptus also produces several major secretory proteins, including groups of isoelectric variants with molecular weights of about 22,000, 30,000 to 40,000, and 65,000 daltons (20). Neither the roles of these proteins nor the roles of conceptus estrogens in maternal recognition of pregnancy have been determined. Although conceptus estrogens are implicated in fixation of the conceptus within the uterine lumen on day 16 of pregnancy and they have not demonstrated to be effective in maintaining the CL as occurs in the pig. It is likely that the conceptus secretory proteins provide the signal for maternal recognition of pregnancy in the mare by inhibiting, directly or indirectly, endometrial $PGF_{2\alpha}$ production. Conceptus effects within the uterine lumen are local and not systemic since conceptus migration appears to play such a critical role in embryonic survival during early pregnancy.

## REFERENCES


1. Pope WF, Maurer RR, Stormshak F. Intrauterine migration of the porcine embryo: interaction of embryo, uterine flushings and indomethacin on myometrial function *In vitro*. J Anim Sci 1982;55:1169–1178.
2. Ginther OJ. Embryology and placentation. In: Reproductive Biology of the Mare. OJ Ginther (ed). Cross Plains, Wisconsin: Equiservices, 1992;345–418.
3. Stroband HW, Van der Lende T. Embryonic and uterine development during early pregnancy in pigs. J Reprod Fert Suppl 1990;40:261–277.
4. Geisert RD, Yelich JV. Regulation of conceptus development and attachment in pigs. J Reprod Fert 1997;52(Suppl): 133–149.
5. Burgdardt RD, Bowen JA, Newton GR, Bazer FW. Extracellular matrix and the implantation cascade in pigs. J Reprod Fert 1997;52(Suppl):151–164.
6. Perry JS. The mammalian fetal membranes. J Reprod Fertil 1981;62:321–335.
7. King GJ, Atkinson BA, Robertson HA. Implantation and early placentation in domestic ungulates. J Reprod Fert 1982;31(Suppl):17–30.
8. McCracken J, Schramm W, Okulicz, W. Hormone receptor control of pulsatile secretion of $PGF_{2\alpha}$ from the ovine uterus during luteolysis and its abrogation in early pregnancy. Anim Reprod Sci 1984;7:31–55.
9. Bazer FW, Spencer TE, Ott TL. Interferon tau: a novel pregnancy recognition signal. Am J Reprod Immunol 1977;37: 412–420.
10. Spencer TE, Becker WC, George P, Mirando MA, Ogle TF, Bazer FW. Ovine interferon-tau inhibits estrogen receptor up-regulation and estrogen-induced luteolysis in cyclic ewes. Endocrinology 1995;136:4932–4944.
11. Thatcher WW, Meyer MD, Danet-Desnoyers G. Maternal recognition of pregnancy. J Reprod Fertil 1995;49(Suppl): 15–28.
12. Gross TS, Thatcher WW, Hansen PJ, Johnson JW, Helmer SD. Presence of an intracellular endometrial inhibitor of prostaglandin synthesis during early pregnancy in the cow. Prostaglandins 1988;35:359–378.
13. Helmer SD, Gross TS, Newton GR, Hansen PJ, Thatcher WW. Bovine trophoblast protein-I complex alters endometrial protein and prostaglandin secretion and induces an intracellular inhibitor of prostaglandin synthesis *in vitro*. J Reprod Fertil 1989;87:421–430.
14. Staples CR, Burke JM, Thatcher WW. Influence of supplemental fats on reproductive tissues and performance of lactating cows. J Dairy Sci 1998;81:856–871.
15. Geisert RD, Thatcher WW, Roberts RM, Bazer FW. Establishment of pregnancy in the pig: III. Endometrial secretory response to estradiol valerate administered on day 11 of the estrous cycle. Biol Reprod 1982;27:957–965.
16. Geisert RD, Zavy MT, Moffatt RJ, Blair RM, Yellin T. Embryonic steroids and the establishment of pregnancy in pigs. J Reprod Fertil 1990;40(Suppl):293–305.
17. Bazer FW, Thatcher WW. Theory of maternal recognition of pregnancy in swine based on estrogen controlled endocrine versus exocrine secretion of prostaglandin F2 alpha by the uterine endometrium. Prostaglandins 1977;14:397–400.
18. Ford SP, Christenson LK. Direct effects of oestradion-17 beta and prostaglandin E-2 in protecting pig corpora lutea from a luteolytic dose of prostaglandin F-2 alpha. J Reprod Fertil 1991;93:203–209.
19. Sharp DC, McDowell KJ, Weithenauer J, Thatcher WW. The continuum of events leading to maternal recognition of pregnancy in mares. J Reprod Fertil Suppl 1989;37(Suppl): 101–107.
20. McDowell KJ, Sharp DC, Fazlaebas AT, Roberts RM. Two-dimensional polyacrylamide gel electrophoresis of proteins synthesized and released by conceptuses and endometria from pony mares. J Reprod Fertil 1990;89:107–115.

CHAPTER 10

# Gestation, Prenatal Physiology, and Parturition

M.R. JAINUDEEN AND E.S.E. HAFEZ

Farm mammals are viviparous. They complete their embryonic and fetal development within the uterus. This period of intrauterine development is termed pregnancy or gestation and is concerned primarily with the nutrition of the growing fetus and the maternal adaptations directed to this end.

This chapter begins with gestation and factors that influence its duration, then maternal adaptations during pregnancy, the mechanism that leads to maternal recognition of pregnancy, and the role of progesterone in the maintenance of pregnancy. The section on the placenta deals with the development of the fetal membranes, the gross and microscopic structures of the placenta, and placental functions. The section on fetal physiology discusses nutrition and growth of the fetus and the role of the fetal fluids. The next section parturition begins with the mechanisms that initiate parturition, the mechanics of delivery, stages of labor, and the fetal responses to an extrauterine life. The chapter concludes with a section on the puerperium and the maternal adjustments necessary to initiate the next pregnancy.

## GESTATION

### Length of Gestation

Length of gestation is calculated as the interval from fertile mating to parturition (Table 10-1). The duration of gestation is genetically determined, although it can be modified by maternal, fetal, genetic, and environmental factors (Fig. 10-1).

MATERNAL FACTORS. The age of the dam influences the duration of pregnancy within a species. For example, the gestation period is extended by about two days in sheep older than eight years. Similarly, young heifers carry their calves for a slightly shorter period than older heifers.

FETAL FACTORS. The duration of gestation is inversely related to litter size in polytocous species except the pig. Multiple fetuses in monotocous species also have shorter gestation periods. Twin calves are carried 3 to 6 days less than single calves. Interaction between fetal and placental sizes may influence gestation in the horse. The sex of the fetus may also determine gestation length; male calves and foals are carried 1 to 2 days longer than females. The duration of pregnancy may be influenced by the endocrine functions of the fetus.

GENETIC FACTORS. The small variations in pregnancy duration among breeds within a species may be due to genetic effects. The influence of fetal genotype on gestation length can be demonstrated in hybrids between the horse and the donkey. In these matings, the gestation length is closer to the paternal than to the maternal component of the fetus. In cattle, the breed of the embryo determines the length of gestation. This has been established by transferring the embryos from breeds with shorter gestation length than the donor's and vice versa.

ENVIRONMENTAL FACTORS. Of the environmental factors, season may influence the duration of gestation, particularly in the horse. Foals conceived in late summer and autumn have significantly shorter gestation periods than those conceived at the start of the breeding season in early spring. Well fed mares have gestation lengths about 4 days shorter than those on a maintenance ration.

TABLE 10-1. *Gestation Length of Farm Mammals*

| ANIMAL | AVERAGE (DAYS) |
|---|---|
| Cattle | 278 |
| Buffalo | 310 |
| Sheep | 148 |
| Goat | 150 |
| Pig | 114 |
| Horse | 335 |

## MATERNAL PHYSIOLOGY IN PREGNANCY

### *Maternal Recognition of Pregnancy*

The close contact between the developing embryo and the mother results in an opportunity for the conceptus to influence maternal physiology through endocrine mechanisms. In both ruminants (sheep, cattle) and nonruminants, the blastocyst, before it attaches to the endometrium, secretes substances which prolong the life span of the cyclic corpus luteum (CL) beyond the period of the estrous cycle. The time at which it occurs is known as maternal recognition of pregnancy (MRP).

In ruminants, the trophoblast of the developing conceptus blocks luteal regression by the production of interferons (IFNs) ensuring MRP (1). In the pig, production of estrogen by the blastocyst was thought to be the signal controlling MRP, but later studies suggest the both IFNs and estrogen may be involved in the pig.

### *Reproductive Organ Changes*

VULVAR AND VAGINAL CHANGES. During the latter half of gestation, changes occur in the genital tract, particularly in the vulva and vagina. The vulva becomes highly edematous and vascular. The vaginal mucosa is pale and dry during most of gestation but is edematous and pliable toward the end of pregnancy.

THE CERVIX. During gestation, the developing fetus is retained within the uterus by tight closure of the external os of the cervix. Highly viscid mucus seals the cervical canal. This so-called mucous plug of pregnancy liquefies and is discharged in strings immediately before parturition.

UTERINE CHANGES. As pregnancy progresses, the uterus undergoes gradual enlargement to accommodate the growing fetus, but the myometrium remains quiescent, thereby preventing premature expulsion. The mechanisms that permit the enormous increase in size are unknown but are probably hormonal.

OVARIAN CHANGES. During pregnancy, the CL of the cycle persists (corpus luteum verum), and as a result, estrous cycles are suspended. Some cows, however, may show estrus during early pregnancy. In the mare 10 to 15 follicles develop between the 35th and 150th day of pregnancy. These follicles luteinize to form accessory corpora lutea. Both the primary as well as the accessory corpora lutea regress by the seventh month of pregnancy.

PELVIC LIGAMENTS. Relaxation of the pelvic ligaments occurs gradually during the course of pregnancy but becomes more rapid with approaching parturition. This relaxation is more noticeable in the cow and ewe than in the mare, and is related to high levels of estrogens in late pregnancy and to the action of relaxin. The caudal part of the sacrosciatic ligament is cordlike in the nonpregnant cow but becomes more relaxed and flaccid as parturition approaches.

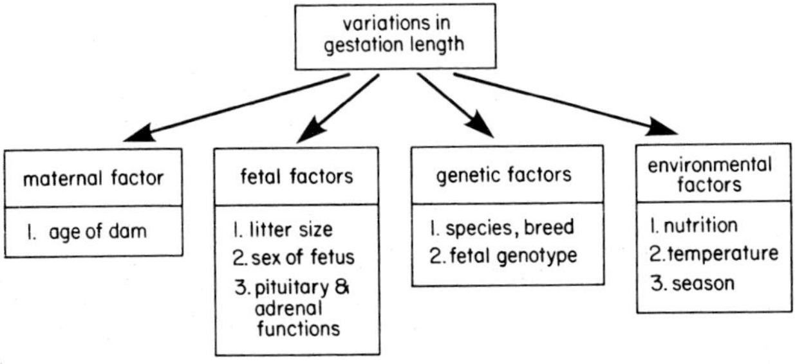


FIGURE 10-1. Schematic representation of variations in length of gestation due to maternal, fetal, genetic, and environmental factors. Whereas many of these factors within a species cause minor variations, hypofunction of the pituitary-adrenal axis of the fetus is associated with prolonged gestation in the ewe and cow.

### *Hormones of Pregnancy*

PROGESTERONE. Progesterone is the key hormone necessary for maintenance of pregnancy. The CL persists throughout pregnancy in all farm animals except the horse. The source of progesterone during the latter half of pregnancy may be from placenta (mare, ewe) or from the CL (cow, goat, and sow) (Fig. 10-2).

The blood progesterone level remains constant throughout pregnancy in the ewe and cow and attains a high level early in pregnancy in the sow. In the mare, progesterone concentration up to day 35 reflects secretion by the primary CL (Table 10-2). The progesterone level then rises with the development of the secondary corpora lutea, and is maintained until the secondary corpora lutea begin to regress by day 150. Beyond this time, the placenta is sufficiently developed to take over the production of a lower level of progesterone. During the last 2 months of gestation, contrary to previous views, the progesterone level

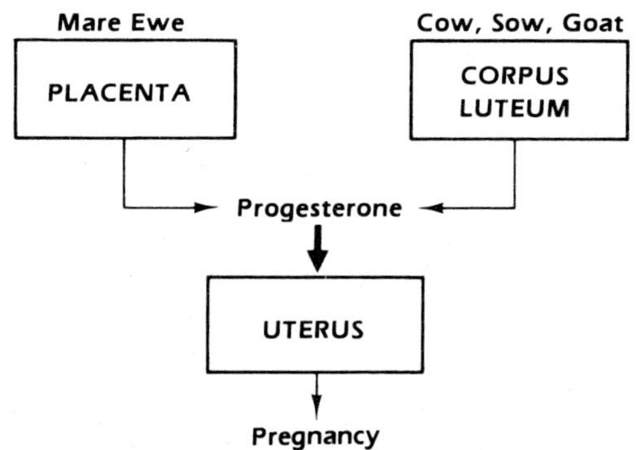


FIGURE 10-2. Progesterone secreted by the CL is essential for the maintenance of early pregnancy in all farm species. The ovaries, however, can be removed (ovariectomy) during the latter half of pregnancy without interrupting pregnancy in the mare and ewe because the placenta produces $P_4$ in these species.

rises steadily to reach a second peak that is significantly higher than previous concentrations.

ESTROGENS. Species differences occur in the urinary excretion of estrogens. In the mare, plasma estrogen concentrations remain low during the first 3 months of pregnancy, then rise steadily to reach a peak between the ninth and eleventh months, thereafter declining rapidly to term. In the sow, total urinary estrogen (estrone) rate shows an increase between the second and fifth weeks of gestation, a decline between the fifth and eighth weeks, and a rapid increase to a peak at the time of parturition, which declines rapidly thereafter. In the cow, maximal excretion of 17$\beta$-estradiol, and to a lesser degree estrone, occurs at 9 months of gestation.

EQUINE CHORIONIC GONADOTROPHIN. Between 40 and 130 days of gestation, high concentrations of equine chorionic gonadotrophin (eCG) (also referred to as pregnant mare serum gonadotrophin, or PMSG) are present in maternal but not in fetal blood. eCG, which is secreted by trophoblastic cells and not by the endometrium as was previously believed, luteinizes follicles and maintains the function of the secondary corpora lutea.

TABLE 10-2. *Endocrinology of Pregnancy in the Mare*

| HORMONE | SOURCE | DAYS OF PREGNANCY |
|---|---|---|
| Progesterone | Ovary | |
| | Corpus luteum (primary) | 1–35 |
| | Corpora lutea (secondary) | 35–150 |
| | Placenta | >150 |
| Equine chorionic gonadotrophin (eCG) | Endometrial cups | 36–140 |
| Estrogen | Placenta | 100–330 |

### *Maternal Adaptations*

During the course of pregnancy, the mother makes metabolic and growth adjustments to provide an adequate supply of nutrients for the development of the fetus. Maternal body composition, feed intake, energy consumption, and metabolism are altered during pregnancy, but the mechanisms responsible are not fully established. Recent evidence has implicated insulin-like growth factors (IGFs) and their binding proteins as playing important roles in maternal adaptation, which guarantees an adequate supply of substrates to the developing fetus (2).

## PLACENTA

A unique feature of early mammalian development is the provision of nutrients from the maternal organism by way of the placenta. The placenta is an apposition or fusion of the fetal membranes to the endometrium to permit physiologic exchange between fetus and mother. The placenta differs from other organs in many respects. It originates as a result of various degrees of fetal–maternal interactions and is connected to the embryo by a cord of blood vessels. The size and functions of the placenta change continuously during the course of pregnancy, and the organ is eventually expelled. For the fetus, the placenta combines in one organ many functional activities that are separate in the adult.

### *Placental Development*

FETAL MEMBRANES. The morphogenesis of the placenta during early gestation is closely related to those extraembryonic or fetal membranes that are differentiated into the yolk sac, amnion, allantois, and chorion (Table 10-3). The fetal membranes participate in the formation of the placenta, either separately or in certain combinations, and give rise to three basic types of placentation which differ in regard to the identity of the fetal membranes involved: chorionic, chorioallantoic, and yolk sac placentation. Among these types, the chorioallantoic placentation derived from the fusion of the allantois with the chorion is characteristic of all farm animals. The rich blood supply in the allantois comes into close apposition to the umbilical arteries and veins located in the connective tissue between the allantois and chorion (Fig. 10-3).

CHORIONIC VILLI. A feature of the chorioallantoic placenta is the highly increased area at the feto-maternal junc-

TABLE 10-3. *The Fetal Membranes of Farm Animals*

| MEMBRANE | ORIGIN | FUNCTIONS |
|---|---|---|
| Yolk sac | Early entodermal layer | Vestigial |
| Amnion | Cavitation from inner cell mass | Encloses fetus in a fluid-filled cavity |
| Allantois | Diverticulum of hindgut | Blood vessels connect fetal with placental circulation<br>Fuses with chorion to form the chorioallantoic placenta |
| Chorion | Trophoblastic capsule of blastocyst | Encloses embryo and other fetal membranes<br>Intimately associated with lining of uterus to form placenta |
| Umbilical cord | Amnion wraps about the yolk stalk | Encloses allantoic vessels and acts as the vascular link between mother and fetus |

tion, either by the formation of chorionic villi protruding into uterine crypts or by the formation of chorionic labyrinths. The chorionic villi consist of vascular mesenchymal cones surrounded by cuboidal trophoblastic and giant binucleate cells. These either penetrate directly into the endometrium or simply interdigitate with vascular foldings of the endometrial surface (e.g., as in farm animals). The function of the villi is to bring the fetal (allantoic) vessels into proximity with the maternal blood vessels.

## *Classification of Chorioallantoic Placenta*

The chorioallantoic placenta may be classified according to gross shape, microscopic characteristics of the maternal-fetal barrier, and loss of maternal tissue at birth (Table 10-4).

GROSS SHAPE. The definitive shape of the placenta is determined by the distribution of villi over the chorionic surface (Fig. 10-4). In ruminants, the fetal cotyledons fuse with caruncles or specialized projections of the uterine mucosa to form placentomes or functional units. The caruncles are convex in the cow and concave in the ewe and goat (Fig. 10-4).

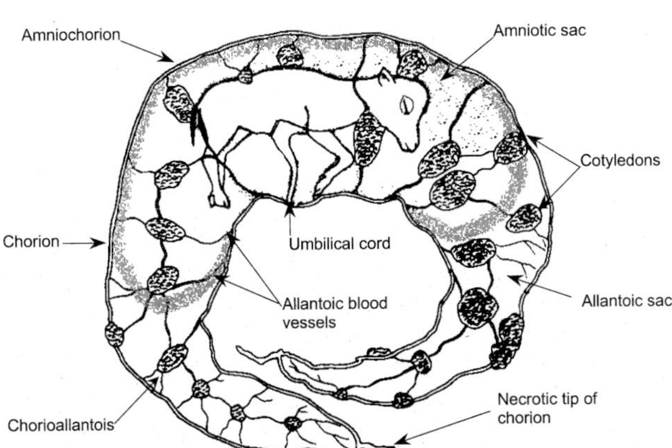


FIGURE 10-3. Diagram of the fetal membranes of a 105-day fetal calf to show the allantoic and amniotic cavities. The cotyledons are distributed over the chorioallantoic membrane and the amniochorion.

In sheep, between 90 and 100 placentomes are evenly distributed between the pregnant and nonpregnant horns. In cattle, 70 to 120 placentomes develop around the fetus and progress toward the distal limit of the chorioallantois in the nongravid horn (Fig. 10-3). During pregnancy, these placentomes enlarge to several times their original diameter. Normally, the chorioallantois extends into the nongravid horn, but the degree to which the caruncles hypertrophy is usually less than that in the gravid horn.

Though there is a high incidence of chorionic fusion during multiple pregnancy, vascular anastomosis between allantoic circulations rarely occurs in sheep. In contrast, a high incidence of vascular anastomosis is encountered between twin bovine fetuses, giving rise to the well known intersexual condition of freemartinism.

In early pregnancy in the mare and sow, the placenta consists of a simple apposition of fetal and maternal epithelia, but between 75 and 110 days of gestation in the mare, the complex folding and branching of the two surfaces give rise to the formation of microcotyledons.

Endometrial cups are a unique feature of the equine placenta. They are discrete, raised areas of a few millimeters to several centimeters in diameter and arranged in a circular fashion at the caudal portion of the gravid uterine horn. These cups are formed by the invasion of the endometrium by a band of specialized trophoblastic cells (chorionic girdle) that peel off the fetal membranes by day 38. The endometrial cups are the source of the eCG present in high concentrations in the blood of mares between 40 and 130 days of gestation (3).

MICROSCOPIC STRUCTURE. The classification of the placenta by microscopic structure is based upon the maternal and fetal tissues that are actually in contact (4). The basic structure comprises on the maternal side blood vessel, connective tissue, and epithelium, and on the fetal side chorionic epithelium, connective tissue, and blood vessel (Fig.

TABLE 10-4. ***Classification of Chorioallantoic Placentas***

| | CLASSIFICATION | | |
|---|---|---|---|
| SPECIES | *Chorionic Villous Pattern* | *Maternal-Fetal Barrier* | *Loss of Maternal Tissue at Birth* |
| Pig | Diffuse | Epitheliochorial | None (nondeciduate) |
| Mare | Diffuse and microtyledonary | Epitheliochorial | None (nondeciduate) |
| Sheep, goat, cow, buffalo | Cotyledonary | Synepitheliochorial | None (nondeciduate) |
| Dog, cat | Zonary | Endotheliochorial | Moderate (deciduate) |
| Human, monkey | Discoid | Hemochorial | Extensive (deciduate) |

From Wooding FBP, Flint APF. Placentation. In: Laming GE, ed. Marshall's Physiology of Reproduction, 4th ed. London: Chapman & Hall, 1994.

10-5). While all layers are preserved in the epitheliochorial (horse and pig) and synepitheliochorial placentas (ruminants,) some layers on the maternal side are lost as in endotheliochorial (cat) and hemochorial (human).

Electron microscopic investigations of the ruminant placenta have demonstrated that fetal chorionic binucleate cells (BCs) migrate to form a syncytium at the junction of the maternal and fetal tissue (3). Thus, these authors have reclassified the ruminant placenta from "epitheliochorial" to "synepitheliochorial." The "syn" prefix refers to the presence of BC-derived syncytium and "epitheliochorial" representing the large areas of simple apposition of maternal tissues.

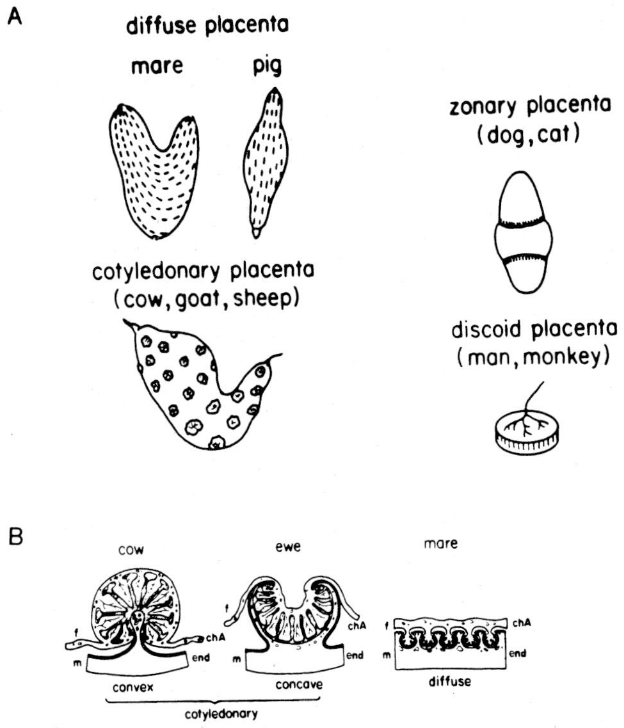

FIGURE 10-4. (A) The distribution of chorionic villi as the basis of classifying placental shape. (B) Epitheliochorial placenta of mare, ewe, and cow. The placenta of mare is diffuse and microcotyledonary; those of the ewe and cow are cotyledonary. *chA*, Chorioallantois; *end*, endometrium; *F*, fetal; *M*, maternal. (Redrawn from Silver In: Comline KS, et al, eds. Proceedings of Sir Joseph Barcroft Centenary Symposium. Cambridge, Cambridge University Press, 1973.)

TISSUE LOST AT PARTURITION. Mammalian species can also be classified as deciduate and nondeciduate. In the deciduate type, maternal epithelium is lost along with fetal membranes at parturition. It is restricted to the hemochorial placenta (human). The nondeciduate type is characteristic of farm animals. The term "placental barrier" connotes a physiological barrier between the fetal and maternal circulations. The thickness of this barrier may range from three to six cells.

## *Placental Circulation*

In the placenta, two circulations are parallel to the fetal and maternal circulations, but the fetal and the maternal blood do not intermingle in the epitheliochorial placentas of farm animals.

The uterine arteries and veins supply the placenta. The umbilical arteries bring blood from the fetus to the placenta, and the umbilical veins return blood from the placenta to the fetus.

Various theoretical models have been proposed to explain the direction of maternal and fetal blood flow in the placenta. Blood flow in adjacent maternal and fetal vascular channels could be countercurrent, concurrent, crosscurrent (multivillous), or pool. In the pool flow, maternal blood enters a large space in which it is exposed to fetal capillaries.

## *Placental Functions*

The placenta performs many functions and substitutes for the fetal gastrointestinal tract, lung, kidney, liver, and endocrine glands. In addition, the placenta separates the mater-

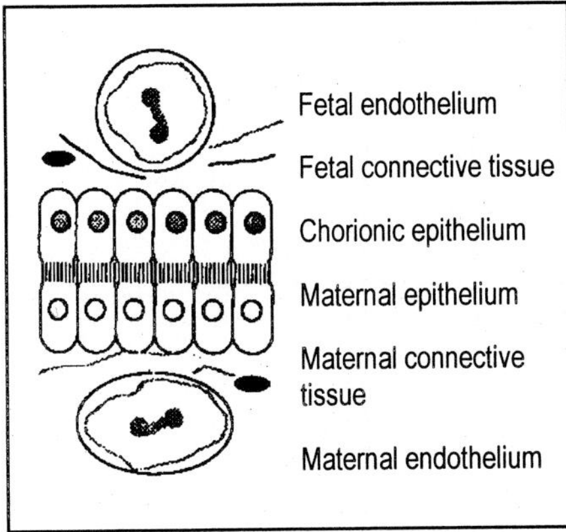


EPITHELIOCHORIAL

e.g. Pig, Horse

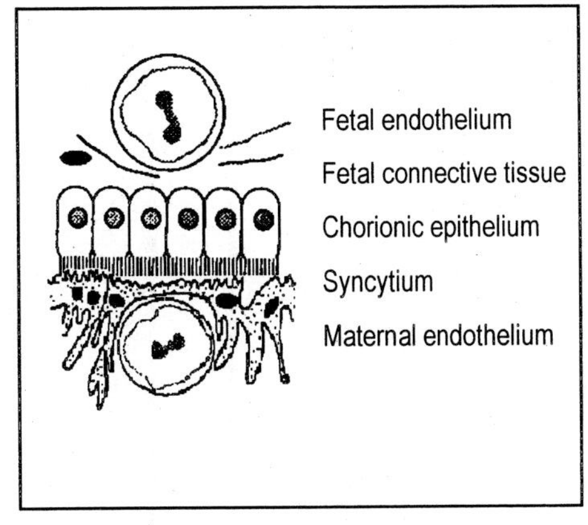


SYNEPITHELIOCHORIAL

e.g. Sheep, Goat, Cattle

FIGURE 10-5. Comparative cytology of fetal/maternal attachment in farm mammals. (Adapted from Broughton-Pipkin F, Hull D, Stephensen T. Fetal Physiology. In: Laming GE, ed. Marshall's Physiology of Reproduction, 4th ed. London: Chapman & Hall, 1994; 769–861.)

nal and fetal organisms, thus ensuring the separate development of the fetus (Fig. 10-6). The blood of the fetus and dam never come into direct contact, yet the two circulations are close enough at the junction of the chorion and endometrium for oxygen and nutrients to pass from maternal to fetal blood, and waste products in the opposite direction.

GASES. Many similarities exist between the gas exchange across the placenta and that across the lungs (Table 10-5). The major difference, however, is that in the placenta it is a fluid-to-fluid system, whereas in the lung it is a gas-to-fluid system. The umbilical arteries carry unoxygenated blood from the fetus to the placenta, while the umbilical veins carry oxygenated blood in the reverse direction.

Carbon dioxide diffuses freely from the fetal to the maternal circulation and is facilitated by certain physiologic mechanisms. For example, fetal blood has a lower affinity for $CO_2$ than maternal blood during placental oxygen trans-

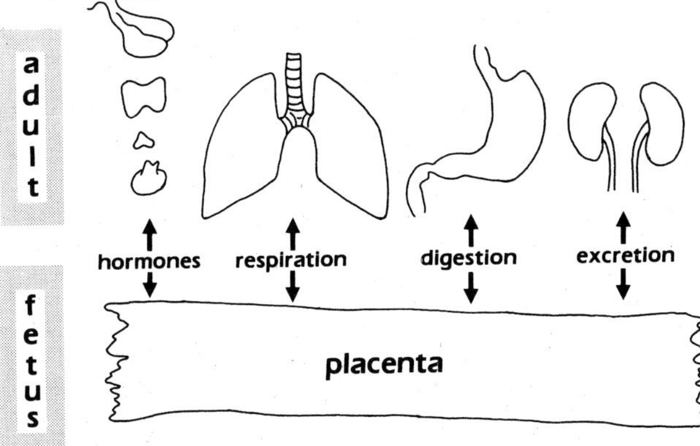


FIGURE 10-6. The functions of the placenta. The placenta combines in one organ many activities of the fetus—hormones, respiration, digestion, and excretion—that are separate in the adult.

TABLE 10-5. *Transfer of Nutrients between Mother and Fetus*

| SUBSTANCE | MECHANISM |
|---|---|
| Water | Diffusion across the placenta either traversing the cells (transcellular) or running between the cells (paracellular). |
| Electrolytes and minerals | Exchange is probably via the paracellular route. |
| Calcium and phosphate | Carrier-mediated and energy-dependent mechanisms. |
| Iron | The major source of fetal iron is the maternal serum transferrin, the carrier protein for iron. After the transferrin enters the placenta by endocytosis it is released into the fetal circulation. |
| Blood gases | Oxygen diffusion depends on partial pressure.<br>Carbon dioxide diffuses readily from the fetal to the maternal circulation. |
| Glucose | Energy supply to fetus. Facilitated transport across the placenta. |
| Fructose | Does not cross the placental barrier. Transplacental osmotic balance. |
| Amino acids | Different mechanisms depending upon the type of amino acid, some of which are actively transported. |
| Free fatty acids | Placenta relatively permeable in some species but not in others, e.g., sheep and pig. |

Adapted from Broughton-Pipkin F, Hull D, Stephensen T. 1994. Fetal Physiology. In: Laming GE, ed. Marshall's Physiology of Reproduction, 4th ed. London: Chapman & Hall, 1994.

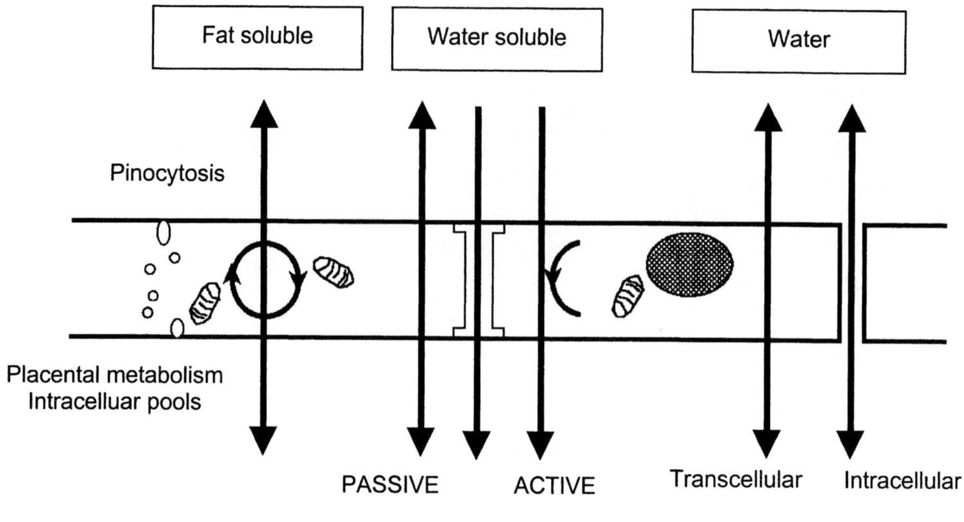


FIGURE 10-7 Placental transport of nutrients as based on net flux from either mother to fetus or in the opposite direction. (Adapted from Broughton-Pipkin F, Hull D, Stephensen T. Fetal Physiology. In: Laming GE, ed. Marshall's Physiology of Reproduction, 4th ed. London: Chapman & Hall, 1994; 769–861.)

fer. This favors the diffusion of $CO_2$ from fetal to maternal blood.

NUTRIENTS. The placenta permits the transport of sugars, amino acids, vitamins, and minerals to the fetus as substrates for fetal growth. Placental transport of nutrients is based on net flux from either mother to fetus or in the opposite direction (4) (Fig. 10-7). It can be due to a concentration difference or of unidirectional carrier-mediated transport. Many nutrients such as glucose, amino acids, electrolytes, and vitamins are transported by carrier systems located in the trophoblast (5).

Free fatty acids (FFA) are transported across the placenta by simple diffusion whereas proteins as such are not transferred (Table 10-5). Immunoglobulins are transmitted in humans and some animals, but not in farm animals. This difference may be related to structural differences in the various placental types.

Water soluble vitamins (B and C) cross the placental barrier more readily than those that are lipid soluble (A, D, E). Polypeptides cross the placenta slowly. Although iodine crosses the placenta readily in sheep, there is little or no transfer of thyroid hormones or thyroid-stimulating hormone. Insulin also probably crosses only slowly and in insignificant amounts. Cortisol is transferred from mother to fetus in many species but not in goat and sheep. The unconjugated steroids, $P_4$ and estrogens cross the placental barrier readily.

FETOPLACENTAL UNIT. The placenta is a transient endocrine organ like the CL. It secretes both trophic and steroid hormones that are released into the fetal as well as the maternal circulations. The concept of a fetoplacental unit was proposed to explain the various mechanisms by which large amounts of progesterone and estrogens are produced during pregnancy. Both the placenta and the fetus lack certain enzymatic functions that are essential for steroidogenesis, but enzymes absent from the placenta are present in the fetus and vice versa. Thus, by sequential integration of the fetal and placental steroidogenic functions, the fetoplacental unit can elaborate most, if not all, hormonally active steroids.

Some species (ewe and mare), but not others (cow, goat, and sow), are capable of synthesizing sufficient amounts of progesterone to maintain pregnancy by using acetate and cholesterol derived from the maternal circulation. During the latter half of gestation, a high rate of estrogen production occurs in the placentas of the mare, cow, sow, and ewe. The placenta relies on fetal cortisol to induce activity of the placental enzyme 17$\alpha$-hydoxylase and thus synthesize estrogen from progesterone.

Placental lactogen (PL), also known as chorionic somatomammotropin, is a peptide hormone of pregnancy found in many mammalian species and reported to have trophic and growth hormone-like effects in both mother and fetus.

## *Mother-Fetus Immunologic Relationship*

The presence of a developing fetus in the intrauterine environment poses a serious problem. The fetus inherits from the father genetic characteristics that are foreign to the mother and therefore may be considered as an allograft or tissue from a different individual of the same species. If the donor has antigens not possessed by the recipient, the recipient will usually reject the transplanted tissue. The failure of maternal tissue to reject the placenta has puzzled immunologists and has led to many theories to explain the unique relationship between mother and fetus. For more on the subject see the Chapter "Immunology of Reproduction."

## Fetal Physiology

The prenatal development of farm animals may be divided into three main periods:

1. The period of the ovum culminates with the initial attachment of the blastocyst but is before the establishment of an intraembryonic circulation.
2. The embryonic period extends from day 15 to day 45 of gestation in the cow, day 12 to about day 34 in the sheep, and day 12 to day 60 in the mare. In this period, rapid growth and differentiation occur, during which the major tissues, organs, and systems are established and the major features of external body form are recognizable.
3. The fetal period extends from about day 34 of gestation in sheep, day 45 in cattle, and from day 60 in horses, until birth. Growth and changes in the form of the fetus characterize this period.

### Fetal Nutrition and Metabolism

Whereas the blastocyst and the early embryo are nourished by endometrial fluid, the fetus receives its supply of nutrients from the maternal circulation across the placenta. The fetus may be regarded as a parasite living within the mother, and it has priority in the event of insufficient maternal nutrition so that its development can proceed unimpaired. It needs carbohydrates, proteins, vitamins, and minerals for maintenance, differentiation, and subsequent development and growth.

The fetus receives a continuous supply of glucose from its mother through the placenta. Glucose is the major metabolic fuel for the fetus. Toward the end of the gestation, the normal fetus accumulates glycogen in its liver and skeletal muscles to assist it in overcoming the transitional period after birth until efficient suckling is established. Although fructose comprises about 70 to 80% of the sugar in the blood of fetal ungulates (cattle, sheep, goats), its use is negligible, except when blood glucose levels are low. In ruminant fetuses, acetate, lactate, and amino acids may be important energy substrates.

The fetus synthesizes all its proteins from the amino acids derived from the mother; proteins are used mainly for synthesis rather than oxidation or gluconeogenesis.

Throughout gestation, the retention of calcium, phosphorus, and iron increases relative to fetal body weight. The fetus has the unique ability to deplete maternal skeletal stores of calcium if feeds are low in calcium. Iron is used for hemoglobin synthesis, but little is known about its distribution and metabolism.

### Fetal Growth

As it grows from the spherical fertilized ovum to the full-term fetus, the embryo not only increases in size and weight but also undergoes many changes in form. The rate of growth—that is, the percentage increase in weight and dimensions per unit of time (relative growth)—is most rapid in the earlier stages and declines as gestation advances. On the contrary, the absolute increment per unit of time (absolute growth) increases exponentially, reaching a maximum during late gestation.

The rate of fetal growth depends primarily on the feed supply and the ability of the fetus to use the feed (Fig. 10-8). Species, breed, and strain differences in fetal size are due to differences in the rate of cell division, which is determined genetically. Thus, there is close integration between the feed supply to the fetus (environmental factors), the rate of cell division (genetic factors), and hence, the rate of growth.

Genetic Factors. Holstein fetuses at birth weigh about 35% more than Jersey calves and about 15% more than the average dairy calf. Similarly, Romney sheep fetuses grow faster than Merino fetuses. The maternal contribution to variability in fetal size is greater than the paternal contribution.

Environmental Factors. These include size, parity, and nutrition of the mother, litter size, placental size, and climatic stress. Of these factors, maternal size is most important. The size of the sire only begins to exert influence on growth after birth. Similar observations have been made in cattle and sheep.

Nutrient supply to the fetus exerts an important influence on fetal growth. However, the direct supply of nutrients for tissue growth may be only a minor component. The indirect effects of nutrition on fetal endocrine and metabolic

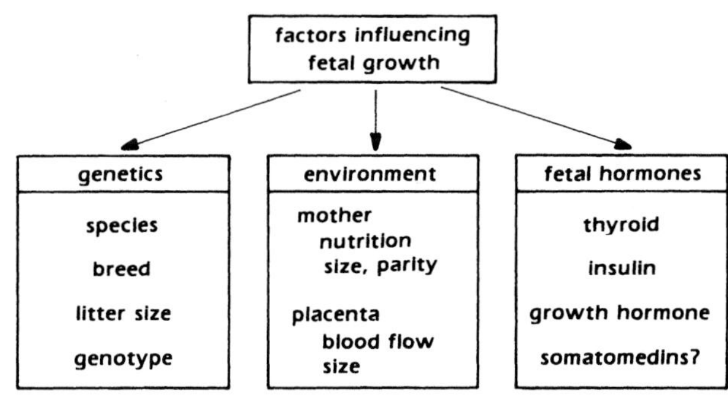


Figure 10-8. Summary of factors influencing fetal growth. Species and breed differences in fetal size are due to differences in the rate of cell division that is determined genetically. The rate of fetal growth depends on the intrauterine environment. Fetal hormones may influence fetal growth. Somatomedins are insulin-like growth factors that stimulate growth of fetal cells *in vitro*, but their role in the fetus is unknown.

status, as well as on the interaction between the fetus, placenta, and mother must be coordinated to permit fetal growth. Birth weight is a poor measure of fetal and the nutritional effects vary with the timing of the insult (6).

In sheep, undernutrition of the ewe during the latter part of gestation leads to the production of stunted lambs, even though a normal level of nutrition was present earlier. Conversely, a reversed type of feeding program results in normal sized lambs.

In polytocous species such as the pig, during early gestation feed and uterine accommodation are adequate, but in the later stages, the number of fetuses sharing the uterine blood supply can have a profound influence on their size at birth. The length of gestation in the pig is not reduced by increases in litter size, suggesting that the small birth weight with large litters must be related to the availability of nutrition to individual fetuses.

High ambient temperature during pregnancy affects fetal size. Exposure of pregnant ewes to heat stress reduces fetal growth, the degree of reduction being proportional to the length of exposure. This dwarfing is a specific effect of temperature and is not due to reduced feed intake during pregnancy.

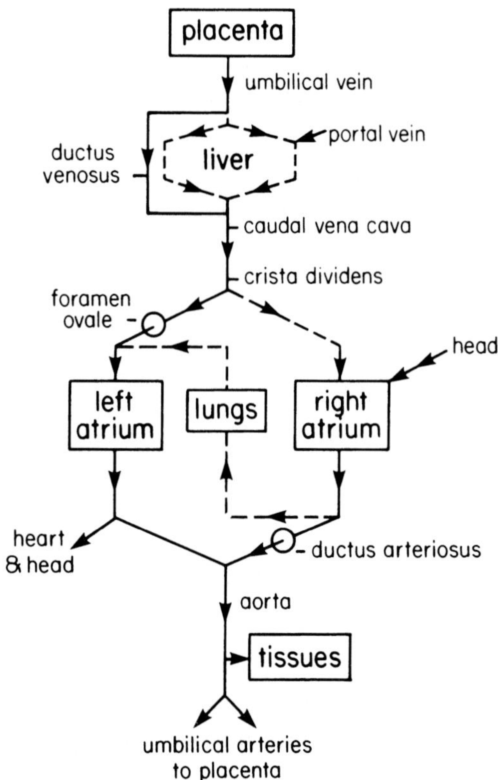


FIGURE 10-9. Schematic representation of fetal circulation. The ductus venosus, crista dividens, foramen ovale, and ductus arteriosus act as shunts directing oxygenated blood away from the liver, right ventricle, and functionless lungs, respectively.

GROWTH HORMONE AND ASSOCIATED FACTORS. Growth hormone can stimulate fetal growth, but there is no evidence that it is essential for fetal growth. Insulin is of importance in fetal growth and exerts its effects through an increase of energy substrate availability and stimulates placental growth. The fetal thyroid is dispensable in some species (rabbit, human), whereas in others (monkey, sheep) its absence results in delayed skeletal and muscular maturation.

The insulin-like growth factors (IGF-I and IGF-II) or sommatomedins are polypeptide hormones similar to insulin. They occur in fetal and placental tissues (7). IGF-II appears not only to mediate fetal growth according to the availability of glucose but also, acting in concert with placental hormones, regulates the metabolic activities of the mother so that a continuous supply of substrates for fetal development is available (2).

### Fetal Circulation

The fetal circulation (Fig. 10-9) is essentially similar to that of the adult except that oxygenation of blood occurs in the placenta rather than in the lungs. The fetal circulation also has several shunts or bypasses that direct oxygenated blood to the tissue.

1. Ductus venosus shunts a major portion of the blood in the umbilical vein from the liver into the caudal vena cava to avoid metabolism. In the pig and the horse, the ductus venosus never develops, and the umbilical venous blood passes through the liver sinusoids.
2. The crista dividens projects from the border of the foramen ovale and separates the caudal vena cava flow into two streams before the atria are reached.
3. Foramen ovale guides the stream from the ductus venosus into the left atrium, thereby directing oxygenated blood to the head and developing the left ventricle in the neonatal period.
4. The ductus arteriosus shunts most of the pulmonary arterial blood flow into the aorta and away from the functionless lungs. The two umbilical arteries originate from the caudal end of the descending aorta and carry blood to the placenta.

The higher blood pressure in the right side of the fetal heart than in the left side keeps the foramen ovale patent. Likewise, this pressure difference causes the blood to flow from the pulmonary artery into the aorta by way of the ductus arteriosus.

### Fetal Fluids

ORIGIN. The origin of fetal fluids (amniotic and allantoic) and the secretions that contribute to them are complex (Table 10-6). There are at least four sites at which absorption and secretion might occur: the respiratory, urinary, and digestive systems, and also the fetal skin. In the fetal lamb,

TABLE 10-6. ***Origin and Functions of Fetal Fluids in Farm Animals***

| FLUID | ORIGIN | FUNCTIONS |
|---|---|---|
| Amniotic | Fetal urine<br>Secretions from respiratory tract and buccal cavity<br>Maternal circulation | Protects fetus from external shock.<br>Prevents adhesion between fetal skin and amniotic membrane.<br>Assists in dilating cervix and lubricating birth passages during birth. |
| Allantoic | Fetal urine<br>Secretory activity of allantoic membrane | Brings allantochorion into close apposition with endometrium during initial steps of attachment.<br>Stores fetal excretory products not readily transferred back to the mother.<br>Helps to maintain osmotic pressure of fetal plasma. |

urine formed by the mesonephros passes into the allantoic cavity through the urachus until about 90 days of gestation. Thereafter, urine passes in increasing quantities into the amniotic sac, which is due to occlusion of the urachus and patency of the urethra. Thus fetal urine forms a major source of amniotic fluid in the latter part of pregnancy in sheep.

Other sources may influence the amount and composition of amniotic fluid in other species, for example: secretions from fetal salivary glands, buccal mucosa, lungs, and trachea; and dynamic interchange between maternal, fetal, and amniotic fluid compartments (Table 10-6).

A rapid exchange of water occurs between the maternal circulation, the fetal circulation, and the amniotic fluid with a new water circulation: mother to fetus to amniotic fluid to mother. The fetus also removes fluid by swallowing or by drawing amniotic fluid into the fetal lungs during respiratory movements.

VOLUME. The relative volumes of fluid in the amniotic and allantoic cavities show much fluctuation during pregnancy. Fetal fluids increase throughout gestation in all species, but in the pig they tend to decline at term. The volume of allantoic fluid is relatively higher than amniotic fluid during pregnancy, the exception being the ewe at midgestation.

FUNCTIONS. Amniotic fluid is not a stagnant pool but rather a vital fluid bathing the fetus and performing several functions (Table 10-6). Allantoic fluid, composed of hypotonic urine, maintains the osmotic pressure of the fetal plasma and prevents fluid loss to maternal circulation.

COMPOSITION. Amniotic and allantoic fluids contain metabolic constituents, electrolytes, enzymes, hormones, cells, and other structures. In ruminants, the inner lining of the amnion, particularly near the umbilicus, contains numerous raised, discrete, round foci called amnionic plaques, which are rich in glycogen and disappear late in gestation. Amniotic fluid also contains cells that may be used for a prenatal diagnosis of sex. Hippomanes are smooth, discoid, rubberlike, amber masses floating in the allantoic fluid and are probably aggregations of fetal hair and meconium.

## PARTURITION

Parturition, or labor, is the physiologic process by which the pregnant uterus delivers the fetus and placenta from the maternal organism.

### *Signs of Approaching Parturition*

Most signs of approaching parturition relate to changes in the pelvic ligaments, enlargement and edema of the vulva, and mammary activity. These signs are useful as a guide, but they are too variable for an accurate prediction of the date of parturition.

Obvious enlargement of the mammary gland occurs in all farm species. The teats become swollen and secretions may escape through the teat orifice. In the mare, colostrum oozes from the teat orifice, forming a bead of waxing material at each teat orifice. Waxing occurs in most mares between 6 to 48 hours before foaling and is replaced by drips or streams of milk 12 to 24 hours later.

Nest building is a feature of impending parturition in polytocous species such as the pig, but an expression of this behavior may be suspended in intensive management systems. Cattle and sheep under grazing systems remain with the herd but seek isolation just before the onset of parturition.

### *Initiation of Parturition*

Parturition is triggered by the fetus and is completed by a complex interaction of endocrine, neural, and mechanical

**TABLE 10-7. *Some Theories on the Initiation of Parturition***

| THEORY | POSSIBLE MECHANISM |
|---|---|
| Fall in progesterone concentration | Blocks myometrial contractions during pregnancy; near term the blocking action of progesterone decreases. |
| Rise in estrogen concentration | Overcomes the progesterone block of myometrial contractility and/or increases spontaneous myometrial contractility. |
| Increase of uterine volume | Overcomes the effects of progesterone block of myometrial contractility. |
| Release of oxytocin | Leads to contractions in an estrogen-sensitized myometrium. |
| Release of prostaglandins ($PGF_{2\alpha}$) | Stimulates myometrial contractions; induces luteolysis leading to a fall in progesterone concentration (corpus luteum-dependent species). |
| Activation of fetal hypothalamic-pituitary-adrenal axis | Fetal corticosteroids cause a fall in progesterone, a rise in estrogen, and a release of $PGF_{2\alpha}$. These events lead to myometrial contractility. |

factors (Table 10-7), but their precise roles and interrelationships are not fully understood.

Several reviews have discussed the control of parturition in sheep, goat, cattle, pig, and horse (Table 10-8) (8). Both fetal and maternal mechanisms play roles in initiating parturition. The fetal endocrine system dominates in ruminants (e.g., sheep, goat, and cattle), whereas it plays a minor role in other species (e.g., horse, human).

**TABLE 10-8. *Possible Mechanisms for Initiation of Parturition in Farm Animals***

| SPECIES | MECHANISM |
|---|---|
| Pig | $PGF_{2\alpha}$ is the luteolysin that induces CL regression. The increase in estrogen reflects increase pituitary-adrenal axis; estrogens increase oxytocin and PG release. |
| Sheep and Goat | Fetal cortisol acts on the placenta to induce the enzyme 17$\alpha$-hydroxylase to decrease plasma $P_4$, while increasing estrogen levels. The increase in E:P ratio enhances the sensitivity of $PGF_{2\alpha}$, $PGF_2$, and oxytocin. |
| Cattle | Parturition is initiated by $PGF_{2\alpha}$-induced luteolysis. Fetal cortisol stimulates the release of $PGF_{2\alpha}$, probably from the uterus. Other endocrine changes are similar to those of sheep and goat. |
| Horse | Oxytocin rises progressively towards the end of pregnancy, then a massive release triggered by a mechanical stimulus stimulates the synthesis of $PGF_{2\alpha}$. The combined actions of these two hormones results in the expulsion of the fetus. |

Adapted from Liggins GC, Thorburn GD. Initiation of Parturition. In: Laming GE, ed. Marshall's Physiology of Reproduction, 4th ed. London: Chapman & Hall, 1994;3:863–1002.

**FETAL MECHANISMS.** One of the exciting discoveries in reproductive biology was the demonstration in the 1960s that hypophysectomy in fetal sheep abolishes the initiation of parturition. This discovery shifted focus from maternal control to fetal control of the onset of parturition. Subsequent studies revealed species differences.

The fetus possesses a number of mechanisms to ensure that the myometrium remains quiescent so that its development in utero is unhindered. The placental production of progesterone imposes a conduction block on the myometrium (Table 10-7). A decrease in maternal progesterone concentration is a prerequisite for the dilation of the cervix and explosive myometrial activity associated with labor. The decrease in progesterone concentrations is induced by a spectacular rise in fetal cortisol during the final stages of gestation in sheep, goat, cattle, and pigs but not in horse. Thorburn (9) has postulated that the increasing metabolic demands on the placenta during the phase of rapid fetal growth (last trimester) stimulate placental production of prostaglandin $E_2$, which in turn activates the fetal hypothalamic-pituitary-adrenal axis, leading to a rise in concentration of fetal cortisol.

The mechanisms that follow the release of cortisol differ among species depending on the source of progesterone maintaining the pregnancy:

1. In sheep, fetal cortisol induces the placental $17_{2\alpha}$ enzyme to catalyse the conversion of progesterone or pregnenolone to oestrogen (8). The elevated levels of estrogen stimulate secretion of prostaglandin and development of oxytocin receptors.
2. In CL-dependent species, cortisol in addition to the

synthesis of estrogen causes a release of prostaglandin from the endometrium, which in turn causes regression of the corpora lutea.

MATERNAL MECHANISMS. The maternal contribution, although less dramatic than those of the fetus, is clearly evident in the timing of birth. For example, the predilection of the mare to foal during the hours of darkness and the ability to postpone birth until she is undisturbed is well recognized. Anxiety, stress, or fear prolongs the act of parturition in several species through a decrease in myometrial contractility induced by a release of epinephrine. Management routines such as feeding may also influence the time of parturition in cattle, horses, and sheep. Thus, it is reasonable to conclude that the fetus determines the day of parturition, whereas the mother decides the hour of parturition.

### *Mechanics of Parturition*

Successful parturition depends on two mechanical processes: the ability of the uterus to contract and the capacity of the cervix to dilate sufficiently to enable the passage of the fetus (Fig. 10-10).

MYOMETRIAL CONTRACTIONS. The activity of the uterine muscle (myometrium) is under the influence of progesterone, which ensures an environment conducive to the developing fetus. Myometrial contractions of low amplitude and frequency occur during the major part of gestation.

At term, the uterus switches from a progesterone dominated to an estrogen-dominated state. As a result, two parallel molecular/biochemical pathways are mobilized within uterine tissues (Fig. 10-11) (10).

1. The first pathway is similar to those in smooth muscle and transforms the uterus from its "relaxed" state during pregnancy to an "activated state."

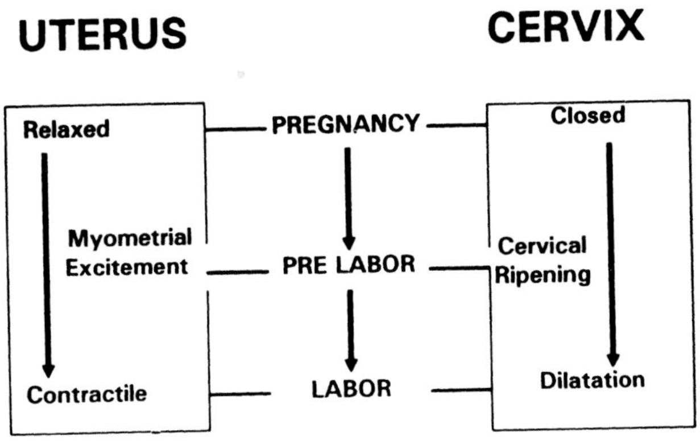

UTERUS

CERVIX

| Relaxed | PREGNANCY | Closed |
|---|---|---|
| Myometrial Excitement | PRE LABOR | Cervical Ripening |
| Contractile | LABOR | Dilatation |

FIGURE 10-10. Roles of the uterus and cervix during pregnancy and labor. During the prelabor stage, the myometrium loses its inhibitions and generates contractility, whereas the cervix "ripens" and dilates, permitting the normal onset of labor. (Redrawn from Calder AA. Reprod Fertil Dev 1990;2:553.)

2. The second pathway that results from an increase of the E/P ratio increases the synthesis or release of uterotonins (e.g., PGF, oxytocin).

These two pathways acting jointly initiate the intense, synchronous myometrial contractions needed to dilate the cervix and effect delivery of the fetus(s). Dilation of the cervix is due more to changes in the physical characteristics of cervical collagen ("ripening") than to increased intrauterine pressure. This is clearly evident in species such as sheep, goats, and cattle that have a rigid cervix. Ripening of the cervix is hormone dependent and may be influenced by factors such as the elevated levels of estrogens, secretion of relaxin (pig), and prostaglandin at the onset of parturition. A few hours before the commencement of labor contractions, the cervix softens, becomes more compliant, and gradually dilates.

### *Labor*

Labor commences with the onset of regular, peristaltic uterine contractions accompanied by progressive dilation of the cervix.

STAGES OF LABOR. For descriptive purposes three stages of labor may be recognized (Table 10-9):

1. Dilation of the cervix,
2. Expulsion of the fetus, and
3. Expulsion of the fetal membranes.

The time required for the expulsion of the fetus is the shortest of the three stages in monotocous species (Table 10-10).

### *Reponse to Birth*

The fetus, which depended on the placenta for respiration, nutrition, and excretion, makes a complex series of structural and physiologic adjustments for extrauterine life. The expulsion of the placenta at parturition deprives the neonate of a source of oxygen, glucose, and heat.

MATURATION OF FETAL ORGANS. To meet the above challenges, several fetal organs undergo maturational changes in late pregnancy that are regulated by fetal cortisol (11). Among these are:

1. Maturation of lungs to overcome the high surface tension with the first breath. Lung expansion is facilitated by secretion of a surface-active material (surfactant), which reduces the surface tension within the alveoli.
2. Glucose production from glycogen reserves and gluconeogenesis to meet the energy supply of the neonate until suckling is established.
3. Increased output of tri-iodothyronine and catecholamines to meet the sharp rise in metablic rate and tem-

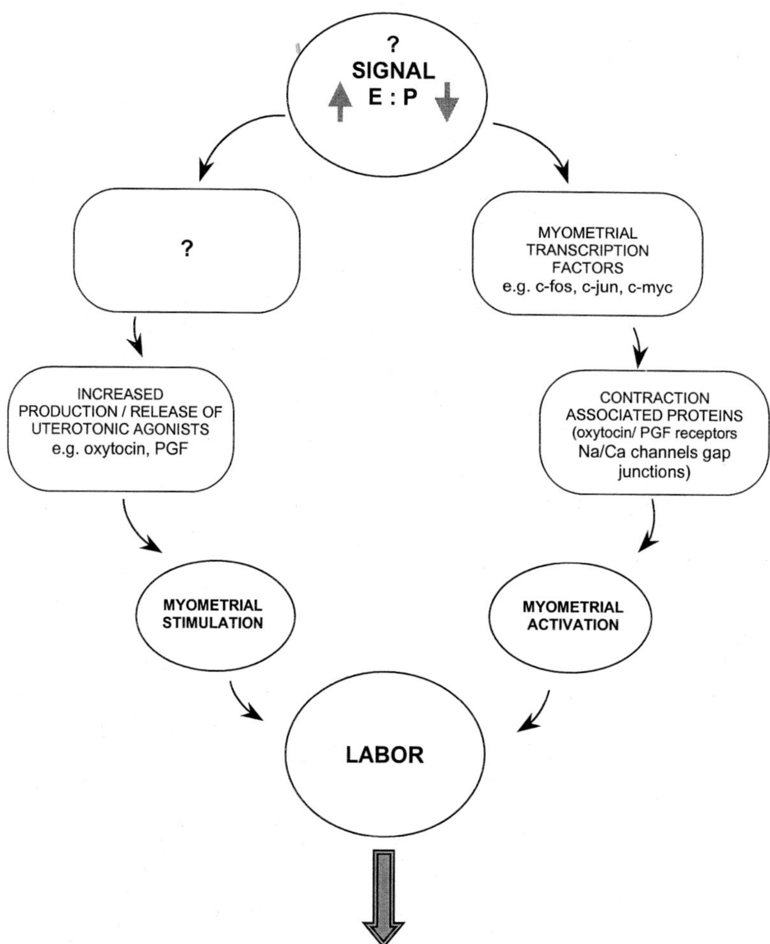


FIGURE 10-11. At term, the uterus switches from a progesterone dominated to an estrogen-dominated state. As a result, two parallel molecular/biochemical pathways are mobilized within uterine tissues. (Adapted from Lye SJ. Initiation of parturition. Anim Reprod Sci 1996;42:495–503.)

perature regulation associated the cold environment. Swine and sheep are particularly susceptible to low ambient temperatures; the rectal temperature of lambs falls 2 to 3°C, while that of piglets declines 2 to 5°C in the first hour after birth.

CARDIOVASCULAR CHANGES. With the cessation of the umbilical circulation and the commencement of lung ventilation at birth, the following changes occur:

1. The closure of the ductus arteriosus is one of the most important adjustments for extrauterine life and allows the flow of blood through the lungs during each circuit of the body.
2. The closure of the foramen ovale within a few hours in the foal and toward the end of the first week of life in the lamb.

IMMUNE STATUS. During prenatal life, the fetus synthesizes little or no antibodies. It acquires antibodies from its mother (passive immunity) while it is still in utero (rat, rabbit, and human), or the antibodies are secreted by the mammary glands and acquired by suckling (farm animals). This difference may be related to the impermeability of the epitheliochorial placenta of farm animals to maternal antibodies. Immediately after birth, however, immunoglobulins are transferred to the newborn through colostrum; the small intestine is permeable to immunoglobulins for a period of 24 to 36 hours after birth.

## PUERPERIUM

While nursing one or more offspring, the postpartum female makes a series of physiologic and anatomic readjustments

TABLE 10-9. *Stages of Labor and Related Events in Farm Animals*

| STAGE OF LABOR | MECHANICAL FORCES | PERIOD | RELATED EVENTS |
|---|---|---|---|
| I. Dilation of Cervix | Regular uterine contractions | Beginning of uterine contractions until cervix is fully dilated and continuous with vagina | Maternal restlessness, elevated pulse and respiratory rates<br>Changes in fetal position and posture |
| II. Expulsion of Fetus[a] | Strong uterine and abdominal contractions | From complete cervical dilation to end of delivery of fetus | Maternal recumbency and straining<br>Rupture of allantochorion and escape of fluid from vulva<br>Appearance of amnion (water-bag) at vulva<br>Rupture of amnion and delivery of fetus |
| III. Expulsion of Fetal Membranes | Uterine contractions decrease in amplitude | Following delivery of fetus to expulsion of fetal membranes | Maternal straining ceases<br>Loosening of chorionic villi from maternal crypts<br>Inversion of chorioallantois<br>Straining and expulsion of fetal membranes |

[a]In polytoccous species (sow) and twin-bearing species (sheep and goat), this stage cannot be separated from the next stage (III).

both in the uterus and ovaries for the restoration of her reproductive capacity (Fig. 10-12). The puerperium, or the postpartum period, is broadly defined as the period extending from delivery until the maternal organism has returned to its normal nonpregnant state. Since early rebreeding is often practiced in horse and cattle, a more suitable definition of puerperium would be the interval between parturition and the occurrence of the first estrus ("open" period) at which conception can occur. In a seasonal breeder such as sheep, postpartum ovarian cycles are suspended until the next breeding season.

### *Involution of Uterus*

Uterine involution is the restoration of the uterus to its normal nonpregnant size and function after parturition. It depends on myometrial contractions, elimination of bacterial infection, and regeneration of the endometrium (Fig. 10-12).

Lochia, the uterine discharge that normally occurs during the puerperium, is composed of mucus, blood, shreds of fetal membranes, and maternal tissue and fetal fluids. Lochia ceases by the first week after parturition. The expulsion of

TABLE 10-10. *Average Duration of the Three Stages of Labor in Farm Animals (hours)*

| | STAGE OF LABOR | | |
|---|---|---|---|
| ANIMAL | *I. Dilation of Cervix* | *II. Expulsion of Fetus(es)* | *III. Expulsion of Fetal Membranes* |
| Mare | 1–4 | 0.2–0.5 | 1 |
| Cow, buffalo | 2–6 | 0.5–1.0 | 6–12 |
| Ewe | 2–6 | 0.5–2.0 | 0.5–8 |
| Sow | 2–12 | 2.5–3.0 | 1–4 |

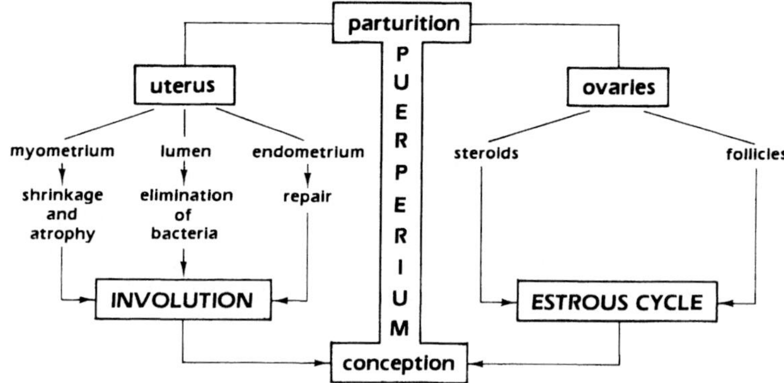


FIGURE 10-12. Diagram depicting the various processes occurring in the uterus and the ovaries. Involution and resumption of the estrous cycle occur during the puerperium before another pregnancy can be established.

lochia and reduction of uterine size are caused by myometrial contractions. This is due to a sustained release of prostaglandin after parturition, which increases uterine tone and thus promotes involution.

The sterile conditions of the uterus that prevailed during pregnancy are disrupted at parturition. Both pathogenic and nonpathogenic bacteria enter the uterus through the dilated cervix and rapidly multiply in a favorable uterine environment. The postpartum uterus depends on three processes to prepare it for the subsequent pregnancy.

1. A defense mechanism that includes a massive infiltration of lymphocytes into the uterine lumen to phagocytize the major pathogens present in the early postpartum period.
2. A massive release of prostaglandin during the first two weeks postpartum induces myometrial contractions and the evacuation of fluids and fetal membrane debris from the uterus. The duration of release of prostaglandin is longer in species with a cotyledonary type of placenta (cow, goat, buffalo) than in those with a diffuse type (horse, pig).
3. Estrogen secreted by the ovaries before the first ovulation makes the uterus more resistant to infection.

The time needed to clear the uterus of bacteria depends on the extent of contamination at parturition, retention of fetal membranes, and the production of estrogen. Regeneration of the endometrium is completed earlier in species with a diffuse placenta than those with a cotyledonary placenta. The endometrium is fully regenerated between the second and third week in the horse and pig, and between the fourth and fifth week in ruminants.

### *Resumption of Estrous Cycles*

Estrus and ovulation are usually suspended during lactation (lactational anestrus) in several mammalian species, but the inhibitory effects of lactation have been partially or completely overcome in farm animals through selection, improvements in nutrition, and weaning. The resumption of estrous cycles has received considerable attention in cattle because of the production target of a calf per cow each year.

By day 50 postpartum, about 95% of dairy cows will resume ovarian cycles, as compared with about 40% of beef cows. The first ovulation is often not preceded by overt estrus. Suckling and increasing the frequency of milking (four milkings vs. two milkings per day) prolong this interval, whereas removal of the calf from the mother shortens it.

Most mares exhibit a foal heat within 6 to 13 days postpartum. It is a routine practice to breed mares at the foal heat despite the lower conception rates and higher incidence of nonviable foals and abortions.

Sows frequently exhibit an anovulatory estrus 3 to 5 days after farrowing, but estrus and ovulation are generally inhibited throughout lactation in most animals. Removing the piglets or weaning them at any time induces estrus and ovulation with 3 to 5 days.

In sheep, a seasonal breeder, births occur at the end of breeding season and the lactational anestrus coincides with seasonal anestrus.

### *Mechanisms of Suckling Induced Suppression of Cyclicity*

Acyclicity during the postpartum period may be due to inhibition at several levels of the hypothalmo-pituitary-ovarian axis (12). Preventing the release of GnRH, FSH, and LH, or failure of ovarian follicles to respond to gonadotrophin stimulation may block ovarian activity.

The most consistent endocrine event preceding the first postpartum ovulation is the appearance of a pulsatile pattern of luteinizing LH in sheep, pigs, and cattle. Also, a small increase in progesterone secretion precedes the first postpartum estrus in cattle and sheep. Suckling apparently inhibits the release of GnRH necessary for restoration of the pulsatile release of LH. In the absence of LH, ovarian follicles fail to grow or secrete low levels of steroids under the influence FSH (13).

## REFERENCES

1. Flint APF. Interferon, the oxytocin receptor and maternal recognition of pregnancy in ruminants and non-ruminants: a comparative approach. Reprod Fertil Dev 1995;7:313–318.

2. Owens JA. Endocrine and substrate control of fetal growth: placental and maternal influences and insulin-like growth factors. Reprod Fertil Dev 1991;3:501.
3. Wooding FBP, Flint APF. Placentation In: Laming GE, ed. Marshall's Physiology of Reproduction, 4th ed. London: Chapman & Hall, 1994;3:235–460.
4. Broughton-Pipkin F, Hull D, Stephensen T. Fetal Physiology. In: Laming GE, ed. Marshall's Physiology of Reproduction, 4th ed. London: Chapman & Hall, 1994;3:769–861.
5. Schneider H. Placental transport function. Reprod Fertil Dev 1991;3:345.
6. Harding JE, Johnston BM. Nutrition and fetal growth. Reprod Fertil 1995;7:539–547.
7. Falconer J, Davies JJ, Zhang HP, Smith R. Release of insulin-like growth factor I by the sheep placenta *in vitro*. Reprod Fertil Dev 1991;3:379.
8. Liggins GC, Thorburn GD. Initiation of Parturition. In: Laming GE, ed. Marshall's Physiology of Reproduction, 4th ed. London: Chapman & Hall, 1994;3:863–1002.
9. Thorburn GD. The placenta, prostaglandins and parturition: a review. Reprod Fertil Dev 1991;3:277.
10. Lye SJ. Initiation of parturition. Anim Reprod Sci 1996;42:495–503.
11. Liggins GC. The role of cortisol in preparing the fetus for birth. Reprod Fertil Dev 1994;6:141–150.
12. Peters AR, Lamming GE. Lactational anoestrus in farm animals. In: Milligan SR, ed. Oxford Reviews of Reproductive Biology. New York: Oxford University Press, 1990;12.
13. McNeilly AS, Forsyth IA. Regulation of Postpartum Fertility in Lactating Mammals. Initiation of Parturition. In: Laming GE, ed. Marshall's Physiology of Reproduction, 4th ed. London: Chapman & Hall, 1994;3:1038–1101.

# Part III

# *Reproductive Cycles*

CHAPTER 11

# Cattle and Buffalo

M.R. JAINUDEEN AND E.S.E. HAFEZ

The domestic cattle (*Bos taurus*, *Bos indicus*) and domestic buffalo (*Bubalus bubalis*), the African wild buffalo (*Syncerus caffer*), and the North American "buffalo" (*Bison bison*) are all in the family Bovidae but belong to different genera and have different chromosome numbers.

Cattle and buffaloes were domesticated for draft, milk, and meat around the same period in history. The domestic buffalo, also known as the water buffalo because its predilection for water, possesses several characteristics that distinguish it from cattle.

Although many similarities in reproduction exist between cattle and buffalo, indiscriminate extrapolation of reproductive phenomena between the two species must be avoided. Therefore, this chapter is presented in two parts: first Cattle, and then Buffalo. Each part focuses on species-specific aspects of the reproductive cycle that include puberty, estrous cycle, postpartum resumption of estrous cycles, and spermatogenesis. Finally, each part ends with a discussion on methods of improving the reproductive performance.

## CATTLE

### Puberty

FEMALE. Heifers attain puberty at the first estrus that is followed by a normal luteal phase. It is now known that puberty and first ovulation are not synonymous in most heifers. After the first ovulation, short cycles and estrus without ovulation (anovulation) often occur before the reproductive system is fully functional.

There is evidence that puberty occurs at a specific physiologic age as opposed to chronologic age. The age at puberty in heifers is influenced by several factors (Fig. 11-1). Historically recommended body size criteria have been based on live bodyweight measurements. Besides live bodyweight, other measurements such as wither height, length, and pelvic area measurements can be used to define body size. A database is available for the Holstein genotype that incorporates measures of skeletal growth and body composition with bodyweight when defining body size (1). It should aid commercial dairy producers to better define replacement heifer growth and management practices.

A low level of nutrient intake and slow growth delay puberty in heifers for weeks and a high level of nutrition and rapid growth hasten puberty. The average age of puberty for heifers on recommended levels of nutrition is 10 to 12 months for dairy breeds and 11 to 15 months for beef breeds. Zebu heifers attain puberty at 18 to 24 months. However, breed differences in age at puberty are not affected by nutrition. Season affects age at puberty. Winter conditions during the prepubertal period delays puberty. If heifers are provided with adequate nutrition, estrus normally recurs regularly after the pubertal estrus.

MALE. Puberty in the male is the age at which the ejaculate contains sufficient spermatozoa to impregnate a cow. One of the earliest changes in the initiation of puberty in the bull is an increase in the frequency of pulsatile release of LH between 12 and 20 weeks. These LH discharges stimulate Leydig cells to secrete testosterone, which is needed for differentiation of Sertoli cells and spermatogenesis. Cellular differentiation occurs gradually in the seminiferous epithelium of the testes during calfhood, with the presence of mature spermatozoa in the seminiferous tubules by about 5 months of age. The testes produce increasing numbers of spermatozoa as puberty nears. A practical definition of puberty in the bull would be the time when the first ejaculate contains 50 million spermatozoa with at least 10% progressive motility.

Breeds differ in age and bodyweight at puberty. Holstein bulls reached puberty earlier than Angus or Hereford bulls, with Charolais bulls falling between the others. Crossbred beef bulls generally reach puberty earlier than straightbred bulls. Zebu bulls reach puberty at a later age than most temperate breeds of cattle. This difference is presumably associated with the more rapid growth rate of crossbred bulls. After bulls reach puberty, the testes continue to grow

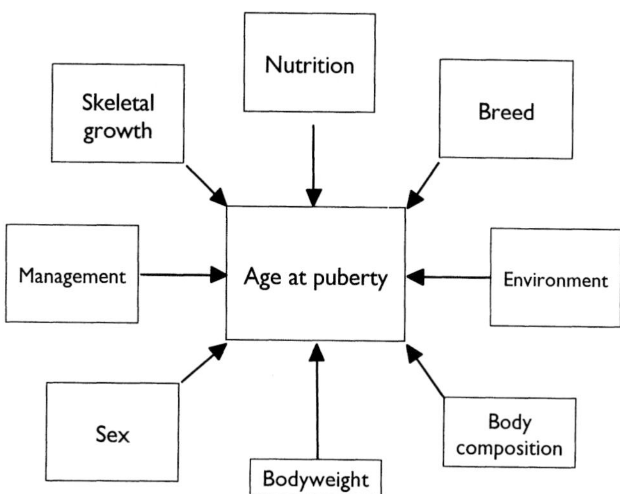


FIGURE 11-1. Factors affecting age at puberty.

and the number of sperm per ejaculate increases until 18 to 24 months of age in both beef and dairy bulls.

## *Estrous Cycle*

**BREEDING SEASON.** Many wild species of bovidae are seasonal breeders with spring and summer being the most suitable times of the year for calving. During the course of domestication, both dairy and beef cattle were selected against seasonality, facilitating them to ovulate and conceive throughout the year. However, beef cows might still be sensitive to photoperiodicity.

**CYCLIC CHANGES.** Morphologic, endocrine, and secretory changes occur in the ovaries and the tubular genitalia of the cow during the estrous cycle (Fig. 11-2). A knowledge of these changes is useful in estrus detection and synchronization, superovulation, and artificial insemination.

*FOLLICULAR DYNAMICS.* Several thousands of follicles are present in each ovary of the cow, but only one follicle ovulates per estrous cycle. Ultrasonic observations have revealed that ovarian follicular development during the estrous cycle in the cow occurs in a wave-like pattern, with as few as one to as many as four; the three-wave pattern is most common (2).

From each wave of growing follicles, a single large "dominant" follicle continues to grow while suppressing the growth of follicles larger than 4 mm in diameter (3). The growth of follicles to diameters greater than 4 mm depends on FSH but large antral follicles (7 to 9 mm diameter) transfer their gonadotrophic requirements to LH. The maintenance and regression of the dominant follicle is associated with changes in $P_4$ and LH environment (4). Thus, at least one large follicle is present in the bovine ovary throughout the estrous cycle, and it apparently controls the fate of other follicles in the ovary.

Only one or two large follicles, present very near the onset of estrus, attain the final spurt of growth leading to mature Graafian follicles, capable of ovulation. The follicle collapses following ovulation. No hemorrhage occurs at this site; instead, the cavity gradually fills with luteal cells. The CL reaches maturity about 7 days after ovulation and functions for a further 8 or 9 days before it finally regresses.

*ACTIONS OF ESTROGENS.* Follicular growth, ovulation, and luteal function are regulated by the hypothalamic-pituitary-ovarian axis. The Graafian follicle secretes estrogens, particularly estradiol-17$\beta$. The rising levels of estradiol induce behavioral estrus and, combined with declining levels of $P_4$, trigger the LH surge. If a mature follicle is present, this LH surge will cause ovulation about 24 hours later.

The actions of estrogens are listed below:

1. Decreases viscosity and maximum ferning of cervical mucus on the day of estrus and a string of clear mucus hanging from the vulva.
2. Dilates the cervix during estrus so that a catheter can be passed into the uterus more readily than at any other stage of the estrous cycle.
3. Improves the contractility or tonicity of the uterus.

Alterations in viscosity, ferning, and electrical resistance are the basis for some methods of detecting estrus in cow (Table 11-1). Since uterine tone is a good indicator of estrus and can be detected by rectal palpation, most inseminators use it to verify if cows submitted for insemination are in estrus.

Estrogen increases vascular growth of the endometrium. The sudden withdrawal of estrogen secretion following ovulation causes the presence of blood in the vulval discharge (metestrous bleeding). Most cows and heifers show bleeding on the second or third day after estrus. Apparently, metestrous bleeding bears no relationship to conception; it is only an indication that a cow has been in estrus. Cows showing blood-stained mucus at the time of insemination are less likely to conceive.

*ACTIONS OF PROGESTERONE.* $P_4$ secreted by the CL acts on the uterus and cervix and has an opposite effect to that of estrogen (Table 11-1). During the luteal phase, cervical mucus is thick and tenacious, the cervical canal is tightly closed, and the myometrium is relaxed. $P_4$ levels in plasma are closely correlated with the growth, maintenance, and regression of the CL.

**ESTRUS DETECTION METHODS.** Most estrous periods can be detected by careful observation of cattle at least twice daily (Table 11-1). During checks for estrus, any distractions to cattle, such as feeding, should be avoided. Detection of estrus is improved by the use of bulls; they may be vasectomized or their penises may be surgically deflected or locked mechanically in the sheath. Other aids to detecting estrus include pressure-sensitive indicators placed on the rump of females and chin-ball markers or marking harnesses on bulls

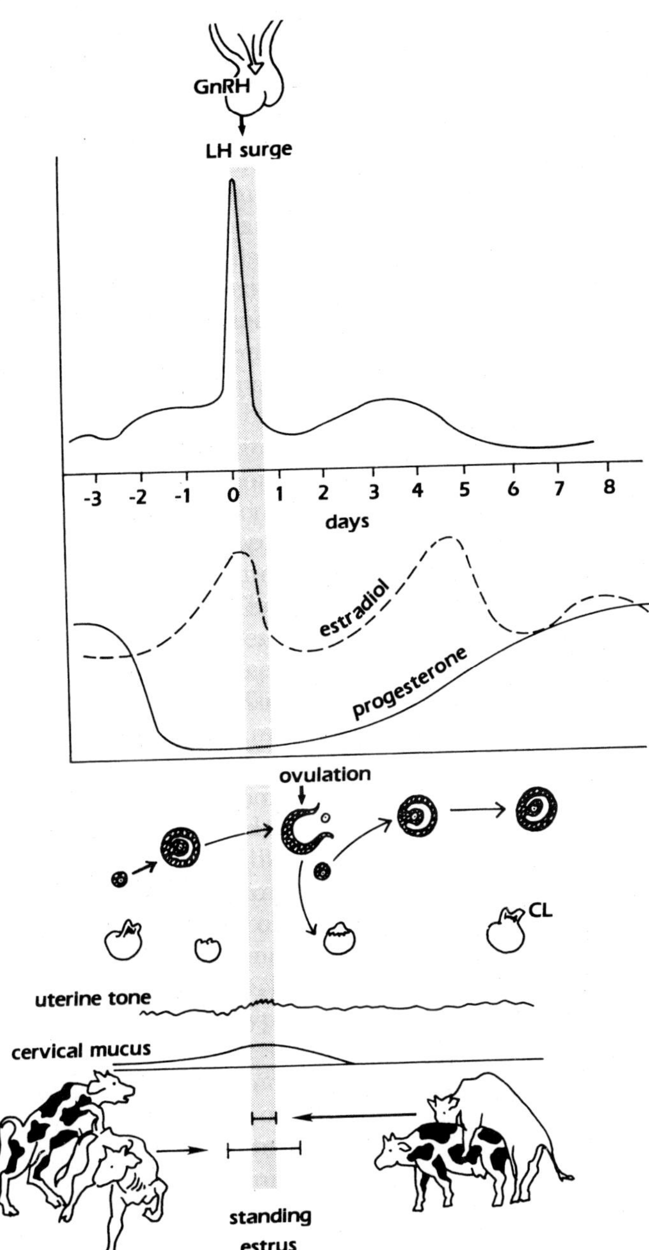


FIGURE 11-2. The endocrine, physiologic, and behavioral changes associated with "standing estrus" (standing to be mounted) in the cow. During proestrus, the preovulatory follicle secretes increasing amounts of estradiol; at this time, the cow may ride other cows and begin to secrete cervical mucus. At the onset of estrus, peak levels of estradiol trigger a surge of LH that causes ovulation to occur about 10 to 12 hours after the end of estrus; uterine tone is maximum, and cervical mucus is copious and watery. While the growing corpus luteum secretes increasing amounts of progesterone, two waves of follicles occur, one at the early phase of the cycle and the other at midluteal phase. (Hormonal levels adapted from Hansel W, Convey EM. J Anim Sci 1983;57(Suppl 2):404.)

(Fig. 11-3) . When bulls equipped with chin-ball markers or harnesses mount an estrous female, an easily visible mark of dye or pigmented grease is left on the rump and tail-head of the female. Although nonestrous cows will occasionally be marked, the marking aids identify cows that should be observed closely for confirmation of estrus.

Efficient and accurate detection of estrus are essential in dairy herds using artificial insemination. Inaccuracies in estrus detection result in insemination of cows that are not in estrus, thus lowering the herd conception rate. Heersche and Nebel (5) have reviewed the methods of measuring the efficiency and accuracy of estrus detection in dairy cattle. These detection criteria may be calculated as follows:

1. Efficiency of detection is expressed as the percentage of possible estrous periods that are observed in a given period of time.
2. Accuracy of detection is the percentage of estrous periods observed that is true estrus. The accuracy can be confirmed by rectal palpation of the uterus for tone and the ovaries for a mature follicle, and basal $P_4$ levels of cows considered to be in estrus.

OVULATION. Cattle are unique among farm animals in that they ovulate 10 to 12 hours after the end of standing estrus, or on the average 30 hours after the onset of estrus (Table 11-2). Except for the first postpartum estrous cycle,

**TABLE 11-1. *Methods of Estrus Detection in Cattle***

| PRINCIPLE | METHOD OF DETECTION | COMMENT |
|---|---|---|
| Sexual behavior (standing to be mounted) | Observations | |
| | Visual | Twice daily observations |
| | Videotape | Night time (limited value) |
| | Teasers fitted with marking devices | Teasers are (a) bulls surgically prepared to prevent release of sperm or copulation; (b) steers treated with testosterone, and (c) cows with cystic ovaries or those treated with androstenedione |
| | Chin-ball mating device | A halter fitted with a reservoir of dye that is released by a ball-type mechanism and marks a line on the back of the cow |
| | Grease | Smeared on brisket |
| | Collar | A pad soaked in dye or grease |
| | Detectors on cows | Applied on point of maximum pressure during mounting—sacral spine (detection is continuous) |
| | Heat mount detector (KaMaR) | Release of dye on pressure (unsuitable in wet weather) |
| | Tail paint | Removes hair at site when mounted |
| Physiologic changes related to estrus | Progesterone | Basal levels in milk or plasma; retrospective confirmation of estrus |
| | Cervical mucus | Alterations in physiochemical properties |
| | Ferning | Maximum on mucus dried on a glass side |
| | Viscosity | Decreased |
| | Electrical resistance | Decreased as measured by a vaginal probe |
| | Vaginal pH | Decreased |
| | Uterine tone | Maximum on rectal palpation |
| | Estrus-related odors | Dogs trained to detect odors in vaginal mucus, milk, or urine |
| | Body temperature | A rise of 0.5 to 0.8°C during estrus but drops on ovulation; radio telemetric measurement of vaginal temperature |
| | Physical activity | Increased as measured by electronic pedometers |

Adapted from Foote RH. J Dairy Sci 1975;58:248; Britt JH. J Dairy Sci 1977;60:1994; Kiddy CA, Mitchell DS, Hawk HW. J Dairy Sci 1984;67:388; Vasquez G, et al. Proc 10th Intl Congress Anim Reprod & AI, III 1984;298; Zartman DL, et al. Theriogenology 1983;19:541.

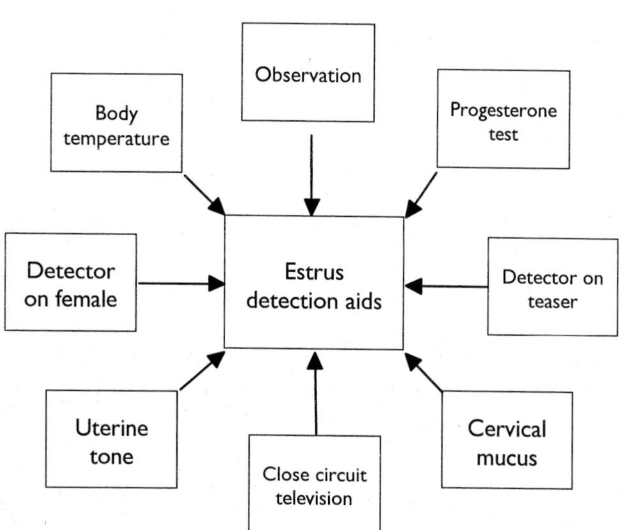


FIGURE 11-3. Estrus detection aids for cattle and buffalo.

ovulations are preceded by behavioral signs of estrus. Cattle are spontaneous ovulators, but ovulation can be advanced by about 2 hours by service with a vasectomized bull. Similarly, manual massage of the clitoris for 10 seconds following artificial insemination of beef cows shortened the interval from beginning of estrus until the LH surge and ovulation by 4 hours, and increased the conception rate by 6%.

Normally, one follicle ovulates per estrous cycle in cattle. Two follicles ovulate about 10% of the time and three follicles infrequently. Follicles ovulate on the right ovary about 60% of the time and on the left ovary about 40% of the time. The first ovulation after parturition occurs more frequently on the ovary opposite to the uterine horn that previously carried the fetus.

## *Sperm Production and Release*

The duration of one cycle of the seminiferous epithelium is 13.5 days for bulls, irrespective of the breed. Approxi-

**Table 11-2. *Female Reproductive Characteristics of Cattle and Buffalo***

| Parameter | Cattle Mean (range) | Buffalo Mean (range) |
|---|---|---|
| Sexual season | Polyestrous | Polyestrous |
| Age at puberty (months) | 15 (10–24) | 21 (15–36) |
| Estrous cycle | | |
| Length (days) | 21 (14–29) | 21 (18–22) |
| Estrus (hours) | 18 (12–30) | 21 (17–24) |
| Ovulation | | |
| Type | Spontaneous | Spontaneous |
| Time from onset (hours) | 30 (18–48) | 32 (18–45) |
| Number of eggs shed | 1 | 1 |
| Life span of corpus luteum (days) | 16 | 16 |
| Fertilizable life of ova (hours) | (20–24) | ? |
| Entry of ova into uterus (hours after ovulation) | 90 (64–96) | ? |
| Gestation length (days) | 280 (278–293) | 315 (305–330) |
| Age at first calving (months) | 30 (24–36) | 42 (36–56) |
| Postpartum intervals (days) | | |
| Uterine involution | 45 (32–50) | 35 (16–60) |
| First ovulation | 30 (10–110) | 75 (35–180) |
| Calving intervals (months) | 13 (12–14) | 18 (15–21) |

mately 61 days (4.5 seminiferous epithelium cycles) are required for completion of spermatogenesis. Thus, an injury to the testes of a bull resulting from fever, heat stress, or transport stress could interfere with spermatogenesis and sperm production; it would take at least 2 months before sperm quality returns to normal.

Daily sperm production, the number of potentially fertile sperm produced per day by the testes, is highly correlated with testicular size, which can be estimated by length and width measurements or scrotal circumference (Fig. 11-4). Both testis size and scrotal circumference, however, are influenced by genotype and age. Thus, it is not possible to have standard measurements for all ages and breeds. Sperm production also varies widely among individual bulls with some variation among breeds.

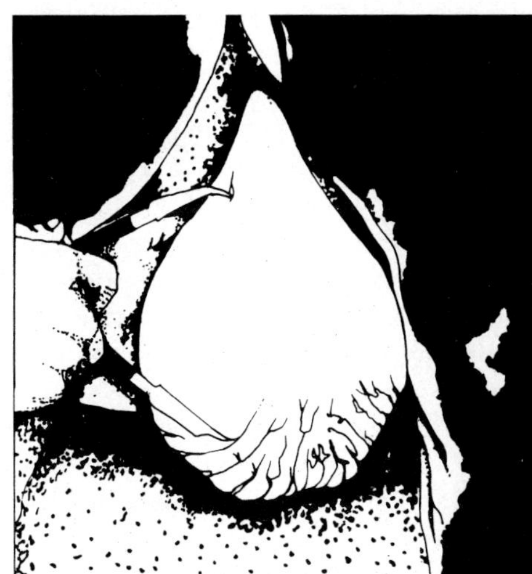

Figure 11-4. Testicular size is estimated by length and width measurements and/or scrotal circumference.

The bull ejaculates 4 to 10 ml of semen containing 0.8 to 2.0 billion sperm per milliliter. Semen output is influenced by the age of bull, season of the year, and frequency of ejaculation. Normally, total sperm per ejaculate increases with the age of bull up to about 7 years, then declines. Large differences exist in semen output characteristics between bulls, between first and second ejaculates, and with intervals between collections.

## *Mating*

Mating Behavior. At rest, the penis of the bull, which is of the fibroelastic type, is relatively small in diameter and rigid. During erection, it undergoes little enlargement. Protrusion is effected by straightening of the S-shaped sigmoid flexure. Vision appears more important than smell in sexual stimulation of a bull. The bull identifies the estrous cow by licking or smelling around her external genitalia and curling his upper lip in a characteristic manner—"Flehmen" behavior. Before mounting, the bull orientates himself behind the cow and rests his chin and throat over the cow's rump. Estrous cows respond to chin-resting pressure by standing.

Mating in cattle is brief (less than 5 seconds) when compared to that in horses and swine. As the partially erect penis protrudes from the sheath and accessory fluid dribbles, the bull mounts and straddles the cow. After the penis penetrates the vagina (intromission), sudden contractions of the abdominal muscles of the bull lead to maximum intromission and ejaculation. The force of the muscular contraction lifts the bull's hind legs off the ground as an active leap forward. This ejaculatory thrust deposits the semen in the anterior vagina near the external os of the cervix.

MATING PRACTICES. Most dairy herds in the United States use an artificial insemination service, but over 90% of beef cattle are bred by natural service. Usually, one bull is assigned to about 30 to 60 cows in either single or multiple-sire mating pastures. Under range conditions, the number of females mated per unit time depends on many interrelated factors such as male to female ratio and the aggressive interactions among bulls.

Social ranking of bulls, largely controlled by age and seniority within groups, can influence their sexual activity. Calves born to cows exposed as a herd to three or four bulls show that the oldest or the second oldest bull in the group sire over 60% of the calves while the youngest bull sired less than 15% of the calves. Breed differences exist in the libido of bulls. Holsteins react more quickly to stimulation at semen collection than most other breeds; Zebu bulls have a slower reaction time than European breeds.

Most beef herds have restricted breeding seasons of 9 to 12 weeks so that cows calve in spring when abundant feed is available. Heifers are bred at an optimum target weight that varies with breed (Table 11-3). Matings should be planned to avoid disproportionately large calves in dams with small pelvic cavities.

TABLE 11-3. ***Optimum Body Weight (and Age) to Breed Heifers***

| BREED | BODY WEIGHT (KG) | AGE (MONTHS) |
|---|---|---|
| Holsteins | 340 | 15 |
| Brown Swiss | 340 | 15 |
| Jerseys | 225 | 13 |
| Jerseys | 225 | 13 |
| Guernseys | 250 | 13 |
| Ayrshire | 275 | 13 |
| Hereford | 270 | 15 |
| Angus | 250 | 13 |
| Charolais | 330 | 14 |

## *Gestation and Parturition*

GESTATION. The length of gestation ranges from 276 to 295 days, and are longest in Brown Swiss and Brahman. Differences in gestation length are associated with twinning, sex of calf, and parity of cow.

IMPENDING PARTURITION. Several clinical changes in the pregnant female indicate approaching parturition. The muscles and ligaments of the rump and tailhead soften and relax, the tailhead is elevated 24 to 48 hours before calving, and the vulva swells. As calving nears, the vulva discharges thick, stringy mucus, the udder enlarges, and the teats appear to be distended with milk. A day or two before calving, the cow may become restless and keep to a small isolated area, which she defends against other cows. Confinement and interference at this time can result in a delay in parturition.

PARTURITION. During the first stage of labor (dilation of the cervix), heifers, but not cows, may be restless and show signs of abdominal pain. As the calf enters the birth canal, abdominal straining commences and the animal lies down in a lateral or sternal position. The amnion or the "second water bag" appears at the vulva. With further straining the calf is delivered; most calves take at least 45 minutes to stand and may take a few hours to suckle for the first time. Cows take about 4 to 6 hours to expel the placenta. They tend to eat the afterbirth more frequently than do sheep.

## *Puerperium*

During the puerperium or postpartum period both uterine involution and resumption of the estrous cycle must occur before conception could occur.

INVOLUTION OF THE UTERUS. Immediately after calving, the gravid horn is considerably larger than the opposite nongravid horn. The bovine uterus is considered to be involuted when on rectal palpation both horns are about equal in size. The uterus involutes faster in primiparous cows and suckled cows than pluriparous cows and nonsuckled cows.

OVARIAN FUNCTION. After parturition, cows enter a period of postpartum anestrus. The end of the anestrus is marked by the first postpartum ovulation, which is not often associated with overt estrus. The incidence of first postpartum ovulation without estrous behavior is relatively high (50 to 95%). Most dairy cows are detected in estrus and ovulate at the second estrus at about 35 days postpartum.

The interval from parturition to first ovulation shows considerable variability. Pluriparous cows ovulate earlier than primiparous cows. Suckling and the plane of nutrition delay the time of the first postpartum ovulation in beef cows. Thus, the first estrus may not reflect the resumption of ovarian cyclicity. The conception rate is lower at first postpartum estrus than at subsequent estrous periods. Dairy cows are bred after 50 days postpartum and should conceive by 80 days to maintain a calving interval of 12 months.

*Effects of suckling.* Suckling-mediated anovulation remains a major problem with the management of beef and dual purpose cattle worldwide. A few studies were conducted on mechanisms through which the suckling calf attenuates gonadotrophin secretion and extend the postpartum anovulatory interval, the maternal-offspring in mediating these effects, including role for maternal visions, olfaction, and calf identity. However, little is known about the physiological regulation of this behavior and its relation to hypothalamic GnRH secretion and GnRH release in cerebrospinal fluid of the third ventricle (6).

*Undernutrition.* Evidence suggests that moderate levels of underfeeding, before or after calving, may interfere with the mechanism(s) of final follicle maturation and ovulation, whereas more pronounced nutritional deficiencies may affect the mechanism(s) regulating dominant follicle and the dynamics of dominant follicle growth and regression (7). Glucose availability, the insulin-like peptides, and uterine prostaglandin $F_{2\alpha}$ play major roles in transition out of the anovulatory state.

## Reproductive Performance

MEASURES OF REPRODUCTIVE EFFICIENCY. The reproductive efficiency of both dairy and beef cattle can be evaluated by several methods (Table 11-4).

**TABLE 11-4. *Measures of Reproductive Efficiency in Cattle/Buffalo***

| TRAIT | DEFINITION |
|---|---|
| First calving | Age (months) |
| Days open | Days calving to conception |
| First-service conception rate (%) | $\frac{\text{No. pregnant first service}}{\text{No. bred first service}} \times 100$ |
| Calving interval (days) | $\frac{\text{Days between successive calving}}{\text{Total cows}}$ |
| Services per conception | $\frac{\text{No. of services in all cows}}{\text{Total conceptions}}$ |
| Pregnancy rate (%) | $\frac{\text{No. of cows pregnant}}{\text{Total cows in herd}} \times 100$ |
| Calving rate (%) | $\frac{\text{No. of calves born}}{\text{Total cows in herd}} \times 100$ |
| Net calf crop (%) | $\frac{\text{Total calves weaned}}{\text{Total cows in herd}} \times 100$ |

1. The 60-to-90–day nonreturn rate evaluates fertility of bulls and efficiency of inseminators in artificial insemination (AI) centers.
2. First service conception rates are based on a rectal diagnosis of pregnancy conducted 6 to 8 weeks after insemination.
3. The calving to conception interval or "days open" is a valuable index reflecting efficiency of estrus detection and the fertility of both females and males in a herd.
4. The percentage of cows pregnant, the index widely adopted in beef herds, has greater significance when the breeding season is short.
5. Calf crop measures pregnancy losses and calf mortality at calving, whereas the percentage of calves weaned reflects the reproductive efficiency of the breeding season, ease of calving, mothering ability, and calf survival.

Although both nonreturn rates and conception rates estimate the proportion of cows estimated to be pregnant, differences between them have long been recognized. The nonreturn rate overestimates the conception rate by about 10 to 15%. Much of this difference is related to failure of estrous detection, anestrus, some early embryonic deaths, sale or death of cows, and the presentation of cows for return insemination beyond a 60-to-90–day period.

Since gestation length is a fixed interval, both calving intervals and days open are usually influenced by similar factors; the latter has the advantage of early detection of problem cows.

A breeding season of about three estrous cycle lengths provides a cow at least two or three matings.

GENERAL FERTILITY. The optimal calving interval for both beef and dairy cattle is 12 months, but 12-month intervals are seldom achieved. Fertility is often measured as the percentage of cows that wean calves each year (net calf crop). For naturally bred beef cattle it is estimated at 70 to 75%. For dairy cattle the percentage of cows calving to first service is only about 50%.

IMPROVING REPRODUCTIVE PERFORMANCE. Because 95% of the beef females in the United States are bred by natural service, the bull must produce semen of high potential fertility and possess sufficient libido and physical stamina to detect estrus and mate repeatedly. Reproductive performance of beef cattle can often be improved considerably by thorough evaluation of bulls for breeding soundness (Fig. 11-5).

Failure of the beef female to express either a pubertal or postpartum estrus early in the breeding season is a serious problem. Conception early in the breeding season for both heifers and cows permits early calving and the weaning of older, heavier calves. Beef cattle must receive adequate nutrition so that heifers attain puberty and maximal pelvic growth at an early age and postpartum females express estrus and have acceptable fertility early in the breeding season.

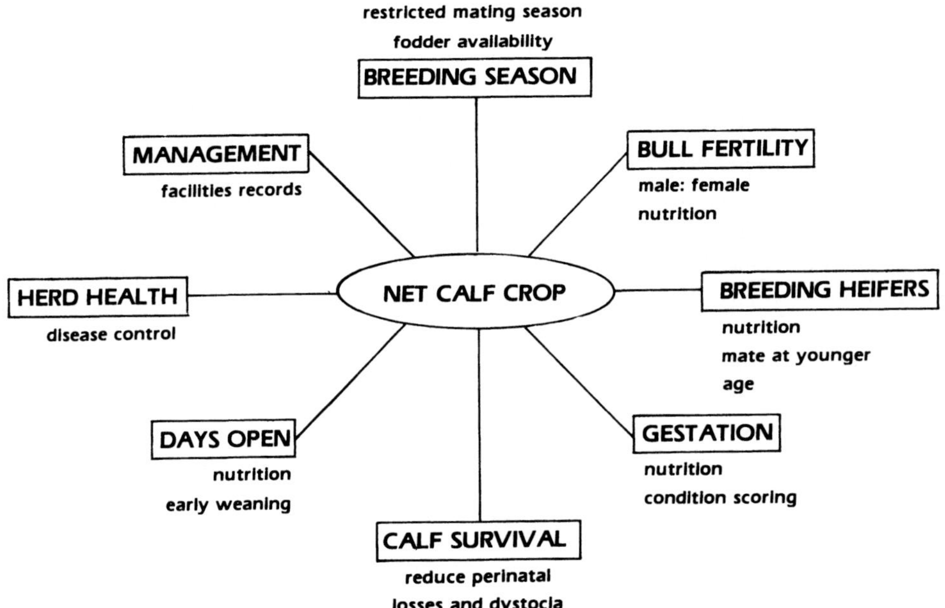


FIGURE 11-5. Methods of increasing the net calf crop in beef cattle.

Current technologies such as traditional calf manipulation, estrus synchronization, targeted nutritional supplementation, and environmentally-optimized breeding programs offer realistic options for minimizing effects of suckling on the postpartum anovulatory period (6, 8).

To maintain a 12-month calving interval in a dairy herd, at least 90% of cows should show standing estrus by day 60 postpartum and conceive by 85 days postpartum (Fig. 11-6). Conception rates are lower when cows were bred earlier than a 60-day postpartum interval than at later intervals. In herds where the incidence of uterine infections, acyclicity, and cystic ovarian disease were reduced by reproductive herd health programs, conception rates were higher and days open were shorter for cows bred at 50 days postpartum than those bred at later postpartum intervals.

Days open can be reduced by increasing efficiency of estrus detection. Thus, a greater number of cows would be submitted for AI between 55 and 85 days postpartum. Most cows in estrus can be detected by careful observation at least twice daily and by using detection aids (Table 11-1) and prediction charts, and by monitoring ovarian activity by milk $P_4$ or rectal palpation. These methods have increased the efficiency of estrus detection in some herds from 50% to about 90%. Also, contact with a bull results in an increased incidence of estrus and may stimulate ovarian activity in beef cattle early in the postpartum period (9).

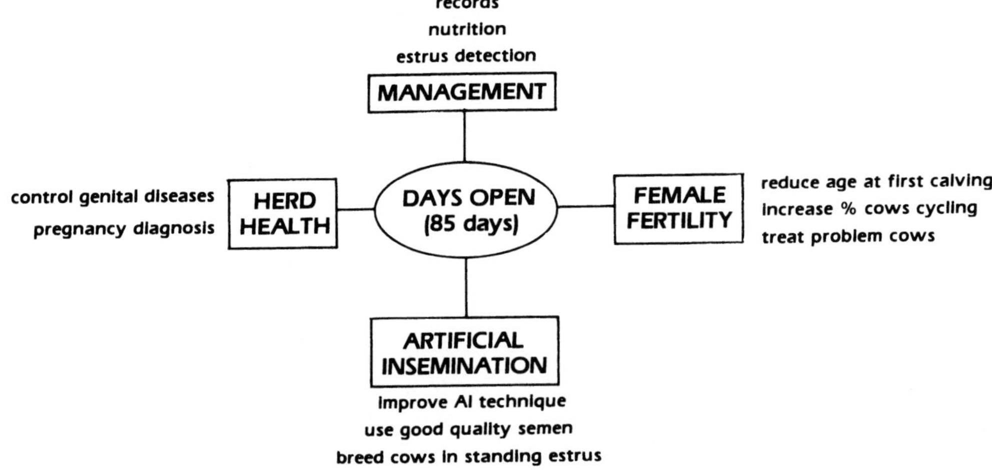


FIGURE 11-6. Methods of improving reproductive efficiency in dairy cattle. For a dairy herd to achieve a 12-month calving interval, at least 90% of cows should be cycling by 60 days postpartum and conceive within 85 days (days open).

Several hormones have been employed to increase the incidence of estrus and ovulation during the second month after calving. Gonadotropin-releasing hormone (GnRH) injections early in the postpartum period or estrus induction techniques have given variable results.

Fertility to AI could be increased by inseminating only cows in estrus, proper semen thawing procedures, placement of semen in the uterus rather than the cervix or vagina, uterine and clitoral massage following insemination, and housing inseminated cows at temperatures below 23°C on the day after insemination.

Treatment with human chorionic gonadotropin (hCG) does not improve the conception rate at the first insemination, but it may be beneficial for cows that require a repeat service. The administration of GnRH or its analogs from 0 up to 6 hours before AI has little beneficial effects on first-service conception rates in dairy cattle. It may even have an antifertility effect and should not be recommended at first services in dairy cattle (10). GnRH, however, may improve the fertility of repeat breeders when administered at time of AI (11).

The effects of nutrition on ovarian function, particularly in lactating dairy cows, have been extensively studied. The problem in feeding high-producing cows is to stimulate their appetite to increase intake to minimize the severity and length of negative energy balance. During the postpartum period, fertility becomes confounded with milk production. Nutritional intake does not influence behavioral estrous traits provided that dietary restriction does not result in body weight loss. High-producing cows that were anestrous or cyclic between day 40 and 60 postpartum obtained more energy from body reserves for milk production during the first 2 weeks of lactation than cows cycling before day 40 postpartum (12). In postpartum beef cows, lipid metabolic status could influence luteal activity with a hyperlipidemia-enhancing luteal activity (13). Reduced luteal activity that is associated with a negative energy balance during the early postpartum dairy cow may be related to the reduced levels of insulin-like growth factor I in serum (14). Recombinant bovine growth hormone (rbSt) used to stimulate lactation may adversely affect reproductive function in the dairy cow if administered before the first postpartum ovulation (15).

## BUFFALO

The world population of 130 million domestic buffaloes, *Bubalus bubalis*, has been broadly classified into the swamp and river types. The swamp buffalo (2n = 48 chromosomes) is the draft animal in the rice fields of the eastern half of Asia and is managed under range conditions similar to beef cattle. The river buffalo (2n = 50 chromosomes) is the dairy animal in countries extending from India and Pakistan to the Mediterranean countries and Egypt.

### *Puberty*

Puberty or age at first mating is difficult to determine due to problems associated with estrous detection. Most estimates have been extrapolated from age at first calving. The buffalo attains puberty at a later age than cattle (Table 11-2). The river type exhibits first estrus earlier (15 to 18 months) than the swamp type (21 to 24 months). First conception occurs at an average bodyweight of 250 to 275 kg, which is usually attained at 24 to 36 months of age (16).

The testes of the buffalo descend into the scrotum at 2 to 4 months of age, although they may be present at birth in some animals. Buffalo testicular quiescence extends from 0 to 7 months of age, followed by a period of rapid testicular growth and considerable androgenic activity (17). Spermatogenesis commences at 12 to 15 months, but the ejaculate contains viable spermatozoa only when animals are about 24 months old (18).

### *Estrous Cycle*

The characteristics of the estrous cycle of the buffalo are summarized in (Table 11-2).

BREEDING SEASON. Buffaloes, like cattle, are polyestrous and breed throughout the year. Seasonal calving patterns reported in many countries have been attributed to ambient temperature, photoperiod, and feed supply. Apparently, the photoperiodic effect on estrous cyclicity is similar in both buffalo and cattle. Buffaloes calving in summer or fall resume ovarian cyclicity earlier than those in winter or spring. Probably decreasing day length and cooler ambient temperatures favor cyclicity. During summer, when ambient temperature and photoperiod are at their maximum, prolactin levels are highest (19) and plasma $P_4$ levels are lowest (20). High ambient temperatures may also contribute to this seasonality by depressing the male libido.

CYCLIC CHANGES. Many cyclic changes in the ovaries, tubular genitalia, and hormonal secretions in the buffalo are comparable to those of cattle. $P_4$ levels in plasma and milk, as in cattle, reflect the endocrine activity of the CL, but levels are lower. Exogenous prostaglandin ($PGF_{2\alpha}$) will cause regression of the cyclic CL; $PGF_{2\alpha}$ of uterine origin, as in cattle, is probably the luteolysin in the buffalo.

ESTRUS AND OVULATION. ESTRUS. Overt signs of estrus are less intense than in cattle. Acceptance of the male is the most reliable sign of estrus in the buffalo. Less than a third of buffaloes in estrus is detected by homosexual behavior. A discharge of clear mucus from the vulva, restlessness, increased frequency of urination, vocalization, and a drop in milk production are not reliable signs of estrus.

Estrus commences toward late evening with peak sexual activity between 6:00 PM and 6:00 AM. Estrus lasts about

12 to 30 hours. Matings continue until late morning in the river buffalo but usually cease during daylight hours in the swamp buffalo.

*ESTRUS DETECTION.* Sexual receptivity toward the male can be determined as in cattle (Table 11-1) by a vasectomized male or an androgenized female buffalo fitted with a chin-ball mating device or the use of heat-mount detectors. The efficiency of these estrus detection aids may, however, be reduced because of the wallowing habits of buffaloes.

*OVULATION.* As in cattle, ovulation occurs 15 to 18 hours after the end of estrus or about 18 to 45 hours after the onset of estrus (Table 11-2). Ovulation is preceded by a surge of LH at the onset of estrus. A single egg is shed during one cycle.

*CORPUS LUTEUM.* The cyclic changes in the ovaries have been studied by in vivo visualization of the ovaries with the use of laparoscopy (21). The CL is smaller than in cattle. At the start of the cycle, it is softer but later becomes larger and firmer. The CL may often fail to protrude above the surface of the ovary and sometimes does not have a clear crown. Such a characteristic may make rectal palpation of the ovarian structures difficult.

## Male

**GENITALIA AND SEXUAL BEHAVIOR.** *GENITALIA.* The testes, accessory sex glands, and the penis of the buffalo are smaller than those of cattle. The sheath of the penis adheres close to the body in the swamp type, but is more pendulous in the river type.

*SEXUAL BEHAVIOR.* Sexual behavior is similar but less intense than in the bull. Libido is suppressed during the hotter part of the day, particularly in the swamp buffalo. Sniffing of the vulva or female urine and the "Flehmen" reaction precede mounting of the estrous female. Mating is brief and lasts only a few seconds, and the ejaculatory thrust is less marked than in the bull. After ejaculation, the male dismounts slowly and the penis retracts gradually into the sheath.

**SPERM PRODUCTION AND RELEASE.** The buffalo has one of the shortest spermatogenic cycles among farm animals, except the boar. The durations of the seminiferous epithelial cycle and spermatogenesis are 8.6 days and 38 days, respectively (22). In general, the frequency of cell stages in the buffalo and cattle are similar.

Scrotal circumference measurement is significantly correlated with number of sperm in the ejaculate and bodyweight in the swamp (23) and river buffalo (24). Also buffalo bulls with higher scrotal circumference produce good quality semen (25).

*EJACULATE.* The normal ejaculate is grayish to milky white, rarely exceeds 5 ml, and has a sperm concentration between 300 to 1500 million cells per milliliter. Sperm motility is lower than in cattle.

**BREEDING.** Artificial insemination in buffalo is similar to that of cattle but is not commonly practiced because of the difficulty of detecting estrus. In countries such as Egypt, India, and Pakistan, however, artificial insemination centers provide a breeding service with either chilled or frozen semen for dairy buffaloes. Frozen semen is now exported from India and Pakistan to upgrade or crossbreed indigenous buffaloes in several countries.

The numerical differences in chromosome numbers in the two types of buffaloes result in crossbreeds having an intermediate karyotype of $2n = 49$. Although both male and female crosses produce unbalanced gametes ($n = 24$ or 25), they are fertile, unlike other hybrids possessing chromosome complements differing from their parents.

## Gestation and Parturition

The CL is maintained throughout gestation, but its role in the maintenance of pregnancy has not been established. Plasma $P_4$ levels remain elevated during pregnancy but decline to basal levels on the day of parturition. Estrus is generally suspended, but a few pregnant animals may exhibit one or more periods of anovulatory estrus.

Buffaloes have a longer gestation period than cattle (Table 11-2). The gestation length ranges from 305 to 320 days for the river buffalo and from 320 to 340 days for the swamp buffalo. A swamp female carrying a fetus sired by a river type has a gestation length that is intermediate (315 to 325 days). Buffaloes producing calves weighing about 35 kg had the shortest (about 308 days) gestation period, whereas those producing heavier or lighter have longer gestation periods. Male calves are heavier at birth than were heifer calves (26).

The signs of approaching parturition, the birth process, and the duration of the various stages of labor are similar to those of cattle. The first stage of labor lasts 1 to 2 hours, being longer in primiparous than in pluriparous buffaloes. During the second stage of labor, lasting 30 to 60 minutes, strong abdominal contractions cause rupture of the amnion and delivery of the fetus in anterior presentation with fully extended limbs. Fetal membranes are expelled 4 to 5 hours after delivery of the fetus. Twins are rare, and their occurrence is less than 1 per 1000 births.

## Puerperium

As in cattle, the female buffalo must undergo both uterine involution and resumption of the estrous cycle must occur before conception could occur.

**UTERINE INVOLUTION.** Uterine involution is completed by 28 days for the suckled swamp buffalo, as compared

TABLE 11-5. *Uterine Involution and Ovarian Activity in the Buffalo*

| | River Buffalo | | Swamp Buffalo | |
|---|---|---|---|---|
| Postpartum Interval (Days) | *Mean* | *Range* | *Mean* | *Range* |
| Uterine involution | 45 | 15–60 | 28 | 16–39 |
| First detected estrus | 75 | 35–185 | 90 | 40–275 |
| First ovulation | 59 | 35–87 | 96 | 52–140 |
| Conception | 125 | 85–150 | 180 | 40–400 |

River buffalo: Chuahan R, et al. Ind J Dairy Sci 1977;4:286; El-Sheikh AS, Mohamed AA. Ind J Anim Sci 1977;47:165; El-Fadaly MA. Vet Med J Egypt 1980;28:399; Swamp buffalo: Jainudeen MR, et al. Anim Reprod Sci 1983;5:181.

with 45 days for the hand-milked river buffalo (Table 11-5). Several factors influence the rate of postpartum uterine involution. Involution occurs earlier in normal than in abnormal parturitions, sooner in suckled than in nonsuckled or milked buffaloes, and earlier in low than in high milk producers, with increasing parity during winter and spring (16).

POSTPARTUM OVARIAN ACTIVITY. The restoration of the estrous cycle after parturition remains a major problem resulting in long calving intervals. As in cattle, pituitary dysfunction is an important factor responsible for postpartum ovarian inactivity. Despite the ability of exogenous GnRH to release LH and FSH characteristic of the preovulatory surge is restored by day 20 postpartum (27), other factors such as the restoration of pulsatile LH release and positive feedback of estradiol may delay the postpartum interval to first ovulation. An increase in follicular activity occurs particularly on the ovary opposite the previously gravid side, between days 30 to 60 postpartum, but only a few animals ovulate.

$P_4$ remains at basal levels in the plasma between parturition and the resumption of ovarian cyclicity. Following the first postpartum ovulation, plasma $P_4$ levels are closely correlated with the morphologic and functional activity of the CL.

The postpartum interval to first ovulation is longer in buffalo than in cattle (Table 11-2). The interval is longer in the suckled swamp buffalo than in the milked river buffalo (Table 11-5). Most first postpartum ovulations are not preceded by estrus. First estrus is observed at 2 to 3 months after parturition (28).

Among the physiologic factors, body condition, lactation, suckling, and age adversely affect ovarian function (Fig. 11-7). Buffaloes in poor body condition and young females in their first lactation possess inactive ovaries and have extended periods of postpartum anestrus. Suckling significantly increases the interval from parturition to first estrus and ovulation in the buffalo. Ovarian cyclicity is restored earlier in non-suckled than suckled river and swamp buffaloes (28).

## *Reproductive Performance*

REPRODUCTIVE EFFICIENCY. Reproductive efficiency of the buffalo can be measured by similar criteria as for cattle, particularly in dairy buffalo herds using AI or hand matings. Conception rates are 50 to 60% with chilled semen, 25 to 45% with frozen semen, and over 60% with natural service. The pregnancy rates following a restricted breeding season of 2 to 3 months in swamp buffalo herds vary from 30 to 75%, depending on the nutritional and lactational status of the females at joining. Calf crops as high as 80% have been reported in elite herds in many countries.

The calving interval is the fertility index widely used at the small farm level. Under range conditions, a buffalo usually produces two calves in 3 years. But in well-managed herds of dairy buffaloes, calving intervals of 14 to 15 months have been achieved. Year and season of conception, and parity all influence the calving interval. Conception during January to March led to the shortest calving interval, and

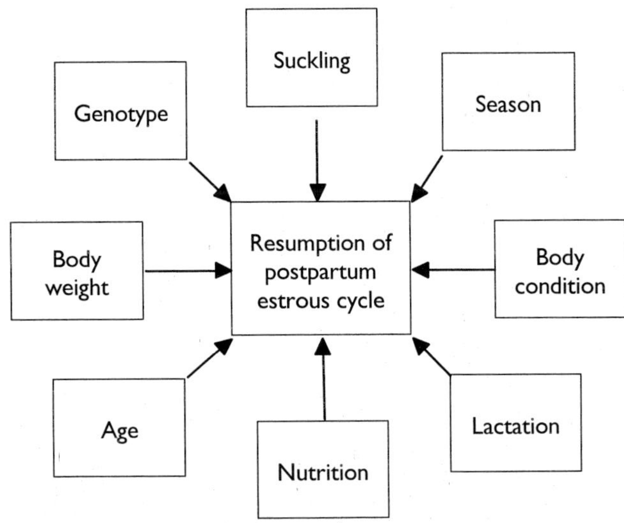


FIGURE 11-7. Physiological factors influencing the postpartum interval to the resumption of the estrous cycle in the buffalo.

during October to December, it led to the longest interval. The highest percentage of conceptions occurred 2 to 5 months after the peak rainfall (29). Parity influences the calving interval, which is longer in primiparous than in pluriparous buffaloes.

**Increasing Reproductive Performance.** Delayed age at first calving, problems related to estrus detection, and days open in the female, and loss of libido in the male are the major constraints to increasing reproductive rates in the buffalo. Improvements in nutrition could increase growth rates and have hastened the onset of puberty. Similarly, management practices such as early weaning, induction of estrus with prostaglandins or intravaginal $P_4$ releasing devices, and better nutrition have hastened the resumption of early postpartum ovarian activity and reduced the days open in the buffalo.

The seasonal nature of the breeding cycle and the long calving intervals under range conditions make it difficult for a buffalo to calve during the peak months of 2 successive years. The marked seasonal fluctuations in libido and semen quality may be overcome by providing cooling facilities for buffaloes during the hot season. Also, semen collected and frozen during the cooler months could be used to inseminate females during periods of high environmental temperatures. Induction of estrus with synthetic analogs of $PGF_{2\alpha}$ and fixed-time insemination with frozen semen may prove useful in restricting mating seasons so that calvings occur when water and green feed are abundant. Reproductive management programs, as for dairy and beef cattle, have been adopted in large buffalo herds worldwide.

Females can be bred either naturally or by AI. Breeding males, as in cattle, should be tested for breeding soundness before assigning them to about 20 to 30 females in single-sire mating paddocks. If AI is planned, then estrus can be synchronized with $PGF_{2\alpha}$ or a progesterone-releasing intravaginal device, and animals can be inseminated at either a fixed time or on detection of estrus. Animals are examined for pregnancy at about 2 months after the end of the mating season or insemination and are separated into pregnant and nonpregnant groups. The adoption of these reproductive management programs combined with herd health service (as for cattle) and improved nutrition have virtually doubled the reproductive rates of the water buffalo.

## References


1. Hoffman PC. Optimum body size for Holstein replacement heifers. J Anim Sci 1997;75:836–845.
2. Ginther OJ, Knopf L, Kastelic JP. Temporal associations among ovarian events in cattle during oestrous cycles with two and three follicular waves. J Reprod Fertil 1989;87:223–230.
3. Savio JF, Thatcher WW, Baldinga L, de la Sota RL, Wolfenson D. Regulation of dominant follicle turnover during the oestrous cycle in cows. J Reprod Fertil 1993;97:197–203.
4. Taylor C, Manikkam M, Rajamahendran M. Changes in ovarian follicular dynamics and luteinizing hormone profiles following different progestagen treatments in cattle. Canadian J Anim Sci 1994;74:273–279.
5. Heersche G, Nebel RL. Measuring efficiency and accuracy of detection of estrus. J Dairy Sci 1994;77:2754–2761.
6. Williams GL, Gazal OS, Guzman Vega GA, Stanlo RL. Mechanisms regulating suckling-mediated anovulation in the cow. Anim Reprod Sci 1996;42:289–297.
7. Jolly PD, McDougall S, Fitzpatrick LA, Macmillan KL, Entwistle KW. Physiological effects of undernutrition on postpartum anoestrus in cows. J Reprod Fertil Suppl 1995;49: 477–492.
8. Short RE, Bellows RA, Staigmiller RB, Berardinelli JG, Cluster EE. Physiological mechanisms controlling anestrus and infertility in postpartum beef cattle. J Anim Sci 1990;68: 799–816.
9. Alberio EH, Schiersmann G, Carol N, Mestre J. Effect of a teaser bull on ovarian and behavioural activity of suckling beef cows. Anim Reprod Sci 1987;14:263.
10. Mee MO, Stevenson JS, Scoby RK. Influence of gonadotropin-releasing hormone and timing of insemination relative to estrus on pregnancy rates of dairy cattle at first service. J Dairy Sci 1990;73:1500.
11. Stevenson JS, Call EP, Scoby RK. Double insemination and gonadotropin-releasing hormone treatment of repeat-breeding dairy cattle. J Dairy Sci 1990;73:1766.
12. Staples CR, Thatcher WW. Relationship between ovarian activity and energy status during the early postpartum period of high producing dairy cows. J Dairy Sci 1990;73:938.
13. Williams GL. Modulation of luteal activity in postpartum beef cows through changes in dietary lipid. J Anim Sci 1989;67:785.
14. Spicer LJ, Tucker WB, Adams GD. Insulin-like growth factor-I in dairy cows: relationships among energy balance body condition ovarian activity and estrous behavior. J Dairy Sci 1990;73:929.
15. Schemm SR, Deaver DR, Griel LC Jr, Muller LD. Effects of recombinant bovine somatotropin on luteinizing hormone and ovarian function in lactating dairy cows. Biol Reprod 1990;42:815.
16. Jainudeen MR. Reproduction in the water buffalo. In: Morrow DA, ed. Current Therapy in Theriogenology. Philadelphia: WB Saunders, 1986.
17. Ahmad N, Shahab M, Khurshid S, Arslan M. Pubertal development in the male buffalo: Longitudinal analysis of body growth, testicular size and serum profiles of testosterone and oestradiol. Anim Reprod Sci 1989;19:61.
18. McCool CJ, Entwistle KW. Reproductive function: age effects and seasonal effects in the Australian swamp buffalo bull. Theriogenology 1989;31:583–594.
19. Kaker ML, Razdan MN, Galhotra MM. Serum prolactin levels of noncycling Murrah buffaloes (*Bubalus bubalis*). Theriogenology 1982;17:469.
20. Rao LV, Pandey RS. Seasonal changes in plasma progesterone concentrations in buffalo cows (*Bubalus bubalis*). J Reprod Fertil 1982;66:57.

21. Jainudeen MR, Sharifuddin W, Bashir A. Relationship of ovarian contents to plasma concentration in the swamp buffalo *(Bubalus bubalis)*. Vet Rec 1983;113:369–372.
22. Sharma AK, Gupta RC. Duration of seminiferous epithelial cycle in buffalo bulls (*Bubalus bubalis*). Anim Reprod Sci 1980;3:217.
23. Bongso TA, Hassan MD, Noordin W. Relationship of scrotal circumference and testicular volume to age and bodyweight in the Swamp buffalo (*Bubalus bubalis*). Theriogenology 1984;22:127–134.
24. Mathroo JS, Chaudhary KC, Bahga CS, Singh MI. Relationship of testicular measurements to seminal traits and fertility in cattle and buffalo bulls. Archiv fur Tierzucht 1994; 37:31–35.
25. Nema SP, Kodagali SB. Transcrotal circumference (TSC) age bodyweight and seminal characters in Surti bulls. Indian J Anim Reprod 1994;15:154–156.
26. Gordon I. Controlled Reproduction in Cattle and Buffalo. New York: CAB International, 1996.
27. Palta P, Madan ML. Alteration in hypophysial responsiveness to synthetic GnRH at different postpartum intervals in Murrah buffalo (*Bubalus bubalis*). Theriogenology 1995;4: 403–411.
28. Jainudeen MR, Bongso TA, Tan HS. Postpartum ovarian activity and uterine involution in the suckled swamp buffalo (*Bubalus bubalis*). Anim Reprod Sci 1983;5:181.
29. Lundstrom K, Abeygunawardena H, de Silva LNA, Perera BMOA. Environmental influence on calving interval and estimates of its repeatability in the Murrah buffalo in Sri Lanka. Anim Reprod Sci 1982;5:99.

CHAPTER 12

# *Sheep and Goats*

M.R. JAINUDEEN, H. WAHID, AND E.S.E. HAFEZ

## INTRODUCTION

Domestic sheep (*Ovis aries*) and goats (*Capra hircus*) are two distinct species in the family Bovidae. They were among the first to be domesticated: sheep for wool and meat, and the goat for milk, meat, and fiber. The goat is important because it can be a major source of animal protein in the tropics. The world population of sheep is about 3 times that of goats. Each species possesses certain unique characteristics (Table 12-1).

## SEXUAL SEASON

### *Female*

In the temperate zone, both sheep and goats are seasonally polyestrous so that the young are born during the most favorable time of the year—the spring. The length of the sexual season varies with day length, breed, and nutrition (Fig. 12-1). This seasonality is governed by photoperiodicity with estrus activity commencing during a period of decreasing day length. In the tropical zones, where variation in day length is less, indigenous sheep and goats tend to breed throughout the year. Therefore, when temperate breeds are introduced into the tropics, they gradually lose their seasonality and follow the breeding patterns characteristic of the new environment. High environmental temperature and lack of feed may restrict sexual activity during some months of the year in the tropics, but shortly after the onset of the rainy season, sexual activity increases.

Genotype influences the sexual season. The Dorset, Merino, and Rambouillet sheep breeds, which originated near the equator, have longer sexual seasons than British breeds such as the Southdown, Shropshire, and Hampshire. Dairy goats such as the Toggenburg, Saanen, French Alpine, and the LaMancha have a restricted sexual season between August and February in most regions of North America. The Anglo-Nubian breed, developed in England by breeding English does with bucks from Nubia in Upper Egypt and Ethiopia, is less restricted to fall breeding, although sexual activity is highest during the fall. The sexual season of the Alpine dairy goat can also be extended under intense management but not beyond April. In the southern part of the United States (30°N latitude), meat-type of goats are anestrous between March and May while less than 40% of Rambouillet sheep are anestrous during the same period (Fig. 12-2).

During summer, the ovaries of anestrous ewes develop follicles and secrete estradiol when stimulated with LH. Follicular activity changes throughout the year in synchrony with the circannual patterns of prolactin secretion and day length, but apparently fluctuations in prolactin are not related to seasonality of mating in sheep. Low progesterone ($P_4$) increases the size of the largest follicles and the age of the oldest ovulatory follicles. Embryos resulting from the ovulation of older and younger follicles in the same ewe do not differ in their ability to survive (1).

The frequency of LH discharges depends on the response to the negative feedback effect of estradiol; the response is low during the breeding season, rises during transition into anestrus, and remains elevated until the onset of the next breeding season, when it diminishes again (Fig. 12-3). Melatonin, a pineal hormone, mediates the response to changes in the photoperiod in sheep. Melatonin levels are high during dark periods and low during light periods; probably these differences in the pattern of melatonin secretion act as a signal indicating day length to the neuroendocrine axis (Chapter 3). There is evidence to suggest that premammillary area of the hypothalamus is an important target for melatonin to regulate reproductive activity (2).

### *Male*

The ram does not show a restricted mating season, but sexual activity is highest in the fall and declines in late winter, spring, and summer. Decreasing (or short) day lengths stimulate the secretion of FSH, LH, and testosterone in rams, while increasing (or long) day lengths inhibit these hormones. The magnitudes of serum gonadotropin and tes-

TABLE 12-1. *Genetic/Physical Characteristics and Reproductive Parameters of Sheep and Goats*

| | PARAMETERS | SHEEP | GOAT |
|---|---|---|---|
| GENETIC CHARACTERISTICS | Chromosome number | 54 | 60 |
| | Taxonomy | *Ovis aries* | *Capra hircus* |
| | Matings | | |
| | Buck x female | Sterile | Fertile |
| | Ram x female | Fertile | Embryonic death |
| PHYSICAL FEATURES | Tail length | Short | Short |
| | Tail carriage | Downward | Upward |
| | Male scent glands | Absent | Present |
| | Face and foot glands | Present | Absent |
| | Lacrimal pits | Present | Absent |
| | Beard | Absent | Present |
| | Body coat | Wool | Hair |
| FEMALE REPRODUCTION | Age at puberty (months) | 6–9 | 5–7 |
| | Estrous cycle | | |
| | Length (days) | 17 (14–19) | 21 (18–22) |
| | Estrus (hours) | 24–36 | 24–48 |
| | Ovulation (No. per cycle) | 1–3 | 2–3 |
| | Life span of corpus luteum (days) | 14 | 16 |
| | Fertilizable life of ova (hours) | 10–25 | ? |
| MALE REPRODUCTION | Age at puberty (spermatogenesis) (months) | 4–6 | 4–6 |
| | Sexual season | none | none |
| | Duration of seminiferous epithelial cycle (days) | 10.3 | ? |
| | Semen | | |
| | Volume (ml) | 0.8–1.2 | 0.1–1.5 |
| | Concentration (billion/ml) | 1.5 | 2–6 |
| | Mating (male : females) | 1:30 | 1:50 |

tosterone secretion of mature rams in response to day length changes show breed differences. These differences are apparent during short days when the hypothalamic-pituitary-testis axis is most active.

The sexual activity of the buck (male goat) is also influenced by day length. Peak sexual activity occurs during the fall and coincides with the sharp rise in plasma testosterone level during the fall breeding season.

## PUBERTY

### *Female*

Puberty, the age at first ovulation, occurs at 5 to 7 months in does, and 6 to 9 months in ewes. Finewool or Merino sheep and the Angora goat fail to reach puberty during the first sexual season. Consequently, they may be 18 to 20 months old at first estrus. Early maturing breeds such as the pigmy goat or the Finn-sheep may reach puberty as early as 3 or 4 months. The onset of puberty in sheep is influenced by genetic and environmental factors such as breed and strain differences, the nutritional planes, and time of birth (Fig. 12-4). First estrus occurs in ewe lambs at 30 to 50 kg body weight (50 to 70% of adult weight).

Many of the endocrine mechanisms leading to ovulation and first estrus are capable of operating long before they are called on to function. Ewe lambs born in the spring have tonic and surge modes of LH secretion and can attain puberty at 20 weeks of age, but the season delays puberty in lambs born in spring until the fall when they are about 30 to 35 weeks of age. By contrast, lambs born in the fall are 30 weeks old during the adult anestrous season, but ovulations are delayed until shortly after the onset of the breeding season at which time they are 50 weeks old. The physiologic events leading to puberty in the ewe lamb are analogous to those that regulate the onset of the sexual season in the adult ewe (Fig. 12-3). Both internal and external cues time puberty, and diet affects the attainment of puberty through changes in LH secretion. Once growth

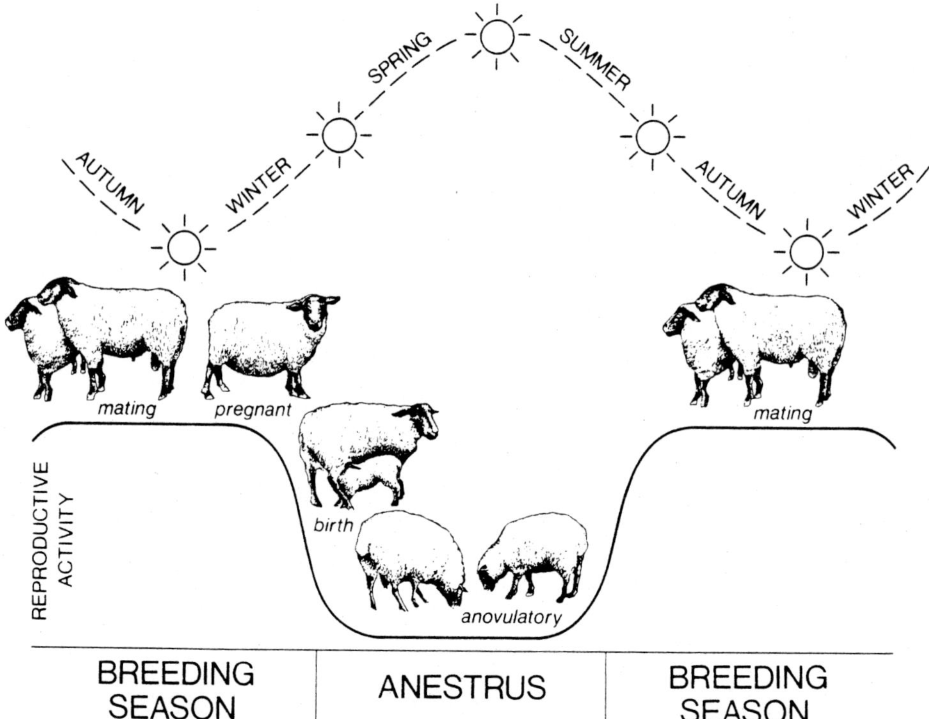


Figure 12-1. Seasonal reproduction in ewe. During the breeding season, ovulations occur at 16-day intervals, with mating and pregnancy; during anestrus ewes do not ovulate until next breeding season. (From Foster DL, Karsch FJ, Olster DH, Ryan KD, Yellon SM. Determinants of puberty in a seasonal breeder. Rec Prog Horm Res 1986;42:331.)

requirements for sexual maturity have been satisfied, photoperiod cues are used to time the onset of puberty to the season of decreasing day length (Fig. 12-5). Only ewe lambs that have been exposed to long hours of daylight, then to short hours of daylight, can accelerate their sexual development.

### *Male*

Puberty in the ram and buck is associated with a marked increase in testosterone secretion, spermatogenesis, and mating behavior (Fig. 12-6). Testis size increases when ram lambs reach 8 to 10 weeks of age at body weights of 16

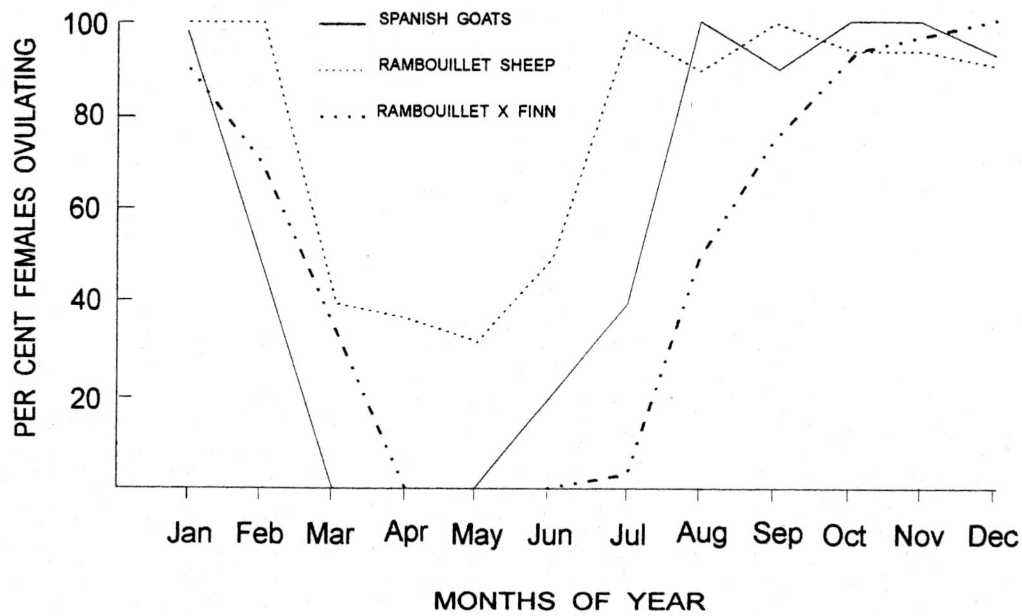


Figure 12-2. Seasonal cycle of reproductive activity in goats and two types of sheep.

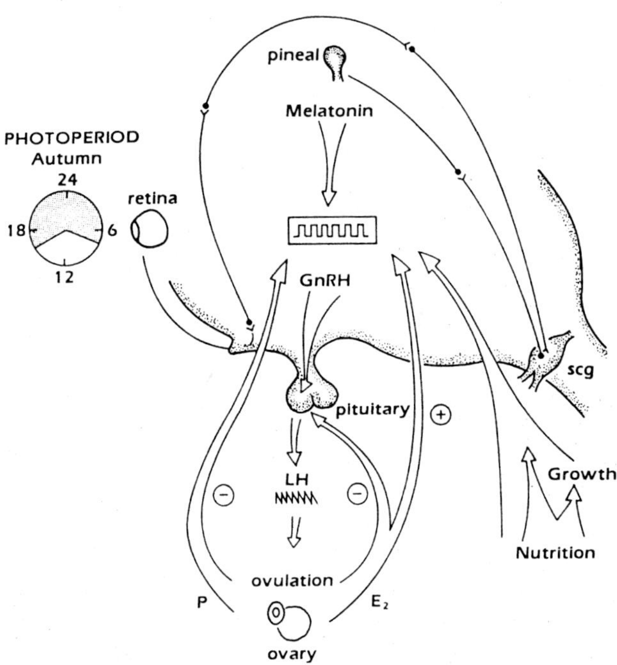


FIGURE 12-3. The events leading to first ovulation in ewe lambs at puberty or in adult ewes at the beginning of the sexual season. (From Foster DL, et al. Neuroendocrine regulation of puberty by nutrition an photoperiod. In: Venturoli S, et al, eds. Adolescence in Females. Chicago: Year Book Medical Publishers, 1985.)

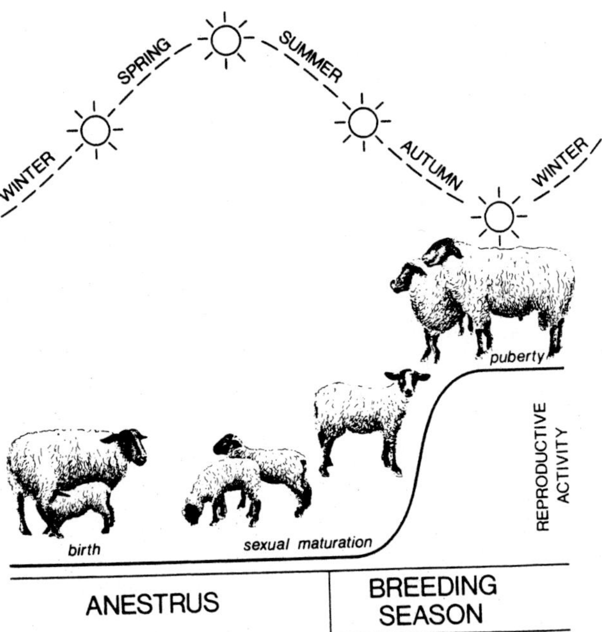


FIGURE 12-5. Onset of puberty in the lamb. Birth and growth occur during long days of the spring and summer (anestrus season). Reproductive cycles and mating begin during the decreasing day length (breeding season). (From Foster DL, Karsch FJ, Olster DH, Ryan KD, Yellon SM. Determinants of puberty in a seasonal breeder. Rec Prog Horm Res 1986;42:331.)

to 20 kg. This coincides with the appearance of primary spermatocytes and the enlargement of seminiferous tubules. In both species, copulation with ejaculation of viable spermatozoa occurs at 4 to 6 months of age with live weights of 40 to 60% of mature weight. As with the ewe lamb, the first exposure of ram lambs born in autumn to long hours of daylight, then to short hours of daylight accelerates their sexual development, depending on the breed. Brief exposures of virgin rams to estrous females can also bring the sexual performance up to levels comparable to that of experi-

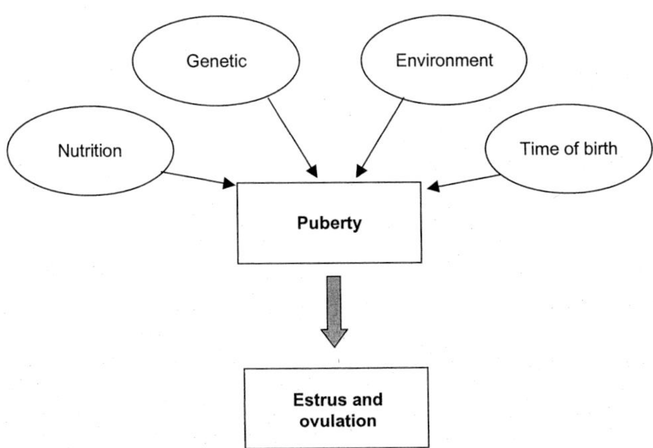


FIGURE 12-4. Factors influencing the onset of puberty in ewes and does.

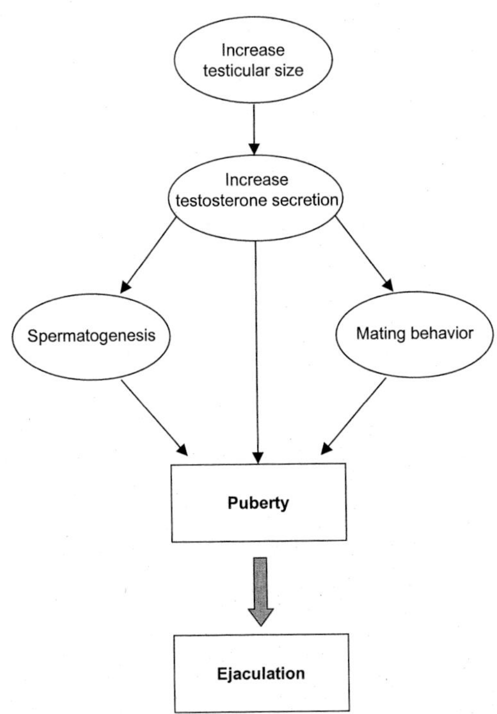


FIGURE 12-6. Factors associated with the onset of puberty in rams and bucks.

enced rams (3). Serum testosterone rises at an earlier age in the goat (17 to 20 months) than in the ram lamb (25 to 28 months) (4). As in cattle, sexual maturity is better correlated with body weight than age.

## FOLLICULOGENESIS

An extensive study has led Scaramuzzi et al (5) to propose a model for follicular growth from the primordial stage to an ovulatory follicle in the ewe (Fig. 12-7). Follicles can be quiescent (primordial), committed to growth (preantral), ovulatory, or atretic. Committed follicles are gonadotropin-responsive but may continue to grow in the absence of FSH and LH. At a later stage of growth, committed follicles are sensitive to gonadotropins. Ovulation occurs following an LH surge or else the atresia occurs.

Daily transrectal ultrasonography of the ovaries of the ewe has provided additional information related to folliculogenesis. The numbers, diameters and position of all follicles ≥2 mm in diameter and the corpora lutea in both ewe ovaries have been recorded (6). A significant increase in the numbers of antral follicles (>2 mm in diameter) emerged on days 2 and 11. The ovulatory follicle (6 to 7 mm diameter) was retrospectively traced to emergence on day 11 and grew over a period of 4 days. The largest nonovulatory follicles of the same period grew at the same rate as ovulatory follicles and regressed over a period of 3 days. In Merino del Pais ewes, number of follicles ≥2 mm per ovary on days 1 through 8 varied with the interaction of ovary by day, being more variable in the non-CL ovary. During the last 7 days, a linear decline in total follicles occurred with a linear increase in number of large follicles (7).

## ESTROUS CYCLE

### *Length of Cycle*

The length of the normal estrous cycle is 17 days for sheep and 21 days for goats, although there is considerable variation due to breed differences, stage of the breeding season, and environmental stress in both species (Table 12-1). The abnormally short cycles that are observed in the ewe and the doe early in the breeding season may be associated with prematurely regressing corpus luteum (CL) or anovulation.

### *Duration of Estrus*

Estrus lasts 24 to 36 hours in the ewe and 24 to 48 hours in the doe (Table 12-1). Breed, age, season, and presence of the male influence duration of estrus. Wool breeds have

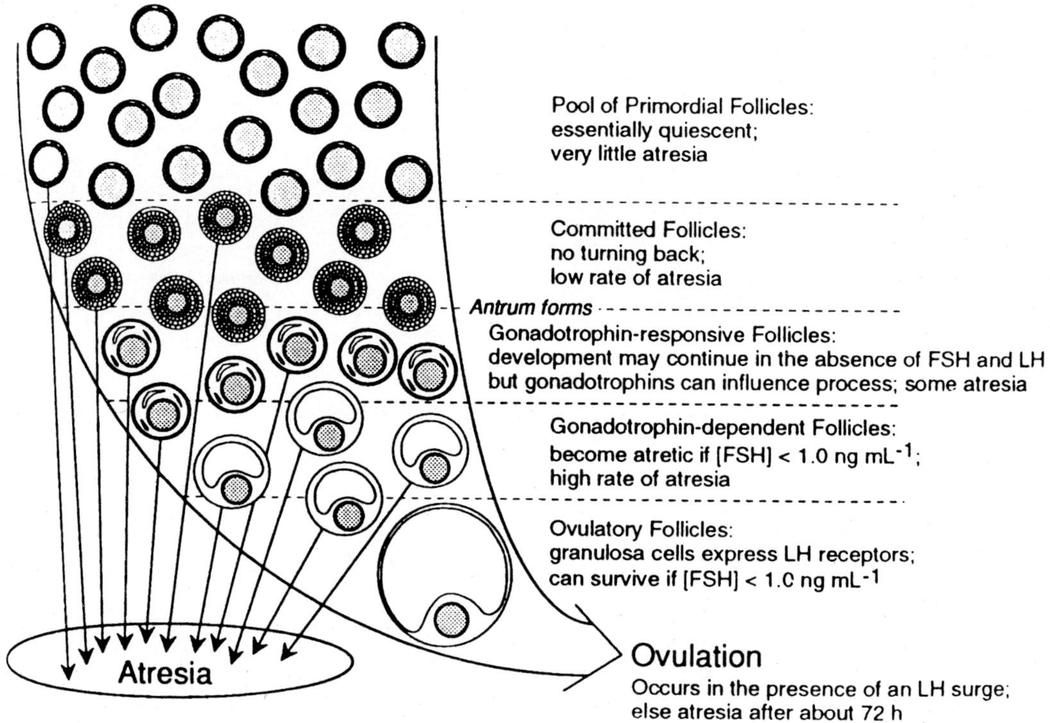


FIGURE 12-7. A model for follicular growth in the ewe. The presence of an ovulatory follicle induces atresia in all gonadotropin-dependent follicles because the estradiol and inhibin it secretes blocks the supply of FSH and increases the amplitude of LH pulses. (From Scaramuzzi RJ, Adams NR, Baird DT, et al. A model for follicular selection and the determination of ovulation rate in the ewe. Reprod Fertil Dev 1993;5:459.)

longer estrous periods than meat breeds. Angora goats have a shorter duration of estrus (22 hours) than the dairy breeds. Estrus is of shorter duration in both species at the beginning and end of the breeding season, in the presence of the male, and in the first breeding season of young females.

### *Signs of Estrus*

Signs of estrus are more conspicuous in does than in ewes. A doe in estrus is restless, bleats frequently, and wags her tail constantly and rapidly; she may have a reduced appetite and a decreased milk production. Estrus in the ewe is relatively inconspicuous and is not evident in the absence of the ram. The vulva may be edematous, and a mucous discharge from the vagina may be evident in both species. A doe may occasionally exhibit homosexual behavior but not the ewe. Ewes and does usually display a strong male-seeking behavior and remain very close to the male. Without the presence of the male, however, estrus is difficult to detect in both the ewe and the doe.

### *Male Influence on Estrus*

The introduction of rams to ewes during the transition from the anestrous season to the breeding season stimulates them to ovulate within 3 to 6 days, and estrous activity occurs 17 to 24 days later. The sexual behavior of ram is also important in initiating ovarian cycle activity (8). The CL of the first ovulation regresses prematurely in about half the ewes and is followed by a second ovulation associated with normal luteal activity. The response of anovular ewes to the ram is due to an androgen-dependent pheromone secreted by the sebaceous glands of the ram.

The introduction of a buck into a group of seasonally anestrous dairy does not only may hasten the onset of the breeding season by several days but can also effectively synchronize them. Most seasonally anestrous does are detected in estrus within 6 days after introduction of the buck, and this is followed by ovulation and normal corpus luteum function. A period of sexual isolation is necessary to obtain a male effect in sheep, but brief contacts of the ewes with rams will not compromise a subsequent use of the male effect (9). The ram effect can be achieved without prior isolation of ewes from rams (10). Thus, ovulation induced by the "male effect" is more effective in the doe than the ewe.

## Ovulation

Both the ewe and the doe are spontaneous ovulators (Table 12-1). The ewe normally ovulates near the end of estrus about 24 to 27 hours after the onset. Most goat breeds ovulate between 24 and 36 hours after onset of estrus, but the Nubian goat ovulates later, which is possibly due to a longer estrous cycle in this breed. Ovulation without estrus occurs before the onset of the breeding season in Nubian and other breeds of goats. The sequence of hormonal events during the estrous cycle is similar in both species, but the doe has a longer progesterone phase than the ewe.

### *Ovulation Rate*

In many breeds of sheep and goat, two or more ova are shed during estrus. The ovulation rate is 1.2 for Merinos and 3 for the Finnish Landrace breed. In both species, the ovulation rate increases with age and reaches a maximum at 3 to 6 years, then declines gradually. Significantly more ovulations occur on the right ovary (53.4%) than left ovary (46.6%) (11). Among the environmental factors influencing ovulation rate, season and level of nutrition are important. Generally, ovulation rates are higher early in the breeding season than later, but factors such as body size, weight, condition, and genotype may also contribute to the increase in ovulation rate.

A nutritional strategy for increasing ovulation rate in Merino anestrous ewes mated in late spring-early summer involved supplementary feeding of lupin grain. Feeding 500 g lupins per head per day for 14 days, commencing 12 days after the introduction of vasectomized rams, increased fecundity (lambs born per ewe lambing) but not fertility (ewes lambing per ewe mated to rams). Net reproductive performance (the product of fertility, fecundity, and lamb survival) was increased by 11 lambs weaned per 100 ewes (12).

The highly fertile breeds of sheep include the Finnish Landrace, Romanov, Booroola Merino, and the D'Man breed. The high ovulation rate of the Booroola Merino is due to the action of a single gene, whereas in the Romanov, ovulation is under polygenic control. In these high fecund breeds, there is a positive association between ovulation rate and plasma FSH in the periovulatory period, but there is no relationship between peripheral FSH concentrations during the late-luteal and follicular phase and subsequent ovulation rates (13). The number of hCG-induced ovulations can be used to identify sheep that are carriers of large ovulatory follicles typical of a breed and are present at stages (prepuberal, anestrus, luteal phase) other than the follicular phase (14). Immunization of Merino sheep with a fraction of bovine follicular fluid containing inhibin activity increases the ovulation rate (15). In the ewe, a single injection of a slow-releasing oxytocin at the onset of estrus results in a higher ovulation rate (16).

## Breeding and Conception

Most of the world population of sheep and goats is managed under free grazing conditions where natural mating is widely practiced. Unlike with cattle, artificial insemination (AI) of sheep and goats has been generally limited, owing to the high cost of labor, difficulty of accurately identifying superior

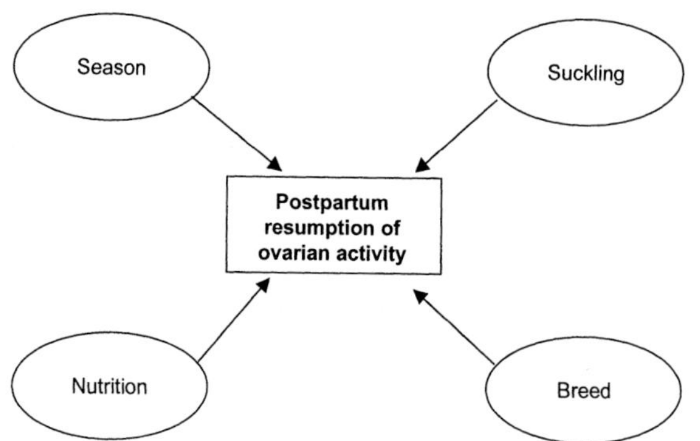


FIGURE 12-8. Factors influencing the resumption of ovarian activity in ewes and does.

sires, and low conception rates, especially with frozen semen. Both the ram and the buck ejaculate a small volume of semen with a high concentration of spermatozoa. Rams may copulate two or three times in a few minutes when first turned with ewes in estrus. They generally mate more frequently when more than one ewe is in estrus. The number of matings per day varies with individual males, and with the climate and time when rams are introduced into breeding. Certain breeds copulate more frequently than other breeds. Normally, one adult ram is assigned to 30 ewes and one buck to 50 does.

Rams continuously bred produce volumes of semen and numbers of spermatozoa per ejaculate that are well below those considered adequate for AI. Ewes mated more than once are more likely to conceive than those mated only once. There is evidence that aggressive behavior of rams directed at ewes was negatively correlated to LH. Effects of the ewe on LH secretion of rams depend on length of the exposure period and sexual activity of the male (17). The sudden introduction of the buck may induce estrus in many does in one day. This can result in many does not being mated. Breeding males may serve does as much as 20 times a day.

Copulation usually occurs before ovulation, and therefore spermatozoa are present in the oviduct by this time. Other spermatozoa are stored in the cervix (up to 3 days) and are continually released into the uterus, where they survive for about 30 hours. Eggs may remain viable for 10 to 25 hours, but abnormal development and lowered viability appear to increase with the age of either the sperm or ovum. In both species, eggs enter the uterus about 72 hours after ovulation.

## GESTATION, PARTURITION, AND PUERPERIUM

### *Gestation*

The normal gestation length for both species is about 150 days; the length varies between breeds and individuals. In sheep, the early maturing breeds and the highly prolific breeds have shorter gestation periods than the slow-maturing wool breeds. Individual gestation periods within a breed vary up to 13 days. Gestation lengths for most breeds of goats are within 2 days of the species average, with the exception of Black Bengal breed, which averages 144 days. Heredity plays an important role in determining gestation length. The genotype of the fetus accounts for almost two-thirds of the variation in gestation length of sheep. Male lambs are carried longer than female lambs, spring-born lambs longer than fall-born lambs, and singles longer than twins. Gestation length also increases with age of the dam.

The CL of pregnancy persists throughout gestation, but the two species differ in the source of progesterone for pregnancy maintenance. The sheep is a placenta-dependent species, whereas the goat is a CL-dependent species. During the first trimester, both species depend on the CL. Later, the placenta becomes the primary source of progesterone in the sheep, whereas the CL continues as the major source in the goat. Therefore, ovariectomy in the goat at any stage of pregnancy causes abortion. The diagnosis of pregnancy is presented in Chapter 28. Hydrometra is the accumulation of fluid in the uterus that mimics pregnancy, but neither fetuses nor placental tissue is detected. Progesterone levels remain elevated. Hydrometra can be diagnosed by ultrasonography and is more common in goat than sheep

### *Parturition*

The fetus plays the key role in initiating parturition in both species, but parturition is preceded by regression of the CL in the goat (Chapter 10). Parturitions are spread throughout the day. Behavior of the ewe largely depends on the ease of parturition, but generally, the initial restlessness is broken by periods of lying down, which are due to abdominal pain. Most lambs and kids are born head and forefeet foremost (anterior presentation). The duration of birth varies widely, particularly with a single oversized lamb or kid, with twins impacted in the birth canal, or with an abnormal presentation. Colostral IgG concentration, total weight of lamb born, lamb mortality, or total weight of lamb weaned are not affected within a body condition score range of 2.5 to 3.5 (18).

Twin births are usually more rapid than single births, but the interval between delivery of twins varies from a few minutes to an hour or more. Goats may be more efficient than sheep in recognizing that they have had twins.

Vigorous licking (grooming) and eating of any fetal membranes adhering to the neonate commence immediately after birth. Fetal fluids appear to play a critical role in attracting the ewe to her lamb. Ewes that have not yet lambed are attracted to the fluids and to the newborn lambs of other ewes, which leads to "lamb stealing." Most lambs are standing within 15 minutes of birth, and within an hour or two most ewes will allow the lamb to move toward the udder. The doe spends more time vigorously grooming and orienting the firstborn, so that the second born, which is usually the weaker of the two, has a greater opportunity to suckle.

The "critical period" of attachment of the ewe to the lamb is short; if the lamb is removed at birth, it will be rejected by the ewe when presented to her 6 to 12 hours later. Some primiparous ewes display little interest and abandon their newborn lambs. Aberrant maternal behavior is more common with twin births, especially among Merinos. Similarly, goats such as Angora show poor mothering ability and may abandon their kids if distracted or frightened soon after kidding (19).

The sheep is a classic example of a "follower" species, as distinct from goats, a "hider" species; that is, the young lambs tend to follow their mothers from birth rather than lie hidden for several days while the dams are absent. Goats appear to be "hiders" for the first few days after birth, as judged by the behavior of feral goats in mountainous country, and there is a clear preference for maternal isolation at the time of birth.

### *Puerperium*

Changes occurring in the reproductive system during the puerperium include uterine involution and resumption of ovarian activity. In sheep, uterine involution is completed by 27 days and precedes the first estrus postpartum. No information is available for the doe. Since ewes and does are seasonal breeders, postpartum intervals to first estrus and ovulation are markedly affected by the season of parturition. The interval may be as short as 5 to 6 weeks in both sheep and goats or as long as 10 weeks in sheep and 27 weeks in some breeds of goats. If parturitions occur during the breeding season, both ewes and does will resume ovarian activity and conceive. The first postpartum ovulation in ewes that lamb during the breeding season occurs within 20 days and is not associated with overt estrus. Factors other than season that influence the resumption of ovarian activity are presented in Figure 12-8.

## REPRODUCTIVE PERFORMANCE

### *Reproductive Efficiency*

Reproductive efficiency depends on conception rate (fertility) or the proportion of ewes mated that conceive, the lambing rate (fecundity) or the number of lambs born of ewes lambing, and the lambing percentage or the number of lambs born per 100 ewes exposed. These rates depend on ovulation rate (number of eggs shed per estrus), which sets the upper limit for lambing percentage. Prolificacy is the relative number of live offspring produced in a given interval, such as a year. Similar methods are used to measure reproductive performance in the doe.

Conception rates are about 85% in mature sheep and goats in temperate zones during midbreeding season. The average lambing rate is about 150%. Marked differences occur in ovulation rate as a result of breed, age, year, season, and nutrition. Fertility is depressed near the equator near the beginning and the end of the breeding season. Fertility is also depressed during hot climates, in undernourished or overly fat females, in young and old females, when the estrogen content of forage is high, and when the females are parasitized or suffering from disease or other stress. Ovulation rate can be increased by changing the plane of nutrition ("flushing"). Ewes in normal body condition respond to flushing during the early part of the breeding season and during the late breeding season, but not during midseason. Crossbreeding with breeds with a high ovulation rate (e.g., Booroola, Finn, and Romanov) may increase lamb crops by 250 to 400% and also may shorten lambing intervals.

Goats in the tropics maintain high fertility and twinning rates. Heat stress and insufficient nutrition depress the reproductive performance of temperate breeds of sheep and goats. This depression in the reproductive performance can be alleviated by crossing them with tropical breeds. Indigenous goat breeds in the tropics kid at intervals of 240 to 390 days, but some Indian breeds of goats such as the Jamnapari and Barbari have more than one kidding per year.

### *Advancing the Breeding Season*

A gestation length of about 150 days makes it possible for a ewe and doe to produce offspring more than once a year. But because of seasonal anestrus in ewes and does in the temperate zone latitudes, they do not cycle after parturition in the spring until the autumn, with the result that only one lamb or kid crop per year is possible. If both species could be induced to breed during seasonal anestrus, they would give birth in the breeding season, thereby producing two crops annually.

Several methods can be used to induce breeding during seasonal anestrus in the ewe. They include a combination of progesterone and eCG, the "ram effect," altering day length by artificial lighting (8 hours light followed by 16 hours of darkness), and with exogenous melatonin (20). The commercial availability of subcutaneous implants of melatonin provides a practical method of obtaining out of season breeding in seasonally anestrous breeds of sheep. The implant exposes the ewe to melatonin for 30 to 40 days, resulting in normal ovarian cyclicity in most ewes. Thus, melatonin will advance the normal breeding season so that ewes can be mated in spring or early summer, but it will not extend the breeding season if it is administered in the middle of the breeding season. One disadvantage of using either photoperiod or melatonin is that animals eventually become refractory to the stimulatory effects of light and melatonin.

In the seasonally anestrous goat breeds, the administration of melatonin to anestrous does will not significantly advance the breeding season. Prenatal lighting treatment of British Saanen dairy goats in late summer was ineffective in the onset of puberty. Testicular development was significantly delayed and plasma testosterone concentrations were lower in autumn-born male kids that experienced a 20 h light and 4 h dark cycle in utero than in kids from mothers in a natural photoperiod (21).

### *Artificial Regulation of Reproduction*

Seasonality in reproduction limits reproductive rate of both the ewe and doe to one parturition per year. Manipulation of reproduction by genetic, physiologic, and environmental methods could increase the frequency of breeding per year and the litter size in these species.

FREQUENCY OF BREEDING. A gestation length of approximately 150 days makes it possible for a ewe and doe to produce offspring more than once per year. Several methods have been investigated to reduce the lambing interval from once per year to three times in 2 years (8-month interval) or twice a year (6-month lambing interval). Altering the day-length pattern by artificial lighting can increase the breeding frequency in sheep but has limited application. Conversely, melatonin can substitute for darkness, which mimics changes in reproductive activity of shortened day length. As previously stated subcutaneous implants of melatonin to seasonally anestrous ewes advanced the onset of the breeding season; this method is being applied in sheep breeding.

LITTER SIZE. Practical methods are available for increasing ovulation rate, which sets the upper limit for litter size. "Flushing" is widely used to increase ovulation rate. Ewes in normal body condition respond to flushing during the early part of the breeding season and during the late breeding season but not during midseason.

Exogenous gonadotropins are employed to induce multiple ovulation in both species, but the response to the dose is highly variable and leads to embryonic losses. An alternative approach to gonadotropin therapy is steroid immunization, which has a consistent response. Immunity to estrone or androstenedione leads to an increased frequency of LH pulses in anestrous ewes and to elevated levels of FSH in the case of estrone; the ovulation rate is increased by 0.6 ovulations per ewe. The technique involves two injections at 3 to 4 week intervals before ram introduction. The increase in ovulation rate was reflected by a 30 to 40% increase in the lambs reared; this technique may have future application in sheep breeding.

Although the heritability of fertility and fecundity appears to be low, prolificacy of sheep has been increased through selection. The most important traits of the Finn sheep and the Romanov ewe are their high prolificacy in lamb crops of 250 to 400%, and their shorter lambing intervals. Therefore, systematic crossbreeding with these breeds could lengthen the natural breeding season and increase litter size of traditional breeds.

## SUMMARY

This chapter deals with the physiology of reproduction in male and female sheep and goat. Initially, it explains various genetic and environmental factors that initiate puberty for both male and female. Puberty normally occurs at 5 to 7 months in does, 6 to 9 months in ewes, and 4 to 6 months for buck and ram. The length of the estrous cycle in sheep and goat is 17 days and 21 days, respectively. Estrus, which is influenced by breed, age, season, and presence of the male, lasts for 24 to 36 hours in the ewe and 24 to 48 hours in the doe. The introduction of rams to ewes during the transition from the anestrous season to the breeding season stimulates them to ovulate within 3 to 6 days, and estrous activity to occur 17 to 24 days later. Most ewes and does normally ovulate near the end of estrus, about 24 to 27 hours and 24 to 36 after the onset of estrus, respectively. The size of preovulatory follicle in ewes is estimated at 6 to 7 mm in diameter and significantly more ovulations occur on the right than the left ovary. Breed, age, season, and level of nutrition influence the ovulation rate.

The male to female breeding ratio is 1 : 30 for sheep and 1 : 50 for goat. Several methods can be used to induce breeding during seasonal anestrus in the ewe. They include a combination of progesterone and equine chorionic gonadotropin, the "ram effect," altering day length by artificial lighting, and with exogenous melatonin. The normal gestation length for both species is about 150 days. In late gestation, the sheep is a placenta-dependent species, whereas the goat is a CL-dependent species (Chapter 10).

## REFERENCES

1. Johnson SK, Dailey RA, Inskeep EK, Lewis PE. Effect of peripheral concentrations of progesterone on follicular growth and fertility in ewes. Domest Anim Endocrinol 1996;13:69.
2. Malpaux B, Daveau A, Maurice-Mandon F, Duarte G, Chemineau P. Evidence that melatonin acts in the premammillary hypothalamic area to control reproduction in the ewe: presence of binding sites and stimulation of luteinizing hormone secretion by in situ microimplant delivery. Endocrinology 1998;139:1508.
3. Price EO, Estep DQ, Wallach SJ, Dally MR. Sexual performance of rams as determined by maturation and sexual experience. J Anim Sci 1991;69:1047.
4. Chakraborty PK, Stuart LD, Brown JL. Puberty in the male Nubian goat: serum concentrations of LH FSH and testoster-

one from birth through puberty and semen characteristics at sexual maturity. Anim Reprod Sci 1989;20:91.

5. Scaramuzzi RJ, Adams NR, Baird DT, et al. A model for follicular selection and the determination of ovulation rate in the ewe. Reprod Fertil Dev 1993;5:459.
6. Ravindra JP, Rawlings NC, Evans AC, Adams GP. Ultrasonographic study of ovarian follicular dynamics in ewes during the oestrous cycle. J Reprod Fertil 1994;101:501.
7. Lopez-Sebastian A, Gonzalez de Bulnes A, Santiago Moreno J, Gomez-Brunet A, Townsend EC, Inskeep EK. Patterns of follicular development during the estrous cycle in monovular Merino del Paris ewes. Anim Reprod Sci 1997;48:279.
8. Perkins A, Fitzgerald JA. The behavioral component of the ram effect: the influence of ram sexual behavior on the induction of estrus in anovulatory ewes. J Anim Sci 1994;72:51.
9. Cohen-Tannoudji J, Signoret JP. Effect of short exposure to the ram on later reactivity of anoestrous ewes to the male effect. Anim Reprod Sci 1987;13:263.
10. Cushwa WT, Bradford GE, Stabenfeldt GH, Berger YM, Dally MR. Ram influence on ovarian and sexual activity in anestrous ewes: effects of isolation of ewes from rams before joining and date of ram introduction. J Anim Sci 1992;70:1195.
11. Scaramuzzi RJ, Downing JA. The distribution of ovulations from the ovaries of merino and Border Leicester × merino ewes and its effect on the survival of their embryos. Anim Reprod Sci 1997;47:327.
12. Nottle MB, Kleemann DO, Grosser TI, Seamark RF. Evaluation of a nutritional strategy to increase ovulation rate in merino ewes mated in late spring-early summer. Anim Reprod Sci 1997;47:255.
13. Fry RC, Driancourt MA. Relationships between follicle-stimulating hormone follicle growth and ovulation rate in sheep. Reprod Fertil Dev 1992;8:279.
14. Driancourt MA, Bondin L, Boomarov O, Thimonier J, Elsen JM. Number of mature follicles ovulating after a challenge of human chorionic gonadotropin in different breeds of sheep at different physiological stages. J Anim Sci 1990;68:719.
15. Cummins LJ, O'Shea TO, Al-Obaidi SAR, et al. Increase in ovulation rate after immunization of merino ewes with a fraction of bovine follicular fluid containing inhibin activity. J Reprod Fertil 1986;77:365.
16. King PR, Coetzer WA. The effect of treatment with a slow-releasing oxytocin preparation at the onset of oestrus on the ovulation rate of Merino ewes. J S Afr Vet Assoc 1997;68:16.
17. Perkins A, Fitzgerald JA, Price EO. Luteinizing hormone and testosterone response of sexually active and inactive rams. J Anim Sci 1992;70:2086.
18. Al-Sabbagh TA, Swanson LV, Thompson JM. The effect of ewe body condition at lambing on colostral immunoglobulin G concentration and lamb performance. J Anim Sci 1995; 73:2860.
19. Bretzlaff K. Special problems of hair goats. Vet Clin North Am Food Anim Pract 1990;6:721.
20. Staples LD, McPhee S, Kennaway DJ, Williams AH. The influence of exogenous melatonin on the seasonal pattern of ovulation and oestrus in sheep. Anim Reprod Sci 1992; 30:185.
21. Deveson S, Forsyth IA, Arendt J. Retardation of pubertal development by prenatal long days in goat kids born in autumn. J Reprod Fertil 1992;95:629.

# CHAPTER 13

# Pigs

L.L. ANDERSON

## SEXUAL DEVELOPMENT AND MATURATION

Genetic sex determines the development of gonadal sex, which in turn determines phenotypic and reproductive capacities. The Y chromosome and genes located on the autosomes are critical to the development of gonads, which are eventually capable of spermatogenesis. These are necessary indirectly for the development of the male reproductive system, body sex, and typical male behavioral characteristics. The porcine embryo has 38 ($2n$) chromosomes.

The gonadal anlage develops on the inner aspect of the mesonephros, which consists of coelomic epithelium, underlying mesenchyme, and primordial germ cells. The germ cells have an extraregional origin. Sex differentiation of the undifferentiated primordium begins when gonads differentiate into genetic males (Table 13-1). In eutherian mammals, evidence suggests that sex determination is equivalent to testis determination. A Y-specific gene is conserved in the pig and encodes a testis-specific transcript.

In testicular organogenesis, the germ cells are attracted to and encapsulated with somatic cells, initially in arrangements as seminiferous cords, which are delineated by connective tissue. The cords of cells eventually hollow into seminiferous tubules with connections to mesonephric tubules. Somatic cells within the seminiferous tubules differentiate into sustentacular cells (supporting or Sertoli cells). Between seminiferous tubules, mesenchymal cells differentiate into interstitial cells (Leydig cells). The testis then produces hormones that induce normal male phenotypic development.

In the female embryo, oogenesis occurs later with the obvious feature being the absence of testicular-inducing patterns of organogenesis. The surface epithelium of the presumptive ovary becomes separated from the central cellular mass. The ovarian cortex proliferates, and germ cells (oogonia) transform into oocytes and enter early phases of premeiosis before they become separated from mesenchyme by a single layer of differentiating follicle (pregranulosa) cells. The primary follicles prevent oocytes from entering meiotic processes beyond the diplotene phase and remain in this resting stage until puberty.

Mesonephric tubules stabilize in the male embryo as the Wolffian ducts (e.g., epididymides, vas deferens, seminal vesicles, and prostate and bulbourethral glands); whereas in the female embryo, the paramesonephric tubules survive as the Müllerian ducts (e.g., oviducts, uterus, cervix, and the upper part of vagina). Both ducts are present in early embryonic development and are capable of developing as male or female internal and external genitalia. Testes are body sex differentiators because they impose masculinity on the developing genital tract and on secondary sexual features and behavior. In their absence, or in the presence or absence of the ovaries, the genital tract and secondary sex characteristics develop as a normal female. The secretion of antiMüllerian hormone (AMH, or Müllerian-inhibiting substance [MIS]) by the testes is essential for inducing the regression of the Müllerian ducts. MIS is a peptide hormone composed of two subunits of 70,000 daltons that is synthesized by Sertoli cells by day 27 and before the appearance of Leydig cells at day 30 of porcine embryonic life.

The gonadal primordium (ridge) in pig embryos at 21 and 22 days is composed of the surface epithelium, proliferating tissue of the primitive gonadal cords, and mesenchyme. Primitive cord cells are derivatives of the epithelial cells. The cords are first found in the posterior part of the gonadal ridge, and by 22 days, their numbers increase and extend into the mesenchyme. Primordial germ cells are round or elongated with diameters of 10 to 20 $\mu$m and a round nucleus (Fig. 13-1**C** and **E**). These germ cells undergo mitotic divisions in the gonadal ridge. The fine morphology of the germ cells is similar in both sexes at 21 and 24 days of embryonic life (Fig. 13-1**E** and **F**).

By 24 days, gonads of both sexes develop primitive cords in continuity with the surface epithelium (Fig. 13-1**C** and **D**). The gonadal blastema occupies space between the surface epithelium and the mesenchyme in the basal part of the gonad. In the central region, the gonadal blastema (*blastema proper*) consists primarily of cells organized irregularly.

**TABLE 13-1. *Gonadal Development of Porcine Embryos***

| DAYS | MALE | FEMALE |
|---|---|---|
| 21 | Gonadal primordium | Gonadal primordium |
| 22–24 | Primitive cord cells<br>Primordial germ cells | Primitive cord cells<br>Primordial germ cells |
| 26 | Surface epithelium<br>Mesenchyme<br>Testicular cords<br>Interstitium<br>Testosterone production | Surface epithelium<br>Mesenchyme<br>Gonadal blastema |
| 27 | Sertoli cells | |
| 29 | AMH production | |
| 30–35 | Leydig cells, 3β-HSD production | Egg nests |
| 40 | | Meiosis of germ cells |
| 60 | Testicular descent | Primordial follicles |
| 70 | | Primary follicles |
| 90 | Testes in scrotum | Secondary follicles |

At 26 and 27 days, the gonads protrude longitudinally along the medial mesonephric surface of both sexes (Fig. 13-1**A** and **B**). The testicular cords and interstitium are derived from gonadal blastema. Sustentacular cells of the testicular cords resemble primitive cord cells, and spermatogonia are similar to primordial germ cells. Interstitial cells have not yet differentiated into Leydig cells. Cells of the surface epithelium, primitive cords, mesenchyme, and primordial germ cells retain ultrastructural features that are similar in both sexes.

Gametogenesis and ovarian development in pig embryos from day 13 to birth and during the early neonatal period indicate mitotic and meiotic activities. The germ cells increase from approximately 5,000 at day 20, peak at 5,000,000 by day 50, and thereafter, germinal mitotic activity decreases and necrosis of germ cells increases. At birth, the population of germ cells is approximately 400,000. Premeiotic DNA synthesis and transformation of oogonia to oocytes continue at least to 35 days of postnatal life. Meiosis begins about day 40 of embryonic development. The premeiotic resting stage (diplotene) of porcine oocytes first appears by day 50, and almost all germ cells are diplotene by 20 days after birth. The paucity of oogonia and absence of oogonial mitoses indicate completion of oogenesis by day 100 of fetal development.

Cellular and nuclear growth of germ cells increases greatly from the oogonial stage (13 μm in diameter) to the oocyte within a primordial follicle (27 μm in diameter) and during early stages of meiotic prophase (leptotene, zygotene, and pachytene). The oocyte in the diplotene stage continues to increase in diameter during follicular maturation; growing follicles increase approximately threefold. The oocyte increases to a maximum diameter of 120 μm in Graafian follicles near the time of ovulation, and the zona pellucida consists of a homogeneous matrix approximately 8.6 μm in thickness. Surface area of the cell membrane (vitelline membrane) is increased by irregularly spaced microvilli in contact with cell processes arising from coronal radiata banding the zona pellucida. Cortical granules about 0.2 μm diameter are numerous immediately beneath the oocyte membrane wall. Other features of the oocyte cytoplasm include yolk globules, mitochondria, and both granular and agranular endoplasmic reticulum. The nucleus consists of an inner and outer nuclear membrane with numerous nuclear membrane pores.

Corona radiata cells are porcine granulosa cells on the outer aspect of the zona pellucida that are arranged in a radial pattern. These granulosa cells adhere to each other and project microvilli through the zona pellucida and perivitelline space that terminate in the oocyte membrane wall. They are nurse cells for the growing oocyte during oogenesis; their nutritive material is conveyed by extensive cytoplasmic processes. These cells disappear soon after ovulation. The cortical granules are extruded through the vitelline membrane on contact with the fertilizing sperm and block polyspermy.

Testicular development from the early fetal period to sexual maturity lags behind body growth. From the late prenatal stage to 3 weeks postpartum, testicular growth exceeds body growth, primarily because of Leydig cell development, but then recedes postnatally as a result of Leydig cell regression. By 7 weeks of age, testicular growth again exceeds body growth because of increasing length and diameter of the seminiferous tubules. From 100 days of fetal life to 3 weeks after birth, the numbers of germ cells per testis show a constant doubling rate. Morphogenesis is nearly complete by 25 weeks after birth.

## HORMONE REGULATION IN THE BOAR

Porcine blastocysts synthesize estrogens by day 12. Fetal pig testes contain $\Delta^3$-3β-hydroxysteroid dehydrogenase (3β-HSD) about day 35 before differentiation of Leydig cells. The fetal testes secrete testosterone during differentiation of the internal and external genitalia. Differentiation of the Wolffian duct and development of the seminal vesicles, prostate, bulbourethral glands, and external genitalia occur between days 26 and 50. By day 29, pig testes produce sufficient AMH to regress the Müllerian ducts, and production of AMH by Sertoli cells lasts until after birth.

Serum testosterone concentrations are low during the later half of fetal development. Testosterone production late

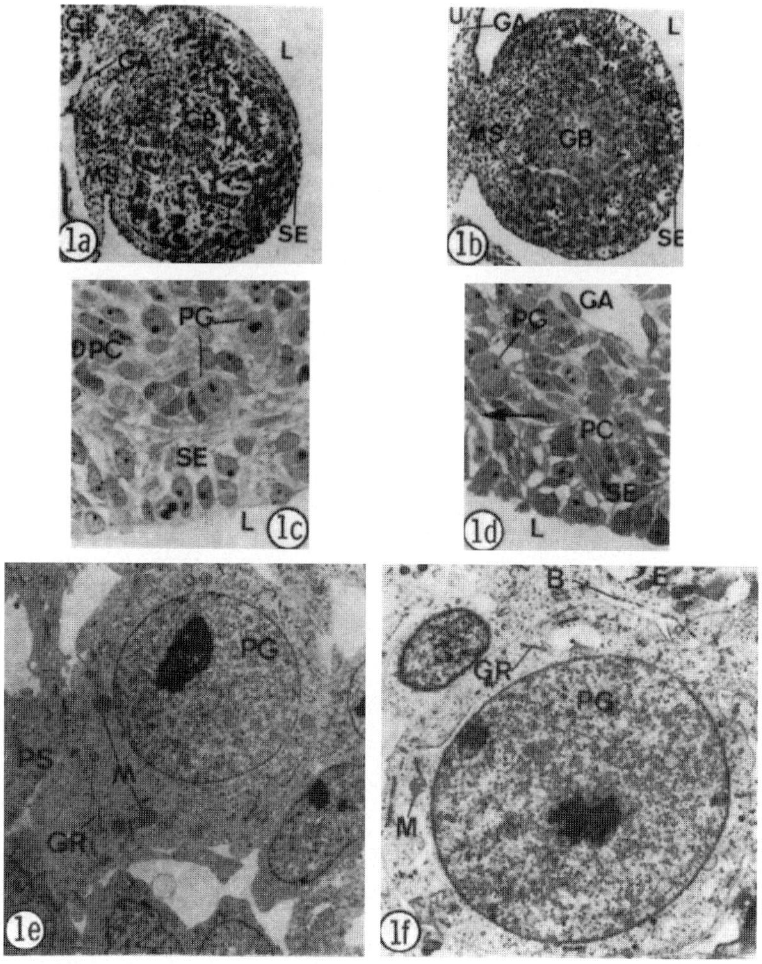

FIGURE 13-1. (**A**) Light micrograph of porcine fetal testis at day 26. (**B**) Light micrograph of porcine fetal ovary at day 27. (**C**) Light micrograph of male gonad in pig embryo at day 24. (**D**) Light micrograph of female gonad in pig embryo at day 24. (**E**) Electron micrograph of a cortical portion of a male gonad in pig embryo at day 24. (**F**) Electron micrograph of a primordial germ cell with a prominent nucleolus of female gonad in pig embryo at day 21. *GA*, surface epithelial basal lamina; *CA*, capillary; *E*, surface epithelial cell; *GB*, gonadal blastema; *GR*, granular endoplasmic reticulum; *IC*, interstitial cell; *IS*, interstitium; *L*, coelomic cavity; *M*, mitochondria; *MS*, mesenchyme; *PC*, primitive cords; *PG*, primordial germ cells; *PS*, pseudopod of cytoplasm; *SE*, surface epithelium. (**A** and **B**: From Pelliniemi LJ. Am J Anat 1975;144:89. **C**, **D**, and **E**: From Pelliniemi LJ. Cell Tissue 1976;8:163. **F**: From Pelliniemi LJ. Anat. Embryol. 1975;147:19.)

in fetal life becomes gonadotropin dependent. Serum LH, FSH, and prolactin reach peak levels during the first week after birth, and then gradually decrease by the seventh week. Elongation of seminiferous tubules is probably increased at this time by FSH stimulation of Sertoli cells.

Testicular descent begins about day 60 of fetal life with growth of the gubernaculum. The testes traverse the inguinal canal (*vaginal process*) about day 85 and move to the base of the scrotum soon after birth. LH and testosterone concentrations parallel testicular development during these prenatal and postnatal periods.

During prepubertal hypertrophy, the Leydig cells reach maximal diameters of 30 $\mu$m with fine structural features of increased numbers of mitochondria, agranular endoplasmic reticulum, and cytoplasmic filaments. These and other cytoplasmic organelles resemble those in adult boars. Hypophysectomy in boars causes regression of the testes, epididymides, prostate, seminal vesicles, and bulbourethral glands, whereas daily injections of human chorionic gonadotropin (hCG) can reestablish the Leydig cells.

From 40 to 250 days of age, the paired testes weight increases markedly from 6 to 120 grams. Testosterone concentrations in peripheral serum increase as pubertal development progresses, and decline near maturity. Estradiol-17$\beta$ serum levels increase steadily throughout pubertal development. Dehydroepiandrosterone sulfate and the 16-androstenes act as precursors to androgenic hormones in the boar. The estradiol-17$\beta$ in the male may play a synergistic role with testosterone in sexual behavior and act on accessory sex glands as well as enhance testicular synthesis of testosterone. Circulating levels of relaxin remain consistently low (less than 0.5 ng/ml) in prepubertal and mature boars (1).

In both pubertal and sexually mature boars, the intravenous injection of LH-releasing hormone (LHRH) causes peak LH release within 10 minutes. Testosterone and its metabolite, 5$\alpha$-dihydrotestosterone (5$\alpha$-DHT), provide both stimulatory and inhibitory effects on LH secretion in the boar. Direct intracerebral implantation of 5$\alpha$-DHT or testosterone into the mediobasal hypothalamus or amygdala inhibits release of LH from the pituitary gland. Thus, androgens modulate the secretion of hypothalamic hormones, which in turn control the release of LH from the adenohypophysis in the boar.

## SPERM PRODUCTION

Mounting activity occurs early (erection by 4 months), but sequential patterns of sexual behavior culminate after 5 months. First ejaculates occur at 5 to 8 months of age; heritability ($h^2$) estimates for age at puberty average 0.32 (2). The number of spermatozoa and the semen volume continue to increase during the first 18 months of life. The duration of one cycle of the seminiferous epithelium requires 8.6 days. The duration of the spermatogenic cycle (spermatogonia to mature spermatozoa) is approximately 34.4 days; thus, four cycles of the seminiferous epithelium occur during one spermatogenic cycle. The duration for transit of the spermatozoa through the epididymis is about 10.2 days. Highest fertilization rates result with spermatozoa obtained from the proximal and distal caudal epididymidis. Testosterone sustains secretory activities of the accessory glands (e.g., seminal vesicles, prostate, bulbourethral glands), and these seminal fluids constitute a large proportion of the total ejaculate in the boar.

## HORMONES AND PUBERTY IN GILTS

The fetal gonad differentiates to an ovary at about day 35 by the appearance of egg nests (Table 13-1). Primary and secondary follicles appear late in gestation. FSH-secreting cells have been identified in fetuses 70 days old and serum levels of FSH, LH, and prolactin increase preceding birth. The amplitude of LH pulses increases, and by 10 weeks, episodic LH release occurs spontaneously. Tertiary follicles develop at 8 weeks after birth and may indicate the period when follicular development becomes dependent on gonadotropins.

In pigs from 10 weeks of age until puberty (i.e., 25 weeks), the frequency and magnitude of serum LH peaks are greatest at 16 weeks. Spikes of FSH and prolactin occur with more than random synchrony throughout this period. The stimulatory estrogen feedback mechanism is essential for onset of cyclic ovarian activity, but the negative feedback control of LH release by ovarian steroids is absent at birth and develops by 8 weeks of age. The sensitivity of the hypothalamic-pituitary axis regulating LH secretion to the negative feedback action of estradiol-17$\beta$ decreases as gilts progress from the prepubertal to the postpubertal state. Intravenous infusion of LHRH induces an immediate increase in serum LH to peak values (greater than 6 ng/ml) within 15 minutes.

### *Ovarian Morphology*

During the prepubertal period, the ovaries contain numerous small follicles (2 to 4 mm diameter) and several (8 to 15) medium-sized follicles (6 to 8 mm). The uterus responds to increasing ovarian steroidogenic activity during the late prepubertal period; the uterus weighs 30 to 60 g during infantile stages, as compared with 150 to 250 g in prepubertal gilts. As ovarian follicles develop in prepubertal gilts, there are corresponding increases in ovarian weights. Puberty is characterized by first estrus, ovulation of Graafian follicles, and the release of ova capable of fertilization.

### *Environment and Hormone Treatment*

The age of puberty ($h^2$ = 0.32) (2) may be influenced by the level of nutrition, social environment, body weight, season of year, breed, disease or parasite infestation, and management practices. Limiting energy intake to half that of the fullfed controls delays puberty more than 40 days. The presence of boars reduces age (191 vs 232 days) and body weight (105 vs 116 kg) to puberty. Puberty also is delayed in gilts penned individually as compared with those maintained in groups of 30 animals.

Since prepubertal gilts have no corpora lutea, low circulating levels (e.g., 2 ng/ml) of progesterone may be at least partly adrenal in origin. Profiles of progesterone during the luteal phase of the first estrous cycle follow a pattern typical of normal cycling gilts. Maturation of ovarian follicles and ovulations can be induced by exogenous gonadotropins in prepubertal gilts after 60 days of age. For example, a single injection of pregnant mare serum gonadotropin (PMSG) followed by hCG induces ovulation in 90% of gilts 90 to 130 days of age, but few of them exhibit estrus or remain pregnant. In gilts 9 to 12 months old who have not exhibited a previous estrus, progesterone remains low (e.g., 2 ng/ml) throughout the proestrus; a similar gonadotropin regimen induces estrus, ovulation, recurrent estrous cycles, and normal fertility in a high percentage. Injection of LHRH also induces ovulations in prepubertal gilts, and the corpora lutea from those ovulations sustain pregnancies.

### *Estrous Cycle*

Onset of estrus is characterized by gradual changes in behavioral patterns (e.g., restlessness, mounting of other animals, lordosis response), vulva responses (e.g., swelling, pink-red coloring), and occasionally a mucous discharge. Sexual receptivity averages 40 to 60 hours. The pubertal estrous period usually is shorter (47 hours) than later ones (56 hours), and gilts usually have a shorter period of estrus than sows. Breed, seasonal variation (e.g., longest estrus in summer and shortest in winter) and endocrine abnormalities affect the duration of heat.

Ova are released 38 to 42 hours after the onset of estrus, and the duration of this ovulatory process requires 3.8 hours. Ovulations occur about 4 hours earlier in mated than in unmated animals. The length of the cycle is about 21 days (range of 19 to 23 days). The pig is polyestrous throughout the year; only pregnancy or endocrine dysfunction interrupts this cyclicity.

**OVARIAN MORPHOLOGY AND HORMONE SECRETION.** There are about 50 small follicles (i.e., 2 to 5 mm in diameter) during the luteal and early follicular phases of the cycle of which 10 to 20 follicles approach preovulatory size (8 to 11 mm), while the number of smaller follicles declines (those less than 5 mm). During the luteal phase of the cycle (days 5 to 16), the number of follicles 2 to 5 mm in diameter (with a few up to 7 mm) increases; whereas after day 18 (proestrous phase), an increase occurs primarily in the growth of preovulatory follicles (those at least 8 mm in diameter).

Soon after ovulation there is rapid proliferation of primarily granulosa and a few theca cells lining the follicle wall. These cells become luteinized to form luteal tissue, thus the corpus luteum (CL). Initially, the corpus is considered a corpus hemorrhagicum because of the blood-filled central cavity, but within 6 to 8 days, the CL is a solid mass of luteal cells with an overall diameter of 8 to 11 mm. The luteal phase (about 16 days) is characterized by the rapid development of the CL to its maximal weight (i.e., 350 to 450 mg) by days 6 to 8, the maintenance of cellular integrity and secretory function to day 16, and then the rapid regression to a nonsecreting corpus albicans.

During luteinization (day 1) granulosa cells at the periphery of the ruptured follicle are cuboidal to columnar and separated by irregular extracellular spaces that contain precipitated liquor folliculi. By day 4, luteinization is essentially complete; the cells are hypertrophied with masses of agranular endoplasmic reticulum. These cells typify the secretory phase (days 4 to 12) by their protein and steroid hormone production. During cell regression (days 14 to 18), there is an increase in cytoplasmic lipid droplets, in cytoplasmic disorganization, and in vacuolation of the agranular endoplasmic reticulum. At the terminal phase of the cycle, there is an increase in the number of lysosomes, vacuolation of agranular endoplasmic reticulum and invasion of connective tissue; these events result in formation of the corpus albicans.

Steroid-secreting activity of the corpora lutea is indicated by concentrations of progesterone and estrogen throughout the cycle (Fig. 13-2**A**). Progesterone levels are low at estrus (day 0), increase abruptly after day 2, reach peak values by days 8 to 12, and then decline precipitously thereafter to day 18. Estrogen concentrations in peripheral plasma increase coincident with the decline and disappearance of progesterone (Fig. 13-2**A**). Peak values occur 2 days preceding estrus and reflect rapid growth and maturation of graafian follicles during late proestrus. Soon after estrus, estrogen declines and remains low during the luteal phase of the cycle. Estradiol secreted by the developing preovulatory follicles stimulates the preovulatory surge of gonadotropins (3). Insulin-like growth factors (i.e., IGF-I) promote differentiation and replication of cultured granulosa cells as well as increase FSH-stimulated production of progesterone, estrogen, cyclic adenosine monophosphate (cAMP), proteoglycans, and LH receptors (4). Epidermal growth factor (EGF) and transforming growth factor-$\beta$ (TGF-$\beta$) can modulate steroidogenesis in porcine theca and granulosa cells. For example, EGF inhibits production of estradiol by theca cells but has little effect on secretion of progesterone or androgens. These growth factors produced by theca and granulosa modulate, in a paracrine or autocrine way, steroidogenesis and follicular differentiation. The life span and secretory function of this ephemeral structure in the pig can be prolonged by pregnancy or hysterectomy.

FSH in peripheral serum peaks on days 2 and 3, after the onset of behavioral estrus (Fig. 13-2**A**). Ovarian follicles depend on secretion of adenohypophyseal gonadotropins for their growth and maturation; hypophysectomy or hypophyseal stalk transection (5) abruptly regresses these follicles. Ovarian follicular fluid of sows contains inhibin, a protein hormone, which suppresses FSH secretion. FSH serum levels are inversely related to inhibin during the late follicular phase; inhibin concentrations decrease with the LH surge. Activin and activin-A are dimers of the $\beta$-subunits of inhibin ($\beta_A\beta_A$ and $\beta_A\beta_B$), and they are equipotent in their ability to stimulate FSH secretion without affecting LH secretion. Follistatin is a single peptide chain of 32,000 to 35,000 molecular weight distinct from inhibin and activin, which can inhibit the release of FSH but not LH.

LH plasma levels show one sharp peak at estrus and drop to low levels during the remainder of the cycle (Fig. 13-2**A**). From days 12 to 15 of the estrous cycle an episodic pattern FSH and LH as well as estradiol secretion occurs (6). Prolactin levels peak during estrus and remain low during the luteal phase of the estrous cycle. Prolactin levels peak when estrogen is highest, and during estrus, prolactin profiles coincide better with the FSH peak than with the preovulatory LH peak. Deafferentation of the anterior hypothalamus and preoptic area abolishes episodic LH secretion, whereas LHRH causes acute release of LH in such animals (7). In contrast, prolactin secretion remains consistently elevated in hypophyseal stalk transected gilts as compared with sham operated controls (8). Thus, the hypothalamus is required for the tonic inhibition of prolactin secretion, and for the regulation of both episodic release and tonic inhibition of basal secretion of LH, FSH, and growth hormone in the pig.

Relaxin remains low in the luteal phase throughout the estrous cycle and shows no relationship to the high levels of progesterone secreted by these same cells during this brief period. Prostaglandin F (PGF) concentrations in uteroovarian venous plasma increase during the estrous cycle to peak values between days 12 and 16, a period coinciding with onset of luteal regression. Porcine endometrium synthesizes $PGF_{2\alpha}$ during the mid- to late-luteal phase whereas indomethacin can block its production.

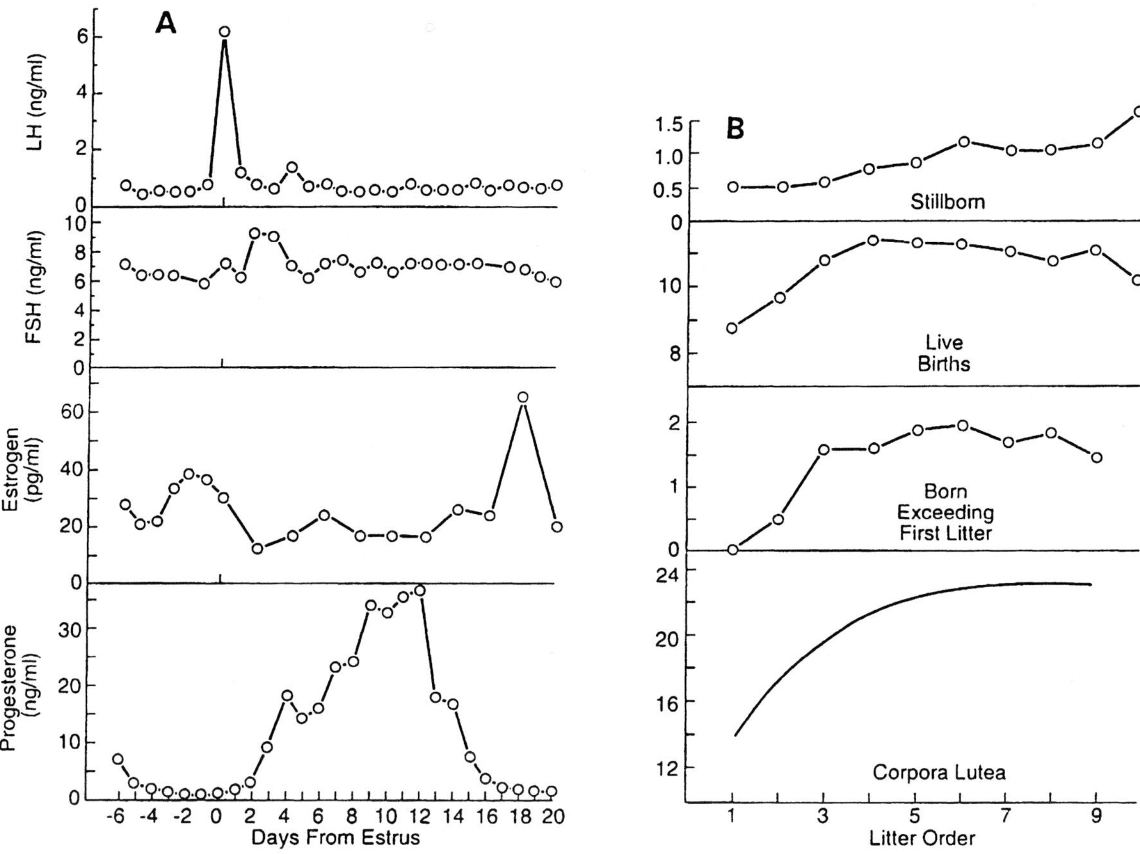


FIGURE 13-2. (A) Peripheral blood plasma concentrations of progesterone, estrogen, FSH, and LH during the estrous cycle in the pig. (B) Reproductive performance in relation to parity in the pig. (A: Adapted from Allrich RD, et al. J Anim Sci 1982;55:1139; Parvizi N, et al. J Endocrinol 1976;69:193; Guthrie HD, et al. Endocrinology 1972;91:675. B: Adapted from Lush JL, Molln AE. Tech Bull US Dept Agric 1942;836; Rasbech NO. Br Vet J 1969;125:599.)

## *Ovulation Rate*

Ovulation rate is associated with breed (lines or crosses), amount of inbreeding, age at breeding, and weight at breeding. In inbred lines there is an average increase of 1.1 ova from the first to third estrus, but little if any additional increase occurs beyond the fourth postpubertal estrus. Reproductive experience correlates with ovulation rate; ovulations increase with parity to seven or more litters (Fig. 13-2**B**). Inbreeding reduces ovulation rate, whereas crossing inbred lines increases the number of ovulations. Selection experiments based on a controlled gene pool over seven generations indicate that heritability of ovulation rate is 0.40 on weighted cumulative selection differential (2, 9).

METHODS TO INCREASE OVULATION RATES. A single injection of PMSG or PMSG followed by an injection of hCG can induce ovulations, and the ovulatory response depends primarily on the dosage of PMSG. HCG induces ovulation in cycling gilts but causes little if any increase in ovulation rate. After an intramuscular injection of hCG (i.e., 500 IU) during the proestrous period, ovulations occur in most of the animals 44 to 46 hours later. The injection of PMSG induces superovulatory responses when given on days 15 or 16 of the cycle. The gonadotropins usually reduce the length of the cycle, increase the duration of estrus, and may increase the incidence of cystic follicles, but the ova shed are capable of acceptable fertilization rates.

NUTRITION AND OVULATION RATE. High energy diets induce a higher ovulation rate in the pig when fed for a restricted duration, but the number of ovulations is predominantly affected by genetic background. The levels of energy restriction (e.g., 3,000 to 5,000 kcal) before feeding the pigs a high energy diet (e.g., 8,000 to 10,000 kcal) are an important factor influencing ovulation rate. The optimal duration of a high energy regimen seems to be 11 to 14 days before expected estrus or mating. Increased protein intake during brief periods has little effect on ovulation rate.

The administration of short- or long-acting insulin in combination with a high energy diet consistently increased ovulation rate and reduced follicular atresia (10). Altrenogest (17$\beta$-hydroxy-17-(2-propenyl)-estra-4,9,11-triene-3-

one) given orally for 14 days to gilts tended to increase ovulation rate, but its effect differed from those of flushing (11).

## Conception Rate

The fertilization rate in pigs is usually high (>90%). Low or high ovulation rates have little or no effect on fertilization rates. Loss of the whole litter may result from fertilization failure or death of all the embryos. Early embryonic death results in resorption of the conceptus, whereas losses occurring after day 50 may result in abortion, fetal mummification, or delivery of stillborns at term.

## Embryo Survival

At least 40% of the embryos are lost before parturition. Within the first 18 days, embryonic survival is reduced by 17%. By day 25, approximately 33% of the embryos die, and this can increase to 40% by day 50. Although sows have greater fecundity than gilts, they lose a greater proportion of their embryos during the first 40 days. With each 10% inbreeding in the dam, there results 0.5 to 0.8 fewer ova, and 0.5 fewer fertilized ova and 0.8 fewer embryos by day 25. Crossing inbred lines causes 0.5 more ova, 0.3 more fertilized ova, and 0.8 more embryos at day 25. Heritability estimates for embryo survival average 0.30 (2).

## Litter Size

Reproductive performance is measured primarily by the number of living pigs at birth or by the total farrowing or weaning weight of pigs produced by the dam within 1 year. Ovulation rates continue to increase with subsequent gestations, but litter size reaches maximal levels by the fourth or fifth parity (Fig. 13-2**B**). The number of pigs farrowed increases between the first and fourth litters, but by the eighth litter, live births decline while the number of stillborn increases. When litter size is related to the age of the dam, reproductive performance begins to decline after 4.5 years. The genetic contribution (heritability) to litter size is estimated as 0.17; most variation is attributed to environmental factors. Breed combinations provide estimates of heterosis and the direct and maternal breed effects. For example, pure lines of Duroc and Yorkshire average 13.8 corpora lutea, but breeding Duroc dams to a boar of another breed increases litter size by 1.4 pigs at farrowing. Survival rates at day 30, and farrowing and weaning of progeny from three-breed crosses exceed those progeny from two-breed crosses.

## Pregnancy

### *Growth of Conceptuses*

Ova are fertilized in the ampulla of the oviduct, and their arrival is aided by the rapid beat, in a downward direction, of cilia on the mucosal surface; in the isthmus of the oviduct, there is an upward ciliary current that may aid sperm ascent. Embryos are usually in the four-cell stage when they enter the uterus. Cleavage advances to morula stage by day 5 and then blastocyst formation by days 6 to 8. Hatching describes at least partial escape of the embryo from the zona pellucida, and it occurs on the sixth day when blastocysts may reach a size of 150 cells or more (Fig. 13-3). Blastocysts are unevenly distributed throughout both uterine horns. Rapid development of conceptuses is indicated by intrauterine migration of the embryos, spacing of the embryos, and transition of blastocysts from spherical to extremely elongated forms and subsequent embryogenesis. By day 11, half the blastocysts rapidly elongate to filamentous forms, often exceeding 60 cm (Fig. 13-4), and by day 13, embryos have completed this process (12). These conceptuses become regularly spaced with no overlap of tubular membranes from other embryos in that horn. Individual conceptuses grow exponentially between days 9 and 18 and independent of the developmental stage or potential loss of those neighbors nearest that conceptus.

Normal embryonic and fetal growth from days 20 to 100 of gestation increase from 0.06 to 1000 g. Fetal wet weight is highly correlated with placental length ($r = .64$), placental surface area ($r = .72$), and total areolae surface per placenta ($r = .65$). Uterine- and conceptus-derived proteins that include mitogens (IGF-I, IGF-II, and EGF);

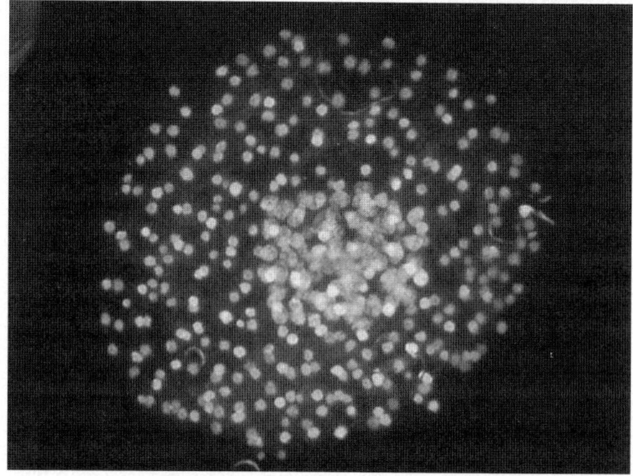

FIGURE 13-3. Photomicrograph of an early blastocyst stage pig embryo on day 6 of gestation. The two cell layers present in the embryo at this time are the inner cell mass (nuclei stained blue) and the trophectoderm (nuclei stained pink). (Photomicrograph courtesy of Stephen P. Ford and Matthew E. Wilson, Iowa State University, Ames.)

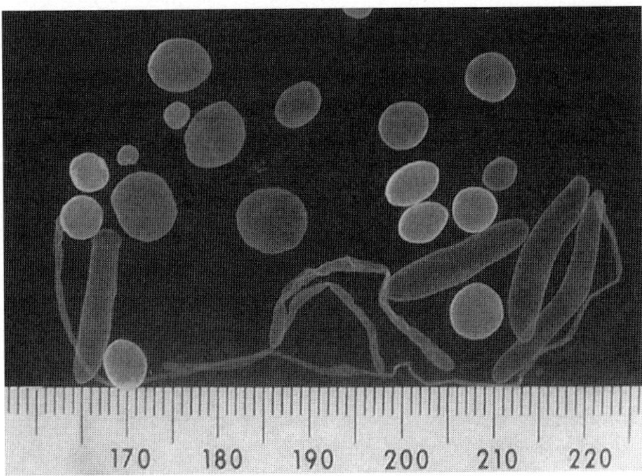


FIGURE 13-4. Picture of the diverse morphologies of pig embryos found on days 11 to 12 of gestation, including spherical, ovoid, tubular, and filamentous forms. The filamentous form can reach lengths of approximately 100 cm. (Photomicrograph courtesy of Stephen P. Ford and Matthew E. Wilson, Iowa State University, Ames.)

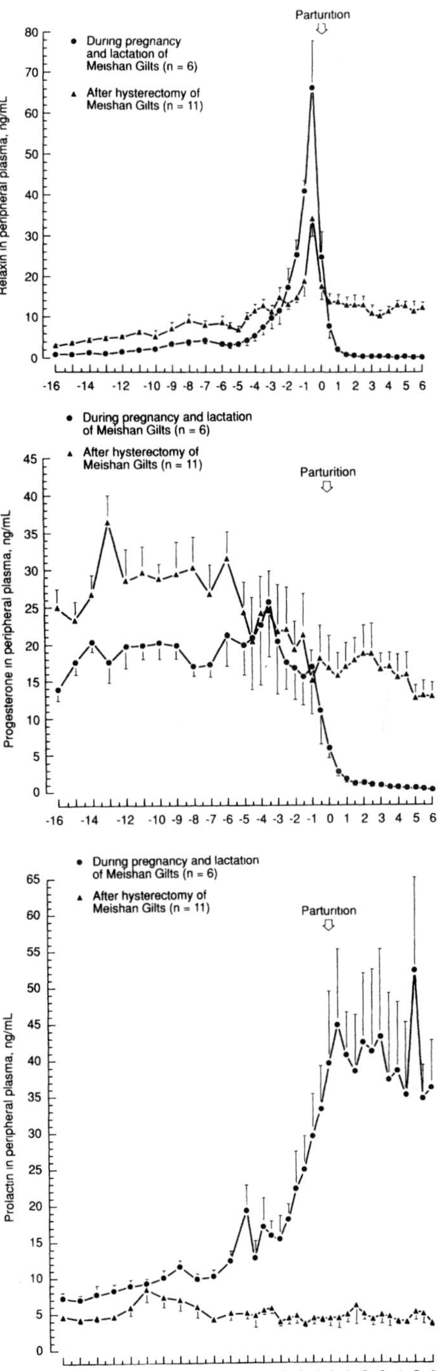


FIGURE 13-5. Relaxin, progesterone, and prolactin concentrations in peripheral plasma of Meishan gilts during pregnancy and lactation compared with those in unmated gilts hysterectomized on days 6 to 8 after estrus. Values are mean ± SE. (Dlamini BJ, et al. J Anim Sci 1995;73:3732.)

binding and transport proteins (uteroferrin, IGF-, and retinol-binding proteins); protease inhibitors (plasmin and trypsin inhibitor); and interferon-related trophoblastic proteins are differentially expressed during the period of maternal recognition of pregnancy and implantation (13, 14).

## *Hormones During Pregnancy*

Corpora lutea are essential for maintenance of pregnancy to term in the pig. The CL develops to maximal weight by day 8 and is sustained to late pregnancy. Two porcine luteal cell populations of 30 to 50 $\mu$m in diameter and 15 to 20 $\mu$m in diameter produce progesterone that seems associated with cell size and stage of pregnancy. After day 114, soon after delivery, there is a precipitous decline in luteal weight. Progesterone concentrations in peripheral blood increase to peak values by day 12, and gradually decrease to levels of 20 to 25 ng/ml by day 104 (Fig. 13-5). Concentrations of unconjugated estradiol-17$\beta$ in peripheral blood increase from 10 pg/ml at days 8 to 60 to peak values (400 pg/ml) just before parturition. Two peaks of estrone sulfate occur at days 30 and 112, respectively, and then drop at onset of parturition. The fetoplacental unit is the major source of estrogen production, as indicated by the finding of similar urinary excretory patterns in intact controls, as seen in sows after ovariectomy, hypophysectomy, or adrenalectomy.

Prolactin is luteotropic in the pig. In hypophysectomized and hysterectomized gilts given daily injections of purified porcine prolactin, both progesterone and relaxin plasma concentrations are maintained throughout a period of 10 days from days 110 to 120 (15). Prolactin plasma levels increase markedly in late pregnancy and remain high during early lactation (Fig. 13-5).

The blastocysts maintain luteal function during critical phases of early pregnancy by overcoming uterine luteolytic action, and they may contribute to the luteotropic effect by their production of estrogen (16). Uterine arterial blood flow increases two to fourfold from days 11 to 13 of pregnancy. In pregnant pigs there is a temporal relationship between blastocyst elongation and increasing quantities of $PGE_2$ and $PGF_{2\alpha}$ as well as estrogens in uterine flushings (17). Porcine blastocysts produce $PGF_{2\alpha}$ and $PGE_2$. When the uterus is removed (hysterectomy), the corpora lutea are maintained for a period exceeding that of pregnancy, and they produce progesterone and relaxin (Fig. 13-5). Exogenous $PGF_{2\alpha}$ is luteolytic and induces abortion from day 23 of pregnancy onward, and unmated hysterectomized gilts can induce abrupt relaxin release and progesterone decrease similar to that seen at normal parturition (18).

During late pregnancy, corticosteroid concentrations increase within 24 hours of parturition and decrease during early lactation. Progesterone levels decline during the last days of pregnancy and drop abruptly to 0.5 ng/ml by day 1 postpartum (Fig. 13-5). Estrone increases to peak concentrations until day 2 prepartum and then falls to basal levels after delivery of conceptuses. The rise in estrone and estradiol is associated with fetal maturity and is primarily of placental origin. Fetal adrenal cortical cells increase markedly from days 105 to 113 to secrete cortisol that may play a role in the timing of parturition.

Relaxin is produced and accumulated in porcine corpora lutea but their concentrations in peripheral blood remain consistently low (up to 2 ng/ml) during the first 90 days, then increase to peak values 2 days before parturition and signal the discharge of accumulated relaxin from the corpora lutea (Fig. 13-5) (19, 20). A programmed peak release of relaxin occurs at day 113 and progesterone decreases by half in unmated hysterectomized gilts, events that mimic hormone changes seen in late pregnancy and parturition (18). Relaxin and estrogen are required for remodeling collagen and dilation of the cervix and for the growth of mammary parenchymal tissue, cervix, and vagina of late pregnant gilts (21–23).

Infusion of antiporcine relaxin during late gestation decreases relaxin plasma concentration and disrupts delivery in late pregnant pigs (24). Premature parturition in intact gilts or sows can be induced by the administration of exogenous $PGF_{2\alpha}$. Dexamethasone injections also decrease progesterone secretion and induce premature delivery, but in hysterectomized gilts they delay relaxin release without altering progesterone secretion (25). The role of the fetal pituitary and adrenal glands in initiating processes of parturition is implicated by the effects of fetal hypophysectomy or fetal decapitation on the prolongation of gestation beyond term. The antiprogesterone RU 486 given orally on days 111 and 112 induces parturition within 31 hours (19). The luteolytic effect of RU 486 likely results from preferential binding to progesterone receptor in the uterus but RU 486 increases progesterone secretion after hysterectomy (19, 26).

## POSTPARTUM ESTRUS

Immediately after delivery, peripheral blood levels of progesterone, estrone, estradiol, and relaxin decline to basal levels during early lactation (Fig. 13-5). Although estrus can occur within 1 to 3 days after parturition, sows fail to conceive because the ovarian follicles are immature and ovulation usually does not occur. Restricting the diet of primiparous sows during lactation had no effect on plasma LH or estradiol concentrations or subsequent reproductive performance (27).

## LACTATION

With the exception of the postpartum estrus, sows rarely exhibit estrus during lactation. Ovarian morphology during the anestrous period indicates an absence of gonadotropic stimulation. The average diameter of the ovarian follicle decreases (i.e., from 4 to 2 mm) during the first week after parturition and then gradually increases (i.e., more than 5 mm) by the fifth week of lactation. Uterine weight and length decline rapidly for 21 to 28 days following parturition; thereafter, both remain constant. The endometrium is thinner and the uterine glands are less numerous, particularly in the basal region near the myometrium.

During lactational anestrus, depressed FSH release and reduced LH synthesis occurs. Prolactin concentrations in peripheral plasma are high at parturition, increase in response to suckling by the piglets, and decline soon after weaning (Fig. 13-5). Prolactin levels, but not LH, increase acutely with suckling or weaning. Estrogen, whether of endogenous or exogenous origin, causes surges in LH, FSH, and prolactin in the postpartum sow.

## SOW AT WEANING

Removal of the litter from the sow after 3 to 5 weeks of lactation results in follicular development, estrus, and ovulation within 4 to 8 days. At weaning, a transient increase occurs in plasma LH and hypothalamic LHRH content. During the postweaning period, plasma concentrations of estradiol-17$\beta$ increase gradually and are terminated by the preovulatory surge of LH at estrus. Increases in plasma FSH levels coincide with the LH surge, but prolactin secretion may be associated more with estrus than the ovulation process.

## REFERENCES


1. Juang HH, Musah AI, Schwabe C, Ford JJ, Anderson LL. Relaxin in peripheral plasma of boars during development copulation after administration of human chorionic gonadotropin and after castration. J Reprod Fertil 1996;107:1.
2. Rothschild MF. Genetics and reproduction in the pig. Anim Reprod Sci 1996;42:143.
3. Kraeling RR, Barb CR. Hypothalamic control of gonadotropin and prolactin secretion in pigs. J Reprod Fertil 1990; 40(Suppl):3.
4. Haseltine FP, Findlay JK, eds. Growth Factors in Fertility Regulation. Cambridge: Cambridge University Press, 1991.
5. Anderson LL, Dyck GW, Mori H, Henricks DM, Melampy RM. Ovarian function in pigs following hypophysial stalk transection or hypophysectomy. Am J Physiol 1967;212:1188.
6. Flowers B, Cantley TC, Martin MJ, Day BN. Episodic secretion of gonadotropins and ovarian steroids in jugular and utero-ovarian vein plasma during the follicular phase of the oestrous cycle in gilts. J Reprod Fertil 1991;91:101.
7. Molina JR, Hard DL, Anderson LL. Hypothalamic deafferentation and LHRH on LH secretion in prepuberal gilts. Biol Reprod 1986;35:439.
8. Anderson LL, Berardinelli JG, Malven PV, Ford JJ. Prolactin secretion after hypophysial stalk transection in pigs. Endocrinology 1982;111:380.
9. Johnson RK, Zimmerman DR, Lamberson WR, Sasaki S. Influencing prolificacy of sows by selection for physiological factors. J Reprod Fertil 1985;33(Suppl):139.
10. Cox NM, Stuart MJ, Althen TG, Bennett WA, Miller HW. Enhancement of ovulation rate in gilts by increasing dietary energy and administering insulin during follicular growth. J Anim Sci 1987;64:507.
11. Rhodes MT, Davis DL, Stevenson JS. Flushing and altrogenest affect litter traits in gilts. J Anim Sci 1991;69:34.
12. Anderson LL. Growth protein content and distribution of early pig embryos. Anat Rec 1978;190:143.
13. Simmen RCM, Simmen FA. Regulation of uterine and conceptus secretory activity in the pig. J Reprod Fertil 1990;40(Suppl):279.
14. Roberts RM, Xie S, Nagel RJ, Low BG, Green J, Beckers JF. Glycoproteins of the aspartyl proteinase gene family secreted by the developing placenta. In: Takahashi K, ed. Aspartic Proteinases: Structure Function Biology and Biomedical Implications. Tokyo: Plenum Press, 1995;231.
15. Li Y, Molina JR, Klindt J, Bolt DJ, Anderson LL. Prolactin maintains relaxin and progesterone secretion by aging corpora lutea after hypophysial stalk transection or hypophysectomy in the pig. Endocrinology 1989;124:1294.
16. Ford SP, Stice SL. Effects of the ovary and conceptus on controlling uterine blood flow in the pig. J Reprod Fertil 1985;33(Suppl):83.
17. Bazer FW, Marengo SR, Geisert RD, Thatcher WW. Exocrine versus endocrine secretion of prostaglandin $F_{2\alpha}$ in the control of pregnancy in swine. Anim Reprod Sci 1984;7:115.
18. Cho S-J, Klindt J, Jacobson CD, Anderson LL. Prostaglandin-$F_{2\alpha}$ induced luteolysis of aging corpora lutea in hysterectomized pigs. Biol Reprod 1998;58:1032.
19. Li Y, Huang CJ, Klindt J, Anderson LL. Divergent effects of antiprogesterone RU 486 on progesterone relaxin and prolactin secretion in pregnant and hysterectomized pigs. Endocrinology 1991;129:2907.
20. Dlamini BJ, Li Y, Klindt J, Anderson LL. Acute shifts in relaxin progesterone prolactin and growth hormone secretion in Chinese Meishan gilts during late pregnancy and after hysterectomy. J Anim Sci 1995;73:3732.
21. Eldridge-White R, Easter RA, Heaton DM, et al. Hormonal control of the cervix in pregnant gilts I Changes in the physical properties of the cervix correlate temporally with elevated serum levels of estrogens and relaxin. Endocrinology 1989; 125:2996.
22. Hurley WL, Doane RM, O'Day-Bowman MB, Winn RJ, Mojonnier LE, Sherwood OD. Effect of relaxin on mammary gland development in ovariectomized pregnant gilts. Endocrinology 1991;128;1285.
23. Huang CJ, Li Y, Anderson LL. Relaxin and estrogen synergistically accelerate growth and development in the uterine cervix of prepubertal pigs. Anim Reprod Sci 1997;46:149.
24. Cho S-J, Dlamini BJ, Klindt J, Schwabe C, Jacobson CD, Anderson LL. Antiporcine relaxin (antipRLX540) treatment decreases relaxin plasma concentration and disrupts delivery in late pregnant pigs. Anim Reprod Sci 1998;52:303.
25. Li Y, Huang CJ, Cho S-J, Anderson LL. Differential effects of dexamethasone and RU 486 an antigestagen and antiglucocorticoid on progesterone and relaxin secretion in hysterectomized pigs with aging corpora lutea. Anim Reprod Sci 1998; 51:131.
26. Rothchild I. The corpus luteum revisited: Are the paradoxical effects of RU 486 a clue to how progesterone stimulates its own secretion? Biol Reprod 1996;55:1.
27. Armstrong JD, Britt JH, Kraeling RR. Effect of restriction of energy during lactation on body condition energy metabolism endocrine changes and reproductive performance in primiparous sows. J Anim Sci 1986;63:1915.

CHAPTER 14

# Horses

E.S.E. HAFEZ AND B. HAFEZ

The various breeds of the domestic horse (*Equus caballus*) are members of the family *Equidae*, which belongs to the order *Perissodactyla*. The horse has several unique aspects of reproductive endocrinology and pregnancy. Whereas other large farm species such as the cattle, swine, and sheep have been highly selected for reproductive efficiency, as well as other productive traits, the only selection practiced with horses has been their ability to walk or run.

Race horses are usually aged from January 1 in the year that they are born, and it has been the practice to breed them as early in the year as possible so that, as 2-year-olds, the offspring have maximal physical advantage.

## BREEDING SEASON

### *Stallion*

The breeding season of stallions is not well marked, and semen can be collected throughout the year. However, remarkable seasonal variations are noted in reaction time, number of mounts per ejaculate, volume of gel-free semen, total number of spermatozoa per ejaculate, sperm agglutination, and motility in fresh and in diluted semen.

The effects of season on seminal plasma are greater than those on spermatozoa. Spermatozoa in first ejaculates are less affected by season than those in second ejaculates. This differential effect on first and second ejaculates is noted for most semen characteristics (1).

### *Mare*

The reproductive cycle of the mare is subject to the greatest variability of all the domestic animals (Table 14-1). Some mares appear to be truly polyestrous; they can produce offspring at any time of the year. However, the great majority of the mare population are seasonally polyestrous. Although many mares in the northern hemisphere show behavioral estrus in February, March, and April, estrus during this time is often unaccompanied by ovulation, and conception rates in mares bred during the period are low. In the northern hemisphere, the best conception rates usually occur in mares bred from May to July. The same trends occur in mares in the southern hemisphere for the corresponding seasons. Although mares who feed primarily on grass normally breed only during summer and go into anestrus in winter, those that are well fed and stabled tend to cycle throughout the year. The onset of the fertile breeding season is closely associated with management.

Mares can be classified into three categories according to their breeding season:

1. Defined breeding season. The wild breeds of horses manifest several estrous cycles during a restricted breeding season that coincides with the longest days of the year; the foals are born during a restricted foaling season.
2. Transitory breeding season. Some domestic breeds and some individual mares manifest estrous cycles throughout the year, but ovulation accompanies estrus only during the breeding season, and the foals are born during a limited foaling season.
3. Year-round breeding. Some domestic breeds and some individual mares exhibit estrous cycles accompanied by ovulation throughout the year.

Thus, it is evident that although some mares, at certain latitudes, may show estrous cycles throughout the year, they do not necessarily conceive during all estrous periods (Table 14-1).

In localities where there is a breeding season, the two transitory periods preceding and following the breeding season are characterized by variability of ovarian activity and sexual behavior. At this time the ovarian follicles develop only to limited degrees and then undergo atresia. Also there is a high frequency of prolonged estrus or estrus of short duration as well as irregular estrous cycles during these periods.

Near the equator, there is little seasonal variation in the length of the estrous cycle. In temperate regions, mares are seasonally polyestrous, with the breeding and nonbreeding seasons occurring during the summer and winter months,

TABLE 14-1. ***Physiological Mechanisms of the Breeding Season, Non-Breeding Season, Non-Ovulatory Season***

| | |
|---|---|
| BREEDING SEASON | Photoperiod/body condition are the main environmental factors to affect reproductive seasonality.<br>Either gradual increase photoperiod or fixed period of 15 hr in December initiate ovulatory season 2 months earlier.<br>Prolonged fixed photoperiods (>20 h) produce an effect intermediate between effects of natural daylength/15-h photoperiod.<br>Photoperiodicity stimulates pineal melatonin during darkness, which in turn, blocks GnRH secretion from the hypothalamus.<br>Hair coat associated temporally with seasonal ovarian activity. |
| NON-BREEDING SEASON | Melatonin-forming activity of the pineal increases in temporal association with decreasing daylength after the fall equinox.<br>Melatonin-activity reaches its zenith in association with quiescence of the hypothalamic-pituitary-ovarian axis.<br>FSH/LH follow seasonal patterns in ovariectomized mares, with FSH decreasing later than LH in fall and increasing earlier than LH in spring.<br>Pineal produces a hypothalamic stimulator when daylength increases. Prolactin may play a role in seasonality.<br>Ovarian follicle become large/competent to produce FSH. |
| PHASES OF NONOVULATORY SEASON | Anovulatory season is divided into 3 phases reflecting hypothalamic-pituitary-ovarian activity:<br>a. recessive b. inactive c. resurgent<br>Some mares exhibit absent or indistinct one, two or three of these phases, diameter of largest follicle is a convenient indicator of phase.<br>Fall transitional season associated with LH deficiency and final growth spurt of a preovulatory follicle.<br>Unseasonable estrus is common even in absence of palpable follicles.<br>FSH/LH levels are minimal during the anovulatory season, except for high levels immediately following/preceding last/first ovulations.<br>Before first ovulation, FSH decreases sooner, estrogen increases sooner, LH and estrogen do not rise as high, and the ovulatory follicle grows slower.<br>Melatonin, GnRH, FSH, LH, estrogen and prolactin interact to terminate anovulatory season.<br>Administration of GnRH can stimulate ovulation during anovulatory season.<br>First ovulation is synchronized by progestins or altrenogest. |

Data from: Ginter OJ. Folliculogenesis during the transitional period and early ovulatory season in mares. J Reprod Fert 1990;90:311–320; Ginther OJ. Prolonged luteal activity in mares-a semantic quagmire. Equine Vet J 1990;22:152–156; Ginther OJ. Reproductive Biology of the Mare. Cross Plains, Wisconsin: Equiservices, 1992; Alexander SL, Irvine CHG, Evans MJ, Taylor TB. Control of the onset of the breeding season in the mare, its artificial regulation by progesterone treatment and subsequent effects on the resistance to uterine infection. Deauville: Abstr Internatl Symp Equine Reprod, 1990;102–103; Aitken WA. The oestrous cycle of the mare. Vet Pract Bull 1926;8:178–189; Bailey JV, Bristol FM. Uterine involution in the mare after induced parturition. Amer J Vet Res 1983;44:793–797; Dinger JE, Noiles EE. Vaginal and cervical mucus ferning as a method of detecting estrus in mares. Theriogenology 1982;18:633–642.

respectively. Photoperiod is perhaps the most important environmental signal and entrains the pituitary-gonadal axis, since artificial photoperiod treatments hasten follicular development and onset of the breeding season. The mare exhibits a photoperiodically entrained seasonal pattern of LH secretion. The cyclic reproductive behavior during the breeding season is mediated by the stimulatory and inhibitory actions of estradiol and progesterone (2).

The arbitrary assignment of January 1 as the birth date for all foals born in a given year has stimulated a demand in the equine industry for the administration of hormones to advance the onset of the natural breeding season in mares by 3 to 4 months; thus, foals would be born nearer to the first of the year. Several hormonal treatments were used with varying success such as: pregnant mare serum gonadotropin (PMSG), human chorionic gonadotropin (hCG), equine pituitary extracts, gonadotropin-releasing hormone (GnRH), progesterone, and prostaglandins.

## REPRODUCTIVE PARAMETERS IN STALLIONS

### *Sexual Maturity*

The testes of the stallion descend into the scrotum at 1 to 3 weeks of age. In a few cases, the testes are already in the scrotum at birth. Postnatal growth of the testes begins during the eleventh month, and the left testis develops earlier and grows faster than the right. At this time, there is also a gradual outward development of the seminiferous tubules around the right testis (Fig. 14-1). The age at which stallions are first used for natural or artificial breeding is determined primarily by managerial conditions (Table 14-1).

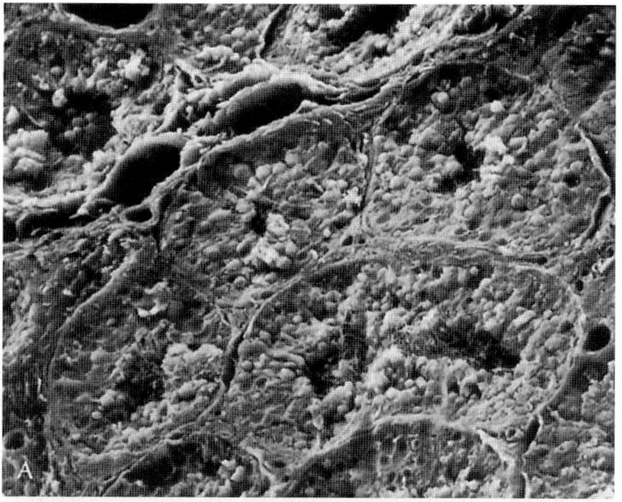


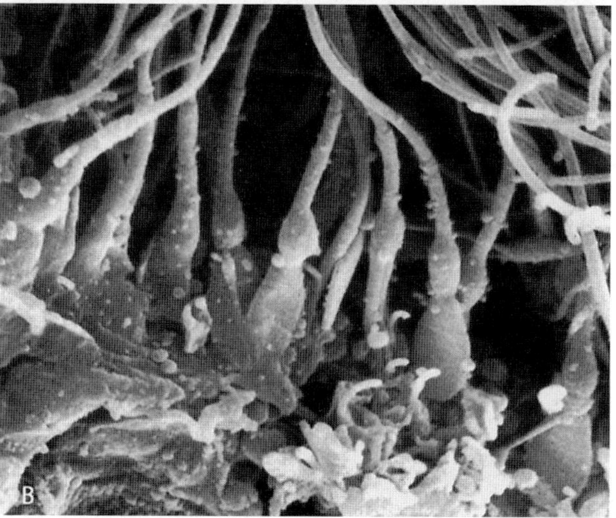


FIGURE 14-1. Scanning electron micrograph of equine testis. (A) Note irregular shape of seminiferous tubules and tails of spermatozoa protruding in the lumen (440×). (B) Spermiation: spermatozoa with cytoplasmic droplets are released from the Sertoli cells (5280×). (From Johnson L. Fertil Steril 1978;17:21.)

### *Semen Production*

The cycle of the seminiferous epithelium can be divided into eight stages on the basis of meiotic divisions, shape of the spermatid nuclei, and location of spermatids with elongated nuclei. The characteristics of semen and spermatogenesis are summarized in Tables 14-2 and 14-3.

The ejaculate is composed of six to nine jets resulting from the contractions of the urethra. The volume of each succeeding jet in the ejaculate reduces to about 50% of its initial value; 70% or more of the spermatozoa and the basic biochemical constituents are contained in the first three jets.

The gelatinous material in semen, secreted by the seminal vesicles, has no effect on the motility or the fertilizing ability of spermatozoa. The volume of gel, composing about one-third of the ejaculate, varies considerably, and is not characteristic of the individual stallion. This is in contrast to gel obtained from boar ejaculates, which is a constant feature of the ejaculates. Ejaculates containing gel seem to require fewer mounts and a shorter reaction time and possess a slightly larger volume of gel-free semen than ejaculates without gel.

Semen characteristics are influenced by the degree of sexual stimulation, frequency of ejaculation, age, testicular size, and method of semen collection. Season of the year influences the physical and biochemical characteristics of semen as well as blood hormone levels, sexual behavior, and fertility of both sexes. Spermatozoal output and libido of stallions are greatest during spring and summer and least during fall and winter. These changes in reproductive capacity coincide with the natural breeding season of mares. The concentration of plasma testosterone of stallions is also influenced by season and may mediate the patterns of seminal and behavioral characteristics.

### *Sperm Motility/Infertility*

Sperm hyperactivation is acquired and required for penetration of the outer investments of the egg. However sperm hyperactivation may not be necessary for traversal of the plasmalemma of the egg.

Sperm with nonprogressive, abnormal, or limited motility may be relatively inefficient in traversing only the outermost barriers of the oocyte. Zona micromanipulation is also applied for sperm with abnormal morphology often associated with inability to penetrate intact zonae.

Severe flagellar deficits and motility disorders in sperm prevent the penetration of the outer egg investments. These sperm cannot penetrate an intact zona pellucida and could fertilize eggs only after zona drilling. It would appear that defects in sperm motility resulting in unexplained infertility can be overcome with zona drilling.

Severe teratozoospermia and other types of sperm morphological anomalies have been clinically treated by application of zona manipulation. Micromanipulation can be

TABLE 14-2. ***Some Reproductive Parameters in the Stallion***

| | REPRODUCTIVE PARAMETERS OR CHARACTERISTICS | VALUES (AVERAGE) |
|---|---|---|
| SEXUAL MATURITY | Postnatal growth of testis | 1 year |
| | Sperm appear in testis | 1 year |
| | Sperm appear in ejaculate | 13 months |
| | Sexual maturity | 2 years |
| TESTICULAR AND EPIDIDYMAL MORPHOLOGY | Testicular weight | 150–170 g |
| | Epididymal weight | 20–30 g |
| | Volume of tubules and testis | 55–70% |
| | Length of tubules and testis | 2300–2600 m |
| SPERMATOGENESIS AND SPERM TRANSPORT IN MALE TRACT | Duration of seminiferous tubule cycle judged by $^3$H-thymidine injection | 13 days |
| | Life span of primary spermatocytes | 19 days |
| | Life span of secondary spermatocytes | 0.7 days |
| | Life span of spermatids with round nuclei | 8.7 days |
| | Life span of spermatids with elongated nuclei | 10 days |

Swierstra EE, Gebauer MR, Pickett MW. Reproductive physiology of the stallion. I. Spermatogenesis and testis composition. J Reprod Fertil 1974;40:113.

useful when the zona pellucida is impenetrable, even by "normal" sperm.

The glycoproteins, a major component of the zona pellucida serve as sperm receptors, and, if masked, will cause the zona to be refractile to sperm binding penetration. Sperm antibodies may be present in the ovarian follicle and may result in unexplained infertility due to interference with fertilization.

### *Ejaculation*

Ejaculation involves complex motor activity which is completed in two phases: emission of sperm and ejaculation of semen.

1. Emission of semen. Sperm from the epididymis/vas deferens as well as secretions from the seminal vesicles and prostate are transported into the posterior portion of the urethra by active concentration of the musculature around the epididymis, vas deferens, and seminal vesicle. Emission is associated with contraction of the internal urethral sphincter and closure of the bladder neck to prevent the ejection of the sperm backward into the bladder.
2. Ejaculation of semen. This phase is triggered by the transport of semen in the prostatic part of the urethra. Afferent impulses stimulate the sacral and lumbar nerves to stimulate spasmodic contraction of bulbocavernosus and perineal muscles. The external urethral

TABLE 14-3. ***Biochemical Characteristics of Semen Fractions of the Stallion***

| SEMEN FRACTION | ORIGIN | PHYSICAL CHARACTERISTICS | BIOCHEMICAL CHARACTERISTICS |
|---|---|---|---|
| Presperm | Urethral glands | Watery | High NaCl content, no ergothioneine, citric acid, or GPC |
| Sperm rich | Epididymal and ampullary glands | Milky, nonviscous | High sperm concentration, ergothioneine and GPC; little NaCl and citric acid |
| Postsperm | Seminal vesicle | Highly viscous | Low sperm concentration<br>High content of citric acid<br>Low ergothioneine and GPC |
| Penile drip | Tail-end sample | Watery | No spermatozoa; lacks any secretory products of epididymis, ampulla, and seminal vesicles (e.g., GPC, citric acid) |

GPC = glyceryl phosphorylcholine diesterase.
From: Mann T, Short RV, Walton A. The "tail-end" sample of stallion semen. J Agric Sci Camb 1957;49:301; Mann T, Leone E, Polge C. The composition of stallion semen. J Endocrinol 1965;13:279.

sphincter relaxes the semen is propelled via the urethra. Semen is ejaculated in several forceful thrusts. Disorders in the ejaculation phase may lead to "retrograde ejaculation" of semen into the urinary bladder.

During ejaculation the urethral diverticulum of the penis is in close apposition to the external cervical orifice of the mare. Semen is ejaculated under high pressure directly into the uterus. The final seminal jets ejaculated when erection is ceasing and the penis is being withdrawn are probably deposited in the vagina. The patterns of ejaculation and emission have been carefully studied (3).

The process of emission is variable because the number of jets per ejaculate varies from 5 to 10, with an average of 8. The early jets occur under high pressure in a stream with characteristic spatter. The later jets, accompanied by declining erection and withdrawal of the penis from the vagina, are associated with low pressure. Of the total time of ejaculation, 24% involves actual emission of semen; the rest comprises intervals between successive seminal jets. The first 3 jets contain 80% of the ejaculated spermatozoa. The total number of spermatozoa and the ergothioneine content gradually decrease in successive jets (3). The terminal jets from 4 to 10, with low concentrations of sperm cells and ergothioneine, consist mostly of the so-called mucous fraction and correspond to fraction 3 (4).

## ESTROUS CYCLES

Table 14-4 shows some of the unique and remarkable characteristics of reproduction in horses (5, 6).

### *Estrus*

During estrus, the vulva becomes large and swollen; the labial folds are loose and readily open on examination. The vulva becomes scarlet or orange, wet, glossy, and covered with a film of transparent mucus. The vaginal mucosa is highly vascular, and thin watery mucus may accumulate in the vagina. The mare assumes a stance characteristic of urination. The tail is raised, urine is expelled in small amounts and the clitoris is exposed by prolonged rhythmic contractions.

The mare's ovulatory cycle is on average 21 days long, consisting of 14 days of diestrus (luteal phase) and 7 days of estrus, when the mare is sexually receptive. Several aspects of the mare's reproductive endocrinology were so surprising to early workers that they hesitated to publish their findings. The mare's ovulatory LH surge is prolonged, with levels rising gradually throughout estrus to peak the day after ovulation. There is no large burst of LH secretion before ovulation as happens, for example, in sheep. FSH surges occur at approximately 10-day intervals, in midiestrus and after ovulation. There are also periods of strikingly differential secretion of FSH and LH; e.g., early estrus when FSH is at its lowest as LH rises, and mid-diestrus when FSH but not LH increases (7).

The size of the preovulatory follicle in mares is such that oocyte retrieval is invariable attempted via puncture through the flank with the ovary manipulated either rectally or abdominally with the hand passed into the abdominal cavity through a vaginal incision. For this reason, laparoscopy techniques do not appear to have been used in mares.

The duration of estrus varies among individuals and also among estrous cycles of the same mare. Long duration of estrus in the mare may be due to the following factors:

1. The ovary is surrounded mostly by a serous coat, and some follicles have to migrate to reach the ovulation fossa to rupture.
2. The ovary is less sensitive to exogenous FSH than that of other species (e.g., cattle, sheep), so that the preovulatory follicle requires a longer time to reach maximal size.
3. The level of LH is low compared with FSH, and this delays ovulation.

### *Corpus Luteum*

Most ovulations occur on days 3, 4, or 5 of estrus, 24 to 48 hours before the end of behavioral estrus (i.e., the time of ovulation is more closely related to the end than to the onset of estrus). The fertility of mating gradually rises to a peak about 2 days before the end of estrus and then falls sharply on the last day. The ruptured follicle can be palpated up to 24 hours after ovulation as a soft fluctuant area. The CL reaches only one-half to three-fourths the size of the follicle at the time of ovulation. The maximal size is attained at 14 days, when luteal cells enlarge and have a peripheral vacuolation (Fig. 14-2). Spontaneous prolongation of the CL, accompanied by follicular activity and without any signs of estrus for periods of 2 to 3 months, is common (8). Corpora lutea that fail to regress at the normal time persist for about 2 months and are characterized by having a white connective tissue core.

A prerequisite for a successful pregnancy is maintenance of a relatively quiescent myometrium. The progestin requirements of equine pregnancy are met by the fetoplacental unit beginning at 70 to 80 days. The placenta of the mare contains 3$\beta$-HSD activity and is able to convert pregnenolone to progesterone. However, the concentration of progesterone in maternal plasma falls to very low levels by midgestation and remains low throughout the second half of pregnancy (9). Progesterone is reduced to 5$\alpha$-pregnancies and pregnancies within the placenta and possibly within

**TABLE 14-4. *Unique Anatomic, Physiologic, and Endocrine Characteristics of Reproduction in the Horse***

| PARAMETERS | UNIQUE REPRODUCTIVE CHARACTERISTICS |
|---|---|
| Development of ovary | During fetal life, cortical tissue entirely surrounds the medullary portion. During neonatal life, cortical tissue becomes confined to one area and is nearly surrounded by medullary tissue. |
| Site of ovulation on the ovarian surface | Follicles can only ovulate through the surface of the ovary adjacent to cortical tissue ("ovulation fossa"). |
| Pattern of follicular growth | A small group of follicles develops during late diestrus, some of which enlarge differentially to ovulate during subsequent estrus; remaining follicles may ovulate during early luteal phase and others regress without ovulation. |
| Primary CL | Primary CL of pregnancy declines in secretory activity 14 to 16 days after ovulation (similar to the time that complete luteolysis would normally occur in the cycling mare). This causes a slow and steady fall in peripheral plasma progesterone concentrations during the next 20–25 days until the initiation of the secondary rise, days 35–45. This coincides with the onset of secretion of equine chorionic gonadotropin (eCG), formerly known as pregnant mare serum gonadotropin (PMSG). |
| Accessory corpora lutea | A secondary progesterone rises from the formation of the first of what eventually becomes a whole crop of secondary corpora lutea that develop in the mare's ovaries between day 40 to 150. By day 120, 3 to 30 accessory luteal structures arise from both normal ovulation and luteinization of unruptured follicles. All primary and secondary corpora lutea regress and leave the ovaries small and completely inactive for the remainder of gestation. |
| Gonadotropins associated with ovulation | Prolonged rise of LH surge during estrus that continues after ovulation. |
| Life span of CL during nonpregnancy | Spontaneous prolongation of CL life span is common; corpora lutea that fail to regress at normal time persist for 2 months. |
| Egg transport in oviduct | Mare can discriminate between fertilized and unfertilized eggs, which may be retained in oviduct during pregnancy and nonpregnancy for up to 7 months. |
| Presence of placental hormone (PMSG) | PMSG found in large quantities; secreted by endometrial cups during early pregnancy. |
| Placental progesterone | Placental tissue contains appreciable quantities of progesterone, and the placenta is secreting sufficient progesterone to maintain pregnancy from about day 100. |
| Endometrial cups | Endometrial cups, a series of small, ulcer-like, endometrial outgrowths form in a circle around the conceptus in the gravid uterine horn. They first appear as pale, slightly raised plaques in the endometrium at day 38 to 40 after ovulation and enlarge steadily during the next 20 to 30 days. They become concave or saucer-shaped on the surface, and they regress in the central regions of the structure. |
| Interspecies breeding | Several equid species can interbreed, producing viable, but infertile, offspring. |

From: Stabenfeldt GH, et al. Unique aspects of the reproductive cycle of the mare. J Reprod Fertil 1975;23:155.

the fetal liver and kidneys (10). The 5$\alpha$-pregnancies may subserve the role of progesterone in maintaining myometrial quiescence in the mare.

### *Endocrine Control of Estrous Cycles*

In normally cycling mares two FSH surges occur, at approximately 20 and 11 days before ovulation. Both FSH and LH concentrations surge around the time of ovulation. The mid-diestrous surge may be important for the subsequent development of follicles destined to ovulate 10 to 13 days later.

The ovary of the mare is less sensitive to FSH than is that of the cow, ewe, and goat. Injection of massive doses of PMSG during the nonbreeding season is ineffective for inducing ovulation of follicles. Injection of PMSG toward

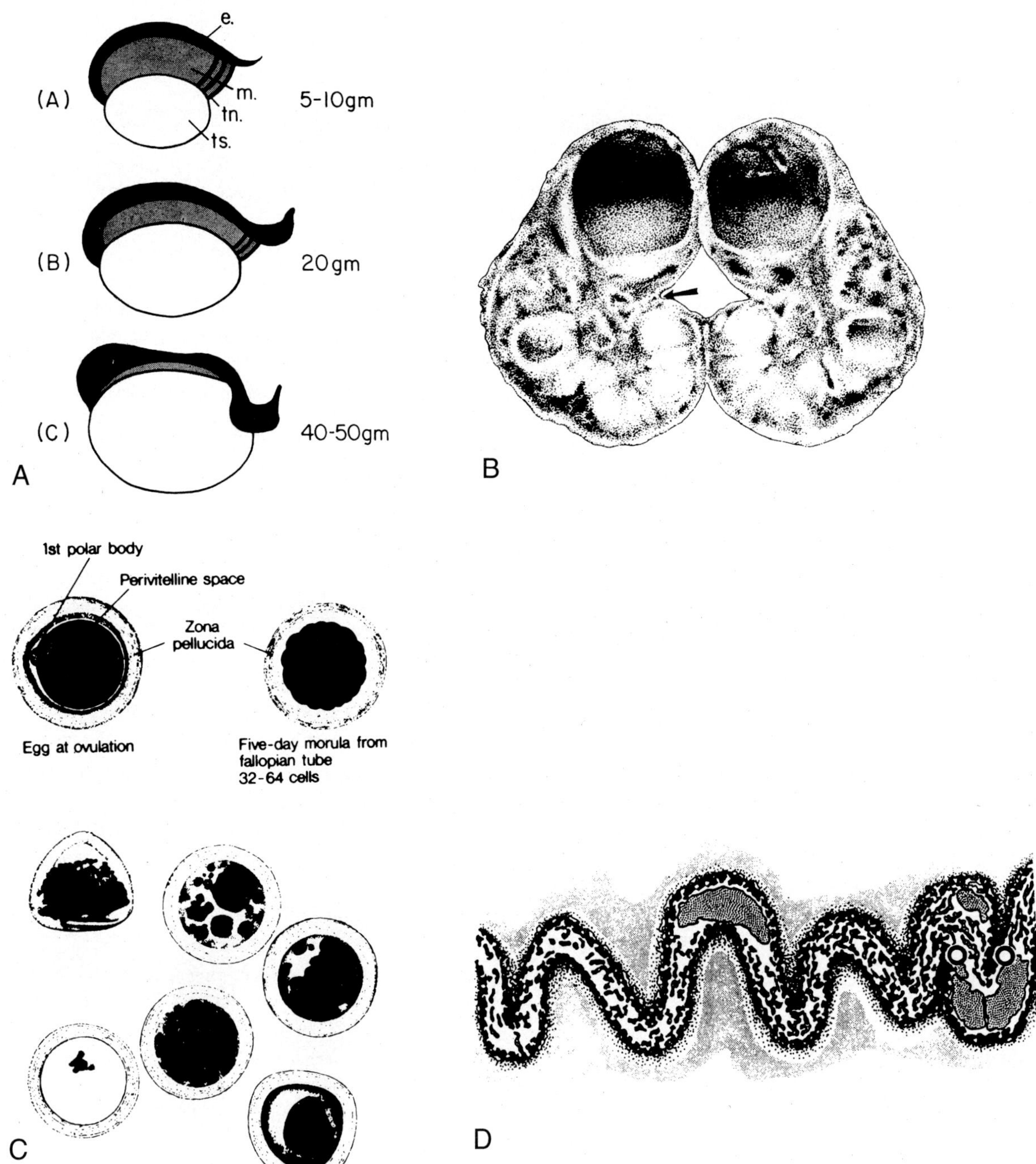


FIGURE 14-2. Ovary, ovulation and ova retention in the oviduct of horses: (**A**) Developmental changes in the attachment of epididymis with the testis in relation to sexual maturity. Figures on right indicate testis weight; *e*, epididymis; *m*, thin membrane; *tn*, tendon; *ts*, testis. *a.* Loose attachment between testis and epididymis: note tendon attachment at head of epididymis. *b.* Elongation of epididymis. *c.* Epididymis fully developed and completely attached to testis. (Adapted from Nishikawa Y. Studies on Reproduction in Horses. Tokyo: Japan Racing Association, 1959.) (**B**) Ovary of the mare cut in halves. Note ovulation fossa (*arrow*). (**C**) A normal horse egg before and after fertilization and degenerating oviductal eggs ranging in age from 1 to 7.5 months. The mechanisms by which the equine unfertilized ova are trapped in the oviduct are unknown. (From van Niekerk, Gerneke. Onderstep. J Vet Res 1966;33:195; redrawn by Short V. In: Austin CR, Short V, eds. Reproduction in Mammals. Cambridge: Cambridge University Press, 1972.) (**D**) Histological characteristics of equine oviduct (one third). Ampulla is to the right. *Sippling* indicates related areas of mesosalpinx. *Coarse line* indicates gelatinous masses lying in oviductal lumen. Positions of retained eggs are shown by *black circles*. (Flood PF, et al. The location of eggs retained in the oviducts of mares. J Reprod Fertil 1979;57:291–294.)

the end of the estrous cycle is also ineffective in promoting follicular development.

The pattern of plasma LH in the mare differs from that in other species, and it is possible that persistence of high concentrations of LH results from a long half-life of the endogenous LH. This in turn may be responsible for the relatively large number of second ovulations detected in many estrous cycles (11). In the mare, the uterus exerts its luteolytic effect on the CL primarily through a systemic utero-ovarian pathway.

Local administration of prostaglandin $F_{2\alpha}$($PGF_{2\alpha}$), a postulated uterine luteolysin, into the uterus did not improve its luteolytic efficacy over systemic administration given intramuscularly. The vascular anatomy of uterus and ovaries provides limited potential for the local transfer of a luteolysin between uterus and ovary through a veno-arterial pathway (12).

### Induction of Estrus and Ovulation

SALINE INFUSION. The technique of intrauterine saline infusion has been used routinely to induce estrus in anestrous mares. Anestrous mares are affected only near the beginning and end of the breeding season when anovulatory heats are induced. Diestrous mares infused between days 5 and 9 return to heat 4 days earlier than expected, and induced estrus is accompanied by ovulation. Mares in prolonged diestrus may show ovulatory heat within 3 to 9 days of infusion (13).

SYNCHRONIZATION OF ESTRUS. Mares are usually mated or artificially inseminated after estrus has been detected with a teaser stallion and follicular development has been assessed by rectal palpation of the ovaries. Synchronization of estrus and ovulation would allow mares to be inseminated at predetermined times without the need to detect estrus or palpate the ovaries.

PROSTAGLANDINS. Of the farm species studied, the mare is most sensitive, on a body-weight basis, to the luteolytic effects of systemically (intramuscular or subcutaneous) administered $PCF_{2\alpha}$. Systemically administered $PCF_{2\alpha}$ is as effective in causing luteolysis in hysterectomized as intact mares, indicating that the principal site of action of exogenous $PCF_{2\alpha}$ is not at the uterine level.

Prostaglandin $F_{2\alpha}$ and its analogues have been used to control the estrous cycle of the mare. The treatment causes a prompt cessation of secretion by the CL as indicated by a rapid fall in plasma progesterone levels. The infusion of 10 mg of $PGF_{2\alpha}$ on days 7 to 9 after ovulation causes a sharp fall in plasma progesterone levels and induces estrus and ovulation. This induced estrus is longer than the natural cycle but the time of ovulation in relation to the end of estrus is normal. The time of return to estrus following luteolysis does not depend on the amount of $PGF_{2\alpha}$. Luteolysis can be induced as early as day 5 following natural ovulation (14). $PGF_{2\alpha}$ and its synthetic analogues are luteolytic in mares and cause abortion.

Intramuscular administration is as effective as subcutaneous administration, and 1.25 mg $PGF_{2\alpha}$ is the minimal effective systemic dose for inducing luteolysis. Administration of $PGF_{2\alpha}$ into the uterus or directly into the CL does not improve the luteolytic efficacy of the intramuscular injection of $PGF_{2\alpha}$.

OVA AND OVA TRANSPORT. At ovulation, the ovum is without corona radiata but is enclosed in a large irregular gelatinous mass of ovarian origin, which separates from the egg within 2 days. Fertilized ova are transported in the uterus, whereas unfertilized ova are trapped for several months in the isthmus of the oviduct. The ovum undergoes degeneration and fragmentation during the ensuing months. If a mare has a succession of sterile estrous cycles followed by a fertile mating, the developing embryo may outrun the unfertilized eggs trapped in the oviduct and enter the uterus.

Nonfertilized eggs may be retained in the oviducts of pregnant and nonpregnant mares for up to 7 months (Fig. 14-2). This indicates that the mare can discriminate between fertilized and nonfertilized eggs, allowing the fertilized egg to pass into the uterus while retaining nonfertilized eggs. Retained eggs are more common in heavy than in light breeds and are found more frequently in early than in late pregnancy.

Little is known about the function of the acellular capsule, which replaces the zona pellucida in the horse and then surrounds the embryo throughout its preattachment life in the uterus. The passage of a substance through the capsule to the embryo is influenced by the size and chemical nature of the substance's molecule.

The time when fertilized ova arrive in the uterus in the mare is much later (more than 144 hours) than in the cow, and the cleavage stage of equine ova at arrival is more advanced than that in cattle. Transuterine migration of ova occurs in 50% of cases.

Extensive investigations conducted on equine reproduction physiology and management included the following: ovarian changes during ovulation and pregnancy (15); endocrine profile in pregnant and postpartum mares and cryptorchid stallions and following increased photoperiods (14, 16, 17); energy undernutrition during weaning (18); and manipulation of the estrous cycle and ovulation luteal function by prostaglandin $F_{2\alpha}$, by hCG and GnRH, and by intrauterine saline infusion (19–22).

## GESTATION

Gestation length in the mare ranges from 315 to 360 days and is influenced by maternal size, fetal genotype, and the stage of the breeding season when conception occurs. Development *in utero* can also be affected by degenerative wear and tear changes of the endometrium such as cystic fibrosis and glandular atrophy (6). Fetal growth is retarded as a result of impaired placental function in mares exhibiting such changes, and gestation may be lengthened as a consequence.

### Pregnancy Diagnosis and Developmental Horizons

Several methods are used for pregnancy diagnosis in the mare (Table 14-5). Diagnosis of pregnancy by rectal palpation of the ovaries and uterus is accurate 40 to 50 days after conception. A mouse biologic test that depends on PMSG to stimulate the ovaries of 21-day-old immature mice is accurate after 35 days of gestation of pregnancy. A qualitative hemagglutination-inhibition test for PMSG in serum is commercially available as a rapid test (MIP test, Diamond Labs). This test must await the serum rise in PMSG; because of that the test is not usable until 35 to 40 days after conception. Early pregnancy diagnosis can be done by ultrasound with 15% false-negative diagnosis. The major development horizona of the equine fetus are summarized in Table 14-6.

### Twinning

Twinning is rare. The natural occurrence of identical twins in the mare is virtually precluded by her general inability to carry twin conceptuses to term. This is primarily due to the competition of the placenta for contact with the maternal endometrium, which results in a net placental insufficiency for both conceptuses (6). The usual outcome is for the more disadvantaged of the two fetuses to die during the second half of gestation and so initiate abortion. Monozygotic (identical) twins are valuable research tools in several types of biologic investigations. While monozygotic twins occur naturally in cattle, sheep, and women, albeit at a low frequency, they have not been reported to date in equids. In 2,673 thoroughbred mares, the spontaneous dizygotic twin conception rate was 2%.

TABLE 14-5. ***Pregnancy Diagnosis in the Mare***

| DAYS AFTER OVULATION | CRITERIA | METHODS | COMMENTS |
|---|---|---|---|
| 16–24 | No behavioral, physical, or hormonal signs of estrus | Estrous detection | Few pregnant mares show estrus (nonpregnant mares may fail to show estrus due to pseudopregnancy or silent estrus) |
| 16–17 | Presence (nonpregnant) or absence (pregnant) of estrus in response to estrogen | Single injection of estrogen detection for estrus | False-positives in pseudopregnancy or early embryonic death |
| 28–term | Changes in stained vaginal mucus | Mucin test | Positive results as early as day 20 effective after day 80; false-positives from pseudopregnancy |
| 45–90 | PMSG in blood | Immunologic and biologic tests | Hemagglutination kits available in some countries<br>Biologic tests: injection of serum into rodents or frogs |
| 60–term | Uterine content | Rectal palpation | Ballottment and palpation of fetus |
| 90–term | Fetal heart beat | Ultrasonography | Transducer placed in rectum; fetal pulse may be detected as early as day 40, consistently days 90–240 |
| 150–term | Estrogens in urine | Chemical (Cuboni) biologic tests | Adding chemicals to urine and observing fluorescence; reliable after day 150 |

PMSG = pregnant mare serum gonadotropin.
From: Ginther OJ. Reproductive biology of the mare: basic and applied aspects. 1st ed. Cross Plains, Wisconsin: Equiservices, 1979.

TABLE 14-6. ***Developmental Horizons of Equine Fetus***

| DAYS OF PREGNANCY | HEAD | LEGS | REPRODUCTIVE ORGANS |
|---|---|---|---|
| 40 | Ears rudimentary<br>Eyelids<br>External nares | Elbows and stifles | Migration of genital tubercle begins |
| 45 | — | — | Sex determinable |
| 55 | Ears-triangle fold cover opening eyelids closed except for 1 mm slit | Hocks and fetlocks | Prominent vulva or penis<br>Mammary papillae (0.25 mm dots) |
| 60 | Eyelids closed or almost closed nares—1 × 0.5 mm slits | Soles and Frogs | — |
| 80 | — | Points of shoulders and hips | Mammary papillae are raised buds<br>Scrotum; pale bulge, 2 cm behind umbilicus |
| 100 | Ears: 1 cm long and curled forward and down<br>Eyes bulging | Hooves: pale yellow, raised coronary band | Clitoris recessed to postnatal position |
| 120 | — | — | Vulval lips meet at ventral commissure<br>Prepuce pendulous |
| 150 | — | Ergots, 5 mm | Glandular shaped mammae in female<br>Palpable gubernaculum in scrotum |
| 180 | — | — | Suspension of mammary gland in female |
| 210 | — | — | Suspension of mammary gland in female |

From: Ginther OJ. Reproductive biology of the mare: basic and applied aspects. 1st ed. Cross Plains, Wisconsin: Equiservices, 1979; Ginther OJ. Intrauterine movement of the early conceptus in barren and postpartum mares. Theriogenology 1984;21:633–644.

Twin pregnancy is unwanted in the horse because of the high rate of abortion and a tendency to poor postnatal development in the few twin foals that survive to term. Thus, most twins that are conceived are deliberately aborted early in gestation, and the mare is remated in an attempt to produce a singleton pregnancy during the same breeding season. In most dizygotic twin pregnancies, there is invagination of the adjacent allantochorions. Identical blood groups are found in twin foals, indicating chimerism and macroscopic or midcroscopic anastomosis between both chorions. Stillbirth is frequent in twin pregnancies, and only one half of the foals born survive. Twin pregnancies are not desirable in view of the high perinatal and postnatal losses and the poor viability and racing performance of twins. Subsequent conception rate is not affected by twin birth if the mare foals at full term, but it decreases following abortion.

### *Ovarian Function*

Four distinct stages of ovarian function are recognized.

1. During early pregnancy, a single CL verum is present; it was believed that this regressed at approximately day 40 of gestation, but according to subsequent observations (15), the primary CL persists beyond day 40.
2. Between day 40 and 150 of pregnancy, ovarian activity occurs. As many as 10 to 15 follicles (over 1 cm in diameter) undergo luteinization to form the accessory corpora lutea. The recovery of recently ovulated ova from the oviducts suggests that some of these follicles ovulate even though unfertilized ova are retained in the oviduct for several months. Usually, each ovary contains 3 to 5 accessory corpora lutea.
3. From the fifth to the seventh month, though both primary and secondary corpora lutea and the large folli-

cles regress completely, the mare does not show signs of estrus, which is due to placental secretion of progesterone until the end of gestation.

4. From the seventh month onward, only vestiges of the corpora lutea and small follicles are present, but during the last 2 weeks of gestation follicular activity commences in preparation for the post-partum estrus ("foaling heat").

The primary and secondary corpora lutea and the placenta all contribute to the total progesterone pool during pregnancy. The corpora lutea progesterone concentration in the peripheral plasma is closely correlated with morphologic changes in the corpora lutea. Similarities and differences in ovarian function observed between pregnant and hysterectomized mares suggest that, while PMSG does not appear to stimulate follicular development, it does prolong the life span and stimulate the secretory activity of the primary CL and induced ovulation and/or luteinization of secondary follicles in pregnant mares (23). Ovariectomy does not terminate pregnancy, if performed after day 70 of pregnancy.

### Placenta

The placenta of the mare is classified as diffuse, microcotyledonary, and epitheliochorial (Table 14-7 and Figs. 14-3 and 14-4). The outer surface of the chorion is closely studded with tufts of branching villi that enter into corresponding invaginations in the endometrium to form small globular structures known as *microcotyledons*. Microcotyledons, which are a distinctive feature of the mature equine placenta, are fully formed by the fifth month of gestation. The primary folds of trophoblast become elaborately subdivided as gestation proceeds. These changes are reflected in the structure of the maternal crypts, which receive the fetal villi. Within each microcotyledon, chorionic and uterine epithelia are in intimate contact, and a microvillous junction is formed at the fetal-maternal boundary.

### Uterine Defense Mechanisms

Breeding or insemination of mare is followed by a transient infection and inflammation. Normal mares eliminate bacte-

TABLE 14-7. ***Physiological/Structural Parameters of Embryology and Placentation of the Horse***

| EMBRYOLOGY | | PLACENTATION |
|---|---|---|
| Fertilization | Sperm penetrate oocyte 10–12 hrs after ovulation | Day 11 endoerm cells encircle blastocoele |
| Cleavage | 1st cleavage occurs after 24 hrs<br>Subsequent cleavage: 3 blastomere/day | Day 16 yolk sac vesicle remains spherical until initial implantation |
| Embryo transport | Day 5 most morulae in oviduct<br>Day 6 morulae/early blastocyst | Day 22 allantoic sac emerges from embryo proper to become dominant over yolks sac |
| Blastocyst hatching | Zona pellucida shed from new inner layer the "capsule" which remains for a few weeks as outer coating | Day 38 fetal cells from chorionic girdle, a belt of tissue surrounding concepts, invade endometrium to form the eCG-producing cells of endometrial cups |
| | | Day 40–150 diffuse placenta involves microcotyledons fitting corresponding microcaruncles |
| | | 7–8 months: fetal gonads are unusually large exceeding size of maternal gonads due to development of interstitial cells similar histologically to luteal cells |
| | | Day 50–95 fetus develops hypothalamic-pituitary portal system |

Data from: Ginther OJ. Folliculogenesis during the transitional period and early ovulatory season in mares. J Reprod Fert 1990;90:311–320; Ginther OJ. Prolonged luteal activity in mares—a semantic quagmire. Equine Vet J 1990;22:152–156; Ginther OJ. Reproductive Biology of the Mare. Cross Plains, Wisconsin: Equiservices, 1992; Casey PL, Wiemer KE, DeVore DC, Youngs CR, Godke RA. The use of computerized image analysis to evaluate the growth and development of equine embryos *in vitro*. Theriogenology 1988;29(Abstract):233; Burns SJ, Irvine CHG, Amoss MS. Fertility of prostaglandin-induced oestrus compares to normal post-partum oestrus. J Reprod Fert 1979;27:245–250; Busch W, Apel M, Schutzler H. Comparison of techniques from inducing abortion and treating endometriosis in mares. Mh Vet-Med 1989;44:134–137; Butterfield RM, Matthews RG. Ovulation and the movement of the conceptus in the first 35 days of pregnancy in Thoroughbred mares. J Reprod Fert 1979;27(Suppl):447–452.

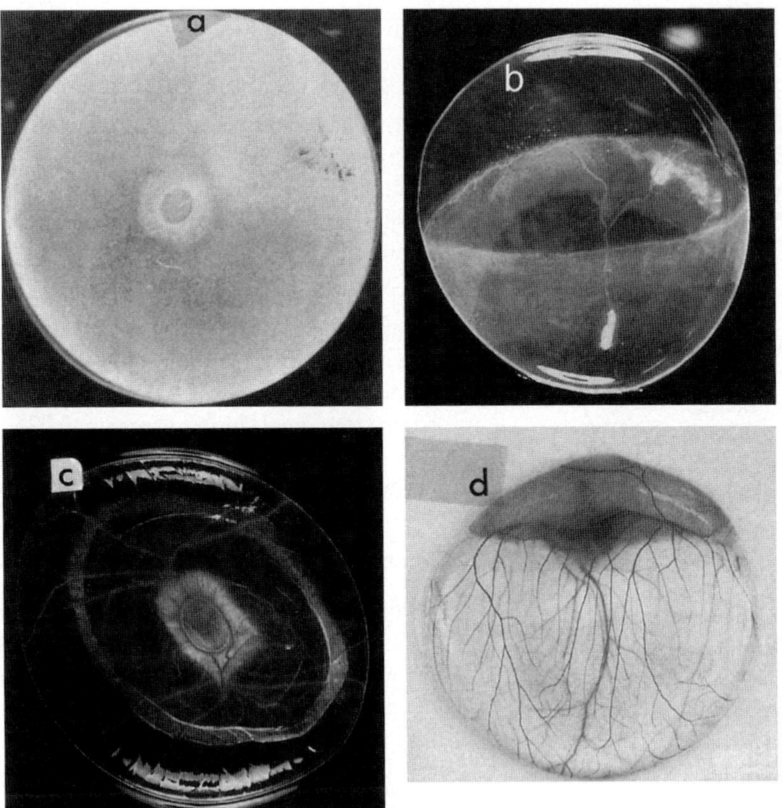


FIGURE 14-3. (A) A day-13 embryo that is 16 mm in diameter. The capsule is clearly visible where it is separated from the trophoblast by a fluid-filled space. The embryonic disc is central in position and roughly elliptical in shape with axes of 1.24 and 1.66 mm. About half of the long axis of the embryonic disc is occupied by the primitive streak. The halo surrounding the disc is created by the developing extraembryonic mesoderm. (**B**) A day 20-embryo measuring 66 by 58 mm. Careful inspection reveals the capsule is still present. The yolk sac vessels are well developed and the sinus terminalis is clearly visible. The sinus terminalis marks the boundary of a cloudy band that extends from the sinus toward the embryonic pole. The caudal end of the embryo shows some expansion, which may be caused by the allantoic primordium. (**C**) A day-24 conceptus seen from the mesometrial pole. It was about 80 mm in diameter when lying on a flat surface but it probably had a slightly smaller diameter in utero where it adopted a more perfect sphere. The sinus terminalis is still visible as a loop surrounding an oval area of bilaminar omphalopleure at the center. Outside the sinus terminalis is a cream-colored zone that is probably associated with the trilaminar omphalopleure. The entire yolk sac is encircled by the pale chorionic girdle that lies about midway between the embryonic pole and the equator of the conceptus. (**D**) The same conceptus as that shown in **C**. Lateral view. The mesometrial side is at the top. The sinus terminalis and the other delicate yolk sac vessels can be seen at the mesometrial pole which is readily recognizable by the yellowish yolk sac fluid. The more open allantoic vascular network is visible over the remainder of the surface. The chorionic girdle is just discernible immediately below the junction of the yolk sac and allantois. The embryo proper can be seen lying between the yolk sac and the allantoic cavity. Its outlines are indistinct, but the left forelimb bud can be seen clearly projecting toward the camera. (From Flood PF. Fertilization, Early Development and the Establishment of the Placenta. Equine Reproduction 1992;56:472–485.)

ria and clear inflammatory by-products rapidly, whereas other mares are not capable of doing this. Differences between these two kinds of mares are best explained by factors involved in uterine clearance, cervical dilation, myometrial activity, and lymphatic drainage (24).

Inflammation related to breeding is induced sooner by spermatozoa than by bacteria. The quantity of bacteria after insemination of normal mares was relatively low and quickly eliminated. However, the intensity of the inflammation depends on the concentration of semen: frozen and centrifuged fresh semen cause the most intensive inflammation (24). The defense mechanism of the uterus against foreign invaders comprises complex interactions between different elements: pneumovagina, urine pooling, and cervical incompetence.

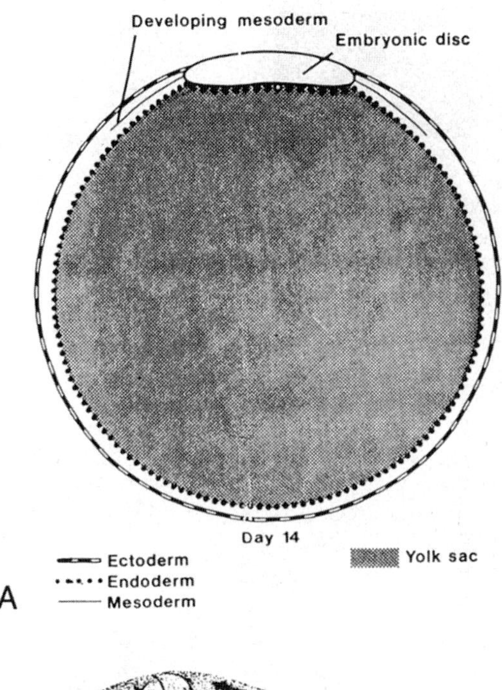


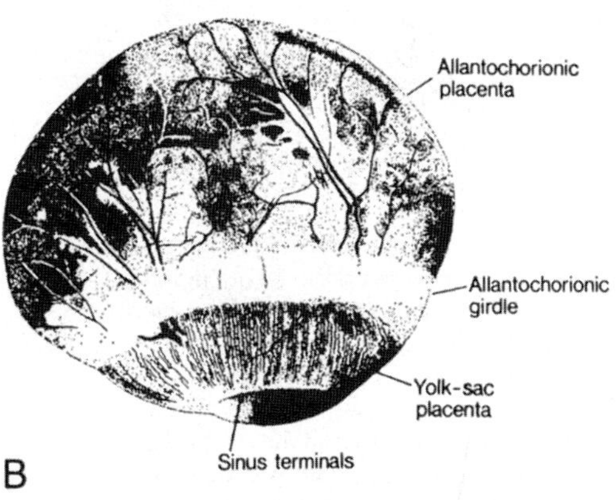


FIGURE 14-4. (A) Equine conceptus of 2 weeks of gestation (diameter, 16 mm) is spherical, located in the uterine body. The conceptus is not attached to its eventual location in the caudal portion of a uterine horn. Mesodermal tissue grows from the embryonic disc into the area between the trophoblast (ectodermal origin) and the endoderm of the yolk sac. The mesoderm gives origin to supportive mesenchyme or connective tissue blood vessels. Some islands of rudimentary vessels are already visible, histologically. (From Ginther OJ. Reproductive Biology of the Mare: Basic and Applied Aspects, 1st ed. Cross Plains, Wisconsin: Equiservices, 1979.) (B) Equine conceptus, 7 weeks of gestation, the size of an orange. Cells become detached around the allantochorionic girdle at this stage to invade the endometrium and form the endometrial cups. (From Short V. In: Austin CR, Short V, eds. Reproduction in Mammals. Cambridge: Cambridge University Press, 1972.)

PLACENTAL BARRIER. The following mechanisms control the passage of gases, nutrients, ions, or hormones across the placental barrier:

1. Those related to diffusion across the placental tissues; i.e., permeability, diffusion distances, total surface area, and concentration gradients between maternal and fetal blood vessels (Figs. 14-5 and 14-6);
2. Rates of supply and removal on either size of the placenta, the presence or absence of specialized exchange areas, the direction of blood flow in these areas, and the existence of shunts or unequal flows;
3. Specialized mechanisms that assist the passage of substances and, in the case of oxygen, differences in hemoglobin $O_2$ affinity and $O_2$ capacity between fetus and mother (25).

The primary CL that develops at the site of the fertile ovulation regresses about day 160 of gestation and is replaced by secondary corpora lutea. The primary and secondary corpora lutea and the placenta all contribute to the total progesterone pool during pregnancy. The luteal progesterone concentration in the peripheral plasma is closely correlated with morphologic changes in the CL.

### *Endocrine Profile*

Plasma progestogen levels decline in midpregnancy and remain low until a few days before parturition, when they increase again. During pregnancy there are two peaks of plasma progestogens. The first, which occurs during the third month, coincides with high levels of PMSG and is probably produced by the endometrial cups or the secondary CL. The second peak occurs in the eleventh month and probably represents the secretion of placental progestogens.

The endometrial cups, which are present from the second to the fourth months of pregnancy, are the source of the gonadotropin PMSG, which circulates in the maternal blood between 40 and 130 days of gestation. The maternal ovaries are thus stimulated, forming ovarian follicles, many of which ovulate and form accessory corpora lutea, while others luteinize without ovulating. The accessory corpora lutea persist until about 180 days of gestation and then degenerate (Fig. 14-7).

Several factors influence PMSG levels: season, maternal size, parity, and fetal genotype. A high level of PMSG occurs in the serum of a mare carrying twin fetuses if a set of endometrial cups develops in both uterine horns.

The fetal genotype has a pronounced effect on PMSG concentration in the mother. Blood serum of mares bred to a jack donkey contains only about 10% of the PMSG concentration in mares bred to a stallion. It appears that the allantochorion may provide a stimulus, possibly chemical in nature, that regulates the secretory activity of the endometrial cups.

## FOALING

The time of foaling, which usually takes place between nightfall and daybreak, seems to be influenced by photoperiods and quietness in the stable. In England, 86% of foalings occur between 1900 and 0700 hours (7:00 PM and 7:00 AM), with a maximal incidence between 2200 and 2300 hours (10:00 PM and 11:00 PM) (Tables 14-8 and 14-9).

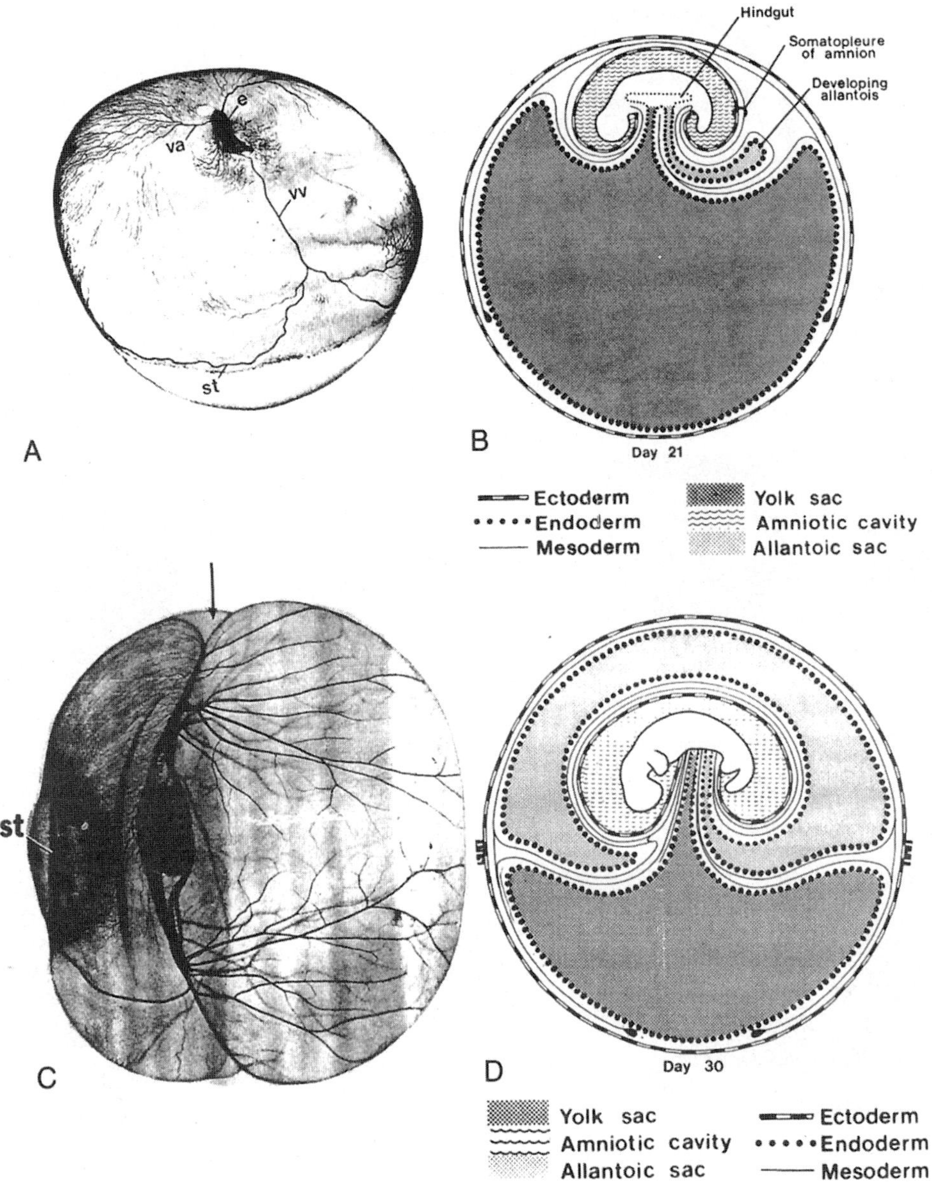


FIGURE 14-5. (**A** and **B**) Spherical conceptus from a pony mare: *e*, embryo; yolk sac vasculature—*vv*, vitelline vein; *va*, vitelline artery; *st*, sinus terminalis; the prominent collecting vein that encircles the vesicle. The vesicle is 2.6 cm in diameter when submerged, and flattened slightly to a diameter of 3.5 cm on removal of the fluid in which it was submerged. Note completion of amniotic cavity and emergency of the allantois from the hind gut. The allantois grows into the exocoelom between the somatopleure and splanchnopleure. (**C** and **D**). The exposed vesicle is viewed from embryonic pole. The dark spot in center of the vesicle is the embryo. Prominent vessels are in the allantochorion. Sinus terminalis is still prominent. Chorion (*arrow*) between allantois (*right*) and yolk sac (*left*) is the location of the chorionic girdle. The mesoderm remains avascular. The allantois continues to grow, and the yolk sac recedes because the yolk sac remains attached at the bilaminar omphalopleure. (From Nishikawa Y, unpublished data.)

The imminence of foaling is suggested by the degree of mammary hypertrophy, waxing of the teats, and possibly the discharge of milk from the udder. The best indication that the first stage has begun is the onset of patchy sweating behind the elbows and about the flanks.

## *Induced Parturition*

Parturition can be induced by various doses of estrogen, prostaglandins $PCG_{2\alpha}$, and oxytocin. The time of appearance and degree of expression of the major clinical signs of

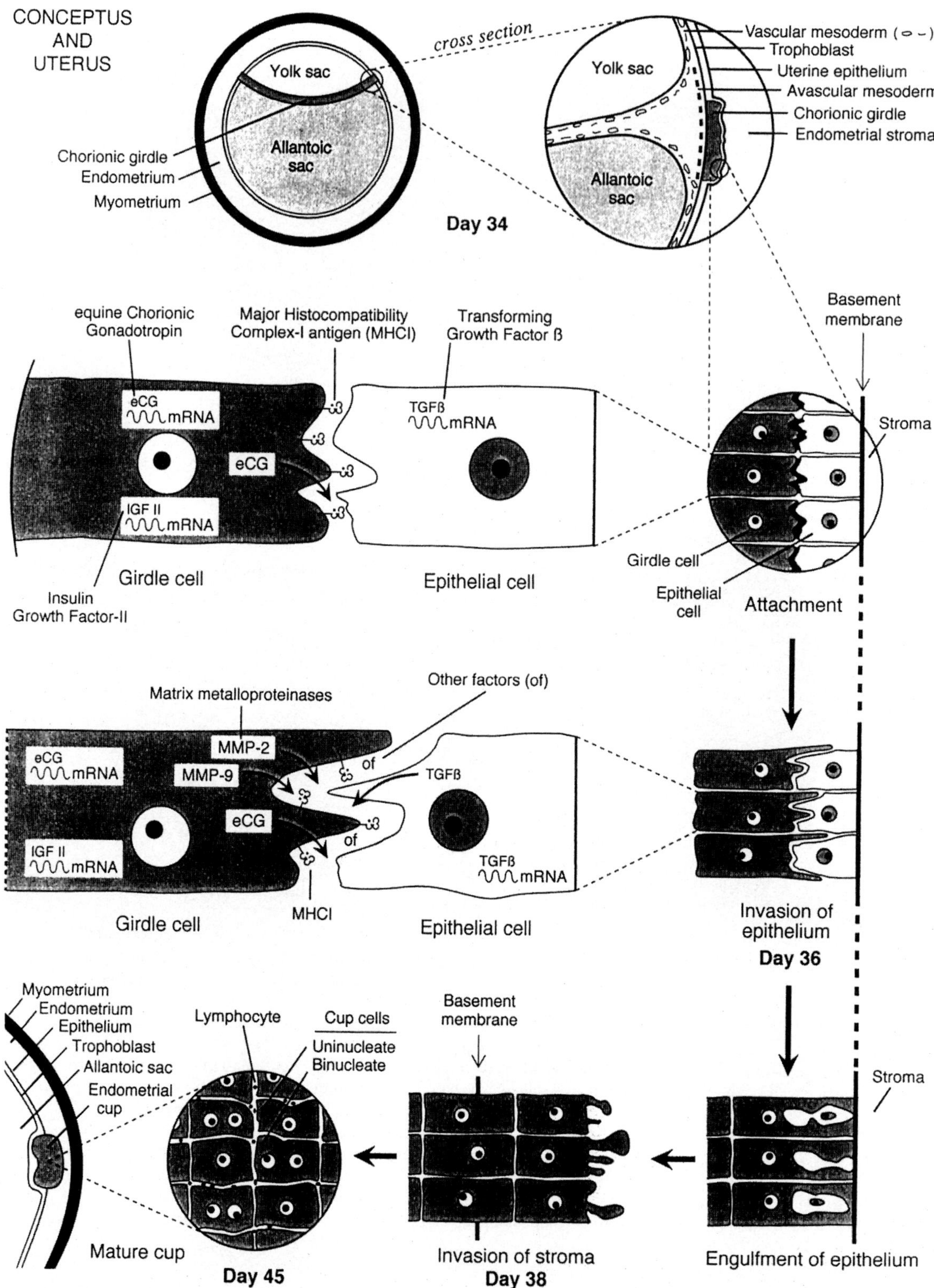


FIGURE 14-6. Embryogenesis/placentation in the horse from 34 to 45 days of gestation showing molecular/physioanatomical parameters of the conceptus/uterus interaction, matrix metalloproteinases attachment/invasion of the epithelium, engulfment of epithelium, invasion of stroma, and maturation of endometrial cups. (Data and diagrams by Dr. Vagonu and Professor OJ Ginther, V.M.D., Ph.D.)

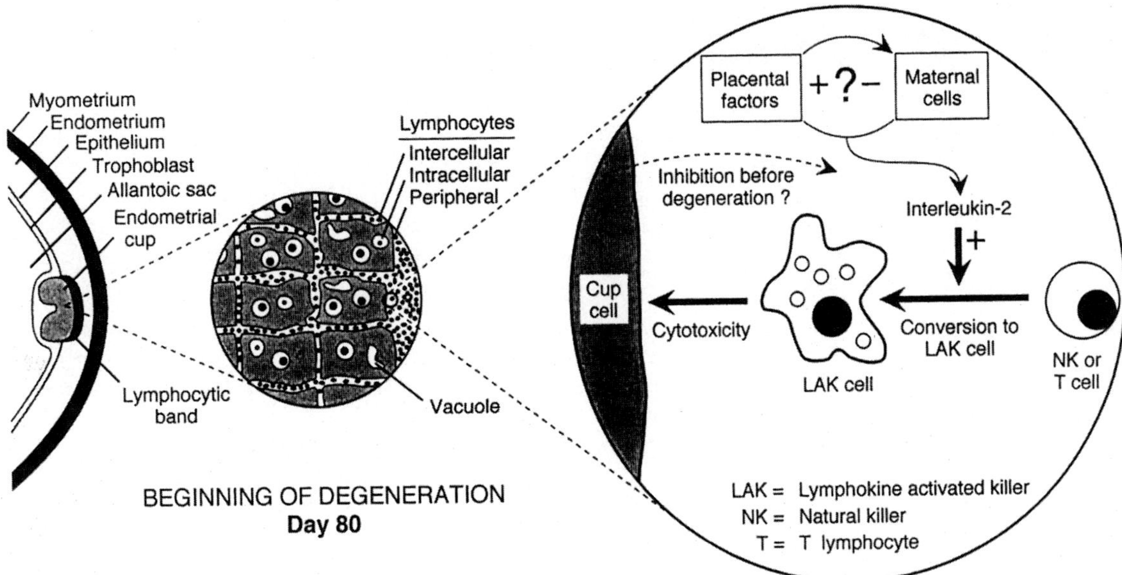


FIGURE 14-7. A diagrammatic representation depicting the onset of the degeneration of endometrial cups. The degeneration process is associated with a dramatic maternal leukocyte reaction to the endometrial cups. Natural cytotoxic maternal leukocytes have been proposed to play a role in regulation of placental development in many species because of their ability to recognize and destroy Major Histocompatibility Complex-I antigen negative cells, such as endometrial cup cells. Cytotoxic leukocytes can be derived from Natural Killer or T-lymphocyte populations and activation by the cytokine Interleukin-2 leading to the formation of lymphokine-activated killer cells. Cultured chorionic girdle cells are susceptible to lymphokine-activated killer cell cytotoxicity. The figure depicts potential placental and maternal interactions in the regulation of lymphokine-activated killer cell interaction with endometrial cup cells. (Data and diagrams by Dr. Vagonu and Professor OJ Ginther, V.M.D., Ph.D. Professor of Veterinary Science, Department of Veterinary Science, University of Wisconsin-Madison, Madison, Wisconsin 53706. Reproductive Biology of the Mare, Basic and Applied Aspects, 1990. Distributed by Equiservices, 4343 Garfoot Road, Cross Plains, Wisconsin 53528, USA. Phone or Fax: 608-798-4910.)

parturition, and the time for completion of delivery and the passage of the placenta are influenced by increasing doses of oxytocin. Parturition can be induced in the mares of large-sized breeds by daily treatment with 100 mg of dexamethasone for 4 days.

Indications for elective induction of parturition include delayed parturition resulting from uterine atony, prolonged gestation, prevention of injury at foaling, preparturient colic, injury to the mare and impending rupture of the prepubic tendon, and obtaining colustrum-deprived foals for research purposes.

### *Postpartum Estrus (Foal Heat)*

Postpartum estrus usually occurs 5 to 15 days after foaling. Some mares, however, may show estrus as late as 45 days after parturition; such estrus may have been preceded by a quiet ovulation. The interval between postpartum estrus and the following estrus may be affected by the milk yield. Breeding at the postpartum estrus may cause an increased percentage of abortion, dystocia, stillbirth, and retained placenta. This may be due to the introduction of bacteria into the uterus before it is completely involved and while it still lacks contractility. Involution of the uterus after normal foaling is rapid. Regression in size is almost complete by the first day of "foal heat" (Table 14-8).

## EQUINE HYBRIDS

There are several equine hybrids:

horse (stallion) × donkey (jenny) = **hinny**
donkey (jack) × horse (mare) = **mule**
zebra × donkey (jenny) = **zebronkey**
zebra × horse (mare) = **zebrorse**

These hybrids of both sexes are infertile because horses, donkeys, and zebras have different chromosome numbers and the hybrids have a number intermediate between their parents. The germ cells of the hybrids proceed through mitosis, but there is a block to meiosis, because pairing of homologous chromosomes is impossible as a result of uneven chromosome numbers (26).

TABLE 14-8. ***Signs, Stages, and Endocrinology of Labor and Post-Partum Ovulation***

| | |
|---|---|
| SIGNS OF IMMINENT FOALING | Assessed by testing mammary secretions for calcium/magnesium using test strips developed for water hardness. 80–90% of foaling occurs at night |
| STAGES OF LABOR | Stage 1 rupture of allantochorion<br>Stage 2 expulsion of foal<br>Stage 3 expulsion of placental membrane within 1 hr<br>In 75–85% of foaling allantochorion is usually discharged inside. |
| ENDOCRINOLOGY OF LABOR | a. fetal adrenal gland: higher levels of cortisol in the umbilical artery than in the umbilical vein.<br>b. $PGF_{2\alpha}$: stimulates myometrical contraction, abrupt increased level at parturition surges on following days.<br>c. Estrogen/progestins: during last 2 weeks of pregnancy estrogens decrease, progestins increase; at parturition both decrease abruptly, during the last day progestins decline, whereas estrogens do not, increasing the estrogen : progestin ratio<br>d. Parturition is induced by massive doses of dexamethasone or by exogenous oxytocin within 1 hour |
| POST PARTUM OVULATION | Occurs in most mares 8–11 days after foaling according to season of year. Some mares do not have a postpartum ovulation or revert to ovarian inactivity after the first ovulation. FSH surge occurs 2–5 days before parturition to peak just before or on day of parturition, accounting for postpartum follicular development.<br>First ovulation for spring-born fillies in good condition occurs during subsequent spring at same time that adults first ovulate; first breeding season (interval between first/last ovulations) is longer in adults.<br>Postpartum uterine involution:<br>day 15: luminal fluid nondetectable<br>day 23: both uterine horns are similar in size |

Data accumulated and adapted from: Ginther OJ. Reproductive Biology of the Mare. Cross Plains, Wisconsin: Equiservices, 1992; Cox JE. Urine tests for pregnancy in the mare. Vet Rec 1971;89:606; Bain AM, Howey WP. Observations on the time of foaling in Thoroughbred mares in Australia. J Reprod Fert 1975;23(Suppl):545–546; Allen WR, Kydd J, Volsen SG, Antczak DF. Equine endometrial cups: maternal uterine responses following extraspecific embryo transfer between horses and donkeys. J Anat 1986;146:9; Allen WE, Kessy BM, Noakes DE. Evaluation of uterine tube function in pony mares. Vet Rec 1979;105:364–366.

## REPRODUCTIVE FAILURE IN MARES

Conception and foaling percentages differ widely. In a few pony studs, conception rate and foaling rates are 100%. In most studs, the foaling rate is much lower than the conception rate. In general, the conception rate is influenced by the breed, nutrition, and age of the dam, and management practices. For example, the conception rate from first service is lower in thoroughbred mares than in most other breeds. The conception rate of foaling mares served during foal heat is lower than the first-service pregnancy rate of foaling mares served after the foal heat. Pregnancy rate, pregnancy loss, and twinning rate are summarized in Table 14-9.

### *Estrous Irregularities*

Irregularities in the estrous cycle are associated with seasonal changes in the photoperiod, nutrition, and climate. Variations in pattens of cyclic behavior include cycle length and estrous behavior, failure of ovulation and follicular development, and spontaneous prolongation of the corpora lutea. "Quiet ovulation," anovulatory estrus, "split-estrus," and prolonged estrus are not uncommon.

### *Anestrus*

There are three forms of anestrus:

1. Winter anestrus that lasts 11 weeks in which follicles rarely reach 35 mm before regressing without ovulation, and plasma levels of progestogen are 1 ng/ml;
2. CL that persists for 5 to 13 weeks with elevated plasma progestogen levels, usually in November and December;
3. Cyclic ovulatory patterns unaccompanied by estrus (8).

A single injection of GnRH in anestrous mares will cause an increase in serum FSH to 3.7 times baseline, which is comparable to the peak increases occurring during the estrous cycle; however, the induced increase in LH is much less than that of the cyclic peak. GnRH in combination with appropriate progesterone treatment in the acyclic mare treated toward the end of the nonbreeding season can con-

TABLE 14-9. ***Reproductive Efficiency in Mares: Percentages of Pregnancy Rate, Pregnancy Loss, and Twinning***

| | |
|---|---|
| % PREGNANCY RATE | Fertilization rate: 90–95% in normal mares<br>Pregnancy rate: 55% per estrus, over all mares<br>78–85% for reproductive healthy mares<br>78–85% live-foal rate for all mares/season<br>Reduced pregnancy rates:<br>18–22% for 1st postpartum estrus<br>45–55% mares with endometritis<br>45–55% mares of advancing age |
| % PREGNANCY LOSS | Breeding at first postpartum estrus may increase embryo and/or fetal-loss rate.<br>Massive uterine cysts (more frequent in old mares) are associated with increased embryo loss but not necessarily with fetal loss in subfertile mares:<br>days 1–10 40–55%<br>days 20–50 minimal loss<br>days >60 no loss<br>Morphological defects of embryos and undersized embryos increases in subfertile mares on 6–10, causing higher pregnancy loss if transferred to recipient mares.<br>Farm pregnancy-loss rates are 4–10% for the last half of the embryo stage (Days 20 to 40) and 10–15% for the fetal stage.<br>Endometritis and infertility have reliable markers: detection of intrauterine fluid accumulation by ultrasonography.<br>Pseudopregnancy: embryo loss followed by luteal maintenance/uterine turgidity: associated with minor losses on days 10–20 progesterone inadequacy during the fetal stage and severe stress may reduce progestins to dangerous levels during pregnancy.<br>Pyometra or chronic severe endometritis associated with loss of $PGF_{2\alpha}$-producing cells/luteral maintenance. Endometritis activate release of luteolytic quantities of $PGF_{2\alpha}$ from endometrium.<br>Luteal insufficiency is not a cause of embryo loss before Day 20, except in mares induced to ovulate when in inactive phase of anovulatory season. |
| TWINNING | Most equine twins result from double ovulations; unilateral fixation occurs in several twin sets.<br>Dissimilarity in size of twin embryos favors unilateral fixation/rapid embryo reduction.<br>Time, incidence, and speed of embryo reduction depends on proportion of vascularized wall of one vesicle in contact with opposite vesicle.<br>Manual correction of twin embryos by transrectal rupture has replaced attempted prevention of twin development.<br>Twins in fetal stage intact seem to undergo abortion not fetal reduction or birth of viable twins. |

Adapted from: Ginther OJ. Using a twinning tree for designing twin-prevention programs. J Equine Vet Sci 1988;8:101–107; Ginther OJ. Reproductive biology of the mare: basic and applied aspects. Cross Plains, Wisconsin: Equiservices, 1990.

sistently induce normal cyclic pituitary and ovarian activity culminating in ovulating (27).

### *Prenatal Mortality*

Prenatal mortality is frequent in lactating mares early in the season or mated after foal heat. Prenatal death is also common in certain horse families. Higher prenatal mortality in yearlings compared to adult mares may be due to inadequate progestogen levels to maintain pregnancy, immaturity of the yearlings, their greater nutritional requirements for growth and maintenance, and the physical stresses imposed on them by the husbandry procedures.

### *Excessive Length of Umbilical Cord*

The length of the umbilical cord is not correlated with gestational age, foal's body weight, sex, or viability, dam's age or parity, or surface area, width, or length of the allantochorion. However, cord length is correlated with weight of the allantochorion and allantoamnion and the length of the nonpregnant horn. Several pathologic conditions of unknown origin cause escessive elongation of the umbilical cord. Reproductive failures associated with these conditions include:

1. Strangulation by the cord around the fetus.
2. Excessive twisting around the amniotic or allantoic

portion of the fetus, causing vascular occlusion and/or urinary retention.
3. Necrosis of the chorioallantois at the cervix.

Strangulation of the fetus may cause abortion, with deep grooves present around the head, neck, thorax, and back with apparent local edema.

Mild urachal obstruction is compatible with normal pregnancy. The umbilical cord may become twisted with multiple urachal dilations that prevent normal sealing of the bladder apex at birth. Excessive twisting of the umbilical cord threatens the integrity of the urachus and umbilical vessels; the effects depend on the completeness, duration, and site of the compression.

### Abortion

The average abortion rate in mares is high (10%). This may be due to peculiarities in the hormonal balance of the mare during pregnancy. Abortion is lowest between 3 and 6 years of age, and most abortions that are due to infection occur during the later stages of pregnancy. During the fifth and tenth months of pregnancy, the mares are endocrinologically susceptible to abortion owing to hormonal deficiencies. It is recommended to avoid sudden changes in the diet or the amount of physical exercise at these times. Postabortion conception rate is low, especially in older mares (Table 14-8).

Abortion in older mares may be due to uterine inadequacies. The normal endometrium is thrown into more or less longitudinal folds that vary in size with the estrous cycle. Implantation ocurs at the junction of the body and horns of the uterus, and the folds in this region can undergo atrophy after several pregnancies. The atrophic areas appear to have a reduced number of endometrial glands, and, in some cases, contain collagen and/or inflammatory cells.

### Neonatal Abnormalities and Neonatal Mortality

Microphthalmos (button eye) and entropion are regular congenital abnormalities in thoroughbreds. The degree of microphthalmos is variable and may be so severe that the globe is obscured behind a well-developed third eyelid. The cornea is often distorted and pigmented, and the palpebral aperture is usually smaller than normal; the condition can be bilateral or unilateral. Entropion is both congenital and hereditary and may lead to corneal opacity and ulceration.

Barker Syndrome (Convulsive Foal Syndrome, or Neonatal Maladjustment Syndrome). This syndrome affects thoroughbred foals, often those that have experienced an easy birth, and occurs from within minutes after birth to 24 hours later. Clinical symptoms include jerking movements of the head, limb, and body musculature; hyperexcitability; inability to stand; convulsions; opisthotonus; and erection of the tail. There may also be collapse of the external nares, deep inspiratory movement, and a barking sound. If able to stand, the foal may walk around aimlessly. Recovery occurs in about 50% of cases and is usually complete.

The syndrome is associated with necrosis of the cerebral cortex, diencephalon, and brain stem, and with severe hemorrhage in the white and gray matter of the cerebral cortex and in the cerebellum.

*Ocular Changes.* The eye of the foal, which is open at birth, has a clear cornea and ocular media. The fundus is differentiated into tapetum lucidum and tapetum nigrum and is similar to the fundus of the adult horse. Ocular changes in the convulsive foal syndrome include asymmetry of pupils, apparent blindness, variable pupil size, scleral splashing, and retinal petechiae. These clinical signs are not always present, even in severe cases. Small round retinal hemorrhages may occur, which are clearly visible as red dots against the background of the tapetal fundus. These hemorrhages occur at 1 and 2 days of age in convulsive foals and persist only a few days.

Perinatology. Equine pregnancy differs from other domestic species in that the equine fetus matures very late in gestation, maternal progestin concentrations rise near term, and the fetal gonads enlarge and produce estrogen precursors. Identification of the compromised equine fetus antepartum is a relatively new approach. The role of the fetal pituitary adrenal axis and thyroid stimulating hormone in the final maturation of the equine fetus is emphasized. Abnormalities in maternal concentrations of progestins and estrogens may signal fetal compromise and their role in the initiation of parturition and fetal maturation are well known (28).

Neonatal Mortality. Neonatal mortality may be a result of weakness of the mother or the foal, or bacterial infection through the umbilical cord of the young. Proper management, clean stables for foaling, and sanitary precautions at foaling are the common preventive methods of neonatal mortality (Table 14-8).

### Recommendations for Breeding Techniques

Careful testing for estrus with the stallion, routine examination of the vagina, and rectal palpation of the reproductive organs may help to improve conception rate. Whenever possible, the time of ovulation should be predicted, because the duration from the onset of estrus may differ between individuals. Conception rate depends primarily on the time and number of inseminations.

On occasion, the mare may strain (as in micturition and defecation) after mating and evacuate most of the semen from the uterus. This may be prevented by having the mare walk for a while after mating. The mare is susceptible to endometritis, especially after foaling, because the cervix of the mare is not a strong barrier to the introduction of bacteria. The mare is more prone to a deficiency in LH than other farm animals; such deficiency may be alleviated by the use of exogenous LH. The intravenous injection of 1500 to 3000 IU of hCG may cause ovulation during anovulatory estrus, provided the ovarian follicle is at least 3 cm in diameter.

### Assisted Reproductive Technology

Artificial insemination (AI), multiple ovulation/embryo transfer (MOET), and *in vitro*-embryo production (IVEP) can produce substantial increases in the rate of genetic improvement, with acceptable rates of inbreeding. In contrast, semen sexing, embryo sexing, and embryo cloning can produce only limited increases in the rate of genetic improvement. However, embryo cloning can produce a once-only substantial boost in the average genetic merit of commercial stock, and can revolutionize breed structure (29).

INTRACYTOPLASMIC SPERM INJECTION (ICSI). Extensive investigations have been conducted on the micromanipulation techniques used to enhance fertilization/successful pregnancy in sheep and goats with special emphasis on the direct sperm injection into the oocytes. Exogenous oocyte activation was not mandatory for fertilization, and subsequent normal fetal development. Lambs were produced from sperm that had been sorted on a flow cytometer and was of the predicted sex. Several techniques have been applied for domestic and exotic mammalian species.

Gamete interaction involves the recognition between a sperm receptor located in plasma membrane, and an oocyte receptor located in zona pellucida (ZP3). ZP3 induces acrosome reaction. Closer interaction occurs between ZP2 and an inner acrosomal membrane receptor. Certain acrosomal proteins are needed for this process. Acrosome is necessary for the correct organization of plasma membrane proteins. The acrosome is necessary for sorting and right organization of plasma membrane proteins (30–37).

EMBRYO CLONING. By making possible the creation of large numbers of identical individuals, embryo cloning has the potential to greatly increase accuracy of selection, because each potential candidate can be evaluated on the average performance of many copies of itself. However, if total testing capacity is fixed, as it usually is in practice, testing of clones can be achieved only at the expense of a reduction in the testing of families of full-sibs or half-sibs (38, 39).

## REPRODUCTIVE FAILURE IN STALLIONS

Reproductive failure in stallions includes abnormal sexual behavior, ejaculatory disturbances, and poor semen characteristics.

### Abnormal Sexual Behavior and Ejaculatory Disturbances

Abnormal sexual behavior of stallions includes:

1. Failure to attain or maintain an erection with poor or excellent libido.
2. Incomplete intromission or lack of pelvic thrusts after intromission, poor libido, or pain from injuries incurred during breeding.
3. Dismounting at onset of ejaculation because of injury or pain.
4. Failure to ejaculate in spite of a complete prolonged erection and repeated intromissions.
5. Good ejaculation for a short time, but no further ejaculation without sexual rest, although libido remains high.
6. Masturbation (1).

Impotent stallions respond well to retraining, and recovery can be achieved without pharmacologic treatment. Masturbation in breeding stallions, an abnormal sexual behavior, may be treated by the use of a stallion ring, but this may cause hemospermia.

Ejaculatory disturbances are manifested differently in individual stallions, from normal copulation with or without occasional ejaculation. In most cases, penile erection is associated with several copulatory movements that terminate in complete or incomplete failure of ejaculation. Ejaculatory disturbances—transitory, intermittent, or permanent—may occur during the first two or three breeding seasons or after several seasons of normal activity. To ensure that ejaculation has taken place after intromission, one holds the hand under the base of the penis. In the absence of ejaculation, a few weak urethral waves may be felt, but when ejaculation takes place it feels like the contents of a 10-ml syringe being transported along the urethra. In a stallion of good fertility, it is usual to feel about five of these waves; in the stallion with lower fertility, only about one to two waves are sometimes felt.

Ejaculatory disturbance may arise from directed blocking of nerve impulses or fatness, poor condition, or exhaustion resulting from frequent services. Stallions usually react strongly to unfamiliar surroundings, and psychic factors of this nature may inhibit the normal stimulation from the supraspinal centers. Ejaculatory disturbance may be due to failure of contraction of smooth muscles in the reproductive tract as a result of refractoriness of these cells to norepinephrine, exhaustion of the norepinephrine depots, or failure to release norepinephrine from the sympathetic nerve endings.

### Poor Semen Characteristics

This may include one of the following: azoospermia, absence of sperm in the ejaculate; oligozoospermia, decreased sperm concentration per milliliter of semen; teratospermia, increased percentage of morphologically abnormal spermatozoa; asthenospermia, decreased sperm motility; or hemospermia, hemorrhage in semen.

Hemospermia results from urethritis in the ejaculatory ducts. Hemospermia may occur occasionally, in isolated instances or in each ejaculate, irrespective of frequency of ejaculation. Affected stallions frequently require several mounts to ejaculate and often exhibit pain on ejaculation. Semen quality is determined by motility, sperm numbers, and morphology is usually unaffected, and the cause of the infertility is unknown. Urethroscopic examination, urethrography, bacterial and viral cultures, biopsy, surgery of the urethra, and histocytologic examination are used for diagnosis (40). The exact cause and location of the hemorrhage should be known before treatment is initiated.

Several species of microflora have been found in the sperm: *Pseudomonas* spp., *Escherichia coli*, *Klebsiella*, *Aerobacter (Enterobacter)*, *Proteus* spp., *Staphylococcus* spp., *Streptococcus* spp., and other gram-positive and gram-negative rods. These microorganisms, however, do not seem to affect the fertility. Most *Streptococcus* spp. in the semen are contaminants from the prepuce.

### *Recommendations for Breeding Techniques*

The detrimental effect of frequent ejaculations on the number of sperm per ejaculate is pronounced in the stallion. In natural breeding, where several mares may exhibit estrus simultaneously, a stallion may copulate several times on one day; this causes a decline in fertility. The use of artificial insemination during such periods of mating will improve the conception rate. The stallion ejaculates directly into the uterus, and in most cases there is little semen left in the vagina. The transfer of semen from the vagina to the uterus following insemination is seldom necessary, but this is recommended with wriggling mares or if a stallion is apt to dismount the mare with the penis still erect, as this pulls semen back into the vagina (Fig. 14-8).

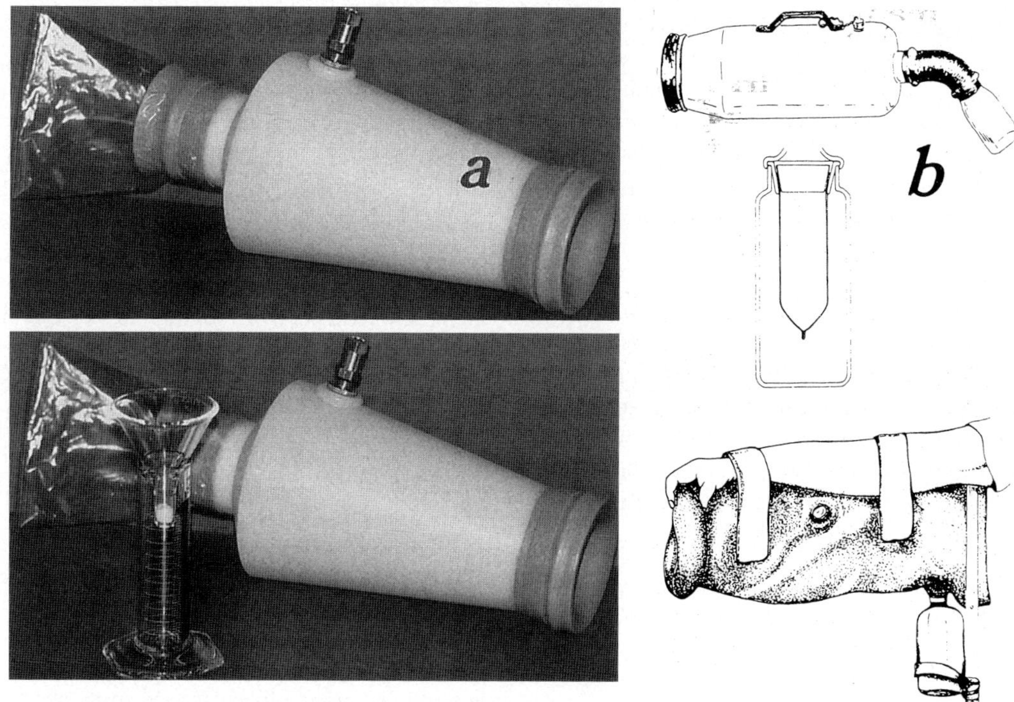


FIGURE 14-8. (**a**) Artificial vagina of the horse. The AV is photographed with graduated cylinder funnel containing a rayon ball which we use for macro filtration of semen to remove any particulates. The AV uses a different principle than the Colorado or Missouri AV for semen collection in that the stallion's penis will "lock" inside it after he "flowers" or "bells" as opposed to the thrusting back and forth in the other models. The stimuli which elicits ejaculation is provided by the operator's hand and thumb on the base of the stallion's penis. This AV is very lightweight when filled with water, about 5 1/2 lbs, as compared with other models. It is particularly well suited for collecting stallions which are standing on the ground on all four feet. It is also used on stallions which have injuries that prevent them from mounting a mare or phantom. (Roanoke AI Laboratories, Inc., 8535 Martin Creek Road, Roanoke, VA 24018 (540) 774-0676.) (**b**) (*Top*) Artificial vagina (modified Japanese model) for stallions. (*Middle*) Enlarged collection bottle fitted with a filter to remove the gel. (Adapted from Komarek R, et al. J Reprod Fertil 1965;10:337.) (*Bottom*) Another type of artificial vagina for horses.

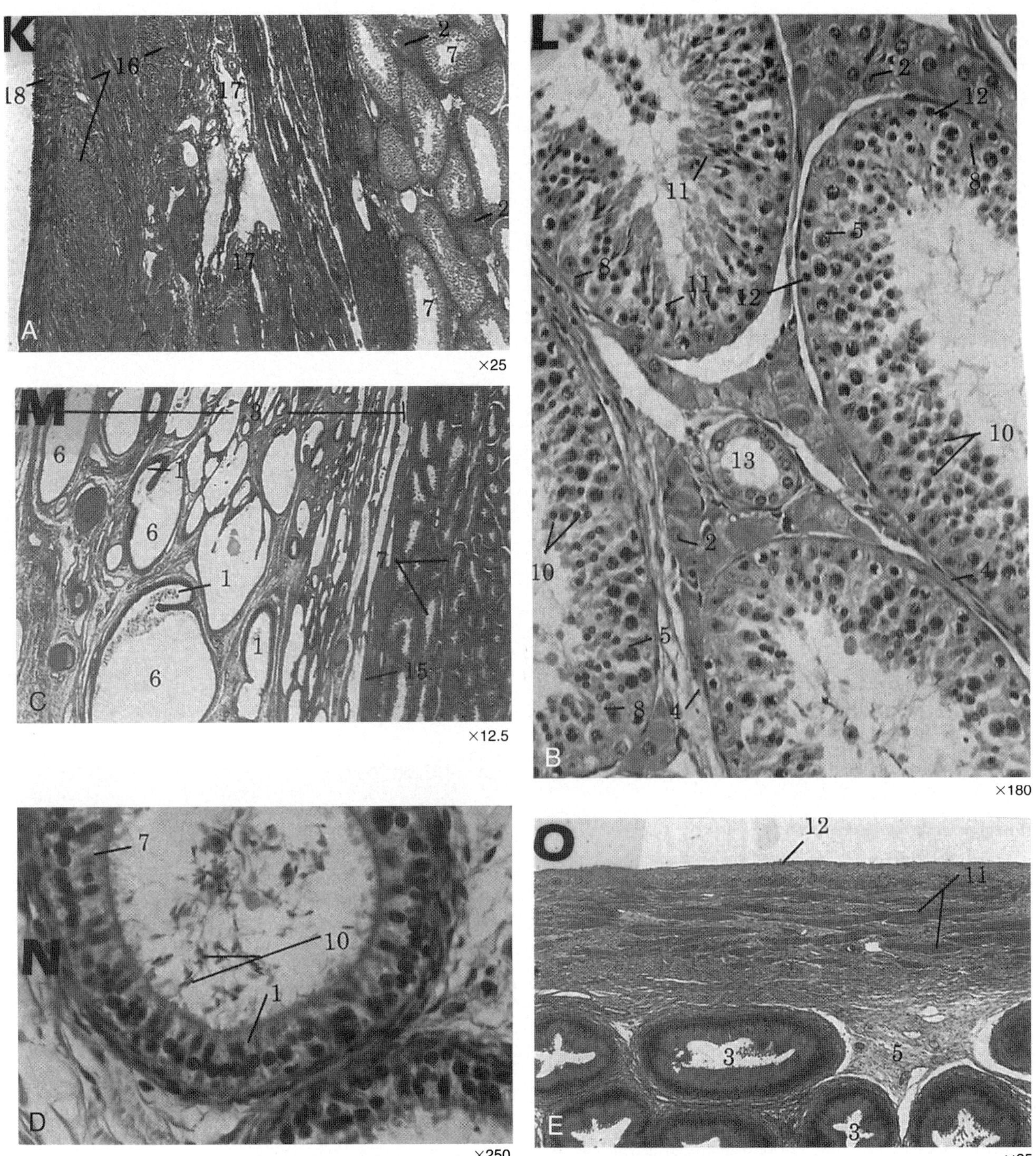


FIGURE 14-9. Histological characteristics of testis and epididymis of the stallion. (From Pacha WJ Jr, Wood LM. Color Atlas of Veterinary Histology. Philadelphia: Lea & Febiger, 1990.) (**A**) Testis, Mallory's. The tunica albuginea of the stallion is characterized by the presence of smooth muscle. (**B**) Seminiferous Tubules, Testis. Four portions of seminiferous tubules are visible. Note the numerous interstitial cells (abundant in the boar and stallion) and the section through a straight tubule. (**C**) Rete Testes. Anastomosing channels form the rete testis, which is surrounded by the loose connective tissue of the mediastinum testis. In the stallion, the rete testis extends through the tunica albuginea and becomes extratesticular, as it is in this micrograph. Note the junctions of rete tubules and efferent ductules. (**D**) Head of Epididymis, Masson's. The epididymis is surrounded by a tunica albuginea of dense irregular connective tissue, which contains smooth muscle in the stallion. Portions of the coiled duct of the epididymis are shown. (**E**) Head of Epididymis. In this region, the pseudostratified columnar epithelium of the duct of the epididymis is thickest. Smooth muscle fibers surrounding the duct are scarce.

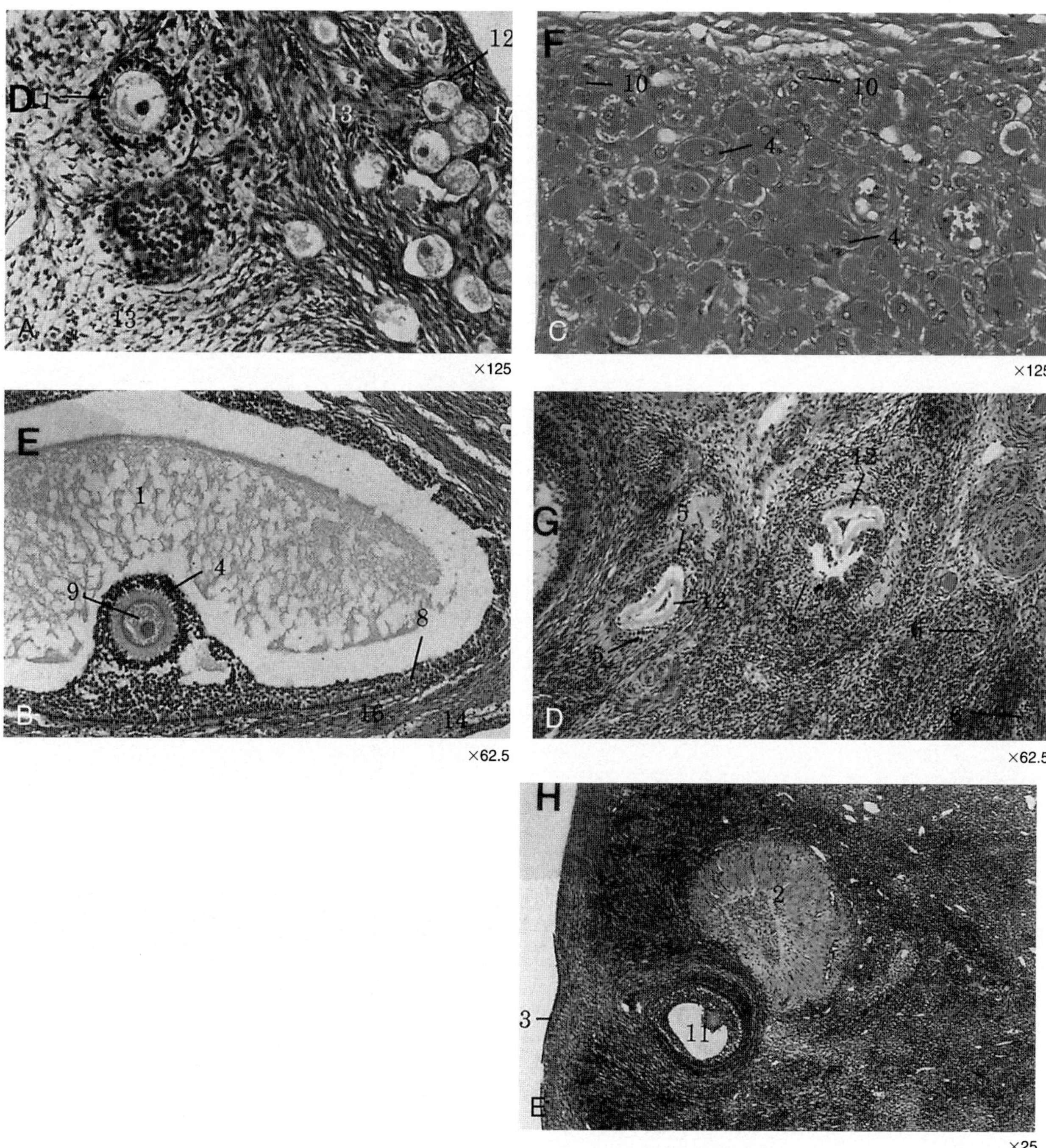


FIGURE 14-10. The histology of mammalian male/female reproductive system. (From Pacha WJ Jr, Wood LM. Color Atlas of Veterinary Histology. Philadelphia: Lea & Febiger, 1990.) (**A**) Ovary, Queen. Early follicles in the outer region of the cortex. (**B**) Ovary, Queen. A young, tertiary follicle. (**C**) Corpus Luteum, Ovary, Sow. Peripheral region of a corpus luteum showing theca lutein cells (*small*) and granulosa lutein cells (*large*). (**D**) Ovary, Bitch. Atretic follicles, each with a swollen zona pellucida. (**E**) Corpus Albicans, Ovary, Cow, Masson's. The scar tissue of the corpus albicans is stained bright blue-green in this preparation.

## CONCLUDING REMARKS

Several studies were conducted on various parameters of equine reproductive physiology: seasonal/lactational anestrus (41); retention of oviductal eggs (42–45); early pregnancy site in consecutive gestations (46); ultrasonographic diagnosis of fetal gender (47, 48); equine embryo manipulation/transfer (49–52); pseudopregnancy in the mare (53); ova transfer between horses/donkeys (52); fertilization (54); histocompatabilities complex antigens (55); immunology of endometrial cups (51, 52). Other studies dealth with clinical parameters: LH levels in cerebrospinal fluid (56); effect of prostaglandin analogues on progesterone-treated ponies (57–63); pregnancy failure induced by human chorionic gonadotropin (41); uterine lavage after insemination (64); rapid progesterone essay (AELIA) (65); oral progesterone for estrus/ovulation induction (5); lack of expression of interferon genes by equine embryos (66); luteolysis after endometrial biopsy (67); and trophoblastic vesicles *in vitro* and in vivo (68–70).

Extensive investigations on ovulation, contractility of the myosalpinx, pre-attachment of the embryo, histochemistry and ultrastructure of the feto-placental unit were conducted by Flood (71–77) (Fig. 14-8). Histological characteristics of the reproductive organs of horses as compared to other farm animals are illustrated in Figures 14-9 and 14-10.

## REFERENCES


1. Pickett BW, Voss LJ. Abnormalities of mating behavior in domestic stallions. In: Rowlands IW, Allen WR, Rossdale PD, eds. Equine Reproduction. Oxford: Blackwell, 1975.
2. Garcia MC, Ginther OJ. Regulation of plasma LH by estradiol and progesterone in ovariectomized mares. Biol Reprod 1978;19:447.
3. Tischner M, Kosianiak K, Bielanski W. Analysis of the pattern of ejaculation in stallions. J Reprod Fertil 1974;40:329.
4. Mann T, Short RV, Walton A. The "tail-end" sample of stallion semen. J Agric Sci Camb 1957;49:301.
5. Allen WR. Hormonal control of early pregnancy in the mare. Anim Reprod Sci 1984;7:283–304.
6. Allen WR, Pashen RL. Production of monozygotic (identical) horse twins by embryo micromanipulation. J Reprod Fertil 1984;71:607–613.
7. Alexander SL, Irvine CHG. GnRH secretion in the mare. Anim Reprod Sci 1996;42:173–180.
8. Hughes JP, Stabenfeldt GH, Evans JW. Clinical and endocrine aspects of the estrous cycle of the mare. Proc A. Meeting Am Ass, Equine Pract 1975.
9. Holtan DW, Nett TM, Estergreen VL. Plasma progestagens in pregnant mares. J Reprod Fertil 1975;23(Suppl):419–424.
10. Holtan DW, Houghton E, Silver M, Fowden AL, Gusty I, Rossdale PD. Plasma progestagens in the mare, foetus and newborn foal. J Reprod Fertil 1991;44(Suppl):517–528.
11. Geschwind II, Dewey R, Hughes JP, Evans JW, Stabenfeldt GH. Plasma LH levels in the mare during the estrus cycle. J Reprod Fertil 1975;23(Suppl):207.
12. Douglas RH, Del Campo MR, Ginther OJ. Luteolysis following carotid or ovarian arterial injectin of prostaglandin F2$\alpha$ in mares. Biol Reprod 1976;14:473.
13. Arthur GH. Influence of intrauterine saline infusion upon the estrous cycle of the mare. J Reprod Fertil 1975;23(Suppl):231.
14. Oxender WD, Noden PA, Hafs HD. Estrus, ovulation and plasma hormones after prostaglandin F2$\alpha$ in mares. 3. J Reprod Fertil 1979;27(Suppl):251.
15. Squires EL, Douglas RH, Steffenhagen WY, et al. Ovarian changes during the estrous cycle and pregnancy in mares. J Anim Sci 1974;38:330.
16. Ganjam VK, Kenney RM, Gledhill BL. Increased concentration of androgens in cryptorchid stallion testes. I J Steroid Biochem 1974;5:709.
17. Ganjam VK, Kenney RM, Flickinger G. Plasma progestagens in cyclic, pregnant and postpartum mares. J Reprod Fertil 1975;23(Suppl):441.
18. Ellis RNW, Lawrence TLJ. Energy undernutrition in the weaning filly foal. Br Vet J 1978;134:205.
19. Kenney RM, Ganjam VK, Cooper WL, et al. The use of prostaglandin F2$\alpha$ THAM salt in mares in clinical anoestrus. J Reprod Fertil 1975;23 (Suppl):247.
20. Neely DP, Hughes JP, Stabenfeldt GH, Evans JW. The influence of intrauterine saline infusion on luteal function and cyclical activity in the mare. J Reprod Fertil 1975; 23 (Suppl):235–239.
21. Neely DP, Stabenfeldt GH, Kindabl H, et al. Effect of intrauterine saline infusion during the late luteal phase on estrous cycle and luteal function of the mare. Am J Vet Res 1979;40:665–668.
22. Michel TH, Rossdale PD. Efficacy of hCG and GnRH for hastening ovulation in thoroughbred mares. Equine Vet J 1986;6:438–442.
23. Squires BL, Ginther OJ. Follicular and luteal development in pregnant mares. J Reprod Fertil 1975;23(Suppl):249.
24. Katila T. Uterine defense mechanisms in the mare. Anim Reprod Sci 1996;47:197–204.
25. Silver M, Comline RS. Transfer of gases and metabolites in the equine placenta: a comparison with other species. J Reprod Fertil 1975;23(Suppl):589.
26. McDonald LB. Reproductive Patterns of Horses. In: McDonald LB, ed. Veterinary Endocrinology and Reproduction, 4th ed. Philadelphia: Lea & Febiger, 1989.
27. Evans MJ, Irvine CHG. Induction of follicular development, maturation and ovulation by gonadotropin in releasing hormone administration to acyclic mares. Biol Reprod 1977; 16:452.
28. LeBlanc MM. Equine perinatology: what we know and what we need to know. Anim Reprod Sci 1996;42:189–196.
29. Nicholas FW. Genetic improvement through reproductive technology. Anim Reprod Sci 1995;42:205–214.
30. Almeida PA, Bolton VN. The effect of temperature fluctuations on the cytoskeletal organization and chromosomal constitution of the human oocyte. Zygote 1996;3:357–365.
31. Dale B, Defelice LJ. Soluble sperm factors, electrical events and egg activation. In: Dale B, ed. Mechanism of Fertilization: Plants to Humans. New York: Springer, 1990.

32. Dale B, Monroy A. How is polysperm prevented? Gamete Research 1981;4:151–169.
33. Danforth RA, Nana SD, Smith M. High purity water: an important component for success in *in vitro* fertilization. American Biotectinofogy Laboratory 1987;5:58–60.
34. Davidson A, Vermesh M, Lobo RA, Paulsen RI. Mouse embryo culture as quality control for human *in vitro* fertilization: the one-cell versus two-cell model. Fertil Steril 1988; 49:516–521.
35. Edwards RG, Brody SA. Human fertilization in the laboratory. In: Principles and Practice of Assisted Human Reproduction. Philadelphia: WB Saunders, 1995;351–413.
36. Fleetharn J, Mahadevan MM. Purification of water for *in vitro* fertilization and embryo transfer. J IVF Embryo Transf 1988;5:147–171.
37. Gianaroli L, Tosti E, Magil C, Ferrarreti A, Dale B. The fertilization current in the human oocyte. Molecular Reprod Develop 1994;38:209–214.
38. De Boer IJM, Brom FWA, Vorstenbosch JMG. An ethical evaluation of animal biotechnology: the case of using clones in dairy cattle. Anim Sci 1995;61:453–463.
39. Villanueva B, Simm G. The use and value of embryo manipulation techniques in animal breeding. Proceedings 5th World Congress. Genet Appl Livestock Proc 1994;20:200–207.
40. Voss JL, Pickett BW. Diagnosis and treatment of haemospermia in the stallion. In: Rowlands IW, Allen WR, Rossdale PD, eds. Equine Reproduction. Oxford: Blackwell Scientific Publications, 1975.
41. Allen WE. Pregnancy failure induced by human chorionic gonadotropin in pony mares. Vet Rec 1975;96:88–90.
42. Betteridge KJ, Mitchell D. Direct evidence of retention of unfertilized ova in the oviduct of the mare. J Reprod Fert 1971;39:145–148.
43. Betteridge/Mitchell, 1975
44. Betteridge KJ, Renard A, Goff AK. Uterine prostaglandin release relative to embryo collection, transfer procedures and maintenance of the corpus luteum. Equine Vet J 1985; 3:25–33.
45. Betteridge et al., 1979
46. Allen WE, Newcombe JR. Relationship between early pregnancy site in consecutive gestations in mares. Equine Vet J 1981;13:51–52.
47. Curran S, Ginther OJ. Ultrasonic diagnosis of equine fetal sex by location of the genital tubercie. 3. Equine Vet Sci 1989;9:77–83.
48. Curran S, Ginther OJ. Ultrasonic detennination of fetal gender in horses and cattle under farm conditions. Theriogenology, 1991.
49. Allen WR, Kydd J, Volsen SG, Antczak DF. Equine endometrial cups: maternal uterine responses following extraspecific embryo transfer between horses and donkeys. J Anat 1986; 146:9.
50. Betteridge KJ. The structure and function of the equine capsule in relation to embryo manipulation and transfer. Equine Vet J 1989;8(Suppl):92–100.
51. Allen WR. Embryo transfer in the horse. In: Adams CE, ed. Mammalian Egg Transfer. Boca Raton, Florida: CRC Press, 1982;135–154.
52. Allen WR. Immunological aspects of the equine endometrial cup reaction and the effect of xenogenic extraspecies pregnancy in horses and donkeys. J Reprod Fert 1982;31 (Suppl):57–94.
53. Allen WE. Some observations on pseudopregnancy in mares. Br Vet J 1978;134:263–269.
54. Wassarman PM, Florman HM, Greve JM. Receptor-mediated sperm-egg interactions in mammals. In: Metz CB, Monroy A, eds. Fertilization, 1985.
55. Donaldson WL, Zhang CH, Oriol JO, Antczak DR. Invasive equine trophoblast expresses conventional class I Major Histocompatibility Complex antigens. Development 1990;11: 63–71.
56. Allen RG, Douglas RH. Luteinizing hormone levels in the cerebrospinal fluid of mares: reflection of ovarian status. East Lansing, Michigan: Ann Meet Amer Soc Anim Sci, 1978.
57. Allen WE. Effect of prostaglandin analogue on progesterone-treated pony mares during early pregnancy. Equine Vet J 1977;9:92–95.
58. Ball BA, Little TV, Hillman RB, Woods GL. Embryonic loss in normal and barren mares. Toronto: Proc Conv Amer Assoc Equine Pract, 1985;535–543.
59. Ball BA, Little TV, Hillman RB, Woods GL. Pregnancy at days 2 and 14 and estimated embryonic loss rates prior to day 14 in normal and subfertile mares. Theriogenology, 1986; 26:611–619.
60. Ball BA, Shin SJ, Patten VH, Garcia MC, Woods GL. Intrauterine inoculation of Candidad parapsilosis to induce embryonic loss of pony mares. J Reprod Fert 1987; 35 (Suppl):505–506.
61. Ball BA, Little TV, Weber JA, Woods GL. Survival of day-4 embryos from young, normal mares and aged, subfertile mares after transfer to normal recipient mares. J Reprod Fert 1989;85:187–194.
62. Ball BA, Miller PG. Viability of equine embryos co-cultured with equine oviductal epithelium from the 4-8 cell to blastocyst stage. Theriogenology, 1991;35(Abstract):183.
63. Ball BA, Woods GL. Embryonic loss and early pregnancy loss in the mare. Compend Equine 1987;9:459–470.
64. Brinsko et al., 1991
65. Allen WR, Sanderson MW. The value of a rapid progesterone assay (AELIA) in equine stud veterinary medicine and management. Sydney: Proc Bain-Fallon Mem Lect, 1987;76.
66. Baker CB, McDowell KJ, Rabb MH, Bailey E. Lack of expression of interferon genes by equine embryos. Deauville: Abstr Internatl Symp Equine Reprod, 1990;138–139.
67. Baker CB, Newton DI, Mather EC, Oxender WD. Luteolysis in mares after endometrial biopsy. Amer J Vet Rec 1981;42:1816–1818.
68. Ball BA, Altschul M, Freeman KP, Hillman RB. Culture of equine trophoblastic vesicles *in vitro*. Theriogenology 1989;32:401–412.
69. Ball BA, Altschul M, Hillman RB. Luteal maintenance in mares after transfer of equine trophoblastic vesicles. Equine Vet J 1989;8(Suppl):21–24.
70. Ball BA, Altschul M, McDowell KJ, Ignotz G, Currie WB. Trophoblastic vesicles and maternal recognition of pregnancy in mares. Deauville: Abstr Internatl Symp Equine Reprod 1990;140–141.
71. Flood PF. The pre-attachment horse embryo: the structure of its capsule and histochemical evidence of steroid metabolism. Information Vet 1975;18:36–38.

72. Flood PF. A method for monitoring contractile activity of the myosalpinx in mares in vivo. Winter Meet Soc Study Fert, London, 1980;11.
73. Flood PF, Betteridge KJ, Irvine DS. Oestrogens and androgens in blastocoelic fluid and cultures of cells from equine conceptuses of 10–22 days of gestation. J Reprod Fert 1979; 27(Suppl):413–420.
74. Flood PF, Jong A, Betteridge KJ. The location of eggs retained in the oviducts of mares. J Reprod Fert 1979;57:291–294.
75. Flood PF, Betteridge KJ, Diocee MS. Transmission electron microscopy of horse embryos 3–16 days after ovulation. J Reprod Fert 1982;32(Suppl):319–327.
76. Flood PF, Marrable AW. Steroid metabolism in the feto-placental unit of the mare: a histochemical study during mid-gestation. J Reprod Fert 1973;35:617–618.
77. Flood PF, Marrable AW. A histochemical study of steroid metabolism in the equine fetus and placenta. J Reprod Fert 1975;23(Suppl):569–573.

## Suggested Reading

Adams TE, Horton MB, Watson JG, Adams BM. Biological activity of luteinizing hormone (LH) during the estrous cycle of mares. Dom Anim Endocr 1986;3:69–77.

Aggarwal BB, Papkoff H. Effects of histidine modification on the biological and immunological activities of equine chorionic gonadotropin. Arch Biochem Biophys 1980;202:121–125.

Alexander S, Irvine CHG. Radioimmunoassay and *in-vitro* bioassay of serum LH throughout the equine oestrous cycle. J Reprod Fert 1982;32(Suppl):253–260.

Alexander SL, Irvine CHG. Secretion rates and short-term patterns of gonadotrophin-releasing hormone, FSH and LH throughout the periovulatory period in the mare. J Endocr 1987;114:351–362.

Allen WR. Maternal recognition of pregnancy and immunological implications of trophoblastendometrium interactions in equids. Ciba Found Symp 1979;64:323–346.

Allen WR, Urwin V, Simpson DJ, et al. Preliminary studies on the use of an oral progestogen to induce oestrus and ovulation in seasonally anoestrous Thoroughbred mares. Equine Vet J 1980;12:141–145.

Alm CC, Sullivan JJ, First NL. The effect of a corticosteroid (dexamethasone), progesterone, oestrogen and prostaglandin F2$\alpha$ on gestation length in normal and ovariectomized mares. J Reprod Fert 1975;23(Suppl):637–640.

Al-Timimi I, Gaillard JL, Amri H, Silberzahn P. Androgen synthesis and aromatization by equine corpus luteum microsomes. J Biol Chem 1989;264:7161–7168.

Antczak DF, Oriol JG. Molecules of early equine trophoblast. Deauville: Abstr Internatl Symp Equine Reprod, 1990; 142–143.

Antzcak DF, Oriol JG, Donaldson WL, et al. Differentiation molecules of the equine trophoblast. J Reprod Fert 1987; 35(Suppl):371–378.
hyn V, 1983. Synchronization of estrus in post-partum mares with progesterone and estradiol-17$\beta$. Theriogenology, 19:779–785.

Channing CP, Batta SK, Condon W, Ganjam VK, Kenney RM. Levels of inhibin activity and an atretogenic factor(s) in follicular fluid harvested from viable and atretic mare follicles. In: Schwartz NB, Hunzicker-Dunn M, eds. Dynamics of Ovarian Function. New York: Raven Press, 1981;73–78.

Conn PM, McArdle CA, Andrews WV, Huckel WR. The molecular basis of gonadotropin-releasing hormone (GnRH) action in the pituitary gonadotrope. Biol Reprod 1987;36:17–35.

Douglas RH. Review of induction of superovulation and embryo transfer in the equine. Theriogenology 1979;11:33–46.

Enders AC, Liu KM. Differentiation, migration, and maturation of equine chorionic girdle cells. Biol Reprod 1991;44(Suppl):6.

Ginther OJ. Internal regulation of physiological processes through local venoarterial pathways: A review. J Anim Sci 1974; 39:550–564.

Ginther OJ. Reproductive seasonality and regulation of LH and FSH in pony mares. Beltsville Symp Agri Res Anim Reprod, Beltsville, 1979;3:291–305.

Ginther OJ. Postfixation embryo reduction in unilateral and bilateral twins in mares. Theriogenology, 1984;22:213–223.

Hughes JP, Stabenfeldt GE, Evans JW. The estrous cycle of the mare. J Reprod Fertil 1973;21(Suppl):161.

Liu IKM, Lantz KC, Schlafke S, Bowers JM, Enders AC. Clinical observations of oviductal masses in the mare. Proc Ann Cony Amer Assoc Equine Pract, Lexington, 1991;41–45.

Squires EL, Garcia MC, Ginther OJ. Effects of pregnancy and hysterectomy on the ovaries of pony mares. J Anim Sci 1974;38:823.

# CHAPTER 15

# *Llamas and Alpacas*

J.B. SUMAR

The family *Camelidae* comprises six species, and they are believed to have originated in the western North America, with two of the species migrating throughout the Bering Strait into Asia, and four into South America. Two of the South American species, the llama (*Lama glama*) and the alpaca (*Lama pacos*), were domesticated around five thousand years ago, while the other two, the guanaco (*Lama guanicoe*) and vicuña (*Lama vicugna*), still exist in the wild.

Most of the present day domestic species and breeds of llamas and alpacas were developed from common ancestors in South America during the past millennia. Many aspects of reproduction are similar in both species, but indiscriminate extrapolation of reproductive phenomena of alpacas to the llama must, if possible, be avoided. Differences between these two domestic species can be attributed to speciacion, and to a physiological variation arising from several hundred years of selection, or to differences in management practices.

## FEMALE

### *Reproductive Anatomy*

Comparisons of the dimensions of alpaca and llama reproductive tracts are provided in Table 15-1. The ovaries are of a globular irregular shape, similar to those of the sow, particularly when they have multiple follicles. In the alpaca, follicles between 5 and 12 mm are considered normal. The uterus of the alpaca is bicornuate and both oviducts are large and convoluted, ending in a bursa which completely surrounds the ovary. The tips of the uterine horns in alpacas and llamas are blunt and rounded, and the oviduct opens into the uterine horn via a small, raised papilla which acts as a well-defined sphincter. Even under pressure, it is not possible to flush liquids from the uterus into the oviduct, but antegrade flushing is possible. The cervix has two or three irregularly annular or spiral folds (Fig. 15-1). The uterine body and horns are readily palpable per rectum (1).

The placenta in the alpaca, as in other camelids, is diffuse and epitheliochorial in type (2). A unique extra fetal membrane encasing the entire fetal body is attached at the mucocutaneous junction and coronary bands in newborn alpacas, llamas, vicuñas (3), and guanacos (4).

### *Puberty*

Young female alpacas of 12 to 13 months of age show behavioural estrous similar to adult alpacas (5), even though ovarian activity begins at 10 months with the presence of follicles of 5 mm or more. In a study carried out in southern Peru with yearling alpaca females, it was determined that a highly significant ($P < .001$) relationship existed between body weight at mating and subsequent birth rates. For each kilogram greater weight, there was a 5% increase in natality, but when body weight exceeded 33 kilograms, the percentage of open females was relatively independent of body weight (6).

In traditional Peruvian production systems, 50% or less of yearling alpacas reach 33 kg of body weight at mating time (1 year); therefore, breeding age is postponed until 2 years of age in alpacas and after three years of age in llamas. It has also been shown that with a better nutritional level after weaning (7 to 8 months of age), almost 100% of yearling alpacas can reach more than 33 kg of body weight (7).

### *Sexual Season*

Studies with alpacas and llamas in their natural habitat in the highlands of southern Peru, where males and females are together all year, showed that the sexual activities are seasonal, and last from December to March (summer months); these are the warmest months of the year, with sufficient rain and abundant green forage (8). Also, the wild species of camelids, the vicuña and guanaco, show this marked seasonality of reproduction (9).

In alpacas, when females are kept separate from males and copulation is allowed only once a month, both sexes are sexually active during the course of the whole year;

**TABLE 15-1. *Comparisons of the Dimensions of Alpaca and Llama Reproductive Tracts***

| | ALPACA | LLAMA |
|---|---|---|
| Length of labia, cm | 2.5 | 5 |
| Vagina (hymen to cervix) | | |
| Length, cm | 13.4 ± 2.0 | 15.0–21.0 |
| Diameter, cm | 3.4 ± 0.7 | 5.0 |
| Cervix | | |
| Length, cm | 2.0 | 2.5 |
| Diamater, cm | — | 2.0–4.0 |
| Rings, n | 2–3 | 2–3 |
| Uterine body | | |
| Length, cm | 3.05 ± 0.71 | 3.0–5.5 |
| Diameter, cm | — | 3.0–5.0 |
| Uterine horns | | |
| Length, cm | 7.9 ± 1.3 | 8.5–15.0 |
| Diameter, cm | — | 3.0–5.0 |
| Oviduct length, cm | 20.4 ± 4.2 | 10.5–18.3 |
| Right ovary | | |
| Length, cm | 1.6 ± 0.3 | 1.3–2.5 |
| Depth, cm | 1.1 ± 0.2 | 1.4–2.0 |
| Width, cm | 1.1 ± 0.2 | 0.6–1.0 |
| Left ovary | | |
| Length, cm | 1.6 ± 0.3 | 1.5–2.5 |
| Depth, cm | 1.1 ± 0.2 | 1.5–2.5 |
| Width, cm | 1.1 ± 0.2 | 0.5–1.0 |

Data from Fowler ME. Medicine and Surgery of South American Camelids. Llama, Alpaca, Vicuña, Guanaco. Ames, Iowa: Iowa University Press, 1989; Sato A, Montoya L. Aparato reproductor de la alpaca (Lama pacos). Anatomía Macroscópica. Rev de Camélidos Sudamericanos 7. Univ Nac M de San Marcos, Lima, Peru, 1990.

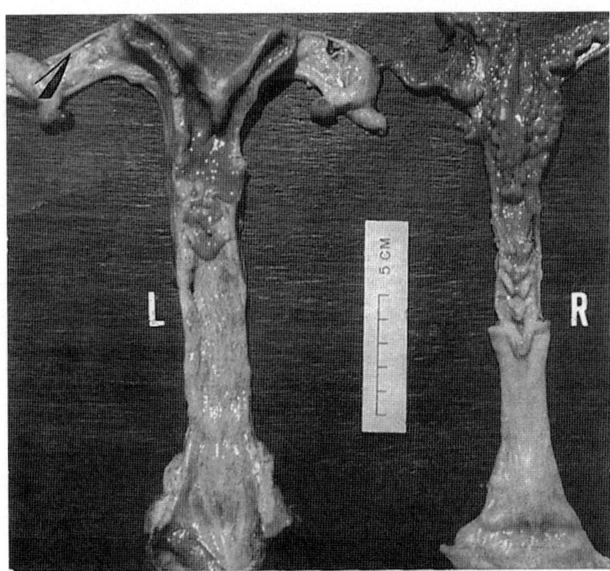


FIGURE 15-1. Reproductive organs of the alpaca (*L*, left) and ewe (*R*, right). The uterine horns in the alpaca are relatively short, not tapered, and come to a blunt utero-tubal junction, unlike those of the ewe, in which the uterine horns are long and taper toward the utero-tubal junction. Also, the alpaca cervix has two irregular annular or spiral folds and a short vagina, compared with five annular folds of the cervix and short vagina in the ewe.

ovulation and fertilization rates, along with embryo survival, were not affected significantly by the season of the year (10).

The continuous association of females and males inhibit sexual activity of the latter and even causes it to disappear altogether (11). Factors responsible for the onset and cessation of sexual activity under natural conditions are unknown. Environmental factors, in addition to visual and olfactory stimulation, could be of influence via the central nervous system.

Records in different zoological parks around the world indicate that camelids, both domestic and wild, are year-round breeders (12). In North America, where llamas are kept under good feeding conditions all year, they are considered non-seasonal breeders. An analysis of the birthing season in the Rocky Mountain area of the United States has been described for the llamas (13). Births were registered all the year round, but most of them (73%) occurred between June and November, the warmest months of the year.

## *Pattern of Ovarian Events*

Since copulation is ordinarily a necessary prelude to ovulation, the alpaca and llama have been classified as reflex or induced ovulators, as opposed to spontaneous ovulators (8, 14). Female alpacas or llamas do not have estrous cycles, unlike other domestic species. Estrous and ovulation are not manifested in a repetitive, cyclic, and predictable fashion.

FOLLICULAR DEVELOPMENT. When not exposed to a male, female alpacas shows periods of long sexual receptivity, and short periods of nonreceptivity to the male that can last 48 hours (8), that may be correlated with rhythmic increases and decreases in serum estrogen levels reflecting successive waves of maturation and atresia of ovarian follicles (Fig. 15-2**A**).

Based on laparoscopic examination of the ovaries of alpacas, it was found that growth, maintenance, and regression of a follicle each required an average of 4 days (total 12 days; range 9 to 17 days) (Fig.15-3) (15). Llamas kept in their natural habit of Peru were examined daily by transrectal ultrasonography (16). Successive dominant follicles emerged at intervals of 19.8 ± 0.7 days in unmated and vasectomized-mated llamas and 14.8 ± 0.6 days in pregnant llamas. Lactation was associated with an interwave interval that was shortened by 2.5 ± 0.05 days compared

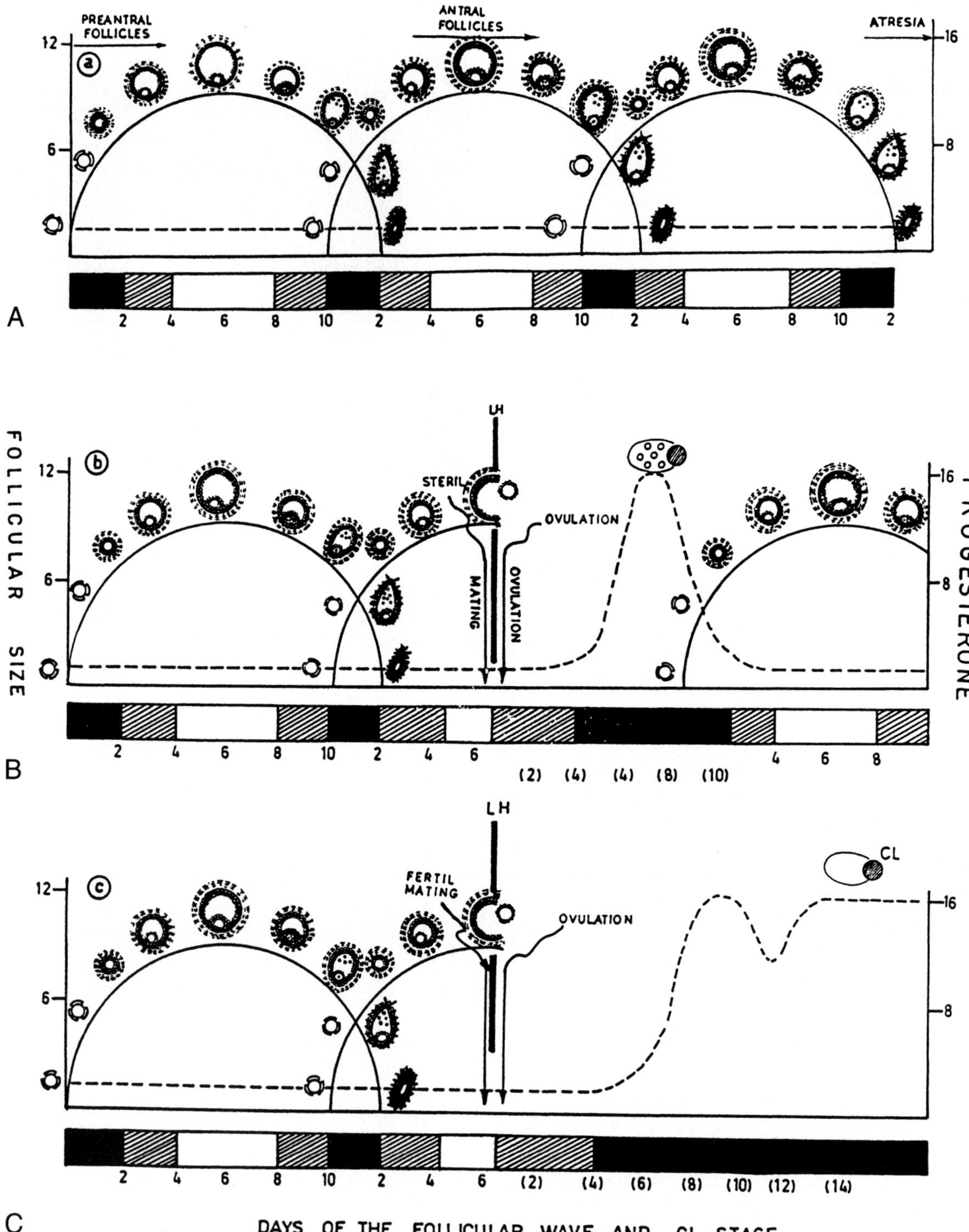


FIGURE 15-2. Diagrammatic representation of the ovarian dynamic in female alpaca. (**A**) Unmated female showing the follicular phase or wave, where follicles grow and wane in a 12-day wave-like fashion. (**B**) Mating at the appropriate time (growing mature follicles) with a sterile male and CL formation lasting 5 to 6 days. (**C**) Mating with a fertile male (at appropriate time ) and establishing pregnancy. *Solid lines*, size of the follicles; *broken lines*, blood progesterone levels; *black bars*, anestrus or female rejection of the male; *hatched bars*, passive receptivity (not true acceptance, nor true rejection); *open bars*, heat or sexual receptivity. Days between brackets, mean CL stage.

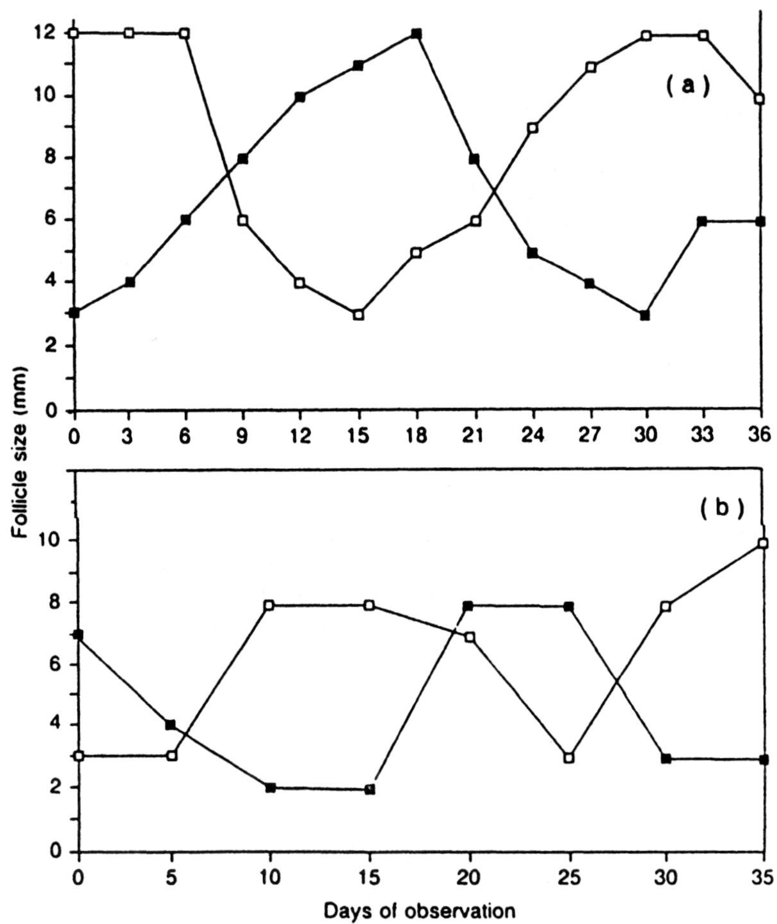


FIGURE 15-3. Alternate follicular growth in left (□) and right (■) ovaries from adult alpacas. Growth, maintenance, and regression of a follicle each require an average of 4 days (total 12 days; range 9–17 days). Panels (**a**) and (**b**) represent individual animals.

with a nonlactating group. It is difficult to explain the differences between studies, but species (alpaca vs. llama), management conditions (poor natural grassland in Peru at 4300 meters altitude vs. intensive management and feeding conditions in the United States at sea level), seasonal variations, the method of examination, and number of animals used in each experiment may be contributing factors. However, a considerable variability between individuals has been observed, regardless of reproductive status (parous vs. nonparous).

The variability that exists in both the duration of sexual receptivity and regularity of its occurrence presumably reflects the fact that in unmated females, the follicular phase is not terminated by ovulation at a predetermined time, and that there is no luteal phase to delineate the timing of events after the end of the estrous.

OVULATION. In the alpaca, the minimum time to ovulation was estimated to be 26 hours after natural mating and 24 hours after treatment with hCG (8). In receptive alpaca females allowed a single mating, 50% ovulated between 26 and 30 hours, 24% ovulated between 30 and 72 hours, and 26% failed to ovulate after mating (17). Forty percent of the animals that failed to ovulate were yearlings and 15% were adults. Using an ultrasonographic technique in llamas, ovulation was detected, on average, 2 days (range 1 to 3 days) after single mating (16, 18). Single service by an intact or vasectomized male resulted in ovulation in 77 to 82% of alpacas, and an increase in the number of services by intact males to three within a period of 24 hours did not significantly affect ovulation rate (19). Ovulation was also induced successfully using 1 mg of LH, and a dose of 4 to 8 $\mu$g of GnRH was also necessary to provide the adequate stimulus for ovulation (20).

A significant increase in serum LH concentration was observed 15 minutes after the onset of copulation, with the peak of the preovulatory surge of LH occurring at 2 hours, and values were basal by 7 hours after copulation (Fig. 15-4). A second release of LH was not detected after a second copulatory period within 24 hours of the first (21). The LH surge observed subsequent to copulation is consistent with the alpaca and llama being induced ovulators.

Females can ovulate without coital stimulation or exogenous hormones, especially when initially isolated from, and then reintroduced to, a male. The rate of expontaneous ovulation was reported to be approximately 5 to 10% in alpacas (20, 22) and 9 to 15% in llamas (14, 16).

The deposition of semen in the vagina of the Bactrian

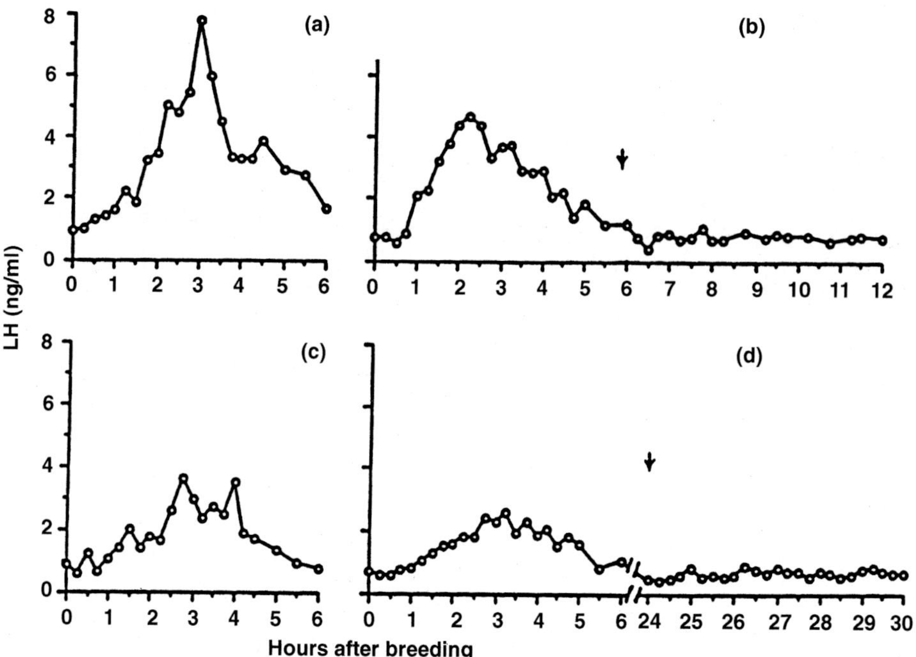


FIGURE 15-4. Time course of LH secretion in llamas after copulation. Panels **a**, **b**, **c**, and **d** represent individual animals.

camel will induce ovulation (23), which has led to the proposition that there may be an "ovulation inducing factor" (OIF) present in the camel and bull semen. Because of the close phylogenetic relationship between Old and New World Camelidae it was considered likely that similar effects would be observed in alpacas and llamas. Ovulation in alpacas and llamas can be induced by deposition of alpaca, llama, or bull semen in receptive alpacas or llamas (24). In the case of camels, the Chinese investigators proposed the presence of a GnRH like effect in the camel or bull semen. Conversely, Paolicchi et al (25) found that the alpaca semen could contain some factor or factors, different to GnRH, that can contribute with LH secretion mechanism in this specie.

No differences were found in the ovulation rate between ovaries. A corpus luteum was detected in the right ovary in 51% of the alpacas, 47% in the left one, and around 2% in both (Table 15-2) (26). In the llama a corpus luteum was detected in the right ovary in 55% of females, 44% in the left, and 1% in both ovaries (27).

CORPUS LUTEUM FUNCTION. Corpus luteum function after sterile and fertile mating has been studied in domestic camelids. After infertile matings in alpacas and llamas, progesterone in blood was elevated from day 5 and reached maximum concentrations of 10 to 20 nmol/L on day 7 to 8, and a rapid decline in progesterone occurred 9 to 10 days, in connection with repeated surge releases of prostaglandin $F_{2\alpha}$ (28). Estradiol-17$\beta$ levels were greater than 100 to 200 pmol/L during estrous when the animals were mated. A temporary increase was detected in connection with the rise in progesterone levels in the early luteal phase (Figs. 15-2**B** and 15-5). With this exception levels of estradiol stayed low, 20 to 40 pmol/L during the luteal phase, but rose in most animals after luteolysis to 40 to 60 pmol/L.

TABLE 15-2. ***Corpus Luteum and Embryo Location in Alpacas and Llamas***

| ANIMAL SPECIES | NO. OF ANIMALS | RIGHT OVARY CL | LEFT OVARY CL | BOTH OVARIES | RIGHT HORN PREGNANCY | LEFT HORN PREGNANCY |
|---|---|---|---|---|---|---|
| Alpaca | 928 | 472 (50.9%) | 440 (47.4%) | 16 (1.7%) | 16 (1.6%) | 913 (98.4%) |
| Llama | 110 | 60 (54.5%) | 49 (44.5%) | 1 (0.9%) | 1 (0.9%) | 109 (99.1%) |

Data from Fernández-Baca S, Sumar J, Novoa C, Leyva V. Relación entre la ubicación del cuerpo luteo y la localización del embrión en la alpaca. Rev Inv Pec (IVITA) Univ Nac S Marcos 1973;2:131–135; Sumar J, Leyva V. Relación entre la ubicación del cuerpo lúteo y la localización del embrión en la Llama (Lama glama). In: Proc III Conv Int sobre Camélidos Sudamericanos. Viedma, Argentina: 1979.

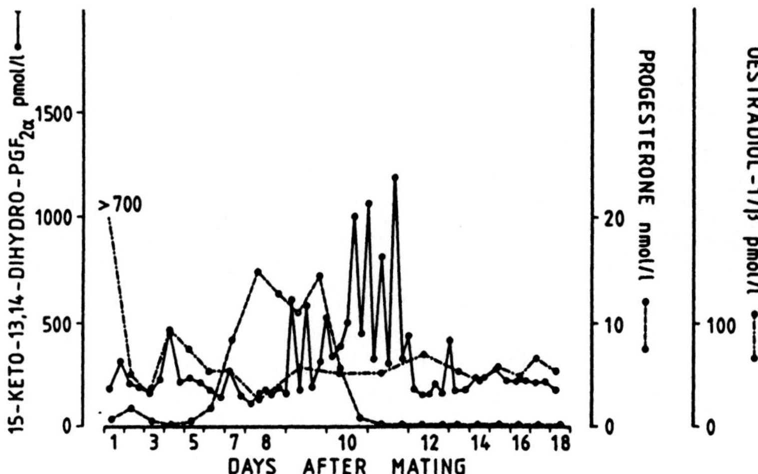


FIGURE 15-5. Levels of 15-keto-13,14-dihydro-$PGF_{2\alpha}$, estradiol-17$\beta$, and progesterone in one llama on day 1 after mating with a sterile male.

During the 3 to 4 days postcoitum, when the corpus luteum is forming and progesterone concentrations are low, most females remain receptive to the male. Plasma progesterone concentrations in female that displayed sexual receptivity at this time were between 0.06 and 0.28 ng/ml (29). In llamas, using ultrasonography, the corpus luteum was first detected on Day 3.1 ± 0.2 (ovulation is Day 0, which occurs on average 2 days after mating) in vasectomy-mated females and reached maximum diameter (13 mm) on Day 5.9 ± 0.3 (equivalent to approximately 8 days after mating) (30). Luteal diameter and plasma progesterone concentration are highly correlated. A prolonged luteal phase was not observed in any sterile-mated (nonpregnant) alpacas or llamas.

A fertile mating results in the formation of a corpus luteum that remains functional throughout gestation (Fig. 15-2C). For the first 60 days of pregnancy, luteal diameter was monitored by transrectal ultrasonography and plasma progesterone concentrations were determined in pregnant llamas (30). The corpus luteum is detected on Day 3.1 ± 0.2, and reach maximum diameter (16 mm) on Day 21 ± 1.2. There was a decrease in mean plasma progesterone concentration between Days 8 and 10, as well as a transient decrease in luteal diameter during this period. A similar decrease in progesterone between Days 8 and 11 has been reported in alpacas (31). The transient drop in progesterone is coincident with the initiation of uterine-induced luteal regression in nonpregnant animals. It has been suggested that the rescue and resurgence of the corpus luteum between 8 and 10 days postmating represent luteal response to pregnancy (maternal recognition). Plasma progesterone concentrations remained elevated until about 2 weeks before parturition (32). Thereafter they began to decline and dropped markedly during the final 24 hours before parturition. Also, progesterone concentrations during sterile and fertile matings have been followed in the milk of alpacas and llamas (31).

### *Sexual Receptivity and Mating Behavior*

In induced ovulators, there is no regular periodic delineation in the timing of events (i.e., no clearly defined estrous cycle). In the absence of copulatory stimulation, female alpacas or llamas display periods of sexual receptivity of up to 36 days, with short periods of nonreceptivity that may last 48 hours (Fig. 15-2A) (8). There appears to be considerable variability in the display of overt receptivity between individuals, regardless of parity. The variability in sexual receptivity may be primarily attributable to the degree of follicle maturity at any given state of the continuous follicular phase; however, no documentation is available in this regard.

The receptive female assumes the prone position (ventral recumbence) after a short period of pursuit by a male, or she may approach a male that is copulating with another female and adopt the prone position (8, 33). Some receptive females may occasionally display mounting behavior with other females of the herd, although such behaviour is much less common than in cattle. If the female is nonreceptive, rejection is shown by running away from and spitting at the male (33). During the very short courting phase and during mating, the males make blowing, grunting, laryngeal-nasal sounds. Copulation takes place in a recumbent position, with the male mounted above and just behind the female (33). The female assumes a very passive attitude during copulation, and in some instances when copulation is prolonged, will appear to tire and may change positions so that she is lying on her side (Fig. 15-6). Compared with other domestic species, coitus is remarkably prolonged in camelids (10 to 50 minutes) (20).

### *Pregnancy*

The length of gestation in alpacas of the Huacaya and Suri breeds has been quoted as 341 and 345 days, respectively

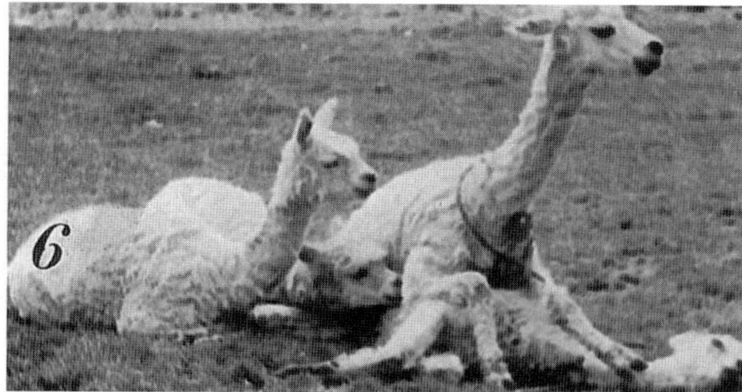


FIGURE 15-6. Copulation takes place in a recumbent position. In some instances when copulation is prolonged, the female will change positions so that she is resting on her side. Note two receptive females lying and standing close by.

(8). In llamas, the gestation length was 346 ± 8 days (327 to 357 days), and neither parity nor sex of the cria was found to influence gestation length (34). Almost all alpaca and llama fetuses occupy the left uterine horn (based on position of the conceptus and site of the umbilical attachment), even though ovulation occurs from both ovaries with equal frequency (Table 15-2) (26, 27). This indicates that embryos originating in the right side migrate to the left horn for attachment (Fig. 15-7). The reason for the right-to-left migration, which is apparently unique to Camelidae, is not well known. One explanation for this phenomenon implicated a differential luteolytic effect of the left vs. right uterine horn. The right horn effects luteolysis via a local pathway, whereas the left horn effects luteolysis via both systemic and local pathways (35).

Multiple ovulations occur in 3 to 10% of alpacas after natural mating and in 9 to 20% after treatment with gonadotropins, but twins born alive are very rare (20, 36). Sumar (37) studied the role of the corpus luteum (CL) during pregnancy in the llama and alpaca, and results indicated that the CL is necessary for the maintenance of pregnancy during the entire gestation period in both species.

PREGNANCY DIAGNOSIS. Several methods of pregnancy diagnosis have been described to assess pregnancy:

1. **Sexual Behavior.** Using teaser alpaca males (vasectomized), those females that showed behavioural receptivity 20 or more days after a previous service were found to be nonpregnant (22). However, not all the females that rejected the male were pregnant. In another study, the accuracy of pregnancy diagnosis was 84% and 95% in the alpaca and llama respectively, within 70 to 125 days of gestation, comparable to the accuracy obtained in sheep (38).
2. **Ballotement or External Palpation** is still used in the traditional breeding system in southern Peru, with an accuracy of about 80%. Pregnancy diagnosis is done by external palpation or ballotement at approximately 8 months of gestation (20).
3. **Rectal Palpation** in alpacas is possible as early as 30 days of gestation, but this method is limited because of the pelvic sizes and fat deposition in the pelvic inlet, particularly in yearling animals (38). Seventy percent of yearlings and 90% of adults alpacas can be palpated rectally. In llamas, almost 100% can be palpated, given adequate restraint, lubrication, and a skilled veterinarian, with a glove size no greater than 7. The accuracy of pregnancy diagnosis by rectal palpation at 2 months postmating was 100% in alpacas and llamas (38).
4. **Circulating Hormones:**

   **Progesterone.** Plasma progesterone change during gestation is determined by standard analytic methods as RIA and EIA. Alpacas or llamas that failed to ovulate, as well as those that failed to conceive, showed basal levels of progesterone on Day 12 and 30 after mating, while pregnant animals were observed at 1.8 ng/mL (39). False positive predictions are related to high blood progesterone concentrations, and are probably due to early embryonic loss (39). From the second to the tenth months, the lower levels of progesterone were 6.29 ± 0.61 and 8.77 ± 0.28 nmol/L in alpacas and llamas respectively.

   **Estrone Sulfate** ($E_1SO_4$). Estrone levels range between 0.02 to 1.2 nmol/L (0.26 ± 1.9) from mating until

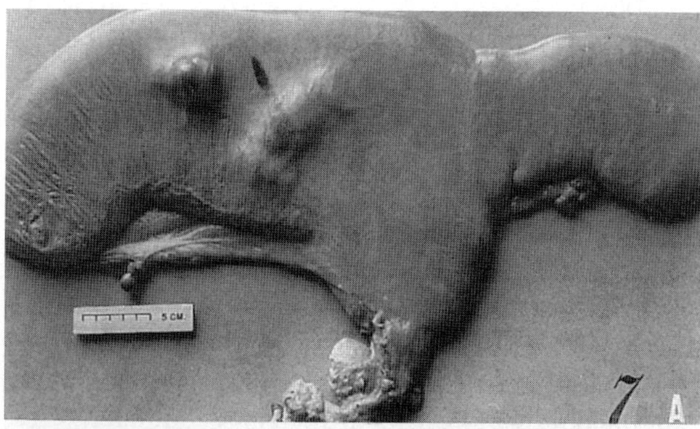


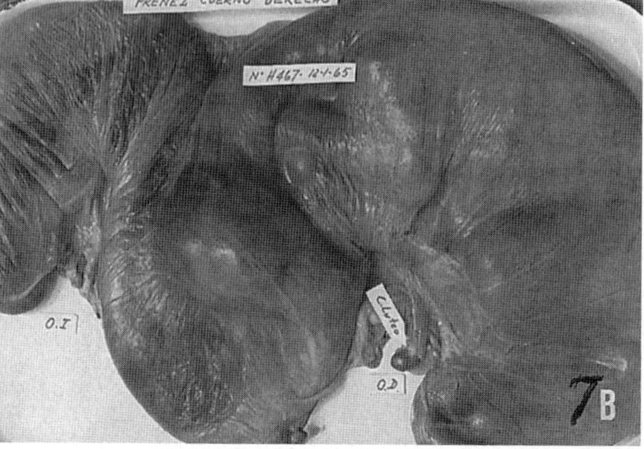


FIGURE 15-7. Site of the pregnancy in the alpaca. (**A**) Left horn pregnancy (98.4% of the cases) and (**B**) right horn pregnancy (1.6% of the cases). However, no differences were found in the ovulation rate between ovaries.

about Days 246 and 262 of gestation in alpacas and llamas (at about 8 months of pregnancy). But thereafter levels increased very rapidly, and the highest levels were monitored 3 days before parturition, at 19 and 16 nmol/L in alpacas and llamas respectively. A sharp decrease of $E_1SO_4$ was observed on Day +1 postpartum in both species, reaching basal levels at 6 to 7 days postpartum. $E_1SO_4$ can be used for advanced pregnancy diagnosis and well being of the fetus.

5. **Milk progesterone** concentration differences between lactating nonpregnant and pregnant alpacas can be observed at 12 Days after mating. These differences might furnish the basis for an early pregnancy test (31, 39).
6. **Fecal Progestagens**. By means of an assay procedure in vicuñas (wild camelids), these have been reported by Schwarzenberger et al (40). This provides a noninvasive approach to investigating reproductive events, in wild camelids.
7. **Ultrasound Techniques,** both A and B Mode, have been used. Detection of fluid filled uterus (A Mode) by means of an ultrasonic Scanopreg, Model 738 (Ithaco Inc, Ithaca, NY), developed specifically for sheep, has been used in alpacas and llamas (38). In alpacas, the highest accuracy (92%) was recorded at a mean fetal age of 80 days, compared to 90% at 70 days of gestation. In llamas, 100% accuracy was obtained at 75 days of gestation. In both species, the accuracy of the test was reduced to 84% and 65% at 165 days in alpacas and llamas.

Using a 3 MHz probe, external ultrasound diagnosis of pregnancy can be performed from 50 days until term, by applying the probe to the bare-skinned area just medial to the stifle (41). The same author reported the use of a small intrarectal probe (5 MHz) in llamas, being able to detect pregnancies as early as 15 days post mating. Transrectal ultrasonography is well suited for characterization of uterine, follicular, and luteal dynamics, ovulatory mechanism, and fetal development from 15 days after mating (16, 18).

### *Parturition*

Unassisted labor in alpacas at 4250 m above sea level in Peru lasted a mean of 203 minutes for primiparous females and 193 minutes for multiparous females (42). In llamas, a mean of 176 minutes has been reported for the three different stages of labour (43). Camelids do not lick their offspring at birth, nor do they abandon the cria, even in the face of extremely poor nutritional status (42). More than 90% of births in alpacas and llamas occur between 07:00 and 13:00 hours. This adaptation gives to the cria the best chance to get warm and dry before the coldness of the night, where even in the summer, freezing temperatures are common at altitudes higher than 4000 m (20). Camelids appears to be able to delay birthing for hours or days to avoid giving birth during the night or on cloudy, sunless, and snowy days (44). Liggins (45) postulated that the fetus may determine the day of birth, but that the mother determines the hour.

CONTROL OF PARTURITION. The arguments for attempting to regulate the onset of parturition are associated principally with managerial or veterinary considerations. Parturition was induced in alpacas, between Days 320 and 351 of pregnancy, using 10 mg of dexamethasone (Group A), dexamethasone 10 mg plus estradiol 10 mg (Group B), $PGF_{2\alpha}$ at 0.12 and 0.25 mg (Groups C and D). One group of pregnant females was considered a control group (Group E) (46). Parturition occurred within 112, 120, 25, and 25 hours, and 29 days for groups A, B, C, D, and E, respectively. The proportion of females giving birth per group were 40%, 60%, 100%, 100%, and 100%, respectively. Adverse side effects (very weak crias) due to prolonged response, were observed in groups A and B only. Not one of the experimental females was observed with retained membranes (46).

INDUCED ABORTION. From time to time the practitioner must apply some treatment to terminate gestation in different animal species. The chosen treatment is dependent on the animal species and time of pregnancy. In alpacas, where pregnancy is entirely dependent on progesterone produced by the corpus luteum, a luteolytic agent is the preferred drug. Following administration of prostaglandins (Dinoprost, Lutalyse) to alpacas and llamas at 2 to 3 and 7 to 8 months of gestation, abortion usually occurs between 26 and 35 hours after injection, showing symptoms of abortion one to four hours before expulsion of the fetus. However, one alpaca and one llama of 7 to 8 months of gestation aborted a dead fetus, without showing any symptoms of abortion, 102 and 126 hours after prostaglandin injection, respectively. In all cases, the serum progesterone levels showed a marked decline (70%) at 6 hours after $PGF_{2\alpha}$ injection and were basal, 12 hours after. No retained fetal membranes were observed.

### *Puerperium*

Up to the fourth day after parturition the female alpaca is submissive and will allow herself to be mounted by the male (47). However, luteal regression, follicular growth, and uterine involution are not complete, and the female will not ovulate or become pregnant from such early matings. Occasional fertilization occurs subsequent to mating at 5 days postpartum. By 10 days postpartum the follicles are 8 to 10 mm in size, the corpus luteum has regressed considerably, and the uterus involuted substantially (weighing only a fifth of what it did 24 hours after birth). Mating of alpaca females is recommended within 15 to 20 days after giving birth to obtain good fertility rates and one offspring per year (47).

## *Reproductive Failures*

The majority of cases of reproductive failures in females domestic camelids are due to (a) anatomical aberrations of the reproductive system and (b) endocrine upsets. Probably both causes are hereditary, so that, at least in domestic camelids, no attempt should be made to correct the anatomic or endocrine causes of sterility lest the condition be spread through a large part of the population.

CONGENITAL AND ACQUIRED DEFECTS. One survey involving large numbers of alpacas of known reproductive history indicate that anatomical abnormalities are frequent and collectively can cause economic losses by increasing perinatal mortality, decreasing maternal productivity, and reducing the value of defective crias (37). Owners should be advised to take appropriate measures to eliminate them. More than 20 congenital reproductive defects have been described in female alpacas, including both slaughterhouse animals and animals whose reproductive histories were known (37). The most frequent defect described was ovarian hipoplasia (16.8%) (Fig. 15-8), segmental aplasia of uterine horns or middle vagina (3.9%), ovarian tumors (3.2%), uterus unicornis (1.3%) (Fig. 15-9), cervix duplex (0.7%), and imperforated hymen (1.3%). Endocrine upsets include follicular cysts (8.4%) (Fig. 15-10), cystic corpus luteum (2.6%), paraovarian cysts (1.3%), hydatids of Morgagni (1.9%), and cystic Gardner's duct (0.7%). Also, large size hemorragic follicular cysts have been described (30) that were not associated with other ovarian irregularities or with infertility.

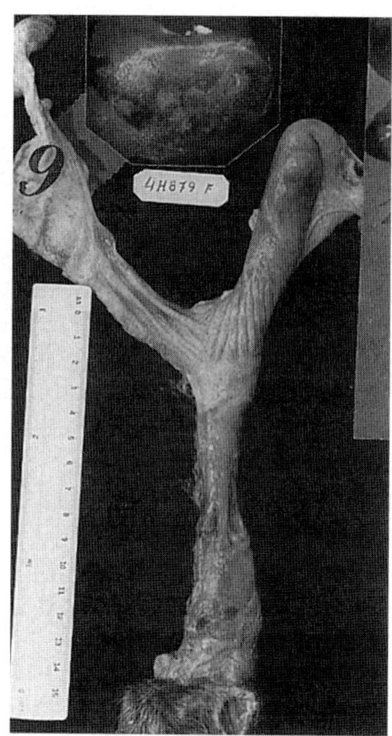


FIGURE 15-9. Uterus unicornis. Aplasia of the left uterine horn in alpaca. Also, the left kidney is missing.

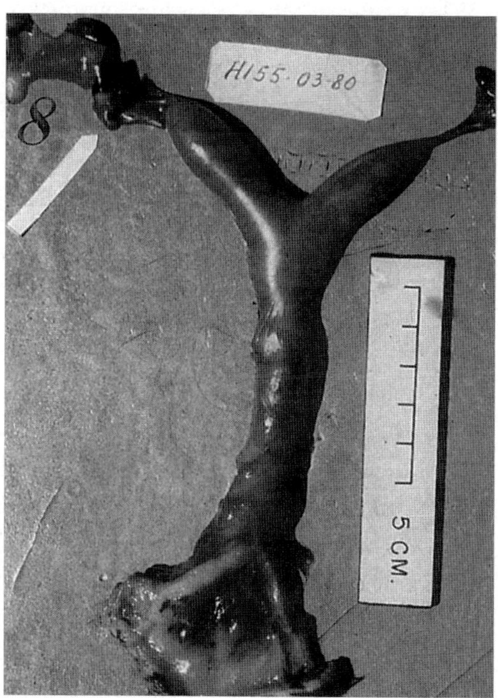


FIGURE 15-8. Bilateral hypoplasia of the ovaries with infantile tubular genitalia in alpacas. Frequent cause of infertility.

ENDOMETRITIS, MUCOMETRA, AND PIOMETRA. Endometritis refers to inflammation limited to the endometrium, and piometra refers to the accumulation of exudate in the uterine lumen (48). Most of the available data on endometritis in alpacas originate in one survey that found 1.3% and 3.4% of cases after postmortem examination (49). *Streptococcus zooepidemicus* and *Staphylococcus aureus* as well as many of the other miscellaneous bacteria, in Peru, and *Corynebacterium pyogenes* and *Escherichia coli* hemolytic in

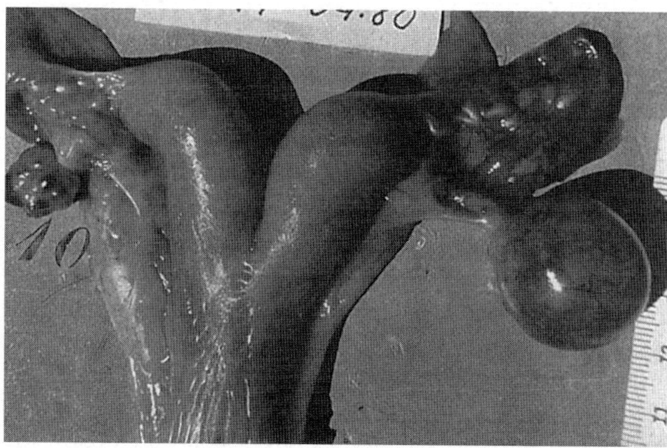


FIGURE 15-10. Follicular cyst in the right ovary of one alpaca, associated with infertility cases.

the United States, have been associated with uterine infections (50, 51). These bacteria gain their entrance more often during the puerperium, and also after mating. Vaginal examination should be conducted in all case of suspected endometritis. Observed purulent discharge from the external os of the cervix remains the only practical evidence of endometritis. A history of conception failure or dystocia, retained placenta, or purulent discharge during the immediate postpartum period, lends support to diagnosis of endometritis.

Endometritis is identified as a cause of infertility in llamas in the United States (52). The problem is associated with a history of repeated unsuccessful breedings in multiparous llamas 20 days or more after parturition. History, clinical examinations, transrectal palpation, ultrasonography, endometrial culture, and biopsy may be indicated to confirm a tentative diagnosis of endometritis (52). A true venereal disease has not been described in Peru. Specific infections of the uterus, as brucellosis, caused by *Brucella melitensis* has been reported only in one single herd in Peru.

In a very large herd with widespread infertility, Ludeña et al (53) described the presence of metritis in alpacas (2.3%), caused by a diverse nonspecific infective agents, but in no case specific infections such as trichomoniasis or vibriosis were found. In general, alpacas are free of diseases such as brucellosis, trichomoniasis, and vibriosis. We do not know if alpacas are resistant to infection of the genital apparatus or other intervening factors that could explain the absence of these diseases.

Mucometra is an accumulation of mucinous fluid in the uterine lumen. There were six cases of mucometra in alpacas, with segmental aplasia of the vagina (49). The uterine content consisted of a pus-like material that ranged in volume from 10 to 50 mL. Where the uterine wall is remarkably thin this may simulate pregnancy. The endometrium became thinner as the volume of uterine fluid increased. Vets should be aware of this condition when transrectal palpation is performed in llamas and alpacas. Piometra has not been diagnosed in alpacas and frequently is confused with mucometra. According to Peter and Smith (52), piometra is rarely observed in llamas and detailed studies are lacking.

**EMBRYONIC AND FETAL LOSS.** Diverse studies have established that prenatal loss attains considerable levels in all farm animals, and that the bulk of this loss occurs during the early embryonic stages. In an early study, more that 80% of the ova recovered 3 days after mating were in process of dividing, and only 50% of the fertilized ova survived for more that 30 days of gestation in alpacas (22). Factors responsible for this high rate of embryonic mortality is unknown, but nutritional constraints, hormonal imbalances, and chromosomal aberrations may be principal etiologies. These studies were conducted in alpacas living in their natural habitat, affected by a harsh natural environment, deteriorating feed supply, and the presence of infectious/parasitic diseases.

Table 15-3 shows the mean level of plasma progesterone in female alpacas and llamas that were mated with fertile males. Progesterone concentration on Day 8 postservice showed a tendency to be higher in pregnant than in non-pregnant animals ($P < .05$) (39). Whether these levels are higher in pregnant animals owing to the presence of a live embryo, or lower in non-pregnant animals because of the incapability of the corpus luteum to secrete progesterone, is still unknown. Peter and Smith (52) speculated that luteal insufficiency and subclinical endometritis might be involved in embryonic loss.

**ABORTION.** Losses occurring from differentiation (42 days) until parturition are termed abortion, and in some cases premature delivery. The causes of abortion include infectious and noninfectious (genetic, thermal, nutritional,

**TABLE 15-3. *Mean Plasma Progesterone Levels (nmol/L) in Female Alpacas and Llamas Mated with Fertile Males***

| | ALPACAS (n = 12) | | LLAMAS (n = 10) | |
|---|---|---|---|---|
| DAY | *Pregnant* | *Non-pregnant* | *Pregnant* | *Non-pregnant* |
| | 0.32 | 0.38 | 0.53 | 0.45 |
| 5 | 2.46 | 1.46 | 1.93 | 1.38 |
| 8 | 18.50 | 12.03 | 16.41 | 10.90 |
| 9 | 16.34 | 3.20 | 17.81 | 14.10 |
| 10 | 13.70 | 0.76 | 20.70 | 6.90 |
| 11 | 12.84 | | 25.13 | 2.90 |
| 12 | 16.00 | | 23.28 | 0.28 |

Data From Sumar J, Alarcón, Echevarría L. Niveles de progesterona periférica en alpacas y llamas y su aplicación en el diagnóstico precoz de gestación y otros usos clínicos. Acta Andina 1993;2:161–167.

toxic, stress). The proportion of abortions due to infectious agents is not known in domestic camelids. However, of those abortions in which the cause is determined, the majority of them were infectious, produced mainly by *Brucella melitensis* (51) and acute attacks of *Fasciola hepatica.*

Brucellosis in alpacas is characterized by abortion in the last trimester of gestation (month 8 through 11.5). Also premature delivery has been observed, the crias dying within in few hours. Large numbers of the organisms are expelled with the fetus and placenta contaminating the environment and allowing transmission to other susceptible camelids and humans. The lesions observed in the fetus and placenta are similar to those observed in cattle. In cases of abortions, no retained placenta has been observed. The diagnostic methods for brucellosis are serologic and bacteriologic. In the United States abortions are due to chlamydial infection, leptospirosis, toxoplasmosis, pine needle ingestion, stress after the use of clostridial vaccines, and also high levels of selenium (13).

In Peru in the last four years, thousands of alpacas has been introduced to other environments, some of them highly contaminated with the liver fluke *Fasciola hepatica.* Approximately 20 days after the introduction to these contaminated areas, advanced gestation alpacas expulsed a normal fetus and placenta, with no recognizable gross lesions. Postmortem studies showed mainly hepatomegalia and abundant yellow fluid in the abdomen. Owners and veterinarians must be aware of this disease when moving animals.

Twinning. Twins born alive are very rare, despite the observation of multiple ovulations (36). Cases of twin pregnancies in alpacas, seen in the early stages of gestation (no longer than 40 days of gestation) are not uncommon (Fig. 15-11) (37). Embryo reduction occurs and probably a single embryo continues to develop. Twins births in llamas may be somewhat more common than in alpacas, and a few cases have been reported in the United States (50). Nearly all alpaca and llama twins are of the fraternal or dizygotic type. Monozygotic twin pregnancies are rare. Similar to the mare, in 95% of alpacas or llamas with twin ovulations one or both ova or embryos are lost early in the gestation period, and this can be another cause of infertility in domestic camelids. In twin pregnancies proceeding to term, one is expelled live and the other frequently small or very weak.

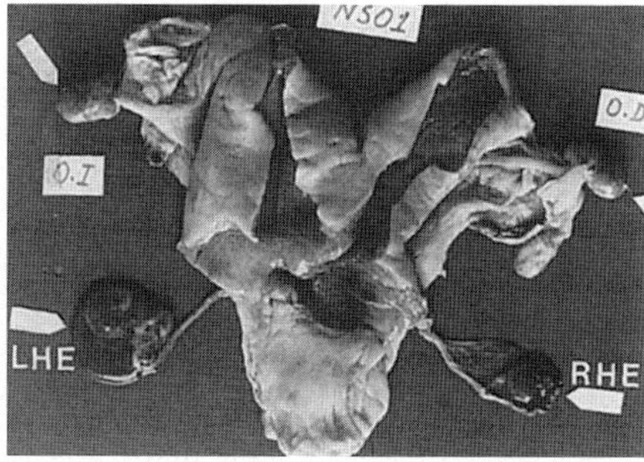


Figure 15-11. Twin pregnancy in alpacas, in early stage of gestation. Note the embryo of the left horn (LHE) is apparently healthy, and dead embryo at the right uterine horn (RHE).

## Male

### *Reproductive Anatomy*

In the adult alpaca the testis are found in a nonpendulant scrotum without a defined neck, and forming a subanal protuberance, Type 5 of the classification of Carrick and Setchell (54). Testis are small and elliptical, located in such a way that the major diameter is oblique with a dorsal and caudal orientation. Normally, both testicles are of the same size, firm, with a free movement inside the scrotum. The small epididymus is firmly connected to the testes, formed of a head, body, and tail. The average weight of one fully developed alpaca testis is approximately 17 g (13–28 g), measuring between 4 and 5 cm in length and 2.5 to 3.0 cm in depth (37).

Llama testis weigh about 12 gm at 2.5 years (83 kg liveweight of the animal), measuring 3.5 cm by 2.2 cm, with a volume of 13 mL. At 5.5 years of age, llama testis weigh about 24 gm, measuring 5.0 cm by 2.7 cm, with a volume of 22 mL. Considerable variation occurs regarding testicle size and liveweight in llamas and alpacas; the weight of each testicle will vary between 0.02 and 0.03% of the body weight. The deferent duct is very thin (2 mm) at its beginning, and thickens (3 mm) when it reaches the abdominal cavity and ends near the bladder, forming what in other species is the ampullae or ampullary glands (42).

The alpaca prostate has an H-shape, lying dorsally and laterally above the neck of the bladder. It is approximately 3 cm by 2 cm by 2 cm in size, not easily palpable per rectum. The bulbo-urethral glands are oval, located at the sides of the urethra in the pelvic outlet. Camelids have no vesicular gland. The penis is fibroelastic, with its end in the form of a curved hook, clockwise direction, and has a small cartilaginous projection of 1 cm in length that could correspond to the "uretral process" (Fig. 15-12). The size of the erect penis in the alpaca is 35 to 40 cm and the sigmoid flexure is prescrotal. The prepuce is small, 15 cm caudal to the umbilicus, with a triangular-shaped opening, and oriented towards the tail (1). During urination camelids direct the stream of urine backward between the hind legs. The protractor prepucial muscle pulls the prepuce forward prior to mating, changing the direction of the prepucial opening and thus allowing for the penis to be directed forward.

### *Puberty*

At birth, the penis is completely adherent to the prepuce. The adherences disappear gradually with growth of the ani-

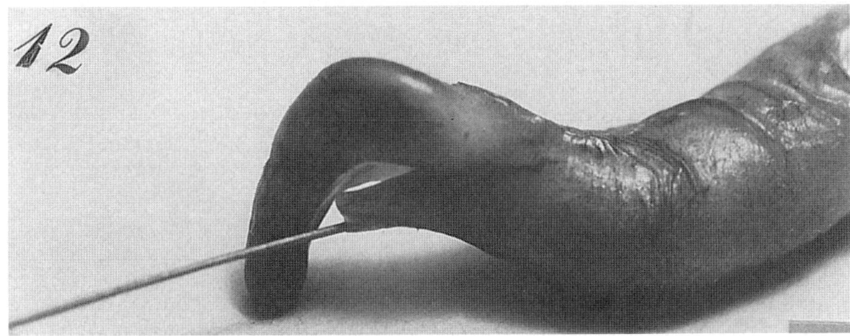


FIGURE 15-12. The *glans penis* of an alpaca, showing a blunt cartilaginous hook, clockwise direction, and a ventral short "urethral process" with a wire in its lumen.

mal under the influence of testosterone (37, 42). At 1 year of age the males show sexual interest in the females; however, only about 8% of the alpaca males show a complete liberation of the penis-prepuce adherences and are capable of performing copulation (Fig. 15-13) (42). At 2 years of age, approximately 70% of the males are free of the adherences, and 100% at three years of age. However, puberty occurs when the male is capable of producing spermatozoa. Postnatal development of spermatogenesis in alpacas was carefully studied by Montalvo et al (55). From 2 to 11 months, the testis grew slowly (infantile stage) showing a sequential increase of the size of the noncanalized sex cords with undifferentiated Leydig cells in the connective tissue. At about 12 months of age, the sex cord starts showing distinct lumen, containing two cell types: the supporting cells and gonocytes. These last cells start to change to give rise to spermatogonias, and the first spermatozoa appears at about 18 months of age with half of the animals having spermatozoa in the caput epididymides. From 18 months the Leydig cell appears very well formed and the number increase considerably. By 20 to 24 months of age the spermatogenesis is more evident, and the diameters of the tubules were greatly increased, with considerable spermatozoa number in the caput epididymides. All alpacas older than

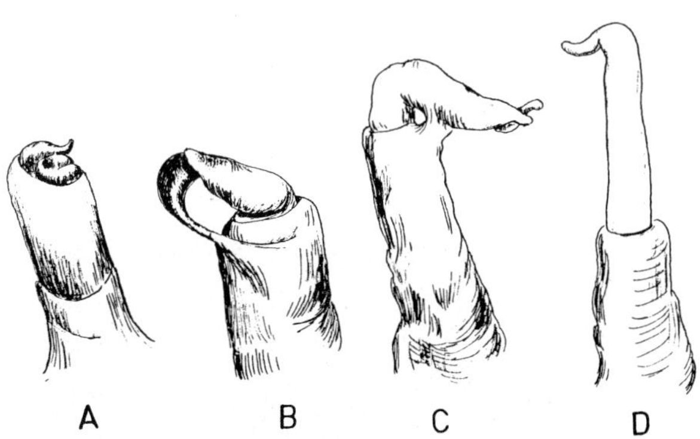


FIGURE 15-13. Penis of an alpaca, showing the different stages of separation of the free end of the penis from its penile prepuce. (**A**) Complete adherences, showing only the tip of the so called "uretral process." (**B**) Beginning of the separation showing the uretral process free of adherences, and the firm hook curved is still adherent. (**C**) The *glans penis* is completely free of adherences, but the posterior part is still adherent. (**D**) Penis totally free from prepuce adherences.

3 years have sperm in both epididymides. Spermatogenesis is initiated in some alpacas as early as 16 months, and in others as late as 26 months (55).

Precocious behavior and early mating are considered desirable traits in genetic selection programs. Future sires are those that do not have prepuce-penis adherences as yearlings. However, the general practice is to use the males for reproduction at 3 years of age (42). In llamas, puberty, based only in penis-prepuce detachment, is attained at an average of 21 months of age (range of 9 to 31 months), having a liveweight of 70 kg (range of 48 to 92 kg) (56). Testosterone concentration starts to increase exponentially at 21 months of age (300 pg/mL), reaching a plateau at 30 months of age (650 pg/mL).

### *Sexual Season*

Alpaca and llama females showed reproductive periodicity under Peruvian climatic and management conditions, but males of these species show much less seasonal variation in libido and testicular function. The male alpaca is capable of producing fertile ejaculates year round, but as in other males domestic species, the seminal quality as well as the libido are affected by the season of the year and the availability of feed (55).

An attempt was made to define the seasonality of reproduction in male alpacas and llamas in the Southern Hemisphere (Peru) by measurement of testosterone concentration in the blood (57). Plasma testosterone content was determined by RIA techniques. Results showed that the two species exhibited a marked elevation of plasma testosterone concentration during spring and summer months (breeding season), while lower levels occurred in autumn and winter months (Table 15-4). These seasonal variations resulted primarily from changes in environmental factors, food availability, temperature, light, and pheromones.

### *Sexual Behavior*

Field observations have shown a sui generis behaviour of the alpaca male. He shows an active, and sometimes aggressive attitude during mating, in contrast to the passive attitude

TABLE 15-4. ***Peripheral Testosterone Levels (pg/mL; mean ± SE) in Alpacas and Llamas in Different Seasons of the Year***

| MONTH | ALPACAS | LLAMAS |
|---|---|---|
| MARCH | 1142 ± 108 | 208 ± 52 |
| JUNE | 992 ± 388 | 37 ± 14.9 |
| SEPTEMBER | 877 ± 91 | 291 ± 74 |
| DECEMBER | 2445 ± 694 | 362 ± 73 |

Data from Sumar J, Franco J, Alarcón V. Niveles de Testosterona circulante en la alpaca (Lama pacos) y llama (Lama glama) en diversas estaciones del año. In: Proc 2nd Jornadas Int de Biopatología Andina, Cusco, Peru, 1990.

of the female (19). The display of mating activity of male alpacas when introduced into a herd of females is rather remarkable. After intense copulatory activity during the first 3 days, there is a considerable decline in spite of the presence of receptive females. Even more remarkable is the observation that when these inactive males are taken to a new herd of females they resume their sexual activity (10). The continuos association of males and females somehow inhibits, after a certain period of time, the sexual activity of the males, a situation that may prevent matings of females returning to estrous after a sterile mating or early embryonic death.

### *Semen Production and Characteristics*

In the only report available, the cycle of the seminiferous epithelium of the llama is divided into eight stages, describing the cell population making up each stage. The relative frequencies of these stages in llamas were different from those described in the camel (*Camelus dromedarius*) (58). Several methods are used for semen collection: intravaginal sacs or condoms, intravaginal sponges or pessaries, electroejaculation, postcoital vaginal aspiration, and fistulation of the urethra (31). The use of an artificial vagina (AV) mounted inside a dummy, more natural and reliable than the other methods, is the method that provides the most natural and physiological sample of semen (Fig. 15-14) (59). This AV, similar to a AV for sheep but simulating a cervix by means of a coil spring, was mounted under and inside a dummy or phantom. The coil spring was a "sine qua non requisite" to obtain semen, because alpacas or llamas penetrate the cervix to deposit the semen in the uterus (60). To maintain the temperature the warm water was changed each 10 minutes or wrapped with a heating pad (called by some authors "modified AV").

The color of the alpaca semen is milky white to crystalline white. The volume is very variable, depending of the collection method. However the best results were obtained with the AV and the uretral fistula. An average of 3.00 mL of alpaca semen was collected with AV in each 10-minute collection, obtaining up to 12.5 mL from one male in 30 minutes of collection, with three changes of water (59). By means of the uretral fistula, Kubicek (61) reported volumes of 8 and 9 mL for two males (range from 1 to 21 mL), and in one male 18 and 21 mL. Recently, llama semen was collected using an AV mounted inside a surrogate, that

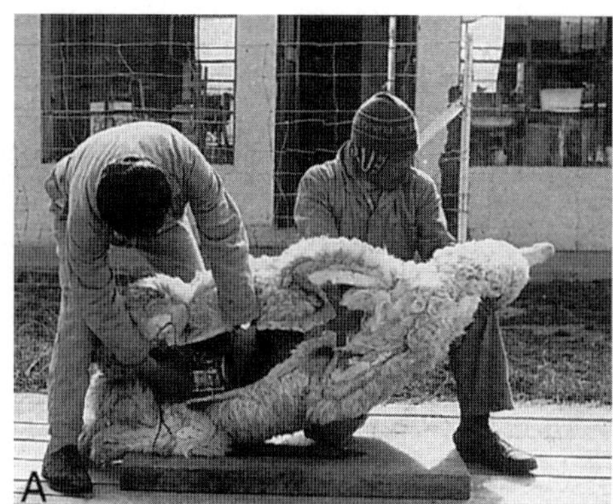


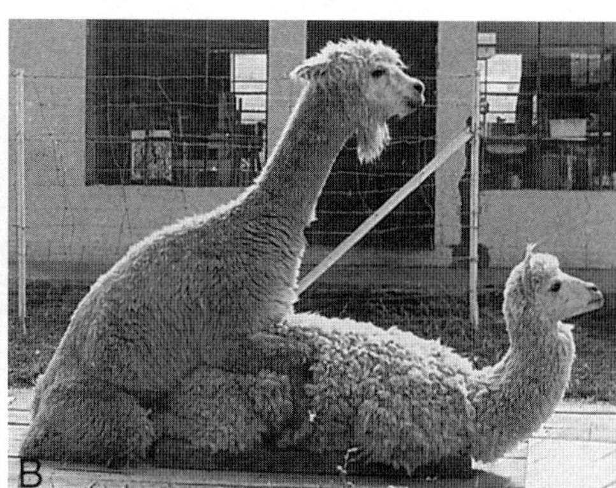


FIGURE 15-14. Semen collection in alpacas. (**A**) Introducing the Artificial Vagina inside a dummy. (**B**) Male in perfect position copulating with the dummy.

consisted of a rigid fiberglass shell which fit over and extended approximately 60 cm caudal to the hindquarters of a recumbent receptive female llama, obtaining an average of 3.0 ± 1.9 mL (62).

In alpacas the pH values given by several authors are very close to neutrality, with some tendency to light alkalinity (31). The pH is increased in urine-contaminated semen, especially after electroejaculation, and appropriate pH paper might be used to test for urine contamination. The semen of the alpaca and llama are highly viscous, making the evaluation of seminal quality very difficult. The spermatozoal motility was assessed with light microscopy. Owing to the high viscosity of the seminal plasma, no "mass motility" exists (no swirls), and the gross or progressive individual motility is very slow (6, 63).

The high viscosity of the alpaca and llama semen makes difficult the assessment of concentration. From the different methods studied, electroejaculation increases tremendously the variability in spermatozoal concentrations. The AV gives the most reliable results, with an average of $0.3 \times 10^6$ sperm per $\mu$L (64). Concentrations of 0.001 to $0.25 \times 10^6$ sperm per $\mu$L was collected with electroejaculations, and with the urethral fistula, concentrations ranging from 0.06 to $0.6 \times 10^6$ sperm per $\mu$L were found.

Grossly abnormal forms of spermatozoa, as proximal cytoplasmic droplets, distal cytoplasmic droplets, bent tails, microheads, twin heads, and broken tails, have been described in the alpaca, with semen collected with an AV (31). In llamas, morphologically abnormal spermatozoa were categorized as abnormal heads (20%), free heads (9%), abnormal acrosomes (13%), abnormal midpieces (1%), cytoplasmic droplets (11%), and abnormal tails (7%) (65). The proportion of the abnormal spermatozoa is very high, indicating that there is no proper semen collection procedure, nor a specific scoring system for camelid semen.

## *Reproductive Capacity*

Reproductive capacity in males can be assessed combining three factors: daily sperm production, extragonadal sperm reserves, and sperm output. One criterion for judging a bull or ram fertility is the daily sperm output. According to Setchell (66), two factors determine the number of spermatozoa produced by the testis: weight of testes and sperm production per unit weight of testis. In bulls, a relatively accurate estimation of sperm output is determined by scrotal circumference and testicular weight is significantly correlated with daily sperm production (67). Thus, daily sperm production can be estimated in a living animal by measuring total scrotal width or calculating testicular volume.

In alpaca males, the average weight of a fully developed testicle is approximately 17 g, with an average body weight of 63 kg (37). Daily sperm production is very low. In one study, one male was allowed up to 8 services per day (Treatment A) while the other was restricted to 4 services per day (Treatment B), on a regimen of two consecutive days of mating followed by a resting period of two days. The results indicate that:

a) Conception rates showed a decreasing tendency with repeated services on the same day, being 34% in treatment A, compared with 59% in treatment B ($P < .01$).
b) The copulatory activity decreased as breeding time progressed, and was more drastic in the male with more copulations per day.
c) The average length of fertile services is significantly longer than services that are not fertile (68).

The extragonadal sperm reserves are the total number of sperm within the epididymis and ductus deferens, and they are probably influenced by the size of the animal and ejaculation frequency. In the alpaca, the epididymis, especially caput, are very small, weighing about 1.7 g, and the ductus deferens very narrow with a 40 cm length (69). The extragonadal sperm reserves in alpacas and llamas are very low. Therefore, breeding males should be used carefully in order to avoid exhaustion of the very low sperm production that can severely impair fertility.

## *Reproductive Failures*

CONGENITAL AND ACQUIRED DEFECTS. One survey involving 3015 breeding males from farms located in the high Andes of Peru revealed that 18.1% were affected by different anomalies of the genital tract (37). Testicular hipoplasia was the most common abnormality (9.9%) with bilateral hipoplasia being more frequent (5.6%) that either left (2.7%) or right unilateral hipoplasia (1.6%) (Fig. 15-15). Cryptorchidism, including cases of ectopic testes, was found in 8.2% of the examined animals. The left side was more affected than right.

In another investigation of the genital organs of 792 male alpacas slaughtered for various reasons, 30% of the organs showed abnormalities. In this material 10.8% has testicular hipoplasia, 4.9% had cryptorchidism or ectopic testes, and 14.5% were found to have cystic formation of the mesonephric tubules. These cysts were similar to those common in stallions and boars, and they are not considered to have an adverse effect in fertility, unless the cyst becomes very large. The majority of the abnormalities encountered are probably hereditary. Abnormalities of infectious origin, like epididimitis and orchitis which are frequent in sheep and cattle, are absent, particularly among males.

DELAYED TESTICULAR DESCENT. During embryonic development, the testes of all mammalian species are located in the abdomen. The descent of the testis occurs through the inguinal canal, so at birth both testicles should be at the scrotum. In the alpaca, at birth or some days latter, the testicles are found in the scrotum, very small and flaccid. At one year of age, which is usually the time when future

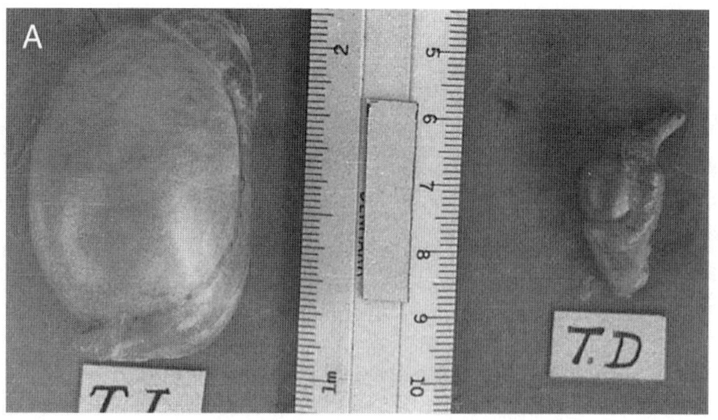


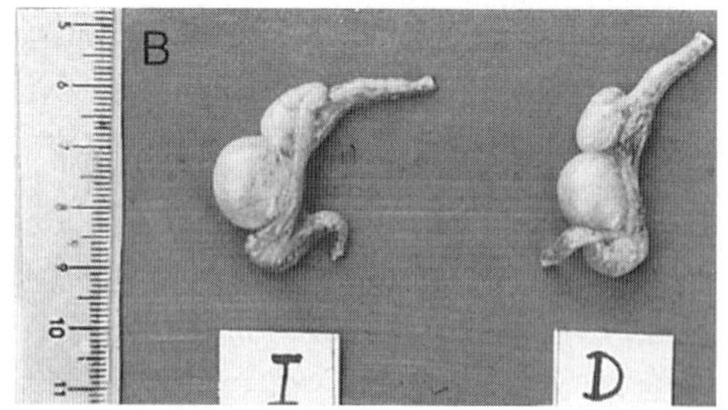


FIGURE 15-15. Testis hypoplasia in alpacas. (**A**) Unilateral right hypoplasia (*TD*), and normal left testicle (*TI*). (**B**) Bilateral hypoplasia (*I*, left testicle; *D*, right testicle).

sires are selected, both testicles should be located in the scrotum, and measure 1.1 cm to 1.4 cm long (37). However, it is very common to find that the descensus of both testicles is delayed, and much more common is to find that only one testicle has entered the scrotum, followed some time later by the other testicle.

A reduction on the plane of nutrition causes a marked delayed in puberty. The breeding of alpacas or llamas in the Peruvian highlands is subject to severe drought, and the caloric and protein intake is reduced, as well as some minerals such as phosphorus and sodium and some vitamins (70). Therefore it is very important to give high priority to nutrition. Not only is it essential to provide adequate feed for the alpacas and llama crias to attain puberty, but the young animal should be provided a diet that will insure adequate postpuberal growth and maximize fertility. As we will see, sperm output is directly related to testicular size in young animals, small testes mean low output and also may mean fewer pregnant females.

PRIAPISM. One disease that frequently is observed in the breeding herds of alpacas is a kind of "priapism." This should be paid close attention, otherwise the male is profoundly affected and discarded as a breeding male. This disease is characterized because the male is unable to retract the penis into the prepuce. The glans penis and about one third of the penis are exposed to the environments, lesions, and contamination with foreign material, ulcers, wounds, and serious infections (31).

The fundamental mechanism of erection is relaxation of smooth muscle cells, namely those of the arteries supplying the cavernous bodies and those of the retractor penis muscle. On the other hand, a principal mechanism maintaining the penis in the relaxed state is contraction of these smooth muscle cells.

## *Artificial Insemination (AI)*

Several studies have been made on the feasibility of AI using fresh semen and using the rectopalpation method, depositing the semen in the corpus uteri or in the right uterine horn (64, 71). Interspecies crosses have also been tested between alpaca and vicuña (the F1 is known as paco-vicuña), and between llama and vicuña (llama-vicuña). In one study conducted to determine the most appropriate time for insemination (after ovulation had been induced with vasectomized males and with hCG), the highest proportion of fertilized ova occurred 35 to 45 hours following induction of ovulation (72). The fertility rates were higher using vasectomized males to induce ovulation than when using hCG.

Further studies using vicuña semen (V) and paco-vicuña semen with female alpacas (A) and llamas (Ll) were conducted (64). The birth rate obtained crossing vicuña with llama was 16.7% (½V-½A), and crossing vicuña with alpaca was 22% (½V-½A). Crossing of the paco-vicuña with llama produced a 60% birth rate (¼A-¼V-½Ll), and 31.1% birth rate for paco-vicuña semen with alpaca (¾A-¼V). Domestic and wild camelids offer advantages over other animal species in the potential use of artificial insemination, since females are in continuous estrus during the breeding season, ovulation can be induced with vasectomized males, synchronization of donor/recipient is possible, and the insemination can be intrauterine (72).

## *Embryo Transfer*

Superovulation, cryopreservation of embryos, embryo transfer, *in vitro* fertilization, and *in vitro* maturation of oocytes for use in domestic South American camelids have been reported (73, 74)

SUPEROVULATION OF DONORS. The first attempt in superovulating three alpacas was reported by Novoa and Sumar (75), using 1200 IU of PMSG subcutaneously (Gestyl, Organon) given in three consecutive daily doses of 400 IU. Twenty-four hours after the last PMSG injection, the females were given endovenously 750 IU of HCG (Pregnyl, Organon), and immediately the female was mated with a fertile male. Seventy-two hours after mating, the females were sedated and three embryos of each female were collected surgically. No accounts were given about the follicular growth and number of CL.

Recent studies reported successful superstimulation with eCG or pituitary FSH in the presence of an induced CL or a progestagen treatment (for the control of the follicular wave) and ovulation has been induced with GnRH and mating or hCG (76–78). Superstimulation was successful with eCG when follicles were 3 mm in size and after a complete follicle wave had been determined by ultrasonography (79). eCG doses of 500 and 1000 IU are appropriate for inducing multiple follicular growth in llamas, and a dose of 2000 IU of eCG hyperstimulated the ovaries, resulting in more cystic follicles than occurred in response to lower doses. As in other species, there is wide variation in individual responses to eCG. The superovulation response of the females varied greatly between animals, and the embryo recovery rate was very low (77, 78).

**RECOVERY PROCEDURES.** Embryos from donor alpacas have been collected either surgically or nonsurgically. Zygotes collected from the oviduct of alpacas by abdominal laparotomy were reported by Novoa and Sumar (75). The zygotes were flushed from the oviduct to the uterus (because is impossible to pass from the uterus to the oviduct due to the presence of a special valve in the utero-tubal junction) and collected through an incision in the uterine wall. The recovery rate in single ovulating alpacas was around 80%.

Nonsurgical techniques used in other domestic animals for the recovery of embryos have been successfully adapted for use in llamas and alpacas (76, 80–82); embryo recovery is usually attempted 7 days after mating or GnRH injection. Alpaca or llama embryos enter the uterus around Day 4 or 5 (day of mating is Day 0). However, the embryo recovery rate was not higher than 50% (78). Brogliatti et al (83), using a transvaginal ultrasound-guided technique for oocyte collection in llamas, reported a 64% collection rate.

**RECIPIENT MANAGEMENT AND EMBRYO TRANSFER.** Recipient females were synchronized with a single injection of hCG in receptive alpaca females (75, 84), or GnRH at mating the female llama donor (85). Embryos were loaded in an inseminating pipette and transferred surgically to the left uterine horn (75), or transcervically manipulated with a Cassou gun, with the embryo loaded in a 0.25 mL straw and deposited in the tip of the uterine horn, ipsilateral to the CL (85). Embryo migration from right to left uterine horn could be a cause of embryo mortality (22); therefore, the embryos must always be deposited in the left uterine horn.

Over the past 26 years, 11 crias have been born throughout the world as a result of embryo transfer techniques (73). Researchers from Peru reported a successful surgical embryo transfer and live birth of one alpaca and three late abortions (84), and the first llama born by nonsurgical collection and transfer technique was done in the United States (82). Later, six live crias were born in the United Kingdom between 1992 and 1995, and in Chile, the birth of one llama cria after two nonsurgical embryo transfers was reported in 1994 (73).

**IVF TECHNOLOGY.** Llama oocytes were collected by mincing the ovary with a razor blade and by aspiration from ovarian follicles 2 to 11 mm in diameter (81); and the first IVF report and development of IVM llama oocytes using epididymal spermatozoa and llama oviductal cell coculture (LLOEC) was reported (86). From a large number of oocytes examined for signs of fertilization, 29.2% were penetrated by spermatozoa with 57.1% of the penetrated oocytes having a male and female pronucleus. There is also evidence to suggest that a longer period of time is necessary for oocyte maturation in alpacas and llamas than in other species such as the cow (36 h vs. 24 h). Llama embryo/trophoblast expansion ranged from a mean of 1.2 mm in diameter on Day 6.5 to 7.5, to 83 mm in length on Day 13 to 14. This accelerated rate of embryo development may be related to the apparent early maternal recognition of pregnancy in these species (30).

## REFERENCES


1. Sato A, Montoya L. Aparato reproductor de la alpaca (Lama pacos). Anatomía Macroscópica. Rev de Camélidos Sudamericanos 7. Univ Nac M de San Marcos, Lima, Peru, 1990.
2. Steven DH, Burton GJ, Sumar J, Nathanielsz PW. Ultrastructural Observations on the Placenta of the Alpaca (Lama pacos). Placenta 1980;1:21–32.
3. Sumar J. Reproduction in llamas and alpacas. Animal Reprod Science 1997;42:405–415.
4. Merk H, Boer M, Rath D, Schoo HA. The presence of an additional fetal membrane and its function in the newborn guanaco (Lama guanicoe). Theriogenology 1988;30:437–439.
5. Novoa C, Fernández-Baca S, Sumar J, Leyva. Pubertad en la alpaca. Rev Inv Pec (IVITA) Univ Nac M S Marcos 1972;1:29–35.
6. Leyva V, Sumar J. Evaluación del peso corporal al empadre sobre la capacidad reproductiva de hembras alpaca de un aão de edad. In: Proc IV Conv Int sobre Camélidos Sudamericanos, Punta Arenas, Chile. (Abstract 1), 1981.
7. Bustinza V, Medina G. Crecimiento de alpacas. In: Proc V Cong Intde Sistemas Agropecuarios Andinos Puno, Peru. 1986.
8. San Martín M, Copaira M, Zúãiga J, Rodríguez R, Bustinza G, Acosta, L. Aspects of Reproduction in the Alpaca. J Reprod Fert 1968;16:395.
9. Franklin WL. Contrasting socioecologies of South America's wild camelids: The vicuña and guanaco. In: Eisenbery JF, Kleinman, eds. Advances in the Study of Mammalian Behaviour. Special Publication of the American Society of Mammalogist 1983;7:573–629.

10. Fernández-Baca S, Sumar J, Novoa C. Comportamiento de la alpaca macho frente a la renovación de las hembras. Rev Inv Pec (IVITA). Univ Nac M S Marcos 1972;1:115–128.
11. Fernández-Baca S, Novoa C, Sumar J. Actividad reproductiva en la alpaca mantenida en separación del macho. Mem ALPA 1972;7:7–18.
12. Schmidt CR. Breeding season and notes on some other aspects of reproduction in captive camelids. Int Zoo Yearbook 1973;13:387–390.
13. Johnson LW. Llama Reproduction. In: Llama Medicine. Workshop for Veterinarians. Fort Collins, Colorado: Colorado State University, 1988.
14. England BG, Foote WC, Matthews DH, Cardozo AG, Riera S. Ovulation and corpus luteum function in the llama (Lama glama). J Endocrinology 1969;45:505–513.
15. Bravo PW, Sumar J. Laparoscopic Examination of the Ovarian Activity in Alpaca. Anim Reprod Sci 1989;21:271–281.
16. Adams GP, Sumar J, Ginther OJ. Effects of lactational and reproductive status on ovarian follicular waves in llamas (Lama glama). J Reprod Fert 1990;90:535–545.
17. Sumar J, Bravo PW, Foote WC. Sexual receptivity and time of ovulation in alpacas. Small Ruminant Res 1993;11:143–150.
18. Adams GP, Griffin PG, Ginther OJ. In situ morphologic dynamic of ovaries, uterus and cervix in llamas. Biol Reprod 1989;41:551–558.
19. Fernández-Baca S, Madden DHL, Novoa C. Effects of different mating stimuli on induction of ovulation in the alpaca. J Reprod Fertil 1970;22:261–267.
20. Sumar J. Reproductive physiology in South American camelids. In: Land RB, Robinson DW, eds. Genetics of Reproduction in Sheep. Butterworths, England, 1985.
21. Bravo PW. Studies on ovarian dynamics and response to copulation in the South American camelid, Lama glama and Lama pacos. Ph.D. Thesis, Univ. of California, Davis, 1991.
22. Fernández-Baca S. Luteal function and the nature of the reproductive failures in alpacas. PhD Thesis. Ithaca, NY: Cornell University, 1970.
23. Chen BX, Yuen ZX, Pan GW. Semen-induced ovulation in the Bactrian camel (Camelus bactrianus). J Reprod Fert 1985;74:335–339.
24. Ríos M, Sumar J, Alarcón V. Presencia de un factor de inducción de la ovulación en el semen de la alpaca y toro. In: Proc VIII Reunión Científica Anual de APPA (Abst. C-27), 1985.
25. Paolicchi F, Urquieta B, Del Valle L, Bustos-Obregón E. Actividad Biológica del Plasma Seminal de Alpaca: Estímulo para la Producción de LH por Células gonadotropas. Rev Arg Prod Anim 1996;16:351–356.
26. Fernández-Baca S, Sumar J, Novoa C, Leyva V. Relación entre la ubicación del cuerpo luteo y la localización del embrión en la alpaca. Rev Inv Pec (IVITA) Univ Nac S Marcos 1973;2:131–135.
27. Sumar J, Leyva V. Relación entre la ubicación del cuerpo lúteo y la localización del embrión en la Llama (Lama glama). In: Proc III Conv Int sobre Camélidos Sudamericanos. Viedma, Argentina: 1979.
28. Sumar J, Fredriksson G, Alarcón V, Kindahl H, Edqvist L-E. Levels of 15-keto-13,14-dihydro-PGF2$\alpha$, progesterone and oestradiol-17$\beta$, after induced ovulations in llamas and alpacas. Acta Vet Scand 1988;29:339–346.
29. Sumar J, García M, Alarcón V, Echevarría L. El celo en la alpaca y llama y los niveles de progesterona plasmática. In: Proc. X Reunión Científica Anual de APPA . Univ Nac del Altiplano. Puno, Peru, (Abstr. 46). 1987.
30. Adams GP, Sumar J, Ginther OJ. Form and function of the corpus luteum in llamas. Anim Reprod Sci 1991;24:127–138.
31. Sumar J. Fisiología de la Reproducción del Macho y Manejo Reproductivo. In: Avances y Perspectivas del Conocimiento de los Camélidos Sudamericanos. Oficina Regional de la FAO para América Latina y el Caribe, Santiago, Chile, 1991.
32. Leon JB, Smith BB, Timm KI, Le Cren G. Endocrine changes during pregnancy, parturition and the early post-partum period in the llama (Lama glama). J Reprod Fert 1990;88: 503–511.
33. England BG, Foote WC, Cardozo AG, Matthews DH, Riera S. Oestrous and mating behaviour in the llama (Lama glama). Anim Behav 1971;19:722–726.
34. Condorena N, Sumar J, Alarcón V. Período de Gestación en Llama. Turrialba 1992;42:112–113.
35. Fernández-Baca S, Hansel W, Saatman R, Sumar J, Novoa C. Differential luteolytic effect on right and left uterine horns in the alpaca. Biol Reprod 1979;20:586–595.
36. Sumar J. Gestación Gemelar en la alpaca. Rev Inv Pec (IVITA) Uni Nac M S Marcos 1980;5:558–60.
37. Sumar J. Removal of the ovaries or ablation of the corpus luteum and its effect on the maintenance of gestation in the alpaca and llama. Acta Vet Scand 1983;83(Suppl):133–141.
38. Alarcón V, Sumar J, Riera GS, Foote WC. Comparison of three methods of pregnancy diagnosis in alpacas and llamas. Theriogenology 1990;34:1119–1127.
39. Sumar J, Alarcón V, Echevarría L. Niveles de progesterona periférica en alpacas y llamas y su aplicación en el diagnóstico precoz de gestación y otros usos clínicos. Acta Andina 1993;2:161–167.
40. Schwarzenberger F, Speckbacher G, Bamberg E. Plasma and fecal progestagen evaluations during and after the breeding season of the female vicuaa (Vicugna vicugna). Theriogenology 1995;43:625–634.
41. Johnson LW. Llama Reproduction. In: The Veterinary Clinics of North America. Food Animal Practice. Llama Medicine, Volume 5, 1989.
42. Sumar J. Algunos aspectos obstétricos de la alpaca. Boletín Técnico No. 2. IVITA, Univ Nac M S Marcos, Convenio CIID-Canada, 1985.
43. Del Castillo M. El parto en la llama (Lama glama). Bach Thesis. Cusco, Peru: Univ Nac S Antonio Abad, 1988.
44. Sumar J, Smith GW, Mayhua E, Nathanielsz PW. Adrenocortical function in the fetal and newborn alpaca. Comp Biochem Physiol 1978;59(A):79–84.
45. Liggins GC. The fetus and birth. In: Austin CR, Short RV, eds. Embryonic and fetal development. Reproduction in mammals, Vol 2. 2nd ed. Cambridge University Press, 1983.
46. Osorio de Valdivia EM, Sumar J, Casas H, Ponce J. Inducción y sincronización del parto en la alpaca. In: Anales VII Reunión de ALPA, Panama, 1979.
47. Sumar J, Novoa C, Fernández-Baca S. Fisiología reproductiva post-parto en la alpaca. Rev Inv Pec (IVITA) Univ Nac M S Marcos 1972;1:21–27.
48. MacEntee K. Reproductive Pathology of Domestic Mammals. Academic Press, Inc, 1990.
49. Sumar J. Studies on reproductive pathology in alpacas. MSc

Thesis. Uppsala, Sweden: Swedish University of Agrarian Sciences, Department of Obstetric and Gynaecology, Veterinary Medicine Faculty, 1983.

50. Fowler ME. Medicine and Surgery of South American Camelids. Llama, Alpaca, Vicuaa, Guanaco. Ames, Iowa: Iowa University Press, 1989.
51. Ramírez A. Enfermedades Infecciosas. In: Fernández-Baca S, ed. Avances y Perspectivas del Conocimiento de los Camélidos Sudamericanos. Santiago, Chile: Oficina Regional de la FAO para America Latina y el Caribe, 1991.
52. Peter AT, Smith CL. Infertility in Female Llamas. In: Youngquist, ed. Current Therapy in Large Animal Theriogenology. Section VI, Llama Theriogenology. Philadelphia: WB Saunders, 1997.
53. Ludeãa H, Barsallo J, Leyva V. Incidencia de Infecciones Genitales en Alpacas. In: Resúmenes de Proyectos de Investigación realizados por la Uni Nac M S Marcos, Tomo III. Período 1980–1981, 1983.
54. Carrick FN, Setchell BP. The evolution of the scrotum. In: Calaby JN, Tyndale-Biscoe CH, eds. Reproduction and Evolution. Canberra: Australian Academy of Science, 1977; 165–170.
55. Montalvo C, Cevallos E, Copaira M. Estudio microscópico del parénquima testicular de la alpaca durante las estaciones del aao. In: Proc V Cong Nac de Cienc Veterinarias, Arequipa, Peru, 1977.
56. Sumar J, Alarcón V, Huanca T. Pubertad en la llama macho. In: Proc XI Cong Panamericano de Ciencias Veterinarias, Lima, Peru, 1988.
57. Sumar J, Franco J, Alarcón V. Niveles de Testosterona circulante en la alpaca (Lama pacos) y llama (Lama glama) en diversas estaciones del año. In: Proc 2nd Jornadas Int de Biopatología Andina, Cusco, Peru, 1990.
58. Delhon GA, Lawzewitsch IV. Reproduction in the male llama (Lama glama) a South American camelid. I. Spermatogenesis and organization of intertubular space of the mature testis. Acta Anat 1987;129:59–66.
59. Sumar J, Leyva V. Colección de semen mediante vagina artificial en la alpaca. In: Proc IV Conv Int sobre Camélidos Sudamericanos, Punta Arenas, Chile, 1981.
60. Franco E, Sumar J, Varela H. Eyaculación en la alpaca (Lama pacos). In: Proc IV Conv Int sobre Camélidos Sudamericanos, Punta Arenas, Chile, 1981.
61. Kubiceck J. Samanentnahme beim Alpaca durcheine Harnrohrenfistel (Semen collection in alpaca with a uretral fistula). Z Tierz Zuechtungsbiol 1974;90:335–351.
62. Lichtenwalner AB, Woods GL, Weber JA. Ejaculatory Pattern of Llamas During Copulation. Theriogenology 1996;46: 285–291.
63. Sumar J, García M. Fisiología de la reproducción de la alpaca. In: Proc of Symp on Nuclear and Related Techniques in Animal Production and Health. Vienna: IAEA, 1986.
64. Leyva V, Franco J, Sumar J. Inseminación Artificial en Camélidos Sudamericanos. In: Proc I Reunión Científica Anual de APPA, Lima, Peru, 1977.
65. Lichtenwalner AB, Woods GL, Weber JA. Seminal Collection, Seminal characteristics and Pattern of Ejaculation in Llamas. Theriogenology 1996;46:293–305.
66. Setchell BP. The Mammalian Testis. Ithaca, New York: Cornell University Press, 1978.
67. Hahn J, Foote RH, Seidel GE. Testicular growth and related sperm output in dairy bull. J Anim Sci 1969;29:41.
68. Condorena N, Fernandez-Baca S. Relación entre frecuencia de servicios y fertilidad en la alpaca. Rev Inv Pec (IVITA) Univ Nac M S Marcos 1972;1:11–19.
69. Obando AG. Complementación al estudio anatomo-histológico del testículo de la alpaca (Lama pacos). Bach Thesis. Puno, Peru: Univ Nac del Altiplano, 1990.
70. Soikes B, Kalinowski J, Velarde CL. Composición Química y Digestibilidad de la Materia Seca y Orgánica de Pastos Nativos Dominantes en la Praderas Alto-Andinas del Perú. Univ Nac Agraria La Molina, Depart de Nutrición, Lima, Peru, 1970.
71. Fernández-Baca S, and Novoa C. Primer ensayo de inseminación artificial de alpacas (Lama pacos) con semen de vicuña (Vicugna vicugna). Uni Nac M Marcos, Revista de la Facultad de Medicina Veterinaria 1968;22:9–18.
72. Calderón W, Sumar J, Franco E. Avances en la Inseminación Artificial de las Alpacas (Lama pacos). Univ Nac M S Marcos, Revista de la Facultad de Medicina Veterinaria 1968;22: 19–35.
73. Del Campo MR. Reproductive Technologies in South American Camelids. In: Youngquist RS, ed. Current Therapy in Large Animal Theriogenology. Philadelphia: WB Saunders Company, 1997.
74. Pugh DG, Montes AJ. Advanced Reproductive Technologies in South American Camelids. In: Veterinary Clinics of North America: Food Animal Practice. Update on Llama Medicine, Vol 10. Philadelphia: WB Saunders, 1994.
75. Novoa J, Sumar J. Colección de Huevos in vivo y ensayos de transferencia en alpacas. Tercer Boletín Extraordinario. IVITA, Univ Nac M S Marcos, Lima, Peru, 1968.
76. Bourke DA, Adam CL, Kyle CE. Successful pregnancy following non-surgical embryo transfer in llamas. Vet Rec 1990; 127:580.
77. Bourke DA, Kyle CE, McEvoy TG, Young P, Adam CL. Superovulatory responses to hCG in llamas (Lama glama). Theriogenology 1995;44:255–268.
78. Del Campo MR, Del Campo CH, Adams GP, Mapletoft RJ. The application of new reproductive technologies to South American camelids. Theriogenology 1995;43:21–30.
79. Bravo WP, Tsutsui T, Lasley BL. Dose response to equine chorionic gonadotropins and subsequent ovulation in llamas. Small Ruminant Research 1995;18:157–163.
80. Correa JE, Gatica R, Ratto M, Ladrix R, Schuler C. Studies on non-surgical recovery of embryos from South American camelids. In: Proc 12th Int Cong Anim Reprod Vol 2. 1992;232:788–790.
81. Del Campo MR, Donoso MW, Del Campo CH, et al. *In vitro* maturation of llama (Lama glama) oocytes. Proc 12th Int Cong Anim Reprod Vol 1. 1992;101:324–326.
82. Wiepz DW, Chapman RJ. Non-surgical embryo transfer and live birth in a llama. Theriogenology 1985;24:251–257.
83. Brogliatti GM, Palasz AT, Adams GP. Ultrasound-guided transvaginal follicle aspiration and oocyte collection in llamas (Lama glama). Theriogenology 1996;45:249.
84. Sumar J, Franco E. Ensayos de Transferencia de Embriones en Alpacas. In: Informe Final (IVITA). Univ N M S Marcos, Lima, Peru, 1974.
85. Bourke DA, Kyle CE, McEvoy TG, Young P, Adam CL.

Recipient synchronization and embryo transfer in South American Camelids. Theriogenology 1995;43:171–177.

86. Del Campo MR, Donoso MX, Del Campo CH, Berland M, Mapletoft RJ. *In vitro* fertilization and development of llama (Lama glama) oocytes using epididymal spermatozoa and oviductal cell co-culture. Theriogenology 1994;41:1219–1229.

## SUGGESTED READING

Adams GP, Sumar J, Ginther OJ. Hemorrhagic ovarian follicles in llamas. Theriogenology 1991;35:557–568.

Bourke DA, Adam CL, Kyle CE, McEvoy TG. Ovarian responses to PMSG and FSH in llamas. In: Proc European Symp on South American Camelids, Bonn, Germany, 1993;75–81.

Bourke DA, Adam CL, Kyle CE, McEvoy TG, Young P. Ovulation, superovulation and embryo recovery in llamas. In: Proc 12th Int Cong on Anim Reprod Vol 1. 1992;57:193–195.

Bravo WP, Stabenfeldt GH, Fowler ME, Lasley BL, Frey RE. Testes Development and Testosterone Concentrations in the Llama (Lama glama). In: Proc 12th Int Cong on Anim Reprod Vol 4. 1992;487:1698–1700.

Leyva V, Sumar J, Franco E. Estudio preliminar de la concentración de espermatozoides de semen de alpaca obtenido por vagina artificial. In: Proc VII Reunión Científica Anual de APPA. Lima, Peru: Univ Agrar La Molina, 1984.

Sumar J. Contribution of the radioimmunoassay technique to knowledge of the reproductive physiology of South American Camelids. In: Isotope and Related Techniques in Animal Production and Health. FAO/IAEA. Vienna, Austria, 1991.

Sumar J. Induction of Abortion in alpacas and llamas with Dinoprost (Lutalyse). 1996.

Sumar J, Edqvist L-E, Kindahl H, Fredriksson G, Alarcón V. Niveles de Sulfato de Estrona periférica durante la gestación y puerperio en la alpaca y llama. In: Proc X Cong Nac de Ciencias Veterinarias, Cusco, Peru, 1990.

# CHAPTER 16

# *Reproduction in Poultry: Male and Female*

D.P. FROMAN, J.D. KIRBY, AND J.A. PROUDMAN

## Male Reproduction

D.P. FROMAN AND J.D. KIRBY

The quality of being *fertile* denotes an ability to reproduce. In the case of male poultry, this ability depends upon:

a) the successful production and maturation of sperm cells within the male reproductive tract,
b) initiation of sperm motility at the time of ejaculation,
c) temporary sequestration of sperm within the hen's sperm storage tubules (SST),
d) passive transport of sperm through the oviduct above the vaginal sphincter,
e) induction of an acrosome reaction in response to sperm contact with an oocyte's perivitelline layer,
f) spermatozoal perforation of the perivitelline layer at multiple sites,
g) introduction of condensed DNA into the oocyte via membrane fusion, and
h) combination of one of several male pronuclei with the female pronucleus.

Therefore, the fertility of any given male entails the successful completion of several critical steps beyond the production of sperm cells by the testis.

As inferred from the criteria listed above, poultry sperm are immotile prior to ejaculation (1). However, sperm become self-propelled DNA delivery vehicles at ejaculation. This attribute is significant because the net *mobility* of sperm populations within the hen's vagina appears to be a critical determinant of fertility in poultry (2). Sperm that ascend the vagina and enter SST (see Bakst et al (3) for a review of sperm sequestration) afford the hen with a resident population of viable sperm that fertilize oocytes over the course of many days (Fig. 16-1). While the phenomenon of sperm sequestration has been known since the 1960s, the mechanism by which sperm exit the SST and re-enter the oviduct has remained a mystery (4). Ironically, sperm efflux from the SST may be explicable in terms of sperm *immobility*. This hypothesis is tenable for the following reasons. First, sperm enter SST with their acrosomes oriented towards the blind end of the tubule and their long axes in parallel (5). Second, sperm mobility under physiological conditions is highly correlated with sperm ATP content (Fig. 16-2). Third, if the SST epithelium secretes a fluid, then a current would be generated within a tubule's lumen. In such a case, viable sperm would be lost from the SST as soon as they failed to maintain position within the tubule due to low intracellular [ATP]. This explanation of spermatozoal efflux is also consonant with the half-life of enzymes and the sperm cell's inability to transcribe nuclear genes.

In any event, poultry reproduction may be best understood as a *process*. In the case of an individual male, this process entails fertilization, the formation of a patent reproductive tract, semen production, and the manifestation of specific behavioral patterns, which include ejaculation. The reader is referred to Froman (6), and Kirby and Froman (7) for a detailed analysis of these phenomena. This chapter will provide an overview of reproductive tract anatomy,

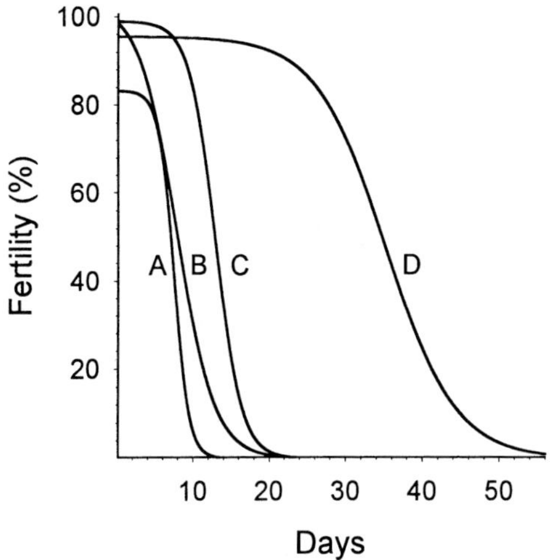


FIGURE 16-1. Duration of fertility in poultry (*A*, Japanese quail; *B*, broiler breeder; *C*, Single Comb White Leghorn; *D*, large white turkey) following a single insemination. The differences in the duration of sperm survival within the oviduct of the female, inferred from the duration of fertility, are due to differences in both sperm physiology and the function of sperm storage tubules within the female's oviduct. Thus, as with domestic mammals the unique attributes of sperm function can vary significantly from species to species as well as within a given species or line. (Data for the quail are from: Reddish JM, Kirby JD, Anthony NB. Analysis of poultry fertility data. 3. Analysis of the duration of fertility in naturally mating Japanese quail. Poultry Sci 1996;75:135.)

spermatogenesis, extragonadal sperm transport, and fertilization as it relates to sperm cells.

## *Reproductive Tract Anatomy*

The gross morphology of the rooster's reproductive tract is shown in Fig. 16-3. The reader is referred to Nickel et al (8), King (9), and Lake (10) for details. Paired tracts lie along the dorsal body wall. The testes are attached to the body wall by a mesorchium. Each testis contains anastomosing seminiferous tubules and associated interstitial tissue surrounded by a connective tissue capsule. The seminiferous epithelium is divided into two distinct compartments, i.e. basal and adluminal, by tight junctions between adjacent Sertoli cells (11, 12).

In essence, the male reproductive tract is an aggregate of seminiferous tubules connected in series with the excurrent ducts of the testis. The latter, in order, include the rete testis, proximal efferent ducts, distal efferent duct, connecting ducts, epididymal duct, and deferent duct (7). While the proximal portion of the deferent duct is referred to as the epididymal duct, there is no significant difference between these two ducts apart from lumenal diameter, smooth muscle content, and the extent to which they are surrounded with dense connective tissue (13, 14). Therefore, the *epididymis*, by convention, is the set of efferent ducts, connecting ducts, and the proximal deferent duct found in association with the hilus of the testis. On a volumetric basis, the efferent ducts constitute the principal duct within the epididymis (Table 16-1).

The deferent duct is the site where semen is stored prior to ejaculation, in particular, the receptaculum of the deferent duct. The highly convoluted deferent duct straightens and widens in proximity to the cloaca to form the receptaculum. Each deferent ducts terminates as a papilla within the cloaca. Each papilla is a small finger-like projection from the lateral wall of the cloaca. A paracloacal vascular body is found in association with each receptaculum. As reviewed by Fujihara (15), these accessory organs are responsible for lymphatic tissue tumescence that accompanies sexual excitement. Specifically, lymph is formed by filtration of arterial blood within the paracloacal vascular bodies. Lymph generation enables eversion of opposing sets of tumescent lymphatic tissue

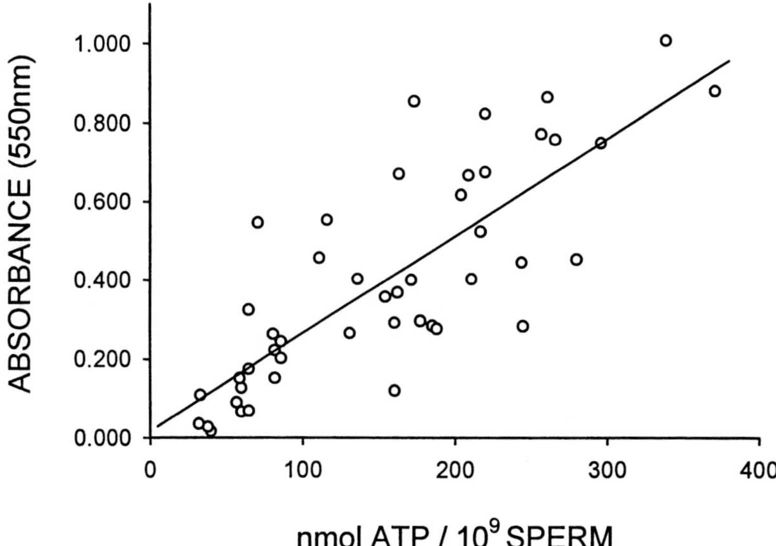


FIGURE 16-2. Correlation of sperm mobility to sperm ATP content. Each open circle denotes a data pair obtained from a single ejaculate (n = 46 roosters) immediately after ejaculation. Sperm mobility was estimated by measuring absorbance of a 6% (w/v) Accudenz solution following overlay with a sperm suspension and incubation at 40°C for 5 min. Sperm ATP content was measured with a bioluminescence assay kit. The solid line represents the regression equation: absorbance = 0.1793 + 0.0025× (ATP). The correlation coefficient was 0.80. (Reproduced from: Froman DP, Feltmann AJ. Sperm mobility: A quantitative trait of the domestic fowl (*Gallus domesticus*). Biol Reprod 1998;58:379. With permission of Society for Study of Reproduction.)

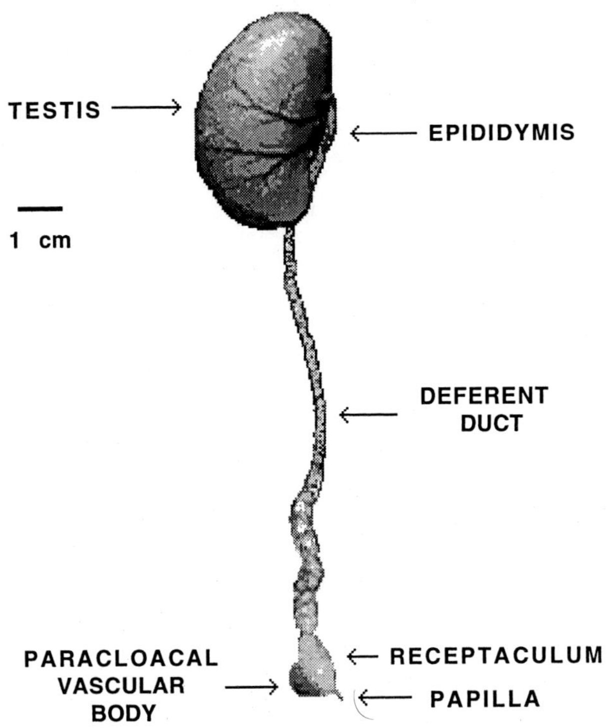


Figure 16-3. Digital image of a rooster's right reproductive tract. Each structure appears as it did in situ with the exception of the testis, which was reflected to the left in order to expose the epididymis. The paracloacal vascular body and receptaculum are found in between the outer surface of the cloaca and the adherent body wall. Thus, these structures must be exposed by blunt dissection. (Reproduced with permission of the Poultry Science Association.)

**Table 16-1. *Comparative Structure of the Galliform Epididymis Based Upon Volumetric Proportions (%) of Component Structures by Species***

| Structure | Chicken | Japanese Quail | Guinea Fowl |
|---|---|---|---|
| Rete testis | 13 | 9.9 | 10.7 |
| Proximal efferent ducts | 27 | 40 | 45 |
| Distal efferent ducts | 7.7 | 15.2 | 16 |
| Connecting ducts | 2.3 | 1.7 | 0.7 |
| Epididymal duct | 7.6 | 2.4 | 1.8 |
| Connective tissue | 38 | 27 | 22 |
| Blood vessels | 2.5 | 2.7 | 2.3 |
| Aberrant ducts | 0.3 | — | — |

Adapted from: Aire TA. Micro-stereological study of the avian epididymal region. J Anat 1979;129:703. Used with permission of Cambridge University Press.

through the vent. The everted tissue forms a nonintromittent phallus (16). Ejaculation occurs when smooth muscle contraction within the wall of each receptaculum accompanies eversion of the phallus.

### *Spermatogenesis*

As in mammalian species, spermatogenesis in poultry is a complex process of cellular proliferation, haploid reduction of the nuclear genome, and cellular differentiation. To date, spermatogenesis in galliform birds has been most fully described from studies of Japanese quail (17–21). Spermatogenesis in all species involves a programmed sequence of steps involving specific types of cells (spermatogonia, spermatocytes, and spermatids) that persist for periods ranging from minutes to days. The temporal associations of specific cell types (stages) within the seminiferous epithelium vary from species to species, with the complete sequence of stages known as the cycle of the seminiferous epithelium. The

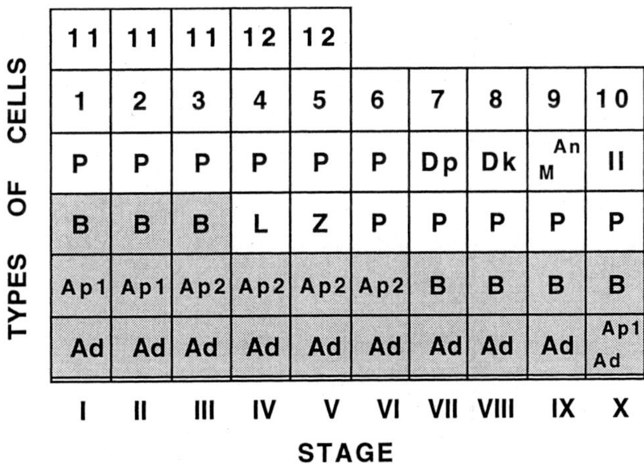


Figure 16-4. Schematic of the cycle of the seminiferous epithelium of Japanese quail: *Ad*, dark type A spermatogonia (stem cell); *Ap1* and *Ap2*, pale type A spermatogonia; *B*, type B spermatogonia; *L*, leptotene primary spermatocytes; *Z*, zygotene primary spermatocytes; *P*, pachytene primary spermatocytes; *Dp*, diplotene primary spermatocytes; *Dk*, diakinesis of primary spermatocytes; M, metaphase primary spermatocytes; *An*, anaphase primary spermatocytes; *II*, secondary spermatocytes; *1–12*, step 1 through step 12 spermatids.

The double line between the Roman numerals and spermatogonial abbreviations represents the periphery of the seminiferous epithelium. The spermatids along the top of the schematic border the lumen of the seminiferous tubule. Thus, as germ cells develop, they pass through the seminiferous epithelium towards the lumen. Germ cells are in contact with Sertoli cells throughout this migration because Sertoli cells span the distance between the periphery of the seminiferous tubule and the lumen.

The blood-testis barrier is found between adjacent Sertoli cells. Shaded boxes denote germ cells within the peripheral compartment of the seminiferous epithelium. Likewise, nonshaded boxes denote germ cells within the luminal compartment of the seminiferous epithelium. (Adapted from: Lin M, Jones RC. Spatial arrangement of the stages of the cycle of the seminiferous epithelium in the Japanese quail, *Coturnix coturnix japonica*. J Reprod Fert 1990;90:361. Reproduced with permission of the Journal of Reproduction/Fertility.)

cycle of the seminiferous epithelium of the Japanese quail is shown schematically in Figure 16-4. In the context of the seminiferous epithelium, approximately 2.69 days would be required for each of the 12 stages to appear at any fixed point within the seminiferous tubule. However, the transformation of a spermatogonial stem cell into 32 sperm would require 4.75 cycles of the seminiferous epithelium. Thus, the duration of spermatogenesis in the Japanese quail is estimated to be 12.8 days.

A complete series of stages juxtaposed in adjacent physical regions of the seminiferous epithelium constitutes a *wave* of spermatogenesis. This phenomenon is manifest as a helix relative to the long axis of the quail's seminiferous tubule (Fig. 16-5). As is true for other species, spermatogenesis in galliform birds entails an extreme reduction in the cytoplasmic content of haploid cells. A reduction of approximately 97% of cell volume accompanies the transformation of spherical spermatids to vermiform sperm in the rooster (22). The efficiency of spermatogenesis in the Japanese quail has been estimated to be $92.5 \times 10^6$ sperm per gram of testis per day (23). This value is comparable to the range reported for the rooster: 80 to $120 \times 10^6$ sperm per gram of testis per day (24–26). Finally, it is noteworthy that while the scrotum provides a cooling apparatus essential for spermatogenesis to occur in domestic mammals at 32 to 35°C, spermatogenesis occurs at core body temperature (40 to 41°C) in poultry with a 1 to 1.5°C circadian rhythm of body temperature (Fig. 16-6) (26).

Gonadotropins and gonadal steroids are essential to galliform spermatogenesis, as they are in other domestic animals (Fig. 16-7). However, apart from LH, the mechanisms by which these hormones exert their effects may differ

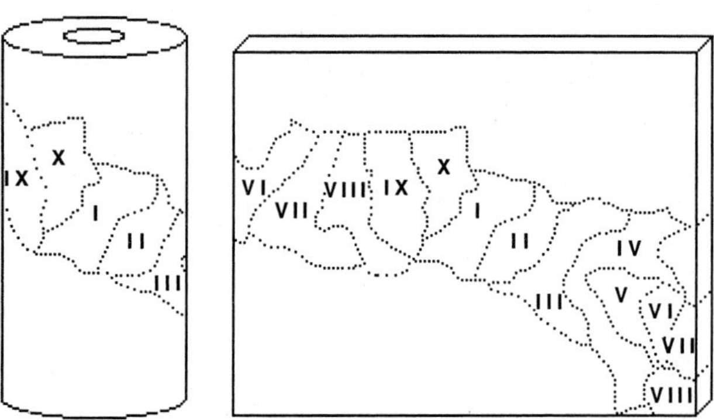


**Figure 16-5.** Spatial arrangement of the wave of spermatogenesis within a seminiferous tubule of the Japanese quail. The cylinder represents a section of a seminiferous tubule. The rectangle to its left denotes the two-dimensional representation of two contiguous cycles of the seminiferous epithelium. The cycle is arranged helically along the length of the tubule. Roman numerals denote stages. (Adapted from: Lin M, Jones RC. Spatial arrangement of the stages of the cycle of the seminiferous epithelium in the Japanese quail, *Coturnix coturnix japonica*. J Reprod Fert 1990;90:361. Reproduced with permission of the Journal of Reproduction/Fertility.)

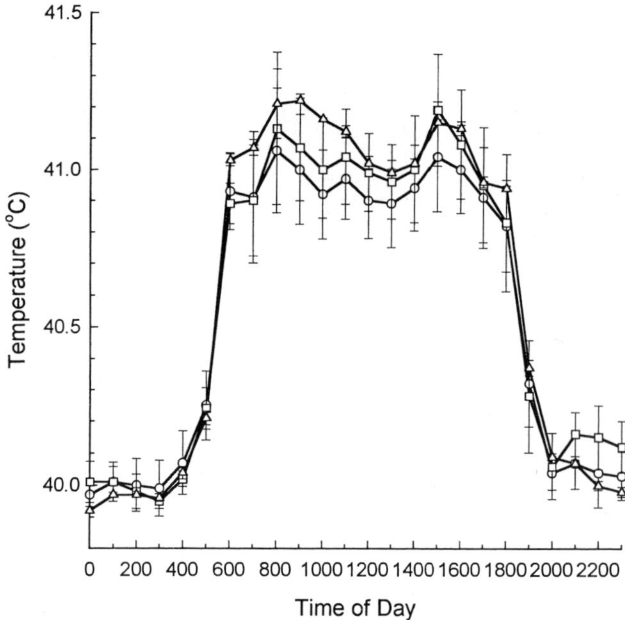


**Figure 16-6.** Testis, liver, and peritoneum exhibit indistinguishable temperature rhythms under a light:dark cycle. Birds were maintained under a 13L:11D cycle. Mean temperature values are presented for this group of birds for individual hour periods during the day. Error bars on the vertical axis are 1 SE around the mean. (Reproduced with permission of the Society for the Study of Reproduction.)

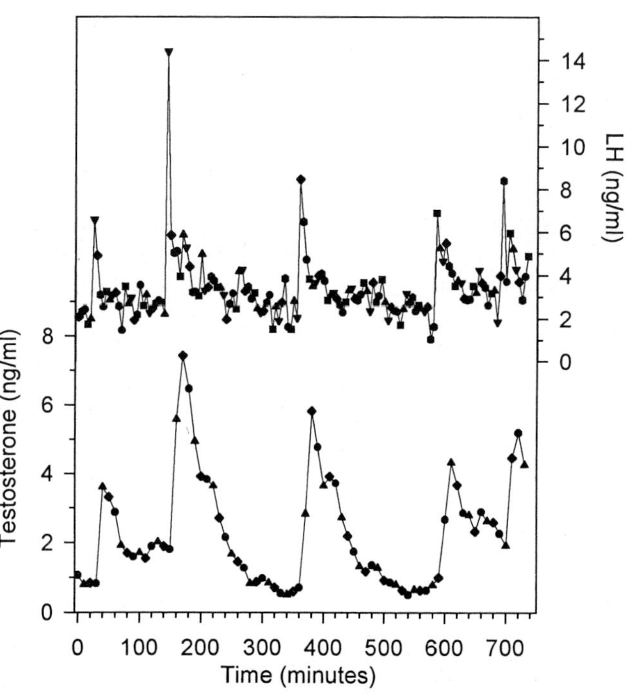


**Figure 16-7.** Patterns of pulsatile changes in circulating LH (*upper panel*) and testosterone (*lower panel*) in an adult male domestic turkey (*Meleagris gallopavo*). The peaks of the discrete LH pulses occur prior to those of testosterone, demonstrating the close relationship between LH secretion and that of testosterone. (Figure and data kindly provided by Dr. Wayne Bacon, Ohio State University.)

between birds and mammals. For example, in mammals the FSH receptor and androgen receptor are expressed in a stage specific manner. In contrast, a similar pattern of expression has yet to be reported for the quail, chicken, or turkey. Furthermore, a direct role of testosterone in the regulation of the seminiferous epithelium of the fowl has been called into question due to the reported absence of androgen receptor-like immunoreactivity within the seminiferous tubule (27). While the sequence of the chicken FSH receptor has been determined (28), the study of the receptor's expression within the rooster's seminiferous epithelium may be complicated by the histological attributes of the seminiferous tubule; preliminary investigations (29, 30) have failed to detect a clearly defined set of spermatogenic stages in the seminiferous epithelium of the fowl testis. Nonetheless, a 4.3 kb mRNA for the FSH receptor has been identified in the rooster testis (31). It is also noteworthy that P450 aromatase has been discovered within germ cells (32) and that estrogen receptors have been found within the excurrent ducts of the testis (33) in domestic fowl. Therefore, while spermatogenesis in galliform males may indeed be dependent upon testosterone secreted by Leydig cells (34), the full biological effect of this hormone on semen production may be mediated, in part, by its conversion to estrogen within the rooster's seminiferous epithelium.

In contrast, the role of estrogen relative to gonadotropin secretion is much more clear. Rozenboim et al. (35) induced precocious puberty in cockerels by treatment with tamoxifen, an estrogen receptor antagonist. As evidenced by the treatment's effect on GnRH-1 and LH, the effect of tamoxifen was exerted at the level of the CNS. Likewise, Kuenzel et al (36, 37) treated chicks with sulfamethazine and induced precocious puberty by modulating circulating gonadotropin levels. Furthermore, circulating FSH levels and a concomitant increase (4-fold) in testis size and sperm production were induced with sulfamethazine in hypogonadotropic adult broiler breeder males (38). Collectively, these experiments illustrate the pivotal role of hypothalamic GnRHergic neurons in controlling spermatogenesis. It is well known that GnRH secretion is affected by somatic and environmental stimuli. Furthermore, the entrainment of reproduction with photoperiod is a well-known phenomenon in birds. Wingfield et al. (39) have developed a model for central integration of environmental stimuli relative to gonadotropin secretion. In the rooster, photoreceptors deep within the ventral forebrain constitute the principal sensory neuron that stimulate hypothalamic GnRHergic neurons (40).

### *Extragonadal Sperm Transport*

Spermatogenesis culminates with the release of immotile sperm from the seminiferous epithelium. In the quail, spermiation is limited to Stage V (Fig. 16-4). Galliform sperm are vermiform with a maximum width of approximately 0.6 μm and a length ranging between 75 and 90 μm (41). Once sperm are released from the seminiferous epithelium, they are carried by a current of seminiferous tubule fluid that flows through the lumena of seminiferous tubules towards the excurrent ducts of the testis. Once again, research with Japanese quail has provided the best assessment to date of the dynamics of sperm transport through the excurrent ducts of the testis. As shown in Table 16-2, the effluent from the seminiferous tubules passes rapidly through the excurrent ducts, and the most evident outcome is the formation of viscous semen due to absorption of seminiferous tubule fluid, particularly at the level of the proximal efferent ducts.

A second outcome of sperm passage through the excurrent ducts is the ability of sperm to become motile when semen recovered from the deferent duct is diluted with a physiologic buffer. This illustrates yet another difference between male poultry and domestic mammals; for testicular sperm from the rooster, while immotile, can nonetheless fertilize oocytes if the sperm are introduced into the oviduct above the vaginal sphincter (42). However that which enables sperm to become motile remains unknown to date even though: (a) apocrine secretion is evident within the efferent ducts (14), (b) the composition of seminal plasma is distinct from that of blood plasma (7), and (c) reproductive tract specific proteins adsorb to the surface of rooster sperm during their passage through the excurrent ducts (43, 44). Likewise, it remains unknown whether extragonadal sperm maturation is dependent upon testosterone, as one might intuit, estrogen (33), or both. In any event, extragonadal sperm transport culminates in semen being moved along the length of the deferent duct by peristalsis. Greater

TABLE 16-2. ***Sperm Transit Through the Excurrent Ducts of the Japanese Quail and Absorption of Seminiferous Tubule Fluid by Region***

| Region | Duration of Sperm Transit | Percentage of Seminiferous Tubule Fluid Absorbed |
|---|---|---|
| Rete testis | 25 s | 6% |
| Efferent ducts | 8 min | 92% |
| Connecting ducts | 22 min | 0.4% |
| Epididymal duct | 80 min | 0.2% |
| Deferent duct | 22.2 h | 0.2% |

Adapted from: Clulow J, Jones RC. Studies of fluid and spermatozoal transport in the extratesticular genital ducts of the Japanese quail. J Anat 1988;157:1. Used with permission of Cambridge University Press.

than 90% of the galliform extragonadal sperm reserve is contained within the deferent duct (7).

### *Fertilization*

Fertilization in poultry occurs within the hen's infundibulum. As illustrated by such phenomena as the acrosome reaction, spermatozoal penetration of an oocyte investment, and the formation of a male pronucleus from condensed DNA, the prerequisites for fertilization in poultry are comparable to those of domestic mammals. And yet, striking differences do exist (45). Based upon the most recent review of mechanisms underlying fertilization in poultry (46), there are two salient differences. First, poultry sperm do not undergo capacitation as do mammalian sperm. Second, polyspermy is the norm. Research conducted since the mid 1980s has focused upon gamete interaction. At ovulation, the oocyte is surrounded by a reticular, noncellular structure several micrometers thick known as the perivitelline layer. Koyanagi et al (47) used dispersed perivitelline layer to induce an acrosome reaction *in vitro*. It is noteworthy that one experimental outcome was lysis of the perivitelline layer. Howarth (48, 49) inhibited sperm induced lysis of the perivitelline layer by pretreating sperm with solubilized glycoproteins derived from the perivitelline layer. The existence of sperm cell surface ligands that bind to receptors associated with the perivitelline layer was demonstrated by these experiments.

Kuroki/Mori (50) demonstrated that sperm binding to the perivitelline layer can occur without subsequent perforation of the perivitelline layer. This was accomplished by including a serine protease inhibitor in their incubation medium. Barbato et al (51) have shown that the ability of sperm to bind to protein derived from the perivitelline layer differs among lines of chickens. Therefore, in addition to sperm mobility (2), it is reasonable to conclude that sperm surface topography is a phenotypic determinant of fertility in male poultry. Thus, fertility in poultry species is a complex process dependent upon the successful completion of a number of critical steps from spermatogenesis, extragonadal maturation, and survival and function within the hen's oviduct.

# Female Reproduction

J.A. PROUDMAN

The reproductive processes in domestic poultry differ substantially from those of other farm animals because the bird must ovulate single ova at frequent intervals, and produce a fertilized egg which fulfills all of the needs of the developing embryo without further maternal input. This chapter provides an overview of the specialized avian egg, the structure and function of the single oviduct, and the unique aspects of the bird's ovary and reproductive endocrine system which permit this highly efficient production of offspring.

### *Reproductive Efficiency*

Although only a few species of birds have been domesticated, these poultry species produce meat, eggs, and other animal products for mankind with remarkable efficiency. The short generation interval and high reproductive capacity of poultry has permitted the rapid genetic selection of breeds and strains which are specialized in the efficient production of meat or eggs (Table 16-3). Supported by sophisticated feeding and management programs, a relatively small population of primary breeding stocks are crossed to produce commercial stock which yield billions of offspring per year.

### *The Egg*

The production of large numbers of offspring from each breeding female is possible, in part, because the bird produces a macroscopic egg which contains all of the nutrients required for the development of the fully formed chick, and because the fertilized egg can be incubated instead of requiring maternal gestation. The egg is formed basically of three components: the yolk, which is equivalent to the microscopic mammalian egg; the albumen, or egg white, which is secreted by the reproductive tract; and the shell, which provides protection and minerals to the developing embryo. Each of these major components is physically and chemically complex (Fig. 16-8).

The yolk, or ovum, comprises about one-third of the mass of the egg and contains the female pronucleus and

TABLE 16-3. ***Comparative Reproductive Performance of Some Birds of Commercial Importance***

| Species | Incubation Period (Days) | Age of Sexual Maturity (Months) | Egg Weight (g) | Number of Eggs in First Laying Year | Fertility (%) | Hatchability of Fertile Eggs (%) |
|---|---|---|---|---|---|---|
| Chicken (*Gallus gallus*) | | | | | | |
| Layer | 21 | 5–6 | 58 | 300 | 97 | 90 |
| Broiler | 21 | 6 | 65 | 180 | 92 | 90 |
| Turkey (*Meleagris gallopavo*) | 28 | 7–8 | 85 | 90 | 90 | 84 |
| Duck (*Anas platyrhynchos*) | | | | | | |
| Layer | 27–28 | 6–7 | 60 | 300 | 95 | 75–80 |
| Meat type | 28 | 6–7 | 65 | 300 | 95 | 75–80 |
| Goose (*Anser anser*) | | | | | | |
| Small type | 30 | 9–10 | 135 | 30–70 | 70 | 70 |
| Large type | 33 | 10–12 | 215 | 30–70 | 70 | 70 |
| Pheasant (*Phasianus colchicus*) | 24–26 | 10–12 | 30 | 50–75 | 95 | 85 |
| Guinea fowl (*Numida meleagris*) | 27–28 | 10–12 | 40 | 80–200 | 90 | 95 |
| Quail (*Coturnix coturnix*) | 15–16 | 1.5–2 | 10 | 300 | 90 | 75–85 |

Only general figures are given since values are greatly affected by breed, location, and nutrition. In particular the values given in the last three columns depend greatly on management practices, and it is unlikely that fertility and hatchability will be the same for all species.

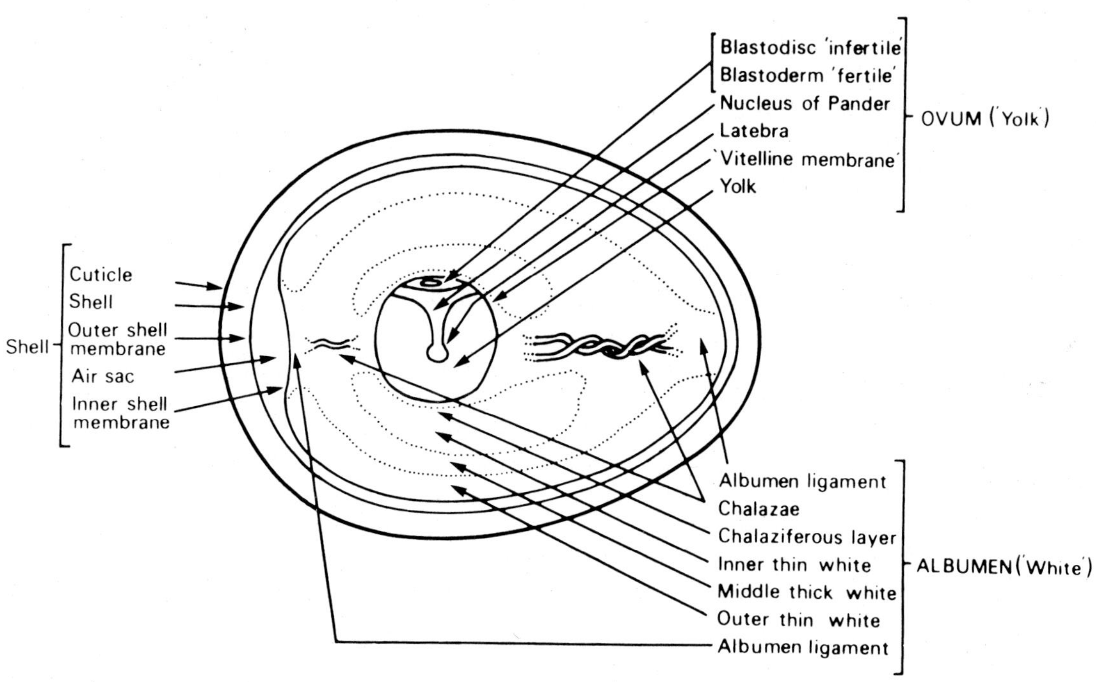


FIGURE 16-8. Diagram of the components of the egg. (From: Gilbert AB. The egg: its physical and chemical aspects. In: Bell DJ, Freeman BM, eds. Physiology and Biochemistry of the Domestic Fowl. New York: Academic Press, 1971.)

most of the nutrients required for embryonic development. The yolk is comprised of 50% water, 32% lipids, and 16% protein, and is surrounded by a four-layer membrane. The outer two layers are derived from the oviduct while the inner two layers are produced by the ovary. The majority of the yolk is a heterogeneous mix of proteins, lipids, pigments, and a variety of minor organic and inorganic components, which provide nutrients for embryogenesis. The yolk also contains immunoglobulin G, which confers maternal immunity to the embryo. The maternal chromosomes are packaged in a small area of the unfertilized ovum called the *blastodisc*. This area is visible on the surface of the yolk as a small, white spot about 3 mm in diameter. The blastodisc floats on a cone of light-colored "white" yolk that forms the Nucleus of Pander and terminates within the ovum in a ball known as the *latibra* (Fig. 16-8). This white yolk contains a larger proportion of proteins than the yellow yolk, and presumably provides the female pronucleus (or the zygote if the egg is fertile) with a normal physiological environment. If the egg has been fertilized, the blastodisc develops during transit down the oviduct into a slightly larger area called the *blastoderm* in the newly-laid fertilized egg.

The albumen surrounds the yolk and positions it in the center of the egg. Comprising 58% of the egg by weight, the albumin has at least seven major regions (Fig. 16-8) containing about 40 proteins, many of which are unique to the laying hen. Since the albumen surrounds the developing embryo, it forms an aqueous mantle that prevents dessication and serves as a major water reservoir for the embryo. It also contributes some proteins, vitamins, and minerals to the embryo during later development. Other functions have been ascribed to specific proteins, since many of the proteins *in vitro* have bactericidal properties, while some have enzymatic activity and some are enzyme inhibitors.

The shell serves to physically protect and contain the embryo during development, to allow gas exchange between the embryo and the environment, and to act as a barrier against microbial invasion and water loss. It is composed of three structures: the membranes, the mineralized shell, and the cuticle. The two shell membranes are sheets of fibrous protein, together about 70 $\mu$m thick. At the large end of the egg, the protein sheets separate to form an air sac. Functionally, the shell membranes provide the surface on which mineralization can occur; fibers of the outer shell membrane serve as the site of growth of calcium carbonate crystals and serve as the organic matrix of the shell. The membranes may also reduce the speed of bacterial entry, allowing the bactericidal properties of egg white to act more effectively.

The egg shell is about 350 $\mu$m thick and is composed of radiating crystals of pure calcium carbonate. Running vertically through the shell are pores that allow gases to pass. The shell forms a physical barrier to substances that might adversely affect the microenvironment of the embryo. It also provides mechanical strength and a rigid support to maintain the orientation of the heterogeneous internal components. The shell's strength is determined mainly by its curvature and thickness, although other factors are involved. It also provides calcium for the developing embryo. The outer covering of the egg, the proteinaceous cuticle, is freely permeable to fluid transfer prior to oviposition, but dries immediately after the egg is laid to become a barrier against bacterial contamination and water loss.

### *Female Reproductive System*

The transformation of an oocyte into a fully-formed egg requires 8 to 10 days from the start of rapid follicular growth to oviposition. The female reproductive system of the bird differs markedly from that of mammals to permit the graded maturation of preovulatory follicles that are then ovulated singly, followed by the successive formation of all other egg components during a one-day passage through the oviduct. The formation of the egg involves the transport of large quantities of material across numerous biological membranes, and the formation of many new substances, particularly specific proteins and lipids. The size and composition of the egg, and the rate at which eggs are produced, are affected by numerous genetic, environmental, and physiologic factors.

OVARY. In birds, as in mammals, two ovaries and oviducts are formed during embryogenesis, but a characteristic feature of birds is the suppression of further development of these organs on the right side (52, 53). Unlike mammals, the embryonic ovary of the bird is much more active in the production of estrogens than is the testis, indicating that the sex of the developing avian embryo is basically male (54). Production of estrogen occurs only in genetic females through expression of the aromatase gene at the time of gonadal differentiation (55). Since the P450 aromatase enzyme converts androgens to estrogens, the gonads of an embryo that is destined to become a female produce more estrogens than those of an embryo destined to become a male. The estrogen receptor is abundant in the cortex of the left ovary but not in the male gonad (56), suggesting that differential expression of both aromatase and estrogen receptor in genetic females may explain many of the unique features of gonadal development in the bird. Müllerian-inhibiting substance (MIS; also called "anti-Müllerian hormone") causes regression of Müllerian ducts in males in both birds and mammals, but unlike mammals, the female embryonic gonad of the bird also produces MIS (57). Since estrogen appears to prevent Müllerian duct regression in females through direct action on the duct (58), the regression of the right duct may result from the combined production of MIS and low expression of estrogen receptor in the right female gonad (55). The functional left ovary (Fig.

16-9) produces ova and acts as an endocrine organ secreting both steroid and protein hormones.

The ovary consists of a medulla, which contains connective tissue, blood vessels, and nerves, and a cortex. The cortex contains the oogonia, which give rise to the oocytes (Fig. 16-10**A**). The pear-shaped, immature chicken ovary is about 15 mm long by 5 mm wide, lying in the body cavity, ventral to the aorta, cranial to the kidney, and close to the two adrenal glands. The blood supply arises from the gonadorenal artery. Two veins drain blood from the ovary. It is extensively innervated from the sympathetic chain by way of the adrenal-ovarian plexus (52).

FOLLICULAR DEVELOPMENT AND GAMETOGENESIS. Ovarian weight increases at the onset of sexual maturity. Of the thousands of oocytes present, many enlarge in size to about 6 to 8 mm in diameter. Once a yellow follicle exceeds 8 mm in diameter, it will normally continue to grow and ovulate. The majority of the follicles in this size range, however, fail to develop or become atretic (Fig. 16-10**F**) (59). In a high-producing chicken, one of the 8 mm follicles will enlarge and enter the follicular hierarchy every 25 to 27 hours. This follicle will continue to grow and will ovulate 5 to 7 days later. This successive maturation of follicles results in the follicular hierarchy that is characteristic of the bird ovary (Fig. 16-9). However, selection of chickens for rapid growth has resulted in an increase in ovarian weight and in the number of developing follicles on the ovary of the meat-type chicken. In contrast to egg-type chickens, the ovaries of the broiler breeder hen contain about twice as many yellow follicles. This increase in the number of developing follicles paradoxically results in a decline in egg production because two or more ova may be ovulated in one day and result in soft-shelled or double-yolked eggs. Some ova are ovulated into the body cavity and reabsorbed without entering the reproductive tract (60). This poor reproduction is typically improved by limiting the body weight of broiler breeders through feed restriction. Turkey hens lay at a lower rate than either egg-type or meat-type chickens (Table 16-3), due in part to a slower rate of follicular growth (9 to 10 days from 8 mm in diameter to ovulation) (61).

The liver, not the ovary, is the major source of yolk proteins and phospholipids (62). The production of yolk precursors in the liver is regulated by estrogen. A chicken that lays each day produces about 19 grams of yolk precursors daily that are transported to the ovary and deposited in growing follicles by receptor-mediated mechanisms. This transport of large quantities of phospholipids results in the extremely lipemic serum that is characteristic of laying hens.

OVIDUCT. The hen's oviduct (Fig. 16-9 and Fig. 16-10**G**) consists of five functionally distinct components. The

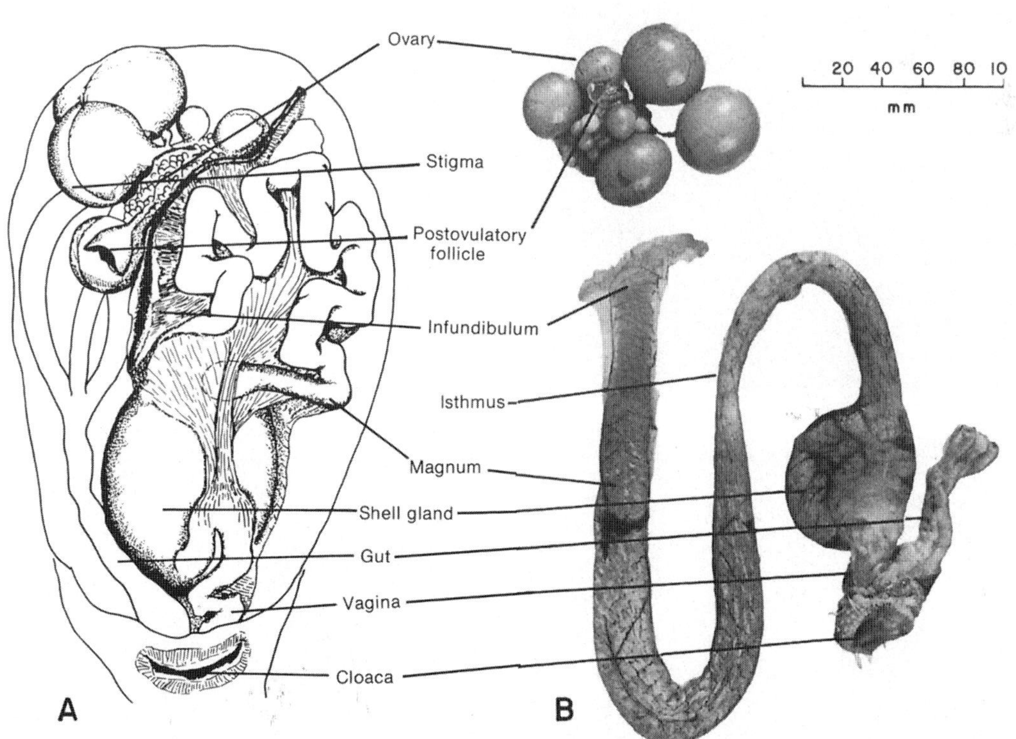


FIGURE 16-9. (**A**) The ovary of the domestic hen in situ. (**B**) The ovary and oviduct of the domestic hen.

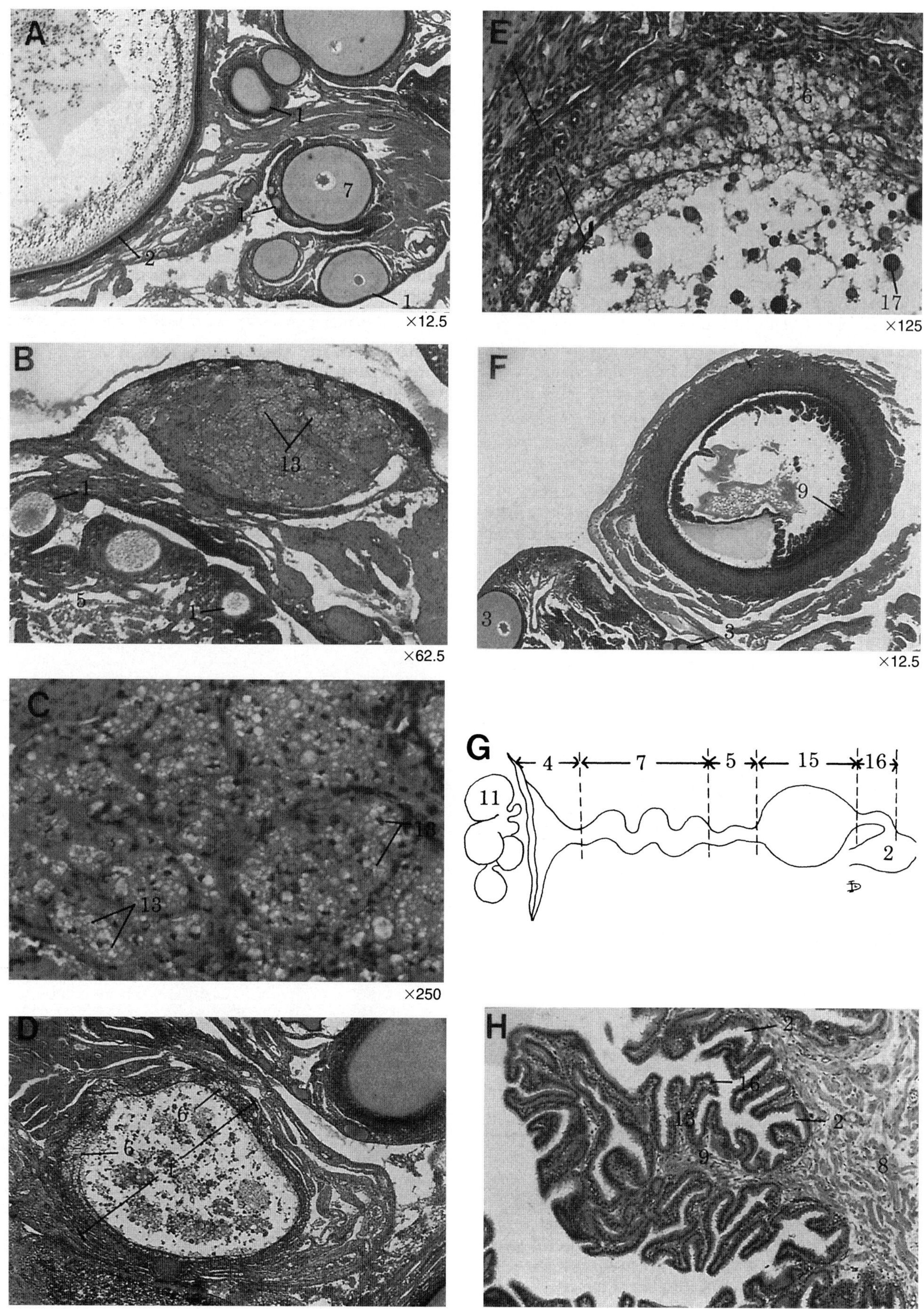
A
1
7
1
2
1
×12.5
B
13
1
5
1
×62.5
C
13
13
×250
D
6
6
1
×25
E
6
17
×125
F
9
3
3
×12.5
G
4
7
5
15
16
11
2
H
2
16
13
2
9
8
×62.5

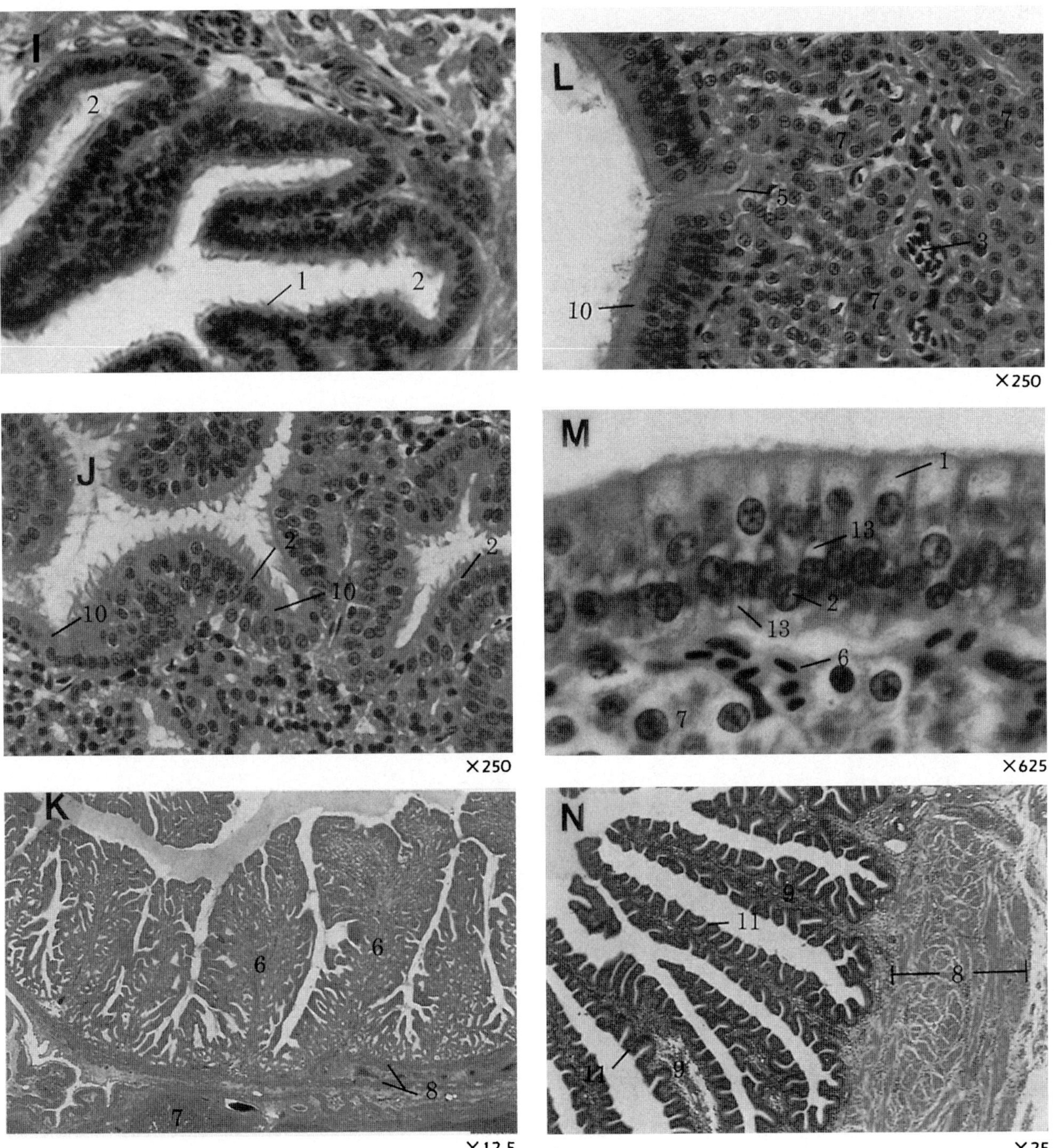


FIGURE 16-10. The histology of the ovary, oviduct, uterus, and vagina of the hen. (From: Pacha WJ Jr, Wood LM. Color Atlas of Veterinary Histology. Philadelphia: Lea & Febiger, 1990. Published with permission from Lippincott Williams & Wilkins, Baltimore, MD.) **(A)** Ovary. A portion of the ovarian cortex with developing follicles. **(B)** Ovary, Vacuolar Cells. A portion of the cortex with a mass of fat-laden vacuolar cells. The latter may represent regressing post-ovulatory follicles. **(C)** Ovary, Vacuolar Cells. Details of **B**. Vacuolar cells have pyknotic nuclei and contain numerous fat vacuoles. Cell boundaries are often indistinct. **(D)** Ovary, Atretic Follicle. In some atretic follicles, interstitial (luteal) cells proliferate, hypertrophy, and migrate inward (see **E**). **(E)** Ovary, Atretic Follicle, detail of **D**. **(F)** Atretic Follicle. Cells of the membrana granulosa have proliferated, forming a thick layer characteristic of many atretic follicles. **(G)** Diagrammatic. The oviduct of the hen is divisible into an infundibulum, magnum isthmus uterus, and vagina. **(H)** Neck of Infundibulum, cross-section, Oviduct. Tall primary mucosal folds bear secondary and tertiary folds. **(I)** Neck of Infundibulum, cross-section, Oviduct. Detail of muscosa showing folds lined by ciliated columnar cells. The bases of the grooves between the folds are lined by nonciliated secretory cells, which collectively line the glandular grooves. **(J)** Magnum Oviductal Epithelium. Cilated columnar and secretory (goblet) cells comprise the epithelium of the magnum. The nuclei of the secretory cells are round and are located close to the base of the cell, whereas the nuclei of the ciliated cells are oval and occupy the central to apical region of the cell. Accordingly, the epithelium is pseudostratified columnar. **(K)** Isthmus, cross-section, Oviduct. The primary folds of the isthmus are not as broad as those of the magnum. They are somewhat angular in appearance. A portion of an adjacent region of the magnum is present in this micrograph. **(L)** Uterus (Shell Gland), Oviduct. Ducts of complex, branched, tubular glands pierce the pseudostratified columnar epithelium at intervals. Ducts are formed from polygonal gland cells. **(M)** Uterus (Shell Gland), Oviduct. Basal cells (nuclei close to the basement membrane) of the pseudostratified epithelium may contain vacuoles above and below their nuclei. Apical cells (nuclei centrally located) contain numerous granules before releasing their secretion. **(N)** Vagina, cross-section, Oviduct. The mucosa of the vagina is characterized by long, slender, primary folds bearing numerous small secondary folds. The muscularis is highly developed.

most anterior is the *infundibulum*, which acts to engulf the ovulated ovum and is the site of fertilization. The narrower, glandular portion of the infundibulum is known as the "chalaziferous region" (Fig. 16-10**H** and **I**), and secretions from this region form an "outer" perivitelline layer and likely contribute to the formation of the chalazae (Fig. 16-8). The chalaziferous region is also one of two known sperm storage sites in the oviduct.

The *magnum* is the albumen-secreting region. It is the longest oviductal segment and is distinguishable from the infundibulum and isthmus by its greater external diameter, thicker walls, and more voluminous folds (Fig. 16-11 and Fig. 16-10**J**). The majority of the 40 proteins which comprise the albumen are produced in the oviductal mucosa. The tubular glands are the source of ovalbumin, which makes up 54% of the egg white, as well as lysozyme, ovotransferrin, and ovomucoid. The cells of the tubular glands appear to produce egg-white proteins continuously and store them in granules, which are released as the ovum passes. The protein avidin is formed in the epithelial goblet cells (Fig. 16-10**J**).

The *isthmus* is a short section of the oviduct which

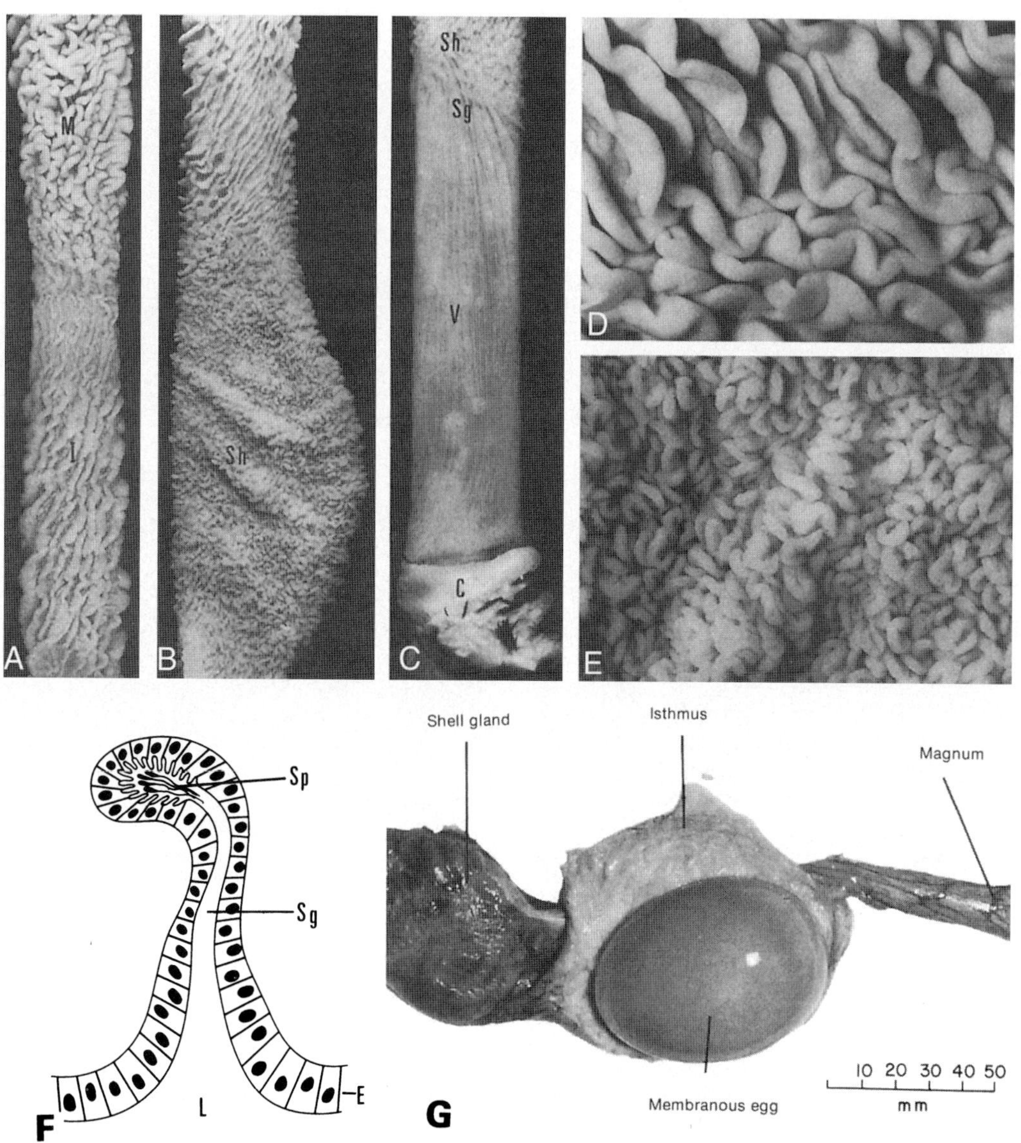


FIGURE 16-11. (**A**) The luminal surface of the magnum and isthmus. (**B**) The luminal surface of the shell gland and its junction with the isthmus. (**C**) The luminal surface of the vagina. (**D**) Higher power view of the mucosal folds of the magnum. (**E**) Higher power view of the mucosal folds of the shell gland. (**F**) Sperm storage tubules located in the junction between the shell gland and the vagina. (**G**) An egg *in situ* in the isthmus. Note the membranous covering only and the typical egg shape. C, cloaca; *E*, epithelium; *I*, isthmus; *L*, lumen of oviduct; M, magnum; *Sg*, sperm storage tubule; *Sh*, shell gland; *Sp*, spermatozoa; *V*, vagina.

forms the shell membrane around the developing egg. The isthmus is characterized by narrower and thinner walls, and by luminal folds less voluminous than those found in the magnum (Fig. 16-10K). Little is known of the mechanisms involved in the formation of the shell membrane proteins or their release and deposition on the egg. It has been observed, however, that while the albumenous egg is entering the isthmus, a membrane is deposited on those parts in contact with the glandular tissue. In the chicken, the typical shape of the egg is produced by the membranes and not by the calcified shell, which is laid down on the already-formed shape (Fig. 16-11). At this stage, the membranes are loosely applied to the egg, which has about 50% of its final mass.

The *shell gland*, often referred to as the uterus, is characterized by a pouch-like section joined to the isthmus by a short "neck" and by extensive muscularization (Fig. 16-9). The egg remains in the shell gland for approximately 20 hours (Fig. 16-12). During the first 6 hours or so, a watery fluid produced by the neck region passes into the egg, resulting in a twofold increase in the mass of egg white. However, this "plumping" may continue throughout the time the egg stays in the shell gland. Thereafter, the main process is calcification. During its stay in the shell gland, rotation of the egg around the polar axis leads to the completion of the formation of the chalazae, which started in the infundibulum, and the stratification of the albumen (Fig. 16-8).

Shell calcification probably starts in the isthmus where small projections from the outer shell membrane, the mammillary cores, are formed. In the shell gland, growth of the calcite crystals continues at a constant rate of mineralization (about 300 mg calcium per hour). The oviduct does not store calcium, and about 20% of the calcium in the blood is removed as the egg passes through the shell gland. The specific cells responsible for transferring calcium into the lumen appear to be the surface epithelial cells and not the tubular gland epithelial cells (Fig. 16-10L). The high-producing hen has an enormous requirement for calcium, depositing 2.0 to 2.5 g of calcium in the egg shell each day. Due to the photoperiodic control of ovulation, deposition of calcium in the shell occurs primarily during the dark period when food and water consumption are normally low. To meet this need, the hen temporarily stores dietary calcium in the bone when demand is low and mobilizes this calcium when needed for shell formation. The calcium is stored as calcium phosphate in medullary bone, initiated by an increase in estrogen secretion at sexual maturity. Calbindin-$D_{28K}$ is an intracellular protein which binds calcium with high affinity and plays an important role in calcium transport in the intestine and shell gland. The production of this protein in the intestine is specifically regulated by $1\alpha,25(OH)_2D_3$, which is the hormonal form of vitamin $D_3$, while calbindin-$D_{28K}$ synthesis in the shell gland appears to be stimulated by the presence of an egg and the calcium flux associated with calcium deposition (63).

The final tasks of the shell gland are pigmentation and the formation of the cuticle. The pigments consist of porphyrin derivatives of hemoglobin metabolism, and are deposited during the last few hours in the shell gland. The cuticle is deposited after the shell is complete, just before oviposition.

The vagina has the appearance of being relatively short, primarily because the cranial half is tightly folded and bound together by connective tissue (Fig. 16-9). The muscular layer is well developed, and the luminal folds are high and

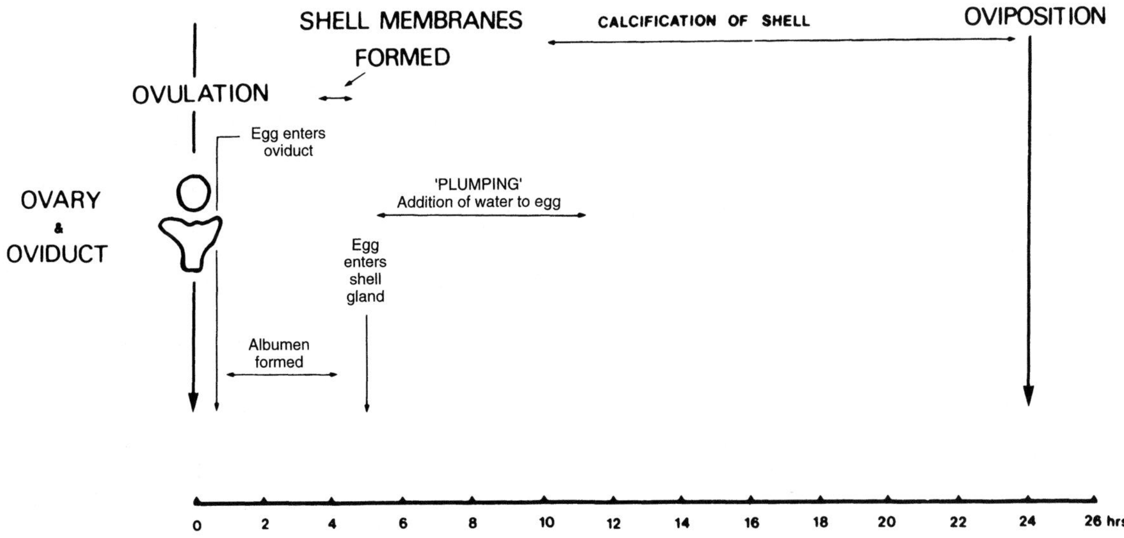


FIGURE 16-12. Egg formation from ovulation to oviposition. (From: Gilbert AB. The female reproductive effort. In: Bell DJ, Freeman BM, eds. Physiology and Biochemistry of the Domestic Fowl. New York: Academic Press, 1971.)

narrow (Fig. 16-10N). The vagina serves as a passage for the formed egg from the shell gland to the cloaca at oviposition. It also serves an important function in the selection, transport and storage of sperm.

EGG TRANSPORT AND OVIPOSITION. The transport of the egg along the oviduct is similar in all domestic poultry. The developing egg spends about 15 minutes in the infundibulum. In the magnum, its speed averages about 2 mm/min and hence takes about 2 or 3 hours to traverse this region (Fig. 16-12). The egg takes about 1 to 1 1/2 hours to pass through the isthmus. About 20 hours of its total time in the oviduct (about 26 hours) is spent in the shell gland. Passage through the vagina takes only a few seconds. Although the mechanism for transport of the egg along the oviduct is not fully understood, egg-induced distention of the oviduct has been shown to excite the smooth musculature and to increase the rate of egg transport in quail.

It is not known precisely how oviposition is initiated, but both hormonal and neural mechanisms are involved. Oviposition, i.e. expulsion of the egg from the oviduct, occurs by vigorous contractions of the shell-gland muscle and relaxation of the uterovaginal sphincter (possibly analogous to the cervix of mammals). Like mammalian parturition, oviposition in birds is regulated, at least partly, by a neurohypophyseal hormone (arginine vasotocin; AVT) and by ovarian prostaglandins. The largest post-ovulatory follicle (the tissue mass remaining after ovulation of the previous follicle) secretes prostaglandin $F_{2\alpha}$, which initiates contraction of the shell gland, where both AVT and prostaglandin receptors are found. Recent studies have shown that galanin, a peptide found widely in the nervous system and various organs in mammals, causes oviposition in quail and may act as a neurotransmitter or neuromodulator in the shell gland (64). Passage of the egg into the vagina and accompanying distention of the vaginal wall brings about the "bearing-down" reflex, which is characterized by a change in respiration and stance, and contraction of the abdominal body muscles.

SPERM STORAGE, TRANSPORT, AND FERTILIZATION. Unlike most mammals in which sperm spend a relatively short time in the female tract, chicken and turkey sperm spend prolonged periods of time (up to 32 days in the chicken, 70 days in the turkey) housed within the oviduct sperm storage tubules located at the uterovaginal junction (Fig. 16-11). How sperm enter, survive, and exit these sperm storage tubules is not known.

Transport of sperm to the uterovaginal junction is rapid, less than an hour; however, only viable sperm enter the sperm storage tubules. Although first thought to be associated with oviposition, current evidence suggests that the release of stored sperm is continuous or episodic. These sperm ascend the oviduct by way of smooth muscle contractions and/or ciliary activity and accumulate in the mucosal folds and short tubular glands at the lower end of the infundibulum. At ovulation, sperm are released (probably by distention of the infundibulum) to fertilize the ovum. Sperm that make contact with the perivitelline layer undergo an acrosome reaction and, presumably by the action of the trypsin-like enzyme acrosin, hydrolyze the perivitelline layer. Polyspermy is observed in the hen ovum, with many holes hydrolyzed in the perivitelline layer. Although theoretically only one sperm needs to penetrate the perivitelline layer surrounding the germinal disc to cause fertilization, a clear relationship exists between the number of such holes present in any egg and the probability of that egg being fertile (65).

## CONTROL OF GAMETE PRODUCTION

### *Initiation of Egg Production*

Most birds, including poultry, are seasonal breeders that initiate reproduction in response to an increase in daylength (photoperiod). When a young bird is hatched, typically in the spring under natural conditions, it is unresponsive to increasing daylength until it has acquired "photosensitivity" by exposure to several weeks of short days (winter). This "photorefractory" period prevents premature reproduction during the winter, when survival of young would be poor. After the female reaches sexual maturity, subsequent exposure to an increasing photoperiod then initiates egg production. The degree of photorefractoriness varies with species. Turkey hens *must* receive a short photoperiod and subsequent photostimulation with at least 11 hours of light per day to lay normally, while young chickens maintained on long days (more than 8 hours of light per day) will begin laying by 24 weeks of age without exposure to a short photoperiod. Environmental light control permits year-round poultry production, and is combined with nutritional manipulations to insure that birds are sufficiently mature, at the time that egg laying commences, to produce adequately large eggs for either hatching offspring or for human consumption. Typically, egg production is initiated at about 18 to 20 weeks of age in chickens and 28 to 30 weeks of age in turkeys by increasing the photoperiod from 6 hours to 12 or more hours. This increase in photoperiod is perceived by photoreceptors in the brain during the first long day and results in an immediate increase in secretion of luteinizing hormone (LH) by the pituitary gland, due primarily to an increase in baseline LH secretion (66). Increased secretion of LH and follicle-stimulating hormone (FSH) results in growth of ovarian follicles and production of estrogen, primarily by the small follicles. These small follicles begin producing estrogens and androgens at an early stage of development in the immature female. Androgens are necessary for the expression of secondary sex characteristics and serve as precursors for estrogen production. Estrogen stimulates development of the oviduct and formation of medullary bone, as discussed earlier. Egg production typically begins

2 to 4 weeks after photostimulation, and will reach a peak within a few weeks. The young egg-type chicken will lay an egg each day for many days before skipping a day. This pattern of daily egg laying followed by a skip day is called a *sequence* or *clutch*. As the chicken ages, the clutch length shortens; e.g., she will drop from 10 to 20 eggs in a clutch to 4 or 5 eggs in a clutch, and the egg production rate will decrease to 60 to 70%. This gradual decrease in the number of eggs laid in a clutch is the result of an increase in the time required for the follicles to become competent to ovulate, and therefore of a greater interval between ovulations. Most hens have a single characteristically long sequence at about the time of peak egg production, and Robinson et al (67) have suggested that the length of this "prime" sequence is a good predictor of that hen's egg production later in life.

### Ovarian Anatomy and Function

As noted earlier, the ovary of the laying hen contains many small white and yellow follicles up to 8 or 10 mm in diameter, plus five to nine (or more) preovulatory follicles arranged in a hierarchy of size. Several postovulatory follicles (Fig. 16-9), representing the regressing ovarian tissue remaining after a prior ovulation, are also found. The preovulatory follicles are numbered according to size, with the $F_1$ being the largest follicle and the next to ovulate; $F_2$, the second largest follicle, will ovulate the day after the $F_1$ follicle ovulates, and so on. The follicle consists of the oocyte and several layers of tissue, namely, the vitelline membrane and zona radiata (the inner-most layers); the perivitelline layer; granulosa layer, theca layer (including theca interna and theca externa); loose connective tissue; and the superficial epithelium (the outermost layer) (Figs. 16-12 and 16-13).

The endocrine function of the avian ovary, like that of the mammal, is critical to reproduction. The granulosa cell layer produces primarily progesterone with low amounts of androgens. The theca interna cells produce some progesterone and principally androgens, whereas the aromatase-containing cells of the theca externa layer are the site of estrogen production (68). As the preovulatory follicles grow ($F_5 \rightarrow F_1$), there is a significant increase in progesterone production by the granulosa layer and a gradual decrease in androgen and estrogen secretion by the theca layer (68–70). These dramatic changes in steroid production are the result of a change in responsiveness to gonadotropins (i.e., the granulosa layer becomes more responsive to LH as the $F_1$ follicle approaches ovulation) and the removal of an inhibition by the theca layer (specifically, androgens and estrogen) on progesterone production by the granulosa layer (71). Thus, the granulosa cells attain their maximum capacity for progesterone production in the $F_1$ follicle.

Other hormones, besides steroids, are produced by the

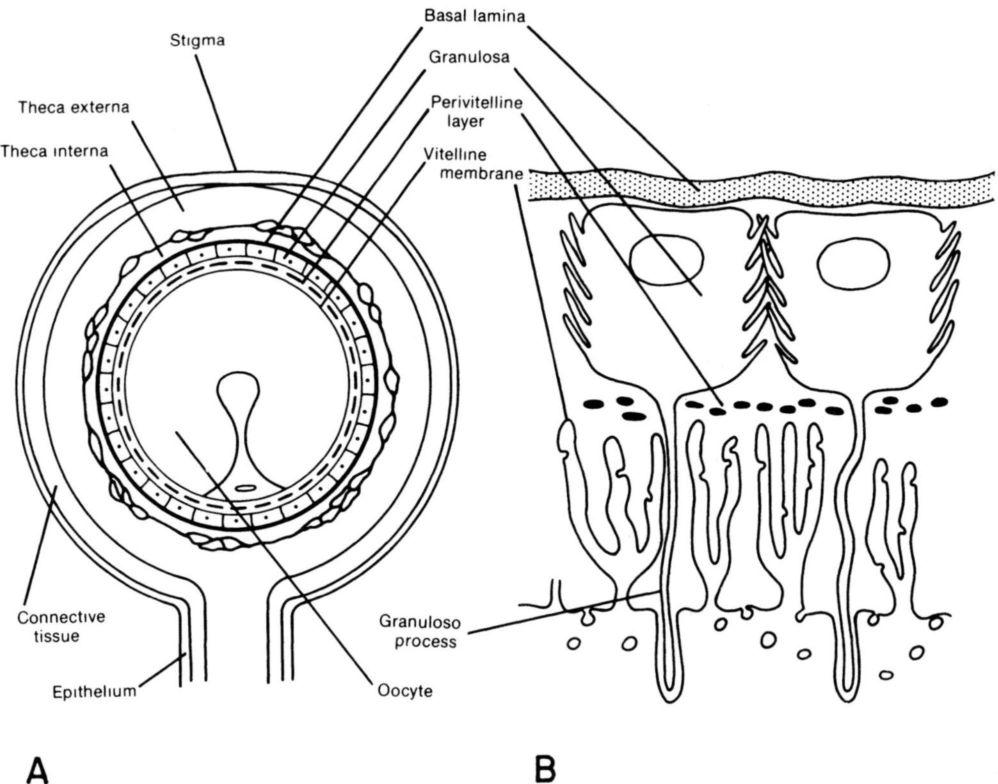


**FIGURE 16-13.** (**A**) Cross section of a maturing follicle. (Redrawn from: Gilbert AB. Female genital organs. In: King AS, McLelland J, eds. Form and Function in Birds. New York, Academic Press, 1979.) (**B**) Diagram of the oocyte surface and the granulosa layer.

ovary. *Prostaglandins*, a class of hormones some of which are involved in the stimulation of uterine contraction and oviposition, are produced by the granulosa cells of the largest follicles (72). Two protein hormones, *inhibin* and *activin*, are also produced by the granulosa cells of large follicles. These hormones each occur in at least two different forms and share a common subunit, but they have opposite biological effects. Inhibin has an endocrine effect on the pituitary, and acts to inhibit FSH release in chickens (73). The endocrine effect of activin in mammals is to stimulate FSH secretion, but this action has not been demonstrated in birds. Both inhibin and activin also exhibit local effects within the ovary in mammals, affecting steroidogenesis, and cell proliferation and differentiation. Rombauts et al. (74) have demonstrated that recombinant human inhibin and activin have opposing actions on steroidogenesis of chicken embryonic gonadal tissue *in vitro*. *Follistatin* is a binding protein for activin, and ovarian expression is most abundant in the small yellow follicles (75). The precise role of these ovarian hormones in regulating follicular development and ovulation in poultry is still largely unknown. Other peptide hormones, including insulin-like growth factors I and II and transforming growth factor alpha, may also be involved in the intraovarian control of ovarian function in the bird.

### *Ovulatory Cycle*

The chicken, unlike the mammal, has only a follicular phase. Because the chicken does not get pregnant, there is no need for a corpus luteum. Therefore, the cycle of follicular growth and hormonal changes that culminates in ovulation is called the *ovulatory cycle*. Approximately every 25 to 27 hours, an egg is laid. During this cycle, a preovulatory surge of LH occurs 4 to 6 hours before ovulation (76). In contrast to the changes in LH, blood levels of FSH are relatively constant throughout the cycle (77).

Ovulation of the second and subsequent ova in a clutch occurs about 30 minutes after oviposition of the preceding egg. Since most hens require more than 24 hours to complete an ovulatory cycle, both oviposition and ovulation occur at later times on successive days. The key factors determining the timing of ovulation (and subsequent oviposition) are the generation of the preovulatory LH surge and the presence of a mature follicle at the time that the LH surge occurs. The timing of the preovulatory LH surge is the result of a circadian rhythm which restricts this surge to an 8-hour "open" period during the 24-hour day. The location of this open period within the light-dark cycle appears to be controlled by the onset of darkness, but the anatomical structures and the exact endocrine interactions among the hypothalamus, pituitary, and ovary which are necessary to define the open period and lead to the preovulatory LH surge are unresolved. The result, however, is that the LH surge occurs at a later time each night until eventually no LH surge can occur because the required neuroendocrine events which culminate in this surge have not occurred during the open period and no egg is laid the next day. This day is called a "pause" day. The hen will then reset her neuroendocrine rhythm, ovulate early in the open period, and lay the first egg of the next clutch early the next day.

### *Termination of Egg Production*

Under natural rearing conditions, egg production is terminated by the onset of incubation behavior or photorefractoriness. Nature's reproductive season is relatively short for most birds, and has been lengthened for commercial poultry through selective breeding and management. High-producing strains of egg-type chickens have been bred to lay an average of 260 to 285 eggs in a year. Use of artificial light provides a constant or increasing photoperiod, and photorefractoriness is minimal in these strains. Similarly, selection for egg production has largely eliminated incubation behavior (broodiness), which is the hen's natural tendency to cease laying and incubate a clutch of eggs. Meat-type strains of poultry have shorter reproductive cycles and produce fewer eggs. Broiler breeder hens average about 180 eggs in a reproductive season of up to 40 weeks, while turkey breeder hens average 90 to 100 eggs in 25 weeks. Flock egg production beyond this period is usually unprofitable and the hens must either be replaced or "recycled"; that is, exposed to a short photoperiod for 10 to 12 weeks and fed to lose body weight so that the reproductive system regresses, the bird 'molts' (replaces its feathers), and the reproductive endocrine system is reset.

PHOTOREFRACTORINESS. The onset of reproduction occurs when light, acting through photoreceptors in the brain, provides neural signals which the bird's reproductive endocrine system perceives as a daylength that is of sufficient length to initiate reproduction. However, as time passes, these neural signals begin to fail to maintain gonadotropin secretion despite continued light stimulation. This "photorefractoriness" is a gradual event characterized by a gradual decline in egg production until, finally, the pituitary is no longer secreting sufficient LH to maintain the gonad and gonadal regression occurs. The mechanism of this ovarian regression appears to reside in the hypothalamus, where the synthesis or secretion of luteinizing hormone releasing hormone (LHRH) declines (78). Photorefractoriness occurs very gradually in egg-type chickens, but often occurs early in the reproductive season of turkey and broiler breeder hens. Only recycling (equivalent to the reproductive "winter") will re-establish the neuroendocrine system at a level that again supports reproduction.

INCUBATION BEHAVIOR. This behavior has largely been eliminated from egg-type chickens, and reduced through breeding in broiler breeder hens, but remains a substantial problem in turkey breeder flocks. Incubation behavior results from a series of neural and endocrine events which lead to a dramatic elevation in pituitary prolactin secretion. High

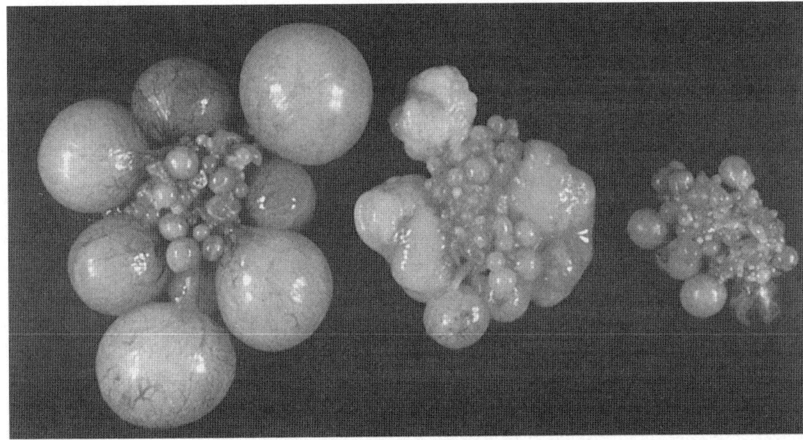

FIGURE 16-14. The onset of broodiness is accompanied by regression of the ovary, beginning with atresia of the larger follicles of the hierarchy and resorption of the yolk. The ovary on the left is from a laying hen. The ovary in the center is from an incubating hen 5 days after lay of the last egg. The ovary on the right is from an incubating hen 10 days after lay of the last egg. (From Proudman JA. Biology of egg production and fertility. In: Bakst MR, Wishart GJ, eds. Proceedings: First International Symposium on the Artificial Insemination of Poultry. Savoy, IL: Poultry Science Association, 1995.)

circulating levels of prolactin cause regression of the ovary and an end to egg laying. A sequence of hormonal and environmental stimuli are necessary to initiate incubation behavior. The increases in estrogen and progesterone secretion which occur with the onset of egg production can also act to prepare the hen for incubation. Progesterone induces nesting activity, while estrogen stimulates the synthesis of *vasoactive intestinal peptide* (VIP), which is the hypothalamic releasing hormone that stimulates prolactin secretion in birds (79). Nesting results in contact of the *brood patch*, a defeathered cutaneous region on the hen's breast, with the nest and eggs, and stimulates eight sensory cutaneous nerves which send impulses to the brain (80). These impulses, through unknown mechanisms, cause increased prolactin secretion which results in persistent nesting behavior. At this time, even though the hen may still be laying eggs at a high rate, the hormonal events which initiate follicular atresia have already occurred, and continued nesting will result in rapid and complete regression of the ovary (Fig.

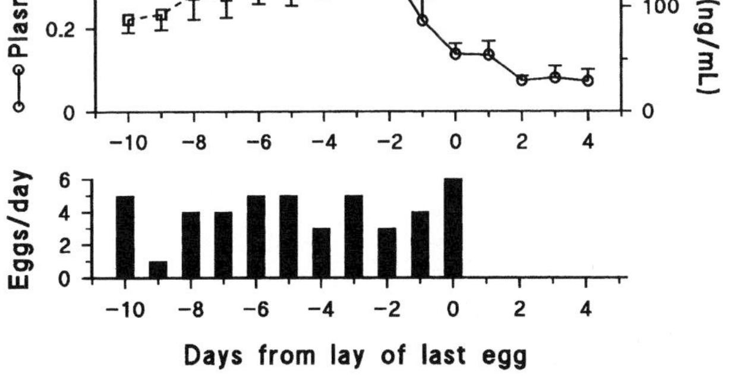

FIGURE 16-15. Changes in plasma prolactin and progesterone concentrations, and egg production in six turkey hens during the transition from egg laying to broodiness. (From Proudman JA. Biology of egg production and fertility. In: Bakst MR, Wishart GJ, eds. Proceedings: First International Symposium on the Artificial Insemination of Poultry. Savoy, IL: Poultry Science Association, 1995.)

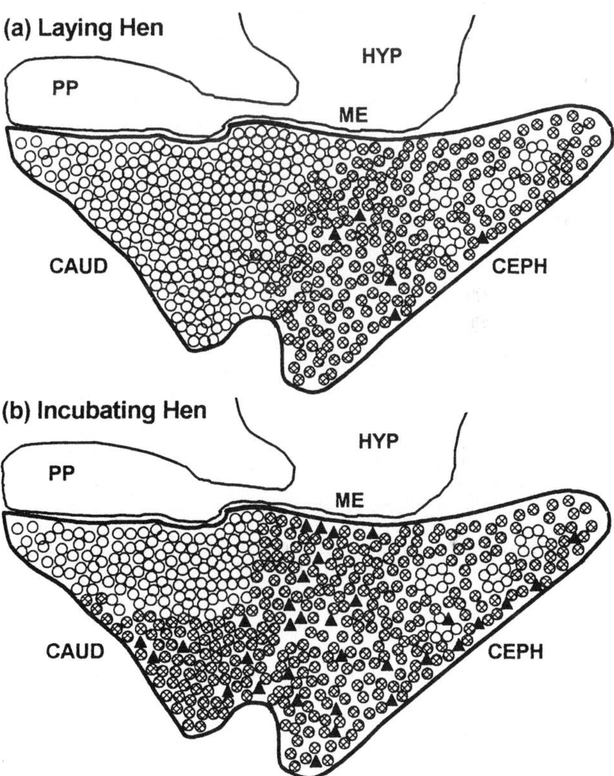


FIGURE 16-16. Diagram of the midsagittal anterior pituitary gland of a laying turkey hen (**A**) and an incubating turkey hen (**B**) showing the distribution of somatotrophs (*open circle*), lactotrophs (*hatched circle*), and mammosomatotrophs (*triangle*). *HYP*, hypothalamus; *PP*, posterior pituitary; *ME*, median eminence; *CEPH*, cephalic lobe; *CAUD*, caudal lobe of the anterior pituitary gland. This diagram is not drawn to scale. (From: Ramesh R, Solow R, Proudman JA, Kuenzel WJ. Identification of mammosomatotrophs in the turkey hen pituitary: Increased abundance during hyperprolactinemia. Endocrinology 1998;139:781.)

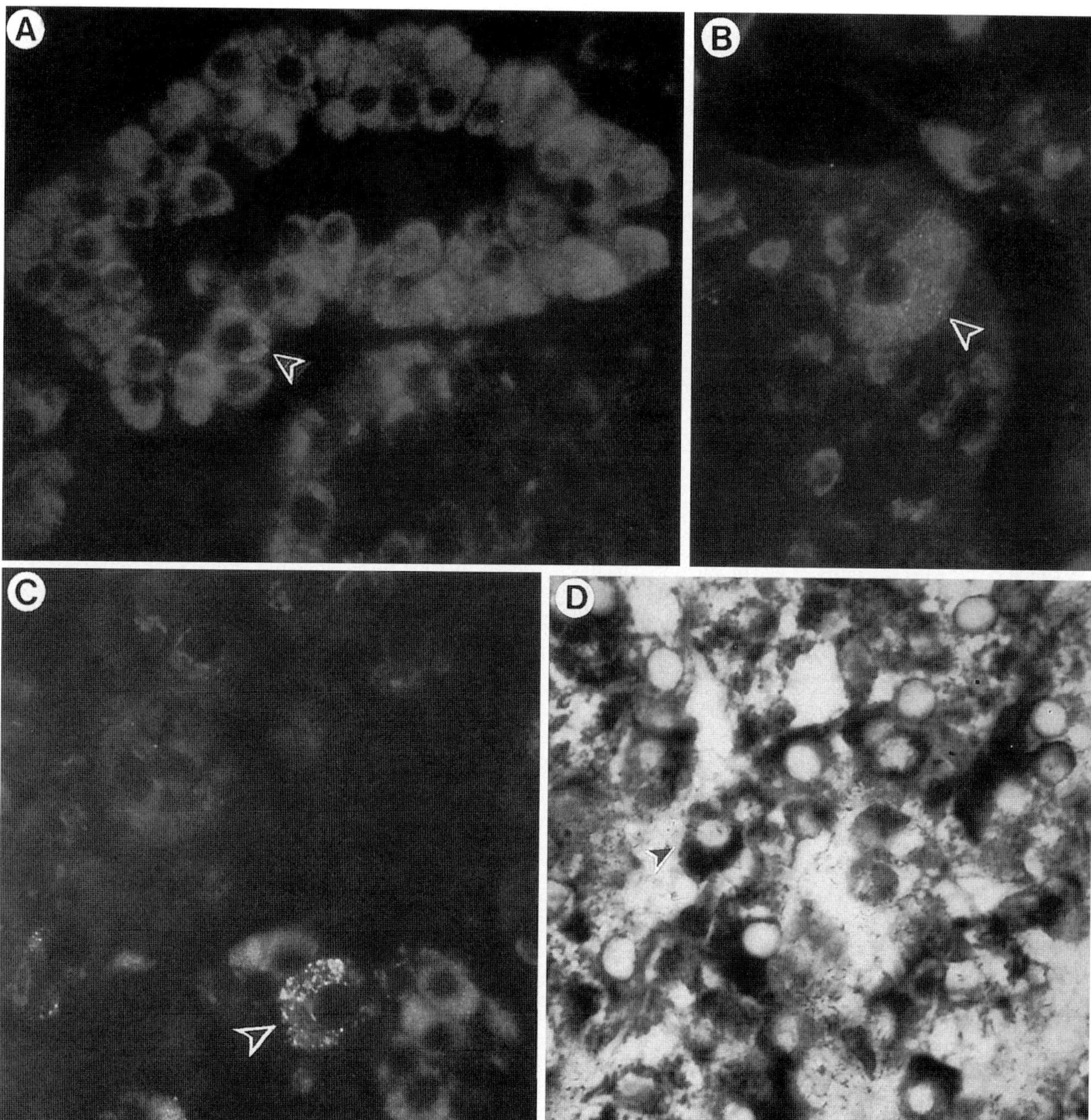


FIGURE 16-17. (A–C) Photomicrographs of midsagittal sections of the anterior pituitary gland of incubating turkey hens showing lactotrophs, somatotrophs, and mammosomatotrophs. *Arrows* in all panels indicate the mammosomatotroph. Original magnification, 1000×. (A) Islets of somatotrophs and lactotrophs in the pituitary cephalic lobe. (B) Hypertrophied mammosomatotroph at the junction of the cephalic and caudal lobes, showing prolactin molecules around the nucleus. (C) Photomicrograph of the caudal lobe, showing mammosomatotrophs containing discrete granules that colocalize prolactin and growth hormone within the same secretory granules. (D) Photomicrograph of a midsagittal pituitary section of an incubating turkey hen stained by *in situ* hybridization and immunohistochemistry. The *arrow* indicates a mammosomatotroph, showing colocalization of prolactin mRNA and growth hormone. Original magnification 1000×. (From: Ramesh R, Solow R, Proudman JA, Kuenzel WJ. Identification of mammosomatotrophs in the turkey hen pituitary: Increased abundance during hyperprolactinemia. Endocrinology 1998;139:781.)

16-14). Figure 16-15 shows that the gradual increase in circulating prolactin levels during the time that nesting frequency is increasing (but while the hen is still laying) is accompanied by a precipitous decline in basal circulating levels of progesterone.

Dramatic changes occur in the pituitary during the onset of incubation behavior to support the need for high and sustained prolactin secretion. *Lactotrophs*, the pituitary cells which produce prolactin, are confined to the cephalic lobe of the anterior pituitary in the laying hen while *somatotrophs*, which produce growth hormone, are mostly found in the caudal lobe (Fig. 16-16). However, as nesting frequency increases lactotrophs become more numerous, first occupying the ventral region of the caudal lobe and subsequently populating the entire pituitary except for the most dorsocaudal region. Simultaneously, somatotrophs quickly disappear from these areas and become localized in the dorsocaudal region (81). This change is associated with a dramatic increase in prolactin secretion (hyperprolactinemia), but growth hormone secretion (which is very low in the adult) is not altered. The mechanism of this change in pituitary cytology is uncertain, but studies have shown the existence of a bihormonal *mammosomatotroph* which contains both prolactin and growth hormone. This cell may be an intermediate in the conversion of cell function from the production of growth hormone to the production of prolactin, and, indeed, the abundance of mammosomatotrophs is 12-fold greater in the incubating turkey hen than in the laying turkey hen (Fig. 16-17) (82). This change in pituitary cytology is readily reversible, since removal of the incubating turkey hen from the nest (and from the tactile stimulation of the brood patch) results in disappearance of lactotrophs and reappearance of somatotrophs within 5 days (83).

In the context of the hen which is permitted to incubate eggs, circulating prolactin levels remain elevated until hatching. Once chicks or poults hatch, incubation behavior ceases and the hen exhibits maternal behavior. This behavioral change is accompanied by a precipitous decline in circulating prolactin levels, and requires the tactile stimulus of the chick. Visual and auditory stimuli alone are not sufficient to terminate incubation behavior (84, 85).

The neuroendocrine events associated with incubation behavior and prolactin secretion are complex (see El Halawani et al (79) for a review), but stimulation of the pituitary by VIP is essential. The increase in plasma prolactin levels which normally occur during egg production and incubation behavior in the turkey hen can be largely abolished by immunization of turkey hens against VIP (86). Immunized hens nest only as needed to lay eggs, incubation behavior is largely eliminated, and flock egg production is improved.

### *Acknowledgement*

Thanks are due to Dr. MR Bakst and Dr. JM Bahr for Figures 16-8, 16-9, 16-11, 16-12, and 16-13 previously published in their respective chapters in the 6th edition of *Reproduction in Farm Animals*.

## REFERENCES

1. Ashizawa K, Sano R. Effects of temperature on the immobilization and the initiation of motility of spermatozoa in the male reproductive tract of the domestic fowl, *Gallus domesticus*. Comp Biochem Physiol 1990;96(A):297.
2. Froman DP, Feltmann AJ. Sperm mobility: A quantitative trait of the domestic fowl (*Gallus domesticus*). Biol Reprod 1998;58:379.
3. Bakst MR, Wishart G, Brillard J-P. Oviducal sperm selection, transport, and storage in poultry. Poultry Science Rev 1994;5:117.
4. Zavaleta D, Ogasawara F. A review of the mechanism of the release of spermmatozoa from storage tubules in the fowl and turkey oviduct. World's Poultry Science J 1987;43:132.
5. Hodges RD. The Reproductive System. In: The Histology of the Fowl. London: Academic Press, 1974.
6. Froman DP. Biology of semen production and ejaculation. In: Bakst MR, Wishart GJ, eds. First International Symposium on the artificial insemination of poultry (Proceedings). Savoy, IL: Poultry Science Association, 1995.
7. Kirby JD, Froman DP. Reproduction in the male bird. In: Whittow GC, ed. Sturkie's Avian Physiology. Orlando: Academic Press, 1998.
8. Nickel R, Schummer A, Seiferle E, Siller WG, Wight PAL. Urogenital System. In: Anatomy of Domestic Birds. Berlin: Springer-Verlag, 1977.
9. King AS. *Systema urogenitale*. In: Baumel JJ, ed. Nomina Anatomica Avium. London: Academic Press, 1979.
10. Lake PE. Male genital organs. In: King AS, McLelland J, eds. Form and Function in Birds, Vol 2. London: Academic Press, 1981.
11. Osman DI, Ekwall H, Ploen L. Specialized cell contacts and the blood-testis barrier in the seminiferous tubules of the domestic fowl (*Gallus domesticus*). Int J Anrol 1980;3:553.
12. Bergmann M, Schindelmeiser J. Development of the blood-testis barrier in domestic fowl (*Gallus domesticus*). Int J Androl 1987;10:481.
13. Tingari MD. On the structure of the epididymal region and ductus deferens of the domestic fowl (*Gallus domesticus*). J Anat 1971;109:423.
14. Bakst MR. Luminal topography of the male chicken and turkey excurrent duct system. Scan Electron Microsc 1980; 3:419.
15. Fujihara N. Accessory reproductive fluids and organs in male domestic birds. World's Poultry Sci J 1992;48:39.
16. King AS. Phallus. In: King AS, McLelland J, eds. Form and Function in Birds. London: Academic Press, 1981.
17. Clulow J, Jones RC. Production, transport, maturation, storage and survival of spermatozoa in the male Japanese quail, *Coturnix coturnix*. J Reprod Fert 1982;64:259.
18. Lin M, Jones RC, Blackshaw AW. The cycle of the seminiferous epithelium in the Japanese quail (*Coturnix coturnix japonica*) and estimation of its duration. J Reprod Fert 1990;88:481.
19. Lin M, Jones RC. Spatial arrangement of the stages of the

cycle of the seminiferous epithelium in the Japanese quail, *Coturnix coturnix japonica.* J Reprod Fert 1990;90:361.
20. Lin M, Jones RC. Renewal and proliferation of spermatogonia during spermatogenesis in the Japanese quail, *Coturnix coturnix japonica.* Cell Tiss Res 1992;267:591.
21. Lin M, Jones RC. Spermiogenesis and spermiation in the Japanese quail (*Coturnix coturnix japonica*). J Anat 1993; 183:525.
22. Sprando RL, Russell LD. Spermiogenesis in the red-ear turtle (*Pseudemys scripta*) and the domestic fowl (*Gallus domesticus*): A study of cytoplasmic events including cell volume changes and cytoplasmic elimination. J Morph 1988;198:95.
23. Clulow J, Jones RC. Studies of fluid and spermatozoal transport in the extratesticular genital ducts of the Japanese quail. J Anat 1988;157:1.
24. de Reviers M, Williams JB. Testis development and production of spermatozoa in the cockerel (*Gallus domesticus*). In: Cunningham FJ, Lake PE, Hewitt D, eds. Reproductive Biology of Poultry. Harlow, UK: British Poultry Science, 1984.
25. Kirby JD, Mankar MV, Hardesty D, Kreider DL. Effects of transient prepubertal 6-n-propyl-2-thiouracil treatment on testis development and function in the domestic fowl. Biol Reprod 1996;55:910.
26. Beaupre CE, Tressler CJ, Beaupre SJ, Morgan JLM, Bottje WG, Kirby JD. Determination of testis temperature rhythms and effects of constant light on testicular function in the domestic fowl (*Gallus domesticus*). Biol Reprod 1997;56:1570.
27. Shanbhag BA, Sharp PJ. Immunocytochemical localization of androgen receptor in the comb, uropygial gland, testis, and epididymis of the domestic chicken. Gen Comp Endo 1996;101:76.
28. You S, Bridgham JT, Foster DN, Johnson AL. Characterization of the chicken follicle-stimulating hormone receptor (cFSH-R) complementary deoxyribonucleic acid, and expression of cFSH-R messenger ribonucleic acid in the ovary. Biol Reprod 1996;55:1055.
29. Tiba T, Yoshida K, Miyake M, Tsuchiya K, Kita I, Tsubota T. Regularities and irregularites in the structure of the seminiferous epithelium in the domestic fowl (*Gallus domesticus*). I. Suggestion of the presence of a seminiferous epithelial cycle. Anat Hist Embryol 1993;22:241.
30. Tiba T, Shimizu Y, Kita I, Tsubota T. Regularities and irregularities in the structure of the seminiferous epithelium in the domestic fowl (*Gallus domesticus*). II. Coordination between germ cell associations. Anat Hist Embryol 1993;22:254.
31. Hsu C-C, Kirby JD. The expression of Follicle Stimulating Hormone receptor during testis development of the domestic fowl. Poultry Sci 1998;(In press)
32. Kwon S, Hess RA, Bunick D, et al. Rooster testicular germ cells and epididymal sperm contain P450 aromatase. Biol Reprod 1995;53:1259.
33. Kwon S, Hess RA, Bunick D, Kirby JD, Bahr JM. Estrogen recptors are present in the epididymis of the rooster. J Andrology 1997;18:378.
34. Rothwell B. The ultrastructure of Leydig cells in the testis of the domestic fowl. J Anat 1973;116:245.
35. Rozenboim I, Snapir N, Arnon E, et al. Precocious puberty in tamoxifen-treated cockerels: hypothalamic gonadotrophin-releasing hormone-I and plasma luteinising hormone, prolactin, growth hormone and testosterone. Br Poult Sci 1993; 34:533.
36. Kuenzel WJ, Abdel-Maksoud MM, Proudman JA, Elasser T. Early sexual maturation induced by sulfamethazine in chicks is mediated by elevated LH and FSH release and transient inhibition of thyroid hormones. Poultry Sci 1995;74(Suppl 1):75.
37. Kuenzel WJ, Paulson OD, Smith DJ. Evidence that stimulation of gonadal development by sulfamethazine involves the central nervous system. Poultry Sci 1996;75(Suppl 1):93.
38. Vizcarra JA, Hernandez AG, Bahr JM, Kuenzel WJ, Kreider DL, Kirby JD. Rescue of impaired spermatogenesis in adult male fowl following unrestricted prepubertal growth and subsequent growth restriction. Biol Reprod 1998;(In press).
39. Wingfield JC, Hahn TP, Levin R, Honey P. Environmental predictability and control of gonadal cycles in birds. J Exp Zool 1992;261:214.
40. Kuenzel WJ. The search for deep encephalic photoreceptors within the avian brain, using gonadal development as a primary indicator. Poultry Sci 1993;72:959.
41. Thurston RJ, Hess RA. Ultrastructure of spermatozoa from domesticated birds: Comparative study of turkey, chicken, and guinea fowl. Scan Electron Microsc 1987;1:1829.
42. Howarth B Jr. Fertilizing ability of cock spermatozoa from the testis, epididymis, and vas deferens following intramagnal insemination. Biol Reprod 1983;28:586.
43. Esponda P, Bedford JM. Surface of the rooster spermatozoon changes in passing through the Wolffian duct. J Exp Zool 1985;234:441.
44. Morris SA, Howarth B Jr, Crim JW, Rodriguez de Cordoba S, Esponda P, Bedford JM. Specificity of sperm-binding Wolffian duct proteins in the rooster and their persistence on spermatozoa in the female host glands. J Exp Zool 1987;242:189.
45. Perrault SD, Kirby JD. Internal fertilization in birds and mammals. In: Knobil E, Neill JD, eds. The Encyclopedia of Reproduction, Vols 1–4. Orlando: Academic Press, 1998.
46. Howarth B Jr. Maturation of spermatozoa and mechanism of fertilisation. In: Cunningham FJ, Lake PE, Hewitt D, eds. Reproductive Biology of Poultry. Harlow, UK: British Poultry Sci, 1984.
47. Koyanagi F, Masuda S, Nishiyama H. Acrosome reaction of cock spermatozoa incubated with perivitelline layer of the hen's ovum. Poultry Sci 1988;67:1770.
48. Howarth B. Avian sperm-egg interaction: Perivitelline possesses receptor active for spermatozoa. Poultry Sci 1990; 69:1012.
49. Howarth B. Carbohydrate involvement in sperm-egg interaction in the chicken. J Receptor Res 1992;12:255.
50. Kuroki M, Mori M. Binding of spermatozoa to the perivitelline layer in the presence of a protease inhibitor. Poultry Sci 1997;76:748.
51. Barbato GF, Cramer PG, Hammerstedt RH. A practical *in vitro* sperm-egg binding assay that detects subfertile males. Biol Reprod 1998;58:686.
52. Gilbert AB. Female genital organs. In: King AS, McLelland J, eds. Form and Function in Birds. New York: Academic Press, 1979.
53. Mittwoch U. Heterogametic sex chromosomes and the development of the dominant gonad in vertebrates. Am Nat 1983;122:159.
54. Tanabe Y, Saito N, Nakamura T. Ontogenic steroidogenesis by testes, ovary, and adrenals of embryonic and postembryonic

chickens (*Gallus domesticus*). Gen Comp Endocrinol 1986; 63:456.

55. Nakabayashi O, Kikuchi H, Kikuchi T, Mizuno S. Differential expression of genes for aromatase and estrogen receptor during the gonadal development of chicken embryos. J Mol Endocrinol 1998;20:193.
56. Andrews JE, Smith CA, Sinclair AH. Sites of estrogen receptor and aromatase expression in the chicken embryo. Gen Comp Endocrinol 1997;108:182.
57. Eusebe D, di Clemente N, Rey R, et al. Cloning and expression of the chick anti-Mullerian hormone gene. J Biol Chem 1996;271:4798.
58. Doi O, Hutson JM. Pretreatment of chick embryos with estrogen in ovo prevents Mullerian duct regression in organ culture. Endocrinology 1988;122:2888.
59. Johnson AL. Regulation of follicle differentiation by gonadotropins and growth factors. Poultry Sci 1993;72:867.
60. Hocking PM. Effects of body weight at sexual maturity and the degree and age of restriction during rearing on the ovarian follicular hierarchy of broiler breeder females. Brit Poultry Sci 1993;34:793.
61. Hocking PM, Waddington D, Walker MA. Changes in ovarian function of female turkeys photostimulated at 18, 24 or 30 weeks of age and fed *ad libitum* or restricted until point of lay. Brit Poultry Sci 1992:33:639.
62. Griffin HD, Perry MM, Gilbert AB. Yolk formation. In: Freeman BM, ed. Physiology and Biochemistry of the Domestic Fowl. London: Academic Press, 1984.
63. Ieda T, Saito N, Ono T, Shimada K. Effects of presence of an egg and calcium deposition in the shell gland on levels of messenger ribonucleic acid of CaBP-$D_{28K}$ and of vitamin $D_3$ receptor in the shell gland of the laying hen. Gen Comp Endocrinol 1995;99:145.
64. Li D, Tsutsui K, Muneoka Y, Minakata H, Nomoto K. An oviposition-inducing peptide: Isolation, localization, and function of avian galanin in the quail oviduct. Endocrinology 1996;137:1618.
65. Wishart GJ. Regulation of the length of the fertile period in the domestic fowl by numbers of oviductal spermatozoa, as reflected by those trapped in laid eggs. J Reprod Fert 1987; 80:493.
66. Bacon WL, Long DW. Changes in plasma luteinizing hormone concentration in turkey hens after switching from short-day to long-day photoperiods. Domest Anim Endocrinol 1995; 12:257.
67. Robinson FE, Hardin RT, Robblee AR. Reproductive senescence in domestic fowl: effects on egg production, sequence length and inter-sequence pause length. Brit Poultry Sci 1990;31:871.
68. Porter TE, Hargis BM, Silsby JL, El Halawani ME. Differential steroid production between theca interna and theca externa cells: A three-cell model for follicular steroidogenesis in avian species. Endocrinology 1989;125:109.
69. Bahr JM, Wang SC, Huang MY, Calvo FO. Steroid concentrations in isolated theca and granulosa layers of preovulatory follicles during the ovulatory cycle of the domestic hen. Biol Reprod 1983;29:326.
70. Etches RJ, Duke CE. Progesterone, androstenedione and oestradiol content of theca and granulosa tissue of the four largest ovarian follicles during the ovulatory cycle of the hen (*Gallus domesticus*). J Endocrinol 1984;103:71.
71. Johnson PA, Stoklosowa S, Bahr JM. Interaction of granulosa and theca layers in the control of progesterone secretion in the domestic hen. Biol Reprod 1987;37:1149.
72. Etches RJ, Kelly JD, Anderson-Langmuir CE, Olson DM. Prostaglandin production by the largest preovulatory follicles in the domestic hen (*Gallus domesticus*). Biol Reprod 1990; 43:378.
73. Johnson PA, Brooks C, Wang S-Y, Chen C-C. Relationship between plasma immunoreactive inhibin and gonadotropins in response to follicle removal in the domestic hen. Biol Reprod 1993;49:1026.
74. Rombauts L, Vanmontfort D, Decuypere E, Verhoeven G. Inhibin and activin have antagonistic paracrine effects on gonadal steroidogenesis during the development of the chicken embryo. Biol Reprod 1996;54:1229.
75. Davis AJ, Johnson PA. Expression pattern of messenger ribonucleic acid for follistatin and the inhibin/activin subunits during follicular and testicular development in *Gallus domesticus*. Biol Reprod 1998;59:271.
76. Wilson SC, Sharp PJ. Variations in plasma LH levels during ovulatory cycle of the hen (*Gallus domesticus*). J Reprod Fert 1973;35:561.
77. Krishnan KA, Proudman JA, Bolt DJ, Bahr JM. Development of an homologous radioimmunoassay for chicken follicle-stimulating hormone and measurement of plasma FSH during the ovulatory cycle. Comp Biochem Physiol 1993;105(A):729.
78. Sharp PJ. Photoperiodic control of reproduction in the domestic hen. Poultry Sci 1993;72:897.
79. El Halawani ME, Youngren OM, Pitts GR. Vasoactive intestinal peptide as the avian prolactin-releasing factor. In: Harvey S, Etches RJ, eds. Perspectives in Avian Endocrinology. Bristol, UK: Society for Endocrinology, 1997.
80. Book CM, Millam JR, Guinan MJ, Kitchell RL. Brood patch innervation and its role in the onset of incubation in the turkey hen. Physiol Behav 1991;50:281.
81. Ramesh R, Proudman JA, Kuenzel WJ. Changes in pituitary somatotroph and lactotroph distribution in laying and incubating turkey hens. Gen Comp Endocrinol 1996;104:67.
82. Ramesh R, Solow R, Proudman JA, Kuenzel WJ. Identification of mammosomatotrophs in the turkey hen pituitary: Increased abundance during hyperprolactinemia. Endocrinology 1998; 139:781.
83. Ramesh R, Proudman JA, Kuenzel WJ. Cellular changes in the pituitary gland following nest-deprivation of incubating turkey hens. Poultry Sci 1997;76(Suppl 1):46.
84. Opel H, Proudman JA. Effects of poults on plasma concentrations of prolactin in turkey hens incubating without eggs or a nest. Brit Poultry Sci 1988;29:791.
85. Richard-Yris MA, Sharp PJ, Wauters AM, Guemene D, Richard JP, Foraste M. Influence of stimuli from chicks on behavior and concentrations of plasma prolactin and luteinizing hormone in incubating hens. Horm Behav 1998; 33:139.
86. El Halawani ME, Silsby JL, Rozenboim I, Pitts GR. Increased egg production by active immunization against vasoactive intestinal peptide in the turkey (*Meleagris gallopavo*). Biol Reprod 1995;44:179.

# PART IV

# *Reproductive Failure*

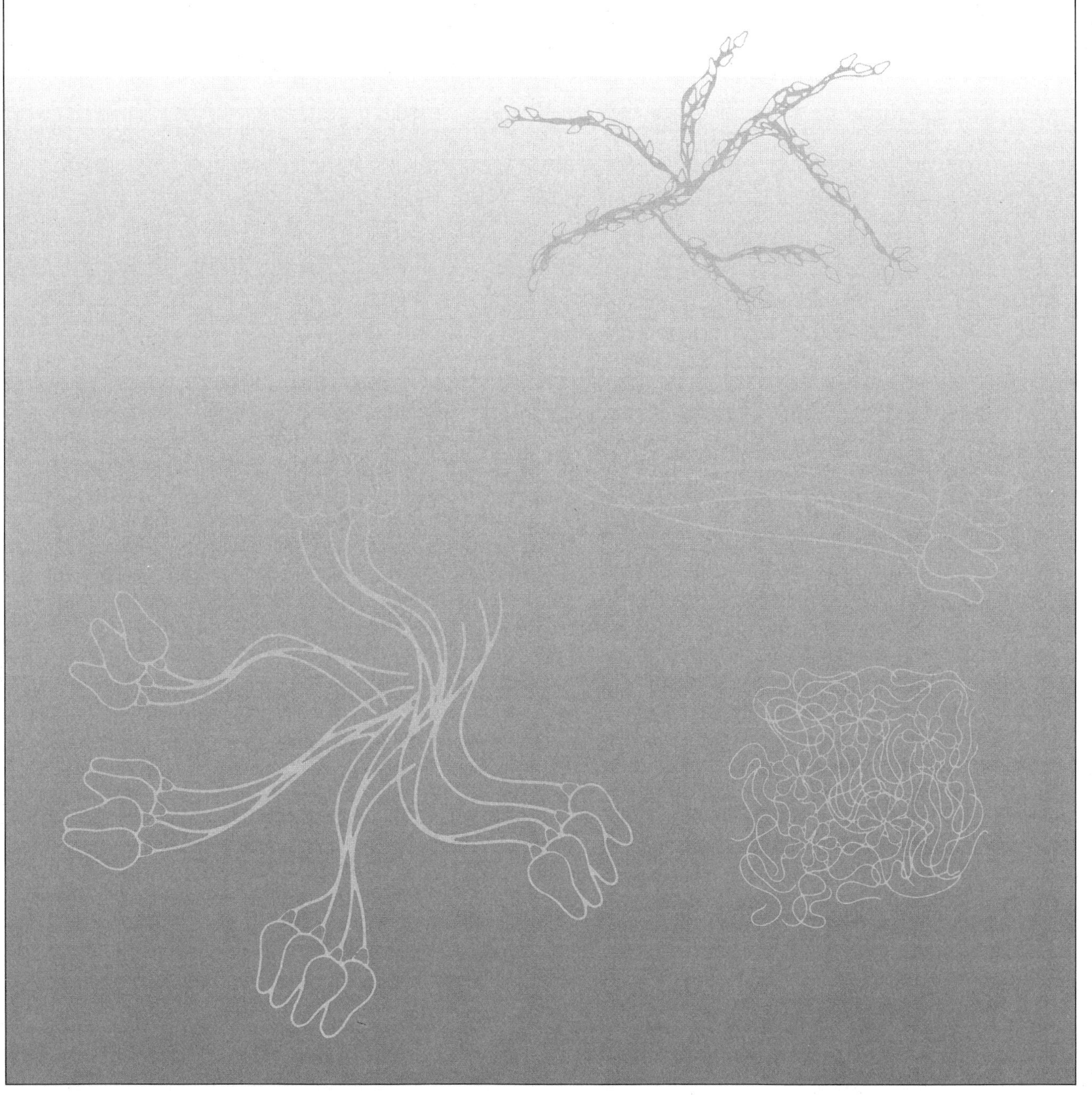

# CHAPTER 17

# *Reproductive Failure in Females*

M.R. JAINUDEEN AND E.S.E. HAFEZ

During domestication, man gradually transformed the reproductive processes of farm animals from a free grazing, seasonal mating system to an intensive production, year-round mating system. As a result, the efficiency of reproduction of farm animals often declined due to environmental factors and the demands of economic production. These factors may result in partial or complete reproductive failure. Sterility is a permanent factor preventing procreation, and infertility or temporary sterility is the inability to produce viable young within a stipulated time characteristic for each species. This chapter examines the phases of the reproductive process that are most vulnerable—estrous cycle, pregnancy, parturition, and shows how hormonal imbalances, infectious diseases, or adverse environmental and genetic factors exert their influences (Fig. 17-1). The chapter discusses ovarian dysfunction, pregnancy wastage, neonatal mortality, and finally the disorders of parturition and the puerperium.

## OVARIAN DYSFUNCTION

The mammalian ovary performs two main functions—the production of ova and secretion of ovarian hormones. These functions are intimately related and directed toward successful reproduction. Reference has already been made to the estrous cycles in different species (see Chapters 10 through 15), particularly to the physiological aspects of puberty, seasonality of breeding, and the postpartum resumption of the estrous cycle. In this section, the discussion will focus on abnormalities of estrus, ovary, and the uterus.

### *Anestrus*

Anestrus denotes a state of complete sexual inactivity with no manifestations of estrus. It is not a disease but a sign of a variety of conditions (Table 17-1). Although anestrus is observed during certain physiologic states—e.g., before puberty, during pregnancy, and lactation, and in seasonal breeders—it is most often a sign of temporary or permanent depression of ovarian activity (true anestrus) caused by seasonal changes in the physical environment, nutritional deficiencies, lactation stress, and aging (Fig. 17-2). Certain pathologic conditions of the ovaries or the uterus also suppress estrus.

### *Ovarian Abnormalities*

Ovarian abnormalities that cause anestrus are of two types (Fig 17-2):

1. Failure of the ovaries to develop. *Ovarian hypoplasia* occurs in Swedish Mountain cattle. Affected animals have infantile reproductive tracts and never exhibit estrus. Ovarian hypoplasia tends to be associated with white coat color, being inherited as an autosomal recessive. Some mares with small inactive ovaries have abnormal sex chromosome complement (e.g., XO) as well as low plasma estrogen and high LH levels. *Freemartins* are heifers born co-twin to bulls, have poorly developed ovaries, and fail to show estrus.
2. Persistence of the CL associated with uterine pathology. The conditions include *pyometra, mucometra, fetal mummification*, or *maceration* in cattle, sheep, and pig (see later in this chapter) and *pseudopregnancy* in the mare, sow, and doe. Functional corpora lutea and a uterus containing either endometrial gland secretions or remnants of embryonic or fetal tissue characterize pseudopregnancy in the pig. Injections of estrogens (embryonic luteotrophin) toward the end of the luteal phase of the estrous cycle also induce pseudopregnancy in the sow.

Pseudopregnancy (hydrometer) in the doe is the accumulation of uterine fluid associated with the persistence of the CL. The abdomen of the doe enlarges as in pregnancy, but udder development and kidding fail to occur. The term

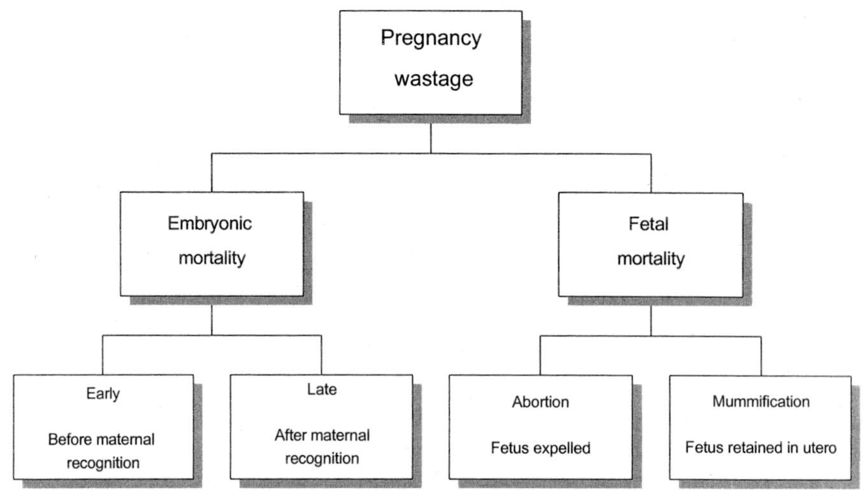


FIGURE 17-1. Manifestations of reproductive failure in female farm animals.

*cloudburst* is used when spontaneous discharge of a cloudy uterine fluid occurs around the expected time of parturition that has been mated. Progesterone levels are elevated, making it difficult to differentiate this state from pregnancy; it can easily be diagnosed by real-time ultrasonography by the lack of placentomes in the fluid-filled uterus (see Chapter 28). The factors causing pseudopregnancy in the goat have not been established, but prolactin plays an important luteotrophic role (1). Both $PGF_{2\alpha}$ and repeated oxytocin treatments result in a decline in progesterone levels, estrous behavior, and the discharge of intrauterine fluid (2).

*Prolonged diestrus*, apparently unique to mares, results from spontaneous prolongation of the life of the cyclic CL beyond the normal 14 to 15 days. It is a major cause of

TABLE 17-1. ***Abnormalities of Estrus***

| SPECIES | ABNORMALITY | CAUSES | PHYSIOLOGIC MECHANISMS |
|---|---|---|---|
| Cattle | Anestrus | Pyometra, mummification | Maintenance of corpus luteum |
| | | Lactation | Suckling stimulus inhibits gonadotropin release |
| | | Cystic ovaries | Deficiency of LH and/or GnRH |
| | | Ovarian hypoplasia and freemartinism | Failure to produce ovarian estrogens |
| | | Nutritional and vitamin deficiencies | Gonadotropin production by anterior pituitary |
| | Subestrus, silent estrus (quiet ovulation) | High lactation | |
| | Nymphomania | Cystic ovaries | Endocrine imbalance |
| Sheep | Anestrus | Season, lactation | Effect of photoperiod on gonadotropin secretion |
| Swine | Anestrus | Lactation | As for cattle |
| Horse | Anestrus | Season, diet, ovarian hypoplasia | As for sheep |
| | Prolonged estrus | Early in breeding season | Failure of follicle beyond 2 cm to develop that is due to inadequate endocrine stimulus |
| | Split estrus, silent estrus | | |
| | Lack of estrus | Pseudopregnancy | Early pregnancy failure with persistence of corpus luteum |
| | | Prolonged diestrus after foaling | Persistance of corpus luteum |

GnRH = gonadotropin-releasing hormone

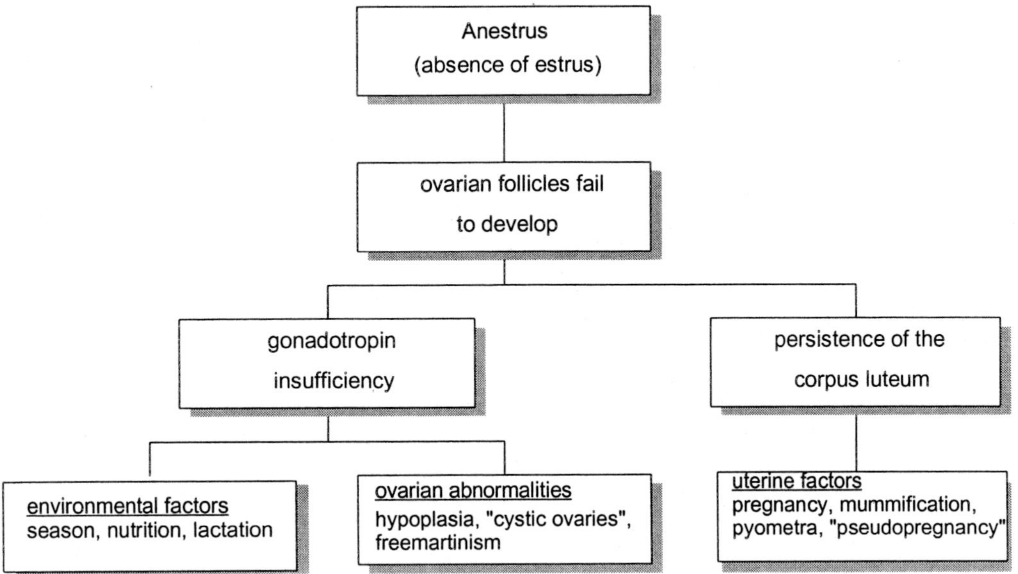


FIGURE 17-2. Possible causes leading to a failure of follicle development in the ovary and anestrus in farm animals. Note that pregnancy is an important cause for an absence of estrus.

anestrus during the natural breeding season. Persistence of the CL may be attributed to a failure of $PGF_{2\alpha}$ release.

## *Ovulatory Failure*

Ovulatory failure may be due to failure of the follicle to ovulate during a normal cycle or to cystic ovaries.

*Anovulatory estrus* is more common in swine and horses than in cattle and sheep. The animal shows normal behavioral estrus and the ovarian follicle reaches preovulatory size but does not rupture. Anovulatory follicles become partly luteinized and then regress during the estrous cycle, as does a normal CL.

*Cystic ovarian disease* or "cystic ovaries" is common in dairy cattle and swine but is rarely encountered in beef cattle or other species. The disease is a common endocrine abnormality in dairy cattle, particularly among high-producing dairy cows. Most ovarian cysts probably develop prior to the first ovulation postpartum since more ovarian cysts are detected in cows examined at 30 days postpartum than after breeding or after abnormal estrous behavior. Although some affected cows may exhibit intense mounting behavior (nymphomania), the majority fails to exhibit estrus (anestrus). One or both ovaries contain one or more large cysts exceeding 2.5 cm diameter. These are either follicular or luteal cysts. Follicular cysts undergo cyclic changes, i.e., they alternately grow and regress but fail to ovulate. Luteal cysts contain a thin rim of luteal tissue, also fail to ovulate, but persist for a prolonged period. In the past, the differentiation of the type of cyst was based on rectal palpation, which was highly subjective. However, with advent of transrectal ultrasonography (Chapter 28), the accuracy of the differentiation has been markedly improved.The available evidence indicates that it may be caused by a failure in the LH-release mechanism. This failure is not due to a deficiency or release of GnRH but more to an insensitivity of the hypothalamic-pituitary axis to elevated levels of estradiol.

The development of cystic ovaries in cattle has been related to high milk production, seasonal changes, hereditary predisposition, and pituitary dysfunction (Fig. 17-3).

1. The cause and effect relationship between milk production and cystic ovarian disease is not clear, but the high milk yield may be a response to hormonal changes in cows with ovarian cysts rather than the cause of the disease.
2. Development of cystic ovaries has been related to postpartum uterine infections. Endotoxins produced by microorganisms in the uterus may trigger the $PGF_{2\alpha}$ release, which in turn stimulates the secretion of cortisol. The elevated cortisol levels suppress the preovulatory release of LH and lead to the development of cysts (3).
3. A relationship exists between cystic ovarian disease and heredity as the incidence has steadily declined in several herds after culling bulls whose daughters had cystic ovarian disease (4).
4. Cystic ovaries are also frequently encountered in dairy cows fed higher levels of nutrients, and during the winter.

Several methods are available for the treatment of cystic ovarian disease in cattle.

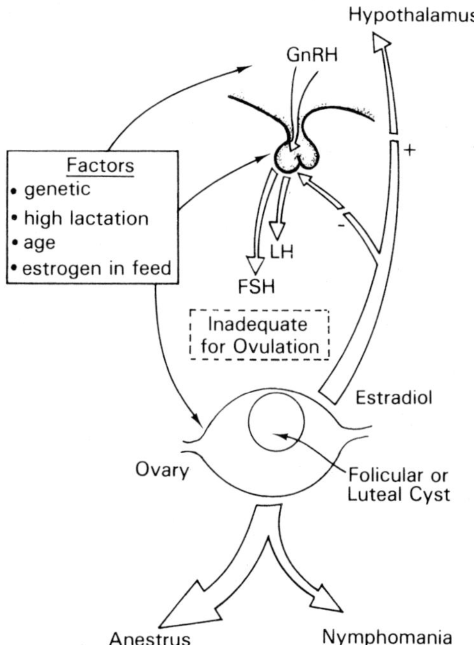


FIGURE 17-3. Endocrine sequence, types of cysts, and behavioral manifestations associated with cystic ovarian disease in the cow. Inadequate secretion of LH results in ovulatory failure and formation of follicular or luteal cysts. Note that affected cows are either nymphomaniac or in anestrus.

1. Manual rupture of the cyst by rectal palpation is one of the oldest methods.
2. hCG and GnRH are equally effective for the treatment of follicular cysts, but GnRH, being of lower molecular weight, is less likely to stimulate antibody formation.
3. Prostaglandin $F_{2\alpha}$ or its analogs are effective for treatment of luteal cysts.
4. Progesterone injections or progesterone intravaginal devices may also restore ovarian cycles in cows with ovarian cysts.

*Cystic ovaries in swine* are an important cause of reproductive failure and a major reason for culling, particularly older sows. Large multiple luteinized follicles are more common than small multiple cysts, and they contain progesterone. Estrous cycles that are irregular with prolonged periods between cycles may be mistaken for pregnancy. Signs of estrus are pronounced, but nymphomania does not occur.

## DISORDERS OF FERTILIZATION

Disorders of fertilization include failure of fertilization and atypical fertilization.

### *Fertilization Failure*

Fertilization failure may result from death of the egg before sperm entry, structural and functional abnormality in the egg or sperm, physical barriers in the female genital tract preventing gamete transport to the site of fertilization, or ovulatory failure (Fig. 17-4).

ABNORMAL EGGS. Several types of morphologic and functional abnormalities have been observed in unfertilized eggs, e.g., giant egg, oval-shaped egg, lentil-shaped egg, and ruptured zone pellucida. Failure to undergo fertilization and normal embryonic development may be due to inherent abnormalities of the egg or to environmental factors. For example, fertilization is lower in animals exposed to elevated ambient temperature prior to breeding. In sheep, some of the conception failures at the beginning of the breeding season are associated with a high incidence of abnormal ova.

ABNORMAL SPERM. The physiologic significance of abnormal sperm in relation to fertilization failure has not been studied in animals other than cattle. Certain forms of male infertility are related to structural defects of the DNA protein complex. Sperm aging and injury may cause:

1. Alterations in the acrosomal cap may prevent defective spermatozoa from fertilizing the egg. In bull, ram, and boar, a good correlation exists between fertility and acrosomal integrity.
2. Leakage of vital intracellular constituents such as cyclic AMP or to the formation of lipid peroxides from sperm plasmalogen when sperm are stored under anerobic conditions.
3. A gradual decrease in the fertilizing capacity of aging of spermatozoa in the female genital tract.

STRUCTURAL BARRIERS TO FERTILIZATION. Congenital or acquired defects of the female genital tract interfere with transport of the sperm and/or the ovum to the site of fertilization (Table 17-2).

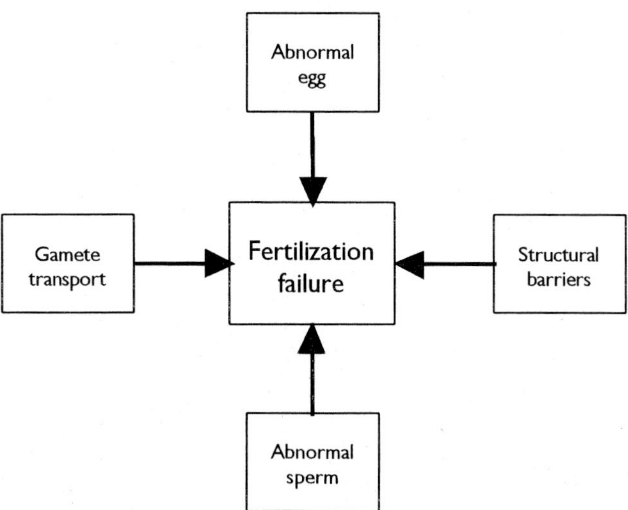


FIGURE 17-4. Causes of fertilization failure.

TABLE 17-2. ***Structural and Functional Causes of Fertilization Failure***

| CAUSE | ABNORMALITY | AFFECTED SPECIES | MECHANISM INTERFERED WITH |
|---|---|---|---|
| STRUCTURAL OBSTRUCTIONS | | | |
| Congenital | Mesonephric cysts | More common in swine, sheep, and cattle than in horses | Sperm transport |
| | Uterus unicornis | | |
| | Double cervix | | |
| Acquired | Tubal adhesions | All species, sheep and swine particularly | Egg pick-up, fertilization |
| | Hydrosalpinx | | Egg transport |
| | Occluded uterine horns | | |
| FUNCTIONAL | | | |
| Hormonal | Cystic ovaries | Cattle and swine | Ovulation |
| | Abnormal cervical and uterine secretions | Cattle; sheep on estrogenic pastures | Gamete transport |
| Management | Delayed insemination | In all species, horses and swine particularly | Death of egg |
| | Insemination too early | Cattle | Death of sperm |
| | Errors in estrus detection | Cattle | Fertilization failure |

1. Congenital defects are the result of arrested development of the different segments of the Müllerian ducts (oviduct, uterus, and cervix) or of an incomplete fusion of these ducts caudally. A classic congenital anomaly associated with the gene for white coat color is "white heifer disease" in cattle, in which the prenatal development of the Müllerian ducts is arrested, and the vaginal canal is obstructed by the presence of an abnormally developed hymen. It can be differentiated from the freemartin syndrome by the presence of normal ovaries, vulva, and labia.
2. Common anatomic abnormalities are adhesions of the infundibulum to the ovary or uterine horns; this interferes with the pick-up of the egg or causes a mechanical obstruction of one part of the reproductive duct system. Bilateral or unilateral missing segments of the reproductive tract also cause anatomic sterility.

PHYTOESTROGENS. Reproductive failure occurs more in sheep than in cattle grazing on plants that contain compounds with estrogenic activity, e.g., subterranean clover (*Trifolium subterranean*) and red clover (*Trifolium pratense*). The estrogenic activity is due to plant isoflavones and related substances with hydroxyl groups. Cows and ewes fed estrogenic forage may suffer impaired ovarian function, often accompanied by reduced conception rates and increased embryonic loss. In cows, clinical signs resemble those associated with cystic ovaries. The infertility is temporary, normally resolving within one month after removal from the estrogenic feed. Ewes grazed on estrogenic pastures around the time of joining shed fewer ova and have a reduced chance of conception. Fertility is improved within 3 weeks, after the ewes are moved into nonestrogenic pastures. The pathologic changes in temporary infertility are due to actions of estrogen on the hypophyseal-ovarian axis and on sperm transport. Ewes grazed for several seasons on estrogenic pastures mate and ovulate, but fertilization rate is depressed as a result of failure of sperm transport caused by severe changes occurring in the cervix (5).

### *Atypical Fertilization*

Atypical fertilization may occur spontaneously as a result of aging of the gametes described below:

1. Aging of the egg is gradual, during which various functions are successively lost. An early effect of egg aging is that the resulting embryo is not viable and is resorbed before birth. Further aging leads to abnormalities in fertilization, particularly involving the pronuclei. The biophysical and biochemical reactions associated with sperm entry into the egg become slower, a condition leading to increased polyspermy (entry of more than one sperm).
2. Polyspermy occurs in several species of laboratory and farm animals. In swine, a delay in copulation or injection of progesterone given 24 to 36 hours before ovula-

tion leads to some eggs having more than two pronuclei. It is not clear whether these potential triploid embryos are caused by failure to extrude the second polar body or to polyspermy, which may result from failure of the block to polyspermy during ovum aging. The incidence of polyspermy increases when mating or insemination is delayed, resulting in triploid embryos that do not survive. This means that in horses and swine with a relatively long estrus, the timing of breeding in relation to ovulation is critical for normal fertilization and embryonic survival.

## PREGNANCY WASTAGE

Pregnancy wastage is responsible for most gestation failures in farm animals. Pregnancy wastage can be divided into *embryonic* and *fetal* mortality (Fig. 17-5). A small percentage of the wastage is involved in the normal reproductive process and may be regarded as unavoidable.

Termination of pregnancy may occur at various stages:

1. Before maternal recognition of pregnancy, in which case length of the cycle is not affected (early embryonic mortality).
2. After maternal recognition of pregnancy, and is associated with a delay in the length of the cycle (late embryonic mortality).
3. During the fetal stage (fetal mortality).

### *Embryonic Mortality*

Embryonic mortality denotes the death of fertilized ova and embryos up to the end of implantation. About 25 to 40% of embryos are normally lost in farm species. It is also noted in large litters of swine and during multiple pregnancies in cattle and sheep. Mortality is more common during the early than the late embryonic period (Table 17-3). Early embryonic mortality should be regarded as a normal process of eliminating unfit genotypes in each generation, particularly in large litters of swine and multiple pregnancies in cattle and sheep.

In the past it was believed that the bovine conceptus was resorbed but transrectal ultrasound examination (6) have demonstrated that that the conceptus and its breakdown products apparently are eliminated by expulsion through the cervix, which either goes unnoticed or appears as a vulval discharge of clear mucus

Embryonic mortality after natural breeding or artificial insemination accounts for the majority of reproductive failures in the cattle, with a mortality rate of up to 40% of all fertilized eggs (7). In cattle, most embryonic deaths occur between days 8 and 16 during hatching of the blastocyst and implantation without affecting cycle lengths. Since most embryos die between days 9 and 15, infertile ewes may experience normal as well as prolonged cycles.

Several methods are used to demonstrate embryonic mortality. In cattle embryonic mortality can be estimated as follows:

1. Calculating the fertilization rate and number of fertilized eggs that fail to continue following slaughter at different intervals after mating.
2. The return to estrus interval following mating is less accurate because an extended cycle length may be due to reasons other than embryonic mortality. Early embryonic deaths before regression of the CL are indistinguishable from failure of fertilization in that both cow and ewe return to estrus at the normal time. Death of one embryo in twin-ovulating ewes may be undetected, as pregnancy will continue.
3. Examining embryos collected by *in vivo* flushing of the reproductive tract at different days after breeding.
4. Determining P4 in blood or milk (see Chapter 28).

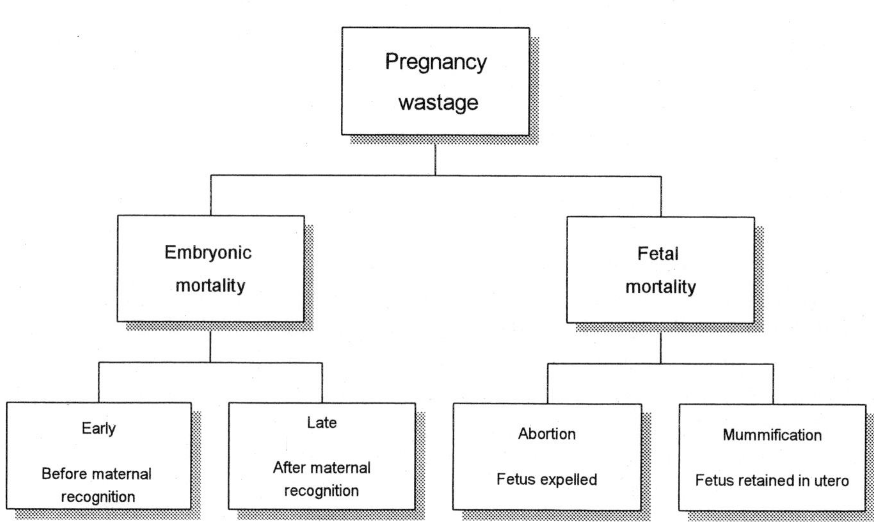


FIGURE 17-5. Pregnancy wastage in farm animals.

TABLE 17-3. *Causes of Embryonic Mortality*

| SPECIES | PERIOD OF MAXIMAL MORTALITY *Days of Gestation* | *Stage of Development* | *Possible Causes* |
|---|---|---|---|
| Cattle | 8 to 16 | Hatching of blastocysts and initiation of elongation and commencement of implantation | Progesterone deficiency; inbreeding; multiple pregnancy; blood group homozygosity; J-antigen in sera; parity; timing of inseminations; chromosomal aberrations |
| Sheep | 9 to 15 | Transition from yolk sac to allantoic placentation | Inbreeding; increasing maternal age; hemoglobin types; overfeeding; multiple pregnancy; high environmental temperatures |
| Swine | 8 to 16 | Spacing of embryos; transuterine migration; maternal recognition of pregnancy | Inbreeding; chromosomal aberrations; overcrowding; overfeeding; increasing maternal age; high environmental temperature; transferrins |
| Horses | 30 to 36 | Corpus luteum of pregnancy regresses and accessory corpora lutea are formed; change from a yolk sac to an allantochorion placentation | Lactation; twinning; nutrition; chromosomal aberrations |

5. Assessment of embryonic heart beat beyond 20 days by real-time ultrasonography (see Chapter 28).
6. Counting the number of ovulations by laparoscopy for the loss of single embryos in sheep.

Several studies have demonstrated the embryonic mortality in swine is 20 to 30%, and that more than two-thirds of the reproductive wastage in the pig occurs between 8 and 18 days of gestation (8). The number of embryos that survive and the stage of pregnancy determine the effects of embryonic mortality on the estrous cycle of swine. For example, if all embryos are lost by day 4 of gestation, the sow returns to estrus after a normal cycle length, but if one to four embryos survive beyond day 4, the pregnancy would still terminate but the next estrous period is delayed by 6 days. For pregnancy to continue beyond day 10 at least a total of 4 embryos must be present in both uterine horns, whereas for it to continue beyond 12 days, as few as 1 embryo is sufficient (9).

Normal and subfertile mares have high fertilization rates, but subfertile mares have a higher embryonic loss rate before day 14 postovulation (10).

## Causes

Embryonic mortality can be due to maternal factors, embryonic factors, or to embryonic-maternal interactions. Maternal failure tends to affect an entire litter, resulting in complete loss of pregnancy. In contrast, embryonic failure affects embryos individually, often leaving others in the litter unharmed. In other cases the maternal environment may be insufficient, allowing the support of only a few strong embryos.

Embryonic loss is influenced by several factors (Fig. 17-6). Chromosomal aberrations and genetic factors contributing to embryonic mortality are discussed in Chapter 28.

ENDOCRINE FACTORS. Accelerated or delayed transport of the egg, as a result of estrogen-progesterone imbalance, leads to preimplantation death. An abnormally undersized conceptus might not be able to counteract the uterine luteolytic effect, with consequent regression of the CL and termination of pregnancy. In swine, as stated previously, at least four living blastocysts are needed by day 10 of pregnancy to counteract the uterine luteolytic effects.

A critical period of embryonic survival is the late blasto-

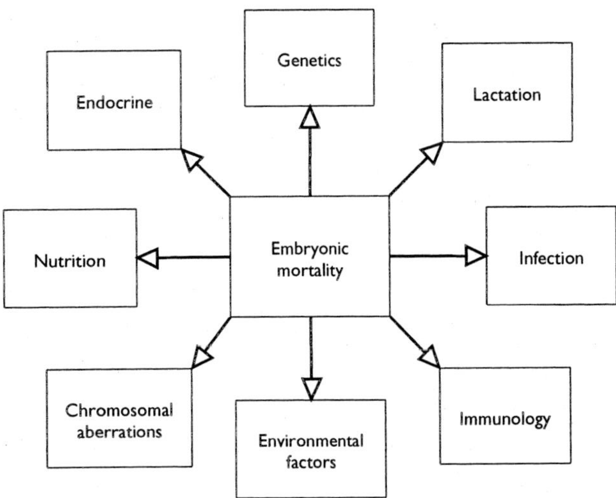


FIGURE 17-6. Causes of embryonic mortality.

cyst stage. Normally, the developing CL secretes progesterone, which acts on the female tract in close synchrony with the development of the embryos. The cause and effect relationship between luteolysis and embryonic deaths is controversial. Apparently, embryonic mortality in cattle is not caused by a progesterone deficiency during the luteal phase of the cycle; luteal regression follows rather than precedes embryonic mortality. However, a diminished response to circulating luteotrophic hormones may contribute to embryo mortality in subfertile cows (11).

LACTATION. Embryonic mortality occurs during lactation in cattle, sheep, and horses and is characterized by prolonged estrous cycles after breeding. Mating of mares at foal heat leads to early embryonic mortality, which has been attributed to reduce effectiveness of uterine defense mechanisms, stress of lactation, and incomplete regeneration of the endometrium. Sows bred after weaning at 7 days of lactation suffer high embryonic losses between days 9 and 20 of pregnancy.

NUTRITION OF THE DAM. Caloric intake and specific nutritional deficiencies affect ovulation rate and fertilization rate, as well as cause embryonic death. Also extremes in the level of feeding are detrimental to embryo survival, so too are extremes in the supply of specific dietary nutrients.

1. In dairy cows, high intakes of rumen degradable protein may lead to embryonic mortality. This effect may be mediated through a reduction in the pH of the uterine environment during the luteal phase of the cycle in which the embryo must grow (12).
2. In swine, high caloric intake or continuous unlimited feeding increases ovulation rate, thereby increasing the incidence of embryonic mortality before implantation. However, following implantation, unlimited feeding decreases fetal death.
3. In sheep, full feeding before breeding also increases ovulation rate as well as embryonic mortality. Poor body condition of ewes at mating increases the incidence of embryonic mortality, whereas moderate feed restriction from day 20 to 100 of pregnancy is less likely to reduce lambing percentages. Undernutrition affects twin ovulators more than single ovulators because both embryos are lost in the former, while a single embryo survives in the latter. Thus, more twin than single ovulating ewes are barren.
4. In the mare, the critical period for embryonic resorption is between 25 and 31 days after ovulation. No resorption occurs if mares are maintained on an adequate plane of nutrition until 35 days after service.

AGE OF DAM. A higher incidence of embryonic mortality is observed in gilts and in sows after the fifth gestation. In the ewe, the incidence of late embryonic loss is higher in ewe lambs and ewes over 6 years than it is in mature ewes, which is due to factors associated with the embryo rather than the uterine environment.

OVERCROWDING IN UTERO. Because the degree of placental development is primarily influenced by the availability of space and vascular supply within the uterus, increasing the number of implantations decreases the vascular supply to each site and restricts placental development. This results in a high embryonic and fetal mortality rate and probably explains the higher incidence of embryonic mortality in cattle and sheep following twin rather than single ovulation. It should be noted, however, that uterine capacity does not limit the ability of the cow and ewe to carry twins, provided they are located in separate uterine horns. In cattle, embryo transfer experiments have shown a higher embryonic mortality rate in recipients which received two embryos in a single uterine horn. This loss may be due to overcrowding and intrauterine competition for nutrients.

In cattle and sheep with multiple ovulations, the number of embryos surviving is reduced to a fairly constant number (2 to 3 embryos per female) within the first 3 or 4 weeks of pregnancy, which implies that embryonic loss increases as the number of eggs shed increases. Mortality does not seem to be due to a deficiency of progesterone. In prolific breeds of sheep, late embryonic deaths occur in ewes with more than five ovulations.

Transuterine migration of embryos is of importance for equal distribution of embryos in the two horns of the uterus in polytocous species such as swine. In its absence, there is a high incidence of embryonic mortality in swine.

THERMAL STRESS. Embryonic mortality increases in a number of species following exposure of the mother to elevated ambient temperatures, especially in tropical areas. The effects of thermal stress on the early embryo are not apparent until the later stages of its development. Fertilized eggs of sheep and cattle, when subjected to high temperatures either *in vitro* or *in vivo*, are damaged but continue to develop, only to die during the critical stages of implantation. Reduced fertility of summer heat-stressed dairy cows may result from decreased viability and developmental capacity of 6-day-old to 8-day-old embryos (13, 14) and may account for the well-documented seasonal reduction in the efficiency of artificial insemination (AI) during summer. Heat stress between days 8 and 17 of pregnancy may also alter the uterine environment as well as growth and secretory activity of the conceptus (15). Apparently heat stress antagonizes the inhibitory effects of the embryo on the uterine secretion of $PGF_{2\alpha}$ (16).

Ealy et al (17) superovulated lactating Holstein cows, artificially inseminated them, and assigned them to be heat stressed on Day 1, 3, 5, or 7 of pregnancy (Day 0 = day of estrus). Embryos were retrieved from the uterus on Day 8 and evaluated for viability and stage of development. Embryos of cows receiving heat stress on Day 1 had decreased viability and development but developed substantial resistance by Day 3. These findings may be useful in designing of environmental modification systems that provide cooling at critical periods of gestation during summer in hot climates.

Several studies have demonstrated that the pig embryo is most susceptible to heat stress before day 18 of pregnancy (8) particularly during implantation. A greater incidence of embryonic deaths was noted among gilts exposed to high temperatures 8 to 16 days postbreeding than among those exposed during 0 to 8 days postbreeding.

SEMEN. A portion of all embryonic mortality is attributable to the male and the mating system. Genetic factors that are transmitted by the male to the embryo may be inherited, may arise from testicular tissue, or may occur in spermatozoa after they are released from the testis. Infertile matings by highly fertile bulls are primarily due to embryonic mortality, while those of bulls with low fertility are due to fertilization failure and embryonic deaths. In swine, semen stored for 3 days before insemination produced zygotes much more susceptible to early embryonic death, presumably owing to the reduced DNA content in aged spermatozoa.

INCOMPATIBILITY. The inherited genotype of the male may include a variety of genetic factors that lead to incompatibility and early embryonic loss. There may be incompatibility between spermatozoa and mother, between spermatozoa and egg, or between zygote and mother. Immunologic incompatibilities may block fertilization (prezygotic selection), or cause embryonic, fetal, or neonatal mortality. In cattle, homozygosity for certain blood groups and certain substances related to transferrin ($\beta$-globulin) and J-antigen in sera are associated with increased embryonic loss as well as decreased fertilization rate.

## *Repeat Breeders*

"Repeat breeder" females return to service repeatedly after being bred to a fertile male. A repeat-breeder cow exhibits normal signs of estrus every 18 to 24 days but requires more than three services to become pregnant. Most embryonic losses occur at a much earlier time than previously believed. Embryos collected nonsurgically from repeat breeder cows revealed that most embryonic abnormalities occur in the oviduct but are not apparent until about 6 to 7 days postservice or the blastocyst stage (18).

Both fertilization failure and embryonic mortality occur at a much higher rate than in normal cows 5 to 6 weeks postinsemination. The cause for loss of approximately 50% of the embryos during the first 3 weeks of pregnancy in repeat-breeder cows is obscure, although several factors have been suspected (Fig. 17-7).

The incidence of repeat breeding is higher in dairy herds using artificial insemination rather than natural service. Errors in estrus detection may also contribute to repeat returns to service in dairy cows. Embryonic mortality decreases with increasing parity up to the fifth pregnancy, then increases. It is likely that the early development of bovine embryos is impaired in the uterine environment of repeat-breeder heifers (19). The higher incidence of embryonic mortality in old cows may be due to a defective uterine environment. Repeat breeding may also be due to numerical chromosomal abnormalities (see Chapter 14).

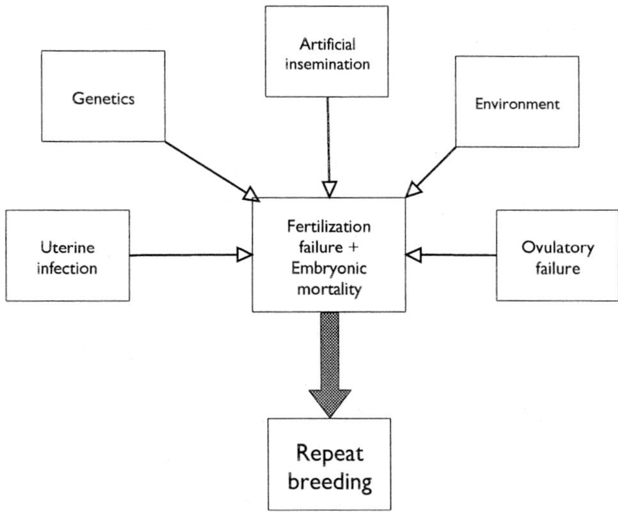

FIGURE 17-7. Causes of repeat breeding in the cow.

Repeat breeding that is due to early embryonic mortality occurs in mares affected by contagious equine metritis. This contagious venereal disease is caused by *Taylorella equigenitalis* and is transmitted by carrier stallions (20).

## *Fetal Mortality*

ABORTION. Abortion is the termination of pregnancy with the expulsion of a fetus of recognizable size before it is viable, which is arbitrarily defined as 260 days for cattle, 290 days for horses, and 110 days for swine. Fetal mortality is not an essential prelude to abortion. Abortions may be *spontaneous* or *induced, infectious* or *noninfectious*.

NONINFECTIOUS ABORTIONS. Noninfectious abortions are more prevalent in cattle, particularly dairy cattle, than in sheep or horses. Noninfectious causes of spontaneous abortion may be due to genetic, chromosomal, hormonal, or nutritional factors (Table 17-4). Spontaneous abortion may also occur in animals bred immediately after puberty or immediately after parturition. Mares seem to be endocrinologically susceptible to abortion between the fifth and tenth months of pregnancy.

Chromosomal abnormalities are known to cause embryonic losses in farm animals (see Chapter 20), but their importance in abortion in farm animals is unknown.

TABLE 17-4. **Noninfectious Causes of Pregnancy Wastage in Farm Animals**

| CAUSES | COW | MARE | SOW | EWE OR DOE |
|---|---|---|---|---|
| Chemicals, drugs, and poisonous plants | Nitrates, chlorinated naphthalenes, arsenic, perennial broomweeds, pine needles | None | Dicoumarin, alfatoxin, wood preservatives (creosote, pentachlorophenols) | Lead, nitrate, locoweeds, lupines, sweet clover, onion grass, veratrum |
| Hormonal | High doses of estrogens, glucocorticoids, $PGF_{2\alpha}$ | High doses of estrogens or cortisone (?) | High doses of estrogens or $PGF_{2\alpha}$ | High doses of estrogens, cortisol or ACTH, $PGF_{2\alpha}$, progesterone deficiency |
| Nutritional | Starvation, malnutrition, deficiencies of vitamin A or iodine | Reduced energy intake | Deficiencies of vitamin A, iron, and calcium | Lack of TDN or energy, deficiencies of vitamin A, copper, iodine, and selenium |
| Genetic or chromosomal | Embryonic mortality, fetal anomalies | Fetal anomalies | Embryonic mortality, congenital or genetic lethal defects | Lethal genetic defects |
| Physical | Douching or insemination of pregnant uterus, stress (transport, fever, surgery) | Manual dilatation of cervix, natural service during pregnancy; rectal palpation of the very young blastodermic vesicle | Stress (transportation, fighting, injury), heat stress | Severe physical stress |
| Miscellaneous | Twinning, allergies, anaphylaxis | Twinning | Poor management | Twinning (?) |

ACTH = adrenocorticotrophic hormone; $PGF_{2\alpha}$ = prostaglandin $F_{2\alpha}$; TDN = total digestible nutrients.

Abortions are occasionally induced with high doses of estrogens, $PGF_{2\alpha}$, or glucocorticoids, particularly in young females bred at an early age and in meat producing animals.

Twin pregnancy is the most common cause of abortion in mares; over two thirds of twin pregnancies terminate in abortions. The inability of a mare to successfully carry twin fetuses to term may be related to placental insufficiency arising from competition between the placentae. This may lead to the death of one fetus and eventually to the abortion of both fetuses.

In the past, habitual abortions at 3 to 4 1/2 months of gestation in Angora goats were attributed to a hereditary defect of the anterior pituitary gland. These abortions are associated with two different syndromes (21). The first of these syndromes is related to nutritional stress. The hypoglycemia that occurs in the doe and fetus activates the fetal hypothalamic-pituitary axis and alters placental endocrine function. $PGF_{2\alpha}$, released by the placenta, causes the regression of the CL of pregnancy and expulsion of one or more recently dead fetuses. Improving the nutritional status of the does may reduce these losses. The other syndrome, resulting from hyperactivity of the maternal adrenal cortex, leads to an excessive accumulation of fetal fluids over a prolonged period. The aborted fetus shows varying degrees of decomposition.

INFECTIOUS ABORTIONS. Infectious abortions account for a major percentage of the pregnancy wastage in farm animals. The major diseases, the organisms, mode of transmission and the clinical findings are summarized for cattle (Table 17-5), sheep and goat (Table 17-6), swine (Table 17-7), and horse (Table 17-8).

CATTLE. *Neospora caninum* is a recently recognized protozoan parasite, which was previously misidentified as *Toxoplama gondii*. It is major cause of bovine abortion in many countries. *N. caninum* was found in fetal tissues of 34 of 688 cases of bovine abortion (22). The aborted fetuses ranged in gestational age from 3 to 8 months. *Neospora sp* has the ability to be transmitted from dam to offspring for several generations. This mode of transmission would explain the maintenance of infection in a population of cattle despite the lack of a definitive host for the parasite (23). Congenitally acquired *N. caninum* infection can cause a substantial number of abortions during the initial pregnancy of heifers, with abortion risk attributable to *N. caninum* decreasing in subsequent pregnancies, possibly because of selective culling. Subsequent abortions can be expected in congenitally infected cows that have aborted previously (24).

TABLE 17-5. ***Summary of Diseases Causing Pregnancy Wastage in Cattle***

| DISEASE | TRANSMISSION | CLINICAL FINDINGS |
|---|---|---|
| **PROTOZOAL** | | |
| Trichomoniasis (*Trichomonas fetus*) | Venereal | Abortion in first trimester; repeat breeding; pyometra |
| Neosporosis (*Neospora caninum*) | Transplacental | Abortions at 3–8 months |
| **BACTERIAL** | | |
| Brucellosis (*Brucella abortus*) | Ingestion | Abortion in last trimester, rate 90% in susceptible herds |
| Vibriosis (*Campylobacter fetus*) | Venereal | Abortion (3–4 months); rate 5–10% infertility |
| Leptospirosis (*Leptospira pomona, Leptospira hardjo*) | Cutaneous, mucosal abrasions | Abortion in last trimester, rate 25–30%; fetal death common |
| Listeriosis (*Listeria monocytogenes*) | Contaminated feed | Low abortion rate associated with septicemia |
| **VIRAL** | | |
| Infectious bovine rhinotracheitis (IBR) | Aerosol infection | Abortion in second half of pregnancy, rate 25–50% |
| Epizootic viral abortion (EVA) | Aerosol infection | Abortion in last trimester, rate 30–40%, mainly in winter |
| **FUNGAL** | | |
| Mycoses (*Aspergillus absidia*) | Inhalation | Abortion at 3–4 months, rate less than 10%; placental disease |

Adapted from: Laing JA, Brinley-Morgan WJ, Wagner WC. Fertility and Infertility in Veterinary Practice, 4th Ed. London: Bailliere Tindall, 1988; Radostits OM, Blood DC, Gay GC. Veterinary Medicine. 8th Ed. London: WB Saunders, 1994; Arthur GH, Noakes DE, Pearson H, Parkinson TM. Veterinary Reproduction and Obstetrics, 7th ed. London: WB Saunders Company Limited, 1996.

Epizootic bovine abortion (EBA, foothill abortion) refers to a well-defined clinical condition that occurred in the 1950s, principally in the foothills and mountain areas surrounding the Central Valleys of California. It is characterized by abortions occurring in the last third of pregnancy, most commonly in beef cattle. The abortion rate may exceed 80% when large numbers of animals are exposed for the first time. The highest incidence is in heifers, but older animals moved into endemic areas for the first time may subsequently abort. Usually a cow aborts only once, makes a complete recovery, and fertility is normal in subsequent gestations.

The cause is suspected to be a virus (*Chlamydia psittaci*). Feeding the tick *Ornithodoros coriaceus* on susceptible cattle during the second trimester of gestation can experimentally produce the disease. No vaccine is available because the causative agent has not been identified. Adjusting the calving season so that the middle trimester of pregnancy does not coincide with the tick season has reduced the incidence of abortion. Animals that have experienced the disease will not abort again, and these should be maintained in the herd. There is no evidence that this disease spreads from cow to cow.

In a 10-year survey of 8995 bovine abortions and stillbirths in South Dakota (25), viruses were associated with 948 (10.58%) and bacteria with 1299 (14.49%). Bovine herpesvirus-1 (IBR) was detected in 485 (5.41%), and bovine viral diarrhea virus (BVDV) was detected in 407 (4.54%). The five bacteria most commonly associated with bovine abortion or stillbirth were *Actinomyces pyogenes*, 378 (4.22%); *Bacillus spp.*, 321 (3.58%); *Listeria spp.*, 121 (1.35%); *Escherichia coli*, 98 (1.09%); and *Leptospira interrogans*, 79 (0.88%) (26).

*SHEEP AND GOAT.* Enzootic abortion of ewes (EAE) occurs in many parts of the world and has been diagnosed in the western United States. The rate of abortion in a newly infected flock may be as high as 30%. In flocks experiencing a reinfection, the rate is less than 5%. Ewes abort during the last month of pregnancy. Abortions continue until normal lambing time, and some fetuses are expelled alive at term but are diseased. The causative agent of EAE is a member of the *Chlamydia* group. This disease must be differentiated from vibriosis. Diagnosis of EAE depends on finding the elementary bodies of the infectious agent in smears from the cotyledon or from placental exudate. The disease produces

**TABLE 17-6. *Summary of Diseases Causing Pregnancy Wastage in Sheep and Goat***

| DISEASE | TRANSMISSION | CLINICAL FINDINGS |
|---|---|---|
| PROTOZOAL | | |
| Toxoplasmosis (*Toxoplasma gondii*) | Ingestion | Late abortion; stillbirth |
| BACTERIAL | | |
| Brucellosis | | |
| (*Brucella ovis*) | Spread from ram to ram through ewes | Late abortion, stillbirths, epididymitis |
| (*Brucella melitensis*) | Infected genital discharges | Abortion; goats are highly susceptible |
| Vibriosis (*Campylobacter fetus* or *jejuni*) | Ingestion | Abortion in last trimester; stillbirths, metritis |
| Salmonellosis (*Salmonella dublin, S. typhimurum*) | Ingestion | Late abortion, neonatal mortality |
| Listeriosis (*Listeria monocytogenes*) | Ingestion (?) | Abortion after 3 months; retained fetal membranes and metritis |
| VIRAL | | |
| Enzootic abortion of ewes (*Chlamydia psittaci*) | Ingestion | Late abortion; stillbirths, weak lambs |
| Rift Valley Fever | Insects | Abortion |

Adapted from: Laing JA, Brinley-Morgan WJ, Wagner WC. Fertility and Infertility in Veterinary Practice, 4th Ed. London: Bailliere Tindall, 1988; Radostits OM, Blood DC, Gay GC. Veterinary Medicine. 8th Ed. London: WB Saunders, 1994; Arthur GH, Noakes DE, Pearson H, Parkinson TM. Veterinary Reproduction and Obstetrics, 7th ed. London: WB Saunders Company Limited, 1996.

**TABLE 17-7. *Summary of Disease Causing Pregnancy Wastage in Swine***

| DISEASE | TRANSMISSION | CLINICAL FINDINGS |
|---|---|---|
| BACTERIAL | | |
| Leptospirosis (*Leptospira pomona*) | Entry of new boar | Abortion in late pregnancy; weak piglets |
| Brucellosis (*Brucella suis*) | Venereal | Abortion; embryonic death; infertility |
| Salmonellosis (*Salmonella dublin, S. typhimurium*) | Ingestion | Abortion during the last month; neonatal mortality |
| VIRAL | | |
| SMEDI | Ingestion | Late abortion, stillbirths, mummified fetus, embryonic death, infertility |
| Porcine reproductive respiratory syndrome (PRRS) | Introduction of infected pigs | Abortions during first half; stillbirths; mummified fetus; embryonic death |
| Aujesky's disease (pseudorabies) | Inhalation or ingestion | Abortions during the first 2 months; stillbirths; embryonic death; mummification |
| Porcine parvovirus (PPV) | Introduction of infected pigs | Possible abortions; embryonic death; mummification; stillbirths |

Adapted from: Laing JA, Brinley-Morgan WJ, Wagner WC. Fertility and Infertility in Veterinary Practice, 4th Ed. London: Bailliere Tindall, 1988; Radostits OM, Blood DC, Gay GC. Veterinary Medicine. 8th Ed. London: WB Saunders, 1994; Arthur GH, Noakes DE, Pearson H, Parkinson TM. Veterinary Reproduction and Obstetrics, 7th ed. London: WB Saunders Company Limited, 1996.
Other viruses may interfere with gestation: Swine fever (hog cholera), foot and mouth disease, swine influenza.

TABLE 17-8. ***Summary of Disease Causing Pregnancy Wastage in Horse***

| DISEASE | TRANSMISSION | CLINICAL FINDINGS |
|---|---|---|
| **BACTERIAL** | | |
| Salmonellosis (*Salmonella abortivo-equina*) | Contaminated feed with uterine discharges | Abortion at 7–8 months of gestation |
| Leptospirosis (*Leptospira pomona*) | | Late abortions |
| Contagious equine metritis (CEM) (*Taylorella equigenitalis*) | Venereal | Endometritis; early embryonic death; repeat breeding |
| **VIRAL** | | |
| Equine herpesvirus (EHV) | Contagious | Abortion in last trimester of gestation |
| Equine viral arteritis (EVA) | Venereal | Abortion in second half of gestation |
| **FUNGAL** | | |
| Mycosis (*Aspergillus spp*, *Candida spp*) | | Sporadic abortion between 4 and 11 months |

Adapted from: Laing JA, Brinley-Morgan WJ, Wagner WC. Fertility and Infertility in Veterinary Practice, 4th Ed. London: Bailliere Tindall, 1988; Radostits OM, Blood DC, Gay GC. Veterinary Medicine. 8th Ed. London: WB Saunders, 1994; Arthur GH, Noakes, DE, Pearson H, Parkinson TM. Veterinary Reproduction and Obstetrics, 7th ed. London: WB Saunders Company Limited, 1996.

immunity. A single infection produces lifetime immunity, and the disease can be prevented by vaccination.

In a 10-year survey of 1784 of ovine abortions and stillbirths in South Dakota (27), infectious agents were found in 39%, noninfectious agents in 5%, and 56% of cases were undiagnosed. Together, *Toxoplasma gondii*, *Campylobacter sp*., and *Chlamydia psittaci* caused about 25% of all abortions and stillbirths.

**SWINE.** A summary of the causes of abortion is listed in Table 17-7. It should be noted that the same diseases cause stillbirth, mummification, embryonic mortality, and conception failure.

**HORSE.** The equine herpesvirus I infection is primarily a disease of the upper respiratory tract. The horse first experiences exposure to this virus as a foal in the fall near weaning time. This epizootic disease in foals produces a massive exposure of mares that are in midpregnancy. Abortion usually occurs after the eighth month of pregnancy, with most abortions occurring between January and April because of seasonal breeding. By far the most frequent cause of epizootics of abortion in mares is the equine herpesvirus I. This infection should be suspected until otherwise eliminated. Abortion from this infection rarely occurs in successive years, and in the absence of other control methods, it may not occur in a single band of mares for several years. Immunization is the best method of prevention.

In a survey of 3514 aborted fetuses, stillborn foals, or foals that died less than 24 hours after birth, and of 13 placentas from mares in Kentucky, fetoplacental infection caused by bacteria (628), equine herpesvirus (143), or fungi (61) was the most common diagnosis. A diagnosis was not established in 16% of the cases seen (585). Leptospirosis (78) was an important cause of bacterial abortion in mares, and that infection by a *Nocardioform actinomycete* (45) was an important cause of chronic placentitis (28).

**FETAL MUMMIFICATION.** Fetal mummification is characterized by mortality of the fetus, but it is not aborted. Instead, resorption of placental fluids, dehydration of the fetus and its membranes lead to a uterus which is tightly wrapped around the fetus. It is more common in cattle and swine than in sheep and horses.

**CATTLE.** The syndrome occurs mainly from the fifth to seventh months of gestation in all breeds of cattle. Affected cows conceive normally in the subsequent breeding period. Occasionally, bovine mummified fetuses are aborted spontaneously, but in most cases they are carried many months beyond the gestation period because the CL persists. It is suspected only when gestation is prolonged. In cases of incomplete abortion, bacteria enter through a partially dilated cervix to autolyze fetal soft tissues leaving fetal bones floating within the uterine lumen. This condition is referred to as *fetal maceration*, which is a septic process unlike mummification. A high incidence of fetal mummification in the Jersey and Guernsey breeds tends to support a hereditary influence.

**SHEEP.** Twin-bearing ewes may abort a mummified fetus during late gestation and maintain the other lamb to full term, or they may deliver a mummified fetus attached to the placenta of a viable offspring.

SWINE. Swine embryos that die in the first 6 weeks of gestation are completely resorbed. The fetuses that die during later stages are retained and expelled as mummified fetuses along with normal piglets at farrowing. Mummified fetuses are more prevalent in large than in small litters, in older sows than in gilts, and in some breeds than in others. Viruses causing stillbirth (S), mummification (M), embryonic death (ED) and infertility (I) in swine are termed *SMEDI viruses*. These viruses are an important cause of mummification in susceptible gilts and young sows. Transplacental infection leads to the establishment of the virus in one or two fetuses. These affected fetuses subsequently die after the infection has been transmitted to adjacent fetuses, which also die later. The retention of a mummified fetus within the uterus could be due to a fetal influence on the endometrium, through suppression of the uterine luteolytic mechanism, causing persistence of the corpus luteum.

## PERINATAL AND NEONATAL MORTALITY

### *Perinatal Mortality*

Perinatal mortality refers to death of the offspring shortly before, during, or within the first 48 to 72 hours of life at normal term. Perinatal mortality, which includes stillbirths (born dead), accounts for most of the losses between birth and weaning. The extent of perinatal losses ranges from 5 to 15% in cattle and horses, up to 20 to 30% in sheep and pigs (29).

Most losses occur within 72 hours of birth. Asphyxia, starvation, chilling, and congenital malformations are major contributing factors (Fig. 17-8). Species differences exist in the relative importance of these stresses. For example, trauma during prolonged or assisted birth occurs more frequently in cattle than in pigs, whereas asphyxiation may be more likely to occur in the pig as a result of premature rupture of the umbilical cord. The use of drugs to induce parturition might adversely affect neonatal survival. For example, induction of parturition in the sow with $PGF_{2\alpha}$ before day 111 of gestation and in the cow with corticosteroids before day 265 of gestation may result in a higher incidence of perinatal mortality.

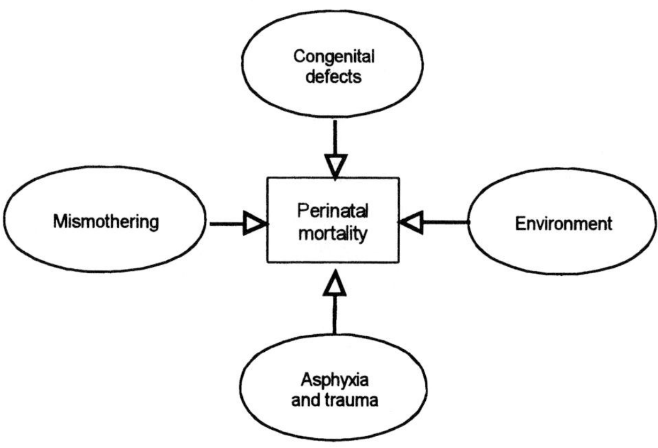


FIGURE 17-8. Factors affecting perinatal mortality.

Stillborn piglets resemble live littermates, but their lungs do not float in water. One to two piglets in approximately one-third of all litters are dead at birth with advancing parity, in extremes of litter size, and in litters in which the gestation period is less than 110 days. Two types of stillbirth occur in swine. In the first type, which is usually due to infectious causes, fetuses die prepartum, whereas in the second type, which is due to noninfectious causes, piglets die during parturition. The presence of meconium on the skin, in the mouth, and in the trachea of the piglet differentiates the latter from the former.

A high incidence of piglet death is observed with uterine inertia, with prolongation of farrowing time or of the interval between births of piglets, in litters that contain less than four or more than nine piglets, and among piglets in the last third of the litter. These intrapartum deaths may be due to the low tolerance of piglets to anoxia and are usually associated with rupture of the umbilical cord prior to delivery. Since piglets suffer irreversible brain damage within 5 minutes after umbilical rupture or impeded umbilical flow, delivery must be completed rapidly.

In sheep, most losses between implantation and weaning occur during the perinatal period, as a result of starvation of the neonate, dystocia among lambs born to maiden ewes, ewes on poor pasture, or ewes with "clover disease."

### *Neonatal Mortality*

Neonatal mortality—death of the neonate during the first few weeks of life—is related to heredity, environmental factors, nutrition, and infection. Several nutritional deficiencies may contribute to neonatal mortality.

*Respiratory distress syndrome* (RDS) is characterized by a failure of the fetal lungs to produce surfactant necessary to maintain the stability of the terminal air spaces of the lung after birth. RDS occurs in premature human infants and is invariably fatal. It has been reported in foals, calves, and piglets. RDS in calves, as in the human infant, is caused by a deficiency of a surfactant (phospholipid), and its diagnosis is based on levels in the amniotic fluid of two phospholipids—lecithin and sphingomyelin.

Neonatal mortality may also result from prolonged labor, poor maternal nutrition, weakness of the mother or the young, bacterial infection of the young through the umbilical cord, poor maternal behavior, or delayed onset of lactation. Exposure of the newborn pig to low environmental temperature leads to hypothermia, hypoglycemia, and death. Heat prostation and some deaths occur in newborn lambs exposed to high environmental temperature. Another source of danger to the neonate is the presence of mammalian or avian predators.

## DISORDERS OF GESTATION, PARTURITION, AND PUERPERIUM

Disorders of gestation, parturition, and puerperium are listed in Table 17-9.

### *Dystocia*

Dystocia, difficult or obstructed parturition, may be due to fetal, maternal, or mechanical causes (Fig. 17-9).

FETAL DYSTOCIA. This results from abnormalities in the presentation or position of the fetus and from postural irregularities of its head or limbs; it may be due to a relatively or absolutely oversized fetus, and to fetal monstrosities. Fetal dystocia is common in certain breeds of dairy cattle, in cattle and sheep with multiple pregnancies, and in sows with small litters. Deviations of the head and flexion of the various joints in anterior presentation, flexion of both hindlimbs (breech) in posterior presentation, or twins may cause dystocia.

MATERNAL DYSTOCIA. It is more frequent in dairy cattle and sheep than in horses and swine. It occurs frequently in primiparous animals and in animals with multiple young. The absence of uterine contractions or inertia may be primary or secondary. Primary uterine inertia that is due to excessive stretching is common in multiple pregnancy in cattle and in large litters in swine. Secondary uterine inertia is due to exhaustion of the uterine muscle secondary to obstructive dystocia. Failure of the cervix to dilate properly leads to "spasm" of the cervix in cattle.

FETOPELVIC DISPROPORTION. This is a disparity between the size of the fetus and the size of the pelvis of the dam. Fetopelvic disproportion is a common cause of dystocia in cows, ewes carrying single lambs, and sows with small litter size. It is uncommon in the mare. Anomalies of the soft parts of the reproductive passages or the bony pelvis are occasional causes of dystocia:

1. Anomalies causing a narrowing of the birth canal (e.g., abnormalities or fractures of the pelvis, and stenosis or obstruction of the cervix, vagina, or vulva).
2. Abnormalities preventing entry of the fetus into the birth passages (e.g., failure of the cervix to dilate or torsion of the uterus).

Fetopelvic disproportion accounts for about 30% of all bovine dystocia. The factors that contribute to fetopelvic disproportion are small pelvic area of the dam and large size of the calf. Dystocia that is due to fetopelvic disproportion may be prevented by:

1. Mating planned to avoid disproportionately large calves in cows with small pelvic areas.
2. Mating heifers by weight rather than age.
3. Reducing birth weights by using bulls of the same breed or a different breed known to sire smaller calves, or selecting dams that have the ability to limit birth weight.

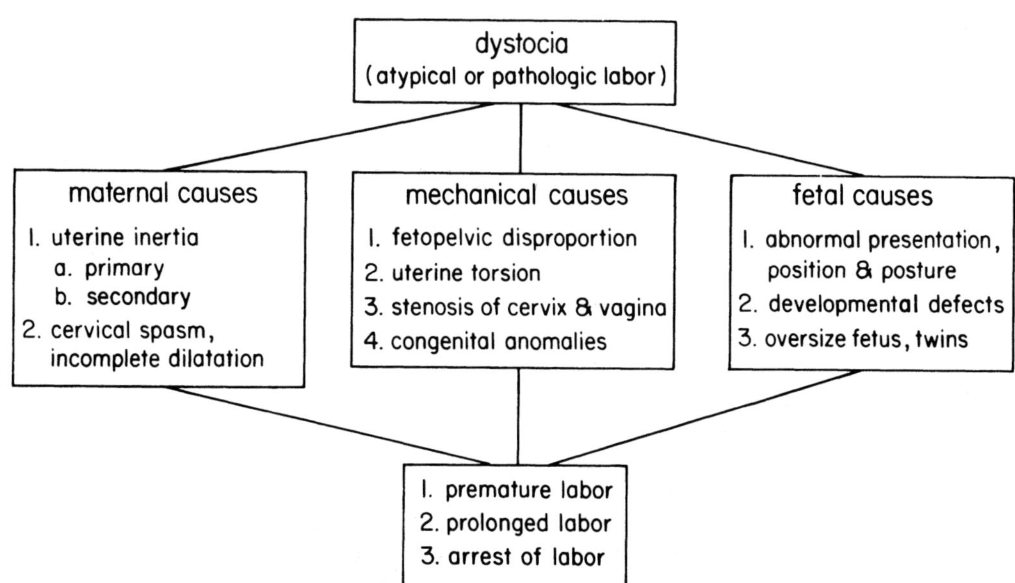


FIGURE 17-9. Maternal, mechanical, and fetal causes that lead to various forms of dystocia that may lead to premature labor, prolonged labor, or arrest of labor.

Calving difficulty affects the future reproductive performance in cattle by increasing days open, days to first breeding, and number of services.

### Retention of Fetal Membranes

RFM is a failure of the fetal membranes to be expelled during the third stage of labor; it is a common postpartum complication in ruminants, particularly in cattle. RFM beyond 12 hours in cattle is considered pathologic and is primarily due to either uterine inertia or an inflammation of the placenta, which in turn results in a failure of the fetal villi to detach themselves from the maternal crypts. RFM invariably accompanies abortions in late gestation due to:

1. infections such as brucellosis, leptospirosis, and infectious bovine rhinotracheitis,
2. premature births associated with twinning, and
3. induced parturition with corticosteroids, obstructive dystocia, and cesarean operation.

RFM occurs more frequently in dairy than beef breeds. Factors such as poor hygiene or the stresses affecting the dairy cow at time of calving, particularly "loose" type of housing, have been implicated. Since RFM leads to an infection of the uterus (metritis and endometritis) and a delay in the involution of the uterus, the future fertility of the animal could be adversely affected.

Controversy exists between removal and the more conservative method of leaving the fetal membranes *in situ*. Bolinder et al (30) reported that manual removal caused an immediate and large but short-lived increase in prostaglandin $PGF_{2\alpha}$ metabolite, which was probably due to the physical damage of uterine tissue. Manual removal also prolonged the interval from calving to first functional corpus luteum by 20 days. The mechanisms and therapy for RFM in the cow have been extensively reviewed (31, 32).

The management of RFM in cattle can be summarized as follows:

1. In uncomplicated cases, no treatment is recommended.
2. Manual removal is the oldest and commonest method of treatment, benefits parlor hygiene but may adversely affect the cow. The use of collagenase may allow manual removal without such side effects.
3. Ecbolic drugs are often ineffective, both as prophylaxis and treatment for the condition. They are most effective within one hour of parturition, particularly after a cesarean section. Endometritis is a very common sequel to RFM.
4. Antibiotics and estrogens have been used to treat, control, or prevent the condition, but they are not routinely effective and may have deleterious side effects. Gonadotrophin releasing hormone and/or prostaglandins have been used to reduce the deleterious effect of RFM on fertility, but the results obtained have been inconsistent.

RFM in other ruminants such as buffaloes, sheep, or goats is less common than in cattle. In the mare, RFM is thought to be a serious problem because it often leads to laminitis. It is usually treated by oxytocin injections with manual removal if it is not expelled by 24 hours after foaling.

### Hydramnios and Hydrallantois

Hydramnios is the excessive accumulation of fluid within the amniotic sac. It is less common than hydrallantois, which is the accumulation of fluid within allantoic sac. Hydramnios is observed more often in cattle than sheep or swine and is associated with certain cranial abnormalities of the fetus. In these defective fetuses, swallowing is impaired, causing the accumulation of amniotic fluid as gestation progresses. Fetuses of the Guernsey and Jersey breeds in prolonged gestation have hydramnios.

Hydrallantois occurs in cattle, especially in twin pregnancies. It is characterized externally by an enormous enlargement of the abdomen after the sixth month of gestation. The syndrome has been attributed to fetal-maternal incompatibility and placental dysfunction. It has also been reported in horses after the seventh month of gestation and was associated with fetal abnormalities.

### Multiple Pregnancy

In cattle, horses, sheep, and goats, the frequency of multiple pregnancies is higher than that of multiple births, owing to the high incidence of abortion and fetal resorption. In the cow, the sequel of twinning includes shortened gestation period, abortion, stillbirth, dystocia, and RFM. Economic losses are related to decreased fertility, neonatal mortality, decrease in birth weights of calves, longer calving intervals, and lower butterfat production. In addition, over 90% of the females born cotwin to a male are sterile (freemartins). Neonatal mortality in sheep is greater among twins than among singles. Ewes carrying twins are more susceptible to pregnancy toxemia (twin-lamb disease). In mares, a high percentage of twin fetuses are aborted.

### Prolonged Gestation

Abnormally long gestation periods occur in cattle, sheep, and swine. These result from genetic and nongenetic factors.

There are two types of prolonged gestation in cattle, and a single autosomal recessive gene governs each.

1. *Fetal gigantism.* This inherited disease occurs in Holstein and Ayrshire breeds. The gestation is prolonged for periods ranging from three weeks to three months. Dystocia usually occurs and the large fetuses have to be delivered by cesarean section. The calves are very large,

TABLE 17-9. ***Disorders of Gestation, Parturition, and Puerperium***

| SYNDROME | SPECIES | CAUSES |
|---|---|---|
| Retention of fetal membranes | Cattle, buffalo, sheep, goat, horse, and pig | Dystocia, infections |
| Vaginal prolapse | Cattle and sheep | Excessive relaxation of pelvic ligaments, restricted exercise, twinning |
| Uterine prolapse | Cattle and sheep | Dystocia, retention of fetal membranes |
| Hydrops of fetal membranes | Cattle, sheep, and horses | Fetal anomalies, placental dysfunction, fetal-maternal incompatibility |
| Twinning | Cattle, sheep, and horses | Spontaneous or induced |
| Prolonged gestation | Cattle | Genetic and fetal abnormalities |
| | Sheep | Ingestion of teratogens in early pregnancy |
| | Swine | Genetic, in certain inbred lines |
| Respiratory distress syndrome | Calves, foals, piglets | Deficiency of lung surfactant (phospholipid) |

show no facial abnormalities, and when delivered die in 6 to 8 hours from severe hypoglycemia. There is hypoplasia of the adenohypophysis and the adrenal cortex. The plasma progesterone level in a cow carrying an affected calf does not fall before parturition as it does in a normal cow.

2. *Craniofacial abnormality*. This type is observed in Guernsey and Jersey breeds. The fetuses are small, many exhibit facial abnormalities and hydramnios, and they lack an adenohypophysis. They survive *in utero* for long periods past term but live for only a few minutes when delivered surgically.

### *Uterine Infections*

Postpartum uterine infections occur commonly in the cow and mare as sequelae to retention of the fetal membranes and dystocia. *Endometritis* is the inflammation of the endometrium, whereas *metritis* involves the entire thickness of the uterus. *Pyometra* is the accumulation of purulent exudate within the uterus.

Most uterine infections affect the dairy cow, and of several bacteria that have been implicated, *Actinomyces pyogenes* is the most frequently encountered organism in the cow. $PGF_{2\alpha}$ is released in postpartum cows with either normal puerperium or uterine infections, but higher levels persist for a longer period in cows with uterine infections. Apparently, bacterial infection and toxins stimulate the uterus to secrete abnormally higher levels of prostaglandins (33), which delay the onset of cyclicity until the infection is cleared and the prostaglandin levels are low. Another possibility is that uterine infection may delay the initiation of folliculogenesis and suppress the rate of follicular growth in dairy cows during the early puerperium (34) by inhibiting LH release. The inhibition is believed to be due to endotoxins produced by Gram-negative bacteria in the postpartum uterus of the cow.

Ovarian activity during the early postpartum period exerts an important influence on the ability of the uterus to resist or eliminate bacterial infections. Both mare and cow can resist uterine infection during the estrogenic phase but are very susceptible during the progesterone phase, which is due to decreased leucocytic activity. If cows with uterine infection resume cyclicity relatively early in the postpartum period, pyometra is likely to occur when elevated levels of progesterone coincide with the presence of high numbers of pathogenic bacteria. Therefore, the practice of injecting cows with GnRH to induce cyclicity early in the postpartum period should be avoided, as it could lead to pyometra.

## REFERENCES


1. Taverne MAM, Lavoir MC, Bevers MM, Pieterse MC, Dieleman SJ. Peripheral plasma prolactin and progesterone levels in pseudopregnant goats during Bromocryptine treatment. Theriogenology 1988;30:777.
2. Pieterse MC, Taverne MAM. Hydrometra in goats: diagnosis with real-time ultrasound and treatment with prostaglandins or oxytocin. Theriogenology 1986;26:813.
3. Bosu WTK, Peter AT. Evidence for a role of intrauterine infections in the pathogenesis of cystic ovaries in postpartum dairy cows. Theriogenology 1987;28:725.
4. Kirk JH, Huffman M, Lane M. Bovine cystic ovarian disease: hereditary relationships and case study. J Am Vet Med Assoc 1982;181:474.
5. Adams NR. Detection of the effects of phytoestrogens on sheep and cattle. J Anim Sci 1995;73:1509.

6. Kastelic JP, Northey DL, Ginther OJ. Spontaneous embryonic death on days 20 to 40 in heifers. Theriogenology 1991;35: 351.
7. Sreenan JM, Diskin MG. The extent and timing of embryonic mortality in the cow. In: Sreenan JM, Diskin MG, eds. Embryonic Mortality in Farm Animals. Boston: Martinus Nijhoff, 1986.
8. Einarsson S, Madej A, Tsuma V. The influence of stress on early pregnancy in the pig. Anim Reprod Sci 1996;42:165.
9. Wettemann RP, Bazer FW, Thatcher WW, Hoagland TA. Environmental influences on embryonic mortality. Proc 10th Int Congr Animal Reprod AI, Champaign-Urbana, IL 1984;4: XIII-26.
10. Ball BA, Woods GL. Embryonic loss and early pregnancy loss in the mare. Compend Cont Ed Pract Vet 1987;9:459.
11. Shelton K, Gayerie De Abreu MF, Hunter MG, Parkinson TJ, Lamming GE. Luteal inadequacy during the early luteal phase of subfertile cows. J Reprod Fertil 1990;90:1.
12. Elrod CC, Butler WR. Reduction of fertility and alteration of uterine pH in heifers fed excess degradable protein. J Anim Sci 1993;71:694.
13. Monty DE Jr, Racowsky C. *In vitro* evaluation of early embryo viability and development in summer heat-stressed, superovulated dairy cows. Theriogenology 1987;28:451.
14. Putney DJ, Drost M, Thatcher WW. Embryonic development in superovulated dairy cattle exposed to elevated ambient temperatures between days 1 to 7 post insemination. Theriogenology 1988;30:195.
15. Geisert RD, Zavy MT, Biggers GG. Effect of heat stress of conceptus and uterine secretion in the bovine. Theriogenology 1988;29:1075.
16. Wolfenson D, Bartol FF, Badinga L, et al. Secretion of PGF2a and oxytocin during hyperthermia in cyclic and pregnant heifers. Theriogenology 1993;39:1129.
17. Ealy AD, Drost M, Hansen PJ. Developmental changes in embryonic resistance to adverse effects of maternal heat stress in cows. J Dairy Sci 1993;76:2899.
18. Linares T, King WA, Ploen L. Observations on the early development of embryos from repeat breeder heifers. Nordisk Veterinaermedicin 1980;32:433.
19. Albihn A, Gustafsson H, Rodriguez-Martinez H, Larsson K. Development of day 7 bovine demi-embryos transferred into virgin and repeat-breeder heifers. Anim Reprod Sci 1989;21: 161.
20. Arthur GH, Noakes DE, Pearson H, Parkinson TM. Veterinary Reproduction and Obstetrics, 7th ed. London: WB Saunders Company Limited, 1996.
21. Wentzel D. Noninfectious abortion in Angora goats. Proc 3rd Int. Conf on Goat Production and Diseases. Tucson, AZ, 1982.
22. Hattel AL, Castro MD, Gummo JD, Weinstock D, Reed JA, Dubey JP. Neosporosis-associated bovine abortion in Pennsylvania. Vet Parasitol 1998;74:307.
23. Bjorkman C, Johansson O, Stenlund S, Holmdahl OJ, Uggla AJ. Neospora species infection in a herd of dairy cattle. Amer Vet Med Assoc 1996;208:1441.
24. Thurmond MC, Hietala SK. Effect of congenitally acquired Neospora caninum infection on risk of abortion and subsequent abortions in dairy cattle Amer. J Vet Res 1997;58:1381.
25. Kirkbride CA. Viral agents and associated lesions detected in a 10-year study of bovine abortions and stillbirths. J Vet Diagn Invest 1992;4:374.
26. Kirkbride CA. Bacterial agents detected in a 10-year study of bovine abortions and stillbirths. J Vet Diagn Invest 1993; 5:64.
27. Kirkbride CA. Diagnoses in 1,784 ovine abortions and stillbirths. J Vet Diagn Invest 1993;5:398.
28. Giles RC, Donahue JM, Hong CB, et al. Causes of abortion, stillbirth, and perinatal death in horses: 3,527 cases (1986–1991). J Amer Vet Med Assoc 1993;203:1170.
29. Randall GCB. Perinatal adaptation. Proc 10th Int Congr Animal Reprod AI, Champaign-Urbana, IL, 1984;4:V-43.
30. Bolinder A, Seguin B, Kindahl H, Bouley D, Otterby D. Retained fetal membranes in cows: manual removal versus nonremoval and its effect on reproductive performance. Theriogenology 1988;30:45.
31. Paisley LG, Mickelsen WD, Anderson PB. Mechanisms and therapy for retained fetal membranes and uterine infections of cows: a review. Theriogenology 1986;26:353.
32. Peters AR, Laven RA. Treatment of bovine retained placenta and its effects. Vet Rec 1996;139:535.
33. Fredriksson G, Kindahl H, Alentus S, et al.Uterine infections and impaired reproductive performance mediated through prostaglandin release. Proc 11th Int Congr Animal Reprod AI, Dublin, Ireland, 1988;5:81.
34. Peter AT, Bosu WTK. Relationship of uterine infections and folliculogenesis in dairy cows during early puerperium. Theriogenology 1988;30:1045.

Chapter 18

# Reproductive Failure in Males

M.R. Jainudeen and B. Hafez

The fertility of a male is related to several phenomena: (1) sperm production; (2) viability and fertilizing capacity of the ejaculated sperm; (3) sexual desire; and (4) the ability to mate. The sterile male is readily identified, but the male with reduced fertility poses serious problems and causes economic losses to breeders and the artificial insemination (AI) industry. The purpose of this chapter is to review the functional aspects of male reproductive failure (Fig. 18-1), and the various techniques to evaluate fertility problems (Fig. 18-2). Genetic factors and chromosomal abnormalities associated with male reproductive failure are discussed in Chapter 20.

There are several causes of male infertility: gonadotropin deficiency, chromosome aberrations, genetic disorders, excurrent duct obstruction, environmental toxins, systemic and genital disease, neurologic disorders, and autoimmune disease (Table 18-1). Stress, any disturbance of homeostasis, has a profound effect on reproductive physiology of male farm animals associated with a decrease in reproductive function. The causes of extreme stress may include high stocking density, new social grouping, poor environments, thermal extremes, and human-animal interactions which cause physical and/or psychological trauma to the animals (1).

This chapter deals primarily with endocrine control of male sexual dysfunction (Table 18-2), etiology of male infertility (Table 18-3), differential diagnosis of azoospermia (Table 18-4), evaluation of sperm morphology (Table 18-5), some biochemical markers (Table 18-6), and therapeutic approaches of male infertility (Table 18-7).

## Congenital Malformations

### Segmental Aplasia of the Wolffian Ducts

In this defect, small or large segments of one or both wolffian ducts (e.g., epididymis, vas deferens, or ampulla) are missing. Males with unilateral tubal deficiencies or occlusions often have normal fertility, but those with the bilateral condition are sterile. It is more common among the offspring of certain bulls that also exhibit this condition. It is characterized in cattle by a total or partial absence of one or both epididymides, but more often the right epididymis. Segmental aplasia of the epididymis is commonly associated with a localized accumulation of sperm within an occluded epididymis, which is known as a *spermatocele*.

### Cryptorchidism

The descent of the testes involves the abdominal migration to the internal inguinal ring, passage through the inguinal canal, and finally migration within the scrotum. In cryptorchidism, one testis or both testes fail to descend from the abdominal cavity into the scrotum. Testicular descent in mammals results from swelling and subsequent regression of the gubernaculum. Early in the process, the gubernaculum extends from the caudal pole of the testis to the external inguinal ring. Traction that develops from swelling of the extra-abdominal portion of the gubernaculum draws the testis into the inguinal canal. Subsequent regression of the gubernaculum enables the testis to descend further into the scrotal position. Abnormal gubernacular development has been associated with cryptorchidism in swine.

The incidence of cryptorchidism is higher in swine and horses than in other farm animals. It is probably a hereditary defect transmitted by the male; it is dominant in the horse and recessive in other species. One or both testes may be located in the abdominal cavity or, more commonly, in the inguinal canal. The left testis is affected more often than the right testis in large type of horses, whereas either testis may be affected with approximately equal frequencies in ponies. The rarity of cryptorchidism in older horses might

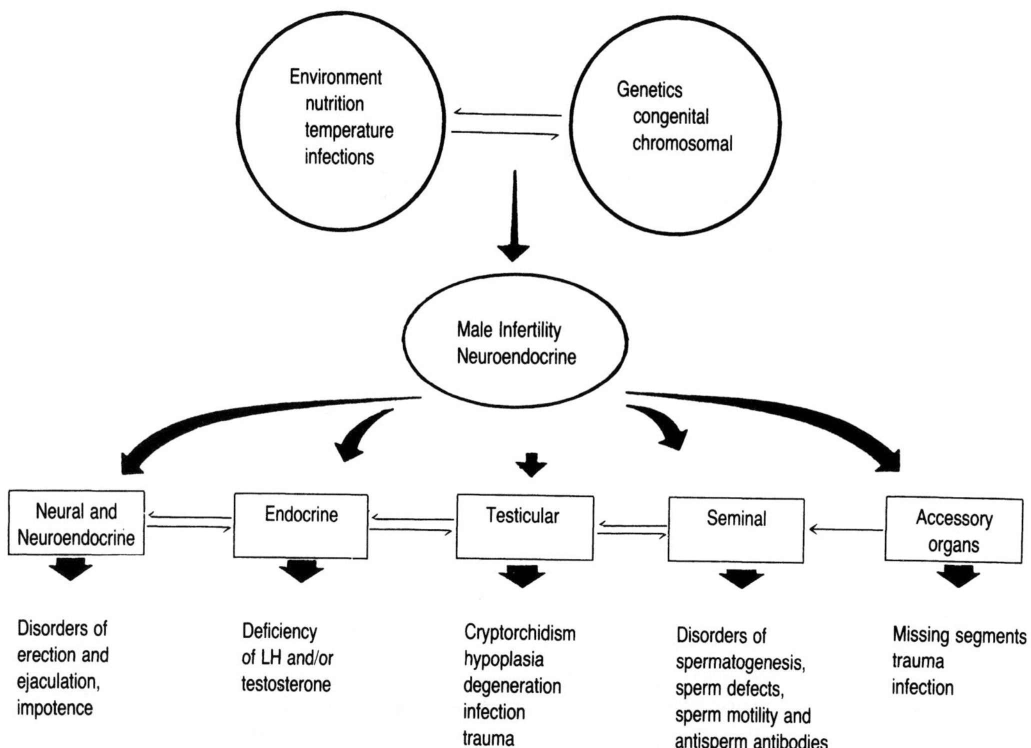


Figure 18-1. The various causes of reproductive failure in male farm animals.

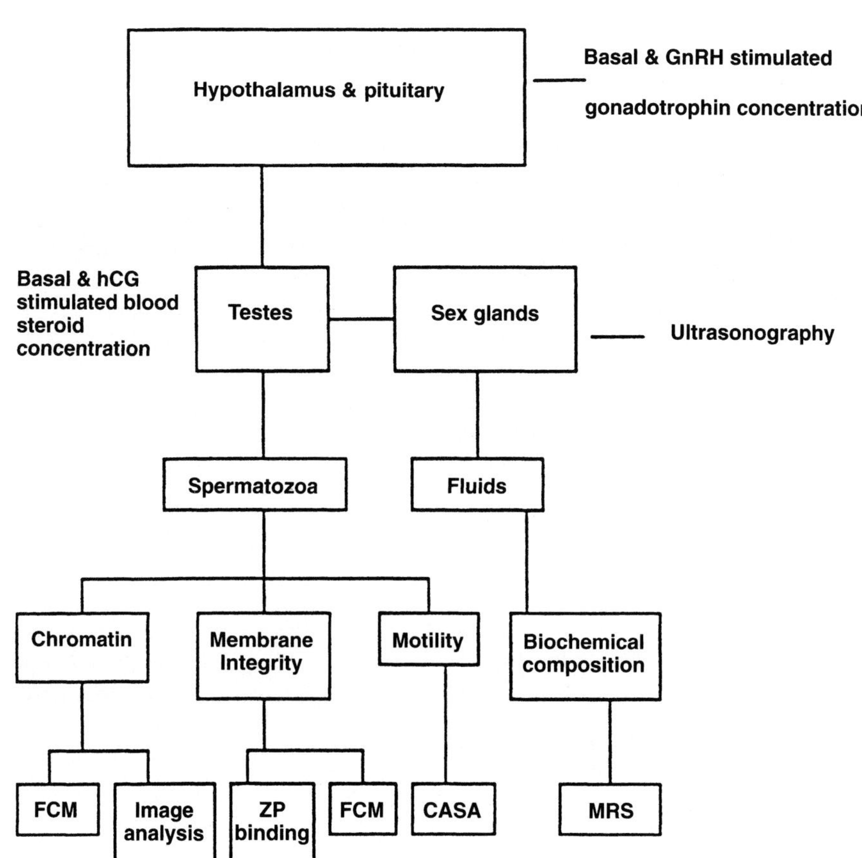


Figure 18-2. Various techniques to evaluate fertility problems in farm mammals: *FCM*, flow cytometry; *CASA*, Computer assisted semen analyses; *ZP*, Zona pellucida binding; *MRS*, Magnetic resonance spectrometry. (From: Magistrini M, Vidament M, Clement F, Palmer E. Fertility prediction in stallions. Anim Rep Sci 1996;42:181–188.)

TABLE 18-1. ***Disorders of Male Reproductive Organs: Species Affected, Causes, Lesions, and Changes in Semen Characteristics***

| SYNDROME | SPECIES AFFECTED | CAUSES | LESIONS | CHANGES IN SEMEN |
|---|---|---|---|---|
| Testicular degeneration | Bull<br>Ram | Thermal, localized or systemic infections; nutrition (vitamin A); vascular lesions; aging; obstructive lesions of the head of epididymis; noxious agents; hormonal factors | Testicular size reduced; fibrosis; disturbances in spermatogenesis; seminiferous tubules destroyed cases | Increase in immature/abnormal sperm with normal motility.<br>Ejaculate is thin/watery due to reduction in sperm concentration.<br>Giant cells; azoospermia or necrozoospermia |
| Orchitis | Bull<br>Ram | Brucellosis, tuberculosis | Inflammatory changes in testis leading to degeneration of seminiferous tubules | Asthenozoospermia; oligozoospermia teratozoospermia.<br>Giant cells; erythrocytes/leukocytes normal semen volume |
| Epididymitis | Bull | Brucellosis viral infections | Inflammation of epididymis.<br>Infiltration of lymphocytes/neutrophils; dead sperm/giant cells | Poor semen characteristics; contaminated by inflammatory exudate |
| Seminal vesiculitis | Bull | Brucellosis | Unilateral inflammation of seminal vesicles; glands enlarged/fibrosed | Purulent exudate in semen.<br>Normozoospermia, asthenozoospermia<br>Fructose content reduced |

Adapted from: Jubb R, Kennedy K. Pathology of Domestic Animals. New York: Academic Press, 1970.; Laing JA, et al. Fertility and Infertility in Domestic Animals. London: Bailliere Tindall/Cassell, 1970.

be because some inguinal testis descend into the scrotum with advancing age.

Bilaterally cryptorchid animals are sterile owing to thermal suppression of spermatogenesis, whereas unilaterally cryptorchid animals have normal spermatogenesis in the scrotal testis. Unilaterally cryptorchid animals are usually fertile but have reduced sperm concentrations; they display normal secondary sexual characteristics because their testes secrete testosterone at nearly normal levels because of elevated levels of LH.

The steroidogenic function of the cryptorchid testis is controversial. The cryptorchid testis has a lower ability than the normal scrotal testis in the ram and bull to secrete testosterone in response to exogenous gonadotropin. On the contrary, steroid production *in vitro* by Leydig cells was similar for both the abdominal and the contralateral scrotal testes in unilateral cryptorchid boars and stallions (2).

Despite the ability of a unilaterally cryptorchid male to reproduce, it should not be used for breeding because the trait can be transmitted to its offspring.

### *Testicular Hypoplasia*

Hypoplasia of the testes, a congenital defect in which the potential for development of the spermatogenic epithelium is lacking, occurs in all farm animals, particularly in bulls of several breeds.

Inherited testicular hypoplasia is best known in Swedish Highland cattle and is caused by a recessive autosomal gene with incomplete (about 50%) penetrance. Testicular hypoplasia also occurs in other breeds of cattle, but a genetic basis has not been well documented even though a familial distribution has been noted (3). Testicular hypoplasia also occurs in *Bos indicus*, particularly the Brahman and Brahman crossbred bulls.

Testicular hypoplasia is suspected only at puberty or later because of reduced fertility or sterility. One or both testes may be hypoplastic. In sterile bulls, the semen is watery and contains few or no sperm. In less severe forms, semen, libido, and the ability to serve are not affected, but sperm numbers may be reduced. Histologically, the seminif-

**TABLE 18-2. *Endocrine Control of Testicular and Neurological Regulation of Male Sexual Function***

ENDOCRINE CONTROL OF TESTICULAR FUNCTION

Hypothalamus → GnRH
↓
Anterior Pituitary
↙ ↘
FSH LH
↓ ↓
Sertoli Cell Leydig Cell
↓ ↓
Androgen-binding protein Testosterone
↘ ↙
Seminiferous tubule

NEUROLOGICAL REGULATION OF MALE SEXUAL FUNCTION

Psychogenic erection
(stimulation from higher center)
↓
SPINAL CORD
(T10–L2) (S2–S4)
↓
Parasympathetic fibres
inpelvic nerve
VASODILATION — EMISSION
↓ ↓
ERECTION — EJACULATION
Pudendal nerve → perineal muscle contraction
Sympathetic Fibers
α receptors in seminal vesicles, prostate, vas, bladder,
↓
close of bladder neck

Adapted from: Acosta AA, Kruger TF, eds. Spermatozoa in Asserted Reproduction. New York: Parmethon Publishing Group, 1996.

erous tubules are characterized by a lack of germinal elements, predominance of Sertoli cells, and a failure of spermatogenesis.

A hypoplastic testis is reduced in size. Although severe cases of testicular hypoplasia may be diagnosed by scrotal and testicular measurements, the less obvious cases are difficult to diagnose. Karyotype analysis may aid diagnosis, since a high incidence of chromosomal secondary constrictions is present in leukocyte cultures from the blood of bulls with testicular hypoplasia (2). As in the bull, testicular hypoplasia in boars and rams is characterized by small testes and semen with low sperm concentration (boar) or with a high percentage of abnormal sperm (ram).

## EJACULATORY DISTURBANCES

Ejaculatory disturbances are of two types: lack of sex drive or libido, and failure to copulate, which encompasses disturbances in erection, mounting, intromission, or ejaculation.

### *Lack of Libido*

Libido or sexual desire is an important aspect of male reproductive function. Lack of libido (*impotentia coeundi*) may be hereditary or may originate from psychogenic disturbances, endocrine imbalance, or environmental factors. Even though seminal characteristics may be satisfactory, fertility may be adversely affected as a result of poor libido.

BULL. Both libido and mating ability in bulls are influenced by genetic factors. Libido was found to be similar between monozygotic twin bulls under different managerial and nutritional systems. Lack of sexual desire is more frequent in some strains and breeds of cattle than in others, e.g., beef breeds and *Bos indicus* cattle. Some bulls become apprehensive about sudden changes in the environment, such as changing the farm, the barn, the herdsman, or the locality of semen location. Since fear and apprehension are inimical to sexual expression, the intensity of sexual behavior declines until the bull becomes accustomed to the new situation. Inhibition may develop as a result of repeated frustration, faulty management, wrong techniques during semen collection, distraction during coitus, and too-rapid

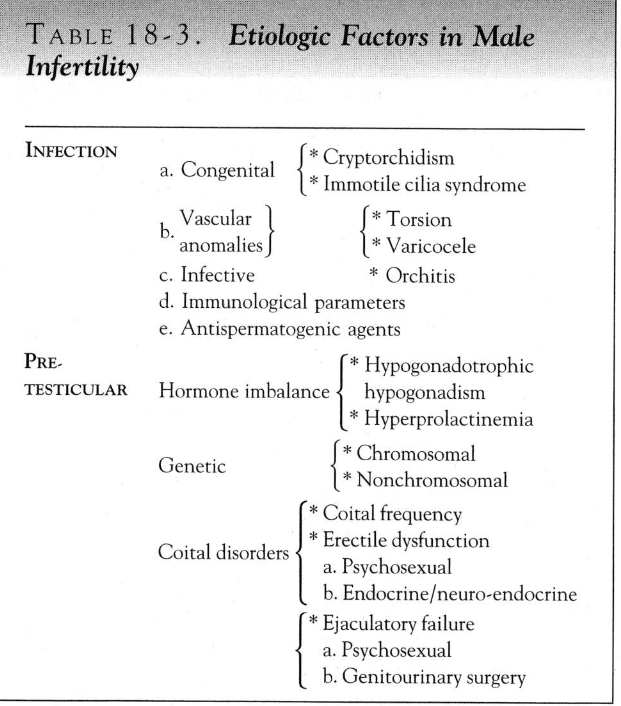

**TABLE 18-3. *Etiologic Factors in Male Infertility***

| | | |
|---|---|---|
| INFECTION | a. Congenital | * Cryptorchidism<br>* Immotile cilia syndrome |
| | b. Vascular anomalies | * Torsion<br>* Varicocele |
| | c. Infective | * Orchitis |
| | d. Immunological parameters | |
| | e. Antispermatogenic agents | |
| PRE-TESTICULAR | Hormone imbalance | * Hypogonadotrophic hypogonadism<br>* Hyperprolactinemia |
| | Genetic | * Chromosomal<br>* Nonchromosomal |
| | Coital disorders | * Coital frequency<br>* Erectile dysfunction<br>a. Psychosexual<br>b. Endocrine/neuro-endocrine |
| | | * Ejaculatory failure<br>a. Psychosexual<br>b. Genitourinary surgery |

TABLE 18-4. ***Differential Diagnosis of Azoospermia/Endocrine Profile***

| CATEGORY | ALGORITHM ENDOCRINE EVALUATION | | | | DIAGNOSIS |
|---|---|---|---|---|---|
| | *LH/nl* | *FSH* | | *Testosterone/nl* | |
| Hypergonadotropic azoospermia | ↑ | ↑ | | ↓ | testicular dysfunction |
| Hypogonadotropic azoospermia | ↓ | ↓ | | ↓ | abnormal hormonal stimulation/endocrine evaluation |
| | nil | nil | | nil | normal testicular unexplained obstruction |
| Eugonadotropic azoospermia | Normal LH<br>Normal FSH<br>Normal Testosterone | | ➡ | Obstruction<br>Maturation Arrest<br>Sertoli Cell Only Syndrome<br>Ejaculatory Dysfunction<br>Sexual Dysfunction | |
| Differential diagnosis of azoospermia based on ejaculate volume/fructose presence | normal semen volume fructose positive | | | | endocrine evaluation |
| | low semen volume and/or fructose negative | | | | postejaculatory urine ↗ (+) sperm ↘ (−) sperm |

withdrawal of the teaser animal after copulation. Inhibition is characterized by refusal to copulate, incomplete erection, or incomplete ejaculation. Bulls exhibit considerable differences in semen characteristics and libido. There is no association between libido and semen quality or scrotal circumference. Good quality semen can be collected with an electroejaculator from low libido bulls, but the method should not be used in AI programs because of the likelihood of disseminating genes associated with low libido. Poor libido is believed to be due to a deficiency in circulating androgens, but in Holstein bulls, the concentration of circulating testosterone is unrelated to libido or semen characteristics.

STALLION. Abnormal mating behavior in stallions is most often due to mismanagement at time of breeding. Overuse, rough treatment at service, or too-frequent ejaculation during winter may exert a detrimental effect on the behavior of young stallions. Pain resulting from injury at copulation or associated with mounting attempts is also a common cause of impotence. Seasonal variations in libido and the secretory and gametogenic activity of the stallion reproductive tract are mediated, at least in part, by the pattern of testosterone secretion. The greatest sperm output in stallions occurs during July, two months after the seasonal peak in plasma testosterone levels.

RAMS. Despite the production of normal numbers of fertile sperm, rams may have low fertility because of their inability to breed sufficient numbers of ewes. This low-service frequency results from a lack of libido, poor dexterity, or interference from other rams. Seasonal factors, such as daylight and temperature, influence the sexual performance of rams of different breeds under a wide variety of both natural and controlled experimental conditions. A decline in the hours of light generally appears to favor enhanced sexual performance, but evidence of such a relationship is conflicting. Ram fertility is also adversely affected during periods of high temperature.

BOAR. Low libido in the boar is associated with obesity, heat stress, or too-high a plane of nutrition. Libido also may be seriously impaired by mismanagement of young boars during service.

### *Inability to Copulate*

Physical disabilities may impede or prevent mating by causing failure in copulation behavior, i.e., mounting, intromission, or ejaculation.

FAILURE TO MOUNT. Inability to mount is a common disorder encountered in older bulls and boars. It is associated

**TABLE 18-5. *Evaluation of Sperm Morphology***

| CATEGORY | TYPES OF ABNORMALITIES |
|---|---|
| Sperm head anomalies | a. Large heads<br>b. Small heads<br>c. Elongated/tapering heads<br>d. Duplicated heads<br>e. Amorphous heads<br>f. Normal sperm heads with neck/midpiece and/or tail and/or cytoplasmic droplet defects. |
| Abnormalities or non-sperm cells counted | a. Precursors<br>b. Tail abnormalities<br>c. Neck/midpiece abnormalities<br>d. Cytoplasmic droplets<br>e. Loose heads |
| Acrosome disorders | TYPE A: Slight disorders where small or missing acrosomes are present. The outline (form) of the sperm is normal or slightly narrowed.<br>TYPE B: Sperm shows the same acrosome defects, but the sperm heads are round with a compact condensation of the chromatin.<br>Combination of TYPE A and TYPE B. |
| Sperm tail defect | TYPE A: Broken tails.<br>TYPE B: Broken tails at neck or midpiece area with coiling of the tails.<br>TYPE C: Short rudimentary (tadpole-like) tails. |
| Structural shaft disturbance of tail based on Shorr staining technique (Dusseldorf Classification) | a. Size defects, too small or too large<br>b. Different degrees of hyperelongation<br>c. Hyperelongation with acrosome defects<br>d. Different degrees of acrosome disorders<br>e. Duplicated forms<br>f. Midpiece and/or tail defects<br>g. Combination of head/tail defects |

Adapted from: Menkveld R, Kruger TF. Evaluation of sperm morphology by light microscopy. In: Acosta AA, Kruger TF, eds. Human Spermatozoa in Assisted Reproduction, 2nd ed. New York: Parthenon Publishing Group, 1996.

with locomotor dysfunction arising from dislocations, fractures, sprains, and osteoarthritic lesions of the hindlimbs and vertebrae. Degenerative changes in the articular surface of the stifle and hock joints and exostoses of the thoracolumbar vertebrae interfere with mobility and ability to mount, particularly in older bulls.

FAILURE TO ACHIEVE INTROMISSION. This is a condition in which the penis fails to enter the vagina. It may result from insufficient protrusion of the penis from the sheath or deviation of the penis.

Phimosis, or stenosis of the preputial orifice that is due to congenital, traumatic, or infectious causes, may prevent the normal protrusion of the penis. The pendulous prolapse that occurs in *Bos indicus* breeds (Santa Gertrudis and Brahman), or the inherent tendency to preputial eversion that occurs in some polled *Bos taurus* breeds (Hereford and Aberdeen Angus), may lead to trauma, inflammatory changes, and eventually to preputial prolapse and phimosis. At service, affected bulls are unable to protrude the penis more than 2 or 3 inches, or even through the preputial orifice in more severe cases. The condition may be corrected by surgical amputation of the prolapsed preputial mucosa. Selective breeding and culling of *B. taurus* bulls with a predisposition to preputial prolapse may help to reduce the incidence.

Another serious cause of inability to protrude the penis is hematoma of the penis as a result of rupture of the corpus cavernosum of the penis. It commonly occurs in bulls during coitus when the penis is thrust against the perineum of the cow. A hematoma develops distal to the sigmoid flexure, although some may be found proximally, and causes swelling, which may be palpated anterior to the scrotum.

Abnormal venous drainage of the corpus cavernosum in the bull could result in a penis too flaccid for intromission despite good libido. This is because erection in the bull is not, as commonly believed, due to the rigidity of the fibroelastic components of the penis and relaxation of the retractor penis muscle but mainly to the high pressures generated

**TABLE 18-6. *Some Biochemical Markers to Identify the Source of Secretion Within the Ejaculate by the Presence of Different Components of Ejaculate***

| SOURCE OF SECRETION | BIOCHEMICAL MARKERS |
|---|---|
| Testes | Androgen binding protein<br>Inhibin<br>Testosterone<br>Transferrin |
| Epididymal Ducts | Carnitine<br>Glycerophosphorylcholine<br>Inositol |
| Seminal Vesicles | Fructose<br>Prostaglandins |
| Prostate | Acid phosphatase<br>Citrate<br>Calcium, zinc<br>Spermine<br>Vesiculase |
| Bulbourethral/Urethral Glands | IgA<br>Mucoproteins |

within the corpus cavernosum penis. This abnormality in the bull appears to be congenital, although it may be due to trauma of the tunica albuginea in older bulls (4).

Tumors of the glans penis may occasionally prevent protrusion of the penis. Fibropapillomas of viral origin are frequently noted on the glans penis of 2-year-old bulls. Affected bulls are reluctant to serve or are incapable of achieving intromission. Although spontaneous regression of the tumor can occur, surgical extirpation or vaccination with a tissue vaccine is employed to control the condition.

**TABLE 18-7. *Therapeutic Approaches of Male Infertility Involving Gamete Micromanipulation***

| | | |
|---|---|---|
| IVF-related | PROST | Pronuclear Stage Tubal-transfer |
| | IVF-ET | *In Vitro* Fertilization and Embryo Transfer |
| | TEST | Tubal Embryo Stage Transfer |
| Other | POST | Peritoneal Ovum and Sperm Transfer |
| | FREDI | Fallopian Replacement of Eggs and Delayed Insemination |
| | ICSI | Intracytoplasmic Sperm Injection |

Congenital deformities of the penis or prepuce may render intromission difficult or impossible. One such deformity is the persistence of the frenulum, commonly encountered in beef Shorthorn and Aberdeen Angus bulls. In this condition, the frenulum attaches the ventral aspect of the glans penis to the preputial mucosa. At coitus, the deformity is noted as a ventral or downward deviation of the penis. Rarely, intromission may be accomplished. The deformity can be corrected by ligating and cutting the band of tissue.

Three distinct types of congenital deviations of the penis are encountered in bulls. A spiral deviation of the penis occurs in most normal bulls after intromission. A similar spiraling occurs with the "corkscrew" type of penile deviation, where the spiraling precedes intromission and prevents coitus. Less common types of deviations of the penis are the ventral or "rainbow" deviation and the mild S-shaped deviation. In the boar, abnormalities of the penis, e.g., persistent frenulum, penile hypoplasia, and enlargement of the preputial diverticulum, frequently result in a failure to achieve intromission and are the major causes of poor mating preference. With these defects, the boar is unable to erect his penis, to penetrate the vagina, or to lock it in the cervix.

FAILURE TO EJACULATE. This condition is occasionally observed with bulls even when accompanied by vigorous thrust at intromission. Poor semen collection techniques, e.g., improper temperature or pressure within the artificial vagina, often cause failure of ejaculation in bulls used for AI purposes. In the stallion, ejaculatory disorders, ranging from intromission without ejaculation to abnormal copulatory pattern with or without occasional ejaculation, are frequently encountered. These disorders are probably caused by a functional disturbance of the nervous mechanisms that regulate the ejaculatory process. Unfamiliar surroundings, obesity, poor condition, or exhaustion resulting from frequent services may exert a detrimental effect on these nervous mechanisms.

## FERTILIZATION FAILURE

Fertilization failure is an important cause of infertility in males that have normal libido and are capable of mating and ejaculating. This capacity or reduced capacity is related to defective semen characteristics or to errors in breeding techniques.

### *Diseases of Testes and Accessory Glands*

Pathologic conditions of the testes, epididymis, and seminal vesicles (Table 18-1) may interfere with fertilization by disturbing spermatogenesis or sperm maturation, causing abnormal semen characteristics, or preventing the passage of sperm from the testes to the urethra.

### Heat Stress

Temperature is one of the important environmental factors modifying reproduction. Elevated body temperatures, during periods of high ambient temperature or pyrexia from disease, lead to testicular degeneration and reduce the percentage of normal and fertile sperm in the ejaculate. In several species, there are seasonal variations in the quality and fertility of semen. Bulls subjected to high environmental temperatures have reduced semen quality. Rams may retain a satisfactory level of fertility throughout the whole year, but in many instances, fertility is depressed when matings occur during the hot months of the year. Conception failure in ewes mated to heat-stressed rams is related more to failure of fertilization than to embryonic mortality.

When the scrotal contents of rams are heated to approximately 40 °C for 1½ to 2 hours, a sharp increase in the proportion of morphologically abnormal sperm occurs in the ejaculate 14 to 16 days later. Sperm that are developing in the testis at the time of heating showed damage (e.g., dead and tailless sperm), whereas epididymal sperm are unaffected. Acrosomal damage is characterized by swelling, vesiculation, and eventual disintegration.

Seasonal variations occur in the fertility of boars, and levels are lowest immediately after the hottest months of the year. Volume of semen and total sperm per ejaculation from boars are greater during cool weather. Boars exposed to elevated ambient temperatures daily for 90 days show decreases in sperm concentration and motility, and increases in sperm abnormalities and acrosomal changes. Exposure of boars for periods of 4 to 5 days to ambient temperatures above 35°C and to the diurnal variations prevailing in subtropical and tropical regions affects their semen quality but not semen volume. The adverse effects are evident 3 to 5 weeks later, particularly on sperm morphology (5). The high incidence of cytoplasmic droplets may be caused by the long-term effect of elevated ambient temperatures on the epididymis which, because of its unique location in the scrotum in the pig, is most sensitive to temperature (6).

Also, infectious diseases resulting in a febrile reaction are likely to affect the subsequent fertility of the boar for a five to six week period. The decrease in conception rate in artificially inseminated gilts maintained under elevated environmental temperatures is apparently due to embryonic mortality.

### Breeding Techniques

Fertilization failure attributed to the male may result from poor breeding management or from faulty techniques in AI. Also, synchronization of estrus in cattle and sheep with progestational compounds, the ingestion of estrogenic pasture grass by sheep, or the imposition of stress during insemination may interfere with sperm transport and cause fertilization failure.

BREEDING MANAGEMENT. Under natural mating programs, the frequency of service and the ratio of females assigned to each breeding male depend on the species, age, libido, fertility, and nutrition of the male; the duration of the mating season; the system of management; and the size of pasture or range.

Spermatogenesis is a continuous process, but frequent and repeated ejaculations adversely affect male libido and semen characteristics. Although libido returns to normal after a week of sexual rest, semen characteristics are not restored to normal for 6 weeks. Similarly, after a period of prolonged inactivity, semen characteristics and fertility remain low for the first few services. Seasonal variations are especially important in seasonally breeding species such as stallions and rams; changes in the ratio of daylight to darkness are reflected in the quality and quantity of semen.

INFERTILITY AND ARTIFICIAL INSEMINATION. The male makes several contributions to reproductive failure in an AI program, e.g., defective semen, improper insemination techniques, or failure of sperm transport in the female tract. These and other factors affecting fertility in AI are considered in other chapters. Changes in the fertility of frozen semen during storage are important in the efficient use and design of AI programs.

### Immunological Factors

The ability of sperm to induce antibodies has been recognized since the beginning of this century. Despite unsuccessful attempts to use immunity to sperm as a method of male contraception, there is sufficient evidence to implicate sperm antibodies as a cause of human reproductive failure (7, 8). In contrast, relatively little is known or understood about immunologic infertility in domestic animals.

Several immunopathologic parameters of sperm antibodies cause several autoimmune responses:

a) Arming macrophages and enhancing of sperm from the male genital tract.
b) Mediating cytotoxic (immobilizing) effects on sperm in the presence of high titer of complement cascade components.
c) Sperm unable to penetrate cervical mucus because of agglutination and related pathologic mechanisms.
d) Interfering with sperm capacitation/decapacitation/ sperm hyperactivation.
e) Direct blocking of penetration of zona pellucida of ova.
f) Influencing sperm selection within the female genital tract.

Several immunopathologic markers are used to detect certain autoimmune responses. IgA sperm-specific antibodies are the main indicators of poor semen penetration.

The antigenic components of semen originate in the testis, epididymis, vas deferens, and accessory glands. They can be broadly classified as those in the seminal plasma and those that are sperm bound. Sperm carry a mixture of antigens, including sperm-specific antigens, histocompatability antigens (i.e., those responsible for the rejection of tissue grafts), blood-group antigens, and other somatic tissue antigens. Sperm antigens may be antigenic within the male (autoantigens) or the female (isoantigens) reproductive system. Of the sperm antigens, those on the surface of the plasma membrane are probably responsible for the reproductive failure. To be effective, antibodies against sperm must enter the seminal fluid or the cervical mucus following deposition in the female tract.

An autoimmune response is normally prevented by the relative isolation of the seminiferous tubules from the rest of the body—*the blood-testis barrier*. If the barrier is breached, antisperm antibodies are produced that might attack sperm. Experimental allergic orchitis is an organ-specific autoimmune syndrome produced in experimental animals, such as the guinea pig, by the injection of autologous or homologous testis or sperm with Freund's complete adjuvant, which potentiates the immune response (6). The testicular damage results in germinal cell destruction and azoospermia (complete absence of sperm in the ejaculate) in the immunized animals. Similar treatment resulted in sperm agglutinins in bulls, but only one showed significant changes in semen characteristics (9). Autoantibodies against sperm have been reported in the serum of infertile men. Antisperm antibodies are also found in the serum and seminal fluid of bulls, but there is no association between their presence and the classification of bulls as satisfactory or unsatisfactory potential breeders (10).

Antisperm antibodies can prevent fertilization by immobilizing sperm, impairing sperm penetration of cervical mucus, inactivating acrosomal enzymes presumed essential for fertilization, inhibiting the attachment of sperm to the zona pellucida, or interfering with embryonic mortality (11). These effects of antibodies have been shown experimentally with isoimmunization of females of several species, including cattle, with sperm or sperm "plasma membrane" preparations. Rabbits inseminated with semen treated with antiserum against a sperm membrane autoantigen experienced a decrease in fertility as a result of the inability of the sperm to penetrate the zona pellucida (12). However, this effect may have been due to more than one mechanism because immune sera could have contained antibodies against different sperm antigens. This problem has been overcome with the development of monoclonal antibodies against sperm surface components of several laboratory species and man. Two such monoclonal antibodies showed a significant inhibition of postfertilization fertility in the rabbit (13).

Sperm antibodies have been implicated as a cause of repeat-breeding in cattle, but there was no evidence to indicate that antisperm antibodies were responsible for the reduced fertility in a group of repeat-breeder cows (14). Egg-yolk and milk used in semen extenders may also act as antigens. Antibodies against egg-yolk antigens have been detected in uterine mucus and tissue from cows that had been inseminated repeatedly (15). When cows were inseminated with extenders containing egg-yolk, the fertility rate was lower in cows showing uterine titers to egg-yolk antigens than in cows not showing uterine titers.

## Nutrition and Male Infertility

The effects of nutritional restrictions on fertility are more notable in the female than in the male. Nutritional deficiencies delay the onset of puberty and depress production and characteristics of semen in the male. The young and growing animal is much more susceptible to nutritional stress than the mature animal. In addition, nutrition affects the endocrine rather than the spermatogenic function of the testis. Common nutritional factors include caloric, protein, and vitamin deficiencies, but minerals or toxic agents may also be important.

### Underfeeding

Despite the ability of a mature male to maintain sperm production and testosterone secretion under low levels of nutrition, the young male shows retarded sexual development and delayed puberty. This is due to suppression of endocrine activity of the testes and, consequently, to retardation of growth and secretory function of the male organs of reproduction. When mature bulls, rams, and boars are fed low-energy rations for prolonged periods, libido and testosterone production are affected much earlier than semen characteristics. The effects of undernutrition may be corrected in mature animals, whereas it is less successful in young animals because of the permanent damage caused to the germinal epithelium of the testis.

Obesity and overfeeding reduce libido and sexual activity in rams, boars, and bulls, particularly during hot weather. Protein deficiency affects the young more than the mature male. Young bulls on a protein-deficient diet show decreases in libido and semen characteristics, whereas mature bulls, rams, and boars are rarely affected. Diets high in protein are not essential for optimal sperm production in the ram.

### Vitamin Deficiencies

Dietary vitamin A or carotene deficiency leads to testicular degeneration in all farm animals. The effect of vitamin A on the testes is probably indirect and due to suppression of the release of pituitary gonadotropins. Injections of gonadotropic hormones or vitamin A will restore spermatogenesis, except in cases in which the damage to the testis is permanent. While bull calves maintained on a low vitamin A diet show degenerative changes in the germinal epithelium of the testis and azoospermia, mature bulls show no adverse effects in spermatogenesis. Cattle are more resistant to vitamin A deficiency than swine. For example, night-blindness and uncoordination of movement precede recognizable reduction in fertility of mature bulls, whereas testicular degeneration is one of the earliest signs of avitaminosis A in the mature boar. Vitamin E (tocopherol or wheat germ oil) is important for normal reproduction, but its role in the fertility of male farm animals is obscure.

### *Mineral Deficiencies and Toxic Agents*

There is a paucity of information concerning the effects of trace mineral deficiencies on male reproductive functions. Iodine deficiency has been suspected as a cause of poor libido and semen characteristics in bulls. Also, improvement in sperm production and fertility have been noted following supplementary feeding of copper, cobalt, zinc, and manganese. Plant estrogens exert adverse effects on male accessory organs, but infertility of sheep and cattle grazing on estrogenic pastures are related to changes in cervical mucus and to a failure of sperm transport in the female tract. Many chemicals, rare earth salts, and ionizing radiations interfere with spermatogenesis in a variety of mammalian species, but their contribution to male infertility remains to be established.

## INFERTILITY AND CHROMOSOMAL ABERRATIONS

Sex differentiation is determined by genetic mechanisms. Genes on the short arm of the Y chromosome determine maleness. The testis determining factor (TDF) is the male specific histocompatibility (H-Y) antigen. Spermatogenesis is regulated by various genetic factors. Chromosomal anomalies are responsible for some 20% of male infertility. Disorders of the Y chromosome include cytogenic anomalies, such as translocations and numerical abnormalities, sex reversal, or ambiguous genitalia caused by mutations in the sex determining region of the Y chromosome (16). Several genes on the long arm play a role in spermatogenesis.

Chromosomal aberrations play an important role in human reproductive failure. From a breeding point of view, it is important to eliminate males that are affected by chromosomal aberrations, particularly those resulting in decreased fertility.

Extensive investigations have been conducted on the etiology, pathophysiology, genetics, biochemistry, biophysical molecular parameters, and therapeutic approaches of male infertility in animals (16–38).

## REFERENCES


1. Varley M, Stedman R. Stress and reproduction. In: Cole DJA, Wiseman J, Varley MA, eds. Principles of Pig Science. Nottingham: Univ Press, 1994;277–296.
2. Ryan PL, Raeside JI. Steroid production in Leydig cells from cryptorchid boars and stallions. Proc 10th Int Congr Animal Reprod AI, Champaign-Urbana, IL 1984;3:177.
3. Galloway DB, Norman JR. Testicular hypoplasia and autosomal secondary constrictions in bulls. 8th Internat Congr Animal Reprod AI 1976;4:710.
4. Ashdown RR, David JSE, Gibbs C. Impotence in the bull: (1) Abnormal venous drainage of the corpus cavernosum penis. Vet Rec 1979;104:423.
5. Cameron RDA, Blackshaw AW. The effect of elevated ambient temperature on spermatogenesis in the boar. J Reprod Fertil 1980;59:173.
6. Stone BA. Thermal characteristics of the testis and epididymis of the boar. J Reprod Fertil 1981;63:551.
7. Jones WR. Immunological factors in male and female infertility. In: Hearn JP, ed. Immunological Aspects of Reproduction and Fertility Control. Lancaster: MTP Press, 1980.
8. Bronson R, Cooper G, Rosenfeld D. Sperm antibodies: their role in infertility. Fertil Steril 1984;42:171.
9. Wright PJ. Serum spermagglutinins and semen quality in the bull. Aust Vet J 1980;56:10.
10. Purswell BJ, Dawe DL, Caudle AB, Williams DJ, Brown J. Spermagglutinins in serum and seminal fluid of bulls and their relationship to fertility classification. Theriogeneology 1983;20:375–381.
11. Menge SM. Clinical immunologic infertility: diagnostic measures, incidence of antisperm antibodies, fertility and mechanisms. In: Dhindsa D, Schumacher GFB, eds. Immunological Aspects of Infertility and Fertility Regulations. New York: Elsevier North Holland, 1980.
12. O'Rand MG. Inhibition of fertility and sperm-zona binding an antiserum to the rabbit sperm membrane autoantigen RSA-1. Biol Reprod 1981;25:621.
13. Naz RK, Saxe JM, Menge C. Inhibition of fertility in rabbits by monoclonal antibodies against sperm. Biol Reprod 1983;28:249.
14. Farhani JK, Tompkins W, Wagner WC. Reproductive status of cows and incidence of antisperm antibodies. Theriogeneology 1981;15:605.
15. Griffin JFT, Nunn WR, Hartigan PJ. An immune response to egg-yolk semen diluent in dairy cows. J Reprod Fertil 1971;25:193.
16. Jainudeen MR, Hafez ESE. Genetics of reproductive failure. In: Hafez ESE, ed. Reproduction in Farm Animals, 6th ed. Philadelphia: Lea & Febiger, 1993;298.
17. Aiken RJ, Irvine DS, Wu FC. Prospective analysis of sperm-oocyte fusion and reactive oxygen species generation as criteria for the diagnosis of infertility. Am J Obstet Gynecol 1991;164:524–551.
18. Allen JF. Separate sexes and the mitochondial theory of aging. J Theor Biol 1996;180:135–140.
19. Brake A, Krause W. Decreasing quality in semen. Br Med J 1992;305:609–612.
20. Elliot OJ, Ma K, Kerr SM, et al. An RMB homologue maps to the mouse Y chromosome and is expressed in germ cells. Hum Mol Genet 1996;5:869–874.
21. Ellis NA, Goodfellow PM. The mammalian pseudoautosomal region. Trends Genet 1989;5:406–410.
22. Foresta C, Ferin A, Garolla A, Rossato M, Barbaux S, De Bortoli A. Y chromosome deletions in idiopathic severe

testiculopathies. J Clin Endocrinol Metab 1997;82:1075–1080.

23. Hollan MK, Storey BT. Oxygen metabolism of mammalian spermatozoa. Generation of hydrogen peroxide by rabbit epididymal spermatozoa. Biochem J 1981;198: 273–280.
24. Lee JD, Kamiguchi Y, Yanagimachi R. Analysis of chromosome constitution of human spermatozoa with normal and aberrant head morphologies after injection into mouse oocytes. Hum Reprod 1996;11:1942–1946.
25. Lovell-Badger R, Hacker A. The molecular genetics of SRY and its role in mammalian sex determination. Phil Trans R Soc Lond B 1995;350:205–214.
26. McLaren A, Simpson E, Tomonari K, Chandler P, Hogg H. Male sexual differentiation in mice lacking H-Y antigen. Nature 1984;312:552–555.
27. Miquel J, Flemming J. Theoretical and experimental support for an "oxygen radical mitochondrial injury," hypothesis of cell aging. In: Johnson JE, Walford R, Harman D, Miquel J, eds. Free radicals, aging and degenerative diseases. New York: Alan R Liss, 1986;51–74.
28. Nohl H, Hegner D. Do mitochondria produce oxygen radicals in vivo? Eur J Biochem 1978;82:563.
29. Overzier C. Die intersexualtat. Stuttgart: George Thieme, 1961.
30. Ozawa T. Mechanism of somatic mitochondrial DNA mutations associated with age and diseases. Biochem Biophys Acta 1995;1271:177–189.
31. Palmer MS, Sinclair AH, Berta P, et al. Genetic evidence that ZFY is not the testis determining factor. Nature 1990;346:240–244.
32. Pichini S, Zuccaro P, Pacifici R. Drugs in semen. Clin Pharmacokinet 1994;26:356–373.
33. Richter C, Park JW, Ames BN. Normal oxidative damage to mitochondrial and nuclear DNA is extensive. Proc Natl Acad Sci 1988;85:6465–6467.
34. Rimini R, Pontiggia A, Spada F, et al. Interaction of normal and mutant SRY proteins with DNA. Phil Trans R Soc Lond B 1995;350:215–220.
35. St. John DC, Cooke ID, Barratt CCR. Mitochondrial mutations and male infertility. Nat Med 1997;3:124–125.
36. Tazaki H, Ikeda N, Omori A. True hermaphrodites in Japan: report of a case and a review of the literature. Kieo J Med 1964;13:143–154.
37. Turrens JP, Boveris A. Generation of superoxide anion by NADPH dehydrogenase of bovine heart mitochondria. Biochem J 1980;191:421–427.
38. Weighardt F, Biamonti G, Riva S. The roles of heterogeneous nuclear ribonucleoproteins (hnRNP) in RNA metabolism. Bioassays 1996;18:747–756.

# Part V

# *Physiopathologic Mechanisms*

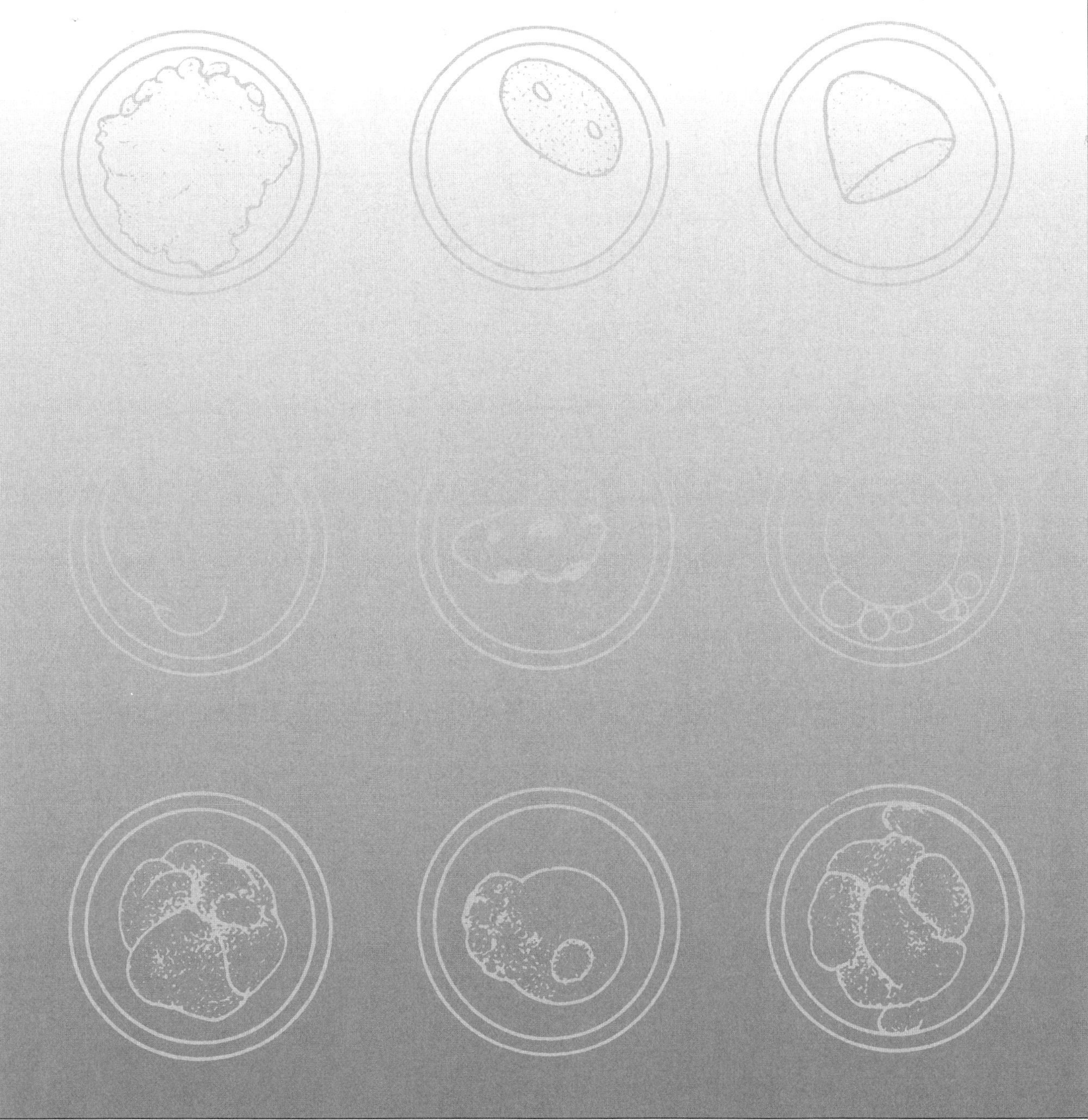

Chapter 19

# Reproductive Behavior

B. Hafez and E.S.E. Hafez

The behavior of animals plays an important role in reproduction, affecting both the success of mating and survival of the young. Behavioral patterns are associated with courtship and copulation, birth, maternal care, and suckling attempts of the newborn (Fig. 19-1). These behavior patterns have been muted by domestication, and restricted or modified by conditions imposed in accordance with husbandry requirements. These requirements include confinement in paddocks, yard, or indoor pens; segregation of sexes; controlled mating; cesarean delivery; enforced weaning; imposed proximity with other individuals; and the inescapable presence of humans, dogs, and machinery.

## Sexual Behavior

Various patterns of courtship, display, motor activities, and postures are directed to bring the male and female gametes together to ensure fertilization, pregnancy, and propagation of the species. The coordination of motor patterns leading to insemination of the female has been achieved by the evolution of an orderly series of responses to specific stimuli. Further, the expression of sexual behaviors are influenced by hormones present in the circulation, and changes in behavior bring about changes in hormone secretion, thus affecting subsequent behaviors. So the chain or sequence of events includes both hormones and behaviors.

Promiscuous sexual behavior in animals is an advantage in domesticating a species and also in carrying out a breeding program based on the use of a few desirable sires. Because any female can be mated to any male, the chances of a suitable pairing are greatly increased over those possible when pair-bonds between male and female must first be established.

### *Psychosocial Aspects of Reproduction*

The encounter of sexual partners is the first step of reproductive behavior. In free-living animals, this occurs largely under the influence of pre-existing social structure and the territorial or home range behavior of males and females, and leads to an organized pattern of reproduction that varies with the sociospatial or territorial characteristics of the species. In the roe deer and muntjak antelope, males and females live in a limited area, the boundaries of which are defended against any intruder of the same sex. The territories of males and females are overlapping, with permanent association between potential sexual partners. In other species, as in the wild rabbit and beaver, the territory is occupied by a permanent couple or harem, and the male avoids any encounter outside his territory. This pattern persists under artificial environments. For example, male rabbits breeding in cages display sexual behavior toward receptive females only after the male occupies the cage for a sufficiently long time to consider it his territory. Territorial behavior is intensified during the season of reproduction, and in fact in many species, such as the seal, it exists only at that time.

Under feral conditions, farm animals do not defend defined territories against intruders, but herds and flocks tend to occupy a "home range." The basic unit is matriarchal, consisting of a female, her adult female offspring, and their immature young. Such a matriarchal herd is remarkably stable. It persists after a temporary dispersion of its members, or mixing in large groups of several hundreds of individuals (African antelopes, bisons). This stability is the consequence of strong interindividual bonds resulting from contacts occurring during infancy. Experimentally, cows reared together from birth form such a stable group even in the middle of a large herd. Such a bond, limited to the dams and their female offspring, could be the basis of the social organization in ungulates.

Increasing population density may lead to abnormal behavior such as tail biting, cannibalism, and an increased level of aggression. Such abnormal behavior may be detrimental in that the performance of individual animals with low social status in the group would decline because of stress (1).

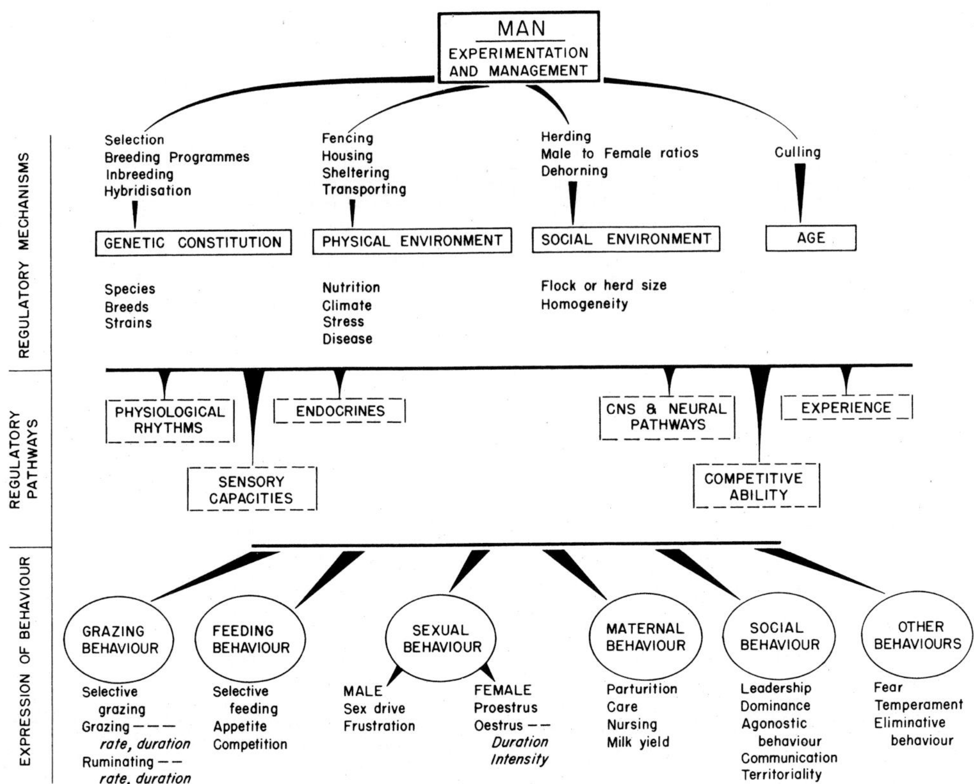


FIGURE 19-1. The interaction between physical and social environment and the development of reproductive and other behaviors in farm animals.

In horses, each matriarchal herd is the permanent harem of a dominant stallion, whereas younger males form a permanent "bachelor" herd (2). In other species, the males either aggregate in groups (feral sheep and goats) or even stay solitary, with occasional contacts with animals of the same species (bisons, wild pigs) (Fig. 19-2). In such cases, the herds of males are only temporary associations in which the interindividual bonds are loose.

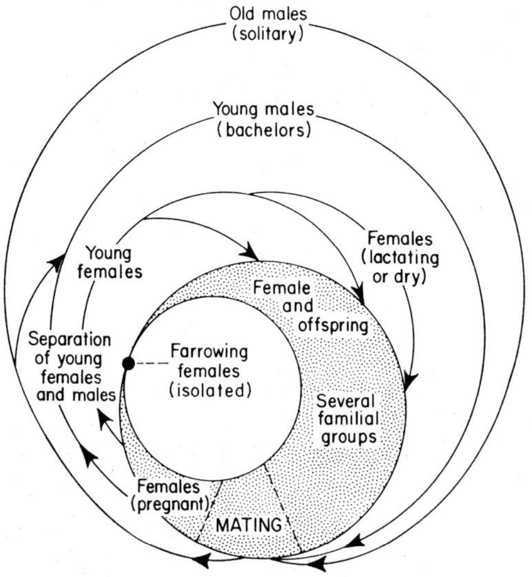

Old males (solitary)
Young males (bachelors)
Young females
Females (lactating or dry)
Female and offspring
Separation of young females and males
Farrowing females (isolated)
Several familial groups
Females (pregnant)
MATING

FIGURE 19-2. Diagram of the evolution of the social organization in pigs. (Courtesy of Dr. J. P. Signoret.)

## *Sequence of Sexual Behavior*

The motor patterns of courtship behavior are stereotyped and are not altered by experience, which acts mainly on the motivation and efficiency of mating (Table 19-1). The components of copulatory patterns are sexual arousal, courtship (sexual display), erection, penile protrusion, mounting, intromission, ejaculation, dismounting, and refractoriness (Fig. 19-3). The duration of courtship and copulation varies with the species; both events are shorter in cattle and sheep than in swine and horses.

MALE. In the male, sniffing and licking the female are the most frequent patterns, suggesting an important function of chemical communication through olfaction. Except in swine, the male of domestic ungulates smells the female's urine and then raises his head, with lips curled, in the ritualized "Flehmen" reaction. In sheep, goats, and cattle, tactile stimulation of the female is made by nuzzling and licking the perineal region, whereas with the horse, the stallion often bites the female's neck, and with swine the boar noses her flanks.

TABLE 19-1. ***Patterns of Male Sexual Behavior***

| ANIMAL | ASPECT MEASURED | TECHNIQUE |
|---|---|---|
| Sheep | Latency of successive ejaculates; total number of ejaculates | Libido measured by time required to produce successive ejaculates and by number of ejaculates in 30 min |
| Cattle | Latency to ejaculation; frequency; reaction to new stimulus situation | Standardized test periods, artificial vagina; constant stimulus animals |
| | Ejaculatory response | Artificial ejaculation using transparent artificial vagina |
| | Variability in sexual performance | Sex drive index devised on basis of performance of sexual pattern |
| Horse | Erection reflex time; effect of elimination of vision and suppression of olfaction on erection | Comparison of young and experienced "old" stallions in tests with blindfold; blindfold, nose mask, and odoriferous substances |

FEMALE. In most species, the estrous female shows increased motor activity, becoming restless and moving at the slightest disturbance. Receptive cows and goats exhibit increased frequency of nonspecific bellows or bleats, whereas the sow utters a typical estrous grunt. Cows, goats, and sows tend to mount and to be mounted by other females, but this is exceptional in ewes and mares. In the presence of a male, the female sniffs at his perineum or scrotal region. Mutual sniffing leads both animals to circling motions in a reverse parallel position. Receptive sows also display interest in the boar's head. Frontal contact between the estrous cow or sow and the boar may be associated with "mock fighting." Estrous mares tend to urinate frequently in the presence of a stallion. Ewes in estrus leave the flock of females to seek out a ram.

When approached and stimulated by the male, the female domestic ungulate assumes a mating posture. This entails immobilization, often accompanied by tail deviation, and some minor species-specific features such as turning the head back in the goat and ewe, cocking the ears in the sow, and exposing the clitoris in the mare.

MATING. The posture of the sexually receptive female terminates courtship behavior by allowing mating to take place. The female stands immobile, and the male mounts and ejaculates (Fig. 19-4).

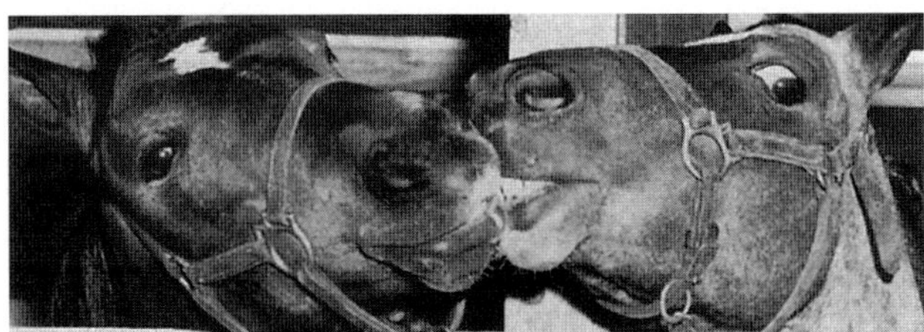

FIGURE 19-3. Patterns of precopulatory courtship in horses.

MOUNTING. In the presence of a proestrous female, the male attempts several mounts; the penis becomes partially erect and protrudes from the prepuce. These mounts are usually unsuccessful. During this activity, the male, especially the bull, excretes "dribblings" of accessory fluid, derived from the Cowper's gland and differing from the seminal plasma emitted from the vesicular glands during ejaculation. If the female is receptive, however, copulation may occur rapidly. The male rests his chin on the female and she in

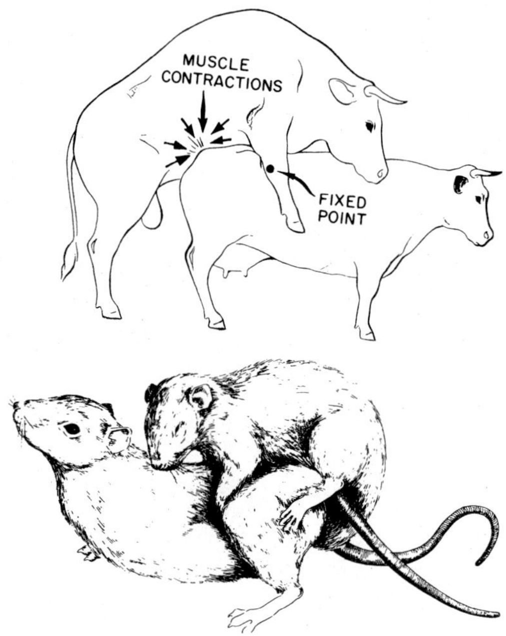


FIGURE 19-4. Species differences: copulatory posture in cattle and rodents.

turn responds by "standing." The male then mounts, "fixes" his forelegs around the female, grasps her firmly and performs rhythmic pelvic thrusts (Fig. 19-4).

The mounting reactions of the male, which are released by a simple visual stimulus, may explain the mounting and homosexuality frequently observed in swine. These mounts are usually unsuccessful, especially in the inexperienced males. Frequently, boars reared in pairs or all-male groups form stable homosexual relationships. Such relationships persist for many months, although members repeatedly copulate with females. The identity of the active and passive partner is maintained. The behavior pattern of the aggressor is the same as the pattern that occurs in normal heterosexual copulation and may include rectal intromission and ejaculation while the passive male stands quietly. If such pairing is well established, homosexual coitus occurs even in the presence of estrous females.

INTROMISSION. At mounting, the abdominal muscles of the male, particularly the rectus abdominis muscles, contract suddenly. As a result, the pelvic region of the male is quickly brought into direct apposition to the external genitalia of the female. The boar, with the penis partially out of the prepuce, thrusts his pelvis until the tip of the penis penetrates the vulva; only then is the penis fully unsheathed and intromission accomplished. When intromission is vaginal, the boar seldom withdraws or dismounts and ejaculation occurs. A series of pelvic thrusts may occur after a rectal intromission, but the penis is most often withdrawn without ejaculation. Abortive ejaculation may take place if the sow refuses intromission or if the boar fails to penetrate either orifice.

Among farm animals, the boar has the longest ejaculation time. Copulation is performed within 3 to 20 min, with an average of 4 to 5 min. The female generally remains completely immobile until the boar dismounts (Fig. 19-5). The female sometimes moves at the end of copulation, but this seldom disturbs ejaculation. After mating, the sow remains by the boar and often licks the flocculent discharge that accumulates on his penis.

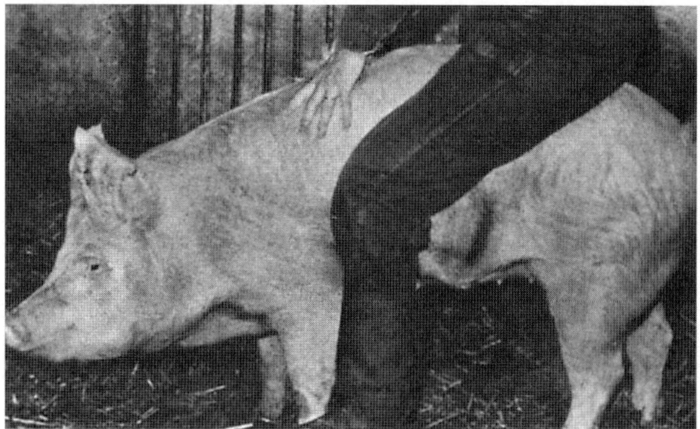

FIGURE 19-5. Among the farm species, sexually receptive female pigs are identified most easily. Those that are in estrus will respond to pressure on the back, especially in the presence of a mature male, by immobility, arching of the back, and "pricking" of the ears.

The stallion oscillates the pelvis several times, resulting in engorgement of the penis with blood and making it rigid for maximal intromission. In contrast, ejaculation in several species of rodents is preceded by a series of mounts and intromissions.

EJACULATION. Semen is ejaculated near the os cervix in the case of cattle and sheep, into the uterus in swine, and partially into the uterus in horses. Abortive ejaculations may occur if the female refuses intromission or the penis fails to penetrate the vulva. In the ram, the goat, and the bull, an intense generalized muscular contraction takes place at ejaculation. Often, the force is so strong in the bull that the hind legs of the male leave the ground, giving the appearance of an active leap. During ejaculation itself, the boar is quiet, presenting only slight rhythmic contractions of the scrotum; such periods of immobility are followed by some thrusts at irregular intervals. After ejaculation, the male dismounts, and the penis is soon retracted into the prepuce.

REFRACTORINESS. Most males show no sexual activity immediately following copulation. The duration of the refractory period is highly variably and increases gradually when several copulations are allowed successively with the same female.

FREQUENCY OF COPULATION. The frequency of copulation varies with the species, the breed, the ratio of males and females present, available space, period of sexual rest, climate, and nature of sexual stimuli. The maximal number of ejaculations is higher in bulls and rams than in stallions and boars; some bulls have been observed to copulate over 80 times within 24 hours, or 60 times within 6 hours; an average of 21 copulations before exhaustion was observed.

After a long sexual rest, a ram may copulate up to 50 times on the first day after joining with the ewes, but this frequency is greatly reduced on subsequent days. The goat, the stallion, and the boar reach exhaustion after a lesser number of ejaculations than in the ram and the bull (Table 19-2).

DURATION OF ESTRUS. The duration of estrus is influenced by species, breed, climate, and management. Estrus is limited to about a day in sheep and cattle but to longer periods in the sow and the mare (Table 19-2). In species in which the period of sexual receptivity is short, ovulation takes place after its end, but in species that remain receptive for long periods, ovulation occurs during estrus.

TABLE 19-2. *Patterns of Mating in Farm Mammals*

| | CATTLE | SHEEP | GOAT | SWINE | HORSE |
|---|---|---|---|---|---|
| Time of ovulation | 4–15 h after onset of estrus | 30 h after onset of estrus | 30–36 h after on set of estrus | 40 h after onset of estrus | 24–48 h before end of estrus |
| MALE ANATOMY | | | | | |
| Penis | Fibroelastic | Fibroelastic with filiform process | | Fibroelastic spiral tip | Vascular-muscular |
| Scrotum | | Pendulous | | Close to body | |
| MATING | | | | | |
| Duration | | Brief (a second or less) | | 5 min | 40 s |
| Site of semen ejaculation | | Near os cervix | | Cervix and uterus | Uterus |
| Number of ejaculations to exhaustion (average) | 20 | 10 | 7 | 3 | 3 |

From: Alexander G, Signoret JP, Hafez ESE. Sexual maternal and neonatal behavior. In: Hafez ESE, ed. Reproduction in Farm Animals, 4th ed. Philadelphia: Lea & Febiger, 1980.

## MECHANISMS OF SEXUAL BEHAVIOR

The physiologic signal that originates sexual motivation is the gonadal steroid balance. Transmitted by the blood flow, the hormones activate the central nervous system. The humoral signal is transformed into sexual motivation, or sex drive. The motor patterns of copulatory activity are programmed according to pre-existing species-specific neuronal circuits.

The behavioral interactions leading to copulation can be divided into four major phases: mutual searching for the sexual partner; identification of the physiologic state of the partner; the sequence of behavioral interactions resulting in the adoption of the mating posture by the female; and the mounting reaction of the male leading to copulation.

The "mating stance" of the sow—clear, long lasting, and easy to release by an experimenter—is especially suitable for a study of releasing mechanism. During the "standing reaction," the receptive sow is absolutely immobile, arches her back, and cocks the ears, and this reaction may be exhibited when an estrous female is touched on the back (Fig. 19-5). Only 48% of estrous gilts, however, will "stand" in the absence of the male. Of those gilts in estrus that do not "stand" in the absence of a male, 60% will show the immobility if presented with the odor of a boar. Broadcasting tape-recorded "courting grunts" is similarly effective in 50% of previously negative females. Thus, the stimuli emitted during precopulatory interactions facilitate the release of the female's postural response.

Females in the mating stance are mounted immediately, and this reaction seems to be released mainly by visual and tactile clues. A restrained female, although not in estrus, is immediately mounted even by a sexually experienced bull or ram. Similarly, a ram does not copulate selectively with an estrous ewe when presented with two restrained anestrous females. Sexual reactions of the male toward stimuli other than those emanating from the female are common. For example, the bull or the boar reacts rapidly to a restrained male or to a dummy.

The sexual releaser for mounting may be the overall shape of the female and her immobility. The other visual, olfactory, or acoustic information from the estrous female may be of minor but complementary importance (Fig. 19-6).

### *Cortex and Sensory Capacities*

Deprivation of sensory capacity can inhibit sexual behavior, reduce the ability to detect the partner, and/or impair orientation. Inexperienced males are impaired to a greater degree than experienced ones. If one sense is inhibited, another sense that is ordinarily used to a lesser degree may be augmented. Thus, elimination of the stimuli to visual receptors in males results in the use of tactile and olfactory receptors. Copulation in domestic mammals is not suppressed with the elimination of vision, smell, or hearing, provided contact with the partner has been established. Tactile stimuli are involved in the organization of postural responses of copulation (e.g., immobilization of the estrous sow and lordosis in the estrous rat in response to flank palpation). Sensory input

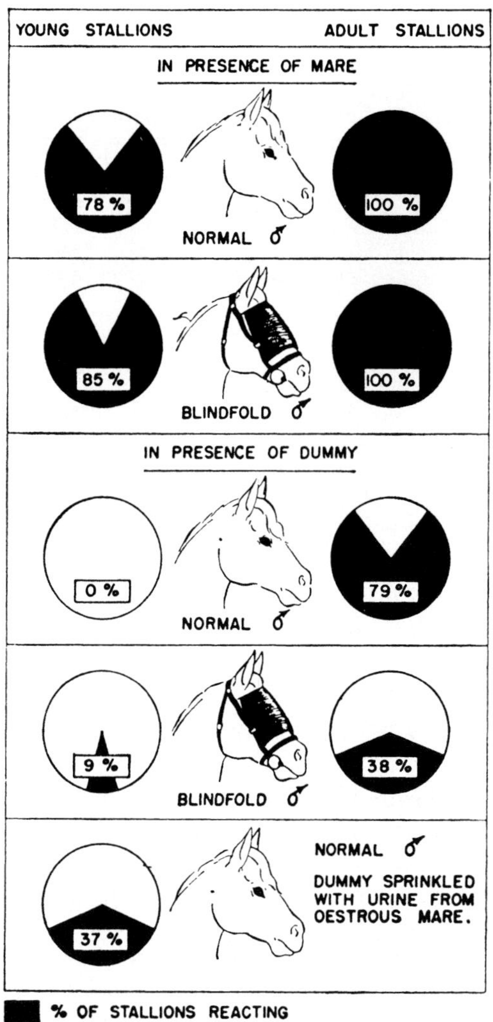


FIGURE 19-6. Effect of sexual experience on copulatory responses of stallions under normal and experimental conditions. Young stallions did not react sexually to the dummy. The percentage of adult stallions that showed sexual responses to the dummy was lower in blindfolded stallions. In young stallions, sexual response was increased toward the dummy when it was sprinkled with urine from an estrous mare. (Adapted from data by S. Wierzbowski.)

from the penis is important for the normal development of mounting and thrusting behaviors in bulls and goats.

### *Neural Mechanisms of Erection and Ejaculation*

Erection is predominantly under the influence of the parasympathetic system. The parasympathetic nerves in the bull, which supply the external genitalia, arise from the sacral segments of the spinal cord.

The copulatory patterns of the male are primarily governed by the neuromuscular anatomy and blood supply of the penis. The bull, ram, and boar have a fibroelastic penis that is relatively small in diameter and rigid when nonerect. Although the penis becomes more rigid on rapid erection, it enlarges little, and the amount of contractile tissue is limited. Protrusion is effected mainly by straightening the S-shaped flexure and relaxation of the retractor muscle.

On the other hand, the stallion has a typical vascular penis with no sigmoid flexure. The function of the penis as an organ of intromission depends on the power of erection as a result of sexual excitement. The size, shape, and length of the penis vary greatly between the flaccid and the erect state (Fig. 19-7).

Intromission and ejaculation are elicited by tactile stimuli (warmth of vagina and slipperiness of mucus) acting on the penile receptors. The penis of the bull and the ram is sensitive to temperature, whereas that of the stallion is more sensitive to pressure exerted by the contractions of the vaginal walls. In the boar, the corkscrew-shaped tip of the penis is engaged in the cervix during mating. The pressure exerted by this is sufficient to elicit ejaculation even without any thermal stimulation.

## FACTORS AFFECTING SEXUAL BEHAVIOR

The patterns and intensity of sexual behavior are affected by genetic, physiologic, and environmental factors as well as previous experience.

### *Genetic Factors*

Breed and strain differences in sexual performance are frequently observed. Males of dairy breeds are more active than beef males, whereas Brahman bulls are sluggish. Yorkshire boars are easier to train for semen collections than Durocs. More differences in the pattern of sexual behavior occur among pairs of identical twin bulls than between members of the pair (Fig. 19-8). Breed differences in the duration of estrus in sheep and pigs may be partly due to differences in ovulation rates. Individual differences in the amount of sexual stimulation required to elicit "immobilization reaction" in the sow are independent of sexual experience.

### *Environmental Factors*

The effect of external stimulation on sexual behavior is more pronounced in the male than in the female.

EFFECT OF NOVELTY OF STIMULUS FEMALES (COOLIDGE EFFECT). Sexual activity of the male increases when new females in the herd become receptive. If four receptive ewes are available, the ram mates three times as much as he does when only one ewe is in estrus. The enhancing effect of a new stimulus animal should be kept in mind under modern husbandry conditions. For instance, changing the teaser

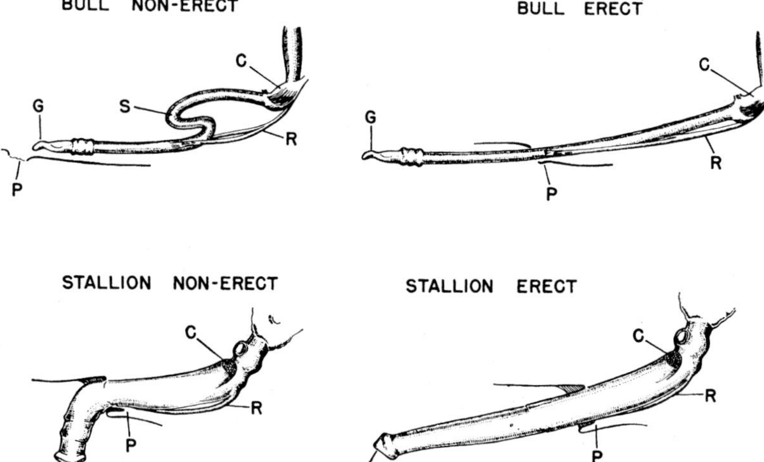


FIGURE 19-7. Diagram of the anatomy of fibroelastic type penis (bull) and a vascular-muscular type penis (stallion) in the nonerect and erect positions. The anatomy of the penis determines, to a great extent, the ejaculatory responses of the species. C, cavernous muscle; G, glans; P, prepuce; R, retractor penile muscle; S, sigmoid flexure.

cow is an effective way to increase sexual behavior of a sluggish male.

NONSPECIFIC STIMULI. Nonspecific external stimuli may lead to sexual activity during the refractory period that follows ejaculation in males of low libido. In the rat, both painful stimuli, such as an electric shock, and gentle handling increase the frequency of ejaculations and reduce the postejaculatory interval. Changing the place of semen collection by moving the teaser animal, or "encouraging" the bull, are all effective in sluggish bulls.

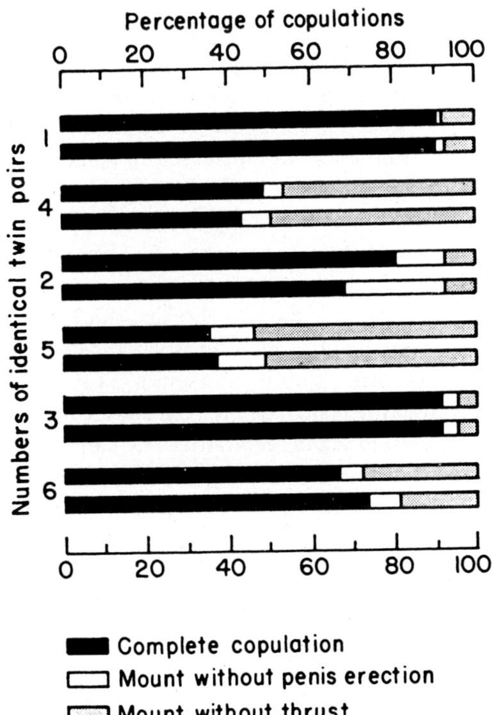


FIGURE 19-8. Ejaculatory behavior in identical twin dairy bulls showing percentage distribution of complete copulations, mounts without penis erection, and mounts without thrust. Note the great similarities in the ejaculatory pattern of the twin brothers and the great variability between the twin pairs. (Adapted from Bane A. Acta Agric Scand 1954;4:95.)

PRESENCE OF OTHER ANIMALS. The presence of other males while teasing a female or copulating improves sexual libido of the male. Social hierarchy, however, may interfere with sexual activity when several males compete for one receptive female. The dominant male performs most of the copulations and restricts the sexual performance of his subordinates. When females are in excess, however, dominant males cannot effectively control the activity of their inferiors. Adult rams usually dominate or "boss" yearling rams, and the degree of their dominance is greater than the dominance of yearling rams over other yearlings. Unfortunately social dominance is not correlated with fertility of males. Thus a "bossy" male who is infertile or diseased may depress the conception rate of the entire breed. The size of the pasture also affects the competition among males and the number of copulations per female.

The sexual performance of males of some species can be improved by providing the animals an opportunity to view other males engaged in sexual activity. Although rams are not stimulated by observing sexual activity, they are aroused when provided the opportunity to smell another male who has just copulated (3).

SEASON AND CLIMATE. Seasonal variations in sexual behavior of sheep, goats, and horses are mostly due to seasonality of hypothalamic/pituitary function controlling the secretion of gonadal hormones. Seasonal changes are also reported in the responsiveness of ovariectomized ewes, does, and sows to exogenous hormones, showing a direct effect of seasons on the response of the CNS. For example, in the ovariectomized female goat (doe) an injection of 30 $\mu$g of estradiol will stimulate the full expression of estrous behavior during the fall, the breeding season. During the spring, however, this dose of estrogen is not effective (4). This finding can be replicated in environmentally controlled rooms, providing evidence for the importance of photoperiod on the expression of sexual behaviors.

The intensity of sexual behavior is reduced in hot climates. The plane of nutrition per se does not seem to affect sexual behavior. However, any physical trouble may seriously affect sexual expression (e.g., inflammation of the hooves or joints, change in teeth, eczema, pains from accidents, or certain diseases).

### *Effect of Experience*

The efficiency of copulation of males and females is improved by experience. Individual contacts before puberty can have an organizing effect on subsequent sexual performance. Social deprivation during infancy drastically impairs adult sexual behavior in primates. In other mammals, the female's sexual behavior does not appear modified by deprivation of social contacts. However, social deprivation during ontogeny may account for some cases of sexual inhibition of domestic males. In boars and rams, rearing in isolation or in unisexual groups has a detrimental effect on subsequent libido. Young, inexperienced males are usually awkward during their first contact with a receptive female: they approach hesitantly, spend a long time exploring the genitalia, mount with erection, descend, and try to mount again. Erection and ejaculation are weak, and the volume of semen is small. After the first ejaculation, the motor patterns are rapidly organized and normal mating efficiency is reached.

UTERINE MOTILITY AND SPERM TRANSPORT. Sterile matings with a vasectomized male stimulate sperm transport in the rabbit but not in sheep. Stimulation of the genitalia or precoital stimuli cause contraction of the cervix and uterus of the ewe and the cow, as a result of the release of oxytocin. Vaginal distention and precoital stimulation cause maximal oxytocin release in sheep and goats. Oxytocin release often occurs before actual coitus has taken place.

EFFECT OF MALE ON ANESTROUS FEMALES. Many domestic females undergo periods of anestrus. By the end of seasonal anestrus in sheep and goats, the introduction of the male results in an earlier and synchronized appearance of estrous cycles. Even the Merino sheep, which is reputed to breed throughout the year, ovulates and breeds spontaneously for only a restricted period during autumn. The peak of estrus observed 17 to 18 days following the introduction of the male represents in fact the second cycle, and this allows normal fertilization. An androgen-dependent pheromone from the male is responsible for similar synchronization of estrus in mice (5), and possibly sheep. Neither sight nor contact is necessary for the synchronization of the first estrus of the breeding season in sheep.

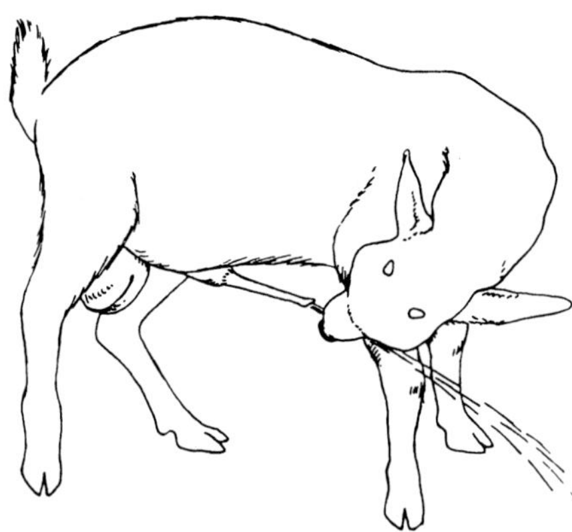

FIGURE 19-9. Self-enurination exhibited by the goat. This behavior, known as urine-marking, scent-urination or self-enurination, is normally accomplished by the animal turning its head and shoulders downward and to the rear and urinating with erect penis onto his face, beard, and front legs. Urine emissions range from a spray to a more concentrated stream and are discharged in spurts or as a steady flow. In most cases the animal actively positions its mouth and nose in the urine flow and laps at the urine with its tongue. By arching its back while in this posture the goat can reach its penis with its tongue and mouth. In this position, the animal often grooms (licks) its penis either with or without any urine discharge. (From: Price EO, Smith VM, Katz LS. Stimulus conditions influencing self-eruniation, genital grooming and flehmen in male goats. Appl Anim Behav Sci 1986;16:371–381.)

Nursing the young delays estrus compared with milking in cows and ewes. The presence of the ram results in an earlier postpartum estrus in nursing ewes, making the postpartum estrus similar in dry and milked females. Male goats exhibit a unique "self-marking" behavior, self-enurination (Fig. 19-9) that likely enhances the odor signal detected by females during the breeding season.

The introduction of the boar shortly before spontaneous puberty in a group of previously isolated gilts results in earlier onset of estrus. This phenomenon is caused by odors emanating from the boar. The pig's characteristic body odor is produced by skin gland secretions. The carpal glands are well differentiated on the front legs. In the male, secretions of the preputial pouch, which give pot its "boar" are involved in sexual behavior.

## ATYPICAL SEXUAL BEHAVIOR

Homosexuality, hypersexuality, hyposexuality, and autoerotic behavior are not uncommon. These syndromes may be due to genetic factors, disturbance in the endocrine or nervous systems, or faulty management. Unadapted sexual reactions are more frequent among domestic animals and under conditions of captivity in the zoo than in the wild. *Homosexuality* refers to sexual behavior among males, particularly at puberty and when young males are housed together. The stimuli eliciting the male's sexual response are essentially visual. A releaser of an appropriate shape and size presented to a highly motivated male may elicit mounting. An immobile anestrous female, another male, or an inanimate object may release sexual reactions. Most homosexual males in sex-segregated groups become heterosexual when placed with females and again homosexual when segregated.

Hypersexuality in males consists of increased sexual excitement, increased frequency of copulation, and attempted copulations with young males and females of the same or different species. Hyposexuality is characterized by abnormalities in the ejaculatory pattern. Certain males may fail to ejaculate in spite of protrusion of erection, whereas others cannot mount or exhibit no sexual desire for varying periods of time.

In Belgian stallions, failure to ejaculate may be manifested in the first breeding season or at the peak of any successive season. In some cases, ejaculation is inhibited when semen is collected by an artificial vagina, but no inhibition occurs with natural mating. Such inhibition is temporary and is mainly due to faulty application of the artificial vagina. Another anomaly is the incomplete intromission and the lack of pelvic oscillations after intromission. This irregularity, which is partly hereditary, may appear in young stallions at the onset of their sexual life and may persist during the following years.

Excessive biting of the mare during copulation may be associated with disturbances in the copulatory mechanisms when the stallion performs the usual pelvic oscillations without ejaculation or with incomplete erection. Excessive biting of the mare may be caused by inhibition.

Autoerotic behavior refers to self-arousal of sexual responses, which is called *masturbation* in males. The motor patterns vary with the species (Fig. 19-9). The stallion rubs his rigid erected penis against the hypogastrium (anterior median of the abdomen) and lowers the loin region rapidly. This is followed by several forward movements of the pelvis, resulting in abortive ejaculation. Masturbation is less common in rams, and most common among bulls on high protein ration (e.g., bulls prepared for shows). As a result of such diets, the peripheral mucosa of the penis become more sensitive to tactile stimulation.

The most common abnormal female behavior is nymphomania in cattle. "Split" estrus and prolonged estrus are common in mares. In split estrus, the manifestation of estrus ceases for a short period followed by recurrence of sexual receptivity during what is evidently one full estrous period. Prolonged estrus may last from 10 to 40 days. The prolonged estrus usually occurs in mares that have failed to conceive or have aborted, and those used for heavy draught.

## MATERNAL AND NEONATAL BEHAVIOR

The behavioral events at birth and shortly afterward (Table 19-3) have an important influence on the survival of the newborn and hence on the successful outcome of reproductive processes. This is especially true when the initial suckling and development of a bond between mother and young occur in the outdoor environment, often under adverse conditions such as inclement weather and the presence of predators, or in artificial conditions of close confinement indoors.

Several experimental approaches have been used to evaluate maternal behavior such as

a) whether each young is suckled,
b) whether each young is groomed (licked) by its mother,

TABLE 19-3. *Maternal and Neonatal Behavior in Domestic Ungulates—Semiquantitative Comparison of Species*

| | SHEEP | GOATS | CATTLE | HORSES | SWINE |
|---|---|---|---|---|---|
| **ABNORMAL MATERNAL BEHAVIOR** | | | | | |
| Desertion of young | + | Probably the same as sheep | + | (P) | + |
| Moves from suckling | + | | + | + | NA |
| Attacks young | + | | + | + | NA |
| Cannibalism | – | | – | – | NA |
| **FREQUENCY OF SUCKLING (TIMES PER DAY APPROXIMATELY)** | | | | | |
| First 4 days | 30 | (?) | 4(?) | (?) | 10 |
| Midlactation | 15 | (?) | 3(?) | (?) | 25 |

NA, not available

c) frequency of suckling or attempting to suckle alien mothers, and
d) other mother-offspring interactions relevant to weaning and development under intensive management conditions (6).

Some standard practices interfere with the formation of maternal bonds between dams and offspring. Early separation of newborn young from the mother, as in dairy cattle practice or in the production of gnotobiotic piglets, induces modifications in the behavior of young animals. In most species of wild bovids, parturient females leave the nursery herd and seclude themselves during parturition and the immediate postnatal period. Most management procedures preclude this possibility and increase the likelihood of interference by other herd members. Lamb stealing is a common and deleterious consequence of housing together large numbers of pregnant ewes. Early weaning and artificial feeding adversely affect the suckling behavior of young lambs and piglets.

### *Suckling*

Milk is let down in response to suckling, massage of the udder, or injection of posterior pituitary hormone. Suckling excites a nervous reflex that augments secretion of hormones from the posterior pituitary. Fright or epinephrine injections inhibit milk letdown.

The young may reach the udder within a few seconds after birth, while the umbilical cord is still attached. They express the suckling response as soon as their noses make contact with other objects. Piglets that are milk-fed and reared in the laboratory must be cared for individually during the first week. If two or more are joined together at birth, they will suckle each other on any available soft part.

### *Parent-Young Interactions*

After birth, the young are able to move about almost immediately and react to a variety of objects as surrogate (substitute) mothers. During this imprinting period, the young normally establish a species-bond to their own species, and as adults direct their sexual behavior toward species members.

Recognition of young is established in sheep and goats soon after parturition, and other young may be adopted at that time. Continuous contact is important and females may reject their own lambs or kids if separated from them for more than a few hours immediately after parturition.

During and immediately following birth, the mothers chew and lick the placenta and its components (a phenomenon called *placentophagy*). The mother may consume parts of it and groom the neonate. Licking or maternal grooming has various functions. The maternal stimulation facilitates the development of successful suckling orientations in the offspring. Suckling by the neonate, in turn, likely has a stimulating influence on the mother in that it reduces tension in the udder and provides the occasion for further licking of the neonate. The response patterns of the mother and offspring rapidly become mutually dependent. At the time of parturition, licking has a hygienic function in addition to stimulating the young to stand and eventually suckle. The mother may "label" her offspring by maternal grooming at this time, thus, providing a mechanism for offspring discrimination. Later, as the young mature, the hygienic significance of grooming is gradually replaced by social functions relating to the establishment and maintenance of a social bond or attachment between mother and young. Removal of the offspring from the maternal animal leads, under some conditions, to the later rejection of the neonate. The mother may reject her own offspring if it is removed at birth and kept away for several hours. A very rapid social attachment is formed between mother and neonate. Kids that have been removed from the dam immediately following parturition and maintained in isolation for a period as brief as one hour are later rejected. Maternal rejection, however, is not an inevitable consequence of early separation of the newborn lamb from its mother. Strong maternal-young attachments form in sheep even when postpartum interaction is delayed for a period of up to 8 hours after birth.

### *Maternal Behavior in Sheep*

PREPARTUM BEHAVIOR. Ewes tend to cease grazing within an hour or so before lambing and wander about as if searching for a lamb. Parturition, at least in Merinos, usually begins while the ewe is with the flock, and the lambing ewe is left behind as the flock grazes on.

ROLE OF FETAL FLUIDS. The birth site appears to be determined fortuitously by where the placental fluids are first spilled. These fluids are attractive to ewes near the time of lambing and the ewe usually remains at the site of spillage, licking and pawing the ground. The fluids appear to play a critical role in attracting the ewe to her newborn lamb. Ewes that have not yet lambed are attracted to the fluids and to newborn lambs of other ewes, leading to "lamb stealing." This adoption sometimes results in lambs being left without maternal care, and the rearing of lambs by ewes that are not their natural mothers.

LAMBING. There is no consistent peak of lambing at any particular time of the day. Behavior during parturition largely depends on the ease of the process, but generally, the initial restlessness is broken by periods of lying with abdominal straining. Most lambs are born with head and forefeet foremost. Lambing usually occurs while the ewe is recumbent, but it can also occur while the ewe is standing; most ewes are on their feet within a minute after birth. The umbilical cord is broken simply by stretching. The fetal placenta, or "afterbirth," is delivered 2 to 5 h later and is frequently eaten by some breeds, but rarely by others.

The duration of birth varies widely within the one flock. Sometimes an extended birth is associated with a single lamb being too large for the vagina, with twins being impacted in the vagina, or with an abnormal presentation resulting in an increase in the effective diameter of the lamb. Birth also tends to be protracted in ewes lambing for the first time or in ewes debilitated by ill-health or undernutrition. Protracted labor can exhaust the ewe and have adverse effects on maternal behavior and the viability of the lamb. Twin births are usually more rapid than single births because twins are usually smaller than singles, but the interval between delivery of twins varies widely from a few minutes to an hour or more.

Postpartum Behavior. Vigorous licking (grooming) and eating of any amniotic and allantoic membranes adhering to the lamb usually commence immediately after birth. During this phase of intense olfactory and gustatory contact, which persists for little more than an hour, the ewe learns to distinguish her own lamb from aliens, which are soon rejected by vigorous butting. Experiments with lambing ewes in which the olfactory bulbs have been destroyed confirms that this attraction is largely olfactory. However, maternal behavior is not abolished by destroying the sense of smell. Other factors, such as warmth and movement, may be important in maintaining the attraction of the mother to the newborn lamb; ewes rapidly lose interest in an immobile, chilled lamb. This "critical period" of attachment of the ewe to the lamb is short; if the lamb is removed at birth, it will be rejected by the ewe if presented to her 6 to 12 h later.

Grooming of the lamb by the ewe may remove some of the 0.5 kg of fluid present in the coat at birth, so reducing heat loss. Grooming may also play an important role in stimulating the lamb to stand and suckle for the first time.

Maternal behavior is under endocrine control; it can be induced in sheep under the influences of a rapidly declining progesterone level and rapidly increasing estrogen level, which occur around birth.

Finding the Teats for the First Time. In goats the teats are found with equal success whether the udder is in the normal position or has been grafted onto the neck. Visual guidance is not essential, as lambs will suckle for the first time in a light-proof room.

Aberrant Behavior. Ewes that are exhausted by a difficult parturition may remain prone for some hours after birth and the lamb may stray. Some ewes lambing for the first time display little interest and abandon their newborn lambs. Other forms of misbehavior in inexperienced ewes include butting the newborn lamb as it moves, and a tendency to move to maintain the initial head-to-head orientation. When these behavioral patterns persist, the lamb's chance of finding the teats and suckling can be reduced, since the teat-seeking activity declines rapidly from about 2 hours after birth in the absence of successful suckling. Some lambs, particularly after poor fetal nutrition, a long birth process, birth injury, or chilling, are slow to stand and suckle.

Aberrant patterns are more common with twin births than with single births, especially among Merinos. For example, if twins are born several meters apart, one lamb may be neglected and become lost or may be repelled as an alien if contact is remade after the critical receptive period of the ewe has passed. Aberrant behavior in the postpartum period is a significant cause of lamb mortality.

Suckling. Ewes with lambs tend to form distinct groups away from the main flock, and for some days after birth, the ewes remain within earshot of their lambs. Accidental separation results in considerable agitation of both ewe and lamb.

Mutual Recognition by Ewes and Lambs. The means whereby ewes and their lambs recognize each other have been the subject of much research. The experiments were largely based on manipulation of the cues to recognition provided by the partner (7). Voices were blocked by local anesthesia, and visual cues were removed by screening, or altered by dusting pigments into the coat or by shearing. Ewes are attracted by a lamb's bleat and the attraction is particularly strong for the lamb's own mother, but it is not essential for a ewe to hear her lamb's voice for her to accept it. The appearance of the lamb is important. If lambs are disguised by blackening or coloring, many ewes actively avoid the approaches of the disguised lamb when initially presented with it, even if the lamb is the ewe's own. Similar experiments with blackening various parts of the lamb show that critical visual cues emanate (Fig. 19-10). The scent of the lamb is also important but only at close quarters. There is nonspecific attraction of ewe's voices initially, but the specificity increases with age. Visual cues become more important than auditory cues by the time the lamb is about three weeks old.

Suckling Behavior. After the newborn lamb has achieved satiety, the frequency of suckling stabilizes at one or twice per hour. During the first week, suckling is usually initiated and terminated by the lamb. Twin lambs may be suckled individually and more frequently than singles.

As the lamb becomes older and mutual recognition improves, ewes and lambs stray farther apart, and the ewe now tends to terminate suckling. With advancing age of the lamb, the frequency and duration of suckling decline. Under natural conditions, these changes culminate in weaning, with maternal solicitude being suddenly replaced by antagonistic behavior.

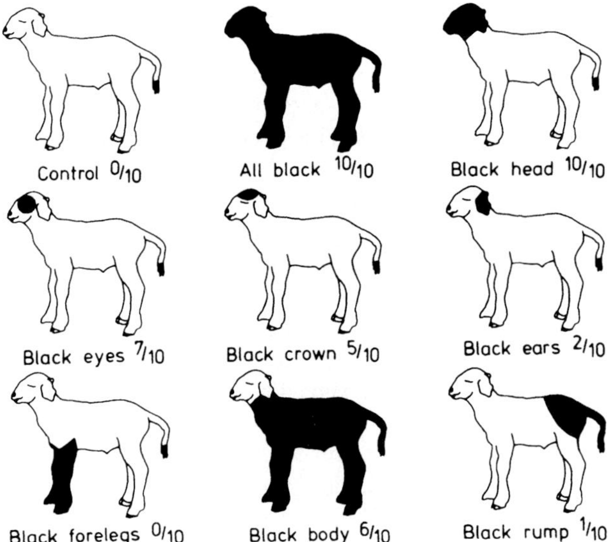


FIGURE 19-10. The effect of blackening various regions of lambs' bodies on the incidence of hesitation or dodging away by their dams when confronted with their partially blackened lamb for the first time. The number of ewes reacting out of the 10 tested with each treatment is indicated. (Adapted from: Alexander G, Shillito R. Appl Anim Ethol 1977;3:137.)

There is no fierce maternal protective behavior in sheep; the mere presence of the ewe appears to act as a deterrent to predators such as foxes and crows. Maternal care consists primarily of supplying milk exclusively for her own lamb.

### *Maternal Behavior in Goats*

Maternal and neonatal behavior of goats is similar to that of sheep. However, goats may be more efficient than sheep in recognizing that they have twins. Also, the doe spends more time vigorously grooming and orienting to the firstborn, so that the secondborn, which is usually the weaker of the two, has the greater opportunity to suckle. Kids' voices are initially similar, when analyzed by a sonagraph, and the does cannot distinguish between kids by auditory means until the sounds begin to diverge at about 4 days of age. Whereas lambs "follow" their mothers from the time they become ambulatory, goat kids are "hiders," lying separated from their mothers for longer periods of time.

### *Maternal Behavior of Cattle*

Both normal and abnormal behavioral patterns of the cow and calf are remarkably similar to those of sheep, although there are differences. A day or two before calving, the cow may become restless and keep to a small isolated area, which she defends against other cows. Confinement and interference at this time can result in prolonged birth and poor calf survival. Cows tend to eat the afterbirth more frequently than sheep. Most new calves take at least 45 min to stand, and may take upward of 4 h to suckle for the first time.

SUCKLING. Newborn calves begin to suckle within 2 to 5 h after birth. Until a teat is located, the calf readily mouths and sucks any protruberance on the mother's body. The mother seems to help the calf find a teat by positioning her body appropriately and by licking, nuzzling, and nudging the calf. Twins are suckled longer than single calves, presumably because of suboptimal milk supply. Twins receive less grooming (licking) from their mothers than single calves.

While the calf suckles, the mother licks its perineal and preputial areas, stimulating it to urinate and or defacate. Cows with calves or those that have recently calved but no longer possess young show little interest in calves that may be present.

Frequently, females may give birth in the close company of pregnant conspecifics and mothers with newborn young. This may increase patterns of aberrant maternal behavior, i.e., abandonment of young, calf stealing, and cross suckling.

Non-nutritional sucking markedly increases in calves fed low-energy, low-protein diets, suggesting that it is related to the diet. Calves suckling their dams drink more than bucket-fed animals, among which the incidence of non-nutritional sucking is high. Non-nutritional sucking has important consequences, particularly if it continues into adult life. Such activity markedly decreases the dry-matter consumption of calves and retards growth. Hair balls commonly occur in the rumina of calves that exhibit non-nutritional licking behavior. These may attain a size of 3788 g and may be fatal if they block the entrance to the rumen and prevent eructation. Like goat kids, calves are hiders, though calves may hide in large group while mothers graze.

### *Maternal Behavior in Horses*

Approaching birth may be indicated by milk ejection and restlessness, but these signs are not confined to the immediate prepartum period. In mares, most births occur at night, but whether this is due to photoperiodic effects or routine husbandry procedures is not clear. Delays in parturition are attributed to human presence and interference, as well as to the presence of spectator groups of mares.

Abnormally long parturition is usually associated with malpresentation of the fetus, though aged mares may not sustain their efforts to foal. Mares tend to remain recumbent longer than sheep, often not standing until more than 10 min after birth. Grooming continues for several hours. Premature young are more common in horses than in ruminants, and the premature foal tends to be weak and slow to progress.

### *Maternal Behavior in Pigs*

Behavior in the pig with its large litters of small, almost naked young contrasts with that in other domestic ungulates. Appropriate behavior patterns are of particular importance in swine because of the susceptibility of the young to starvation, chilling, and accidental injury by the sow.

**PREPARTUM BEHAVIOR.** In the field the approach of parturition is indicated by characteristic nest-building activity, but in practice, sows are so restricted by the lack of nest-building materials and by modern farrowing pens designed to protect the piglets that this activity is inhibited and the sows may become disturbed. As parturition approaches, characteristic vocalizations become evident and the "nest" area is defended as if piglets are present.

Parturition in the sow is most frequent after sunset. Though most domestic sows tolerate the presence of an observer at farrowing, some become highly disturbed. Sows normally farrow lying on one side, and delivery is accomplished with much less apparent effort than in other farm animals.

The rupture of the membranes and the voiding of the fetal fluids is not well-defined as in other ungulates. Most piglets are born partly covered with fetal membranes, and in contrast with the larger young of other ungulates, the piglet must escape from these without maternal aid, or perish. The umbilical cord is broken by the piglet moving away from the vulva. At the end of delivery, the sow usually stands to urinate, and in the process of lying down again and also during earlier bouts of restlessness, the piglets are prone to be overlain and injured.

The average duration of farrowing is about 3 h, but can range from 30 min to 8 h or more. The interval between birth of individual piglets ranges from less than a minute to three or more hours. Piglets in the last half of the litter are prone to be stillborn, perhaps because of premature rupture of the cord and prolonged hypoxia.

**POSTPARTUM BEHAVIOR.** Newborn piglets are almost immediately mobile. They rapidly find their way to the udder and may be suckling within 5 min; most have obtained milk within half an hour of birth. At this early stage, milk is available on demand, possibly because of continuous milk letdown due to circulating oxytocin associated with the birth process. Behavior of litters immediately after birth is variable, and piglets may be attracted to infrared heaters before moving to the udder. Attraction to heaters is probably undesirable at this early stage when a teat-order is being established but may be desirable subsequently in keeping piglets from being overlain by the sow. In the search for the teats, the piglets tend to concentrate on the pectoral region of the udder and explore vertical surfaces with their noses until a teat is contacted, grasped, and suckled. Piglets that do not find a functional teat soon after birth rapidly deplete their energy reserves in cold weather and die from hypothermia.

**SUCKLING.** Having suckled initially, the piglets tend to sample several teats in the same row as the teat first sucked; they locate these teats readily, having rapidly learned the appropriate orientation and teat height.

**TABLE 19-4. *Nursing and Suckling Behavior in Swine***

| SUCKLING PATTERN | VALUES |
|---|---|
| Suckling frequency (periods/d) | 18–28 |
| Interval between sucklings (min) | 51–63 |
| Duration of nursing (min) | 4–8 |
| Duration of suckling (s) | |
| NOSING PHASE | 55–140 |
| Quiet phase | 16–23 |
| True suckling | 13–37 |
| Milk consumption of piglet/suckling period (g) | 24–28 |
| Milk consumption of piglet/day (g) | 600–700 |
| Milk consumption of piglet/lactation period (kg) | 30–37 |

The teat order tends to be unstable with large litters or with a poor milk supply. Identification of teats by piglets does not seem to be based on taste or smell. In small litters, some piglets have the regular use of adjacent teats, though one is usually preferred. There is clear preference for the anterior teats. Although their control is usually gained by the larger, dominant piglets, there appears to be no major advantage in suckling from them.

Suckling bouts are initiated by the sow, either spontaneously or by the piglets squealing or attempting to suckle. There is a distinctive food call, a series of soft grunts to which the litter rapidly becomes conditioned, and which initiates suckling. The bouts can be stimulated by a disturbance in the farrowing house or by suckling by a neighboring sow (Table 19-4). Suckling positions tend to be characteristic of the individual sow; the standing position is more common in feral than domestic pigs.

The food call initiates a period of intense udder massage lasting several minutes by the nose of the piglet; at the same time, a recumbent sow rotates her body to expose the teats. The grunt frequency increases to a peak, and the phase of active movement by the piglets is suddenly replaced by a quieter phase of milk letdown and suckling that lasts for only a minute or two. Piglets do not appear to discriminate between sows. Fostering is not difficult, and litters can be reared together, with piglets suckling more than one sow. Lactating sows may become aggressive if piglets are disturbed or threatened.

**BEHAVIORAL ANOMALIES, THERMOREGULATION AND NEONATAL MORTALITY.** Newborn piglets, with their small body size, sparse pelage, and skin wet with fluids, are prone to chill in air temperatures as high as 20°C with a 5 km/h wind, despite a vigorous thermogenic response (8). Young piglets huddle together or against the sow to minimize heat loss; feral piglets appear to be more cold-resistant than domestic piglets.

Improved thermoregulation in newborn wild pigs is partly due to extra pelage and to a more mature metabolic response to cold. Piglet mortality is attributed to infection, chilling, poor nutrition, and crushing. These ultimate causes of death may be secondary to inadequate development of energy stores prenatally and inactive metabolic pathways postnatally (9). Deaths from direct or indirect effects of chilling are common in unheated farrowing houses, but the resistance to cold increases during the two or three days that piglets would remain in the nest. Piglets exposed to cold spent more time in behavioral thermoregulation than in suckling. Behavioral thermoregulation causes a reduction in the amount of colostrum consumed. This phenomenon would represent a cold-induced decrease in the ingestion of colostral immunoglobulins. Alternatively, cold exposure may also reduce the capability of piglets to localize, internalize, and transport colostral immunoglobulins through the intestinal epithelial cells and into the blood (10).

Sows occasionally kill and eat their young during parturition. If aggressive behavior is detected as farrowing approaches, the piglets can be removed at birth and returned in relative safety after farrowing is complete, but cannibalism can also occur later in lactation.

Starvation accounts for nearly half of the 10% mortality in liveborn domestic piglets. Young piglets will suckle anything that contacts their noses, including the maternal vulva and other piglets. The number of teats available is effectively reduced in some sows, particularly in older animals in which the teats can be hidden beneath the udder. Piglets that are displaced from their established position at the udder after the first day or two do not readily accept a vacant teat and may die.

## REFERENCES


1. Randolph JH, Cromwell GL, Stahly TS, Kratzer DD. Effects of group size and space allowance on performance and behavior of swine. J Anim Sci 1981;53:922–927.
2. Klingel H. Soziale Organization and Verhalten freilebender Steppenzebras. Z Tierpsychol 1967;34:580.
3. Maina D, Katz LS. Exposure to recently mated conspecific may enhance ram sexual performance. Appl Anim Behav Sci 1997;51:69–74.
4. Billings HJ, Katz LS. Progesterone facilitation and inhibition of estradiol-induced sexual behavior in the female goat. Horm Behav 1997;31:47–53.
5. Bronson FH. Energy allocation and reproductive development in wild and domestic house mice. Biol Reprod 1984;31:83–88.
6. Price EO, Thos J, Anderson GB. Maternal responses of confined beef cattle to single versus twin calves. J Anim Sci 1981;53:934–939.
7. Alexander G. Role of auditory and visual cues in mutual recognition between ewes and lambs in Merino sheep. Appl Anim Ethol 1977;3:65.
8. Alexander G. Body temperature control in mammalian young. Br Med Bull 1975;31:62.
9. Kasser TR, Martin RJ, Gahagan JH, Wangsness PJ. Fasting plasma hormones and metabolites in feral and newborn pigs. J Anim Sci 1981;53:420–426.
10. Kelley KW, Blecha F, Regnier JA. Cold exposure and absorption of colostral immunoglobulins by neonatal pigs. J Anim Sci 1982;55:363–368.


## SUGGESTED READING


Denenberg VH, Banks EM. Techniques of measurement and evaluation. In: Hafez ESE, ed. The Behavior of Domestic Animals. London: Bailliere, Tindall & Cassell, 1969.

CHAPTER 20

# Genetics of Reproductive Failure

Y. ROSNINA, M.R. JAINUDEEN, AND E.S.E. HAFEZ

Infertility and anomalous sex differentiation of domestic animals are of great economic importance. These problems are also of interest to veterinarians and scientists because of the avenues explored on basic mechanisms of reproductive processes. Several abnormalities of the reproductive system in farm animals are known to be of genetic origin, but only some specific types of reproductive anomalies are really characterized as genetic anomalies. Some of these include cryptorchidism and testicular hypoplasia which occur in all farm species. In this chapter, a review of some basic genetic concepts precedes depiction of certain genetic factors leading to abnormalities in the structures and functions of the reproductive system (see also Chapters 17 and 18).

## BASIC GENETIC CONCEPTS

### Chromosomes

The total number of chromosomes is constant in all normal individuals within a particular species, and when arranged in pairs the chromosomes are identical for all members of that species. The paired chromosomes in mammalian somatic cells are called *autosomes*. An exception to these autosomes is the *sex chromosomes*, which are paired in mammalian females (XX; *homogametic sex*) and unpaired in males (XY; *heterogametic sex*). The mammalian X chromosome is usually larger than the Y chromosome. In birds, however, it is the female that is the heterogametic sex (ZW) and the male is the homogametic sex (ZZ). Thus, unlike in mammals, the female bird determines the sex of the offspring.

The normal chromosome number for a somatic cell is called the diploid number (2n) and is constant in normal individuals within a species. On the other hand, the gamete has one-half the diploid number and is known as the haploid number (n). When a male and a female gamete unite at fertilization, the diploid number is restored.

Chromosomes, when photographed, cut out, and arranged systematically according to cytogenetic conventions, is called a karyotype (1). Chromosomes can be classified according to the length of the chromosome and the position of the centromere seen at metaphase stage. The centromere is a heterochromatic region (nonstaining) which tends to constrict the chromosome at a specific position (primary constriction). If the centromere is situated half-way between the chromosome arms it is known as metacentric, and when located towards one end of the chromosome it is called submetacentric. However, if the centromere is located at the very end, the chromosome is referred as acrocentric. The morphologic features of the different types of chromosomes are shown in Figure 20-1.

### Genes and Patterns of Inheritance

Genes, located in a fixed position (locus) on a chromosome, are the basic units of inheritance. Each gene governs a specific trait (phenotype) and is recognized by alteration (mutation) of that particular gene which changes the phenotype of an individual who carries the mutant gene. Genes which control the alternative in expression for specific traits are called alleles. Thus, the genotype of an animal is its complete set of genes, and the phenotype is the expression of these genes, whether as physical, biochemical, or physiologic traits.

A trait determined by a gene can be inherited either as an autosomal or sex-linked trait, and also can either be dominant or recessive. Traits that are governed by dominant genes express themselves when these genes are present on both chromosomes of a homologous pair (homozygous condition), or on only one of the chromosome pair (heterozygous condition). On the other hand, a trait may only be expressed when both parents have contributed the mutant genes. Such mutations are known as recessive mutations and traits governed by these genes are called recessive traits.

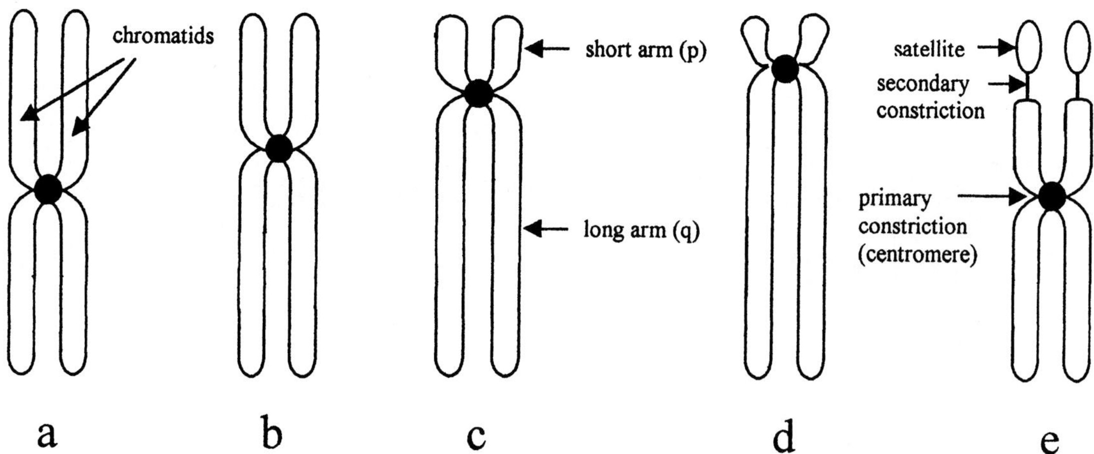


FIGURE 20-1. Types of chromosomes based on centromeric position: **a**, metacentric; **b**, submetacentric; **c**, acrocentric; **d**, telocentric; and **e**, metacentric with satellited arms. Metacentric and submetacentric are also called biarmed chromosomes. Adapted from Basrur PK. Veterinary Medical Genetics. Guelph: University of Guelph Press, 1994.

Autosomal dominant traits affect both males and females. They tend to vary considerably in their severity (expressivity), and rarely skip a generation (nonpenetrance). Autosomal recessive traits affect brothers and sisters (sibs), but parents are phenotypically normal.

Abnormalities of both structure and function of the reproductive system may be genetically determined. As most anomalies are the result of an interaction between environment and genotype, it is difficult to classify them strictly into inherited or acquired disorders. It may take breeding trials, for example, daughter groups of sires under different environmental conditions, to determine whether the defect is inherited or acquired. Most inherited abnormalities follow simple Mendelian inheritance, a few are acquired as sex-linked, and others as polygenic traits.

## ABNORMAL KARYOTYPES

### *Chromosomal Aberrations*

Aberrations of chromosome structure and number are important because of their association with reproductive problems such as birth defects and embryonic or fetal death. Changes in chromosomes may be an alteration in the total number of chromosomes, involving either addition to or loss of one or more chromosomes or set of chromosomes. It also may be structural changes associated with rearrangement of chromosome segments within a chromosome or between two chromosomes (Table 20-1).

NUMERICAL ABERRATIONS. Modification in the chromosome number of an animal from that of the diploid number of that species is a prerequisite for a numerical aberration. This type of abnormality may affect a whole set of chromosomes such that, instead of the normal diploid (2n) number of chromosomes, triploid (3n), tetraploid (4n), or even pentaploid (5n) animals may result. This condition is known as *polyploidy*.

There are various mechanisms leading to these numerical changes. Mechanisms resulting in polyploidy include errors during meiosis (failure in the reduction of chromosome number) or at the time of fertilization (polyandry or polygyny) (Fig. 20-2), and abnormalities of the mitotic spindles at critical stages during fetal development (2). Thus, polyploidy is considered as a cause of embryonic mortality in domestic animals.

Triploidy, however, has been found in spontaneously aborted fetuses of domestic animals. Fertilization of a diploid ovum by a haploid sperm, fusion of the polar body nucleus with the nucleus of the fertilized ovum, or fertilization of a haploid ovum by a diploid sperm are some major etiologies of production of a triploid conceptus. Nevertheless, fertilization of the ovum by two sperms (polyspermy) is believed to be the most common cause of triploidy.

Delayed fertilization resulting in a triploid conceptus is seen in many species of animals. Polyspermy in normal ova is prevented by the presence of a protease-like enzyme present on the zona pellucida of an ovum. The enzyme is denatured or becomes ineffective with aging of the egg, allowing polyspermy to occur. This mechanism was supported by observations in sows bred long after the onset of estrus, whereby a relatively large proportion of embryos were triploids.

Chromosome numbers of inexact multiples of the haploid number are also observed in domestic animals. *Nullisomy* (2n − 2) refers to the absence of both chromosomes of a homologous pair, while *monosomy* (2n − 1) occurs when one chromosome of a pair is absent. *Trisomy* denotes one set of homologous chromosomes present in triplicate,

TABLE 20-1. ***Basic Types of Chromosomal Alterations***

| TYPE OF ALTERATION | DEFINITION | EXAMPLE | ANIMAL |
|---|---|---|---|
| **Numerical** | Alteration in chromosome number | | |
| Aneuploidy | Inexact multiples of haploid number eggs. 2n ± 1; 2n ± 2 | 39,XXY—Klinefelter-like syndrome<br>63,XO—Turner-like syndrome | Cat<br>Mare |
| Euploidy (Polyploidy) | Exact multiples of the haploid number, e.g., 3n, 4n, 5n | 180,XY | |
| Mosaic | An animal with two or more cell populations (different karyotypes) derived from a single zygote which differ in chromosome number and/or structure | 60,XY/59,XYrob(1,29) | Bull |
| Chimera | An animal or its tissues having two or more populations of cells derived from two or more zygotes | 60,XX/60,XY | Freemartin heifer |
| **Structural** | Alteration in structure of the chromosome | | |
| Deficiency | A segment of a chromosome is lost | 38,Xyt(7q−;11q+) | Boar |
| Duplication | A chromosome segment exists in excess of the normal | | |
| Inversion | A segment is in a reverse sequence | | |
| Translocation | A segment or a whole arm of one chromosome is transposed to another chromosome | 59,XY rob (1,29)<br>38,XY rcp (13q−;14q+) | Bull<br>Boar |

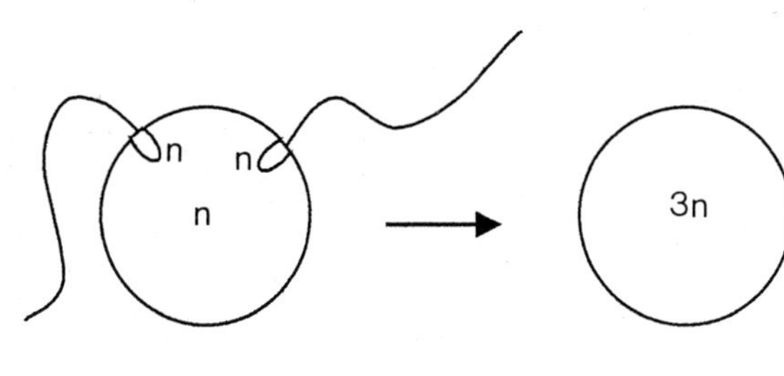


a. polyandry

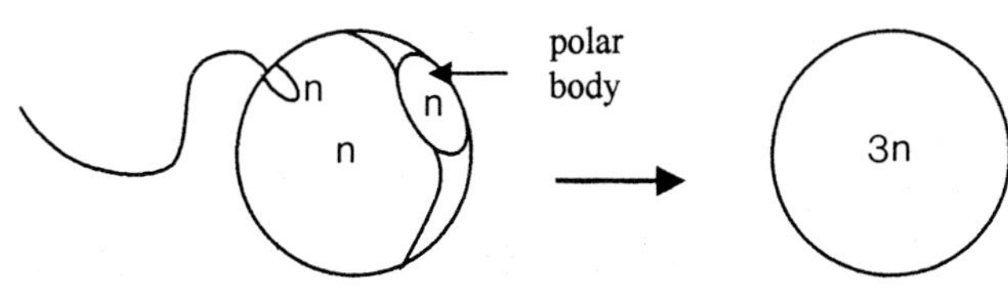


b. polygyny

FIGURE 20-2. Mechanisms resulting in triploidy by (a) polyandry and (b) polygyny. (Adapted from Basrur PK. Veterinary Medical Genetics. Guelph: University of Guelph Press, 1994.)

e.g., trisomy 21, and in *tetrasomy* one set of homologues has four chromosomes. Thus trisomy, monosomy, and nullisomy are some examples of *aneuploidy*.

Aneuploidy results from errors during cell division at gametogenesis (meiosis I or meiosis II), or during mitosis in the fertilized ovum, either during early cell cleavage or embryogenesis. Errors of these kind are associated with unequal segregation (*nondisjunction*) or failure of a chromosome to move to the nearest pole (*anaphase lag*) at mitotic or meiotic anaphase (Fig. 20-3).

In nondisjunction, both chromosomes move to the same pole, resulting in both daughter cells becoming aneuploid, since one of them will have a chromosome in excess of normal (2n + 1) while the other will have one less than normal (2n − 1). In anaphase lag, one of the chromosomes falls behind and thus fails to be included into the nucleus gene of the daughter cells. This results in only one of the daughter cells being aneuploid.

In general, lacking a chromosome in the whole complement set is incompatible with life, while the presence of an extra chromosome disrupts the normal process of embryogenesis. When a large chromosome is associated in aneuploidy, the conceptus dies early in the embryonic stage of fetal development regardless of the type of aneuploidy involved. However, an exception to this rule is the aneuploidy of the X chromosome.

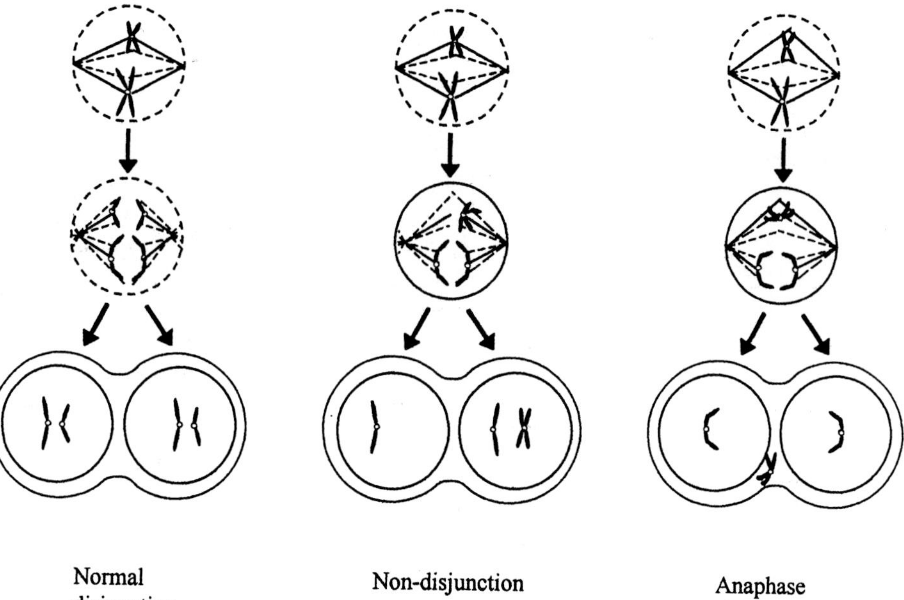


FIGURE 20-3. Diagrammatic illustrations on the mechanisms of nondisjunction and anaphase chromosome lag leading to aneuploidy. (Adapted from Basrur PK. Veterinary Medical Genetics. Guelph: University of Guelph Press, 1994.)

STRUCTURAL CHANGES. A change in the structure of a chromosome is a result of one or more segmental breaks on that chromosome, with or without reunion of the broken segments. These can be divided into four major categories: deletion, duplication, inversion, and translocation. In addition to these, misdivision of the centromere may occur occasionally, leading to the formation of an isochromosome (Fig. 20-4).

A chromosomal *deletion* is a consequence of one or two breaks and the loss of a chromosome segment, and may be either terminal or intercalary. A *terminal deletion* occurs when there is a break and the loss of the terminal segment or two breaks and the reunion of the broken ends to form a ring. On the other hand, *intercalary (or interstitial) deletions* involve the loss of a chromosome segment between two breaks. A chromosome segment devoid of a centromere (acentric fragment) is lost during cell division as it cannot orient itself on the mitotic spindle. Deletions involving large chromosome segments are not seen in animals because cells from which the chromosome segments are deleted are not viable. Nevertheless, if the segment deleted is small or genetically inactive (heterochromatic), the cell with the deletion may be maintained. For instance, a cell containing a deleted chromosome may be viable and capable of reproduction. However, its phenotype (or tissues containing cells with deletions) may be adversely affected. In a majority of cases, deletions can be identified using banding techniques, which enable segmental delineation of the chromosome.

*Duplications* involve addition of an extra segment to a chromosome, through abnormal replication or unequal crossing over in meiotic cells of the parent. A duplicated segment can be terminal or intercalary, and at times shifted to another region. However, duplications are more common and less harmful than deletions. Instead, duplications of genes and segments of chromosomes are considered to be more important in evolution as they are believed to potentially provide material for new gene combinations.

*Inversion* involves two breaks on a chromosome and the rotation of the broken segment prior to reunion of the broken ends, resulting in the reversal of a gene sequence. Inversions can be either pericentric or paracentric. In *pericentric inversion*, the centromere is included in the inverted segment, but for a *paracentric inversion* the centromere is not involved and is confined to one arm of the chromosome only. Paracentric and pericentric inversions interfere with gametogenesis and may be causally related to reduced fertility in all domestic animals.

*Isochromosomes* represent misdivision of the centromere and are always metacentric with identical but reversed gene sequence. For example, the metacentric bovine X chromosome when misdivided would give rise to a long and a short chromosome, each with two identical arms which are actually two chromatids.

*Translocation* occurs when a portion of one chromosome is attached to a nonhomologous chromosome. It often involves a reciprocal exchange of a segment between chromosomes. *Reciprocal translocation* is a result of an exchange between a segment of one chromosome and a segment of another chromosome (Fig.20-5). This translocation is relatively rare in humans and domestic animals. Interchange between segments of different chromosomes involving small segments of autosomes will be overlooked in farm animals such as cattle and goats, since the autosomes are all acrocentric in these species. Thus, the identification of the translocated chromosomes is only possible with the aid of techniques such as banding. An interchange which results in

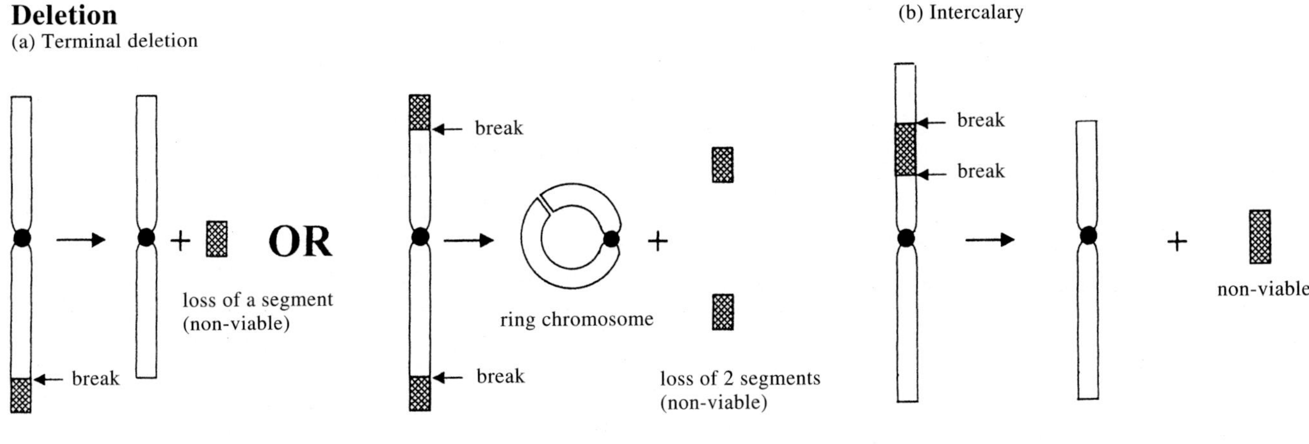


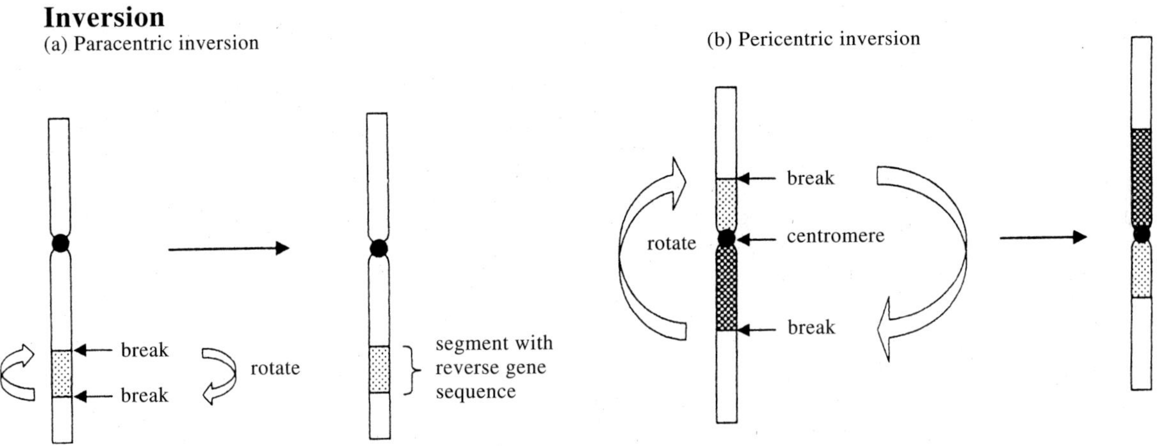


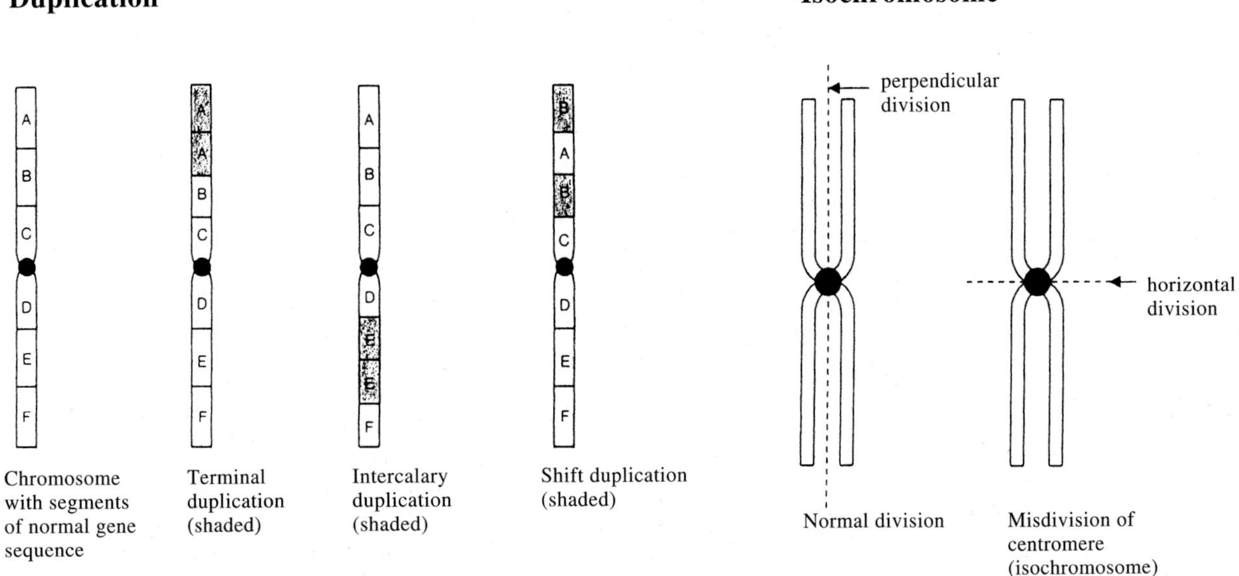


FIGURE 20-4. Diagrammatic illustrations on various structural aberrations: deletion; inversion; duplication; isochromosome. (Adapted from Basrur PK. Veterinary Medical Genetics. Guelph: University of Guelph Press, 1994.)

Reciprocal translocation

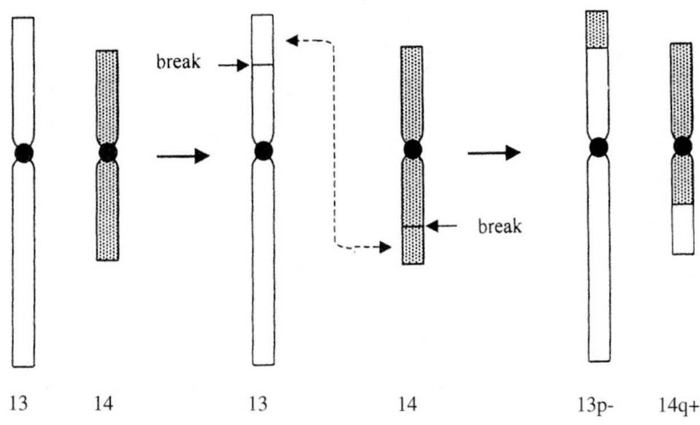


Robertsonian translocation

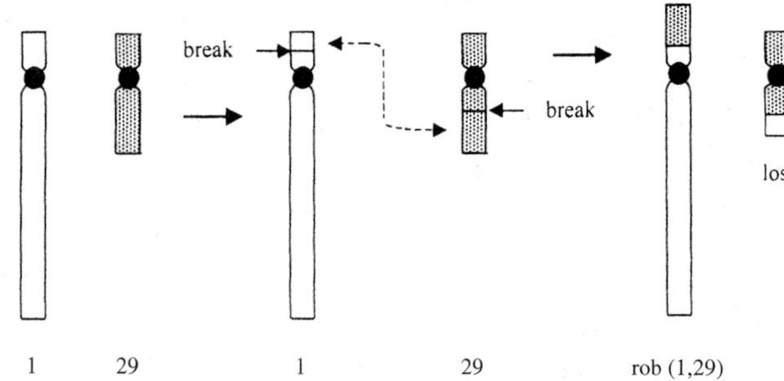


FIGURE 20-5. Diagrammatic illustrations on reciprocal translocation and Robertsonian translocation. (Adapted from Basrur PK. Veterinary Medical Genetics. Guelph: University of Guelph Press, 1994.)

an extremely long or short chromosome which has no morphologic pair in the karyotype will be possible to identify by karyotypic examinations.

Reciprocal translocations have been reported in farm animals including cattle, sheep, and pigs. In cows, this type of rearrangement involved an autosome and one of the X chromosomes, whereas in pigs, three translocations of this manner involving three different sets of autosomes have been described. Boars heterozygous for this translocation exhibit reduced fertility when bred to normal sows. On the other hand, such translocations in the sows have a more adverse effect on fertility.

Several different types of *Robertsonian translocations* associated with reduced fertility have been observed in ruminants and other farm animals. The commonest of these is the submetacentric translocation first reported in the Swedish Red and White cattle by Gustavsson in 1969. This type of translocation involved the largest and the smallest of the bovine chromosome complement whereby the entire arm of one chromosome is transposed to another chromosome (Fig. 20-5).

In this classical rob(1,29) translocation, the smaller segments are generally lost during subsequent divisions because of their minute size and they are not easily accommodated on the mitotic spindle. Although this type of rearrangement involved the loss of the centromere and subsequently a reduction in the total number of chromosomes, most of the genetic materials of the original chromosome complement is preserved in the rearranged chromosome. Therefore, a bull or a cow with such a translocation has 59 instead of 60 chromosomes in all the cells, and generally displays a normal phenotype. The probable reason for the normal physical appearance of these carriers is attributed to the fact that most of the genetic materials of chromosomes 1 and 29, which are essential for normal development, is contained in the translocated chromosomes (1/29T). Since the centromeric region is generally devoid of genetic material, the loss of a centromere would not interfere with the normal growth of the animal. This type of rearrangement, where essentially both chromosomes are retained to assure genic balance in carriers, apparently arise spontaneously and relatively frequently in animal populations. It is also believed to have played an important role in evolution and speciation.

## GENETICS OF INFERTILITY

### *Genetic Infertility in Males*

ABNORMAL SPERMIOGENESIS. A high incidence of abnormal spermatozoa observed are found to be linked with testicular hypoplasia in mammals. Interval occurrence of testicular hypoplasia is a normal phenomenon in seasonal animals. However, an increased frequency of a specific type of abnormal spermatozoa is encountered in nonseasonal species in association with normal testicles, and in these cases the condition is believed to be inherited. An example associated with this type is the "knobbed acrosome" sperm defect found in the bull (Table 20-2). The acrosome of the defective spermatozoon exhibits acentric thickening due to differentiation failure of the proacrosome, and subsequently is unable to adorn over the nucleic surface. Generally, the affected bull is sterile. This condition is caused by a single autosomal recessive gene. However, in boars with a similar defect, affected spermatozoa were able to reach the ova but failed to attach themselves to the ova for fertilization. It is thought that these defective spermatozoa are unable to undergo capacitation and acrosome reaction. The mode of inheritance in these boars suggest a dominant pattern of transmission, since in a pedigree study of a Swedish Yorkshire breed, five full sibs were found to be sterile.

Other forms of abnormalities observed in spermatozoa include decapitated sperm seen in sterile Guernsey bulls, the dag defect found in Danish Jersey bulls of very low fertility, and the "pseudo-droplet" defect (Table 20-2).

TABLE 20-2. ***Some Inherited Sperm Defects Affecting Fertility***

| DEFECT | DESCRIPTION OF DEFECT | FERTILITY |
|---|---|---|
| Knobbed sperm | Acentric thickening of acrosome | Sterility |
| Decapitated | Head and tail separated at the neck region | Sterility |
| Dag defect | Folding of tail over the midpiece, giving an impression of a swollen midpiece | Infertility |
| Pseudodroplet | Rounded or elongated thickening of the midpiece | Sterility |
| Corkscrew | Tail defect | Infertility |
| Diadem effect | Nuclear pouch formation | Infertility |
| Sterilizing tail stump | Tail defect | Sterility |

WOLFFIAN DUCT APLASIA. Several structures arising from the Wolffian duct, such as segments of the epididymis, ductus deferens, and the seminal vesicles, which are not fully developed are occasionally observed in males of some domestic animals. The malformation may be either unilateral or bilateral despite the gonads being well-developed. This condition is hereditary but the mode of inheritance is yet to be established.

Another defect is epididymal stenosis, resulting in spermatocoele. Stenosis of the epididymis generally has a higher incidence in bucks, rams, and bulls. In this defect, the spermatozoa which accumulate in the ductus efferentes lead to the formation of a spermatocoele in the epididymal head of sexually mature males.

IMPOTENCY. A type of impotency has been reported among Friesian bulls in which they are unable to extend the Sigmoid curve of the penis during erection; the defect was identified in the paired retractor penis muscle. Other types of malformations leading to impotency include persistence of the penile frenulum in Aberdeen Angus and Shorthorns, and retroversion of the penis in Chianina bulls. Although these conditions can be corrected surgically, the elimination of the defective gene is difficult since females do not exhibit these traits. Thus, the hereditary nature of these traits should be analysed carefully.

TESTICULAR HYPOPLASIA. Testes of subnormal size which exhibit inadequate growth and development are considered as hypoplastic. Although cryptorchid testes are hypoplastic, testicular hypoplasia also occurs with normal descended testes in some animals (Tables 20-3 and 20-4).

Testicular hypoplasia is commonly found in cattle, goats, and pigs and is inherited as a sex-limited recessive trait. Removing affected bulls from the herd is, however, ineffective in eliminating testicular defects. Nevertheless, to reduce the incidence, bulls with gross testicular defects are not used in natural services, and also breeding parents who had produced offspring with testicular defect are also avoided.

CRYPTORCHIDISM. Cryptorchidism is the failure of the testes to descend into the scrotum or to its normal position. It is the commonest type of defective differentiation of the male genital system and is very common in pigs, goats, and horses, and occasionally occurs in cattle (Table 20-3). Although this condition is sporadic with a high degree of variability in manifestation, only one testis is affected. The position of the undescended testis may be in any part of the descent path, including the inguinal region or diverted to an ectopic position after traversing the inguinal canal. The affected testicles remain smaller than normal since the germ cells fail to undergo normal prepubertal development. Orchidectomy of the maldescended testis is advised since tumors are common among cryptorchid animals.

Cryptorchidism is inherited in pigs and is observed in certain families in high frequency because of selective breeding. Line breeding experiments showed that this condition is controlled by two pairs of recessive autosomal genes in goats. In sheep, however, the incidence of cryptorchidism is low, and in the Australian Merinos is associated with hornlessness. Cryptorchidism occurs in almost all cattle breeds but at low frequency. Bilateral cryptorchidism has been reported in Shorthorns and in some Hereford bulls. It is believed that the variable manifestations, wide distribution, and the low incidence of occurrence may suggest that two or more pairs of recessive genes are involved in many cryptorchid farm animals.

## *Genetic Infertility in Females*

OVARIAN HYPOPLASIA. Hypoplasia of the ovary, the counterpart of testicular hypoplasia, occurs in certain breeds of cattle. Commonly, the left ovary is affected and only about 9% are bilaterally hypoplastic, resulting in juvenile ovary. The common manifestations of cows with hypoplastic ovaries are failure of estrous cycles and poorly developed secondary sex characteristics. In partial ovarian hypoplasia, cows exhibit varying degrees of functional impairment and infertility (Tables 20-3 and 20-4). Like testicular hypoplasia, this defect is inherited as a sex-limited recessive trait and

TABLE 20-3. *Some Inherited Abnormalities of Male and Female Reproductive Systems*

| ABNORMALITY | ANIMAL AFFECTED | MODE OF INHERITANCE | REPRODUCTIVE PROBLEM |
|---|---|---|---|
| Sperm defects | Bull | Inherited | Infertility |
| | Boar | Inherited (?) | Infertility |
| Testicular hypoplasia | Bull | Recessive autosomal gene with incomplete penetrance | Sterility/Infertility |
| Ovarian hypoplasia | Cow | | |
| Cryptorchidism | Boar<br>Stallion | Sex-limited trait | Disturbance in spermatogenesis |
| Cystic ovaries | Cow | Polygenic trait | Anestrus/nymphomania |
| Defects of Müllerian Duct system (white heifer disease) | Cow | Single recessive sex-limited gene for white coat | Sterility |

is generally associated with white coat color phase, although other coat color phases may show this trait occasionally.

CYSTIC OVARIES. Cystic ovarian disease is a common cause of infertility in dairy cows. In this disease, one or more follicles become enlarged but fail to ovulate, and the enlarged follicle persist with accompanying granulosa and theca cell degeneration. Animals with ovarian cysts exhibit irregular or continuous estrus, and eventually become virilized. This condition is associated with an increase in FSH production and a reduction in the LH concentration. A lack of ovarian receptors to LH, which normally facilitates the release of mature ova, may also be associated with ovarian cysts. However, in early stages the condition may be remedied with LH injection, combined with progesterone. This condition is inherited as a polygenic trait in cattle (Table 20-3).

DEFECTIVE DEVELOPMENT OF THE MÜLLERIAN DUCTS. An example of abnormal development to Müllerian ducts is the segmental aplasia of the duct system which occurs in all farm animals. In less severe cases, only the hymen is affected whereby it becomes thick so as to occlude the vagina or area located anterior to the external urinary meatus. The anterior vagina and the uterus are distended with secretions if the hymen is totally imperforated, causing continuous distress to the affected cow. However, in more severe forms, mucometra could be mistaken for pregnancy and in some cases, one or both uterine horns may exhibit embryonic features of the Müllerian duct. Although no satisfactory

TABLE 20-4. *Reproductive Failure Associated with Chromosomal Aberrations*

| REPRODUCTIVE FAILURE | SPECIES | CHROMOSOME ABERRATION | KARYOTYPE |
|---|---|---|---|
| Testicular hypoplasia | Cattle | Disomy-X | 61,XXY |
| | | Chimera | 60,XX/60,XY |
| | Sheep | Disomy-X | 55,XXY |
| | Pig | Disomy-X | 39,XXY |
| Ovarian hypoplasia | Horse | Monosomy-X | 63,XO |
| | | Trisomy-X | 65,XXX |
| | | Mosaic | 63,XO/64,XX |
| | Cattle | Trisomy -X | 61,XXX |
| Repeat breeding | Cattle | Mosaic | 60,XX/60,XY |
| | | Mosaic | 59,XO/60,XX |
| | | Mixoploid | 59,XO/60,XX/61,XXX |
| Infertility | Cattle | Robertsonian translocation | 59,XY rob(1,29) |
| Embryonic mortality | Pig | Reciprocal translocation | 38,XY,t(7q−;11q+) |
| | | | 38,XY,t(13q−;4q+) |

genetic explanation has been found, an association between the gene for reduced or absent coat colour pigment and segmental aplasia is apparent (Table 20-3). A pleiotropic effect of the codominant gene for white colour phase has been often used as an explanation.

### Sex Anomalies in Domestic Animals

HERMAPHRODITISM. A hermaphrodite or an intersex refers to an animal of equivocal sex, since the physical characteristics including the external genitalia are inconclusive. In farm animals, hermaphroditism is most common in cattle, pigs, and goats.

Hermaphroditism can be categorized into three groups:

a) true hermaphrodite
b) male pseudohermaphrodite
c) female pseudohermaphrodite, based only on the presence of gonads but not the sex chromosome constitution or external genitalia.

The degree of intersexual modifications depends on when the sexual differentiation process was retarded or interrupted.

TRUE HERMAPHRODITES. A true hermaphrodite has the gonads of both sexes, either separately (ovary on one side and testes on the other side) or as ovotestes, and an animal is only diagnosed as a true hermaphrodite when both male and female gonadal tissues are present and functional in that animal. This condition is rather frequently seen in pigs (Table 20-5). The hermaphroditic pigs may resemble a sow, but in many cases either the clitoris is enlarged or the penis is short. They may even carry functional ovaries and nonfunctional testes, either a bilateral ovotestes, or testis and ovary on each side. The testicular tissue is devoid of germ cells but the interstitial cells are active in hermaphrodite pigs. The ovary or the ovarian part of the ovotestes in a hermaphrodite pig may have normal follicles and may even produce offspring. The sex chromosomes of true hermaphrodites are variable. The majority apparently have normal female karyotype, while others exhibit the coexistence of male and female cells. Many of the XX/XY hermaphrodites are probably chimeras which arise from double fertilization, or vascular anastomosis following fusion of fetal membranes of male and female embryos.

MALE PSEUDOHERMAPHRODITES. The prefix "male" in male pseudohermaphrodite refers to an individual with testes as the gonads; however, the sex chromosomes may be either XY, or XX with a translocated portion of the Y. The genital ducts and external genitalia generally exhibit varying degrees of female sex characteristic, ranging from hypospa-

TABLE 20-5. ***Reproductive Abnormalities in Intersexes***

| SYNDROME | SPECIES[a] | GONADS | EXTERNAL GENITALIA | SEXUAL BEHAVIOUR |
|---|---|---|---|---|
| TRUE HERMAPHRODITE | Goat | Ovotestes | Female | Female |
| | Pig | Ovotestes | Female | Female |
| | | Ovotestes | Female | Female |
| | | Ovotestes | Female | Female |
| | Horse | Ovotestes | Underdeveloped penis | Lack of male behaviour |
| | | | Penis | Male |
| | Cattle | Ovary and ovotestes | Penis | |
| PSEUDOHERMAPHRODITE | | | | |
| Male | Goat | Hypoplastic testes | Female | Male |
| | Pig | Testes | Female | Male |
| | Horse | Retained testes | Enlarged clitoris and rudimentary penis | Male |
| | Cattle | Cryptorchid testes | Enlarged clitoris | Male |
| | Cattle[b] | Abdominal testes | Female | Anestrus |
| | Sheep (rare)[b] | Testes | Female | Anestrus |
| Female | | Ovary | Male | ? |
| Freemartin | Cattle | Ovotestes | Enlarged clitoris | Anestrus |

Data from: Bishop, M.W.H. (1972). Genetically determined abnormalities of the reproductive system. J Reprod Fertil Suppl. *15*, 51; Dunn, H.H., Smiley, D., Duncan, J.R. and McEntee, K. (1981). Two equine true hermaphrodites with 64,XX/64,XY and 63,XO/64,XY chimerism. Cornell Vet *70*, 137; Hare, W.C.D. and Singh, E.L. (1979). Cytogenetics in animal reproduction. Animal Breeding Abstracts. Commonwealth Agriculture Bureaux, Farnham Royal, Slough, UK; Marcum, J.B. (1974). The freemartin syndrome. Animal Breeding Abstracts *42*, 227.

[a]Species are arranged in descending order of incidence for each syndrome.

[b]Testicular ferminization syndrome.

dias in mild cases to total feminization. The causal agents leading to varying degree of male pseudohermaphroditism are many such as chimerism, sex chromosomes aneuploidy, translocation of the Y chromosome either to an autosome or the X chromosome, and also gene mutations. In mutation of the gene, testosterone secretion of the gonad of the male fetus is blocked due to a defective enzyme in the steroidogenetic pathway or failure of Leydig cells to respond to endogenous gonadotropins (Table 20-5).

**FEMALE PSEUDOHERMAPHRODITES.** This condition is less common in farm animals than male pseudohermaphroditism. In female pseudohermaphrodites, the sex complement is XX, the gonadal ducts are of female type but the urogenital sinus and external genitalia are virilized. This aberration develops through a gene mutation and is transmitted by an autosomal recessive gene. In cattle, female pseudohermaphroditism arising from virilization of the adrenal glands resulted in hypertrophy of the glands. In some instances, the affected cow, known as a "buller," in the advanced stage exhibits nymphomania. Some of the genetic etiological factors leading to female pseudohermaphrodites is sex chromosome monosomy (e.g., XO or Turner-like syndrome in horses), and gene mutation which interferes with hormonal influence on development of the reproductive tract (Table 20-5).

**TESTICULAR FEMINIZATION.** This condition is caused by an X-linked recessive gene, resulting in the failure of the target organs to respond to testosterone. The affected animal is a genetic male but has female external phenotypes and abnormal testes. This "female" shows no signs of estrus and although the undescended testes secrete androgens, the accessory sex glands and skin of the genital region are nonresponsive to the androgens because these target tissues are unable to convert testosterone to dihydroxytestosterone. Since this condition is sex-linked, it is inherited through the dam, and thus it is advisable to cull the animal accordingly.

### *Freemartinism*

**BOVINE FREEMARTINISM.** Freemartinism is a form of intersexuality known to exist since the first century BC. The first anatomical description was documented in the late eighteenth century. It occurs mostly in cattle bearing heterosexual twins, but may occur in pigs, goats, sheep, and horses. The events leading to a freemartin are development of anastomosis between days 30 and 50 of gestation, which coincides with the sensitive phase of reproductive organogenesis. Anastomosis provides a physical basis for the exchange of blood cell precursors and hormones between fetuses. The earlier the anastomosis occurs, the greater the degree of masculinization of the female cotwin.

The characteristic features of a bovine freemartin are those affecting the genital system. The external genital is that of a normal female with variable masculinization of the internal reproductive organs. Sometimes, there is clitoromegaly and the gonads are rudimentary and are located intra-abdominally. These gonads are referred to as ovotestes (Table 20-5). The affected animal does not show estrus, and on palpation through the rectum the reproductive tract is underdeveloped. Vaginal probing with a speculum reveals a short (about one-third the normal length), blind-ended vagina (*cul-de-sac* vagina). A definitive diagnosis by karyotyping the suspected individual reveals chimerism (XX/XY) with varying percentages of male cell populations found in freemartins. The male cotwin is also affected but without structural abnormalities. However, fertility decreases with age.

Two theories have been advanced to explain freemartinism: the hormonal theory and the cellular theory. According to the hormonal theory, hormones from the male twin that reach the female through vascular anastomoses between the fused placentas cause masculinization of the female gonad. However, attempts to experimentally induce the freemartin syndrome have failed.

The cellular theory for the induction of freemartinism is based on the exchange of blood forming cells and germ cells between the fetuses. As a result of this reciprocal exchange between dizygotic twins, identical erythrocyte antigen types occur in both twins, and sex chromosome chimerism (60,XX/XY) appears in peripheral blood mononuclear leukocytes. The incidence of twinning in cattle is low. Approximately 92% of heterosexual twin females are freemartins. In the other cases, chorioallantoic vascular anastomose either fail to develop or occur after the critical stage in organogenesis.

Occasionally, a single-born animal is a chimera. It is possible that one of the twins degenerates during early gestation and the surviving twin exhibits chimerism. The freemartin syndrome generally refers to cattle, but has also been described in other farm animals such as goats, sheep, and pigs.

## MAMMALIAN HYBRIDS

Hybrids are the offspring resulting from the breeding of two closely related species, e.g. horse and donkey, cattle and bison, or sheep and goat, in the hope of obtaining the desirable traits of both species. Some interspecific hybrids are fertile, others are subfertile, and many are sterile. The hybrids of interest are those resulting from the crossing of domestic cattle (*Bos taurus*) with Zebu cattle (*Bos indicus*), cattle with bison (*Bison bison*), cattle with yak (*Bos grunniens*), and the river-type buffalo (*Bubalus bubalis*) with the swamp-type buffalo (*B. bubalis*).

One distinctive feature shared by hybrids of the bovids is that the female hybrids exhibit normal fertility and the male hybrids show sterility. Both *B. taurus* and *B. indicus* have diploid chromosome numbers of 60, consisting of 58 acrocentric autosomes and the sex chromosomes. However, there is one apparent morphologic difference between the Y chromosomes of the two species: the Y chromosome is a small acrocentric in *B. indicus* and a small submetacentric in *B. taurus*. Two forms of Y chromosomes are found in the hybrid, depending on the breed of sire used to establish the foundation stock. The hybrid "line" based on Brahman bulls has an acrocentric Y chromosome, while that based on European bulls has a submetacentric Y chromosome. The F1 hybrid female is fertile, whereas the male is sterile.

The diploid number of the swamp-type and river-type of water buffaloes are 48 and 50, respectively. The reduction in the diploid number in the swamp-type by 2 is due to a tandem fusion of chromosome 9 to chromosome 4. The F1 swamp X hybrid possesses the intermediate karyotype of 2n = 49 with one of the fused chromosome (4/9). Chromosomal anomalies appear to occur at different developmental stages (Table 20-6). However, unlike other interspecific hybrids possessing chromosome complements different from the parent species, both F1 males and females are fertile.

Hybrids belonging to *Equidae*, such as the mule, the hinny (cross between the horse and the donkey), and the zebronkey (offspring of grevy zebra and donkey), have been studied in detail. Most of these interspecific hybrids are sterile. The hybrid mule (*Equus mulus mulus*, 2n = 63), produced by mating a male donkey (2n = 62) to a female horse (2n = 64), is usually sterile in both sexes.

A hybrid pregnancy that usually does not develop to term is that between domestic sheep (*Ovis aries*, 2n = 54) and domestic goat (*Capra hircus*, 2n = 60). Attempts to fertilize sheep oocytes with goat spermatozoa are rarely successful, and if conception is achieved, the zygote never continues after the first few cleavage divisions. On the other hand, does impregnated by rams either naturally or by artificial insemination readily conceive, but gestation does not extend beyond the second month. The possible underlying cause of pregnancy failure between these two species is immunological rejection.

**TABLE 20-6. *Chromosomal Abnormalities at Different Developmental Stages***

| STAGE | CYTOGENETIC ANOMALIES |
|---|---|
| Maternal gametogenesis | Somatic division of oogonia before onset of meiosis or during first or second meiotic division |
| Paternal gametogenesis | Mitotic divisions while male is *in utero*, or during postpuberty first or second meiotic division after puberty |
| Fertilization | Normal chromosomes with errors during fertilization; fertilization of a normal egg by two normal sperm |
| Zygote | Improper division of one or more chromosomes, anaphase lag, or nondisjunction; failure of cleavage of blastomeres or mosaic embryo |

## REFERENCES


1. McFeely RA. Domestic animal cytogenetics: Introduction. In: Cornelius CE, Marshak RR, Melby EC, eds. Advances in Veterinary Science and Comparative Medicine. New York: Academic Press, 1990;34:1.
2. Basrur PK. Veterinary Medical Genetics. Ontario, Canada: University of Guelph Press, 1994.


## SUGGESTED READING


Basrur PK, Yadav BR. Genetic diseases of sheep and goats. Vet Clin NA Food Anim Prac 1990;6:779.

Basrur PK. Congenital abnormalities of the goat. Vet Clin NA Food Anim Prac 1993;9:183.

Basrur PK, Pinheiro LEL, Berepubo NA, Reyes ER, Pospecu PC. X chromosome inactivation in X autosome translocation carrier cows. Genome 1992;35:667.

Gustavsson I, Jönsson L. Stillborns partially monosomic and partially triosomic, in the offspring of a boar carrying a translocation: rcp (14;15)(q29;q24). Hereditas 1992;117:31.

Khan MZ, Foley GL. Retrospective studies on the measurements, karyotyping and pathology of reproductive organs of ovine freemartins. J Comp Pathol 1994;110:25.

King WA, Gustavsson I, Popescu CP, Linares T. Gametic products transmitted by rcp(13q−;14q+) translocation heterozygous pigs, and resulting embryonic loss. Hereditas 1981;95:239.

King WA. Chromosome abnormalities and pregnancy failure in domestic animals. Adv Vet Sci Comp Med 1990;34:229.

Long SE. Chromosomes of sheep and goats. In: Cornelius CE, Marshak RR, Melby EC, eds. Advances in Veterinary Science and Comparative Medicine. New York: Academic Press, 1990;34:109.

McEntee K. Reproductive pathology of domestic animals. New York: Academic Press, 1990.

Pinheiro LEL, Guimaraes SEF, Almeida IL Jr, Mikich AB. The natural occurrence of sheep × goat hybrids. Theriogenology 1989;32:987.

Pinheiro LEL, Mikich AB, Bechara GH, Almeida IL, Basrur PK. Isochromosome Y in a fertile heifer. Genome 1990;33:690.

Singh B, Fisher KRS, Yadav BR, Basrur PK. Characterization of a translocation and its impact on fertility in the pig. Genome 1994;37:280.

Weber AF, Buoen LC, Terhaar BL, Ruth GR, Momont HW. Low fertility related to 1/29 centric fusion anomaly in cattle. JAVMA 1989;195:643.

CHAPTER 21

# Genetic Engineering of Farm Mammals

C.A. PINKERT

Our ability to manipulate the genome of whole animals, and the production of transgenic animals, has influenced the sciences in a most dramatic fashion. In less than 15 years, manipulations of the genetic composition of animals have allowed researchers to address fundamental questions in fields ranging from production agriculture to biomedical research. In a host of transgenic animal models, basic research into the regulation and function of specific genes forged the way to *in vivo* genetic modifications that resulted in either the gain-of-function of a transferred gene or the ablation of an endogenous gene product. Pioneering efforts in transgenic animal technology have markedly influenced our appreciation of the factors that govern gene regulation and expression, and have contributed significantly to our understanding of the genetic bases of reproduction and development.

## DEVELOPMENT OF TRANSGENIC ANIMALS

The ability to introduce functional genes into animals provides a very powerful tool for dissecting complex biological processes and systems. Transgenic animals represent unique models that are custom tailored to address specific biological questions. Furthermore, classical genetic selection cannot engineer a specific genetic trait in a directed fashion. For identification of interesting new models, genetic screening and characterization of chance mutations remains a long and arduous task. Thus, gene transfer in farm animals can surpass classical breeding practices where long life cycles slow the rate of genetic improvement.

Although the entire procedure for microinjection into living cells was described in the late 1960s, it took 15 years before transgenic animals were created (Table 21-1). Following the description of a microinjection process by T.P. Lin in 1966 (1), the first technological shift toward production of a transgenic vertebrate occurred in 1977, when Gurdon transferred mRNA and DNA into Xenopus embryos and observed that the transferred nucleic acids could function (2). Then, in 1980, Brinster and his colleagues reported on similar studies in the mouse (3). They found that an appropriate translational product was produced following transfer of a specific messenger RNA (mRNA) into embryos. Sequentially, these studies laid the groundwork for the development of the first transgenic mammals.

From late 1980 through 1981, six research groups reported success at gene transfer and the development of transgenic mice. In gene transfer, animals receiving new genes (foreign DNA sequences integrated into their genome) are referred to as *transgenic*, a term first coined by Gordon and Ruddle in 1981. As such, transgenic animals are recognized as specific strains or even species variants, following the introduction and integration of new gene(s), or *transgenes*, into their genome. More recently, the term transgenic has been extended to embryonic stem cell technology including "knock-out" mice in which gene(s) have been selectively removed from the host genome.

Production of transgenic mice marked the convergence of previous advances in the areas of recombinant DNA technology and the manipulation and culture of animal germplasm. Transgenic mice provide powerful models to explore the regulation of gene expression as well as the regulation of cellular and physiological processes. Experimental designs have taken advantage of our ability to direct specific (e.g., cell, tissue, or organ specificity) as well as ubiquitous (whole-body) expression *in vivo*. From embryology to virology, transgenic technology provides unique animal models for studies in various disciplines that would

**TABLE 21-1. *Transgenic Animal Milestones***

| YEAR | MILESTONE |
|---|---|
| 0000 | Genetic selection to improve animal productivity |
| 1880 | Mammalian embryo cultivation attempted |
| 1891 | First successful embryo transfer |
| early 1900s | *In vitro* embryo culture develops |
| 1961 | Mouse embryo aggregation to produce chimeras |
| 1966 | Zygote microinjection technology established |
| 1973 | Foreign genes function after cell transfection |
| 1974 | Development of teratocarcinoma cell transfer |
| 1977 | mRNA and DNA transferred into Xenopus eggs |
| 1980 | mRNA transferred into mammalian embryos |
| 1980–1981 | Transgenic mice first documented |
| 1981 | Transfer of ES cells derived from mouse embryos |
| 1982 | Transgenic mice demonstrate an enhanced growth (GH) phenotype |
| 1983 | Tissue-specific gene expression in transgenic mice |
| 1985 | Transgenic domestic animals produced |
| 1987 | Chimeric "knock-out" mice described |
| 1989 | Targeted DNA integration and germ-line chimeric mice |
| 1993 | Germ-line chimeric mice produced using coculture |
| 1994 | Spermatogonia cell transplantation |
| 1997 | Nuclear transfer using ES and adult cell nuclei in sheep |
| 2000 | ? |

otherwise be all but impossible to develop spontaneously (Table 21-2) (4–10).

## DEFINITIONS

Some key terms at this juncture will help in understanding some of the underlying technologies associated with genetic engineering efforts. *DNA microinjection* is a gene transfer technique where DNA constructs (transgenes) are directly injected (or microinjected) into pronuclei or nuclei of fertilized ova. DNA microinjection is the most commonly used gene transfer technique for creating transgenic mammals. In contrast, *embryonic stem (ES) cell transfer* involves the transfer of pluripotent embryonic stem cells into a developing embryo. *Gene transfer* can be defined as one of a set of techniques directed toward manipulating biological function via the introduction of foreign DNA sequences (genes) into living cells (Table 21-3). Today, a *transgenic*

**TABLE 21-2. *Application and Use of Transgenic Animal Models***

Transgenic animals have provided models in biomedical, veterinary, agricultural and biotechnology disciplines in the study of gene expression and developmental biology, as well as for modeling:

- In many fields including: embryology, endocrinology, genetics, immunology, neurology, oncology, pathology, physiology, toxicology, virology. . . .
- Genetic bases of human and animal disease and the design and testing of strategies for therapy.
- Gene therapy.
- Disease resistance in man and animals.
- Drug and product efficacy testing/screening. Toxicological screening protocols can now incorporate transgenic technology.
- Novel or improved products ("molecular farming"), ultimately targeting products or productivity of domestic animals. Models range from enhancing production traits of interest to "foreign" protein production and human organ replacement (xenotransplantation).

**TABLE 21-3. *Gene Transfer Methodologies***

Mouse modeling techniques evolved from procedures for nonspecific (whole genome) transfer to the transfer of discreet genes and the modification of endogenous genes.

- Blastomere/embryo aggregation
- Teratocarcinoma cell transfer
- Retroviral infection
- Microinjection
- Electrofusion
- Nuclear transplantation
- Embryonic stem (ES) cell transfer
- Spermatozoa-mediated transfer and spermatogonial-cell–mediated transfer
- Particle bombardment and jet injection

*animal* can be an animal either integrating foreign DNA segments into its genome following gene transfer, or resulting from the molecular manipulation of endogenous genomic DNA. A *transgenic line* is a direct familial lineage derived from one or more transgenic founders, characterized by the passing of the transgene(s) to successive generations as a stable genetic element. The line includes the founder and any subsequent offspring inheriting the specific germline manipulation.

## APPLICATIONS OF TRANSGENIC ANIMALS

A number of methods exist for gene transfer in mammalian species (Table 21-3). Transgenic technology was reported in a variety of animal species including mice, rats, rabbits, swine, ruminants (including sheep, goats, and cattle), poultry, and fish. With advances in the characterization of factors that control gene expression (including promoter-enhancer elements and transcription-regulatory proteins), gene transfer technology has become a proven asset as a means of dissecting gene regulation and developmental pathways *in vivo*.

Normally, gene function is influenced by cis-acting elements and trans-acting factors. For transferred genes, the cis-activators and trans-activators, in conjunction with the gene integration/insertion event within the host genome, influence gene function. Using genes that code for reporter proteins (e.g., oncogene, lac Z/$\beta$ *gal* or fluorescent protein gene, or GH gene constructs), analysis of transgenic animals has revealed the importance of such factors in determining developmental timing, tissue distribution, and relative efficiency of gene expression. Additionally, transgenic animals have also proven quite useful in determining *in vivo* artifacts of other model systems or techniques.

There are a number of strategies in the development of transgenic mouse models, including systems designed to study aspects such as dominant gene expression, homologous recombination/gene targeting and the use of ES cells, efficiency of transformation of eggs or cells, disruption of gene expression by antisense transgene constructs, gene ablation or knockout models, reporter genes, and marking genes for identification of developmental lineages.

## PRODUCTION OF TRANSGENIC LABORATORY ANIMALS

### *The Mouse and Other Laboratory Animal Models*

The relative importance of using particular strains or breeds of animals in gene transfer experimentation will vary dramatically according to the species under consideration. Probably the most complex system is encountered in the production of transgenic mice, simply because so much work has been done with this species. Here, well-documented differences in reproductive productivity, behavior, related husbandry requirements, and responses to various experimental procedures influence the efficiency and degree of effort associated with production of transgenic founder animals. A general discussion of these factors therefore serves as an appropriate starting point for understanding the many processes and procedures that must be evaluated and monitored when considering production of transgenic animals.

DNA microinjection, the most direct and reproducible method for producing transgenic animals, necessitates that several "pools" of animals be maintained for specific purposes (Fig. 21-1). Equipment and supplies used for this procedure, as well as other gene transfer methods in various species, are outlined in Fig. 21-2. Most commonly, donor females are induced to superovulate by using a regimen of gonadotropin injections. These donor females are then mated to fertile males and large numbers of zygotes are surgically obtained. Alternatively, ova may be collected from donor females and then subjected to *in vitro* maturation (IVM) and/or *in vitro* fertilization (IVF) to obtain viable ova. In either case, the DNA construct, in a buffer solution, is microinjected into the male pronuclei of pronuclear zygotes, or into the nuclei of later stage ova. Ova that survive microinjection are then surgically transferred to the reproductive tracts of hormonally synchronous pseudopregnant female recipients that carry the embryos to term (pseudopregnancy is induced by mating with vasectomized males, since in rodents cervical stimulation is required to maintain pregnancy).

Beyond the mouse model, other laboratory animal species may be necessary to study a particular biological phenomenon. The significance and critical importance of optimized protocols cannot be underestimated. In any given species, selection and management of donor females that respond well to hormonal synchronization and superovulation, embryo transfer recipients that are able to carry fetuses to term and then care for neonates appropriately, and the effective use of males in a breeding regimen will all add to the relative experimental efficiency that one might encounter. However, methods used for hormonal synchronization, selection of proestrus females, and to evaluate other forms of reproductive behavior may differ significantly from those identified for mice. Transgenic animal protocols developed in mice have been modified to accommodate production of other transgenic species.

### *DNA Microinjection*

DNA microinjection generally involves the use of micromanipulators and an air-driven or oil-driven microinjection apparatus to physically inject the DNA construct solution

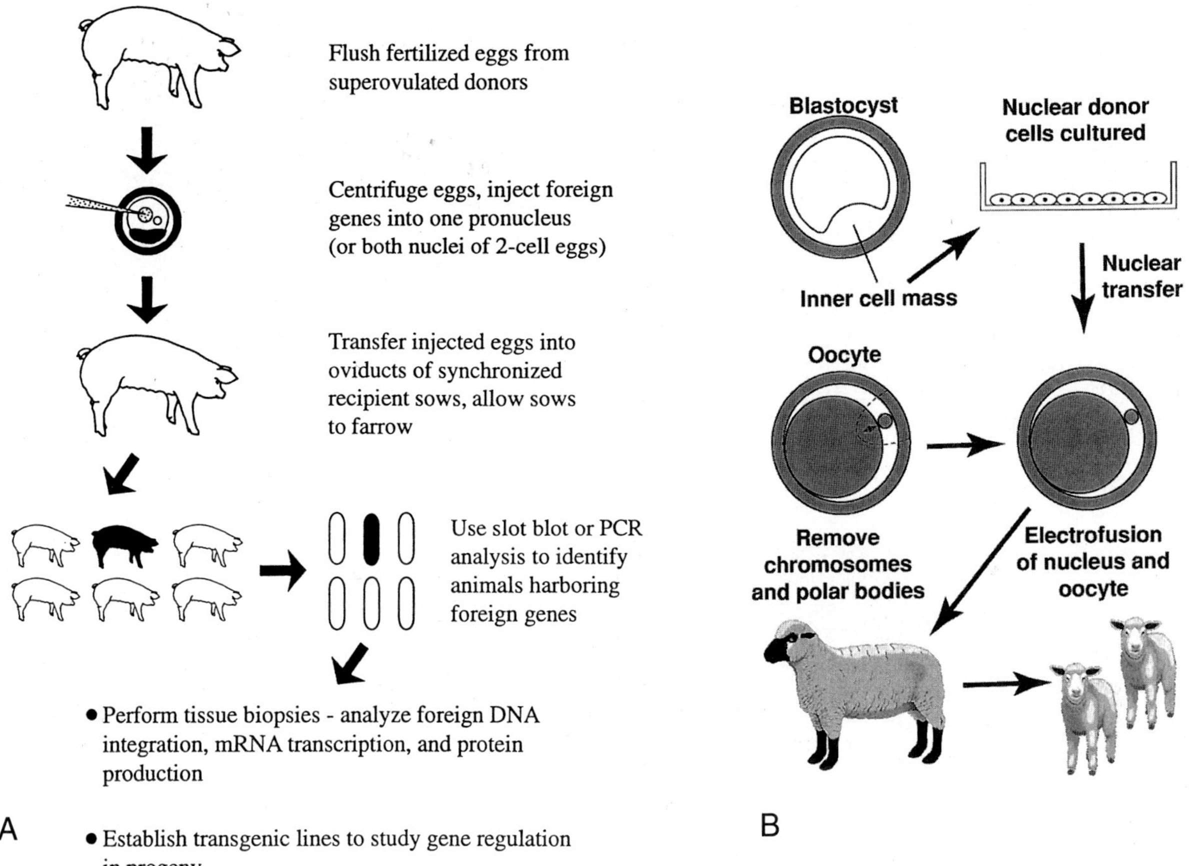


FIGURE 21-1. (**A**) DNA microinjection. The methodology used in the production and evaluation of transgenic pigs by DNA microinjection. Note for microinjection into zygotes (or later-stage ova), visualization of the pronuclei (or nuclei) is necessary. This is accomplished by centrifugation of the ova to stratify the opaque (lipid) material, making pronuclei or nuclei readily visible. Reprinted with permission from Pinkert CA. Transgenic swine models for xenotransplantation. Xeno 1994;2:10–15. (**B**) Nuclear transfer and cloning. Cells from blastocysts (e.g., inner cell mass cells) or other somatic tissues are obtained and grown in culture. These cells are used as nucleus donors for transfer into enucleated oocytes. In contrast to DNA microinjection, this genetic-engineering process includes an electrofusion step to fuse the transferred nuclei and enucleated oocytes. The fused "couplets" (transferred nucleus + oocyte) are transferred to recipients and liveborn offspring are then evaluated for the genetic modification.

into ova (Fig. 21-2). Virtually any cloned DNA construct can be used. With few exceptions, microinjected gene constructs integrate randomly throughout the host's genome, but usually only in a single chromosomal location (the *integration site*). This fact can be exploited to simultaneously co-inject more than one DNA construct into a zygote. The constructs will then co-integrate together at a single, randomly located, integration site.

The integration process itself is also poorly understood, but it apparently does not involve homologous recombination. During integration, a single copy or multiple copies of a transgene (actually as many as a few hundred copies of the particular sequence) are incorporated into the genomic DNA, predominantly as a number of copies in head-to-tail concatemers. Regulatory elements in the host DNA near the site of integration, and the general availability of this region for transcription, appear to play major roles in affecting the level of transgene expression. This "positional effect" is presumed to explain why the levels of expression of the same transgene may vary dramatically between individual founder animals as well as their offspring (or lines). It is therefore prudent to examine transgene expression in offspring from at least three or four founder animals in order to determine what might be a result of the integration location, and what might reflect the activity of the transgene.

Host DNA near the site of integration frequently undergoes various forms of sequence duplication, deletion, or rearrangement as a result of transgene incorporation. Such alterations, if sufficiently drastic, may disrupt the function

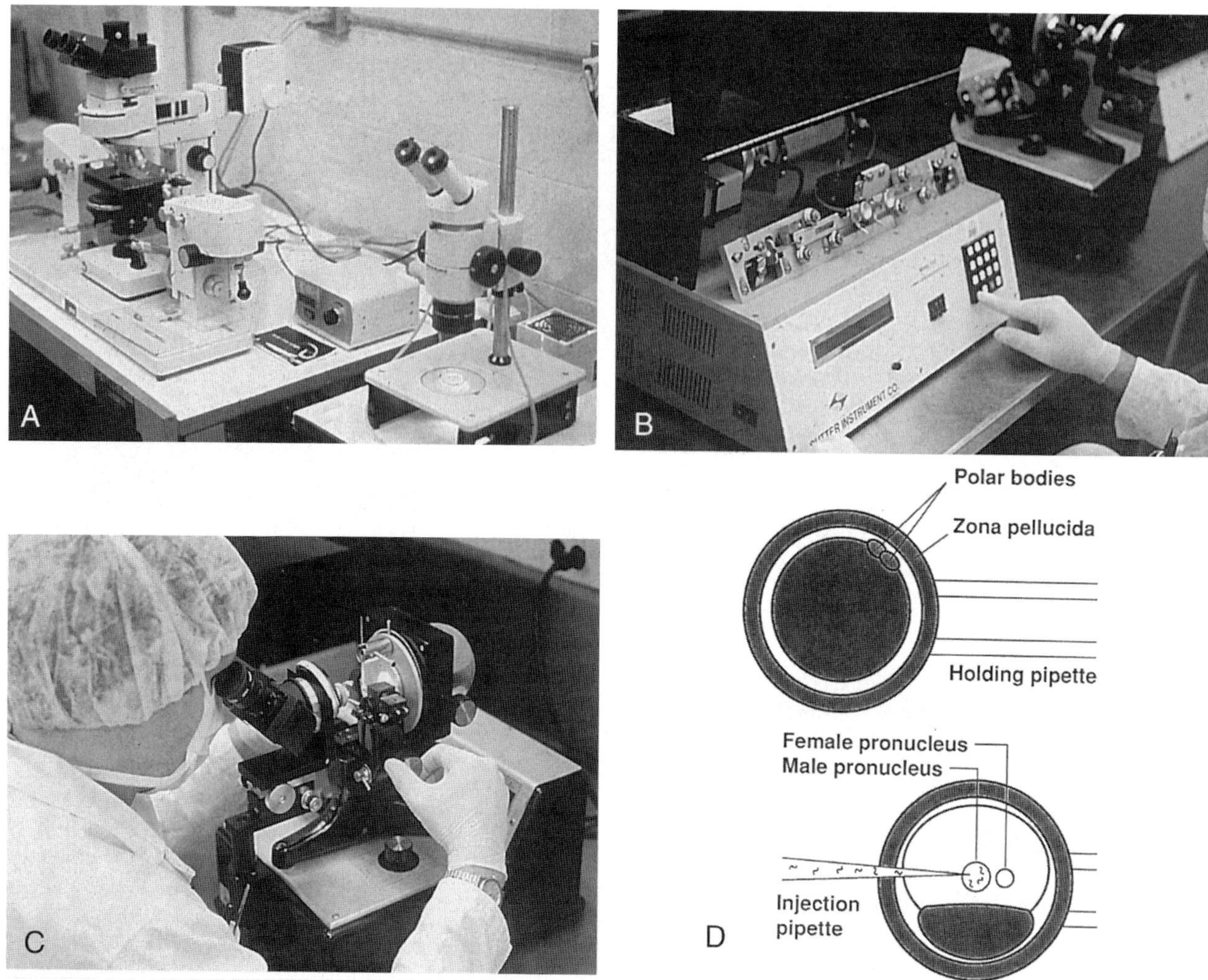


FIGURE 21-2. Micromanipulation station, microforge, pipette puller, and microinjection. (A) A microinjection station includes a dissecting microscope (*right*) used for batch preparation of embryos and cells (and embryo transfer in mice) and microinjection microscope (*left*). Flanking the microinjection microscope, micromanipulators aid in the precise manipulations with embryos, cells, and buffers. (B) Pipette puller. Microneedles can be prepared with uniform tapers and shapes using an electronic or gravity-driven pipette puller. (C) Microforge. Needles may be fire-polished or bent to desired specifications using the microforge assembly that includes a microscope assembly for visualization of the finished product. (D) Microinjection of a pig zygote. Many farm animal embryos, including those from pigs, are lipid-rich and relatively opaque (*top*). To make nuclear structures readily visible, one-cell and two-cell eggs are centrifuged to stratify lipids in the cytoplasm (*bottom*). After centrifugation, the eggs are placed in a drop of medium, with silicone oil to prevent evaporation of the medium. The eggs are held in place, sequentially, using the large-bore holding pipette. A small-bore injection pipette containing DNA in a buffer solution is inserted through the zona pellucida and plasma membrane into a pronucleus (or nuclei of a two-cell egg) that readily expands (~50% increase in volume) as the DNA solution is delivered. The diameter of the egg is ~125$\mu$m. Adapted from Pinkert CA. The history and theory of transgenic animals. Proc US Anim Health Assoc 1987;91:129–141.

of normally active host genes at the integration site and constitute *insertional mutagenesis*, wherein an aberrant phenotype may result. Such events cannot be purposefully designed, but have led to the serendipitous discovery of previously unsuspected genes and gene functions. Because DNA microinjection is usually accomplished in ova at the one-cell stage, transgene incorporation occurs in essentially every cell that contributes to the developing embryo. Incorporation of the transgene into cells that will eventually contribute to development of germ cells (sperm or ova) is a common occurrence with this method, and makes heritability of the transgene by offspring of founder animals likely within one generation. In such cases, the transgene has been said to be germ-line or the animals are referred to a *germline-competent*. However, integration of the microinjected DNA construct into the host's genome occasionally may be inexplicably delayed. In such a case, if cells of the early embryo (blastomeres) undergo mitosis before the transgene-integration event occurs, some but not all of the cells will contain the transgene, and the founder animal, although still considered to be transgenic, will be classified as a mosaic or chimera.

Advantages of the DNA microinjection method are:

a) Relatively high frequency of generating transgenic animals (20 to 30% of liveborn offspring).
b) High probability of germ-line transmission of the transgene.
c) Relative lack of constraints on the size or type of DNA construct used.
d) Relative stability of the transgene as it is transmitted from generation to generation.
e) Low frequency of mosaicism or double integrations (combined estimate of 10 to 30% of founders).

In contrast, disadvantages of this method include:

a) Random and potentially significant influence that the site of integration may exert on transgene expression (positional effects).
b) Potential for undesired insertional mutagenesis.
c) Occasional production of mosaic founders.
d) Occasional lack of germ-line incorporation.
e) Time and expense required to obtain micromanipulation and microinjection skills.

### *Retrovirus-Mediated Gene Transfer*

Transfer of foreign genes into animal genomes has also been accomplished using retroviruses. Although embryos can be infected with retroviruses up to midgestation, early eggs, usually at the 4-cell to 16-cell stages, are used for infection with one or more recombinant retroviruses containing a foreign gene. Immediately following infection, the retrovirus produces a DNA copy of its RNA genome using the viral enzyme, reverse transcriptase. Completion of this process requires that the host cell undergoes the S phase of the cell cycle. Therefore, retroviruses effectively transduce only mitotically active cells. Incomplete infections, in which not all embryonic cells acquire the retrovirus, occur more frequently when using embryos after the 4-cell stage, with resultant chimeric embryos. Modifications to the retrovirus frequently consist of removal of structural genes, such as gag, pol, and env, which support viral particle formation. Additionally, most retroviruses and complementary lines are ecotropic in that they infect only rodents, such as rats and mice, and rodent cell lines rather than humans.

The DNA copy of the viral genome, or provirus, integrates randomly into the host cell genome, usually without deletions or rearrangements. However, as is the case for gene transfer by microinjection, because integration is not by way of homologous recombination, this method is not used effectively for site-directed mutagenesis.

Very high rates of gene transfer are achieved with the use of retroviruses. However, disadvantages include:

a) Low copy number integration.
b) Additional steps required to produce retroviruses.
c) Limitations on the size of the foreign DNA insert (usually 9 to 15 kb) transferred.
d) Potential for undesired genetic recombination that may alter the retrovirus.
e) High frequency of mosaicism.
f) Possible interference by integrated retroviral sequences on transgene expression.

### *Embryonic Stem Cell Technology*

Gene transfer has been used to produce both random and targeted insertion or ablation of discrete DNA fragments into the mouse genome. For targeted insertions, where the integration of foreign genes is based on a recombinant gene insertion with a specific homology to cellular sequences (termed homologous recombination), the efficiency of DNA microinjection is extremely low (11). In contrast, the use of ES cell transfer into mouse embryos has been quite effective in allowing an investigator to preselect a specific genetic modification, via homologous recombination, at a precise chromosomal position (Fig. 21-1). This preselection has led to the production of mice that:

a) Incorporate a novel foreign gene into their genome.
b) Carry a modified endogenous gene.
c) Lack a specific endogenous gene following gene deletion or "knock-out" procedures.

Technologies involving ES cells, and more recently primordial germ cells, have been used to produce a host of mouse models. Pluripotential ES cells are derived from early pre-implantation embryos and maintained in culture for a sufficient period for one to perform various *in vitro* manipulations. The cells may then be injected directly into the blastocoel of a host blastocyst or incubated in association with a zona-free morula. The host embryos are then transferred into intermediate hosts or surrogate females for continued development. Currently, the efficiency of chimeric mouse production results in about 30% of the live-born animals containing tissue derived from the injected stem cells. This ability to produce chimeric animals using ES cells has given researchers another tool in their armamentarium to produce transgenic animals. In this set of techniques, the power of gene transfer technology has been catapulted forward because such processes allow for targeted insertions into the genome. Such targeting is extremely important, particularly in areas of gene therapy and correction, wherein previous technologies allowed only for random integration events.

The genome of ES cells can be manipulated *in vitro* by introducing foreign genes or foreign DNA sequences by techniques including electroporation, microinjection, precipitation reactions, transfection, or retroviral insertion. The use of ES cells to produce transgenic mice faced a number of procedural obstacles before it became competitive with DNA microinjection as a standard technique in mouse modeling. Within the last few years, the addition of coculture techniques involving tetraploid host embryos (8-cell stage to morulae), has resulted in founders that can be derived completely from the cocultured ES cells (Fig. 21-1) (12). Hence, the founders are no longer chimeras, as all the cells come from the same progenitor cells and the founder animals will breed true (and faithfully transmit the genetic modification in the first generation offspring).

Yet, while ES cell lines have been identified for species other than the mouse, the production of germline-competent ES cell-derived/chimeric farm animals has not been reported. With the advent of nuclear transfer-related technologies, the need to identify and use ES or primordial germ cells (PGCs) to effect genetic change, may become of lesser consequence.

### *Other Technologies: From Spermatozoa to Cloning*

In contrast to progress in embryo manipulation, a completely different tact was taken with the advent of sperm-related transfer procedures. In 1989, sperm-mediated gene transfer was reported but hotly disputed when many laboratories around the world were unable to duplicate the outlined procedures. Yet, by 1994, the sperm-mediated story generated interest that resulted in the development of spermatogonial cell transplantation procedures as a potentially feasible alternative for *in vivo* gene transfer (13). However, whole animal and somatic-cell techniques (including liposome-mediated gene transfer, particle bombardment, and jet injection), coupled with novel vector systems, will continue to evolve in order to genetically engineer animals in an efficient and effective manner.

In the early 1980s, a number of laboratories reported on nuclear transfer experiments in laboratory animals. While some of these studies were controversial, most work of late has tended to focus on domestic animals and nonmammalian vertebrates. As seen in the next section, nuclear transfer has now taken on much greater emphasis as a vehicle for genetic engineering experimentation.

## PRODUCTION OF TRANSGENIC DOMESTIC ANIMALS

### *Overview*

The success of transgenic mouse experiments led a number of research groups to study the transfer of similar gene constructs into the germ-line of domestic animal species. With one exception, these efforts have been directed primarily toward either of two general endpoints: improving the productivity traits of domestic food animal species, or development of transgenic animals for use as "bioreactors" (i.e., producers of recoverable quantities of medically or biologically important proteins). Since 1985, the vast majority of transgenic farm animals were created using growth-related gene constructs. Unfortunately, for the most part, ideal growth phenotypes were not achieved because of an inability to coordinately regulate gene expression and the ensuing cascade of endocrine events that unfolded.

### *Methodology*

Today, DNA microinjection and the recently reported nuclear transfer procedures are the only methods used to successfully produce transgenic livestock. Although involved and at times quite tedious, the steps in the development of transgenic models are relatively straightforward. For either DNA microinjection or nuclear transfer, once a specific fusion gene is cloned and characterized, sufficient quantities are isolated, purified, and tested in cell culture. If *in vitro* mRNA expression of the gene is identified, the appropriate fragment is linearized, purified, and readied for preliminary mammalian gene transfer experiments. In contrast to nuclear transfer studies, DNA microinjection experiments are first performed in the mouse. While the transgenic mouse model will not always identify likely phenotypic expression patterns in domestic animals, we have not observed any gene constructs that would function in a farm animal when there had been no evidence of transgene-encoded expression in a pilot mouse model.

The successful "cloning" of a sheep, followed by the use of nuclear transfer to produce transgenic sheep and cattle, has captured the imagination of researchers around the world (14). Within the next few years, these and subsequent technological breakthroughs should play a significant role in the development of new procedures for genetic engineering in a number of mammalian species. It should be noted that nuclear transfer, with nuclei obtained from either mammalian stem cells or differentiated adult cells, is an especially important development in nonmouse species. This is because a technological barrier was surpassed that allows for specific *in vitro* manipulations that will lead to targeted genetic modifications in many first generation ($G_0$) animals. Previously, it was not possible to produce germline-competent transgenics in mammalian species (other than in mice), using any technique other than DNA microinjection (that only allowed for random and imprecise integration of transgenes in founder animals). Thus, with the exception of nuclear transfer experiments in sheep and cattle, there has been little change in the methods used to produce transgenic mammals, birds, and fish over the last few years. Unfortunately, relative efficiencies for nuclear transfer experimentation pale in comparison to conventional DNA microinjection. However, while nuclear transfer might be considered inefficient in its current form, major strides in enhancing experimental protocols within the next few years are envisioned, comparable perhaps to the early advances in DNA microinjection technology.

### *Experimental Considerations*

Using DNA microinjection, the types of genes introduced into livestock species become important considerations. Pursel and Rexroad (15) provided a comprehensive list of gene constructs used in the production of transgenic cattle, goats, pigs, and sheep that has not materially changed—a reflection of the enormous resources necessary for such endeavors. The major scientific limitations to the wide scale application of transgenic technology to improve farm animals have not basically changed over the last decade. Those limitations include:

a) Lack of knowledge concerning the genetic basis of factors limiting production traits.
b) Lack of temporally and spatially controllable or inducible sequences for use in developing gene constructs, expression vectors, and in gene targeting.
c) Establishment of novel methods to increase efficiency of transgenic animal production.

In order to optimize genetic engineering efforts, gene regulation and expression can be evaluated in mice, as a prelude to the more labor, cost, and time-intensive gene transfer experiments in other species. In mouse studies, less than two months is required from the time the DNA construct is ready for microinjection through weaning of founder pups. In contrast, for pig experiments, a much longer time line follows from synchronizing embryo donors and microinjecting equivalent numbers of ova, the generational interval, and the time necessary to identify, breed, and characterize transgenic pigs—illustrating the extended requirements associated with the production of transgenic farm animals. Hence, there is an obvious advantage to characterizing transgenic mice to expedite what will ultimately be a lengthy undertaking.

### *Traits Affecting Domestic Animal Productivity*

Interest in modifying traits that determine productivity of domestic animals was greatly stimulated by the first experiments where body size and growth rates were dramatically affected in transgenic mice expressing growth hormone (GH) transgenes driven by a metallothionein (MT) enhancer/promoter (16). From that starting point, similar attempts followed in swine and sheep studies to enhance growth by introduction of various GH gene constructs under control of a number of different regulatory promoters. Use of these constructs was intended to allow for tight regulation of individual transgene expression by dietary supplementation. However, although resulting phenotypes included altered fat composition, feed efficiency and rate of gain, and lean : fat body composition, they were accompanied by undesirable side-effects (e.g., joint pathology, skeletal abnormalities, increased metabolic rate, gastric ulcers, and infertility). Such problems were attributed to chronic over-expression of the growth-related transgenes and could be mimicked, in several cases, in normal animals by long-term treatment with elevated doses of GH. Subsequent efforts to genetically alter growth rates and patterns have included production of transgenic swine and cattle expressing a foreign *c-ski* oncogene or GDF-8 (myostatin) gene, which target skeletal muscle, and studies of growth in lines of mice and sheep that separately express transgenes encoding growth hormone-releasing factor (GRF) or insulin-like growth factor I (IGF-I). Cumulatively, it has become apparent from these studies that greater knowledge of the biology of muscle growth and development will be required in order to genetically engineer lines of domestic animals with desirable growth characteristics.

Other productivity traits that are major targets for genetic engineering include altering the properties or proportions of caseins, lactose, or butterfat in milk of transgenic cattle and goats, more efficient wool production, and enhanced resistance to viral and bacterial diseases (including development of "constitutive immunity" or germline-transmission of specific antibody genes).

### *Domestic Animals as Bioreactors*

The second area of significant interest in genetic engineering of farm animals has been related to the development of animal bioreactors to direct expression of transgenes encoding biologically active (human) proteins. In such a strategy, the goal was to economically recover large quantities of functional proteins, that have therapeutic value, from serum or from the milk of lactating females. To date, expression of foreign genes encoding $\alpha_1$-antitrypsin, tissue plasminogen activator, clotting factor IX, and protein C were produced with varying efficiency (as high as gram/liter quantities) within the mammary glands of a number of farm animal species. Additionally, lines of transgenic farm animals were created that produced human hemoglobin or specific circulating immunoglobulins, with an ultimate goal of harvesting serum proteins, for use as important constituents of blood transfusion substitutes, or for use in diagnostic testing.

### *Pig Models*

In contrast to gene transfer in mice, the efficiency associated with the production of transgenic livestock, including swine, is quite low. However, two advantages offered by swine over other domestic species include a favorable response to hormonal superovulation protocols (20 to 30 ova can be collected on average), and as a polytocous species, they have a uterine capacity to nurture more offspring to term.

An initial problem encountered during the creation of transgenic farm animal species concerned the visualization of the pronuclei or nuclei within the ova. As swine ova are lipid-dense, the cytoplasm is opaque and the nuclear structures are not discernable without some type of manipulation. Fortuitously, centrifugation of pig ova resulted in stratification of the cytoplasm rendering pronuclei and nuclei visible under the microscope (Figs 21-1**A** and 21-2**D**).

The proportion of transgenic swine that develop from microinjected ova is still low, approaching 10 to 20% of liveborn pigs (Table 21-4). The survival of microinjected pig embryos is related to several factors, including the developmental stage of ova injected, the duration of *in vitro* culture, synchrony of ova donors and recipients, the number of ova transferred, and donor age. Other factors which have been shown to influence transgenic mouse production—including technician proficiency and embryo handling/transfer, pipette dimensions, DNA preparation, and the viability of manipulated ova—are also factors that readily influence transgenic production efficiency for all other species.

Following DNA microinjection, surgical embryo transfer is necessary. However, the mechanical insult to the embryos is severe and only 15 to 25% of them will still be viable 5 days after transfer. Therefore, 30 to 50 microinjected embryos are routinely transferred per recipient sow with the expectation that 50% of the recipient females will maintain pregnancy (Table 21-5). While the number of embryos transferred may seem excessive, the basis is derived from classical studies that establish a requirement of four viable embryos at the time of implantation for a sow to initiate and maintain a successful pregnancy.

For studies targeting pigs, the use of outbred domestic pigs is the most practical way to produce transgenic founders. However, miniature or laboratory swine are now used with increasing frequency in biomedical research, where their well-characterized background genetics make them more suitable for human modeling studies (e.g., xenotransplantation research). Reproductive efficiency in miniature swine is low compared to commercial swine and is characterized by a low ovulation rate, low birth weight, and small litter size. Average litter size is between 4 and 7 pigs at birth, with each breeding sow producing 12 to 18 pigs per year. Estrous cycles and gestation length are similar to standard commercial swine, however sexual maturity in males and females occurs between 4 and 6 months of age in some breeds, which is sooner than the 6 to 9 month norm of commercial swine. Breeding requirements for transgenic pigs are critical and management warrants expertise from record keeping to animal husbandry.

TABLE 21-4. ***Superovulation and Zygote Recovery in Farm Animals***[a]

| | PIGS[b] | CATTLE[c] | SHEEP[c] |
|---|---|---|---|
| Ova recovered/donor | 25 | 10 | 10 |
| Fraction of fertilized ova recovered | >90% | 60% | 90% |
| Pronuclear/injectable ova | 20 | 4 | 7 |
| Number of ova transferred/recipient | 35 | 1–3 | 1–3 |
| Average litter size after embryo manipulation [normal litter size] | 5 [10] | <1 [1] | <1 [1] |
| Fraction of transgenic offspring obtained from total born | 15% | 10% | 6% |
| Fraction of transgenic offspring obtained from total ova transferred | 1% | <1% | <1% |

[a]In contrast to DNA microinjection, nuclear transfer experiments result in a 10 to 100-fold **lesser** efficiency.
[b]From a recent collaborative study (C.A. Pinkert, F.F. Bartol, D.F. Wolfe, W.F. Owsley et al., unpublished data).
[c]Data from: Wall RJ, Hawk HW, Nel N Making transgenic livestock: genetic engineering on a large scale. J Cell Biochem 1992;49:113–120.

### *Ruminant Models*

In contrast to swine modeling, the relative experimental efficiencies associated with the production of transgenic ruminants (goats, sheep, and cattle) are even lower (Table 21-4). While the different techniques from DNA microinjection to nuclear transfer require a large number of embryos to ensure success, other factors play significant roles in experimental yields and success. Such factors include the low rate of embryo survival following manipulation, uterine capacity (generally these species are monotocous—one to at most three offspring would be feasible), long generational interval, and relative cost of hormonal induction/ova recovery/ova transfer and animal maintenance, all negatively affecting experimental costs and efficiencies. In many laboratories, *in vitro* maturation (IVM), *in vitro* fertilization (IVF), and culture of ova (in surrogate hosts or incubators, although culture conditions are not optimal for embryo survival at this time) prior to final transfer aide in maximizing resources for production of genetically engineered ruminants. Many of these steps are timely, as the ability to biopsy individual blastomeres for analysis of specific genetic modifications (by PCR) can minimize the number of animals used and maintained in these studies.

For cattle, ova can be collected surgically (by laparoscopy or laparotomy, either by flank incision or transvaginally, and with or without the aid of ultrasonography) or

TABLE 21-5. ***Influence of Number of Manipulated Ova Transferred on Embryo Survival in Pigs***

| NUMBER OF OVA TRANSFERRED PER RECIPIENT | NUMBER OF TRANSFERS | PREGNANCY RATE | PIGS BORN PER LITTER | PIGS BORN PER TRANSFER |
|---|---|---|---|---|
| <30 | 48 | 25% | 5.0 | 1.3 |
| 31–40 | 57 | 32% | 4.6 | 1.4 |
| >41 | 77 | 47% | 4.4 | 2.0 |

Reprinted with permission from Brem G, Springmann K, Meier E, Krausslich H, Brenig B, Muller M, and Winnacker E-L. (1989). Factors in the success of transgenic pig programs. In: Transgenic Models in Medicine and Agriculture (R.B. Church, ed.), Vol. 116, pp. 61–72. Wiley–Liss, New York.

from ovaries at necropsy. The most common procedure at this time is to collect large numbers of ova from slaughterhouse ovaries and subject them to IVM/IVF. If slaughterhouse ovaries are not available, standard superovulatory regimens using various gonadotropins can be employed to obtain oocytes, zygotes, or later stage ova (17). For sheep and goat studies, reproductive cycles and seasonality can limit the use of either males or females, and the selection of specific breeds to establish appropriate modeling should be carefully evaluated. Most sheep and goats are seasonally polyestrous, although as outlined in Chapter 12, there are breeds of sheep and goats that can reproduce throughout the year, if photoperiod and temperature are controlled. While sheep and goat ova are transferred surgically into the oviduct, cattle ova can be transferred surgically, or after culture to the morula or blastocyst stage, they can be transferred transvaginally or transcervically using established embryo transfer protocols. One problem that currently exists is that *in vitro* culture results in lowered survival rates than what would be comparable in *in vivo* culture. Rabbits have been used as intermediate hosts to maintain ova at various stages of development, for the most part using a ligated oviduct as the storage depot. Others have used cows, sheep, goats, rabbits, and mice as intermediate hosts in such cross-species "culturing." However, *in vitro* culture conditions are still improving, and will probably become the most efficient method of intermediate culture, once survival rates become comparable to *in vivo* results. Currently, use of coculture techniques (where ova are maintained on a bed of supportive cells; e.g., oviductal cells, follicular cells, or fibroblasts from other sources such as buffalo rat liver cells), conditioned media preparations, or various defined media preparations with specific growth factors have all been used to enhance embryo survival rates.

Lastly, with the rather long gestation lengths in ruminants, if blastomere biopsy is not used prior to embryo transfer, then a number of techniques may help decrease the long experimental time lines. Early pregnancy diagnosis following implantation is routine today, and can be determined by onset of behavioral estrus, ultrasound, hormonal profiles (progesterone or placental hormones), or in cattle by palpation. In addition to pregnancy diagnosis, analysis of the specific genetic modification can be performed using a number of fetal biopsy techniques as well as determining if a transgene-encoded product is present (if appropriate to the particular modification). For confirmation in liveborn animals at birth, blood samples, tail tissue (from tail docking), umbilicus samples, or other biopsies can be used to confirm the presence of the genetic modification from nucleic acid analyses to mRNA and protein expression as described in the next section.

## ANALYSIS OF GENETIC MANIPULATIONS: TRANSGENES AND OTHER MODIFICATIONS

### *Presence of the Genetic Modification of Interest*

Representative tissues for analysis of transgene integration and expression can be obtained at birth. For integration analysis, typically blood or tail tissue are obtained. Preliminary determination of transgene integration by the PCR technique can be very useful when the target sequence (the transgene) possesses unique sequences (not endogenous to the genome of the animal). However, given the extreme sensitivity of PCR, other more informative techniques (either DNA slot blot or Southern blot hybridization) should be used to confirm the presence of a transgene. Southern blotting is the most useful as it can indicate transgene copy number, length of a given target sequence, and possible sequence mutation (where the identified sequence is not present and completely intact). Additionally, a transgene can be constructed to include a molecular *tag*—a unique sequence that is easily detected and has minimal similarity to any endogenous sequence. This strategy is especially useful when the transgene itself is similar or nearly identical to an endogenous gene. In such cases, another strategy that may be helpful is the introduction of new restriction sites into the transgene, without perturbing function, so that restriction fragment length polymorphism (RFLP) analysis can be used to distinguish the genetic modification from its endogenous counterpart (should one exist). Finally, in some instances phenotypic screening is possible for both gain-of-function and loss-of-function studies, if the genetic modification leads to an identifiable change in the appearance of the animal. Phenotypic screening by co-transfer of a second transgene or marker that gives rise to a specific phenotype can also be useful, particularly in those models where the marker co-integrates with the sequence of interest in DNA microinjection, or the marker can be associated with the particular cell line used in nuclear transfer. However, in either scenario, the integration of the desired genetic modification must subsequently be confirmed by other direct means.

Other concerns related to analysis of the genetic modification vary as to gain-of-function or loss-of-function models. In gain-of-function, or where a suppressor gene is used to induce loss-of-function, it is important to characterize copy number of the transgene per cell, orientation of tandemly-arranged copies, the presence of multiple integration sites, and possibly methylation state (or identifying other post-translational events). These questions can be addressed by Southern blot hybridization following digestion of the genomic DNA with appropriate restriction enzymes. In contrast, in loss-of-function studies where a targeted disruption or conditional knock-out is predicated on a secondary event (e.g., Cre-lox targeting vectors where a particular sequence is excised from the genome), analyzing the modified chromosomal locus is warranted to characterize the specific targeting event. Lastly, the critical question of whether the gene modification is stably heritable must be answered.

### *Transgene-Encoded mRNA Expression*

While absence of mRNA expression is likely for loss-of-function models and may only represent a confirmatory step of minor significance, the analysis of expression of the transgene is absolutely essential in determining the usefulness of a particular transgenic animal. Technically, the most critical step in analyzing transgene expression is the isolation of RNA. Care must be taken to avoid contamination of RNA preparations with ribonucleases (enzymes that degrade RNA). The presence of a specific mRNA is usually determined by RNA slot-blot or northern blot hybridization. Northern blotting is more informative as it confirms not only the presence but also the size of the mRNA transcript of interest.

Additional techniques exist for determining the presence or relative levels of mRNA transcripts from transgenic animals. In a nuclease protection assay, a labeled probe is allowed to hybridize to the RNA in solution, followed by nuclease digestion of non-hybridized RNA. The sample is then resolved on a polyacrylamide gel. This technique is very useful in determining the steady-state levels of RNA in a given tissue. In the reverse transcription-PCR (RT-PCR) assay, the RNA of interest is transcribed into a cDNA molecule by use of a specific primer and the enzyme, reverse transcriptase. A second primer is added and a standard PCR amplification is performed. The advantage of RT-PCR lies in its extreme sensitivity—theoretically, one mRNA molecule can be amplified to a quantity sufficient for visualization on an agarose gel. Lastly, in an *in situ* hybridization technique, a labeled probe is hybridized to a target mRNA transcript in sections of tissue so that individual cells containing the transcript can be identified. This technique is particularly useful in identifying a small subset of cells within a given tissue that would be too few to detect by other means.

### *Transgene-Encoded Protein Expression*

Various techniques are often employed to identify the unique protein itself or perhaps a specific enzyme activity. The immunoblotting technique, in which proteins are resolved on a polyacrylamide gel, transferred to a membrane, and detected with a labeled antibody, is useful in verifying the appropriate molecular weight of the protein product of interest. To identify which cells within a tissue contain the protein product of the transgene, immunohistochemical staining of tissue sections with a labeled antibody can also be employed. Additionally, the use of "reporter genes" (e.g., an oncogene, or a growth hormone or fluorescent protein gene) can often simplify determination of expression levels by producing a protein that is easily and unequivocally detectable.

In analyzing the expression of any transgene, it is always important to evaluate at least two separate lines of transgenic animals in order to show that the expression patterns are consistent and reproducible. It is not uncommon for the site of integration within a given line of transgenic animals to have a profound influence on transgene expression, independent of any transcriptional control sequences in the transgene itself.

## CONCLUSIONS AND FUTURE DIRECTIONS

### *Gene Transfer and Genetic Engineering Today*

The expertise and effort associated with gene transfer experimentation in animal biology are quite significant and challenging. Innovative technologies to enhance experimental gene transfer efficiency in different species are desperately needed. Such enabling techniques would not only bring the cost of individual projects into a reasonable realm but would also increase the likelihood of new innovations in many disciplines. The outlined efficiencies for the production of transgenic animals represent what is considered current state-of-the-art technology. It is envisioned that procedures will be modified and enhanced as new research breakthroughs are reported. As such, there are a number of specific achievements that would significantly enhance experimental productivity. Enabling technologies would center on the following areas:

a) Development of alternative DNA delivery systems (e.g., liposome-mediated gene transfer, or targeted somatic cell techniques).
b) Identification of optimal conditions for a given gene transfer procedure and identification of breeds best suited to the specific technologies.
c) Complete animal genome mapping and identification of homologies to human genes.
d) Establishment of routine and efficient germplasm culture and preservation systems (from preservation of gonadal tissue to culture and cryostorage of gametes).
e) Development of a means to reduce the number of animals and embryos required (e.g., use of PCR amplification of blastomere DNA, or fluorescence-activated cell sorter [FACS] analyses and gating of genetically-modified germplasm).

Primary considerations for genetic manipulations and gene transfer are not limited to animal management (including surgical manipulations and embryo handling), but also to expertise in tissue/cell culture and molecular biology techniques. For most species, husbandry considerations are extensive, running the gamut from animal and record-keeping management to female-specific (e.g., controlled estrus cycles/synchronization) and male-specific (e.g., sperm analysis/quantitation) requirements. Harvest of embryos and the trauma associated with most manipulations are significant factors. The refinement of nonsurgical techniques for embryo collection and transfer would bypass the huge financial and labor requirement necessary to maintain an ongoing transgenic farm animals program. More importantly, fewer experimental animals would be necessarily subjected to significant surgical manipulations. Lastly, and equally critical to experimental design, are the ethical considerations and regulatory requirements associated with genetic engineering experimentation.

### *Future Directions*

Recent advances in nuclear transfer may provide a ready alternative to developing pluripotential ES cell technology—the effort that has become the "Holy Grail" of farm animal geneticists and biotechnologists. However, with the complexity of the mammalian genome, determination of appropriate genes to engineer and transfer will remain critical. What are the appropriate genetic targets in different species and how will gene targeting manipulations influence mammalian development? If genetic polymorphisms (indicative of related genes that code for different isoform proteins) or pseudogenes are present, targeting efforts can be long and arduous. For well-characterized genomes, the identification of specific genetic variation may only provide a glimpse of the effort necessary to develop in other species. Yet, it is hoped that with current efforts focused on a number of mammalian genomes, accumulating data will prove quite informative and adaptable to different species, as conserved linkage groups are highly probable and exploitable.

Much has been learned about various physiologic processes in transgenic farm animals that were created to date. Even if a "better production animal" has not reached the marketplace as yet, the pioneering studies were not unsuccessful. Various transgenic animals have provided far reaching insights in redefining many regulatory and developmental processes previously misunderstood in agricultural species. While studies of transgene expression in farm animals may not always correlate exactly, the utility of transgenic animal models to scientific discovery cannot be overestimated. The use of nuclear transfer procedures or related methodologies to provide efficient and targeted *in vivo* genetic manipulations offers the prospects of creating profoundly useful animal models for agricultural and biomedical applications. However, the road to such successes will continue to be an arduous but exciting challenge for animal scientists in the 21st century.

## REFERENCES

1. Lin TP. Microinjection of mouse eggs. Science 1966;151:333–337.
2. Gurdon JB. Egg cytoplasm and gene control in development. Proc R Soc London B 1977;198:211–247.
3. Brinster RL, Chen HY, Trumbauer ME, Avarbock MR. Translation of globin messenger RNA by the mouse ovum. Nature 1980;283:499–501.
4. Hogan B, Beddington R, Costantini F, Lacy E. Manipulating the Mouse Embryo: A Laboratory Manual. Cold Spring Harbor, New York: Cold Spring Harbor Laboratory, 1994.
5. Pinkert CA. Transgenic Animal Technology: A Laboratory Handbook. San Diego: Academic Press, 1994.
6. Pinkert CA. Transgenic swine models for xenotransplantation. Xeno 1994;2:10–15.
7. Monastersky GM, Robl JM. Strategies in Transgenic Animal Science. Washington, DC: American Society for Microbiology Press, 1995.
8. Houdebine LM. Transgenic Animals: Generation and Use. Amsterdam: Harwood Academic Publishers, 1997.
9. Pinkert CA, Irwin MH, Moffatt RJ. Transgenic animal modeling. In: Meyers RA, ed. Encyclopedia of Molecular Biology and Molecular Medicine. New York: VCH, 1997;6:63–74.
10. Pinkert CA, Murray JD. Transgenic farm animals. In: Murray JD, Anderson GB, McGloughlin MM, Oberbauer AM, eds. Transgenic Animals in Agriculture. Wallingford, UK: CAB International, 1998.
11. Cappechi MR. Altering the genome by homologous recombination. Science 1989;244:1288–1292.

12. Wood SA, Allen ND, Rossant J, Auerbach A, Nagy A. Non-injection methods for the production of embryonic stem cell-embryo chimaeras. Nature 1993;365:87–89.
13. Brinster RL, Avarbock MR. Germline transmission of donor haplotype following spermatogonial transplantation. PNAS 1994;91:11303–11307.
14. Wilmut I, Schnieke AE, McWhir J, Kind AJ, Campbell KH. Viable offspring derived from fetal and adult mammalian cells. Nature 1997;385:810–813.
15. Pursel VG, Rexroad CE Jr. Status of research with transgenic farm animals. J Anim Sci 1993;71(Suppl. 3):10–19.
16. Palmiter RD, Brinster L, Hammer RE, et al. Dramatic growth of mice that develop from eggs microinjected with metallothionein-growth hormone fusion genes. Nature 1982;300: 611–615.
17. Rexroad CE Jr, Hawk HW. Production of transgenic ruminants. In: Pinkert CA, ed. Transgenic Animal Technology: A Laboratory Handbook. San Diego: Academic Press, 1994;339–355.

## SUGGESTED READING

Brinster RL. Stem cells and transgenic mice in the study of development. Intl J Devel Biol 1993;3:89–99.

Matsui Y, Zsebo K, Hogan BL. Derivation of pluripotential embryonic stem cells from murine primordial germ cells in culture. Cell 1992;70:841–847.

Pinkert CA. The history and theory of transgenic animals. Lab Anim 1997;26:29–34.

Pinkert CA. Transgenic Animal Technology: A Laboratory Handbook. San Diego: Academic Press, 1994.

Houdebine LM. Transgenic Animals: Generation and Use. Amsterdam: Harwood Academic Publishers, 1997.

# CHAPTER 22

# *Pharmacotoxicologic Factors and Reproduction*

A.E. ARCHIBONG AND S.E. ABDELGADIR

Livestock must be managed for optimum reproductive performance, and therefore maximum economic returns, if the industry must survive in today's economy. In cattle, and presumably in other livestock, it has been suggested that the principal economic factors, ranked from highest to lowest (10 being the highest) are: reproduction, 10; yearling weight, 3; carcass quality, 1. The correctness of these values can be debated, but if there is no reproduction, the other values have no meaning (1); thus, reproductive efficiency is one of the most important economic factors in livestock production. This section will discuss the effects of pharmacologic and toxicologic (contributing the pieces of the title word, "pharmaco" and "toxicologic") substances on livestock reproduction. At this juncture, it is important to place a distinction between toxins and toxicants. Toxins are poisonous substances of plant or animal origin, while toxicants are poisonous substances not necessarily of animal or plant origin. In short, toxins are toxicants but toxicants are not necessarily toxins.

## PLANTS THAT AFFECT MALE REPRODUCTION

Certain plants produce toxins/toxicants that perturb reproduction in sheep and presumably other grazing livestock (Table 22-1). The toxin swainsonine, from locoweed, directly inhibits testosterone synthesis and release in rams as confirmed by increased systemic LH (2). Inhibition of testosterone can delay puberty in juvenile animals and decrease libido in adult animals. Furthermore, reduced systemic testosterone impacts on spermatogenesis and epididymal sperm maturation as manifested by low sperm count and motility, respectively, in ejaculates of rams fed locoweeds (3). Plant and plant products, e.g., cotton and cotton seeds, produce gossypol which causes delayed testis development that culminates in delayed puberty (4). In adult animals, gossypol also causes a reduction in spermatogenesis which subsequently results in low sperm count and motility. Toxins in snakeweed cause a reduction in testis weight probably due to a reduction in spermatogenesis. It is not known whether these toxins act directly on the germinal epithelium to reduce spermatogenesis. However, it is possible that swiansonine-induced testosterone reduction contributes to reduced spermatogenesis. While swainsonine causes testicular degeneration, gossypol and toxins in snakeweed cause the production of morphologically abnormal forms of sperm in rodents fed diets containing toxins from snakeweed (5) or gossypol (6). Sperm with head and tail abnormalities penetrate cervical mucus poorly. Cervical mucus penetration by sperm is the first significant safeguard towards the transportation of sperm to the fertilization site (oviduct).

## PLANTS THAT AFFECT FEMALE REPRODUCTION

Plant toxins also perturb the reproductive efficiency of female animals (Table 22-2). Age at puberty is negatively correlated with growth rate, and any agent that retards growth will increase age at puberty. Mimosine, a toxin in a tropical leguminous shrub, can increase age at puberty in female animals. It acts by limiting iodine entrapment by the thyroid gland, which eventually results in goiter, reduced systemic thyroid hormone secretion, reduced appetite, and reduced growth rate (7, 8). Gossypol also increases age at puberty by reducing growth rate by rendering animals anorexic (6).

Pasture legumes (Red clover, Subterranean clover, Berseem clover, Soybean, Native American legume, Birdfoot trifoil) produce plant estrogens called *phytoestrogens*. These plant estrogens have certain similarities with 17$\beta$-estradiol, which presumably enable them to interact with nuclear

TABLE 22-1. *Effect of Toxic Plants on the Hormonal Milieu and Reproductive Characteristics of Male Animals*

| TOXIC PLANT/PRODUCT | HABITAT | TOXIN | EFFECT | LITERATURE SOURCE (REFERENCE NUMBER) |
|---|---|---|---|---|
| **Locoweeds** *Oxytropis sericea*, *Astragalus lentiginosis*, *A. pubentisimisus* | Western US | Swainsonine (an indolizine alkaloid) | Increased serum LH; decreased testosterone; decreased libido; low sperm count; low sperm motility | Ortiz et al. (2) Panter et al. (3) |
| **Snakeweed** *Gutierrezia microcephalia*, *G. sarothrae* | Desert ranges of Las Cruces, NM | Monoterpenes and diterpenes, triterpinoid saponins, highly oxygenated flavonal methyl esters, and unidentified alkaloids | Decreased testis weight; increased fraction of abnormal sperm | Edrington et al. (5) |
| **Cotton/cotton seed** *Gossypium spp.* | Southern US | Gossypol | Delayed puberty; low sperm count; sperm tail lesion; low sperm motility | Kramer et al. (4) Randel et al. (6) |

receptors for estrogen in target organs to exert estrogen-dependent processes in the brain, pituitary, and female reproductive system. The continuous grazing on phytoestrogen producing plants by livestock creates a syndrome called estrogenism that results in various forms of infertility. They cause a reduction in ovulation rates in animals probably by limiting the release of LH as well as reducing conception rates by maintaining continuous uterine contractility as a result of estrogen dominance. Toxins in snakeweed also cause inhibition in ovulation and consequently a reduction in circulating progesterone concentrations (9, 10). Other contributory factors to infertility due to phytoestrogenic activity include: prolapse of the vagina, an abnormal morphology of the vagina; irregular estrous cycles, and total anestrous in grazing animals; nymphomania accompanied by the swelling of the vulva, continuous cervical mucus discharge; enlargement of uterus; cystic endometrium; and mammary development (11–17).

Gossypol and toxins in snakeweed reduce ovulation and circulating progesterone concentrations probably because of their ability to inhibit the responsiveness of the ovaries to pituitary gonadotropins. Elevated LH and FSH have been demonstrated in animals exposed to gossypol (18–23), an indication of a compromise in the steroid biosynthetic regulatory mechanism and as a consequence, increased estrous cycle length and irregular estrous cycles. Swainsonine also contributes to infertility among grazing animals by inhibiting oogenesis and fertilization (1).

### *Plant Toxins That Have Teratogenic Effects on the Fetus*

Plant toxins have been shown to cross into the placenta and perturb embryonic and fetal development (Table 22-3) (1). Facial, skeletal, and trachial defects have been observed in ewes consuming false hellebore during the first trimester of gestation (24, 25). Cows consuming certain species of lupine during early and late first trimester of pregnancy can deliver calves with skeletal abnormalities and midline defects (cleft palate) (26). Consumption of poison hemlock and tree tobacco by ewes and does have produced fetal deformities similar to those described for cows ingesting lupine (27). Diagnostic ultrasound has been useful in the detection of fetotoxic effects of poisonous plants on fetal physiology; growth, and development (27, 28). By the use of this diagnostic tool, it was possible to detect the effects on the fetuses of the consumption of locoweed by pregnant ewes. Locoweed caused skeletal defects, and fetal edema enlargement of the right ventricle of the heart, indicative of congenital heart failure (1). Furthermore, consumption of selenium-accumulating species of pasture plants and ponderosa pine causes deformed hooves and low birth weight offspring, respectively.

### *Plants That Cause Embryonic Death and Abortion in Livestock*

Several plant toxins have the potential to cause embryonic or fetal wastage, or induce abortion in livestock. In many cases, abortion can occur in 100% of the animals consuming some of these plants (Table 22-4) (1). Locoweed has the potential to cause embryonic death, induce abortion, or cause delayed implantation if grazed by pregnant cattle, sheep, and horses. The incidence can range from low, rather insignificant levels to very high levels (1, 29). Snakeweed and ponderosa pine cause abortion and premature birth when cattle are grazed during the last trimester of gestation

TABLE 22-2. ***Effect of Toxic Plants on the Hormonal Milieu and Reproductive Characteristics of Female Animals***

| TOXIC PLANT | TOXIN | EFFECT | LITERATURE SOURCE (REFERENCE NUMBER) |
|---|---|---|---|
| **Tropical leguminous shrub** *Leucaena leucocephala* | Mimosine (alkaloid) | Altered plasma thyroxine | Quirk et al. (7) Jacquemet et al. (8) |
| Red clover *Trifolium pratense* **Subterranean clover** *T. subterraneum* **Berseem clover** *T. alexandanrinum* | Formononectin, genistein, biochanin A (phytoestrogens) | Reduced ovulation rate; reduced conception rate; prolapse of the vagina; discharge of cervical mucus; irregular estrus; anestrus; nymphomania | Alder and Trainin (11) Lockhart (13) Kallela et al. (15) Adam (17) |
| **Soybean** *Glycine spp.* | Isoflavones, mainly genistein, diadzein, glycetin, and coumestrol (phytoestrogens) | Infertility due to estrogenism—mammary development, vulvar swelling, discharge of cervical mucus, and enlargement of the uterus | Drane et al. (14) Sharma et al. (16) Adams (17) |
| **Native American legumes** *Vicia americana, Astragelus srotinus* | Phytoestrogen | Cystic endometrium | Gammie and Kitts (12) Adams (17) |
| **Birdfoot trifoil** *Lotus corniculatus* | Phytoestrogen | Cystic endometrium | Gammie and Kitts (12) Adams (17) |
| **Snakeweed** *Gutierrezia microcephalia, G. sarothrae* | Monoterpenes and diterpenes, triterpinoid saponins, highly oxygenated flavonal methyl esters, and unidentified alkaloids | Reduced ovulation rate; reduced circulating progesterone | Flores-Rodriguez et al. (9) Smith et al. (10) |
| **Cotton/cotton seed** *Gossypium spp.* | Gossypol | Anorexia; reduced growth rate; increased serum FSH; increased LH; reduced estrogen; reduced progesterone; increased estrous cycle length; irregular estrous cycles | Wu et al. (18) Gu and Anderson (19) Lagerloof and Tone (20) Lin et al. (21) Bender et al. (22) Gu et al. (23) |
| **Locoweeds** *Oxytropis sericea, Astragalus lentiginosis, A. pubentisimisus* | Swainsonine (an indolizidine alkaloid) | Inhibited oogenesis; reduced fertilization | James et al. (1) |

(30, 31), whereas locoweed can induce abortion at any stage of pregnancy (1). Toxin(s) in false hellebore causes embryonic and fetal death if grazed by pregnant ewes, (32) while that in little leaf horsebrush has the potential to induce abortion (1). In vivo and *in vitro* exposure of swine and bovine embryos, respectively, to gossypol reduced blastocyst formation (6, 33). The reduced litter size observed in pigs fed a gossypol containing diet was attributed to reduced conception rates (34).

## MYCOTOXINS AND MALE REPRODUCTION

Molds are parasitic plants that thrive on pasture grasses and common livestock feedstuffs. Not only do molds reduce the quality of grains, they also produce toxins called mycotoxins which impair growth and reproductive efficiency. Molds capable of synthesizing mycotoxins have been identified on tall fescue grass, ryegrass, American tropical morning glory, sleepy grass, corn, cereal grains, and peanuts. The effects of the various types of mycotoxins and their effects are summarized in Table 22-5. Endophytic molds that infect the aforementioned pasture crops and grains produce toxins called ergot alkaloids, among whose effects (ergotism) include perturbation of reproductive efficiency. In rams, ergot alkaloids caused a reduction in systemic prolactin (PRL) (35, 36) through their action on doperminergic and antiserotonergic activities (37). The ergot-induced reduction in systemic PRL causes the reduction of precusors (e.g. cholesterol) available for conversion to testosterone by the Leydig cells (38). These alkaloids also cause reduced testicular

TABLE 22-3. ***Plants That Have Teratogenic Effects on the Fetus***

| TOXIC PLANT | TOXIN | EFFECT | LITERATURE SOURCE (REFERENCE NUMBER) |
|---|---|---|---|
| **False hellebore** *Veratrum californicum* | Jervine, cyclopamide (steroidal alkaloid) | Facial defects; skeletal defects; tracheal defects | Keeler et al. (24) Keeler and Stewart (25) |
| **Lupine** *Lupinus spp.* | Anagyne (quinolizine alkaloid), ammodendrine (piperidine alkaloid) | Skeletal defects; cleft palate | Shupe et al. (26) |
| **Poison hemlock** *Conium maculatum* | Coniine, $\gamma$-coniceine (piperidine alkaloid) | Skeletal defects | Panther et al. (27) |
| **Locoweeds** *Oxytropis sericea, Astragalus lentiginosis, A. pubentisimisus* | Swainsonine (indolizidine alkaloid) | Skeletal defects; fetal edema; enlarged right ventricle of the heart | James et al. (1) |
| **Tree tobacco** *Nicotiana spp.* | Anabasine (piperidine alkaloid) | Skeletal defects; cleft palate | Panther et al. (27) |
| **Selenium accumulating species** | Selenium | Deformed hooves | James et al. (1) |
| **Ponderosa pine** *Pinus ponderosa* | Unknown | Low birth weight | James et al. (1) |

growth (35). Alamer and Erikson (39) reported that endophyte produced alkaloids reduced gonadotropin-releasing hormone (GnRH)-stimulated testosterone secretion, via the inhibition of gonadotropin secretion, and also cause a reduction in the population of Sertoli cells in 3-month-old beef bulls. Taken together, ergot alkaloids inhibit the release of GnRH from the hypothalamus, thereby preventing anterior pituitary gonadotropin secretion and testicular steroidogenesis, which in turn results in delayed puberty in juvenile animals and infertility in adult male animals. Reduced feed intake and reduced weight gain (ADG) in juvenile animals caused by ergot alkaloids (36), and other mycotoxins like

TABLE 22-4. ***Plant Toxins That Cause Embryonic Death and Abortion in Livestock***

| TOXIC PLANT | TOXIN | EFFECT | LITERATURE SOURCE (REFERENCE NUMBER) |
|---|---|---|---|
| **Locoweeds** *Oxytropis sericea, Astragalus lentiginosis, A. pubentisimisus* | Swainsonone (indolizidine alkaloid) | Abortion; embryonic death; delayed placentation | James et al. (29) |
| **Snakeweed** *Gutierrezia microcephalia, G. sarothrae* | Monoterpenes and diterpenes, triterpinoid saponins, highly oxygenated flavonal methyl esters, and unidentified alkaloids | Abortion; premature birth | Kingsbury (30) |
| **Ponderosa pine** *Pinus ponderosa* | Unknown | Abortion; premature birth | James et al. (29) |
| **Little leaf horsebrush** *Tetradymia glabrata* | Unknown | Abortion | James et al. (31) |
| **False hellebore** *Veratrum californicum* | Jervine, cyclopamide (steroidal alkaloid) | Embryonic death; fetal death | Binns et al. (32) |
| **Cotton/cotton seed** *Gossypium spp.* | Gossypol | Reduced blastocyst formation and retarded embryo growth; abortion; reduced conception rates; reduced litter size | Randel et al. (6) Lin et al. (21) Ziekle et al. (33) Eisele (34) |

TABLE 22-5. *Effect of Mycotoxins on the Hormonal Milieu and Reproductive Characteristics of Male Animals*

| TOXIC FUNGUS | HOST | MYCOTOXIN | EFFECT | LITERATURE SOURCE (REFERENCE NUMBER) |
|---|---|---|---|---|
| *Acremonium coeniphialum,* tall fescue endophyte<br>*A. lolii,* ryegrass endophyte<br>*Claviceps purpurea* | *Festuca armundinacae*<br>**Tall fescue grass**<br>*Lolium perenne*<br>**Ryegrass, grains (corn, wheat)**<br>*Ipomoea violacae, Rivea corymbosa*<br>**American tropical morning glory**<br>*Stipa robusta, S. vaseyi*<br>**Sleepy grass** | Ergot alkaloids | Low systemic PRL; low systemic GnRH; low serum cholesterol; low serum testosterone; delayed testis growth; reduced Sertoli cells; reduced feed intake; reduced ADG; increased rectal temperature | Barenton and Pelletier (35)<br>Erikson (39)<br>Porter and Thompson (36)<br>Aldrich et al. (42) |
| *Fusarium roseum, Aspergillis flavus* | **Corn** | Zearalenone (phytoestrogens) | Low serum testosterone; reduced testis, epididymis, and vesicular weight; azoospermia; reduced libido | Dieckman and Green (40) |
| *Gibberella zaea* | **Cereal grains, corn, peanuts** | Aflatoxins | Reduced feed efficiency and growth rate | Dieckman and Green (40) |
| *Aspergillis ochraceus, Penicillium viridicatum* | **A variety of foodstuffs** | Ochratoxins | Poor ADG | Harvey et al. (41) |

aflatoxins (40) and ochratoxins (41), can also cause delayed puberty as previously explained. Aldrich (42) showed that Holstein steers maintained on endophyte diet suffered from hyperthermia because of ergot-induced compromise in their thermoregulatory mechanism, particularly in the summer months. A rise in body temperature normally results in a rise in testicular temperature accompanied with infertility resulting from temperature influenced reduction in spermatogenesis and the production of abnormal morphologic forms of sperm.

Consumption of corn containing zearalenone (ZEN; phytoestrogens) by immature boars results in reduced testis weight (43), and in conjunction with ZEN's ability to reduce testosterone production (44), this mycotoxin can delay puberty. Reduced testis weight was observed in boars that received ZEN diet (45), an indication of infertility resulting from ZEN-induced cessation in spermatogenesis (46). Zearalenone also causes a reduction in epididymis, vesicular gland weights, and libido (44, 45), further indices of infertility, due to a concomitant reduction in testosterone secretion.

## MYCOTOXINS AND FEMALE REPRODUCTION

As in male animals, mycotoxins also impact on reproduction in female livestock (Table 22-6). Consumption of ergot alkaloids from endophyte-infected tall fescue has been observed to reduce ADG in beef heifers (47), and consequently to delay puberty. Other consumable mycotoxins not of endophyte sources that cause a delay in puberty by reducing feed efficiency and growth rate are deoxynivalentol (DON) (48–50) and aflatoxins (40).

The consumption of endophyte-infected fescue inhibits the release of PRL from the pituitary and as a result, a reduction in plasma PRL in ewes (51), beef cows (52), and mares (53–55), which in turn reduces the stimulatory effect of PRL on follicular steroidogenesis (56) and corpora lutea function (57). Because of altered follicular and luteal steroidogenesis, animals exhibit delayed estrus, reduced conception rates, embryonic mortality, and reduced birth rates (58–63).

Despite their structural dissimilarities with steroidal estrogens, ZEN and several of its derivatives possess estrogenic activity to which the prepubertal gilt is the most sensitive of domesticated animals (40). The genital tracts of immature gilts undergo gross and histologic changes after exposure to ZEN. Gross changes include tumefaction of the vulva, increased size and weight of the uterus, and mammary enlargement (64). In extreme cases, rectal and vaginal prolapses do occur (64, 65). Microscopic changes include edema and thickening of the uterus caused by a combination of hypertrophy and hyperplasia of both endometrium and myometrium. The hyperestrogenism imposed by ZEN has been

Table 22-6. ***Effect of Mycotoxins on the Hormonal Milieu and Reproductive Characteristics of Female Animals***

| Toxic Fungus | Host | Mycotoxin | Effect | Literature Source (Reference Number) |
|---|---|---|---|---|
| *Acremonium coeniphialum*, tall fescue endophyte<br>*A. lolii*, ryegrass endophyte<br>*Claviceps purpurea* | *Festuca armundinacae*<br>**Tall fescue grass**<br>*Lolium perenne*<br>**Ryegrass, grains (corn, wheat)**<br>*Ipomoea violacae*, *Rivea corymbosa*<br>**American tropical morning glory**<br>*Stipa robusta*, *S. vaseyi*<br>**Sleepy grass** | Ergot alkaloids | Reduced ADG; delayed puberty; low systemic PRL; delayed onset of estrus; reduced conception rate; embryonic mortality; decreased calving rates | Bond and Bolt (47)<br>Washburn and Green (63)<br>Bolt et al. (51)<br>Bond et al. (59)<br>Beer and Piper (60)<br>Gay et al. (61)<br>Mizinga et al. (62) |
| *Fusarium roseum*, *Aspergillis flavus* | **Corn** | Deoxynivalenool | Reduced ADG | Forsyth et al. (48)<br>Long and Diekman (49)<br>Trenholm et al. (50) |
| *Fusarium roseum*, *Aspergillis flavus* | **Corn** | Zearalenone (phytoestrogens) | Gross histologic changes in reproductive system of immature gilts; delayed pubertal estrus; extended estrus cycles; pseudopregnancy and inferility | Young et al. (64)<br>Blaney et al. (65)<br>Edwards et al. (66, 69)<br>Flowers et al. (68) |
| *Gibberella zaea* | **Cereal grains, corn, peanuts** | Aflatoxins | Reduced feed efficiency and growth rate | Dieckman and Green (40) |

shown to delay pubertal estrus (66). Exposure of cycling gilts to ZEN causes multiple reproductive dysfunctions. Chang et al. (67) reported that feeding ZEN from the time of weaning continuously throughout the next gestation produced constant estrus, peudopregnancy, and ultimately, infertility. Flowers et al. (68) extended the interval between estrus by administering ZEN on day 6 to 10 or day 11 to 15 of the estrous cycle. Similar results were observed when ZEN was fed to gilts between days 5 and 20 of the estrous cycle (69). Furthermore, luteal function was maintained as manifested by high serum progesterone concentrations on day 19 to 21 for those gilts with extended cycles. The persistent corpora lutea regressed 30 days after ZEN was removed from the diet.

## Mycotoxins and Embryonic Death, Fetal Death, and Abortion in Livestock

Gilts fed low doses of ZEN from day 2 to 15 postmating had normal embryonic development. However, those that received a higher dose of ZEN had no fetuses at day 40 to 43 postmating (70), and sows that consume ZEN from breeding until expected parturition failed to maintain their pregnancy (71). Zearalenone added to diets of pregnant sows caused them to farrow small litters with smaller than normal offspring (67). Also intramuscular injection of this mycotoxin in sows and a gilts each day during the last month of pregnancy caused stillbirths and splayed legs in live piglets (72).

## Agricultural Pesticides and Male Reproduction

Agricultural pesticides, intended for preventing, destroying, repelling, or mitigating any pests that infest livestock and crops have adverse effects on reproduction. Dibromochloropropane (DBCP) is a brominated organochloride used as a nematocide, for the protection of cash crops, particularly soybeans (73), which is a major component of livestock and poultry feed. Exposure of male animals to DBCP causes degenerative changes in the seminiferous tubules and epi-

TABLE 22-7. *Effect of Agricultural Chemical on Male Reproduction*

| CHEMICAL | USE | EFFECT | LITERATURE SOURCE (REFERENCE NUMBER) |
|---|---|---|---|
| Dibromochloropropane | Nematocide | Increased Sertoli cell numbers; degeneration of seminiferous tubules; oligospermia; increased population of abnormal morphologic forms of sperm; inhibition of sperm motility | Torkelson et al. (74)<br>Kluwe (75)<br>Kluwe et al. (76) |
| Chlordecone | Insecticide and fungicide | Increased serum testosterone; irregular LH profile; reduced seminal vesicle weight; reduced sperm motility; reduced sperm viability | Hammond et al. (77)<br>Linder et al. (78) |
| Ethylene dibromide | Feed and corn fumigant | Impaired spermatogenesis; Leydig cell metabolism of compound may produce metabolites that compromise its function; reduced seminal vesicle weight | Hurtts and Zenick (79)<br>Kowalski et al. (80) |

didymal dysfunction (Table 22-7). Degenerative changes caused by this toxicant include an increase in Sertoli cells, oligozoospermia, and an increase in the population of abnormal morphologic forms of sperm (74, 75). The aspects of epididymal function disrupted by exposure of animals to DBCP include the reduction of sperm motility, and therefore infertility (76).

Chlordecone, better known by the trade name Kepone, was manufactured for use as insecticide. Consumption of this compound by animals causes a disruption in endocrine milieu and epididymal function (Table 22-7). Increased systemic concentrations of testosterone, irregular LH profile, reduced seminal vesicle weights (77), and reduced sperm motility and viability (78) followed consumption of chlorde-

TABLE 22-8. *Effect of Agricultural Chemical on Female Reproduction*

| CHEMICAL | USE | EFFECT | LITERATURE SOURCE (REFERENCE NUMBER) |
|---|---|---|---|
| DDT | Insecticide | Precocious puberty; increased uterine weight; thickened, vacuolated uterine epithelium; cornified vaginal epithelium; reduced LH; reduced granulosa progesterone production; nymphomania with anovulation | Heinrichs et al. (81)<br>Gellert et al. (82)<br>Ottoboni et al. (83)<br>Haney et al.(84) |
| Methoxychlor | Insecticide | Decreased fecundity | Cummings and Gray (87) |
| Organophosphates | Insecticide | Reduced LH; reduced conception | Rattner and Michael (88) |
| Carbamates | Insecticide | Reduced gonadotropins; prolonged estrous cycle; inhibition of oocyte maturation; reduction in ovarian and uterine weight; reduced embryo numbers per pregnancy | Ghizelea and Czeranschi (90)<br>Krylova et al. (91)<br>Bentue-Ferrer et al. (89) |
| Chlordecone | Insecticide and fungicide | Increased uterine weight; thickened, vacuolated uterine epithelium; cornified vaginal epithelium; enhancement of uterine protein synthesis; nymphomania | Uphouse et al. (85)<br>Heinz et al. (86) |
| Hexachlorobenzene (HCB) | Fungicide | Decreased litter size; increased incidence of stillbirth | Grant et al. (92) |

cone. Mating of females with chlordecone-exposed males was observed to result in small litters (77).

Ethylene dibromide (EDB), a fumigant for feed and corn, also adversely affects the male reproductive system (Table 22-7). The consumption of high doses of this fumigant impairs spermatogenesis by causing a decrease in testicular spermatid count and epididymis weight and subsequently, a reduction in the weight of the seminal vesicles (79). The decreased seminal vesicular weight implies the effect of EDB either on the hypothalamo-pituitary-Leydig cell pathway controlling testosterone secretion or on the sex accessory gland itself. At least some involvement of the Leydig cells has been suggested, based on the ability of this tissue to activate EDB to metabolites that become bound to the same tissue (80). Whether or not these metabolites interfere with the ability of the cells of Leydig to produce and secrete testosterone remains a question that needs to be answered.

## AGRICULTURAL PESTICIDES AND FEMALE REPRODUCTION

DDT, an organochloride, and chlordecone, a cyclodiene, are insecticides with estrogenic properties in mammals, thus creating hyperestrogenism and adverse female reproductive outcomes similar to those described for phytoestrogens (Table 22-8) (81–86). Another effect exerted by DDT, apart from those similar to phytoestrogens, is the initiation of precocious puberty in juvenile female animals. Methoxychlor is an insecticide with much lower acute toxicity than DDT but also has estrogenic properties with adverse effects on the uterus. It is conceivable that this toxicant decreases fecundity by preventing implantation (87).

Organophosphates and carbamates affect female reproduction by causing a reduction in serum concentrations of pituitary gonadotropins (Table 22-8). Organophosphates selectively cause a reduction in serum LH which in turn reduces ovulation and conception rates (88). Carbamates, however, cause a reduction in serum concentrations of both FSH and LH (89) and consequently cause reduced ovarian weight due to reduced follicular development. Furthermore, estrous cycles become prolonged and oocyte maturation ceases. If ovulations occurred at all, their rate, number of embryos, and pregnancy remain low (90, 91). Because of the reduction in folliculogenesis, it is conceivable that the reduced uterine weight resulting from exposure of animals to carbamates (90) is due to reduced exposure of the uterus to ovarian estrogens.

Hexachlorobenzene, a pre-emergence fungicide, affects reproduction in the female. It is embryotoxic in pregnant females, and as a consequence reduces litter size and increases the incidence of stillbirth in animals (Table 22-8) (92).

## REFERENCES


1. James LF, Panter KE, Nielsen DB, Molyneux RJ. The effect of natural toxins on reproduction in livestock. J Anim Sci 1992;70:1573.
2. Ortiz AR, Hallford DM, Galyean ML, Schneider FA, Kridli RT. Effect of locoweed (*Oxytropis sericea*) on growth, reproduction and serum hormone profiles in young rams. J Anim Sci 1997;75:3229–3234.
3. Panter KE, James LF. Transient testicular degeneration in rams fed locoweed (*Astragalus lentiginosus*). Vet Hum Toxicol 1989;31:42.
4. Kramer RY, Garner DL, Erisson SA, Wesson DA, Downing TW, Redilman D. The effect of cottonseed component on testicular development in pubescent rams. Vet Hum Toxicol 1991;33:11.
5. Edrington TS, Flores-Rodriguez GI, Smith GS, Hallford DM. Effect of ingested snakeweed (Gutierrezia microcephala) foliage on reproduction, semen quality and serum clinical profiles of male rats. J Anim Sci 1993;71:1520.
6. Randel RD, Chase CC, Wise SJ. Effect of gossypol and cottonseed products on reproduction of mammals. J Anim Sci 1992; 70:1628.
7. Quirk MF, Bushnell JJ, Jones RJ, Megarrity RG, Butler KL. Live-weight gains on leucaena and native grass pastures after dosing cattle with rumen bacteria capable of degrading 2,3-DHP, a rumenal metabolite of leucaena. J Agric Sci (Camb) 1988;111:165.
8. Jacquemet N, Fernandez JM, Sahlu T, Lu CD. Mohair and metabolic profile of angora goats during acute mimosine toxicity. J Anim Sci 1990;68(Suppl 1):400 (Abst).
9. Flores-Rodriguez GI, Smith GS, McDaniel KC. Effects of ingested snakeweek (*Gutierrezia microcephala)* herbage on reproduction, serum progesterone and blood constituents of female albino rats. Proc West Sec Am Soc Anim Sci 1989; 40:217.
10. Smith GS, Ross TT, Flores-Rodriguez GI, Oetting BC, Edrington TS. Toxicology of snakeweeds, *Gutierrezia microcephala* and G. *sarathrae*. In: James LF, Evans JO, Ralphs MH, Child RD, eds.. Noxious Range Plants. Boulder, CO: Westview Press, 1991;23:236–246.
11. Adler JH, Trainin D. A hyperestrogenic syndrome in cattle. Rafuah Vet 1960;17:115.
12. Gammie JS, Kitts WD. Phytoestrogen activity of two species of native B.C. legumes. J Anim Sci 1972;43:914(abstr).
13. Lookhart GL. Analysis of coumestrol, a plant estrogen, in animal feeds by high-performance liquid chromatography. J Agric Food Chem 1980;28:666.
14. Drane HM, Wrathall AE, Patterson DSP, Hebert CN. Possible estrogenic effects of feeding soyameal to prepubertal gilts. Br Vet J 1981;137:283.
15. Kallela K, Heinonen K, Saloniemi H. Plant estrogens: the cause of decreased fertility in cows. A case report. Nord Veterinaermed 1984;36:124.
16. Sharma OMP, Adlercreutz H, Strandberg JD, Zirkin BR, Coffee DS, Ewing LL. Soy of dietary source plays a preventive role against the pathogenesis of prostatitis in rats. J Steroid Biochem Molec Biol 1992;43:557.

17. Adams NR. Detection of the effects of phytoestrogens on sheep and cattle. J Anim Sci 1995;73:1509.
18. Wu YM, Chappel SC, Flickinger GL. Effects of gossypon on pituitary-ovarian endocrine function, ovulation and fertility in female hamsters. Contraception 1981;24:259.
19. Gu Y, Anderson NO. Effects of gossypol on the estrous cycle and ovarian weight in the rat. Contraception 1985;32: 491.
20. Lagerloof RK, Tone JA. The effect of gossypol acetic acid on female reproduction. Drug Chem Toxicol 1985;8:469.
21. Lin YC, Fukaya T, Rikihisa Y, Walton A. Gossypol in female fertility control: ovumimplantation and early pregnancy inhibited in rats. Life Sci 1985;37:39.
22. Bender HS, Saunders GK, Misra HP. A histopathologic study of the effects of gossypol on the female rats. Contraception 1988;38:585.
23. Gu Y, Lin YC, Rikihisa Y. Inhibitory effect of gossypol on steroidogenesis pathways in cultured bovine and luteal cells. Biochem Biophys Res Commun 1990;169:455.
24. Keeler RF, Young S, Smart R. Congenital tracheal stenosis in lambs induced by maternal ingestion of *Veratrum californicum*. Teratology 1985;31:83.
25. Keeler RF, Stuart LD. The nature of congenital limb defects induced in lambs by maternal ingestion of *Veratrum californicum*. Clin Toxicol 1987;25:273.
26. Shupe JL, Binns W, James LF, Keeler RF. Lupine, a cause of crooked calf disease. J Am Vet Med Assoc 1967;151:198.
27. Panther KE, Keeler RF, Bunch TD, Callan RJ. Congenital skeletal malformations and cleft palate induced in goats by ingestion of Lupinus, Conium and Nicotiana species. Toxicon 1990;28:1377.
28. Panther KE, Bunch TD, James LF, Sisson DC. Ultrasonographic imaging to monitor fetal and placental developments in ewes fed locoweed (*Astragalus lentiginosus*). Am J Vet Res 1987;48:686.
29. James LF, Shupe JL, Binns W, Keeler RF. Abortive and teratogenic effects of locoweed on sheep and cattle. Am J Vet Res 1967;28:1379.
30. Kingsbury J. Poisonous plants of the United States and Canada. Englewood Cliffs, NJ: Prentice-Hall, 1964.
31. James LF, Short RE, Panter KE, Molyneux RJ, Stuart LD, Bellows RA. Pine needle abortions in cattle: a review and report of 1973-1984 research. Cornell Vet 1989;79:39.
32. Binns W, James LF, Shipe JL, Everett G. A congenital cyclopian-type malformation in lambs induced by a range plant, Veratrum californicum. Am J Vet Res 1963;24:1164.
33. Ziekle SM, Lin YC, Gwazdauskas FC, Canseco RS. Effect of gossypol on bovine embryo development during the preplantation period. Theriogenology 1988;30:575.
34. Eisele GR. A perspective on gossypol ingestion in swine. Vet Hum Toxicol 1986;28:118.
35. Barenton B, Pelletier J. Prolactin, testicular growth and LH receptors in the ram following light and 2-Br-alpha-ergocryptine (CD-154) treatments. Biol Reprod 1980,22:781.
36. Porter JK, Thompson FN. Effects of fescue toxicity on reproduction in livestock. J Anim Sci 1992;70:1594.
37. Berde B, Schild HO. The ergot alkaloids and related compounds. In: Handbook of Experimental Pharmacology. Vol 49. New York: Springer-Verlag, 1978.
38. Bartke A. Pituitary-testis relationships: role of prolactin in the regulation of testis function. In: Hubinont PO, ed. Progress in Reproductive Biology. Basel: Karger, 1976;1:136.
39. Almar MA, Erickson BH. Effect of fungus-infested fescue on testicular development and hormonal secretions in beef bulls. J Anim Sci 1990;68(Suppl 1):402(Abstr).
40. Diekman MA, Green ML. Mycotoxins and reproduction in domestic livestock. J Anim Sci 1992;70:1615.
41. Harvey RB, Huff WE, Kubena LF, Phillips TD. Evaluation of diets co-contaminated with aflatoxin and ochratoxin fed to growing pigs. J Am Vet Res 1989;50:1400.
42. Aldrich CG, Paterson JA, Tate JL, Kerley MS. The effects of endophyte-infected tall fescue consumption on diet utilization and thermal regulation. J Anim Sci 1993;71:164.
43. Christensen CM, Mirocha CJ, Nelson GH, Quast JF. Effect on young swine of consumption of rations corn invaded by *Fusarium roseum*. Appl Microbiol 1972;23:202.
44. Berger T, Esbenshade KL, Diekman MA, Hoagland, J Tuite. Influence of prepubertal consumption of Zearalenone on sexual development of boars. J Anim Sci 1981;53:1559.
45. Palyusik M. Effect of zearalenone Fusareum toxin on the prostate gland of swine. Acta Microbiol Acad Sci Hung 1977; 24:104.
46. Vanyi A, Szeky A. Fusariotoxicisis 6. The effect of F-2 toxin (zearalenone) on the spermatogenesis of male swine. Magy Allatorv Lapja 1980;35:242.
47. Bond J, Bolt DJ. Growth, plasma prolactin and ovarian activity in heifers grazing fungus-infected fescue. Nutr Rep Int 1986; 34:93.
48. Forsyth DM, DeUriate LA, Tuite J. Improvement for swine in Gibberella zeaedamaged corn by washing. J Anim Sci 1977;42:1202.
49. Long GG, Diekman MA. Characterization of effects of zearalenone in swine during early pregnancy. A J Vet Res 1986; 47:184.
50. Trenholm HL, Hamilton RM, Friend DW, Thompson BK, Hartin KE. Feeding trials with vomitoxin (deoxynivalenone)-contaminated wheat: effects on swine, poultry and dairy cattle. JAMA 1984;185:527.
51. Bolt DJ, Bond J, Lynch CP, Elsasser T. Concentrations of PRL, LH, FSH, GH and TSH in plasma and pituitary of ewes grazing tall fescue and orchardgrass pastures. J Anim Sci 1982;55(Suppl 1):4(Abstr).
52. Christopher GK, Salfen BE, Schmidt SP, et al. Effects of grazing Kentucky-31 tall fescue infected with Acremonium coenophialium on endocrine function in ovariectomized beef heifers. J Anim Sci 1990;68(Suppl 1):469(Abstr).
53. Monroe JL, Cross DL, Hudson LW, Hendricks DM, Kennedy SW, Bridges WC. Effects of selenium and endophyte contaminated fescue on the performance and reproduction in mares. Equine Vet Sci 1988;8:148.
54. McCann JS, Caudle AB, Thompson FN, Stuedeman JA, Heusner GH, Thompson DL. Hormonal and behavioral responses of gestating mares to low and highly infected tall fescue. Stillwater, OK: Equine Nutr And Physiol Symp 199, 1989.
55. McCann JS, Caudle AB, Thompson FN, Stuedeman JA, Heusner GH, Thompson DL. Influence of endophyte-infected tall fescue on serum prolactin and progesterone in gravid mares. J Anim Sci 1992;70:217.
56. Veldhius JD, Klase PA, Hammond JM. Divergent effects of prolactin upon steroidogenesis by porcine granulosa cells

in vitro: Influence of cytodifferentiation. Endocrinology 1980; 107:42–46.

57. Smith SM. Role of prolactin in regulating gonadotropin secretion and gonadal function in female rats. Fed Proc 1980; 39:2571.
58. Bond J, Hawk HW, Lynch GP, Jackson C. Lower fertility in ewes grazing tall fescue pastures. J Anim Sci 1982;55(Suppl 1):46(Abstr).
59. Bond J, Lynch GP, Holt JD, Hawk HW, Jackson C. Reproductive performance and lamb weight gains for ewes grazing fungus-infected tall fescue. Nutr Rep Int 1988;37:1099.
60. Beer KW, Piper EL. Effects of grazing endophyte infected fescue on heifers growth, calving rate and calf birth weight of first calf heifer. Arkansas Farm Res 1987;36:7.
61. Gay N, Boling JA, Dew R, Miksch DE. Effects of endophyte-infected tall fescue on beef cow-calf performance. Appl Agric Rec 1988;3:182.
62. Mizinga KM, Thompson FN, Stuedeman JA, Kizer TE, Smith CK, Powell RG. Effect of endophyte infected seed on endocrine function, body weight and milk production in postpartum beef cows. J Anim Sci 1990;68(Suppl 1):402(Abst).
63. Washburn SP, Green JT. Performance of replacement beef heifers on endophyte infected fescue pastures. In: Proc 40th Annu Conf North Carolina Cattlemen's Assoc. February 25–26, 1991. Raleigh, NC: North Carolina State University, 1991.
64. Young LG, Vesonder RF, Funnel HS, Simmons I, Wilcock B. Moldy corn in diets of swine. J Anim Sci 1981;52:1312.
65. Blaney BJ, Bloomfield RC, Moore CJ. Zearalenone intoxication in pigs. Aust Vet J 1984;61:24.
66. Edwards S, Cantley TC, Day BN. The effect of zearalenone on reproduction in swine. II. The effect of puberty attainment and postweaning rebreeding performance. Theriogenology 1987;28:51.
67. Chang K, Kurtz HJ, Mirocha CJ. Effects of the mycotoxin zearalenone on swine reproduction. Am J Vet Res 1979; 40:1260.
68. Flowers B, Cantley BT, Day BN. A comparison of effects of zearalenone and estradiol benzoate on reproductive function during the estrous cycle in gilts. J Anim Sci 1987;65: 1576.
69. Edwards S, Cantley TC, Rottinghaus GE, Osweiler GD, Day BN. The effect of zearalenone on reproduction in swine. I. The relationship between ingested zearalenone dose and anestrus in non-pregnant, sexually mature gilts. Theriogenology 1987;28:43.
70. Long GG, Diekman MA. Effect of purified aearalenone on early gestation in gilts. J Anim Sci 1984;59:1662.
71. Christensen CM. Zearalenone. In: Shimoda, ed. Conference on Mycotoxins in Animal Feeds and Grains Related to Animal Health. Rockville, MD: Food and Drug Administration, 1979;35–45.
72. Miller JK, Hacking A, Gross VJ. Stillbirths, neonatal mortality and small litters in pigs associated with the ingestion of Fusarium toxin by pregnant sows. Vet Res 1973;93:555.
73. Whorton MD, Foliart DE. Mutagenicity, carcinogenicity, and reproductive effects of dibromochloropropane (DBCP). Mut Res 1983;123:13.
74. Torkelson TR, Sadek SR, Rowe VK, et al. Toxicologic investigation of 1,2-dibromo-3-chloropropane. Toxicol Appl Pharmacacol 1961;3:545.
75. Kluwe WM. Acute toxicity of 1,2-dibromo-3-chloropropane in the F344 male rat. II. Development and repair of the renal, epididymal, testicular, and hepatic lesions. Toxicol Appl Pharmacol 1981;59:84.
76. Kluwe WM, Gupta BN, Lamb JC IV. The comparative effects of 1,2-dibromo-3-choloropropane (DBCP)-induced infertility in male rates mediated by post-testicular effect. Toxicol Appl Pharmacol 1983;71:294.
77. Hammond B, Bahr J, McConnei J, Metcalf R. Reproductive toxicology of mirex and Kepone. Fed Roc 1978;37:501.
78. Linder RE, Scotti TM, McElroy WK, Laskey JW, Strader LF, Powell K. Spermatoxicity and tissue accumulation of chlordecone (Kepone) in male rats. J Toxicol Environ Health 1983;12:183.
79. Hurtts M, Zenick H. The spermatotoxic effects of ethylene dibromide (EDB). Toxicologist 1985;5:114.
80. Kowalski B, Brittebo EB, Brandt I. Epithelial binding of 1,2-dibromoethane in the respiratory and upper alimentary tracts of mice and rats. Cancer Res 1985;45:2616.
81. Heinrichs WL, Gellert RJ, Bakke JL, Lawrence NL. DDT administered to neo-natal rats induces persistent estrus syndrome. Science 1971;173:642.
82. Gellert RJ, Heinrichs WL, Swerdloff RS. DDT homologues: Estrogen like effects on the vagina, uterus and pituitary of the rat. Endicronology 1972;9:1095.
83. Ottoboni A, Bissell GD, Hexter AC. Effects of DDT on reproduction in multiple generations of beagle dogs. Arch Environ Contam Toxicol 1977;6:83.
84. Haney AF, Hughes SF, Hughes CL. Screening of potential reproductive toxicants by use of porcine granulosa cell cultures. Toxicology 1984;30:227.
85. Uphouse L, Eckols K, Sierra V, Kolodziej M, Brown H. Failure of chlordecone (Kepone) to induce behavioral estrus in adult ovariectomized rats. Neurotoxicology 1986;7:127.
86. Heinz GW, Rourke AW, Bradley TM. The influence of chlordecone and estrogen on the secretion of proteinaceous molecules of the mouse uterus. Environ Pollut 1987;46:297.
87. Cummings AM, Gray LE Jr. Methoxychlor affects the decidual cell response of the uterus but not other progestational parameters in female rats. Toxicol Appl Pharmacol 1987;90:330.
88. Rattner BA, Michael SD. Organophosphorus insecticide induced secrease in plasma luteinizing hormone concentration in white-footed mice Peromyscus-leucopus-noveboracensis. Toxicol Lett 1985;24:65.
89. Bentue-Ferrer D, Allain H, Reymann JM, Van Den Driessche J. Study of 3 biocides—bimethoate, parathion-ethyl and zineb—on female rat neuro-endocrinological balance. Toxicol Eur Res 1981;3:279.
90. Ghizelea G, Czeranschi L. Influence of the carbamate pesticides zineb and thiram on the estrous and reproductive capacity of white rats. Stud Cercet Endocrinol 1973;24:491.
91. Krylova TV, Shilova SA, Krylov DG, Denisova AV, Smirnov AA. Consequences of using a pesticide affecting the reproductive function of mammals. Zool Zh 1975;54:1874.
92. Grant DL, Phillips WEJ, Hatina GV. Effect of hexacholorobenzene on reproduction in the rat. Arch Environ Contam Toxicol 1977;5:207.

CHAPTER 23

# Immunology of Reproduction

P.J. HANSEN

The inner lining of the female reproductive tract is continuous with the external environment of the animal. Thus, like other organ systems such as the respiratory and gastrointestinal tracts, tissues of the reproductive tract are repeatedly subjected to invasion by microbiologic organisms. Mating leads to microbial contamination because the penis and sometimes the seminal plasma contains microorganisms. At parturition, the cervix is distended and placental tissues can provide a passage for movement of microorganisms into the uterus. Other mechanical or environmental insults may also lead to introduction of microbes into the reproductive tract. Despite these microbial invasions, microorganisms can be rapidly removed from the reproductive tract (Fig. 23-1) and the tract usually remains free from infection. A sterile environment in the reproductive tract is maintained by the presence of an effective antimicrobial defense system that includes physical barriers, **phagocytes** that engulf and kill microorganisms, B **lymphocytes** that produce antibodies against invading microbes, and T lymphocytes that can kill virus and bacteria-infected host cells. Immunologically, the reproductive tract shares many features in common with the mucosal immune system found in the tissues lining the gastrointestinal and respiratory tracts.

Immune function in the reproductive tract is regulated by hormones to maximize antimicrobial function during estrus, when the likelihood of microbial challenge is high, and to reduce immune function during periods of elevated progesterone secretion, when deposition of microbes as part of the mating process is unlikely and when the **conceptus** is present in the uterus. The foreign nature of the conceptus, caused by inheritance of genes from its father that encode for proteins foreign to its mother, poses a unique problem for species that are viviparous since the mother's immune system can potentially destroy the conceptus. That this does not usually occur is a consequence of modification in maternal immune cells as well as unique features of the fetal placenta that limit its foreignness to the mother. There is great plasticity in the maternal immune system to allow for fetal survival despite wide disparity in genetic makeup (1). In some cases, interspecific matings lead to live offspring; examples include mules (donkey jack × horse mare), and gaur × cattle (*Bos gaurus* × *Bos taurus*). Also, embryo manipulation technologies can result in live births from chimeric fetuses that include cells from two separate species.

Sometimes immunologic defense mechanisms in the reproductive tract are not sufficient to prevent microbial colonization, and the resultant infections can temporarily or permanently cause infertility or sterility, and even compromise the life of the female. Thus, immune function in the reproductive tract is important for health and for maintaining a high rate of fecundity. The extent to which pregnancies in domestic animals sometimes become compromised by failure of the maternal immune system to be properly regulated is unknown. However, such effects could potentially lead to embryonic loss or fetal stunting. Paradoxically, certain types of maternal immunologic recognition of the placenta may be beneficial to pregnancy.

## AN IMMUNOLOGY PRIMER

Cells of the immune system function to prevent establishment of infection from microorganisms, and to clear cancerous or damaged cells in the host. These cells are organized into specialized tissues such as the thymus, spleen, and lymph nodes, circulate in the blood, and are present in various tissues of the body, especially those in contact with the external environment. A wide array of cells participate in the immune system and each has a specific function—a list of the major cells and their properties is in Table 23-1. In addition, the organism is protected from microorganisms by physical barriers, such as the skin, as well as by proteins such as complement that circulate in the blood and can bind to microorganisms to promote their **phagocytosis** and lysis.

Once a microorganism penetrates the physical barriers

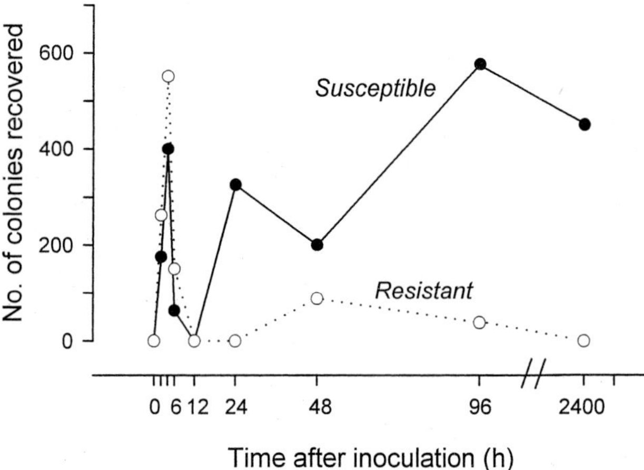


FIGURE 23-1. Example of uterine defense mechanisms. Data shown here, which represent the numbers of bacteria recovered from the uterus of mares following intrauterine inoculation of β-hemolytic *Streptococcus*, illustrate the effectiveness of the uterus in removing bacteria in mares having effective uterine immune function (see line labeled as resistant.) Uterine immune defense mechanisms can be compromised, however, so that the reproductive tract becomes unable to clear microorganisms and infection results. Compare the bacterial numbers for mares diagnosed as clinically susceptible to endometritis with those diagnosed as resistant to endometritis. (After Williamson P, Penhale JW, Munyua S, Murray J. The acute reaction of the mare's uterus to bacterial infection. Proc 10th Int Congr Anim Reprod AI Champaign–Urbana, 1984;3:477.)

of an animal, there are two general types of responses by cells of the immune system. Responses mediated by the innate immune system occur rapidly but do not provide any long-term adjustments for improving the effectiveness of **immune responses** upon subsequent exposure to a microorganism. Cells participating in acquired immune responses often take longer to exert their functions but responses are specific for individual foreign molecules (**antigen**) and result in a process called immunologic memory so that subsequent exposure to the same antigen will lead to a stronger response to that antigen.

### *Innate Immune System*

The most immediate responses to invasion of foreign organisms are those mediated by phagocytic cells of the innate immune system. **Macrophages** and **neutrophils** engulf foreign particles and then kill the organism. This process, called phagocytosis, can be stimulated by other components of the immune system. For example, phagocytes have receptors for antibodies (produced by B lymphocytes) and complement (produced by the liver) and more easily recognize microorganisms coated with these molecules. Also, various regulatory molecules called **cytokines** produced by T lymphocytes can activate phagocytes and make them more effective. One such cytokine is tumor necrosis factor.

**Natural killer (NK) cells** are a type of lymphocyte but, unlike other cells of this lineage, they do not have receptors that recognize specific antigens. Rather, NK cells kill cells that

a) do not display proteins called class I **major histocompatibility complex (MHC)** antigens on their cell surfaces, or
b) have class I MHC, but without the self-peptide usually present in association with the MHC protein.

The most common type of cell with either of these conditions are those infected with virus. Like phagocytes, activity of NK cells can be increased by certain cytokines from other lymphocytes. One such molecule is interferon-γ. Also, NK cells contain **immunoglobulin** receptors and have increased killing activity against cells that have **antibody** on their cell surfaces. Clear proof that NK cells

TABLE 23-1. *Some Key Cellular Components of the Immune System*

| CELL TYPE | KEY FUNCTION |
|---|---|
| *Phagocytes* | |
| Macrophage | Phagocytosis; antigen presentation |
| Dendritic cell | Endocytosis and phagocytosis; antigen presentation |
| Neutrophil | Phagocytosis |
| *Lymphocytes* | |
| B lymphocyte | Secretion of antibody; antigen presentation |
| $T_H1$ T helper lymphocyte | Secretion of cytokines that stimulate macrophages and cytotoxic T cells |
| $T_H2$ T helper lymphocyte | Secretion of cytokines that stimulate B cells and antibody responses |
| Cytotoxic T lymphocyte | Lysis of target cells |
| Gamma-delta (γδ) T lymphocyte[a] | Lysis of target cells; secretion of cytokines and growth factors |

[a]T-cell receptor is of the γδ type; other T lymphocytes have alpha-beta αβ type.

exist in ruminants such as sheep and cattle does not yet exist.

In addition to cellular components, the innate immune system also includes proteins such as complement, which promotes phagocytosis and lysis of microbes, and lactoferrin, which can inhibit bacterial growth.

### *Acquired Immune System*

The two main types of cells of the acquired immune system are B and T lymphocytes. B cells derive their name because in chickens they differentiate in an organ called the Bursa of Fabricius. In mammals, they are derived from the bone marrow. T lymphocytes also are formed from precursors in the bone marrow but undergo a period of differentiation in the thymus before seeding various lymphoid tissues. Both T and B cells express receptors on their cell surfaces that are specific for a particular antigen. For B cells, the antigen receptor is an immunoglobulin molecule, while for T cells, the receptor is a protein called the **T-cell receptor**. Two types of T cells can be identified. Some T cells have a receptor made of an alpha and beta subunit. These cells, called $\alpha\beta$T cells, predominate in lymphoid organs such as the spleen and lymph node and are the major cells in blood. Other lymphocytes have a T-cell receptor made of a gamma and delta subunit. These $\gamma\delta$T cells are numerous in epithelia such as the skin and lining of the intestinal and reproductive tract.

One key feature of lymphocytes is their capacity for immunologic memory. When a lymphocyte recognizes an antigen specific for its receptor, it undergoes a process called activation whereby the cell proliferates. Some of these daughter cells differentiate into effector cells that perform various activities such as antibody production or lysis of target cells. Other cells, however, become memory cells which persist in the animal for long periods of time. Exposure of the animal to a second exposure to antigen results in a heightened immune response because the number of cells specific for that antigen (i.e., the memory cell) has been increased. This phenomenon forms the basis for vaccination.

### *Recognition of Antigen By T Lymphocytes*

One property of T lymphocytes is that the T-cell receptor can only recognize antigen if it is expressed on the surface of a cell in association with a protein of the major histocompatibility complex. Thus, most T cells cannot recognize antigen themselves, but require so-called **antigen-presenting** cells that can process foreign proteins in such a way as to place the processed antigen within an MHC protein. Cells that can function as antigen-presenting cells include macrophages, **dendritic cells** (phagocytic and **endocytic** cells located in many tissues), B lymphocytes, and certain epithelial cells, perhaps including the epithelium of the uterus and vagina (2).

Antigen-processing cells process antigens one of two different ways. Antigens that are phagocytosed by antigen-presenting cells (i.e., bacteria and protozoa) are placed with one form of the MHC called MHC class II. Only one class of T cells, the **CD4** T cell, can recognize antigen bound to MHC class II. Antigens from intracellular pathogens (viruses and intracellular bacteria) are processed to be bound to MHC class I. Only a class of T cells called **CD8** recognize these antigens.

While the major role of MHC proteins is to present antigen to T cells, these proteins were originally described based on their role in tissue rejection responses. It is MHC antigens that provoke the strongest tissue rejection response in the host when a foreign tissue such as a kidney or liver is transplanted. This is because either the MHC proteins contain self peptides from the foreign donor that provoke an immune response in the host, or because slight genetic differences in the structure of the MHC molecule itself are sufficient to be recognized as foreign by the host.

### *Role of T Lymphocytes*

The actions of T lymphocytes are collectively termed cell-mediated **immunity**. This term came about because transfer of T-cell dependent immunity from an immunized animal to a nonimmunized one requires transfer of T cells themselves. There are two classes of T cells. The first class is the **cytotoxic** T cell. These lymphocytes, which are CD8 T lymphocytes, kill cells expressing antigen recognized by the lymphocyte's cell T receptor. Lysis is caused by secretion of toxic proteins such as perforin and the granzymes. CD8 lymphocytes are activated by antigen that is bound to MHC class I antigens, i.e., intracellular antigens such as virus. Thus, cytotoxic T cells kill cells that contain intracellular antigens that would not be found by antibody or phagocytosed by macrophages or neutrophils. The second class of lympyocyte, the **helper T cell**, regulates the activity of other lymphocytes by providing "help" in the form of secretion of various cytokines. This activity is exerted primarily by CD4 T cells (those that recognize extracellular antigens). In rodents, there are at least two types of helper T cells. The $T_H1$ cell functions to romote cell-mediated immunity. $T_H1$ cells produce cytokines such as interferon-$\gamma$ that preferentially stimulates bacterial killing by macrophages; lymphotoxin, which stimulates neutrophils; and interleukin-2, which promotes growth of cytotoxic T cells. The $T_H2$ cell promotes primarily antibody-dependent immunity. The characteristic cytokine produced by $T_H2$ cells is interleukin-4, which stimulates B lymphocytes to produce antibody.

Most of what is known about T cells comes from studies of those having $\alpha\beta$T cell receptors. The role of $\gamma\delta$ T cells is less widely studied. Some subpopulation of $\gamma\delta$ T cells are involved in regulating function of other cells that participate in innate and acquired immune responses (3). Other $\gamma\delta$ T cells can kill target cells in a manner reminiscent of NK cells. Some $\gamma\delta$ T cells may exert a relatively novel function for lymphocytes—promotion of proliferation of epithelial cells (4).

## B Lymphocytes

Immunity mediated by B lymphocytes is referred to as humoral immunity because transfer of immunity from one animal to the next can be achieved via transfer of blood plasma or serum. B cells inhibit microbial growth by secreting soluble proteins called antibodies that circulate in the blood and are present in extracellular fluids. Antibodies exert a variety of actions that inhibit microbial growth. Some activated B cells secrete antibody and are called **plasma cells**. Others do not secrete antibody but persist in the animal for months or years. Thus, subsequent exposure to the same antigen can result in heightened immune response.

Structurally, antibodies are members of a family of proteins called immunoglobulins. Each immunoglobulin is made up of four separate protein subunits (two heavy chains and two light chains) organized to give the molecule two sites for binding antigen, and one site called the Fc portion that is involved in binding to specific cells and to complement (Fig. 23-2). There are several types of immunoglobulin molecules secreted by B cells including IgG, IgM, IgA, IgD, and IgE. Each activated B cell secretes only one immunoglobulin type specific for one antigen. The most common immunoglobulin in blood is IgG. Another immunoglobulin molecule of particular interest for the reproductive tract is IgA, which is a major antibody in several mucosal sites such as the gastrointestinal and reproductive tracts. Immunoglobulin A exists as two separate antibody molecules joined by a short protein called J-chain. In addition, IgA secreted across epithelia contains an additional protein called secretory component that is added as IgA crosses epithelial cells on its passage to the mucosal surface.

Antibody binding to a microorganism can result in several actions that lead to the clearance of the microbe. For many microbes, successful colonization of a host requires binding of the microbe to cell membranes of the host. This can be made more difficult when the bacteria are coated with antibody. In addition, the Fc portion of IgG and IgA can be bound by specific receptors on macrophages and neutrophils so that the rate of phagocytosis can be enhanced when bacteria are coated with antibody. Proteins of the complement system, too, can bind to the Fc portion of IgG and lead to complement-mediated lysis of the microbial cell. Cells infected with virus or bacteria can be destroyed in a process called antibody-dependent cell cytotoxicity, which occurs when NK cells or **eosinophils** release toxic granules upon binding of their surface Fc receptors to antibody attached to infected cells. Receptors for the Fc portion of immunoglobulins also exist on T and B cells, and this provides for additional regulation of lymphocyte function by antibody-bound particles.

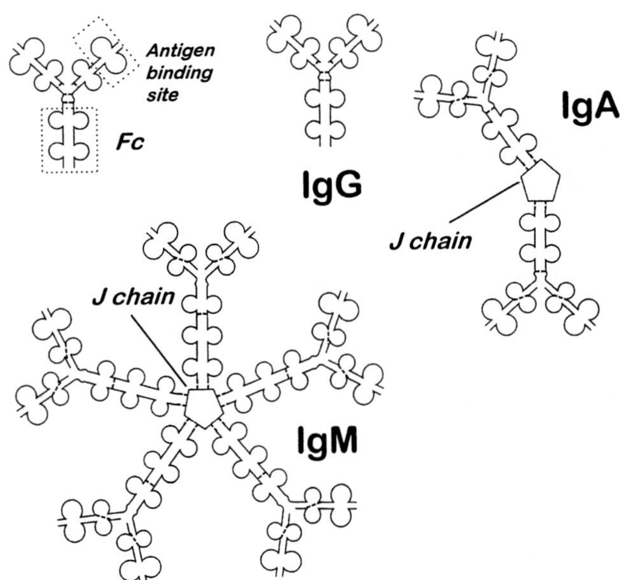


FIGURE 23-2. Schematic representations of the structure of IgG, IgA, and IgM. Each immunoglobulin is formed by two heavy chain molecules and two light chain molecules held together by disulfide bonds (indicated by *dashed lines*). The loops in each chain are formed by intramolecular disulfide bonds. There are two antibody sites for each immunoglobulin monomer. The Fc portion of the protein is responsible for binding to complement, and to immunoglobulin receptors on neutrophils, macrophages, and other cells. IgG is secreted as a monomer, whereas IgA is a dimer and IgM exists as a pentamer. Multimeric forms of immunoglobulin are held together by a protein called J-chain. In addition, IgA secreted across epithelial surfaces (not shown here) contains another protein called secretory component. (Adapted from Abbas AK, Lichtman AH, Pober JS. Cellular and Molecular Immunology, 3rd ed. Philadelphia: WB Saunders, 1997.)

## Anatomic Sites for Immune Responses

Activation of immune responses can occur at several levels in the body, including the site of entry of microorganisms (skin, lungs, etc.). Antigens that enter the blood stream are concentrated in the spleen where T and B cell responses can be initiated. Similarly, another circulatory system, the lymphatic system, drains extracellular fluid from tissues. Antigen collected in the lymphatic vessels is captured in lymph nodes, which also contain both T and B cells. Activated effector and memory T cells leave the spleen and lymph nodes, circulate throughout the body, and home specifically to sites of antigen entry. B cells also can be present in peripheral organs, particularly mucosal tissues such as the intestine and reproductive tract. However, many activated cells remain in the spleen and lymph nodes, perhaps because the actions of B cells are dependent upon antibodies which circulate in the blood.

## COMPONENTS OF THE IMMUNE SYSTEM IN THE REPRODUCTIVE TRACT

### *Anatomic Considerations*

The vagina is in contact with the outside air and is thus a portal for microorganisms to enter the body. The vulva and vulvar sphincter muscle limit entry of microorganisms into the vagina, while the vestibular sphincter muscle reduces microbial movement into the anterior reaches of the vagina. Nonetheless, resident microflora are typically present in the vagina although at levels that do not lead to overt clinical problems. The cervix is the major physical barrier to movement of organisms further into the reproductive tract. The function of the cervix is mediated in part by the secretions of this organ; these form a thick plug in the cervical lumen during pregnancy. Cervical secretions also contain molecules such as lactoferrin that inhibit bacterial growth.

In addition to the physical barrier afforded by the cervix, the reproductive tract contains macrophages, T lymphocytes, B lymphocytes, neutrophils, and other cells that participate in maintaining the reproductive tract in a sterile state. Moreover, the reproductive tract is drained by the lymphatic system. Lymph vessels draining the uterus join with similar vessels from the ovary so that concentrations of progesterone in utero-ovarian lymph on the side ipsilateral to an ovary with a functional corpus luteum can be 10 to 1000 fold higher than concentrations in jugular blood (5). The major lymph nodes filtering lymph derived from the reproductive tract are the medial iliac lymph nodes and the lumbo-aortic lymph nodes (Fig. 23-3). These lymph nodes also collect lymph from other organ tissues in the abdominal and pelvic areas.

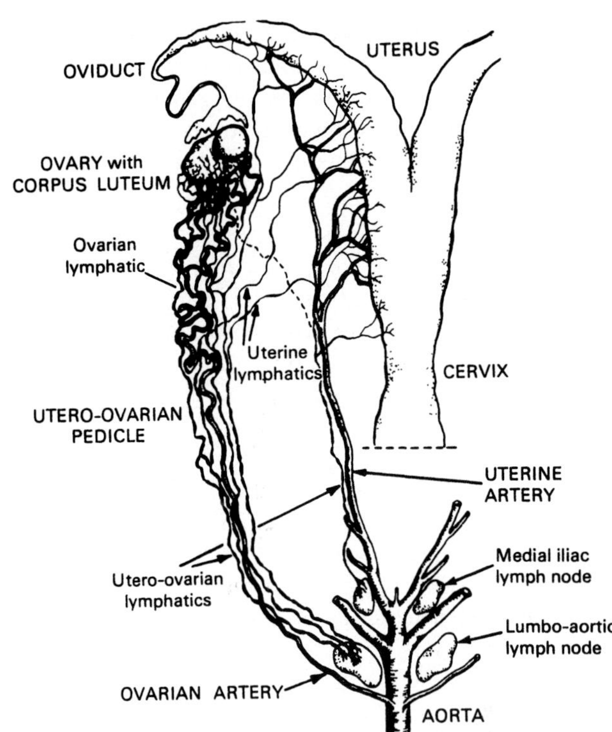


FIGURE 23-3. Lymphatic drainage of the reproductive tract of the ewe. Note that lymph vessels draining the uterus join with similar vessels from the ovary. The major lymph nodes filtering lymph derived from the reproductive tract are the medial iliac lymph nodes and the lumbo-aortic lymph nodes. These also collect lymph from other organs and tissues in the abdominal and pelvic areas. (Staples LD, Fleet IR, Heap RB. Anatomy of the utero-ovarian lymphatic network and the composition of afferent lymph in relation to the establishment of pregnancy in the sheep and goat. J Reprod Fertil 1982;64:409–420.)

### *Innate Immune System*

When antigens are placed in the reproductive tract, initial removal is accomplished by phagocytic cells of the innate immune system. Macrophages and dendritic-like cells are located in the reproductive tract. There are usually few neutrophils present in the reproductive tract in the absence of infection although, in gilts, these cells can be seen in the base of the uterine endometrial epithelium lining the uterus, especially near estrus (6). Microbial infection, deposition of semen, or other inflammatory stimuli cause the release of chemotactic molecules that stimulate the movement of neutrophils out of the blood and into the lumen of the uterus. For example, the number of neutrophils recovered from the uterine lumen of cows receiving intrauterine infusion of oyster glycogen, a stimulator of neutrophil recruitment, varied from $10^8$ to $10^9$ cells, as compared to only $10^5$ cells for cows not receiving oyster glycogen (7).

Opsonins (from the Greek, *opsonein*, to prepare food) are molecules that bind to particulate antigens and increase the affinity of phagocytes for that antigen. For example, serum contains complement C3b which can cause **opsonization** by binding to microorganisms; neutrophils and macrophages have receptors for C3b on their cell surfaces. There seems to be little active complement in uterine fluid, at least in the mare, but immunoglobulins, which are also in uterine fluid, can act as opsonins. IgG was the major opsonin in uterine fluid of mares (8). Enhancement of phagocytic function by the addition of serum to uterine fluid has been recommended as a therapy for treating uterine infections in mares, although not all studies have yielded positive results (9).

Microbial infection is also associated with inflammation accompanied by vasodilation, increased vascular permeability, movement of serum proteins into the uterine lumen, and production of a uterine discharge. These effects may be mediated by **mast cells**, **basophils**, and eosinophils which release vasoactive molecules upon activation. During uterine infection, physical clearance of microorganisms via movement of inflammatory fluids through the cervix and vulva may be an important mechanism for reducing the likelihood of infection. Indeed, certain mares that are very susceptible to developing **endometritis** have reduced capacity for physical clearance (10). The reproductive tract also secretes proteins that are involved in limiting bacterial growth. These include lysozyme, identified in the pig uterus, and lactoferrin, found in uterine fluid of the cow.

### *Lymphocytes*

The location of T lymphocytes in the uterus varies with species. In cows (11) and ewes (12, 13), CD4 cells are limited to the stroma and are not very abundant. In contrast, CD8 lymphocytes are located primarily in the epithelium, or in the stroma immediately adjacent to the epithelium. Most CD8 cells in the sheep uterus have cell surface markers indicating that they are naive rather than memory cells formed as a result of previous exposure to antigen. About a third of the CD8 cells in the luminal epithelium of the nonpregnant ewe sheep are $\gamma\delta$T cells (13). In the gilt, both CD4 and CD8 cells are located primarily in the epithelium or in the immediately-adjacent stroma (6), while in the mare, both CD4 and CD8 are located primarily in the stroma (14). The number of T cells likely increases in response to microbial challenge since mares that had endometritis had higher numbers of endometrial T cells, often present in large aggregates (14).

B cells are present in the reproductive tract in the endometrial stroma, often closely apposed to glandular or luminal epithelia. Lymphoid nodules can sometimes be observed in the stroma of the vagina and uterus. These structures are circular clusters of lymphoid cells that contain large numbers of B and plasma cells. The predominant immunoglobulin produced by plasma cells varies with species and region of the reproductive tract. Like tissues of the mucosal immune system, IgA producing cells are a major type but IgG and IgM producing cells are also present. Depending on the species and specific tissue type, IgG-producing cells can outnumber IgA-producing cells (Table 23-2).

**TABLE 23-2. *Numbers of Plasma Cells per 100 Fields in the Reproductive Tract of the Sow***

| TISSUE | STAGE OF THE ESTROUS CYCLE | IgG | IgA | IgM |
|---|---|---|---|---|
| Oviduct | Estrus | 25 | 33 | 9 |
| | Diestrus | 3 | 3 | 1 |
| Endometrium | Estrus | 181 | 79.5 | 40 |
| | Diestrus | 19 | 7 | 2 |
| Cervix | Estrus | 87 | 212 | 30 |
| | Diestrus | 21 | 48 | 3 |
| Vagina | Estrus | 56 | 187 | 35 |
| | Diestrus | 18 | 59 | 7 |

Data from: Hussein AM, Newby TJ, Bourne FJ. Immunohistochemical studies of the local immune system in the reproductive tract of the sow. J Reprod Immunol 1983;5:1–15.

Immunization with antigen placed in the reproductive tract can lead to production of antibody in the reproductive tract and confer some protection from specific infectious agents (15). In addition to the local secretion of immunoglobulins by plasma cells, there is exudation of circulating antibodies from the blood into the lumen of the reproductive tract. As a result, the major immunoglobulin class in reproductive tract secretions is IgG. Also, systemic immunization can lead to appearance of antibodies within the reproductive tract and protection against establishment of infection (16).

## REGULATION OF CELLULAR IMMUNE FUNCTION IN THE REPRODUCTIVE TRACT

Changes in physiologic state place different demands upon immune defenses of the reproductive tract. During estrus, the process of mating leads to introduction of microorganisms into the reproductive tract, and the cervix is open to allow sperm transport. Thus, there is special need at this time to efficiently clear microorganisms entering the reproductive tract. Moreover, the large numbers of sperm present in the tract following mating must be removed in a manner that does not lead to permanent immunity of the female against these cells. Successful mating is followed by the growth within the reproductive tract of a conceptus that is itself genetically foreign to the mother. Changes in maternal immune function and placental antigenicity are necessary to prevent this organism from being immunologically rejected by the mother. During and after parturition, the reproductive tract is again subject to massive bacteriologic insult, and reestablishment of a sterile uterus is one of the requirements for pregnancy to be reestablished in the subsequent postpartum period. The immune network in the reproductive tract and associated lymph nodes is capable to adjusting to these differences in requirements because lymphoid cells in the reproductive tract are regulated by ovarian steroid hormones, regulatory molecules in seminal plasma, and locally-produced factors from the reproductive tract and conceptus.

### *Steroid Hormone Regulation*

The major hormones regulating function of the immune system in the reproductive tract are estradiol-17$\beta$ and progesterone. Ovariectomized females, in which steroid hormone concentrations are low, can often readily clear bacteria placed experimentally in the uterus (Table 23-3). Estradiol-17$\beta$ can facilitate removal of microorganisms

TABLE 23-3. *Effect of Steroid Hormone Treatment on Development of Uterine Infections in Ovariectomized Mares Following Intrauterine Inoculation with Bacteria*

| PHYSIOLOGIC STATE AT INOCULATION | TIME AFTER INOCULATION (d) | BACTERIA IN UTERUS ($\log_{10}$ COLONY COUNTS) |
|---|---|---|
| Control | 7 | 5.4 ± 0.4 |
| Estradiol cypionate | 7 | nondetectable |
| Progesterone | 7 | 5.7 ± 0.8 |
| Control | 10 | nondetectable |
| Estradiol cypionate | 10 | nondetectable |
| Progesterone | 10 | 5.1 ± 0.3 |

Data from Washburn SM, Klesius PH, Ganjam VK, Brown BG. Effect of estrogen and progesterone on the phagocytic response of ovariectomized mares infected in utero with β-hemolytic streptococci. Am J Vet Res 1982;43:1367–1370.

while treatment with progesterone often leads to establishment of uterine infection (Table 23-3).

Actions of steroid hormones on bacteria may be due in part to effects on physical clearance of microorganisms through discharge of inflammatory fluids via the cervix and vagina (17). Greater physical clearance at estrus may be a consequence of changes in cervical tone. Also, estrogen may increase migration of cells that promote inflammation in the reproductive tract. One of these, the eosinophil, accumulates in the reproductive tract (especially the oviduct) at estrus, at least in the cow (18). Vascular porosity, as determined by migration of trypan blue dye from the blood into the uterus, was increased by estradiol in sheep (19).

The local production of antibody is also regulated by ovarian steroids in some species. For example, the number of plasma cells in the sow reproductive tract increases in number at estrus (Table 23-2). In the mare, concentrations of IgA in uterine fluid (but not IgG) have been reported to be greater at estrus than during the luteal phase (20).

Steroid hormones can regulate neutrophil function in the uterus—the nature of the effect depends on species and the nature of the agent used to attract neutrophils to the uterus. In cows, for example, the number of **leukocytes** invading the uterus after intrauterine injection of *Escherichia coli* was greater at estrus (21), but no differences in neutrophil migration were seen due to stage of the cycle or steroid treatment in another study in which oyster glycogen was used to induce neutrophil migration (7). In the mare resistant to endometritis, uterine neutrophils collected at estrus were more active than those collected during the luteal phase (22).

In addition to affecting antibacterial mechanisms, progesterone appears to have a major role during pregnancy in inhibiting uterine immune responses. Thus, treatment of ewes with progesterone caused a decrease in lymphocyte numbers in the endometrium (23) and allowed prolonged survival of skin grafts placed within the uterus (24). At least in the sheep, progesterone appears to inhibit lymphocyte function by inducing the secretion of a protein from the uterine endometrium variously called ovine uterine serpin or uterine milk protein, which itself is immunosuppressive. In ewes, withdrawal of progesterone in early pregnancy leads to movement of neutrophils into the endometrium (25). Perhaps the reduction in progesterone near the end of pregnancy may allow for movement of neutrophils into the uterus and cervix to facilitate parturition and removal of the placenta.

### Responses to Sperm

Sperm are antigenic when injected subcutaneously into females. Therefore, mechanisms must be found to remove spermatozoa from the reproductive tract following mating in a way that will not lead to the development of humoral or cellular immunity to sperm. The major fate of spermatozoa in the reproductive tract is phagocytosis by neutrophils; deposition of sperm induces influx of phagocytic cells (neutrophils, macrophages, and dendritic-like cells) into the reproductive tract. In the stallion, components of seminal plasma coat the sperm and act as opsonins to further promote sperm phagocytosis (26). Seminal plasma also contains various molecules that can inhibit lymphocyte activation. There is a decrease in T lymphocytes in the endometrium of gilts following mating with a vasectomized boar (27), indicating that components of seminal plasma can reduce lymphocyte numbers in the uterus. In contrast, lymphocytes in the lymph nodes draining the uterus can become activated by seminal plasma, perhaps because immunosuppresants are inactivated as sperm antigens reach the lymph nodes.

Despite the presence of mechanisms to prevent immune responses to sperm, females can develop anti-sperm immunity, and antibodies directed towards sperm can be occasionally recovered from the reproductive tract. The incidence of anti-sperm antibodies in female domestic animals has not been accurately established, however; nor is it known to

**TABLE 23-4. *Effects of Deposition of Killed Semen into the Uterus, Prior to Mating, on Litter Size of Gilts Following a Subsequent Mating with Fertile Boars***

| TRAIT | SALINE INFUSION | KILLED SEMEN |
|---|---|---|
| Litter size at birth | 8.8 ± 0.88 | 10.8 ± 0.98 |
| Live pigs at birth | 8.7 ± 0.80 | 10.1 ± 0.90 |

Data from Murray FA, Grifo AP, Parker CF Jr. Increased litter size in gilts by intrauterine infusion of seminal and sperm antigens before breeding. J Anim Sci 1983;5:895–900.

what extent female domestic animals with naturally-occurring anti-sperm antibodies are infertile.

Experiments in pigs suggest that some aspects of immune stimulation by semen may be beneficial to subsequent pregnancy. In some studies (although not all), deposition of killed semen in the uterus prior to mating led to increased litter size (Table 23-4). The mechanism by which spermatozoa or seminal plasma exerts this effect is unknown. However, deposition of seminal fluid in the uterus increased proliferation of the endometrial luminal epithelium (27). Thus, growth factors released in response to semen deposition may affect endometrial growth.

### *Changes During Pregnancy*

Pregnancy is associated with changes in lymphocyte numbers in the uterus. While some cell populations decrease in number, others apparently become activated. In the pig, for example, early pregnancy is associated with a decrease in number of T lymphocytes in the endometrial epithelium and underlying stroma at days 2 to 4 postestrus (28). Numbers of lymphocytes remain relatively unchanged until days 18 to 21, when there is an increase in numbers of CD4 lymphocytes in the endometrial stroma. There is also appearance of NK cells in the porcine endometrium from days 10 to 20 of pregnancy; NK cells are not present in cyclic animals, and return to nearly nondetectable levels by day 30 (29). The signal for activation of NK cells is not known, but may be one or more of the interferon molecules produced by the porcine conceptus at this time of pregnancy. After days 18 to 21, the numbers of lymphocytes in the luminal epithelium decline, becoming rare except at **areolae**, the sites where glands open (28). Stromal lymphocytes also appear to decline in number from day 45 of pregnancy.

In cows, there is also a decrease in intraepithelial lymphocytes in early pregnancy—numbers of lymphocytes during this time are half that found in cyclic cows (30). This decrease may be caused by interferon-$\tau$, which is secreted by the bovine **trophoblast** around this time (maximal secretion about day 17), and which can inhibit lymphocyte proliferation. Thereafter, formation of the placenta is associated with regional patterns of distribution of lymphocytes in the uterus—there are few lymphocytes present in the placentomes although lymphocytes persist in regions of the endometrium between placentomes (31).

A similar pattern of lymphocytes exist in the sheep endometrium during pregnancy, with lymphocytes being confined primarily to the intercaruncular regions. There are also marked changes in numbers of lymphocytes in the intercaruncular endometrium during pregnancy (32). The number of lymphocytes in glandular epithelium and stroma decrease as pregnancy proceeds. In the luminal epithelium, in contrast, the number of lymphocytes in the luminal epithelium increases dramatically during late pregnancy, so that lymphocytes comprise about 10% of the cellular population of the luminal epithelium by days 127 to 134 of pregnancy. These lymphocytes belong to the $\gamma\delta$T class, and become activated as indicated by increased granularity and expression of markers of activation such as the interleukin 2 receptor (33). Activation is caused by some local product of the conceptus.

## IMMUNOLOGIC IMPLICATIONS OF PREGNANCY

Changes in lymphocyte numbers in the uterus during pregnancy, which have been described in the previous section, reveal some of the adjustments the maternal immune system makes to the presence of the conceptus during pregnancy. The conceptus is at risk to be immunologically rejected by the mother since the paternal genes it inherits make it a foreign tissue. Placement of other foreign tissues such as skin grafts into the uterus results in prompt rejection of the foreign tissue, but the conceptus usually thrives within this same environment without suffering any deleterious immunologic attack from the mother. Thus, the evolution of viviparity has been accompanied by the development of mechanisms to prevent the immunologic destruction of the fetus. These mechanisms include altered antigenicity of the placenta itself, as well as regulatory processes mediated by placental and maternal molecules that direct maternal lymphocytes away from anti-fetal cytotoxic responses.

Pregnancy loss can occur when the mother mounts an anti-fetal immune response, because heifers that were immunized against day 32 to 38 conceptuses subsequently were more difficult to get pregnant (Fig. 23-4). Moreover, porcine trophoblast cells can be lysed *in vitro* by maternal NK cells from the endometrium (34). In rodents, various pathologies have been described to occur as a consequence of altered immunologic responses to the conceptus, including damage to the vascular bed nourishing the placenta, increased fetal resorption rate, and decreased birth weights. The degree to which these problems occur naturally in

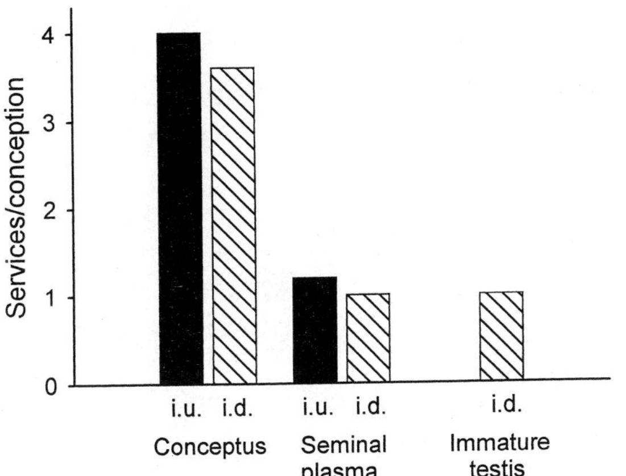


FIGURE 23-4. Effects of immunization against conceptus tissues on fertility on heifers. Heifers were immunized via intradermal (i.d.) or intrauterine (i.u.) routes with conceptus tissues from 32 to 38 days of pregnancy. Controls were immunized with seminal plasma or immature testis. Fertility was measured as the number of services required to achieve pregnancy. (After Menge AC. Early embryo mortality in heifers isoimmunized with semen and conceptus. J Reprod Fertil 1969;18:67–74.)

domestic animals is not known. Moreover, there is some evidence in rodents that certain types of immune recognition of the conceptus by the mother may be beneficial to the conceptus, perhaps through the secretion of locally acting cytokines which can promote placental function, or because such recognition leads to other alterations in immune function that limit anti-fetal immunity. The evidence for similar phenomena in domestic animals is only now being accumulated.

Several theories have arisen to explain the nature of the maternal-conceptus immunologic relationship. A summary of those for which there is some experimental support is provided in Table 23-5. These theories are based primarily on work in mice and humans, which are the two most studied subjects of immunologic research. Our understanding of the immunology of domestic animals has lagged behind knowledge of immunology in mice and humans. Nonetheless, there is good evidence to support two of the theories for survival of the fetal allograft. These are the ideas that 1) the placenta is made less antigenic than other tissues because of selective inhibition of gene expression for MHC antigens, and 2) lymphocyte activation is inhibited at the maternal-fetal interface because of the production of immunoregulatory molecules by maternal and placental tissues.

### *Regulation of MHC Antigens on Trophoblast*

As mentioned earlier, MHC antigens serve as antigen presenting molecules to allow lymphocytes to recognize a foreign antigen. Additionally, MHC molecules are the major molecules that evoke a tissue rejection response when tissue grafts are placed in a host. The host immune system recognizes as foreign those self-antigens of the graft that are associated with the graft MHC molecules as well as small genetic variations in the structure of the MHC molecule itself. MHC class II molecules have a limited tissue distribution, being primarily expressed by lymphoid tissues, but MHC class I molecules are produced by most cells. In several species, the genes for MHC antigens are turned off in the outer layers of placental trophoblast. In the cow, for example, the early blastocyst expresses MHC class I antigens. Once the placenta is formed, however, there are no detectable MHC class I molecules in the placentomal region of

TABLE 23-5. ***Theories to Explain Survival of the Fetal Allograft During Pregnancy***

| THEORY | ALTERATION IN IMMUNE FUNCTION/CONSEQUENCES FOR CONCEPTUS SURVIVAL |
|---|---|
| Immunosuppression | Placental and maternal tissues produce molecules that prevent generation of maternal anti-conceptus lymphocytes. |
| Blocking antibody | Maternal system produces anti-fetal antibodies that do not fix complement and which mask fetal antigens. |
| Reduced antigenicity | MHC antigens are not expressed on regions of trophoblast in contact with the mother to prevent activation of maternal anti-fetal MHC lymphocytes. |
| Fas ligand | Trophoblast and endometrium express Fas ligand to induce programmed cell death in activated maternal T cells. |
| Temporary tolerance | The number of maternal T cells against fetal MHC antigens decreases during pregnancy to cause temporary tolerance to fetal MHC antigens—could be related to actions of Fas. |
| $T_H1$-$T_H2$ shift | During pregnancy, antibody responses are favored instead of cell-mediated immunity because of preferential activation of $T_H2$ helper T cells over $T_H1$ helper T cells. |
| Immunotrophosism | Trophoblast growth and hormone secretion is stimulated by maternal lymphocytes that secrete growth factors for trophoblast. |

the trophoblast and only limited expression of MHC class I molecules by the interplacentomal chorion (31). Thus, the potential antigenicity of the conceptus is greatly reduced at the site where maternal immunologic surveillance occurs. Experiments in mice indicate that viral infection may compromise placental function by increasing expression of placental MHC antigens (35).

Work in the human suggests that, in place of classical MHC class I molecules, the trophoblast produces an unusual MHC class I molecule called HLA-G that is less genetically variable between individuals but which can prevent NK cells from lysing the placenta (NK cells preferentially lyse targets without MHC). It is not known whether a similar phenomenon occurs in other species. In any case, reduced expression of MHC antigens on the placenta is probably not the only mechanism by which the conceptus escapes maternal immunologic attack, because the conceptus expresses other paternally-derived gene products which are antigenetic to the mother. The importance of other transplantation antigens is indicated by the observation that grafts from mice that lack MHC class I and II antigens are still readily rejected by their hosts (36).

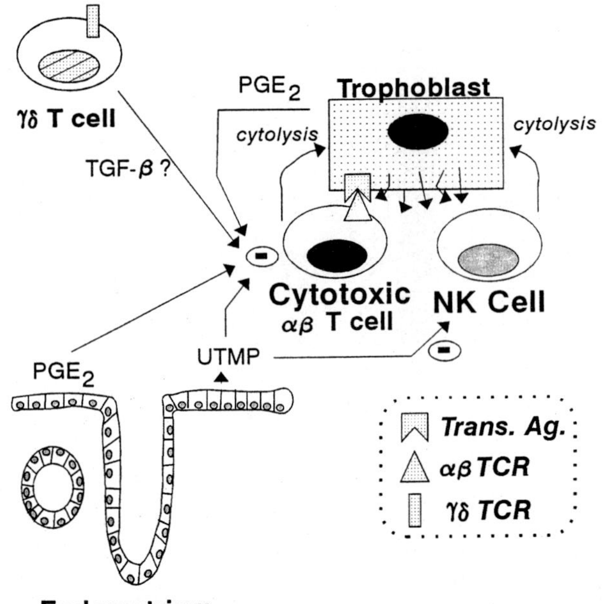


FIGURE 23-5. Model illustrating how lymphocyte inhibitory molecules from the endometrium and trophoblast inhibit activation and effector functions of maternal lymphocyte in the sheep. There are at least two cells that could potentially cause cytolysis of trophoblast cells. These are $\alpha\beta$ cytotoxic T cells that possess T cell receptors (*TCR*) specific for trophoblast transplantation antigens (*Trans. Ag.*), and natural killer (*NK*) cells, which recognize trophoblast without major histocompatibility antigens. These cells are inhibited by molecules secreted from the trophoblast and endometrium. Among the lymphocyte-inhibitory molecules at the fetal-maternal interface are prostaglandin $E_2$ (*$PGE_2$*), secreted by trophoblast and endometrial stroma, and uterine milk protein (*UTMP*), produced by endometrial epithelial cells. Endometrial $\gamma\delta$T cells also become activated in late pregnancy. These cells may secrete transforming growth factor-$\beta$ (*TGFβ*), which also inhibits lymphocyte functions. (Modified after Hansen PJ, Liu WJ. Immunological aspects of pregnancy: concepts and speculations using the sheep as a model. Anim Reprod Sci 1996;42:483–493.)

### *Immunosuppression*

The fetal maternal interface is bathed with molecules that can inhibit activation of T lymphocytes. The abundance and diversity of such molecules in the sheep is illustrated in Figure 23-5. Secretion of lymphocyte-inhibitory molecules may represent a mechanism to nonspecifically inhibit local immune responses against conceptus antigens while avoiding suppression of systemic immune function.

Lymphocyte inhibitory molecules in the reproductive tract come from a variety of sources. Several cellular compartments of the endometrium produce molecules capable of inhibiting lymphocyte function. Endometrial epithelial cells secrete the cytokine TGF-$\beta$ while stromal cells are a major source of prostaglandin $E_2$; both these molecules can inhibit T cell proliferation. In the sheep, a major product of endometrial epithelial cells during pregnancy is uterine milk protein (now called ovine uterine serpin), which is induced by progesterone and can inhibit T cell proliferation in culture and antibody responses in vivo, and can block abortion in mice induced by activation of NK cells (37). There also appear to be suppressor cells that appear in the uterus at specific times in pregnancy. Cells that secrete TGF-$\beta$2 and which are primarily eosinophils accumulate near the endometrial cups of the horse conceptus (38). A suppressor cell that failed to express conventional lymphocyte markers was identified in the sheep uterus (39).

The conceptus also contributes immunosuppressive substances to the maternal-fetal interface. The peri-implantation (about day 15 to 25) ruminant conceptus secretes two molecules that can inhibit lymphocyte function: interferon-$\tau$, and a 800,000 molecular weight glycoprotein secreted by the cow and sheep embryo (40). The pig conceptus at a similar stage of development also secretes interferon molecules. Once placentation is complete, the placenta secretes additional lymphocyte-inhibitory factors. These include progesterone, which inhibits lymphocytes at high concentration, and which may reach such inhibitory concentrations in species such as the sheep in which placental progesterone synthesis becomes sufficient by midgestation to maintain pregnancy. Prostaglandin $E_2$ is also produced by placental tissues.

Other partially characterized lymphocyte-inhibitory molecules have been described in uterine fluid, and in embryo or placenta conditioned culture medium. The chemical and immunomodulatory properties of most lymphocyte-inhibitory molecules at the fetal-maternal interface have not been completely described, and few studies have been done to evaluate the effects of these molecules on uterine lymphocytes, which are different functionally from the peripheral blood lymphocytes usually used to identify lymphocyte-inhibitory molecules.

That some uterine immunosuppression exists is supported by studies that progesterone can delay skin graft rejection in the sheep uterus (24), that lymphocyte numbers in the uterine epithelium of cattle decrease in number coincident with secretion of interferon-$\tau$ by the peri-implantation conceptus (30), and that there is a reduction in uterine lymphocyte numbers in one of more regions of the uterine endometrium during the course of pregnancy in sheep (32) and pigs (6). Uterine immunosuppression must be selective because certain populations of lymphocytes appear to become activated at specific stages of pregnancy, for example, NK cells at days 10 to 20 of pregnancy in pigs (29) and $\gamma\delta$T cells in late pregnancy in sheep (13, 33).

### *Other Mechanisms to Prevent Immunologic Rejection*

While evidence is not available for domestic animals, a few additional theories to explain maintenance of the fetal allograft outlined in Table 23-5 are of importance enough to justify some additional discussion. Among these is the idea that there is a redirection of T-cell responses during pregnancy from those driven by helper T cells secreting $T_H1$ cytokines (i.e., favoring inflammatory and cell mediated responses deleterious to the conceptus) to those driven by $T_H2$ cytokines (i.e., favoring antibody production which is not harmful to the conceptus). The switch from $T_H1$ to $T_H2$ may be caused by secretion of cytokines such as IL-10 from the placenta. In support of this theory is the finding that infection of mice with the protozoan *Leishmania* can cause a shift in the $T_H1/T_H1$ cytokine ratio and result in pregnancy failure (41).

In some species, the placenta and endometrium can express a molecule on cell surfaces called Fas ligand (42, 43). Binding of Fas ligand to the membrane receptor Fas on the surface of activated lymphocytes leads to programmed cell death of the activated lymphocyte. Such a phenomenon would prevent movement of maternal lymphocytes into the placenta and reduce the number of activated maternal T cells specific for placental antigens. Mice lacking a functional gene for Fas ligand experienced extensive leukocyte infiltration into the uterus and reduced litter sizes (43). Whether because of Fas ligand or other mechanism, experiments using transgenic mice indicate that pregnancy is accompanied by temporary tolerance of the mother against paternal antigens, and that this tolerance is associated with a selective and temporary reduction in maternal T cells that have receptors specific for paternally-inherited antigens (44).

### *Equid Pregnancy—An Example of Limited Immunologic Destruction of Placental Tissue?*

As compared to many species, interspecific pregnancies among equids are easy to establish. The product of one of these matings, the mule, has been used for centuries as a draft animal. Pregnancy in equids also differs from some other species in that specific regions of the placenta express MHC antigens and appear to be destroyed by a maternal immune response without the survival of the conceptus being compromised.

Like other species, the noninvasive regions of the horse trophoblast generally do not express MHC class I molecules except at regions next to endometrial glands (45). However a structure on the pre-attachment conceptus called the chorionic girdle strongly expresses MHC class I antigen. This structure forms as a band around the embryo at about days 25 to 36 of pregnancy in the mare. The cells of the girdle express MHC class I antigens at this time and antibodies to MHC class I antigens are regularly seen in the blood of mares by day 60 of pregnancy. The chorionic girdle cells subsequently invade the uterine endometrium at about day 36 to 38 of pregnancy in the mare to form a ring of endometrial cups that secrete the hormone equine chorionic gonadotropin (eCG) into the maternal circulation (Fig. 23-6).

Soon after invasion of the endometrium, MHC class I on endometrial cup cells becomes down-regulated (45). Nonetheless, maternal leukocytes accumulate in the endometrial stroma near the site of the cups (Fig. 23-6). These cells include CD4 and CD8 lymphocytes, some B cells, and especially towards the end of the cup lifespan, eosinophils and neutrophils (46). The endometrial cups are destined for destruction, presumably by the maternal leukocytes, and this occurs by days 100 through 140 of pregnancy in the mare, and is accompanied by a decrease in maternal concentration of eCG. The stimulus for leukocyte recruitment and destruction of the endometrial cups may be transplantation antigens other than those of the MHC complex because elimination of the endometrial cups occurs even when the fetus's sire has the same MHC type as the mother (47). The development of immune responses towards endometrial cups may be limited somewhat by maternal leukocytes that secrete the immunosuppressive molecule transforming growth factor-$\beta_2$ (38).

### *Positive Aspects of Immunological Recognition of the Conceptus*

Not all facets of immunologic recognition of the conceptus by the maternal immune system are necessarily harmful. Some recognition does occur because some populations of lymphocytes in the uterus become activated during pregnancy. For example, there is an increase of NK activity in the uterus of the pig during early pregnancy. Also, $\gamma\delta$T cells accumulate large granules in their cytoplasm (13) and it has been suggested that they may release cytokines that promote placental growth or hormone secretion. Indeed, $\gamma\delta$T cells at other sites (i.e., skin) promote cellular growth.

Growth of the preimplantation embryo can be stimulated by many products of immune cells including IL-1,

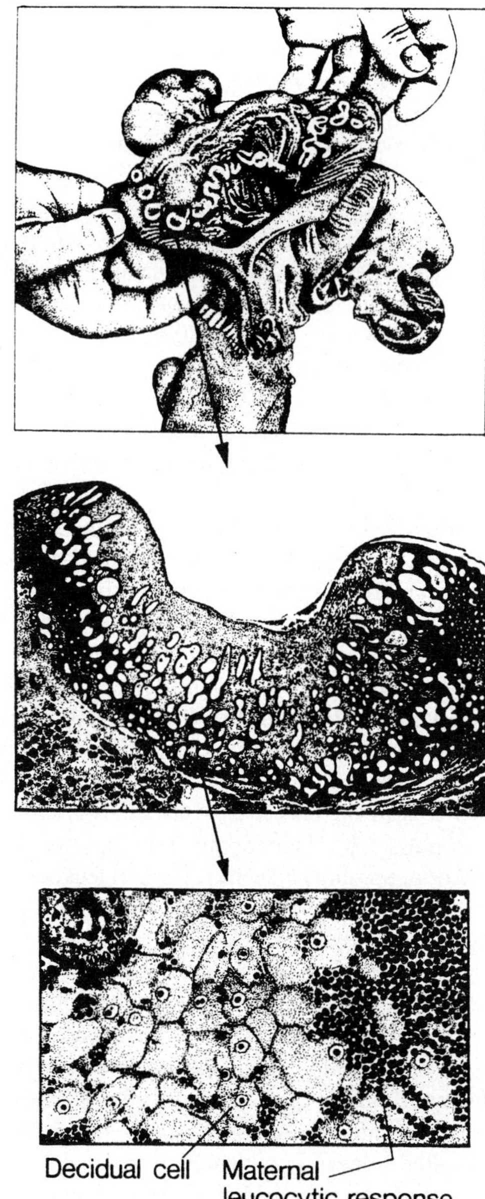


FIGURE 23-6. The endometrial cup reaction in the mare. The *top* panel shows the appearance of the uterus at day 60 of pregnancy after removal of the conceptus to reveal the ring of endometrial cups imbedded in the endometrium. The *middle* and *lower* panels represent the histologic appearance of the cups. Note the large number of maternal leukocytes that accumulate around the cups. Cells labeled as decidual cells are actually fetal in origin. (Short RV. Species differences. In: Austin CR, Short RV, ed. Reproduction in Mammals, Cambridge University Press, London, 1972;4:1–33.)

granulocyte-macrophage colony-stimulating factor, and leukemia inhibitory factor. Passive immunization to neutralize leukemia inhibitory factor tended to reduce pregnancy rate in sheep (48). The degree to which cytokine regulation of early embryonic development involves the maternal immune system is unclear because some of these cytokines are produced by nonlymphoid cells of the reproductive tract.

Remodeling of the cervix coincident with parturition involves actions of proteases produced by neutrophils. The process of shedding of the placenta after birth may also involve actions of leukocytes, and the degree to which the mother and conceptus share histocompatibility antigens may affect this process. In cattle, retention of the placenta following calving was more likely when dam and calf shared MHC class I antigens (49).

## REFERENCES


1. Anderson GB. Interspecific pregnancy: barriers and prospects. Biol Reprod 1988;38:1–15.
2. Wira CR, Rossoll, RM. Antigen-presenting cells in the female reproductive tract: influence of sex hormones on antigen presentation in the vagina. Immunology 1995;84:505–508.
3. Boismenu R, Havran WL. An innate view of $\gamma\delta$T cells. Curr Opin Immunol 1997;9:57–63.
4. Boismenu R, Havran WR. Modulation of epithelial cell growth by intraepithelial $\gamma\delta$T cells. Science 1994;26:1253–1255.
5. Staples LD, Fleet IR, Heap RB. Anatomy of the utero-ovarian lymphatic network and the composition of afferent lymph in relation to the establishment of pregnancy in the sheep and goat. J Reprod Fertil 1982;64:409–420.
6. Bischof RJ, Brandon MR, Lee CS. Studies on the distribution of immune cells in the uteri of prepubertal and cycling gilts. J Reprod Immunol 1994;26:111–129.
7. Lander Chacin MF, Hansen PJ, Drost M. Effects of stage of the estrous cycle and steroid treatment on uterine immunoglobulin content and polymorphonuclear leukocytes in cattle. Theriogenology 1990;34:1169–1184.
8. Hansen PJ, Asbury AC. Opsonins of *Streptococcus* in uterine flushings of mares susceptible and resistant to endometritis: control of secretion and partial characterization. Am J Vet Res 1987;48:646–650.
9. Hussain AM, Daniel RCW. Bovine endometritis: current and future alternative therapy. J Vet Med Ser A 1991;38:641–651.
10. LeBlanc MM, Asbury AC, Lyle SK. Uterine clearance mechanisms during the early postovulatory period in mares. Am J Vet Res 1989;50:864–867.
11. Cobb SP, Watson ED. Immunohistochemical study of immune cells in the bovine endometrium at different stages of the estrous cycle. Res Vet Sci 1995;59:229–237.
12. Lee CS, Gogolin-Ewens K, Brandon MR. Identification of a unique lymphocyte subpopulation in the sheep uterus. Immunology 1988;63:157–164.
13. Meeusen E, Fox A, Brandon M, Lee CS. Activation of uterine intraepithelial $\gamma\delta$T cell receptor-positive lymphocytes during pregnancy. Eur J Immunol 1993;23:1112–1117.
14. Watson ED, Thomson SR. Lymphocyte subsets in the endometrium of genitally normal mares and mares susceptible to endometritis. Equine Vet J 1996;28:106–110.
15. Corbeil LY. Vaccination strategies against *Tritrichomonas foetus*. Parisitol Today 1994;10:103–106.
16. Corbeil LY, Anderson ML, Corbeil RR, Eddow JM, BonDurant RH. Female reproductive tract immunity in bovine trichomoniasis. Am J Reprod Immunol 1998;39:189–198.

17. Evans MJ, Hamer JM, Gason LM, Graham CS, Asbury AC, Irvine CHG. Clearance of bacteria and non-antigenic markers following intra-uterine inoculation into maiden mares: effect of steroid hormone environment. Theriogenology 1986;26: 37–50.
18. Matsuda H, Okuda K, Imori T. Tissue concentrations of eosinophils in the bovine oviduct and uterus at different stages of the estrous cycle. Res Vet Sci 1983;34:369–370.
19. Brinsfield TH, Hawk HW, Righter HF. Interaction of progesterone and oestradiol on induced leucocytic emigration in the sheep uterus. J Reprod Fertil 1964;8:293–296.
20. LeBlanc MM, Hansen PJ, Buhi WC. Uterine protein secretion in postpartum and cyclic mares. Theriogenology 1988;29: 1303–1316.
21. Hawk HW, Brinsfield TH, Turner GD, Whitmore GW, Norcross MA. Effect of ovarian status on induced acute inflammatory response in cattle uteri. Am J Vet Res 1964;25:362–366.
22. Asbury AC, Hansen PJ. Effects of susceptibility of mares to endometritis and stage of cycle on phagocytic activity of uterine-derived neutrophils. J Reprod Fertil Suppl 1987; 35:311–316.
23. Gottshall SL, Hansen PJ. Regulation of leukocyte suppopulations in the sheep endometrium by progesterone. Immunology 1992;76:636–641.
24. Hansen PJ, Bazer FW, Segerson EC. Skin graft survival in the uterine lumen of ewes treated with progesterone. Am J Reprod Immunol Microbiol 1986;12:48–54.
25. Staples LD, Heap RB, Wooding FBP, King GJ. Migration of leukocytes into the uterus after acute removal of ovarian progesterone during early pregnancy. Placenta 1983;4: 339–350.
26. Hansen PJ, Hoggard MP, Rathwell AC. Effects of stallion seminal plasma on hydrogen peroxide release by leukocytes exposed to spermatozoa and bacteria. J Reprod Immunol 1987;10:157–166.
27. Bischof RJ, Lee CS, Brandon MR, Meeusen E. Inflammatory response in the pig uterus induced by seminal plasma. J Reprod Immunol 1994;26:131–146.
28. Bischof RJ, Brandon MR, Lee CS. Cellular immune responses in the pig uterus during pregnancy. J Reprod Immunol 1995;29:161–178.
29. Yu Z, Croy BA, Chapeau C, King GJ. Elevated endometrial natural killer cell activity during early porcine pregnancy is conceptus-mediated. J Reprod Immunol 1993;24:153–164.
30. Vander Wielen AL, King GJ. Intraepithelial lymphocytes in the bovine uterus during the oestrous cycle and early gestation. J Reprod Fertil 1984;70:457–462.
31. Low BG, Hansen PJ, Drost M, Gogolin-Ewens KJ. Expression of major histocompatibility complex antigens on the bovine placenta. J Reprod Fertil 1990;90:235–243.
32. Lee CS, Meeusen E, Gogolin-Ewens K, Brandon MR. Quantitative and qualitative changes in the intraepithelial lymphocyte population in the uterus of nonpregnant and pregnant sheep. Am J Reprod Immunol 1992;28:90–96.
33. Liu WJ, Gottshall SL, Hansen PJ. Increased expression of cell surface markers on endometrial $\gamma\delta$T cell receptor intraepithelial lymphocytes induced by the local presence of the sheep conceptus. Am J Reprod Immunol 1997;37:199–205.
34. Yu A, Croy BA, King GJ. Lysis of porcine trophoblast cells by endometrial natural killer-like effector cells *in vitro* does not require interleukin-2. Biol Reprod 1994;51:1279–1284.
35. Vassiliadis S, Athanassakis I. Two novel colony-stimulating factor-1 (CSF-1) properties: it post-transcriptionally inhibits interferon-specific induction of class II antigens and reduces the risk of fetal abortion. Cytokine 1994;6:295–299.
36. Grusby MJ, Auchincloss H, Lee R, et al. Mice lacking major histocompatibility complex class I and class II molecules. Proc Natl Acad Sci USA 1993;90:3913–3917.
37. Hansen PJ, Liu WJ. Biology of progesterone-induced uterine serpins. Adv Exp Biol Med 1997;425:143–154.
38. Lea RG, Stewart F, Allen WR, Ohno I, Clark DA. Accumulation of chromotrope 2R positive cells in equine endometrium during early pregnancy and expression of transforming growth factor-$\beta 2$ (TGF $\beta 2$). J Reprod Fertil 1995;10:339–347.
39. Segerson EC, Li H, Talbott CW, Allen JW, Gunsett FC. Partial characterization of ovine intrauterine suppressor cells. Biol Reprod 1998;58:397–406.
40. Newton GR, Vallet JL, Hansen PJ, Bazer FW. Inhibition of lymphocyte proliferation by ovine trophoblast protein-1 and a high-molecular-weight glycoprotein produced by the peri-implantation sheep conceptus. Am J Reprod Immunol Microbiol 1989;19:99–107.
41. Krishman L, Guilberg LJ, Wegmann TG, Belosevic M, Mossmann TR. T helper 1 response against *Leishmania major* in pregnant C57BL/6 mice increases implantation failure and fetal resorptions. Correlation with increased IFN-$\gamma$ and TNF and reduced IL-10 production by placental cells. J Immunol 1996;156:653–662.
42. Guller S. Role of Fas ligand in conferring privilege to non-lymphoid cells. Ann NY Acad Sci 1997;828:262–272.
43. Hunt JS, Vassmer D, Ferguson TA, Miller L. Fas ligand is positioned in mouse uterus and placenta to prevent trafficking of activated leukocytes between the mother and the conceptus. J Immunol 1997;158:4122–4128.
44. Tafuri A, Alferink J, Moller P, Hammerling GJ, Arnold B. T cell awareness of paternal alloantigens during pregnancy. Science 1995;27:630–633.
45. Kydd JH, Butcher GW, Antczak DF, Allen WR. Expression of major histocompatibility complex (MHC) class I molecules on early trophoblast. J Reprod Fertil 1996;44(Suppl): 463–477.
46. Grünig G, Triplett L, Canady LK, Allen WR, and Antczak DF. The maternal leukocyte response to the endometrial cups in horses is correlated with the developmental stages of the invasive trophoblast cells. Placenta 1995;16:539–559.
47. Allen WR, Kydd J, Miller J, Antczak DF. Immunological studies on feto-maternal relationships in equine pregnancy. In: Crighton DB, ed. Immunological aspects of reproduction in mammals. London: Butterworths, 1984:183–193.
48. Vogiagis D, Salomonsen LA, Sandemann RM, Squires TJ, Fry RC. Leukemia inhibitory factor in ovine blastocyst implantation: its endometrial expression and the effect of passive immunization. Proc 13th Int Congr Anim Reprod, Sydney 1996;2:11.
49. Joosten I, Sanders MF, Hensen EJ. Involvement of major histocompatibility complex class I compatibility between dam and calf in the aetiology of bovine retained placenta. Anim Genet 1991;22:455–463.

CHAPTER 24

# Molecular Biology of Reproduction

R. JUNEJA AND S.S. KOIDE

Deoxyribonucleic acid (DNA) is the molecule that contains and transfers genetic information from one generation to the next. The DNA molecules in association with histones and various proteins are organized to form complex intracellular structures called "chromosomes." Each species is endowed with a fixed number of pairs. Mammalian gametes are the direct products of reductive division of chromosomes termed meiosis, and thus contain the haploid number (abbreviated n) of the hereditary determinants. Both gametes contribute equally to the genetic makeup of a new progeny by transmitting haploid number (n) of chromosomes to the newly formed diploid zygote (2n) of the next generation (Figure 24-1). Sex steroids allow the female to carry the growing embryo over a prolonged period until parturition (viviparity), and to nurture the young after birth through an extended period by supplying milk and protection (Figure 24-2).

Farm animals show marked differences in the time of onset of puberty, sensitivity in reproductive function to environmental factors, estrus cycle, gestational period, and number of offspring born. Recent advances in genetics and molecular biology have made it possible to select and take advantages of the genetic makeup of farm animals. Although there are considerable variations in the pattern of reproduction, the general mechanisms and genes expressed during ovulation, spermatogenesis, fertilization, and implantation remain common to all the farm animals (Table 24-1). This chapter is focused on the molecular biology of different aspects of reproduction.

## GENETIC DETERMINANTS IN REPRODUCTION

DNA contains within its helical structure the hereditary information, and also provides the basis for the evolutionary process. DNA directs cellular growth and proliferation, and also regulates the differentiation of fertilized egg to form the multitude of specialized cells required for organogenesis and proper functioning of mature animals. The majority of the DNA is located within the nucleus in the form of coiled rods and is an integral part of chromosomes. Each species of farm animal has a fixed number of chromosomes, and each chromosome occurs as duplicates (homologous chromosomes). During the formation of gametes (sex cells), reductive division designated as meiosis occurs, whereby the number of chromosomes in the cells is reduced to a haploid number (n), or half the diploid number (2n), found in somatic or nonsex cells.

Each species of farm animals possesses a definite number of autosomes (nonsex chromosomes) and one pair of sex chromosomes. Female mammals are the homogametic sex because both sex chromosomes are of the X type and all the oocytes are haploid possessing a single X chromosome. Conversely, the male is termed the heterogametic sex, since one pair of sex chromosome consists of an X and a Y type. This produces two distinct populations of spermatozoa, one bearing an X and the other a Y chromosome (Figure 24-3).

Fertilization of an egg by a sperm containing an X chromosome generates female (XX) progeny, whereas fertilization by a sperm having a Y chromosome yields male (XY) progeny. Thus, male gametes determine the sex of the new progeny. Following advances in genetics and *in vitro* fertilization techniques, X or Y bearing sperm can be selected and used to fertilize an egg and obtain progeny having the desired sex. However, there are no known inherent advantages of fertilizability between X and Y bearing gametes.

## DEVELOPMENT OF THE GONADS

The fetal gonads arise from the indifferent primordial anlage and develop into a testis or an ovary. In mammals, the direction of sex development is controlled genetically; fe-

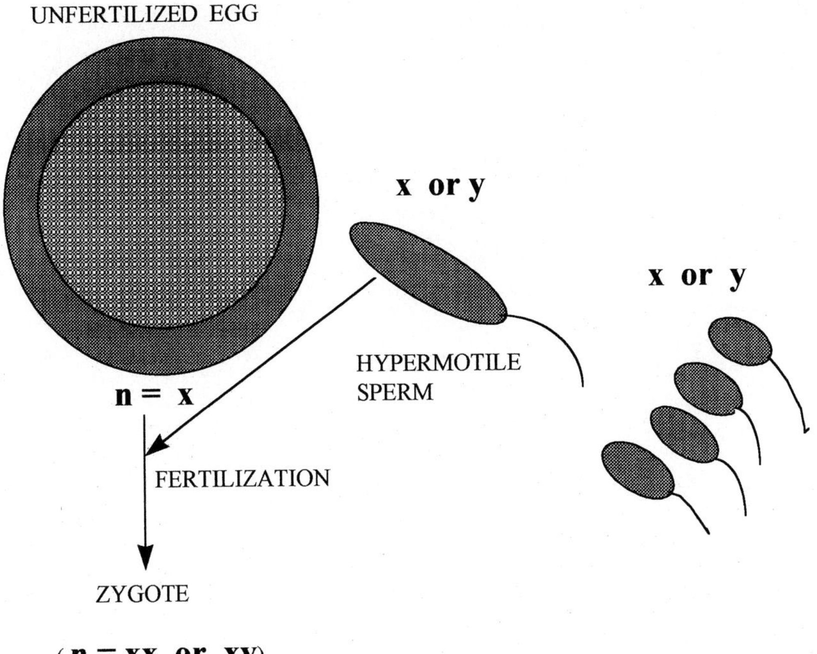


FIGURE 24-1. Fertilization of haploid gametes and generation of a diploid zygote.

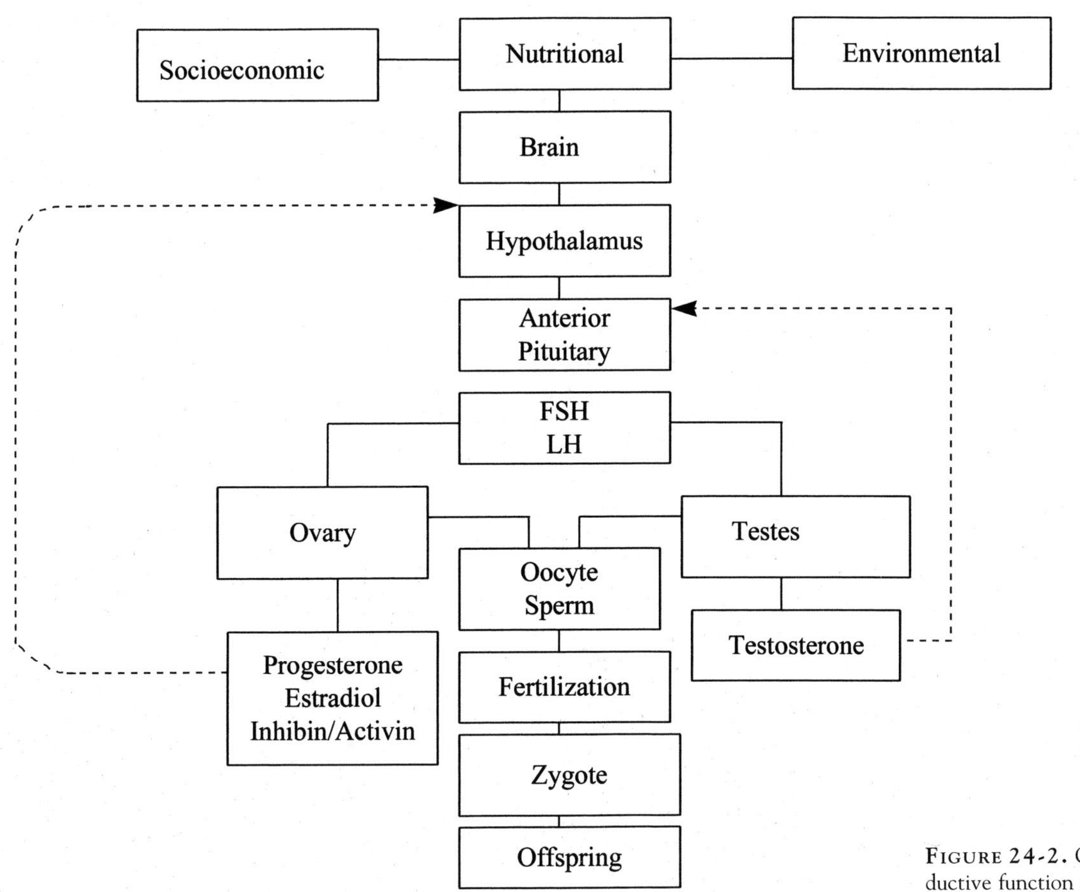


FIGURE 24-2. General aspects of reproductive function and control.

TABLE 24-1. *Genes Expressed in Reproduction*

| REPRODUCTIVE PROCESS | GENE |
|---|---|
| Spermatogenesis | Proacrosin gene[a]<br>Smcy, Hya, Sdma, CRES[b,c]<br>Spx1, MSH2, HSF2[d,e,f]<br>Pgk-2, ApoA1, Oct-3/4[g] |
| Oogenesis | RLF gene, oxytocin gene[h,i] |
| Fertilization | BE-20[j] |
| Preimplantation and implantation | Cytokines, Sry[k,l]<br>Myc, Sp1[m,n]<br>Oct4, Oct6, PIBF[o,p]<br>EGF[q] |

[a]Nayernia K, Adham I, Kremling H, et al. Stage and development-specific gene expression during mammalian spermatogenesis. Int J Dev Biol 1996;40:379–383.
[b]Agulnik AL, Mitchell MJ, Lerner JL, et al. A mouse Y chromosome gene encoded by a region essential for spermatogenesis and expression of male-specific minor histocompatibility antigens. Hum Mol Genet 1994;3:873–878.
[c]Cornwall GA, Hann SR. Transient appearance of CRES protein during spermatogenesis and caput epididymal sperm maturation. Mol Reprod Dev 1995;41:37–46.
[d]Branford WW, Zhao GQ, Valerius MT, et al. Spx1, a novel x-linked homeobox gene expressed during spermatogenesis. Mech Dev 1997;65:87–98.
[e]Vani RG, Rao MR. Cloning of the cDNA encoding rat homologue of the mismatch repair gene MSH2 and its expression during spermatogenesis. Gene 1997;185:19–26.
[f]Sarge KD, Park-Sarge OK, Kirby JD, et al. Expression of heat shock factor 2 in mouse testis: potential role as a regulator of heat-shock protein gene expression during spermatogenesis. Biol Reprod 1994;50:1334–1343.
[g]Ariel M, Cedar H, McCarrey J. Developmental changes in methylation of spermatogenesis-specific genes include reprogramming in the epididymis. Nat Genet 1994;7:59–63.
[h]Bathgate R, Balvers M, Hunt N, Ivell R. Relaxin-like factor gene is highly expressed in the bovine ovary of the cycle and pregnancy: sequence and ribonucleic acid analysis. Biol Reprod 1996;55:1452–1457.
[i]Furuya K, Mizumoto N, Makimura N, et al. A novel biological aspect of ovarian oxytocin: gene expression of oxytocin and oxytocin receptor in cumulus/luteal cells and the effect of oxytocin on embryogenesis in fertilized oocytes. Adv Exp Med Biol 1995;395:523–528.
[j]Xu WD, Miao SY, Zhang ML, et al. Expression of the BE-20 epididymal protein gene: in situ hybridization. Arch Androl 1997;38:1–6.
[k]Gerwin N, Jia GQ, Kulbacki R, Gutierrez-Ramos JC. Interleukin gene expression in mouse preimplantation development. Dev Immunol 1995;4:169–179.
[l]Cao QP, Gaudette MF, Robinson DH, Crain WR. Expression of the mouse testis-determining gene Sry in male preimplantation embryos. Mol Reprod Dev 1995;40:196–204.
[m]Domashenko AD, Latham KE, Hatton KS. Expression of myc-family, myc-interacting, and myc-target genes during preimplantation mouse development. Mol Reprod Dev 1997;47:57–65.
[n]Worrad DM, Schultz RM. Regulation of gene expression in the preimplantation mouse embryo: temporal and spatial patterns of expression of the transcription factor Sp1. Mol Reprod Rev 1997;46:268–277.
[o]Abdel-Rahman B, Fiddler M, Rappolee D, Pergament E. Expression of transcription regulating genes in human preimplantation embryo. Hum Reprod 1995;10:2787–2792.
[p]Check JH, Szekeres-Bartho J, O'Shaughnessy A. Progesterone induced blocking factor seen in pregnancy lymphocytes soon after implantation. Am J Reprod Imunol 1996;35:277–280.
[q]Tamada H, Kai Y, Mori J. Epidermal growth factor-induced implantation and decidualization in the rat. Prostaglandin 1994;47:467–475.

males have two X chromosomes whereas males have one X and one Y chromosome. Animals with a single X chromosome and no Y chromosome (XO) are phenotypically females, indicating that the Y chromosome dictates male development.

### *Development of the Testis*

A particular region of the Y chromosome must encode a dominant inducer of testis formation. The Y-linked genes controlling this process have been named the "testis determining factor" (TDF) which instructs the undifferentiated genital ridge to develop into a testis. The gonad is composed of cells derived from four lineages: supporting cells, steroid-producing cells, connective tissue cells, and germ cells. The repression of the Y-chromosome in determining gonadal sex becomes discernible at the time of completion of germ cell colonization, during the sixth week in human embryo development.

### *Development of the Ovary*

The differentiation of a gonad into an ovary is not dependent on the expression of Sry. The primitive sex cords of

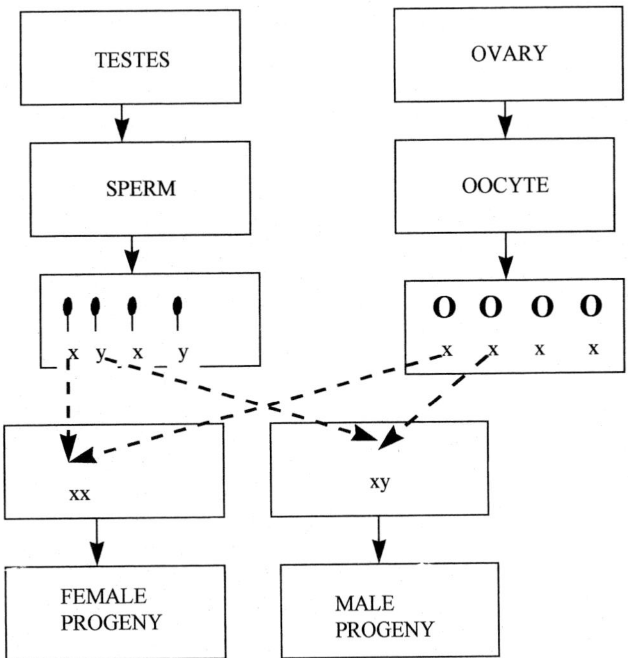


FIGURE 24-3. Schematic representation of generation of two different progenies by fertilization between two distinct populations of sperm with eggs.

the human female are morphologically ill-defined, although in some farm animals, e.g. sheep and pigs, the cords are well delineated. The normal development of the ovary and follicles depends on the presence of germ cells. The absence or an excess of X chromosome (XO or XXX) results in nonviable oocytes. Many genes coding for important factors and receptors are expressed during the development of the testis (Table 24-2) and the ovary.

The relaxin-like factor (RLF) gene is highly expressed in the follicular theca interna and in the corpus luteum of the female cow and in the bovine male gonads. RLF in the cow retains relaxin binding receptor motif and seems to substitute functionally for relaxin in the cow. A recent study demonstrates that the gene encoding for oxytocin is detected in both mouse and human cumulus cells, whereas the oxytocin receptor gene is expressed in human cumulus cells. These studies suggest that ovarian oxytocin may have some physiologic role in cell cleavage.

**TABLE 24-2. *Genetic Control of Testis Determination***

| GENES | ROLE DURING TESTIS DEVELOPMENT |
|---|---|
| Tdy (testis determining factor in mice) | Act on supporting cell lineage and inducing differentiation of supporting cells to Sertoli cells. |
| Sry (a Y-chromosome specific gene) | Different homologues of Sry have a common open reading frame which has a 41% homology to a DNA binding motif HMG-box; Sry encoded protein might have DNA binding activity. |
| Sox6 (Sry related gene), Sox5 | Overlapping functions in the regulation of gene expression during spermatogenesis in the adult mouse. |
| Sox9 | A critical Sertoli cell differentiation factor. |
| TAZ83 | Coding at early to mid-pachytene germ cell stage. |
| TAZ4 | Testis specific gene located on chromosome 11. |
| TNZ1 | Expressed in neonatal Leydig cells. |

## MOLECULAR PARAMETERS OF SPERMATOGENESIS

Spermatogenesis is a process of cell differentiation and development that occurs in three phases: mitotic, meiotic, and postmeiotic (Figure 24-4).

### *Mitosis*

Germ cells present in immature testes are reactivated at puberty and undergo mitosis while situated in the basal compartment of the tubule. These generated spermatogonial stem cells give rise to cells with a distinct morphological characteristic, classified as A1 spermatogonia. The emergence of these cells marks the beginning of spermatogenesis. Each spermatogonia undergoes a defined number of mitotic divisions unique to the species, giving rise to a "clone" of cells which differ morphologically from their parents. The nuclear division during mitosis (karyokinesis) is complete, whereas the cytoplasmic division (cytokinesis) is incomplete, resulting in primary spermatocytes connected by thin cytoplasmic bridges. This interconnecting syncytial state of germ cells exists throughout the entire process of spermatogenesis.

### *Meiosis*

During meiosis, a number of genes present on autosomes are expressed; however, genes located on sex-chromosomes remain inactive. Later during spermatid formation, the autosomes cease RNA production and their DNA becomes highly condensed or heterochromatic.

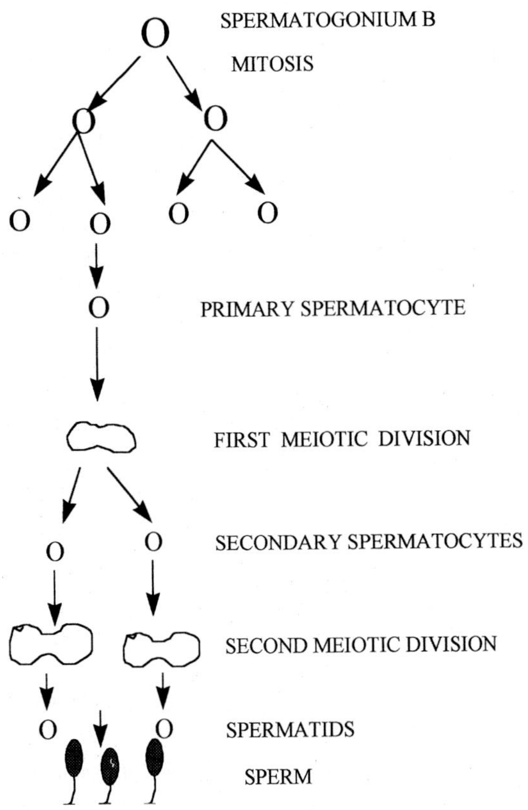


FIGURE 24-4. A series of events occurring during spermatogenesis.

### *Postmeiotic Phases*

Spermiogenesis involves major remodeling of the structure of spermatids to form spermatozoa, which are composed of three distinct parts; head, midpiece, and tail. The nucleus present in head region contains compact packaged haploid chromosomes. Upon completion of spermatogenesis, the spermatozoa are released into the lumen of the seminiferous tubules by spermiation. Different species have varying periodicity in the spermatogenesis cycle. Nonetheless, within a given species the rate of progression of germ cell differentiation through various stages of spermatogenesis is remarkably constant (Table 24-3).

TABLE 24-3. ***Duration of Spermatogenesis in Different Species***

| SPECIES | TIME (DAYS) |
|---|---|
| Bull | 54 |
| Boar | 39 |
| Ram | 47 |
| Man | 74 |

TABLE 24-4. ***Genes Involved During Spermatogenesis and Their Function***

| GENES | ROLE DURING SPERMATOGENESIS |
|---|---|
| Smcy | A Y-chromosome gene; isolated from the region encoding a spermatogenesis gene Spy. |
| Hya, Smda | A regulatory role in the espression of the male specific minor histocompatibility antigen H-Y. |
| CRES (cystatin-related epidydimal and spermatogenic) gene | Specialized role during sperm development and maturation. |
| YRRM (Y-located RNA recognition motif) gene | A candidate for azoospermia factor. |
| Spx1 (X-linked homeobox gene), MSH2 (mismatch repair gene), HSF2 (heat shock factor 2) | A regulatory role during spermatogenesis. |
| Pgk-2, ApoA1, Oct-3/4 | Role in sperm maturation process. |
| Gene encoding T-type $Ca^{2+}$ channel | The voltage-sensitive calcium-channel sensitive to blocking agents dihydropyridine and Nifedipine. |

Spermatogenesis provides an interesting system for examining the regulation of gene expression during development and differentiation. The genes expressed during spermatogenesis can be divided into two main groups: (a) diploid, e.g. the proacrosin gene, and (b) haploid expressed genes, e.g. the gene encoding the transition protein 2, a novel gene from the rat protamine gene cluster (Prm3), and a spermatid located calpastatin gene. A number of novel genes playing a role during spermatogenesis have been identified (Table 24-4).

## MOLECULAR PARAMETERS OF OVULATION

In females, the production and differentiation of oocytes occur by three different processes: (a) cell proliferation by mitosis, (b) genetic restructuring and chromosome reduction by meiosis, and (c) packaging of chromosomes during maturation. Oogonia, the primordial cells, undergo mitotic proliferation during fetal development that ceases during the prenatal period in human beings and in some animals (cow, sheep, goat, and mouse), or shortly after birth (pig, cat, hamster, rabbit, and rat).

### *Primary Oocytes*

Oogonia differentiate into primary oocytes which commence meiotic division and become surrounded by a layer of granulosa cells. The basement membrane "membrana propria" is produced by the follicular cells. The oocytes are arrested at the first meiotic prophase, the "dictyate stage," where chromosomes are retained within the nucleus of the germinal vesicle. The arrested oocytes remain in this stage until reactivated to resume maturation.

### *The Antral Phase*

The oocytes are surrounded by a single layer of cells to form the primordial follicle. At puberty, a few follicles resume growth periodically so that a continuous wave of developing follicles is produced. The growth of each primordial follicle is accompanied by the biosynthesis of a large amount of ribosomal ribonucleic acid (rRNA) and messenger RNA (mRNA) reflecting expression of the dictyate chromosomes. These newly synthesized RNAs are translated to generate proteins required for the metabolic processes, occurring during later stages of oocyte maturation. During this period, the oocyte reaches its final size and becomes surrounded by a translucent acellular layer called the zona pellucida. The surrounding granulosa cells divide and the follicle enlarges, while layers of theca cells are laid down around the granulosa cells. During subsequent development, theca cells differentiate into an inner glandular, highly vascular theca interna, surrounded by a fibrous capsule, the theca externa. Fluid begins to accumulate in the spaces between the granulosa cells and coalesce to form a fluid-filled antrum. The appearance of the follicular antrum marks the beginning of the antral phase of development. Although the oocyte does not increase in size during the antral period, synthesis of RNA and turnover of proteins continues to occur with an increase in the size of follicular antrum, and the oocyte becomes surrounded by a dense mass of granulosa cells (cumulus oophorus) and becomes suspended in fluid.

### *Ovulation*

In species that usually undergo a single ovulation, one dominant follicle will progress to ovulation. In species that produce litters, a preovulatory cohort of follicles progresses to ovulation. At ovulation (in most species), the oocyte completes the first meiotic division, culminating in an extraordinary cell division in which half the chromosomes, and almost all the cytoplasm, goes to one cell called the secondary oocyte. The remaining chromosomes are extruded as a small bag of cytoplasm called the first polar body. This unequal division of cytoplasm ensures that all the essential materials synthesized during the earlier phases are retained by the secondary oocyte.

The chromosomes in the secondary oocyte immediately enter the second meiotic division and progress to the metaphase stage. Then, suddenly, meiosis arrest occurs, and the arrested oocyte is ovulated in the metaphase stage. These oocytes can be activated by spermatozoa or by various chemical stimuli. Similar to spermatogenesis, the periodicity of the ovarian cycle is constant for a particular species, but varies somewhat among species.

## FERTILIZATION AND IMPLANTATION

The immotile and immature spermatozoa undergo a series of changes during their transit through the rete testes, ductuli efferentia, and epididymis to become motile and mature. Expression of the BE-20 epididymal protein gene is detected in the cauda epididymis and the proximal segment of the ductus deferens, suggesting a role in sperm maturation and its capacity to fertilize ova.

### *Sperm-Egg Interactions*

Sperm-egg binding between the outer membrane of the sperm and outermost glycoprotein covering (zona pellucida 3, ZP3) of the egg occurs initially as a species-specific interaction. The sperm-receptor present on the surface of the unfertilized egg involved in the sperm-egg binding has been identified as ZP3. The sperm-egg binding triggers the acrosome reaction in the sperm head, which involves fusion of the outer acrosomal membrane with the overlying sperm plasma membrane. The net result of the acrosome reaction is the release of hydrolytic enzymes and exposure of the inner acrosomal membrane. Together with increased motility (hyperactivation), and the liberated hydrolytic enzymes, the acrosome-reacted sperm has the potential to penetrate its way through the zona pellucida and enter the perivitelline space. The sperm head next sinks into the oocyte, triggering the second meiotic division, which leads to the formation and extrusion of the second polar body.

### *Conceptus Development*

The conceptus undergoes cell proliferation to form blastomeres. During early stages of development, the conceptus' own chromosomes are inactive and dependent upon maternal cytoplasmic products, which makes maternal cytoplasmic inheritance a crucial determinant. A deficiency in oocyte maturation may result in abnormal growth. At a specific stage of development, which is characteristic for the species, conceptus genes become active and encode for newly synthesized proteins. At this point all maternal mRNA are destroyed. Several growth factors seem to act as autocrine and paracrine agents in promoting early development.

The zona pellucida surrounds the dividing conceptus until it reaches the fully expanded blastocyst stage, and may play two important roles: (a) protecting the dividing blastomeres from the deleterious agents in the environment and, (b) preventing two distinct conceptuses from making a chimeric conceptus.

### *Embryo Development*

Cleavage of the embryo is a period of transitions; protamines are replaced by histones, maternal control of development is succeeded by zygotic control, a diploid genome is formed after a wave of demethylation of the haploid paternal genome. The embryo can be manipulated during the preimplantation stage by transferring, cryopreserving, cloning, or microinjecting with transgenic constructs for improvement in animal production. Several genes, cytokines (polypeptide growth factors released by a variety of activated immune and nonimmune cells), and growth factors are expressed during specific stages of cleavage. Expression of the testis-determining factor gene, Sry, in a male blastocyst-stage embryo indicates the possibility that sex determination begins during early embryonic development. First, maternally inherited Myc proteins and the corresponding mRNA, and subsequently stage-specific expression of Myc genes and its target genes, play a crucial role in cleavage. The amount of a transcription factor, Sp1, which regulates the expression of a number of genes involved in cell proliferation and differentiation, increases eight-fold during preimplantation. The expression pattern of two transcription regulators, Oct4 and Oct6, indicates that these two genes play a differential role in embryogenesis and are conserved in evolution.

### *Implantation*

The implantation of the blastocyst involves complex local embryo-uterine interactions in which embryo proteins, steroid hormones, and other signals play important roles. Soon after implantation there is an increase in the percentage of lymphocytes expressing the gene coding the progesterone-induced blocking factor (PIBF) during pregnancy. It would appear that PIBF may play an important role in implantation by inhibiting the destructive activities of natural killer lymphocytes. The epidermal growth factor plays an important role in blastocyst implantation (1).

## PREGNANCY AND PARTURITION

The fetus determines the time of parturition via the secretion of adrenal cortical factors. Glucocorticoids stimulate the production of prostaglandin $F_{2\alpha}$ ($PGF_{2\alpha}$) by the placenta, which in turn incites luteolysis or regression of luteal cells leading to a reduction in progesterone levels. The low level of progesterone will promote contraction of the myometrium and the resulting increase in the estradiol : progesterone ratio will facilitate oxytocin release from the posterior pituitary promoting uterine contractions. This in turn will enhance further release of $PGF_{2\alpha}$ as parturition progresses. The low levels of uterine oxytocin receptor mRNA during pregnancy, the subsequent rise at term, and a further marked increase at parturition suggests a significant role of oxytocin in the expulsion of the neonate.

## LACTATION AND MATERNAL BEHAVIOR

Lactation plays an important role for the final success in reproduction of perpetuating the species, since it ensures the survival of the newborn by providing the essential nutrients contained in milk. Although the basic structure of the breast is the same, the number of mammary glands, size, location, and shape vary by species. The sow has nine pairs of mammary glands (total eighteen), the cow has two pairs, and sheep has one pair of mammary glands.

At the onset of puberty, successive exposure of the mammary glands to estrogen and progesterone induces breast growth. During pregnancy, milk secreting capacity is influenced by the steroids secreted by the adrenal, ovary, and placenta. High levels of prolactin stimulate milk secretion; estrogen and progesterone suppress milk production. Suckling of the teats promotes the prolactin receptor gene expression and promotes the continuous production of milk. Termination of breast feeding eventually leads to a suppression of milk production. Fertility is usually suppressed in lactating mothers for approximately six weeks postpartum. The hypothesis proposed to explain the infertile condition is that the continued production of high levels of prolactin during lactation suppresses the cyclic production of gonadotropins which are required for initiating ovulation and progression of the menstrual cycle.

Maternal behavior is critically important throughout pregnancy and also after birth to provide protection, warmth, and food required for the survival of the newborns. Maternal behavior plays an important role starting with the preparation for the arrival of the newborn, to the immediate feeding and protection of the young, and to instill independence in her young ones. In contrast to general belief, pregnancy hormones appear not to promote development of maternal behavior, although exposure to hormones, e.g., estradiol, during late pregnancy modifies maternal behavior. Cervical stimulation appears to play an important role in the performance of maternal behavior and this finding has had a major impact on sheep farming. The most important event that governs maternal behavior is still the continuous contact of the mother with her growing newborn.

In February 1997, a lamb named Dolly was successfully cloned from an adult cell. This technology has opened new vistas to create genetically tailored livestock (a) to churn out medically useful proteins in their milk, (b) to harvest organs to transplant in humans, (c) to serve as better animal models for genetic diseases, and (d) to produce possibly leaner, faster growing livestock. The scientific breakthrough—cloning animals from adult mammalian cells—has changed science fiction into reality and will electrify both the research community and the general public for years to come.

## REFERENCES

1. Tamada H, Kai Y, Mori J. Epidermal growth factor-induced implantation and decidualization in the rat. Prostaglandin 1994;47:467–475.

## SUGGESTED READING

Chandley AC, Cooke H J. Human male fertility-Y-linked genes and spermatogenesis. Hum Mol Genet 1994;3:1449–1452.

Fuchs AR, Ivell R, Balvers M, Chang SM, Fields MJ. Oxytocin receptors in bovine cervix during pregnancy and parturition: gene expression and cellular localization. Am J Obstet Gynecol 1996;175:1654–1660.

Harley VR. Genetic control of testis determination. In: d' Krester D, ed. Molecular Biology of Male Reproductive System. San Diego: Academic Press, 1993;1–20.

Harvey MB, Leco K J, Arcellana-Panlilo MY, Zhang X, Edwards DR, Schultz GA. Roles of growth factors during peri-implantation development. Hum Reprod 1995;10:712–718.

Hutchinson JSM. Background in Reproductive Biology. In: Hutchinson JSM, ed. Controlling Reproduction. London: Chapman and Hall, 1993.

Johnson MH, Barry JE. Essential Reproduction. Oxford: Blackwell Science Ltd, 1995.

Lamb DJ. Genes involved in testicular development and function. World J Urol 1995;13:277–284.

Lievano A, Santi CM, Serrano CJ, et al. T-type $Ca^{2+}$ channels and alpha1E expression in spermatogenic cells, and their possible relevance to the sperm acrosome reaction. FEBS Lett 1996; 388:150–154.

# Part VI

# Assisted Reproductive Technology

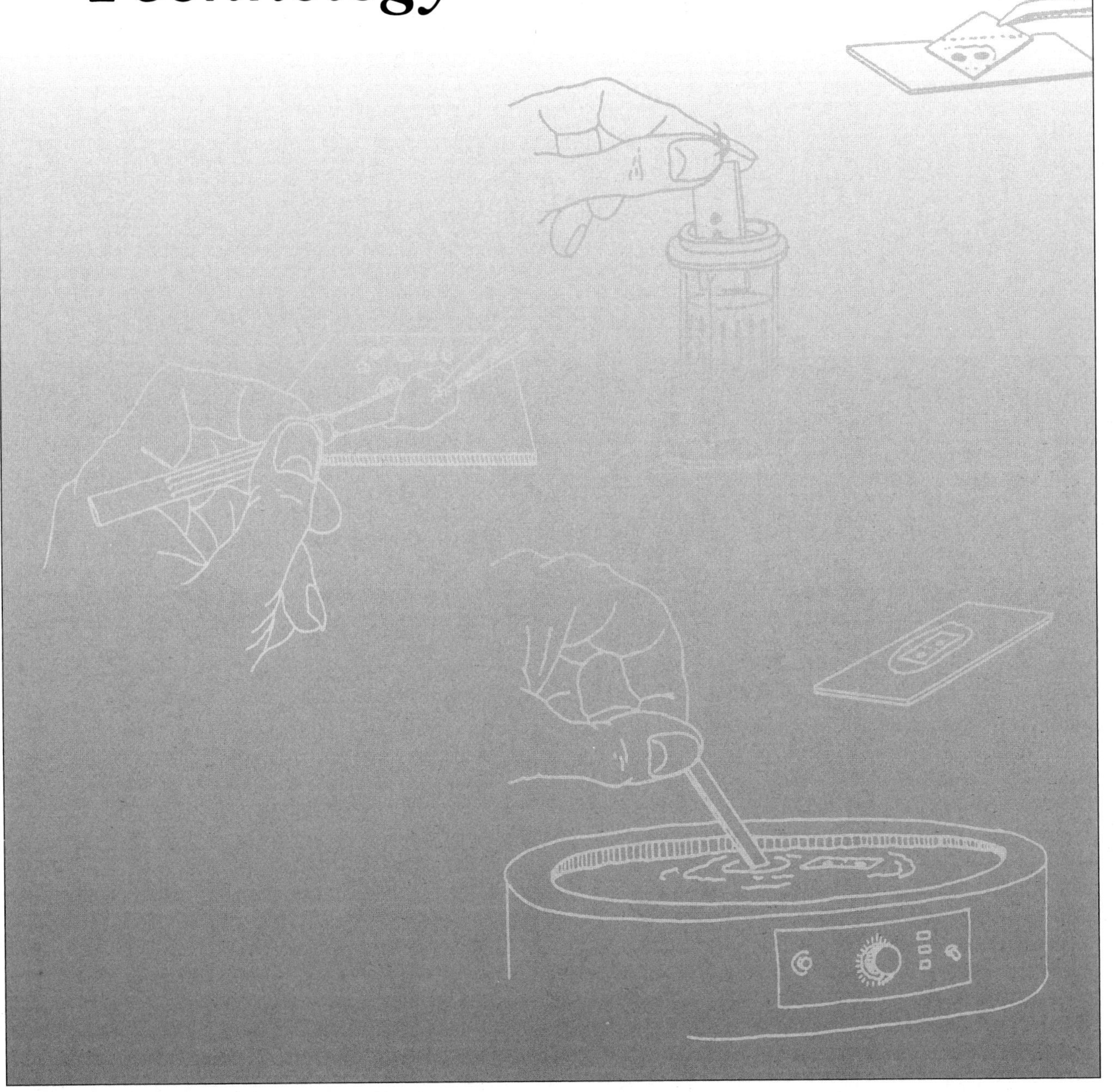

# Chapter 25

# Semen Evaluation

R.L. Ax, M. Dally, B.A. Didion, R.W. Lenz, C.C. Love,
D.D. Varner, B. Hafez, and M.E. Bellin

Sperm are unique among cells in form and function. Mature sperm are terminal cells, the end products of complex developmental processes, that cannot undergo further division or differentiation. The standard method of evaluating the fertility of breeding males, other than directly evaluating their ability to produce a pregnancy, is by examination of semen.

## Evaluation and Fertility

No single test accurately predicts fertility of a sperm sample, however examining various physical characteristics of semen can determine greater fertility potential. The guidelines of Society for Theriogenology represent minimal acceptable thresholds for semen characteristics that must be met for a bull to pass a breeding soundness evaluation, which includes physical examination and perhaps a vaccination/health certification (1). In general, the minimal standards for a classification of a specimen of bull semen are as follows:

- Over 500 million sperm per mL are present;
- More than 50% of motile sperm make forward progression;
- More than 80% of the spermatozoa conform to normal morphology.

Only when motile sperm are totally absent and the reproductive system has been carefully examined for disease can it be stated that a bull is sterile.

Diagnostic analysis of boar semen involves obtaining maximum information about the physiologic status of testicular and epididymal function by examining one or several ejaculates. In general, the minimum requirements for a **probable fertile** boar semen sample would include:

- At least 65% motility;
- Less than 20% morphological abnormalities;
- At least 100 million sperm per mL, with at least 60 to 75 mL produced per ejaculate.

## Appearance and Volume

### Bull

Semen should have a relatively uniform, opaque appearance indicative of high sperm cell concentration. Translucent samples contain few sperm. The sample should be free from hair, dirt, and other contaminants. Semen with a curdy appearance, containing chunks of material, should not be used; this indicates infection. Bulls can produce yellow semen, owing to the harmless presence of riboflavin. This should not be confused with urine, which has its own distinctive odor. Young animals and those of smaller size within a species produce smaller volumes of semen. Frequent ejaculation results in lower average volume, and when two ejaculates are obtained consecutively, the second usually has the lower volume. Small volume is not harmful, but if accompanied by a low sperm concentration, total output declines.

### Boar

The ejaculate from a boar is collected in several fractions. The first fluid to appear is the **pre-sperm fraction**. It is translucent and easily identified. The next thick, whitish, opaque fluid is referred to as the **sperm-rich fraction**. This is followed by a **post-sperm fraction** similar in appearance to the pre-sperm fraction, but it is less translucent with greater concentrations of sperm. Ordinarily, the total volume of the ejaculate is recorded.

The average expected parameters are 240 to 250 mL of total volume, with approximately 20% of this volume consisting of gelatinous like fluid, 20 to 30% consisting of sperm, and the difference being pre-sperm and post-sperm fluids. Total volume and sperm concentrations are influenced by age, environment, health status, semen collection procedure, season of the year, frequency of collection, and breed differences. A wet mount of the sample is placed on a clean glass slide and is observed for the following: white

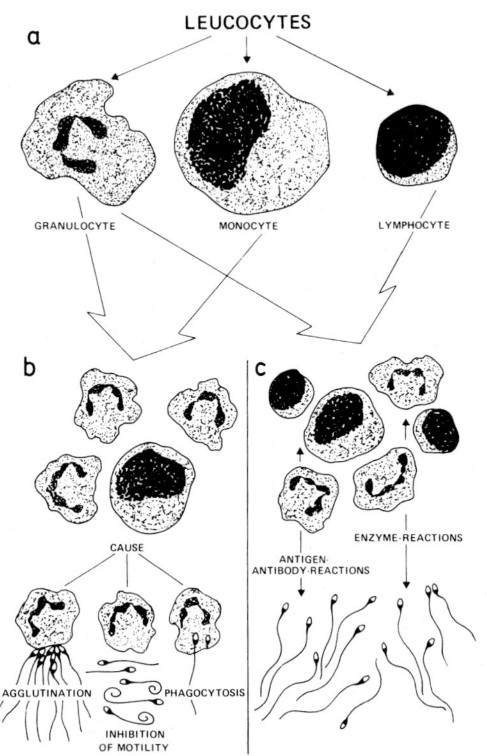


FIGURE 25-1. Cellular interactions among granulocytes, monocytes, lymphocytes, and spermatozoa.

blood cells, red blood cells, spermatogenic cells, crystals, debris, and agglutination (Fig. 25-1).

### *Stallion*

Sperm quality and quantity should be assessed immediately after collection. Gel is separated from the gel-free fraction by aspiration with a syringe, if a filter was not placed in the artificial vagina before collection. Filtration also is required to help remove extraneous debris, such as smegma, hair, and dirt, from the gel-free semen. Volumes of gel and gel-free semen are then measured, noting color and consistency of the sample. Although volume, by itself, is not important to fertility, it is used in calculation of total sperm number contained in an ejaculate. Consequently, accurate measurement of volume is essential. Semen volume can be increased by excessive precopulatory teasing, but total sperm numbers remain unchanged. Semen volume is also affected by season, with less produced in winter compared to summer. Gross evaluation of a semen sample provides a rough estimate of its sperm concentration and permits detection of contaminants.

### *Ram*

Ram semen is milky-white or a pale creamy color. Pink color indicates blood, likely due to injury of the penis at collection. Contamination or an infection of the ram reproductive tract is suggested by gray or brown semen. When an electroejaculator is used, rams may urinate. This is indicated by a strong odor, with yellow and dilute semen. Contaminated samples should be discarded. Semen volume varies according to collection method. Larger volumes result from electroejaculation compared to artificial vagina (AV) collections. Ejaculate volume is affected by ram age and condition, season, skill of collector, and frequency of collection. When using an AV, false mounts may increase ejaculate volume. If rams are collected three or more times per day or for lengthy periods, ejaculate volume declines. The ejaculate volume ranges from 0.5 to 2.0 mL mature animals, and 0.5 to 0.7 mL in young rams.

### *Buck*

Buck semen is grayish white to yellow and color varies more than ram semen. In fact, color varies between bucks, and between ejaculates from the same buck. Ejaculate volume is 1.0 mL with a range of 0.5 and 1.2 mL.

## SPERM CONCENTRATION

The terminology for semen is listed in Table 25-1. Accurate determination of the number of sperm and volume of the

**Table 25-1. *Semen Analysis Nomenclature***

| PARAMETER | EVALUATION CRITERIA | NOMENCLATURE |
|---|---|---|
| Volume | None | Aspermia |
| | Reduced | Hypospermia |
| | Increased | Hyperspermia |
| Sperm concentration | Zero | Azoospermia |
| | Reduced | Oligozoospermia |
| | Normal | Normozoospermia |
| | Increased | Polyzoospermia |
| Sperm motility | Decreased | Asthenozoospermia |
| Sperm viability | All dead | Necrozoospermia |
| Abnormal sperm | High percentage | Teratozoospermia |

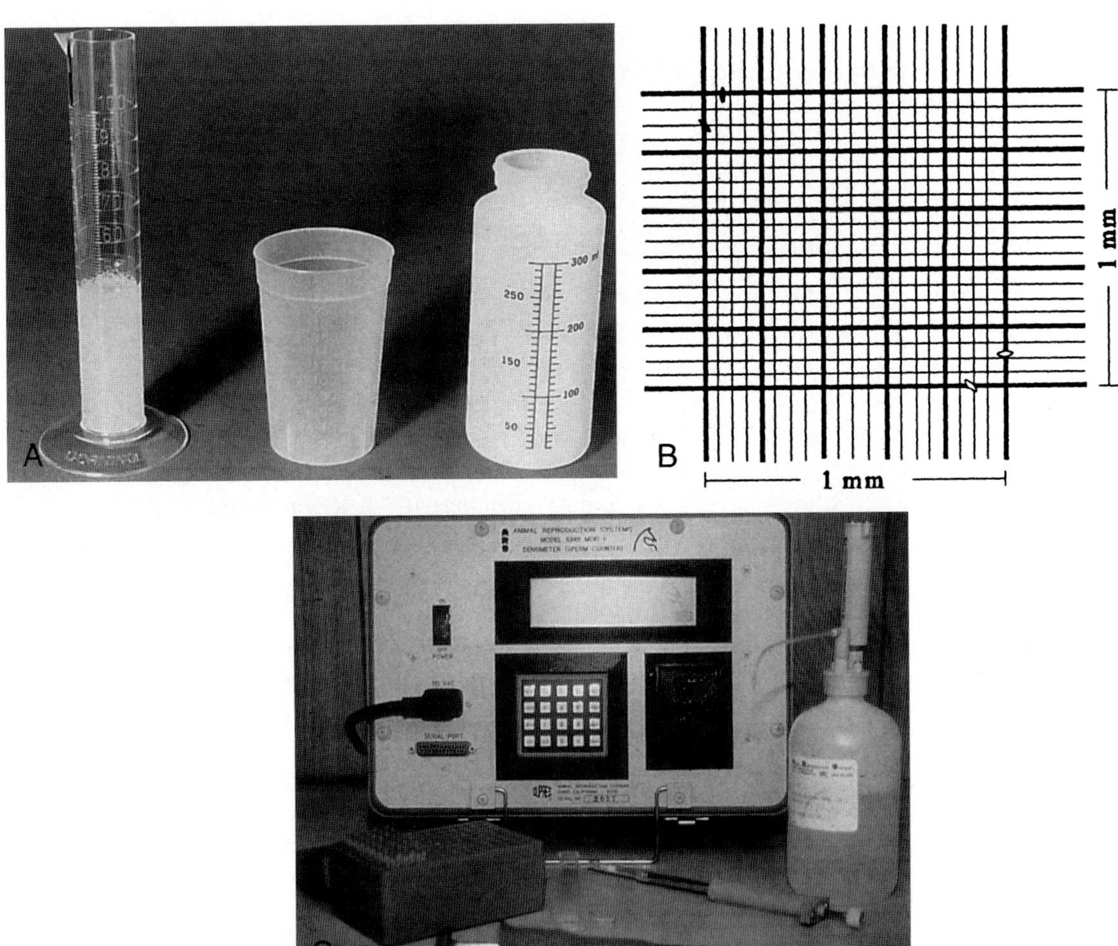


FIGURE 25-2. (A) A graduated cylinder (*left*) is superior to a specimen cup (*center*) or semen collection receptacle (*right*) for measuring semen volume. (B) Technique for determining sperm concentration using a hemacytometer. (C) Photometric instruments such as this densimeter (Animal Reproduction Systems, Chino, California) can accelerate measurement of sperm concentration. These units should be properly calibrated using hemacytometer measurements.

ejaculate determines how many females can be inseminated (Fig. 25-2**A**). Concentration is measured using a hemacytometer, colorimeter, or spectrophotometer (Figs. 25-2**B** and 25-2**C**). A hemacytometer is a microscope slide with precisely scored chambers. The number of sperm per chamber are manually counted. This is very time consuming, however, it is very accurate. This time-consuming method can be replaced with either a spectrophotometer or colorimeter that has been calibrated to a hemacytometer. They have the advantage of being precise and fast. A spectrophotometer is preferred for determining sperm concentrations. The machine is calibrated at 550 nm. The solution used for dilution of the ejaculate is 2.9% sodium citrate and 5 mL of 10% formalin per liter. A standard curve measuring concentration versus 0.5% increments of light transmittance gives a range needed to measure concentration. However, photometers are not accurate with contaminated semen, and addition of cloudy extenders prior to estimation of concentration can confound results.

### Bull

Sperm concentration ranges from $2 \times 10^8$ sperm/mL in young bulls to $1.8 \times 10^9$ sperm/mL in mature bulls.

### Boar

The concentration in the sperm-rich fraction of the sperm approaches 6 to $10 \times 10^8$ sperm/mL, with final concentration due to volumes of pre-sperm and post-sperm fractions being lower.

### Stallion

Sperm numbers range in tha stallion from $100 \times 10^6$ to $150 \times 10^6$ sperm/mL, with a total fluid volume of 60 to 100

TABLE 25-2. ***Concentration of Ram Semen Assessed for Consistency***

| | | NUMBER OF SPERM ($\times 10^9$) | |
|---|---|---|---|
| SCORE | CONSISTENCY | *Mean* | *Range* |
| 5 | Thick creamy | 5.0 | 4.5–6.0 |
| 4 | Creamy | 4.0 | 3.5–4.5 |
| 3 | Thin creamy | 3.0 | 2.5–3.5 |
| 2 | Milky | 2.0 | 1.0–2.5 |
| 1 | Cloudy | 0.7 | 0.3–1.0 |
| 0 | Clear (watery) | insignificant | |

mL, yielding 7 to 15 billion total sperm per ejaculate. Total sperm number per ejaculate is subject to seasonal variation. It is also affected by frequency of ejaculation, age, testicular size, size of extragonadal sperm reserves, and various reproductive diseases (2–5).

### *Ram*

The normal concentration ranges from $3.5 \times 10^9$ to $6.0 \times 10^9$ sperm/mL in the ram. Rams with fertility score of 0 to 2 should not be used (Table 25-2).

### *Buck*

A colorimeter cannot be used to measure buck sperm due to the variation in color. Sperm concentration is lower than the ram. Buck sperm concentration ranges from $2.5 \times 10^9$ to $5.0 \times 10^9$ sperm/mL.

## SPERM MOTILITY

Motility assessment involves subjective estimation of the viability of spermatozoa and the quality of the motility. Light microscopic analysis of sperm is most commonly used. Evaluation of sperm motility is conducted with raw and extended semen.

Evaluation of raw semen is an indicator of sperm performance in its own accessory gland fluid. Measuring motility in the raw form can be hampered by higher sperm concentrations, making it difficult to discern individual motility patterns. To overcome this limitation, an aliquot of semen should also be extended (concentration of $25 \times 10^6$ sperm/mL) in a good quality extender (5).

Sperm motility is extremely susceptible to environmental conditions (such as excessive heat or cold), so it is necessary to protect the semen from injurious agents or conditions prior to analysis. To further enhance the reliability of motility estimation, an experienced person using a properly equipped microscope is needed. A drop of extended semen is placed on a glass slide and smeared with another slide, then observed using a microscope with a built-in stage warmer and phase-contrast optics. Magnification of 200× to 400× is generally used to estimate sperm motility (Fig. 25-3).

Parameters of motility include:

a) percentage of sperm which are motile (normal is 70 to 90% motile),
b) percentage of sperm which are progressively motile,
c) sperm velocity (based on an arbitrary scale of 0 [stationary] to 4 [fast]),
d) longevity of sperm motility in raw semen (at room temperature: 20 to 25°C), and in extended semen (at room temperature, or refrigerated temperature: 4 to 6°C).

Various patterns of motility are visualized. General patterns of sperm motility in diluted semen appear in a long semiarc pattern. The degree of vigor is used to score a sample (Table 25-3). Many factors influence sperm motility (Fig. 25-4). The extender may slightly alter motility, usually by increasing velocity measures. After initial extension, a high percentage of sperm may exhibit a circular motility pattern, which usually resolves after 5 to 10 minutes in the extender. If there is excessive fluid between the slide and coverslip it will appear that the sperm cells are reflecting light as they spiral (rolling over) moving forward. In the case of less fluid the cells may appear to move in a two-dimensional pattern. Sperm with hyperactivated motility make an X-pattern reac-

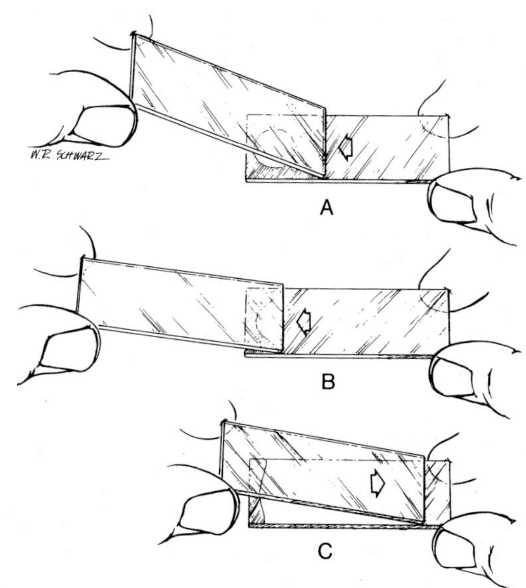


FIGURE 25-3. Preparation of a semen smear to evaluate motility. **(A)** A drop of semen is placed on a glass slide. **(B and C)** Another slide is used to prepare the smear without damage to the sample.

**TABLE 25-3. *Determination of the Score for Vigor of Wave Motion of Sperm***

| SCORE | ASPECTS OF WAVE MOTION |
|---|---|
| 0 | Total immobility |
| 1 | Individual movement |
| 2 | Very slow movement |
| 3 | General wave movement, slow amplitude of waves |
| 4 | Rapid wave motion, no eddies |
| 5 | Rapid wave motion, eddies present |

tion. If sperm are swimming in a tight circular motion, this signifies that they could have been subjected to cold shock. Oscillatory motion could be defined as aged or drying cells (6). Motility patterns are also correlated with infertility or subfertility of males (Table 25-4).

Several procedures have been developed for objective (unbiased) evaluation of sperm motility; time-lapse photomicrography, frame-by-frame playback videomicrography, spectrophotometry, and computerized analysis. Computer-assisted semen analysis (CASA) systems are used in reference laboratories as an objective means of assessing sperm motion (Fig. 25-5) (7). Motility descriptions with CASA include:

1. curvilinear velocity
2. average path velocity
3. straight line velocity
4. amplitude of lateral head displacement
5. linearity
6. beat cross frequency
7. mean angular displacement
8. area of tracked sperm head
9. time each spermatozoa is tracked

Flow cytometry can detect viable sperm based on binding of fluorescent dyes (SYBR-14 and propidium iodide) (8). Time lapse photomicrography permits visualization of sperm tracks (Fig. 25-6). Automated systems are accurate, but their relatively high costs limit routine use in commercial labs.

## SPERM MORPHOLOGY

Every semen sample contains some abnormal sperm cells (Figs. 25-7 and 25-8). Morphologic abnormalities of sperm have the greatest relationship to fertility of livestock. Heat stress causes high numbers of damaged sperm. Periods of high ambient temperature combined with high humidity may render a male sterile for up to six weeks. Large numbers of abnormal sperm appear in ejaculates collected during the recovery period. Providing adequate shade and clean cool water will help minimize effects of heat stress.

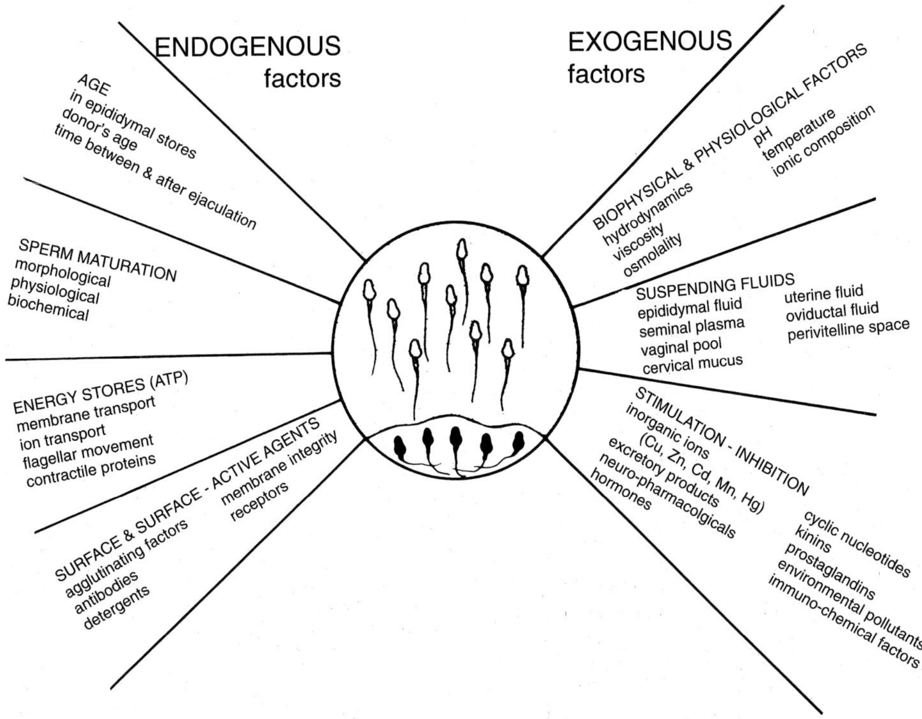


FIGURE 25-4. Some endogenous and exogenous factors influencing sperm motility.

TABLE 25-4. *Motility Patterns of Sperm From Subfertile and Infertile Males*

| PATTERNS OF MOTILITY AND MORPHOLOGY | SPERM TAIL | SPERM HEAD | SPERM MOVEMENTS AND PROGRESSION |
|---|---|---|---|
| Vibratory circular | Slow or rapid quivering from side to side; vibrations of various types and frequency bent in a curved shape; immotile | Immotile or vibrating in one place | Motility without progression; perpendicular, oblique, or horizontal clockwise or counterclockwise motion |
| Darting | Vibration with high velocity | Irregular; propelling; no rotation | Minimal and erratic; wandering path |
| Rotating | Undulations of small amplitude pass down tail | Whole sperm rotates around its axis; periodic "flashing" effect | Rapid forward progress in a straight line |
| Asymmetric head and/or flagella | Amplitude of tail wave is asymmetric at both sides | Irregular; propelling; usually no rotation | Circular orbits if rotation is absent |
| Sperm with cytoplasmic droplet | Amplitude of tail waves is unequal; rapid vibrations | Irregular, often rocking; seldom rotational | Perpendicular, oblique, seldom progressive |
| Agglutinated sperm | Decreasing, vibrating motion; slow, vibrating motion | Slow; irregular propelling; rocking | Depends upon the type of agglutination |

### *Bull*

When abnormal sperm cells exceed 20%, fertility typically declines. The types of abnormality being evaluated determines microscopic magnification (9). Morphologic abnormalities are categorized as primary, secondary, or tertiary. Primary abnormalities are associated with sperm heads and the acrosome; secondary abnormalities refer to the presence of a droplet on the midpiece of the tail; and tertiary abnormalities refer to other tail defects. A reference for performing wet mounts, using conventional staining techniques, and identifying morphological abnormalities has been compiled (10).

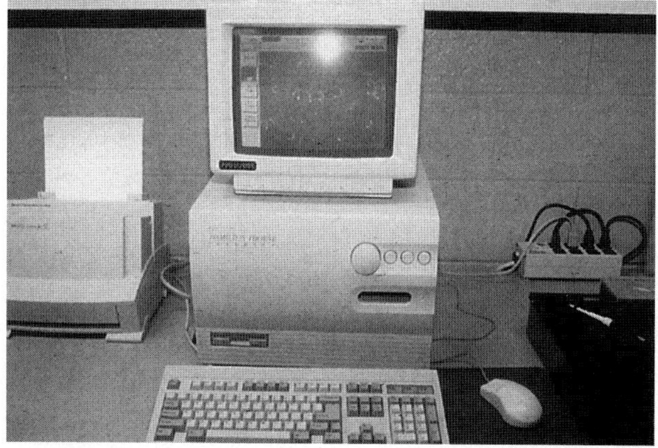

FIGURE 25-5. Computerized sperm motility analyzers, such as this Hamilton-Thorne model, are commonly used by reference laboratories to provide objective analysis of numerous sperm motility parameters.

### *Boar*

The percent of sperm possessing an intact acrosomal membrane is regarded as an important parameter of semen quality. Several staining procedures are used for sperm morphology assessment. Sperm membrane integrity is evaluated by phase-contrast microscopy with gluteraldehyde fixed boar sperm (11). The apical ridge of the acrosome can be easily seen and classified relative to intactness. Wet mounts of fixed boar sperm examined with phase-contrast in conjunction with cell membrane integrity (using fluorochrome H33258) is another method to assess morphology/viability (12). Often Giemsa stain is used for morphological assessment. Higher resolution sperm quality assessment was conducted on twelve semen samples from two healthy, sexually mature Landrace boars using scanning electron microscopy (SEM), and 16 new types of aberrant sperm were identified (13).

### *Stallion*

The morphology of stallion sperm is examined with air-dried semen smears using a light microscope (1000×). Specific sperm stains include those developed by Williams and Casarett. General purpose cellular stains (e.g., Wright's, Giemsa, hematoxylin-eosin) also have been used to accent

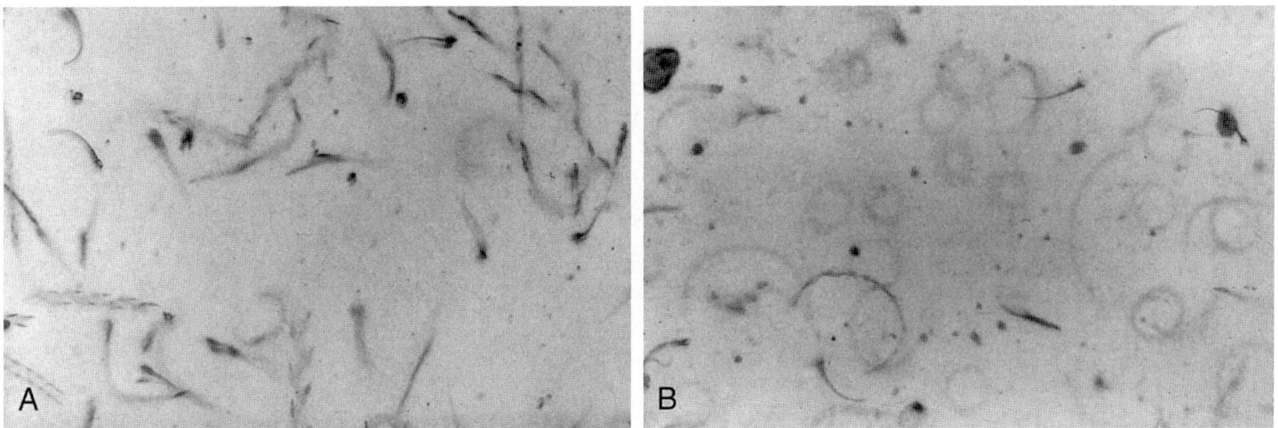


FIGURE 25-6. Time-lapse photomicrography of sperm permits visualization of sperm tracks. (**A**) Note the stationary (nonmotile) and progressively motile sperm. (**B**) Indicates a high percentage of sperm with circular tracks.

both germinal and somatic cells in semen smears (Fig. 25-9). Background stains (e.g., eosin-nigrosin, India ink) probably are the most widely used stains because of their ease of use. Visualization of sperm structural detail are enhanced by fixing the cells in buffered formol-saline or buffered glutaraldehyde solution, then viewing the unstained cells as a wet mount with either phase-contrast or differential interference-contrast microscopy. Sperm fixation is simplified by this method and the incidence of artifactual changes is reduced in comparison with stained smears.

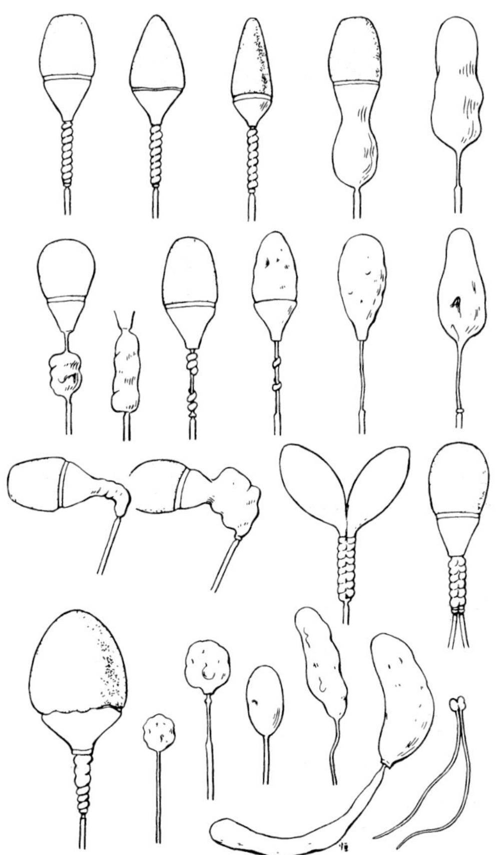

FIGURE 25-7. Drawings of major morphologic abnormalities in mammalian sperm.

At least 200 spermatozoa are evaluated for the presence, type, and incidence of each morphologic defect. Specific morphologic defects, such as knobbed acrosomes, proximal protoplasmic droplets, swollen midpieces, and coiled tails are recorded (Fig. 25-10). This classification is ideal since it reveals more specific information regarding a population of sperm while avoiding erroneous assumptions about the origin of these defects. Some morphologic abnormalities like detached heads can be primary, secondary, or tertiary in nature, thereby introducing the possibility of error when using this classification system exclusively. The total number of morphologically normal sperm in ejaculates may provide more information regarding the fertility of a stallion than the percentage or absolute number of morphologically abnormal sperm. The percentage of morphologically normal sperm in a semen sample is similar to the percentage of progressively motile sperm. If sperm motility is low and the percentage of morphologically normal sperm is high, it suggests that laboratory errors occurred which led to a lowering of sperm motility.

### *Ram*

There is a positive correlation between morphologically normal sperm and sperm motility. All ejaculations contain some abnormal sperm. However, when 20% or more are abnormal, the ram's fertility is questionable. Semen with more than 15% abnormal sperm should not be used for AI. The percentage of abnormal sperm varies with the season; higher numbers of abnormal sperm are seen in the spring, with the number declining as the breeding season advances.

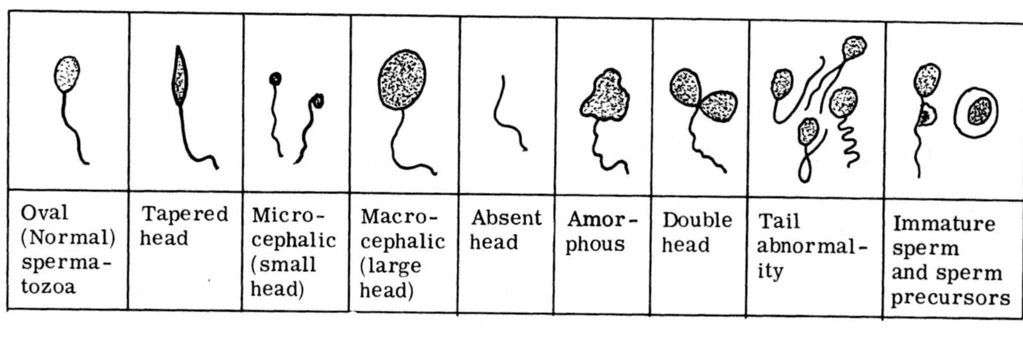


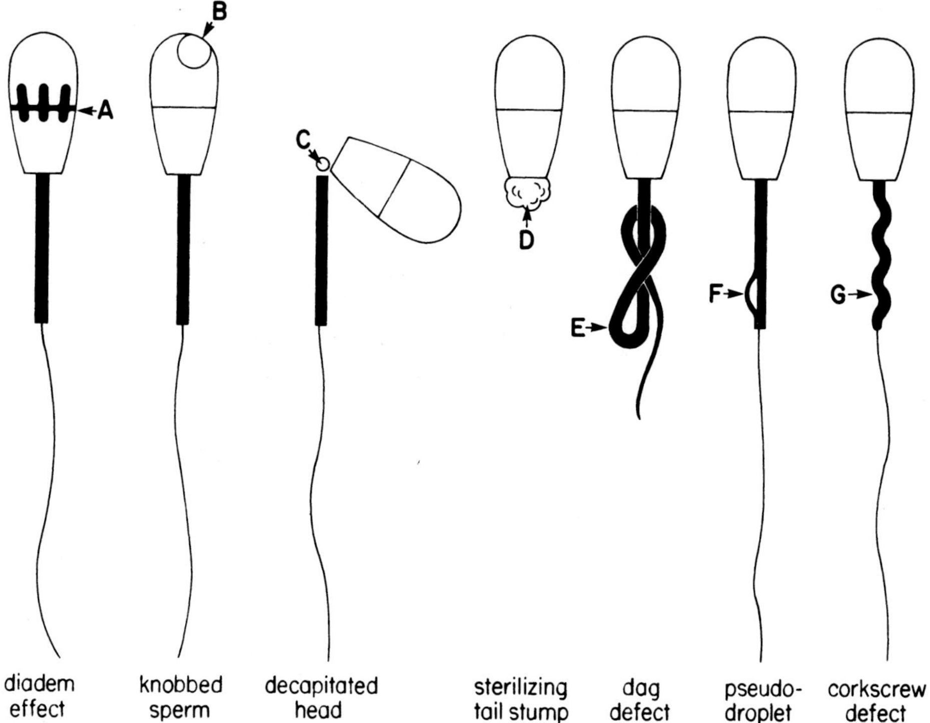


FIGURE 25-8. Morphologic anomalies of sperm.

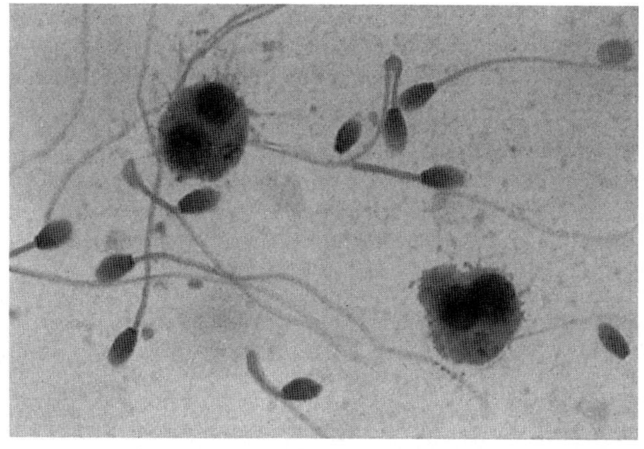

FIGURE 25-9. Semen sample stained with hematoxylin-eosin, revealing two premature (round) germ cells in among a group of mature sperm.

Sperm morphology is examined by using eosin-nigrosin stain. Wright's and Williams' stains can also be used.

Stained slides are examined using a high microscopic magnification (400×). At least 150 spermatozoa are examined, with abnormal sperm classified into 5 categories:

a) tailless,
b) abnormal heads,
c) abnormal tail formations,
d) abnormal tail formations with a proximal cytoplasmic droplet,
e) and abnormal tail formations with a distal droplet.

## SEMEN QUALITY

### *Bull*

The methods of evaluating sperm quality from frozen semen are associated with motility and intact acrosomes. Two

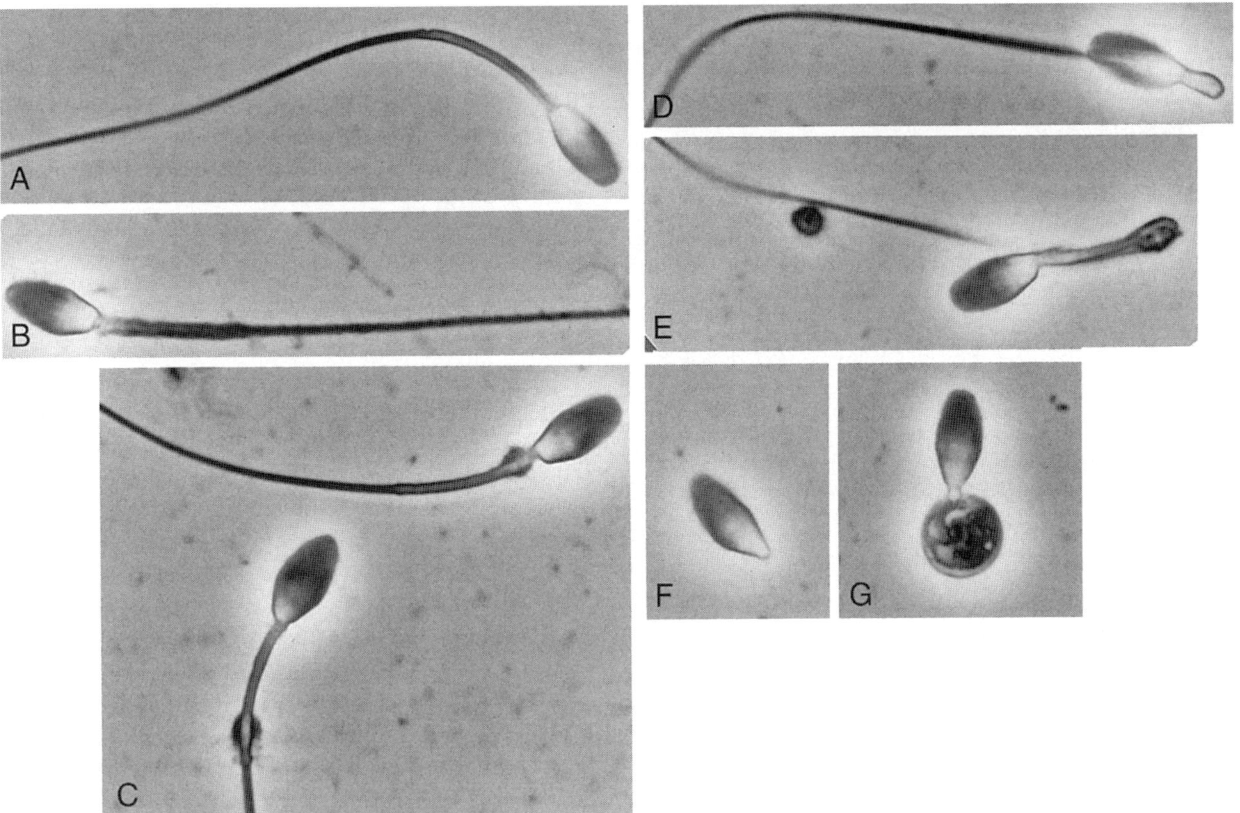


Figure 25-10. Equine sperm morphology characteristics using phase-contrast microscopy. (A) Normal sperm. (B) Abnormal midpiece. (C) Proximal and distal droplets. (D) Bent midpiece. (E) Reflexed (bent) tail. (F) Detached (tailless) head. (G) Coiled tail.

straws (0.5 mL or 0.25 mL) are thawed in a 95°F water bath; after 45 seconds, one straw is removed and dried with a paper towel, because water can be hazardous to sperm. The contents within the straw are shaken toward the cotton plug end. The other end of the straw is cut off, and semen is released into a small clean disposable test tube by cutting a small opening just below the cotton plug. A small drop of semen is placed on a warm slide with a cover slip. Initial motility readings can be performed using microscopic analysis (160×).

A microscope with interference (Nomarski) optics (1000×) and oil immersion is used to examine percentage of intact acrosomes and abnormalities of sperm, after incubating the second straw for 3 h at 95°F. The acrosome covers the anterior two-thirds portion of the sperm head. The acrosome contains enzymes that allow capacitated sperm to penetrate the egg. There is a direct correlation with the percent intact acrosomes after this 3 h incubation and fertility (14). Figure 25-11 illustrates a dual-staining procedure for viability and acrosomal integrity (15). Several other procedures are used to stain for acrosomes (16, 17).

### Boar

The most accurate assessment of boar fertility is to determine pregnancy and the birth of live young. Although semen from boars can meet several criteria to suggest a high quality status, the fertilizing potential of that specimen may be suboptimal. The search for a single *in vitro* parameter which predicts boar fertility continues (Table 25-5).

### Ram

Ram semen with greater than 85% motility and less than 10% abnormal sperm is considered of high quality. Unfortunately, fertilizing ability does not rely solely on these two parameters. The total number of live sperm per insemination is more important than the percent abnormal sperm. The inability of a single sperm to penetrate the zona pellucida of the ova is believed to be one of the limiting factors in semen fertility.

## Ancillary Tests

### Electron Microscopy

Light microscopy affords limited magnification and, therefore, limited appraisal of sperm morphology. Subtle abnormalities in sperm structure can be detected using scanning and/or transmission electron microscopy (SEM/TEM). Al-

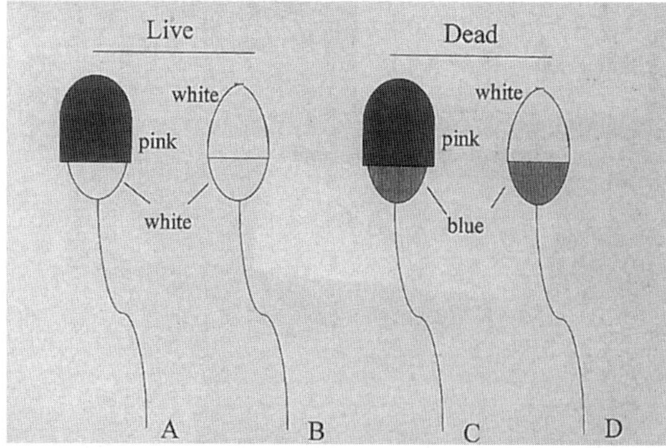


FIGURE 25-11. Patterns of sperm stained with the dual stain technique. (**A**) Live sperm with intact acrosome. (**B**) Live sperm without acrosome (true acrosome reacted). (**C**) Dead sperm with intact acrosome. (**D**) Dead sperm without acrosome (false acrosome reacted).

though expensive, these two microscopic methods offer high-resolution detail and permit closer examination of sperm morphology. Three-dimensional visualization of the entire sperm is observed with SEM, and TEM permits cross-sectional viewing of sperm revealing ultrastructural detail.

### *Sperm Chromatin Structure Assay (SCSA)*

A flow cytometric procedure has been developed to evaluate the structural integrity of sperm chromatin by measuring the relative amounts of double-stranded and single-stranded DNA in sperm populations. SCSA has been useful for identifying some forms of subfertility in bulls and stallions. SCSA can screen 5,000 to 10,000 sperm within a few minutes.

### *Other Fluorescent Probes*

New fluorescent probes are being investigated to evaluate their reliablity for sperm function tests using a microscope or flow cytometer. These assays may become very valuable adjunctive tests because of their ability to provide detailed information on specific sperm features such as acrosomal integrity, plasma membrane integrity, and mitochondrial membrane potential.

### *Antisperm Antibody Assay (AAA)*

Sperm maturation is completed in an immunologically privileged site, the adluminal compartment of the seminiferous tubules, to circumvent immunologic attack. Escape of sperm (or their haploid precursors) from the adluminal compartment of the seminiferous tubules can provoke an immune response, with formation of antisperm antibodies. Precipitating factors for this immunologic attack of sperm might include lacerations, biopsies, neoplasms, trauma, or degenerative changes of the testes. Antisperm antibodies interfere with the fertilization process in humans, but the specific mechanism(s) of action remain unresolved. There is indirect evidence that antisperm antibodies can play a role in reduced fertility of stallions. Subfertility of some stallions cannot be explained on the basis of a standard breeding soundness examination. It would appear that autoantibody response to sperm is primarily of the IgG type in serum and of the IgA type in seminal plasma. Evaluation of serum, seminal plasma, and sperm of stallions for presence of autoantibodies is currently being investigated. Tests which evaluate actual binding of antibodies to sperm provide the best predictive fertility index.

TABLE 25-5. ***Reported Assays Used to Predict Fertilizing Potential of Boar Spermatozoa***

| METHOD |
|---|
| Zona-free hamster ova penetration assay[a] |
| Percoll gradients separate high velocity sperm associated with fertility[b] |
| Sperm chromatin structure assay detects integrity of sperm DNA[c] |
| Specific sperm membrane proteins correlated to sperm penetrated zona-free hamster eggs[d] |
| Hemizona binding assay suggests that more sperm bound correlated with increased fertility[e] |
| Male pronuclear formation rate for discriminating among boars[f] |

[a]Clark RN, Johnson LA. Effect of liquid storage and cryopreservation of boar spermatozoa on acrosomal integrity and the penetration of zona-free hamster ova *in vitro*. Gamete Res 1987;1:193–204.
[b]Grant SA, Long SE, Parkinson TJ. Fertilizability and structural properties of boar spermatozoa by percoll gradient centrifugation. J Reprod Fert 1994;10:477–483.
[c]Evenson DP, Thompson L, Jost L. Flow cytometric evaluation of boar semen by the sperm chromatin structure assay as related to cryopreservation and fertility. Theriogenology 1994;4:637–51.
[d]Ash KL, Berger T, Hurner CM, Famula TR. Boar sperm plasma membrane protein profile: correlation with the zona-free hamster ova assay. Theriogenology 1994;4:1217–1226.
[e]Fazeli AR, Holt C, Steenweg W, Bevers MM, Holt WV, Colenbrander B. Development of a sperm hemizona binding assay for boar semen. Theriogenology 1995;4:17–27.
[f]Xu X, Foxcroft GR. IVM/IVF technology for assessment of semen quality and boar fertility. Reprod Dom Anim 1996;3:37–47.

### *Biochemical Analysis of Seminal Plasma/ Secretions of Female Reproductive Tract*

Electrolyte concentration, protein concentration, or specific protein composition of seminal plasma do not provide good predictive information on post-thaw motility of cryopreserved sperm. Two proteins of epididymal origin which serve as markers of bull fertility potential are **osteopontin** and **lipocalin-type prostaglandin D synthase** (18, 19). **Deoxyribonuclease-1-like enzyme** and **type 2 tissue inhibitor of metalloproteinases** (TIMP-2) are secreted by the accessory glands at ejaculation and bind to sperm as they traverse the male reproductive tract, and are also associated with greater bull fertility (20). **Glycosaminoglycans**, which are components of the female reproductive tract secretions, bind to bull sperm and cause acrosome reactions *in vitro*. There is a high correlation between percent acrosome reacted sperm stimulated by glycosaminoglycans and a bull's 60 to 90 day field nonreturn days (21).

## References


1. Chenoweth PJ, Spitzer JC, Hopkins FM. A new bull breeding soundness evaluation form. Proc Ann Mtng Soc Theriogenology, San Antonio, TX, 1992.
2. Blanchard TL, Varner DD, eds. Stallion Management. Veterinary Clinics of North America - Equine Practice. Philadelphia: WB Saunders, 1992.
3. Blanchard TL, Varner DD, Schumacher J. Manual of Equine Reproduction. St. Louis: Mosby, 1998.
4. McKinnon AO, Voss JL, eds. Equine Reproduction. Philadelphia: Lea and Febiger, 1993.
5. Varner DD, Schumacher J, Blanchard TL, Johnson L. Diseases and Management of Breeding Stallions. St. Louis: Mosby-Year Book, 1991.
6. Herman HA, Mitchell JR, Doak GA. Evaluation of semen: general considerations, appearance and viability. In: Thè Artificial Insemination and Embryo Transfer of Dairy and Beef Cattle. Danville, IL:Interstate Publishers, 1994;59–72.
7. Holt WV. Can we predict fertility rates? Making sense of sperm motility. In: Rath D, Johnson LA, Weitze KF, eds. Reproduction in Domestic Animals. Blackwell Science, 1996;3:37–47.
8. Johnson LA, Maxwell WMC, Dobrinsky JR, Welch GR. Staining sperm for viability assessment. In: Rath D, Johnson LA, Weitze KF, eds. Reproduction in Domestic Animals. Blackwell Science, 1996;3:37–47.
9. Barth AO. The relationship between sperm abnormalities and fertility. Proc 14th Tech Conf AI Reprod 1972;47-63.
10. Herman HA, Mitchell JR, Doak GA. Evaluation of semen: live-dead staining and morphology. In: The Artificial Insemination and Embryo Transfer of Dairy and Beef Cattle. Danville, IL:Interstate Publishers, 1994;81–92.
11. Pursel VG, Johnson LA, Rampacek GB. Acrosome morphology of boar spermatozoa incubated before cold shock. J Anim Sci 1972;3:278–283.
12. Woelders H.. Overview of *in vitro* methods for evaluation of semen quality. In: Johnson LA, Rath D, eds. Boar Semen Preservation II. Berlin and Hamburg: Paul Parey Scientific Publishers, 1990.
13. Bonet S, Briz M. New data on aberrant spermatozoa in the ejaculate of Sus domesticus. Theriogenology 1991;3:725–730.
14. Saacke RG, White JM. Semen quality tests and their relationship to fertility. Proc 14th Tech Conf AI Reprod. 1972;22–27.
15. Didion BA, Dobrinsky JR, Giles JR, Graves CN. Staining procedure to detect viability and true acrosome reaction in spermatoza of various species. Gamete Res 1989;2:51–57.
16. Cross NL, Meizel S. Methods for evaluating the acrosomal status of mammalian sperm. Biol Reprod 1989;4:635–641.
17. Kovacs A and Foote RH. Viability and acrosome staining of bull, boar and rabbit spermatozoa. Biotech Histochem 1992;67:119–124.
18. Cancel AM, Chapman DA, Killian GJ. Osteopontin is the 55-kilodalton fertility-associated protein in Holstein bulls seminal plasma. Biol Reprod 1997;5:1293–1301.
19. Gerena RL, Irakura D, Urade Y, Eguchi N, Chapman DA, Killian GJ. Identification of a fertility-associated protein in bull seminal plasma as lipocalin-type prostaglandin D synthase. Biol Reprod 1998;5:826–833.
20. McCauley TC. Identification of seminal proteins related to fertility of bulls. Ph.D. dissertation. Tucson, AZ: University of Arizona, 1998.
21. Lenz RW, Martin JL, Bellin ME, Ax RL. Predicting fertility of dairy bulls by inducing acrosome reactions in sperm with chondroitin sulfates. J Dairy Sci 1987;7:1073–1077.

# Chapter 26

# *Artificial Insemination*

R.L. Ax, M.R. Dally, B.A. Didion, R.W. Lenz, C.C. Love, D.D. Varner, B. Hafez, and M.E. Bellin

Artificial insemination (AI) is the most important single technique devised for the genetic improvement of animals, because a few select males produce enough sperm to inseminate thousands of females per year. In contrast, relatively few progeny per female can be produced per year even by embryo transfer. The earliest carefully documented use of AI was in 1780 when Spallanzani, an Italian physiologist, obtained beagle puppies. Other reports appeared in the 19th century, but it was not until 1900 that extensive studies with farm animals began in Russia and shortly thereafter in Japan. Major advantages of AI are: a) genetic improvement, b) control of venereal diseases, c) availability of accurate breeding records, d) economic service, and e) safety through elimination of dangerous males. AI is facilitated with estrous synchronization programs, and it has been proposed as a means of gender control through separation of spermatozoa containing X and Y chromosomes.

When properly done, there are few disadvantages to using AI. However, it is necessary to have trained personnel to provide proper techique, and to have appropriate arrangements for corralling females for hormone therapy or detection of heat and insemination, particularly under range conditions.

Advantages of AI are:

a) Enables the widespread use of outstanding sires with valuable genetics to any livestock operation.
b) Facilitates progeny testing under a range of environmental and managerial conditions, thereby further improving accuracy of selection.
c) Leads to improved performance and potential of the national herd.
d) Permits crossbreeding to change a production trait.
e) Accelerates introduction of new genetics.
f) Enables use of deep-frozen semen after a donor is dead, aiding in the preservation of select lines.
g) Permits use of semen from incapacitated or oligospermic males.
h) Reduces risk of spreading sexually transmitted diseases.
i) Is usually essential after synchronization of estrus in large groups of animals.
j) May permit males with desirable genetic markers to be used in specific genetic matings.
k) Provides a useful research tool for investigating many aspects of male and female reproductive physiology (1).

The genetic improvement achieved by AI of dairy cattle has resulted from the use of progeny-tested sires. Obtaining semen at the earliest possible age from potential valuable sires being tested is desirable to hasten identification of superior sires. Ultimately, the genetic impact of a superior sire is limited by the number of sperm produced, which is a direct function of testicular size.

Carefully selected young males should be sampled as soon as possible after puberty. Performance and progeny test programs are important to make maximal genetic progress with meat-type farm animals. AI facilitates crossbreeding, requiring that only one breed be maintained on the farm. Development of AI in beef cattle has been slower in the United States and some other countries, because of the difficulty of heat detection and insemination under range conditions. It is also possible to have considerable genetic improvement for highly heritable traits, using performance-tested bulls, without AI.

## Management of Males/Semen Collection

When young males are properly fed and managed, semen can be collected successfully at the following approximate ages: bulls, 12 months; rams, goats, and boars, 7 to 8 months; and stallions, 24 months. Of major importance to an AI program is the correct collection of semen (Table 26-1).

### *Mounts and Teasing Procedures*

Live mounts—such as a teaser female, another male, or a castrated male—are the most successful techniques for routine semen collection. The exception is that teaser animals

TABLE 26-1. ***Frequency of Semen Collection and Preparation of Artificial Vagina***

| SPECIES | FREQUENCY OF COLLECTION | PREPARATION OF ARTIFICIAL VAGINA |
|---|---|---|
| Cattle | Collect semen twice a day 2 or 3 days per week to harvest more sperm to freeze at one time. | The temperature of the AV is more important than the pressure it exerts on the penis. Water is used to control both, but final pressure may be adjusted by pumping in air. Temperature inside the AV is near 45°C, but from 38–55°C has been employed. |
| Sheep | Rams are ejaculated many times a day for several weeks before severely depleting epididymal reserves of sperm. Bucks are ejaculated less frequently than rams. | AV temperature and technique of collection is similar to cattle. Forward thrust of the ram is less vigorous but more rapid. Semen collector must coordinate movements swiftly with those of the ram. |
| Swine | Large numbers of sperm are expelled in each ejaculate and deplete epididymal reserves quickly. Collections not more than every other day are recommended. If daily ejaculates are required for several days, sexual rest for 2–3 days is recommended. | Pressure is especially important for collecting semen. The boar ejaculates when the curled tip of penis is firmly engaged in the sow's cervix, the AV, or the operator's hand. When using the AV or gloved hand, pressure is exerted on the coiled distal end of the penis throughout ejaculation. The boar remains quiet for the few minutes required for ejaculation. Ejaculate consists of three fractions: (1) presperm fraction, (2) the sperm-rich fraction, and (3) postsperm fraction. Presperm fraction is discarded before sperm-rich fraction is collected. |
| Horse | Males expel large numbers of sperm in each ejaculate and deplete epididymal reserves quickly. Collections not more than every other day are recommended. If daily ejaculates are required for several days, sexual rest for 2–3 days is recommended. | Wash the penis with warm soapy water and rinse with clean water to remove smegma and other debris on the surface of the penis. The mare should be hobbled. AV is larger than it is for other animals to accomodate the stallion's erect vascular penis. |

for stallions are mares rather than males. Some males, especially boars, can be trained to mount dummies equally well, which avoid disease transmission and provide stability for physical collection (Fig. 26-1).

## CATTLE

### *Semen Collection*

A general routine to follow for mature bulls is a Monday, Wednesday, and Friday schedule. The bull can be collected twice daily for optimal sperm output. The average ejaculate contains 8 to 16 billion total sperm. A weekly average to strive for is a total of 30 billion sperm cells. Young bulls can be collected on Tuesdays and Thursdays (2). There are three stimulatory approaches: the introduction to a different mount animal(s) in the original locale; change the locale with the same mount; or change both locale and mount. If a bull does not mount after 5 min, then it will require more stimulation to provide a satisfactory ejaculate (3). The artificial vagina (AV) is made of a cylindrical rubber tube (radiator casing), a thin rubber liner, a thin-walled rubber cone, and a collection vial encased in an insulated jacket. The space between the wall of the rubber casing and the inner rubber liner is filled with hot water (60°C). A rubber cone is fitted on the end of the rubber casing. To the other end of the cone, a 15 mL graduated test tube is attached. An insulated jacket is used to ensure that the entire AV is kept at approximately 45°C for the time of collection (Figs. 26-2, 26-3, and 26-4). A sterile lubricant is applied to the inner liner (4, 5).

After precollection stimulation, consisting of 3 to 5 false mounts and active restraint, the bull is allowed to mount the teaser animal (Figs. 26-5 and 26-6). The collector diverts the bull's penis into the AV, which is held alongside the flank of the mount. Immediately on contact with the warm and lubricated surface, the bull ejaculates into the AV. Upon ejaculation, the AV is immediately tilted downward toward the test tube. The semen drains into the collection tube, which is then removed and placed in a water bath maintained at 34°C, before measurement of sperm concentration.

The method of electro-ejaculation is reserved for lame or old bulls, and for bulls that have temporarily lost their desire to serve the AV. The technique involves introducing either a probe or finger electrodes into the rectum, where the nerves suppling his reproductive organs are electrically

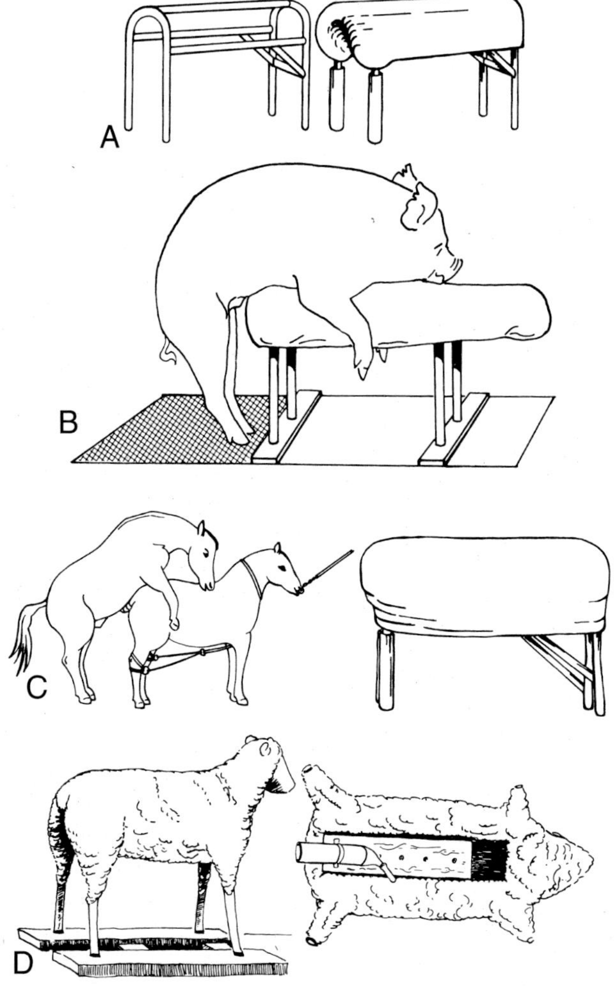


FIGURE 26-1. Dummies and mounts used for collecting semen from farm animals.

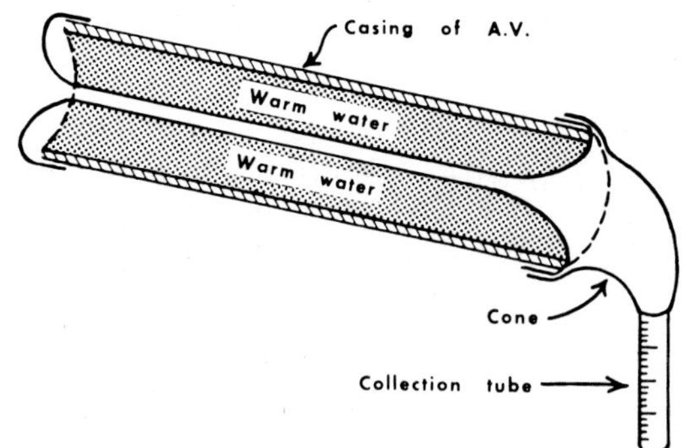


FIGURE 26-2. Artificial vagina for bulls shown in longitudinal section to illustrate construction.

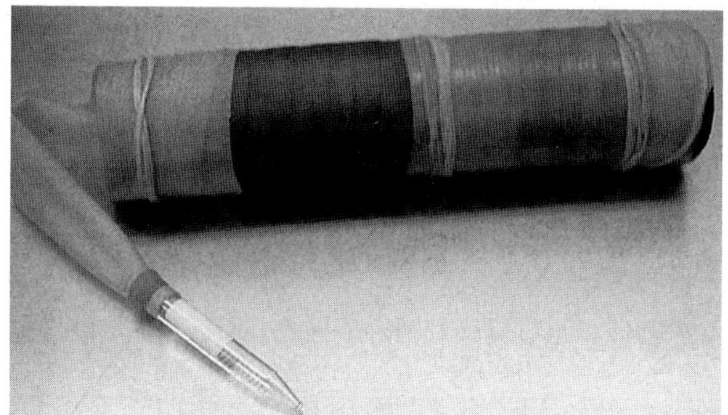

FIGURE 26-3. Artificial vagina exposed.

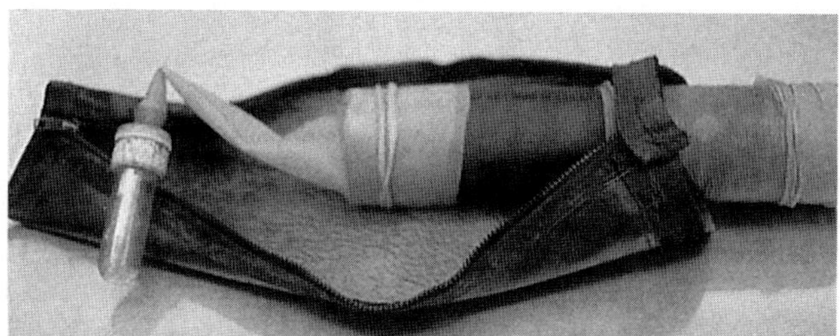

FIGURE 26-4. Artificial vagina in case.

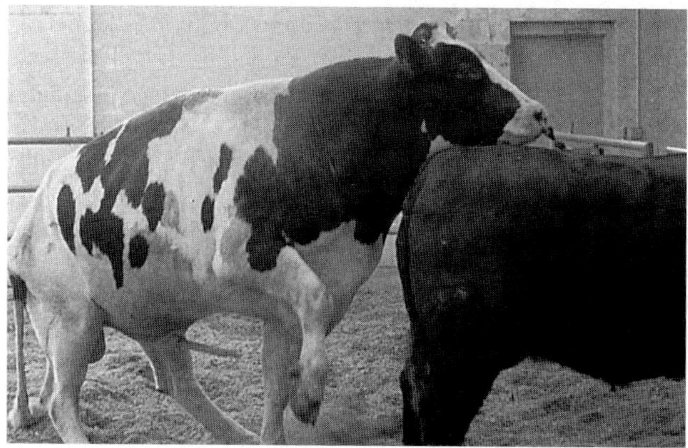

FIGURE 26-5. Bull mounting teaser animal.

stimulated. Voltage is gradually increased with repeated rhythmic stimulation pulses. Experience is necessary to cause erection followed by ejaculation. Ejaculates from this procedure have large volumes (4). It is not unusual for a bull to ejaculate 7 to 10 mL of semen which contains 1.0 to 1.5 billion sperm/mL, with an average progressive motility of 60 to 75%. A semen packaging machine and a large storage tank for semen in frozen inventory are shown in Figures 26-7 and 26-8, respectively.

The best indicator of estrus is when the female stands to be mounted by other females. There are many aids in detecting estrus, typically pressure sensitive devices mounted on the cow's back. They can change color or activate electronic devices which send a signal to a computer from the pasture (Table 26-2 and Fig. 26-9) (6).

### *Thawing Semen*

Thawing 2 or 3 mL straws is accomplished in a 37°C water bath (45 seconds). The inseminator must be able to provide

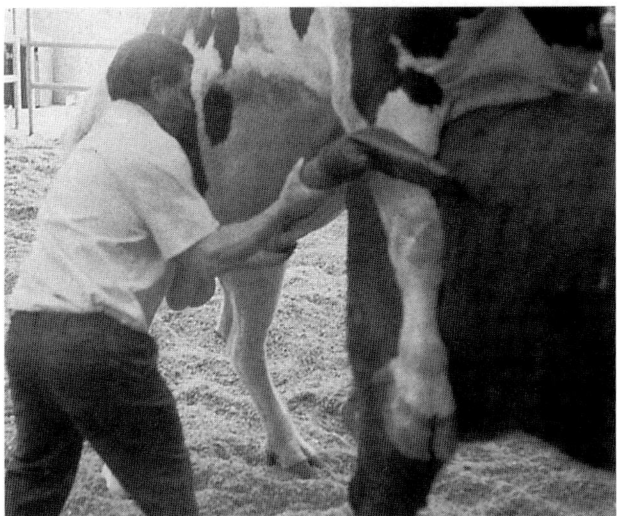

FIGURE 26-6. Placement of artificial vagina for semen collection.

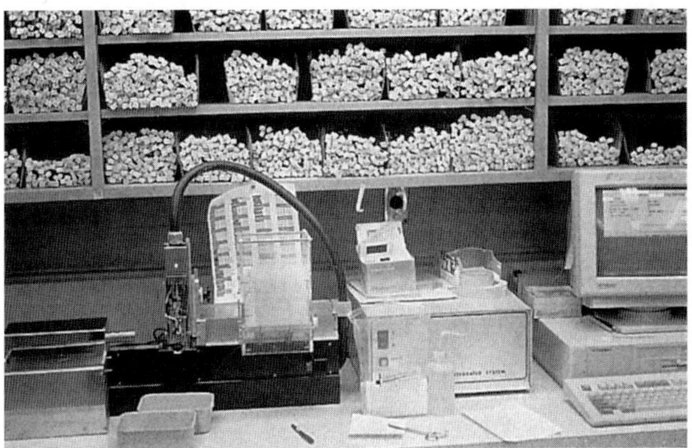

FIGURE 26-7. Equipment used for holding semen in straws to assure accurate identification.

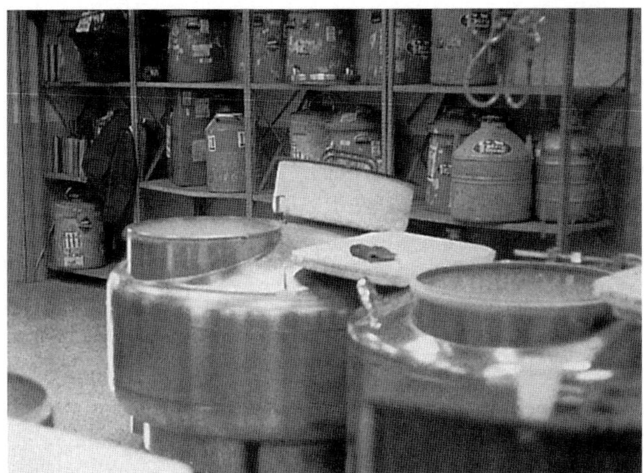

FIGURE 26-8. Liquid nitrogen storage tanks for packaged semen.

some protection for thawed semen on cold days. Never allow semen to cool down or refreeze. Try to dry the straw and maintain the 37°C temperature while loading the insemination gun in cold weather. Prewarm the gun by vigorous rubbing several times.

### *Insemination Technique*

The rectovaginal technique of artificial insemination in cattle is one of the most widely used methods and is taught by every AI company. Excess fecal matter can be removed by a series of gentle raking motions of the inserted hand. Once excess fecal matter has been expelled, the vulva is wiped clean and dried with an absorbent paper towel to prevent contamination. If rectal constrictions persist, press down with the palm of the hand and massage back and forth on the floor of the pelvic cavity. This will also help to locate the cervix, which has been described as feeling like a turkey's neck. The insemination gun should be held at a 30° angle with the end containing the semen uppermost when entering the reproductive tract; this is necessary to prevent the inseminating instrument from entering the suburethral diverticulum or urethra, which is located on the floor of the vagina a short way inside the opening of the vulva.

The gun is forward along the roof of the vagina and at the same time the cervix is pushed forward to straighten out any vaginal folds which might otherwise be encountered with the tip of the gun. The cervical os or opening is usually in the center of the cervix, but one may have to probe very lightly with the gun tip until the opening is found.

To work the cervix onto the gun, keep the first two fingers and the thumb on the gloved hand just behind the tip of the gun to manipulate the cervix. Having gone through the cervical rings, the gun will slip forward with little resistance. When this happens, the tip of the gun will be in the uterine body, or perhaps may have slipped even further into the uterine horn. One will be able to feel the tip since the uterine wall is quite thin. Next, rotate the gloved hand around the cervix until the hand lies on top. It will be possible to use the forefinger as an indicator of where the gun tip is located. Slowly pull the gun back until it is flush with the cervical opening (7). Keeping the gun steady with the outside hand, raise the index finger of the gloved hand away from the gun tip. Be certain to push with the thumb and pull the gun out of the cervix with your fingers. Slowly deposit the semen, taking at least 5 seconds to push the plunger in. Depositing semen slowly helps get the maximum distribution of semen. Following correct insemination procedures will help one achieve better breeding efficiencies. If the cervical mucus of a cow previously inseminated feels thick or sticky, she may have become pregnant from the previous insemination. In that case, go halfway through the cervix and deposit semen. Inspect the tip of the gun for signs of infection. Make notes for the veterinar-

TABLE 26-2. ***Detection of Estrus and Procedures of Insemination***

| SPECIES | DETECTION OF ESTRUS | PROCEDURES FOR INSEMINATION |
|---|---|---|
| Cattle | Cows are observed early in the morning and evening every day for standing when mounted by other cows. | Insemination while standing in a stanchion or stall is recommended. Beef cows in estrus are penned and a squeeze chute provided to restrain the animal during insemination. Stress should be avoided. Semen is deposited in the uterus. |
| Sheep | Difficult to detect. Vasectomized rams with paint appliet to brisket or contained in a harness. | Ewe is held by putting hind legs over a rail or placing her in an elevated crate during insemination. Insemination with aid of a speculum and light permits semen to be deposited into or through the cervix rather than the vagina. A laparascope can also be used. |
| Swine | Sound, sight, and smell of a vasectomized or intact boar are helpful. Sows in heat seek the boar and assume a rigid stance (lordosis), ears become erect when mounted or, similarly, when pressed firmly on their back. The vulva swells and reddens as blood flow increases. Sows come into estrus 3–8 days after weaning their litter. Weaning time is used as a method of synchronized estrus. | Insemination can occur without restraining the sow. With some rubbing and pressure on the back, the sow stands calmly during AI. The insemination tube is guided into the cervix because the vagina tapers directly into the cervix, which itself tapers. Large semen volume and high sperm numbers are required. |
| Horse | Mares are teased daily with a stallion in special teaser paddocks. Indications of acceptance of stallion are elevation of tail, spreading of lags, standing, frequent urination, and contraction of the vulva—"winking." | The mare is restrained by hobbles, backed against baled hay or a board wall, or put in a breeding chute to protect the inseminator. The area around the vulva is scrubbed before insemination to minimize contamination. Arm placed in a plastic sleeve, lightly lubricated, is inserted into vagina and index finger inserted into cervix. Inseminating catheter is guided into the uterus to deposit semen. |

ian. Bend the sheath and straw as one removes it from the insemination gun. Record the bull's identity, collection code, date of breeding, and registration number. Keep all equipment clean by washing and wipe down prior to use.

## SWINE

### *Semen Collection*

The boar is led to the dummy sow in a collection area with a nonslip surface (i.e., wood-shavings, sawdust, or perforated rubber matting) and the dummy sow should be stabilized by fixing to the floor or wall. Once the boar has mounted the dummy sow, he will begin thrusting movements. If possible the preputial fluid retained in the prepuce should be emptied and the prepuce dried with a paper towel. The penis will emerge and the technician should grasp the end of the penis allowing the boar to lock in it. Pressure is the stimulus which allows the boar to ejaculate and pressures will vary (slight to hard squeeze) for each boar. The technician would note the various fractions of the ejaculate taking care to collect the sperm-rich fraction.

Training a new boar to mount a dummy sow is best attempted immediately after another boar has already worked on it. Boars observing other boars mounting live or dummy sows have enhanced libido or sexual drive, and sexual stimulation of the boar prior to semen collection has been shown to increase the number of sperm in the ejaculate (8).

### *Frequency of Collection*

Too frequent collection in the case of AI boars, or overuse of boars for natural mating, is one of the greatest factors causing temporary loss of fertility. Gerritts et al. (9) found that over a 20-day period, 5, 10, and 20 ejaculations gave an average total yield of spermatozoa of $55 \times 10^9$, $40 \times 10^9$, and $23.7 \times 10^9$, respectively. The effect of increased collection frequency would be more dramatic in young boars. Young boars should not serve more than two sows per week (10).

### *When to Inseminate*

Successful AI in swine is influenced by the variation that exists in the onset of heat after weaning, duration of estrus,

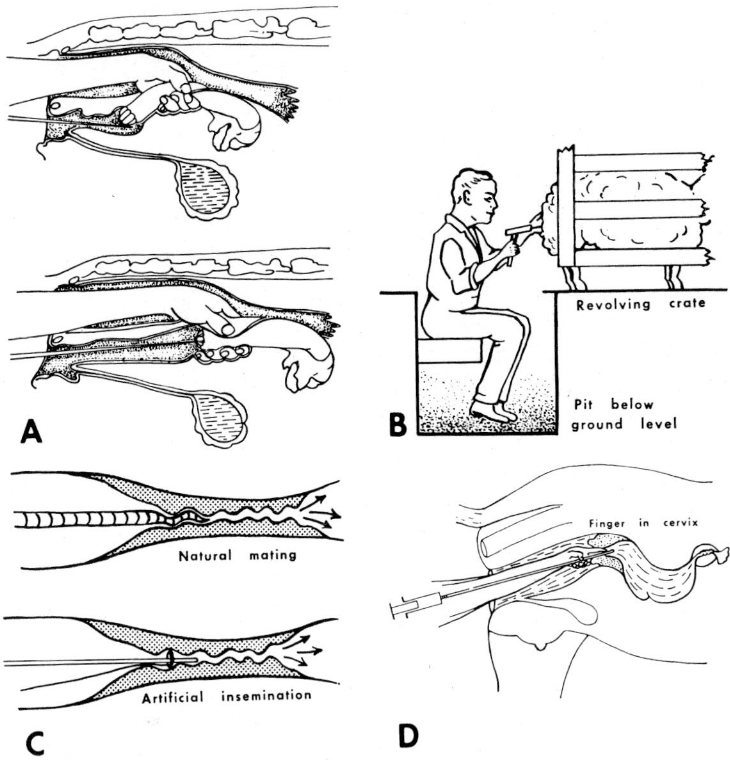


FIGURE 26-9. Artificial insemination procedures.

and the time between estrus onset and ovulation. Using transcutaneous sonography of weaned sow ovaries, Weitze (11) was able to identify ovulation times relative to estrus onset on 427 sows. The following recommendations were made with respect to insemination time:

AI sows that show estrus early post-wean: on second and third day of estrus once every 12 h.

AI sows that show estrus at usual time post-wean: at 24 h after detection and once every 12 h later.

AI sows that show estrus late post-wean: as early as possible after detection.

### *Insemination Techniques*

Several methods are used to impregnate swine: natural service; transcervical (Figure 26-10) with fresh, extended, or frozen semen; and surgical insemination (Figure 26-11) with fresh, extended, or frozen semen. Farrow rates average 70 to 85% for transcervical insemination with fresh and extended semen; 40 to 70% for transcervical insemination with frozen semen; and 30 to 55% for surgical insemination with fresh, extended, and frozen semen (12–16).

For AI the technician inverts the semen dose (plastic bottle/vial/cochette) several times slowly to mix the semen. The end of the catheter is lubricated beforehand (with K-Y jelly, semen, or extender). The vulva is wiped clean and the vulva lips are opened to allow the catheter to be inserted in an upwards/forwards motion (Figure 26-12). The technician will feed the end of the catheter **lock** into the cervix. Attach the semen dose to the catheter and allow semen to flow by gravity into the female. The normal uterine contractions (1 to 2 per minute) will assist in drawing semen into the uterine horns.

Surgical insemination into the oviduct (Figure 26-13), or tip of uterine horn, is effected by using a Tomcat Catheter pushed through a hole made in the upper 1.5 cm of the uterine horn. This procedure is invasive but has merit in situations using semen that has high economic merit.

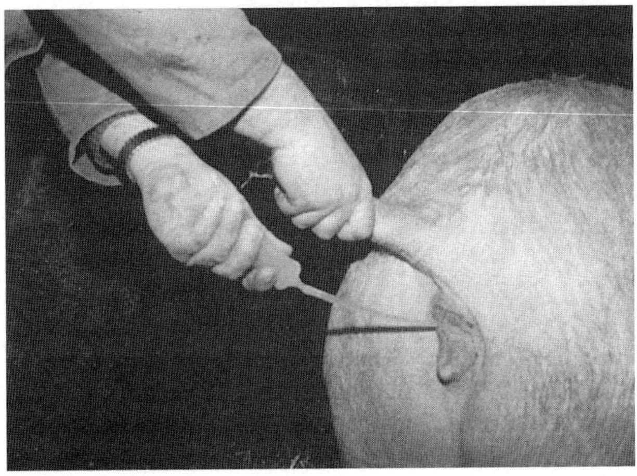

FIGURE 26-10. Transcervical AI procedure in swine.

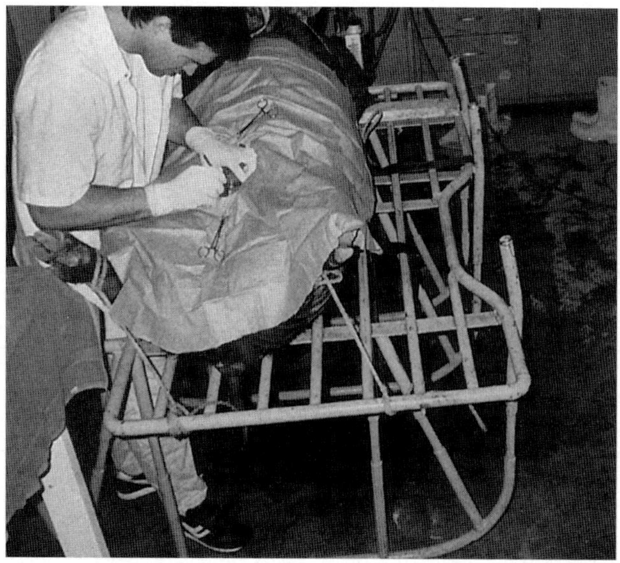

FIGURE 26-11. Surgical insemination AI procedure in swine.

### *Semen Diluents and Dilutions for AI*

There are a variety of semen diluents available for extending boar semen. The diluents can be supplied in a powder form. Extended semen would be stored at 18°C if an on-farm diluent is used, and sperm are viable for up to three days.

The concentration of sperm in one insemination dose should be somewhere between $2.0 \times 10^9$ and $3.0 \times 10^9$ cells for optimal fertility. Although the sperm concentration of an ejaculate can be assessed with instruments, if a sample displays at least 65% motility and less than 20% abnormalities, it can be extended by 1 part semen to 8 parts diluent for an appropriate concentration for AI.

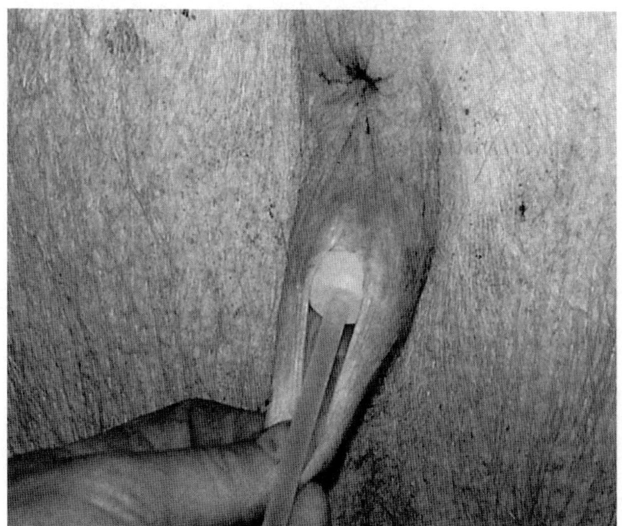

FIGURE 26-12. Placement of catheter in vulva for transcervical AI in swine.

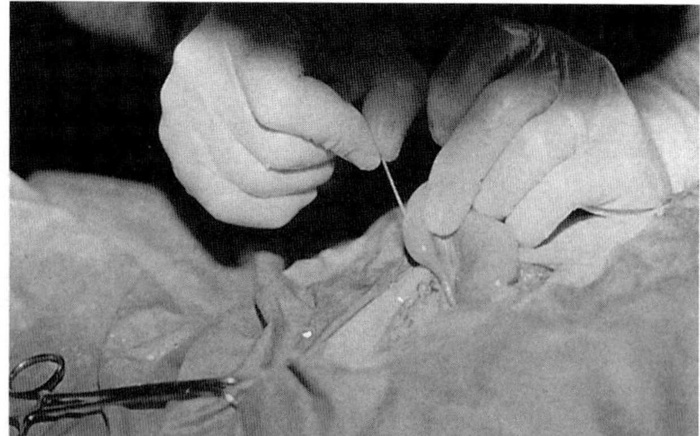

FIGURE 26-13. Placement of catheter in oviduct for surgical insemination in swine.

## HORSES

### *Collection of Semen*

Ejaculated semen is collected from stallions for artificial insemination of mares, or for assessment of semen quality (refer to Chapter 25, Semen Evaluation). To ensure protection of the sperm, semen should be collected using an artificial vagina which has been properly prepared. Quality of semen collected in a condom is generally inferior to that obtained with an artificial vagina, because spermatozoa can be adversely affected by debris from the penis or toxicants in the condom.

### *Artificial Vaginas*

Several models of artificial vaginas are available commercially (Table 26-3). Homemade artificial vaginas may also be constructed to meet any specific needs of the user. It is imperative that all components of an artificial vagina which come in contact with semen are nontoxic to sperm. For disinfectant, rubber liners can be submerged in 70% isopropyl or ethyl alcohol for 20 minutes. Rubber liners of some artificial vaginas can be toxic to spermatozoa. If possible, sterile, nontoxic disposable equipment should be used to avoid contamination of semen with toxic chemicals, and to minimize transmission of venereal diseases (Figs. 26-14 and 26-15). Some stallions resist ejaculation when the penis is placed in an artificial vagina fitted with a plastic liner.

A filter should be installed in the artificial vagina prior to collection of semen. This filter allows the sperm-rich portion of an ejaculate to pass into the semen receptacle, but retains the gel fraction. In stallions with suspected inflammatory conditions (seminal vesiculitis), or plugged ampullae or urospermin, the filter should be carefully inspected, since evidence of these conditions can be trapped in the filter. The result is a higher usable sperm harvest because far fewer spermatozoa become entrapped in the gel during

TABLE 26-3. *Some Models and Sources of Equine Artificial Vaginas*

| MODEL | SOURCE |
|---|---|
| Missouri | NASCO<br>901 Janesville Ave.<br>Ft. Atkinson, WI 53538-0901<br>(414) 563-2446 |
| C.S.U. | Animal Reproduction Systems<br>14395 Ramona Ave.<br>Chino, CA 91710<br>(909) 597-4889 |
| Lane | Lane Manufacturing Co.<br>2075 S. Valentia<br>Denver, CO 80231<br>(303) 745-2603 |
| Roanoke | Roanoke A.I. Labs<br>Route 7<br>Box 320<br>Roanoke, VA 24018<br>(703) 774-0676 |

collection. Nylon-micromesh filters are preferable to conventional polyester matte filters.

The internal temperature of the artificial vagina normally should not exceed 45 to 48°C at the time of semen collection, because irreversible damage to spermatozoa can result from exposure (even short-term) to temperatures above this level. If the glans penis is beyond the water jacket of the artificial vagina at the time of ejaculation (as typically occurs when using the Missouri-model artificial vagina), the temperature of the water jacket can be adjusted to 50 to 60°C without any temperature-related injury incurred by ejaculated spermatozoa. Only lubricants which are nonspermicidal should be used in the interior of the artificial vagina.

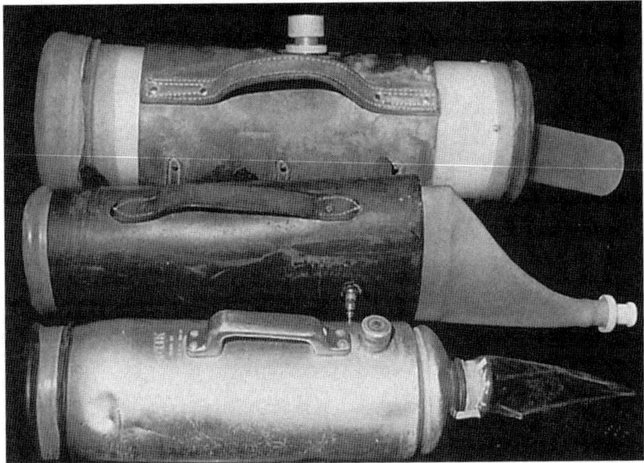

FIGURE 26-14. Three commonly used artificial vaginas for collection of stallion semen. From top to bottom: Colorado model, Missouri model, Japanese model.

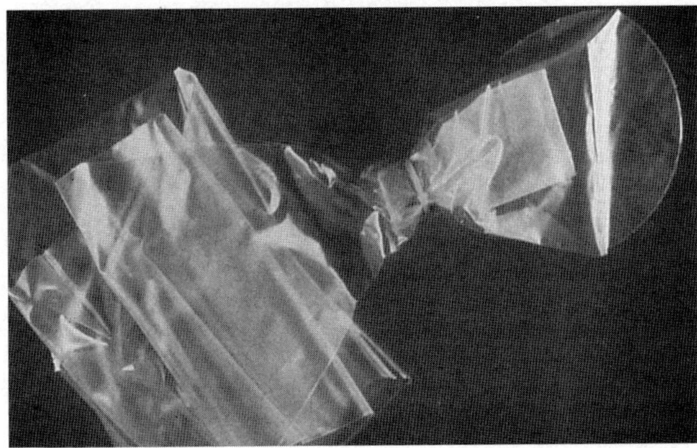

FIGURE 26-15. Plastic liner for artificial vagina that is fitted with an in-line filter to remove gel and extraneous debris from the gel-free portion of a stallion's ejaculate.

### Other Considerations

Prior to collecting semen, the stallion's penis (particularly the distal portion) should be cleansed with water, then thoroughly dried. Semen is generally collected after allowing the stallion to mount a breeding dummy, or a receptive and properly-restrained mare. Stallions can also be trained to ejaculate while standing. Ejaculated semen is promptly transported to the laboratory (maintaing 35 to 37°C) for evaluation and further processing. Upon arrival the semen should be promptly placed in an incubator adjusted to 37 to 38°C, then mixed with an appropriate extender.

### Semen Extenders

Semen collected for artificial insemination should always be placed in a semen extender, which may be purchased commercially, or prepared in the laboratory (Table 26-4) (17, 18). If semen is to be used for insemination soon after collection, it should be mixed with semen extender at a 1:1 to 1:3 ratio (semen to extender). More extensive dilution is recommended if semen is to be stored for a prolonged period of time prior to insemination.

### AI Technique

Artificial insemination is permitted by the vast majority of United States breed associations. Only sterile, nontoxic, disposable equipment should be used for the procedure. All inseminations should be performed using a minimum-contamination technique. With the mare adequately restrained, and the tail wrapped and elevated, the area be-

TABLE 26-4. ***Commonly Used Equine Semen Extenders***

| NAME | FORMULA[a] |
|---|---|
| Kenney extender | 1. Mix nonfat dry milk solids (2.4 g) and glucose (4.9 g) with 92 mL deionized water.<br>2. Add: (a) crystalline streptomycin sulfate (150,000 μg) or (b) gentamicin sulfate (100 mg) mixed with 2 mL of 7.5% sodium bicarbonate. |
| Modified Kenney extender (Texas A&M University formula) | 1. Mix nonfat dry milk solids (24 g), glucose (27 g), and sucrosoe (40 g) with 907 mL of deionized water.<br>2. Add potassium penicillin G (1,000,000 units) and amikacin sulfate (1 g). |
| Skim milk extender | 1. Heat 100 mL nonfortified skim milk to 92–95°C for 10 min in a double boiler. Cool.<br>2. Add polymyxin B sulfate (100,000 units). |
| Cream-gel extender | 1. Dissolve 1.3 g unflavored gelatin in 10 mL sterile deionized water. Sterilize.<br>2. Heat Half & Half cream to 92–95°C for 2–4 min in a double boiler. Remove scum from surface.<br>3. Mix gelatin solution with 90 mL of heated Half & Half cream (100 mL total volume). Cool.<br>4. Add crystalline penicillin G (100,000 units), streptomycin sulfate (100,000 μg), and polymyxin B sulfate (20,000 units). |
| Modified cream-gel extender (Neely formula) | 1. Heat Half & Half cream (1 pt) to 85–92°C in a glass flask for 10 min. Remove scum from surface.<br>2. Dissolve 6 g unflavored gelatin in 40 mL 5% dextrose and heat to 65°C in a water bath.<br>3. Add hot gelatin solution to cream, cover, and allow to cool to 35–40°C.<br>4. Add potassium penicillin G (1,000,000 units), or potassium penicilllin G (1,000,000 units) and amikacin sulfate (0.5 g). |

[a] Many different antibiotics and antibiotic dosages have been used with these basic extenders, including: potassium penicillin G (1000–2000 units/mL), streptomycin sulfate (1000–1500 μg/mL), polymyxin sulfate (200–1000 units/mL), gentamicin sulfate (100–1000 μg/mL), amikacin sulfate (100–1000 μg/mL), or ticarcillin (100–1000 μg/mL). Use of gentamicin sulfate or amikacin sulfate may require the addition of sodium bicarbonate to adjust the pH of the extender to 6.8–7.0. The extenders can be stored in small packages at −20°C and thawed immediately prior to use.

tween the base of the tail and ventral commissure of the vulva is thoroughly scrubbed, rinsed, and dried. Semen contained within a syringe is deposited into the anterior uterine body through a 22-inch sterile insemination pipette. A sterile or clean plastic shoulder-length sleeve should be worn when passing the pipette through the cervix to the uterine body where the semen is to be deposited (Figure 26-16).

Mares are generally inseminated with $250 \times 10^6$ to $500 \times 10^6$ progressively motile spermatozoa, contained in a semen extender. The volume of the inseminate typically ranges from 5 to 20 mL. For maximum pregnancy rates, it is best to inseminate mares within 12 to 24 h prior to ovulation, although pregnancies have been achieved at a similar rate when mares are inseminated within 12 h following ovulation. Using semen from highly fertile stallions, mares may sometimes be inseminated 48 to 72 h prior to ovulation with no depression in pregnancy rate. Containers for transporting stallion semen and straws for packaging stallion semen are illustrated in Figures 26-17 and 26-18.

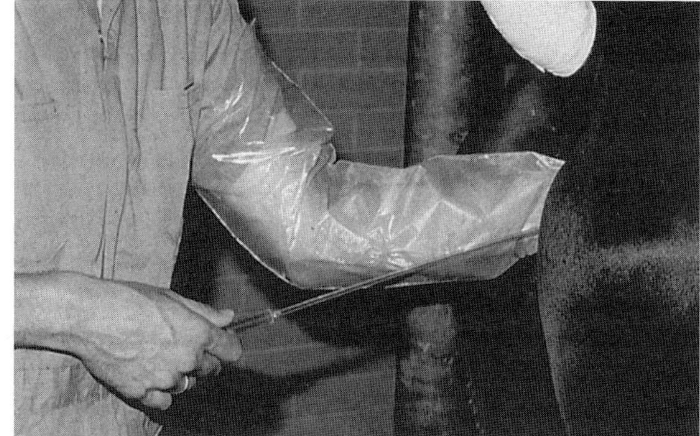

FIGURE 26-16. A 22-inch plastic insemination pipette is being passed into the uterine body of the mare in preparation for artificial insemination. The perineal area of the mare should be properly cleaned prior to attempting this procedure.

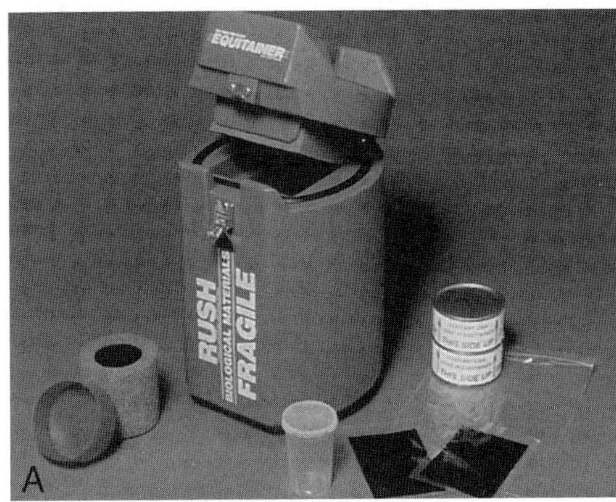


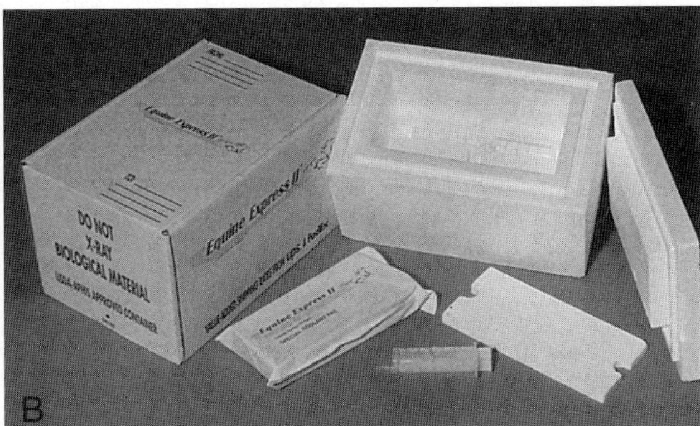


FIGURE 26-17. Two types of semen transport containers that are available commercially. (**A**) Hamilton-Thorne Equitainer II is a reusable container that is quite durable and reliable. The semen is stored in plastic bags. (**B**) Equine Express is a disposable container in which the semen is stored in all-plastic syringes.

Post-thawed spermatozoa are considered to have lowered longevity in comparison to freshly ejaculated spermatozoa. Therefore, insemination of mares with frozen/thawed semen should be reserved for the periovulatory period. As ovulation approaches, the ovaries should probably be examined two to four times daily by transrectal ultrasonography to more closely predict the exact time of ovulation. Mares should be inseminated within 6 to 12 h prior to ovulation, or within 6 h post-ovulation. Administration of human chorionic gonadotropin (hGC; 2000 to 2500 I.U.) to mares with a dominant follicle of specific size (35 to 40 mm in diameter) provides additional predictive power regarding timing of ovulation because most of these mares will ovulate 36 to 40 h following injection of hCG.

## SHEEP

### *Semen Collection*

There are two methods by which semen may be collected from the ram: electro-ejaculation (EE), or using an artificial vagina (AV). The EE procedure is performed by inserting a bipolar electrical probe into the ram's rectum. Low voltage electrical stimulation is given for 2 to 4 seconds at 10-second to 20-second intervals until an ejaculation occurs. EE collections are highly variable in both sperm concentrations and volume. Contamination with urine can be a problem when semen is collected by EE. EE is stressful on the ram, so it should only be used in extreme cases.

The AV is the preferred method for collecting semen. Rams must be trained to use the AV, but this is not difficult and most rams can be trained within a week. It is best to collect semen during the peak of the breeding season. The AV consists of a hose 20 to 25 cm in length and 5 to 7 cm in diameter, with a rubber liner. It is critical to have the interlining lubricated, with a temperature of the AV between 42 and 46°C. As the ram mounts the ewe, his penis is gently guided inside the AV. The amount of inter-AV pressure will vary among rams. It is also important to have the glass collecting tube warm (37°C) to avoid cold shock. After the ram ejaculates, the glass tube containing the semen is removed and placed in a waterbath at 30°C until the semen reaches that temperature.

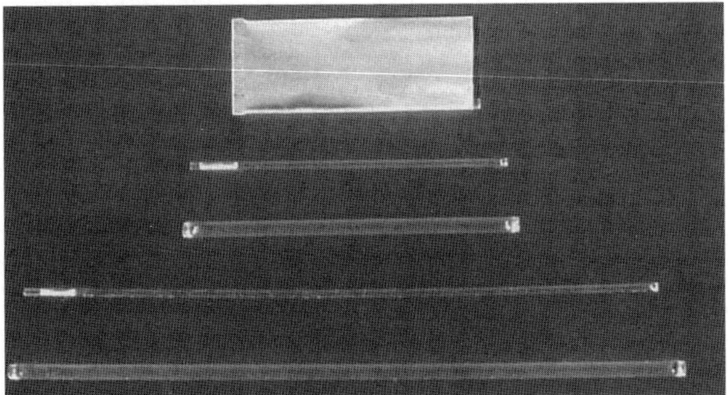

FIGURE 26-18. Various packages used for packaging equine semen for cryopreservation. From top to bottom: Aluminum packet, 0.5 mL PVC straw, 2.5 mL PVC straw, 1 mL PVC straw, and 5 mL PVC straw.

### *Semen Diluents and Dilutions*

Motility and concentration govern the ratio which semen is diluted. Semen which score 5 in both motion and concentration may be diluted as high as a 4 : 1 ratio. Most ejaculates are diluted at a 2 : 1 ratio. Semen scoring 2 should not be diluted and should only be used in the fresh, undiluted state.

Natural or synthetic diluent can be used. Cow milk is the most commonly used natural diluent. When whole, skim, or powdered milk is used, it must be heated to 92 to 95°C in a water bath for 8 to 10 min. If ultra-heat-treated milk is used, no additional heating is required. Table 26-5 lists a commonly used synthetic diluent. Diluent and semen

**TABLE 26-5. *Egg Yolk-TRIS Fructose Diluent for Ram Semen***

| COMPONENT | AMOUNT |
|---|---|
| Tris(hydroxymethyl)aminomethane | 3.634 g |
| Fructose | 0.50 g |
| Citric acid, monohydrate | 1.99 g |
| Egg yolk | 14 mL |
| Glass-distilled water | add to make up 100 mL |

should be at the same temperature (30°C) when dilution is performed; adding the diluent to the semen will reduce shock to the sperm. Never add the semen to the diluent. The mixture should be gently mixed, with evaluation of semen after dilution, to confirm sperm viability.

### *Buck*

Buck semen is less concentrated than ram semen, therefore the dilution ratio is lower. When egg yolk is used in a diluent, amount added is significantly less than in a ram's diluent (14 mL vs 2.5 mL). Buck semen's seminal plasma is removed by centrifuging the semen. This method also requires the sperm concentration to be determined in the centrifuged sample before dilution.

### *Estrus Synchronization for AI*

AI can be successful only if it is performed during the last half of the estrous period. Synchronizing the ewe's estrus with that of other ewes permits the AI technician to inseminate a group in one session and facilitates insemination during the period of optimal conception. Synchronization can be accomplished naturally or pharmacologically. The natural method involves the use of a teaser ram or testosterone-treated wether checking for estrus twice daily at 12-hour intervals. Ewes found to be in estrus are artificially inseminated 12 and 24 h after detection. If checked only once a day, insemination would be performed 13 to 17 h after detection. This method is labor intensive but does not incur any drug costs.

There are two commonly used pharmacologic procedures to synchronize ewes: progesterone and prostaglandin therapy. Progesterones can be administered by several means. They can be fed daily, implanted, injected intramuscularly, or inserted into the ewe in the form of a vaginal pessary or sponge. The pessary method is the most widely used and convenient one. A pessary impregnated with progesterone is inserted into the ewe's vagina and remains in place for 12 to 14 days. Any naturally occurring corpus

**TABLE 26-6. *Summary of Various Insemination Methods for Sheep***

| PROCEDURE | CONSIDERATIONS |
|---|---|
| VAI | 1. Simple, little training required.<br>2. Only fresh or fresh-diluted semen is used (0.2 mL).<br>3. $200 \times 10^6$–$400 \times 10^6$ sperm are used.<br>4. Ewe is in standing position.<br>5. Pipette is inserted 13 cm.<br>6. Conception rate is 40–65%. |
| CAI | 1. More skill than VAI, less semen required, higher conception rates.<br>2. Chilled semen can be used.<br>3. $100 \times 10^6$–$200 \times 10^6$ sperm are used.<br>4. $450 \times 10^6$ frozen sperm results in 30–35% conception rate.<br>5. Speculum is used to open cervix, inserted 10–14 cm.<br>6. Semen is deposited 1–3 cm beyond the cervix.<br>7. Conception rate is 60–70%. |
| TAI | 1. Cryopreserved semen can be used.<br>2. 90% conception rate with fresh semen.<br>3. 22–51% conception rates with cryopreserved semen.<br>4. Vaginoscope is required for technique (Fig. 26-19).<br>5. Cervical penetration is accomplished in 70–90% of ewes.<br>6. Recommended on large, multipurpose ewes 4 months post-lambing.<br>7. 0.5 mL volume of semen required.<br>8. Ewe is restrained on her back for AI. |
| LAI | 1. Cryopreserved semen can be used.<br>2. Conception rate 65–80% with cryopreserved semen.<br>3. Food and water withheld for 18 h.<br>4. Placed in laparoscopic cradle (Fig. 26-20).<br>5. Local anesthetic given 14 cm anterior to udder and 6 cm on both sides of the ventral midline.<br>6. Ewe lying on back at 40° angle.<br>7. Trocar is used to puncture abdominal wall.<br>8. Trocar removed, manipulating probe and endoscope are placed through cannulus into abdominal cavity.<br>9. Fiber optic light in endoscope reveals reproductive tract.<br>10. $CO_2$ injected in abdomen (mild anesthetic).<br>11. Probe is used to properly position uterus.<br>12. Semen (~1 mL) is deposited into uterine lumen, both horns (Fig. 26-22).<br>13. Topical antibiotic spray applied on incisions.<br>14. Ewe is placed in holding pen, eats in a few minutes, infection rates extremely low. |

luteum on the ovaries will regress during this period, leaving the exogenous progesterone as the only progesterone source. At pessary removal, the ewes are given a intramuscular injection of pregnant mare serum gonadotropin (PMSG). PMSG causes a closer synchronization and increases ovulation rate. PMSG doses of 400 to 500 IU or 600 to 750 IU are commonly recommended during the natural breeding season and nonbreeding season, respectively, except in small-bodied breeds when PMSG doses of as little as 250 IU are recommended. As PMSG dosages increase, ovulation rates increase; however, at levels above 800 IU the conception rate may decrease.

Another intravaginal device, the **controlled internal drug release** (CIDR) dispenser, is used to synchronize ewes. The CIDR contains 9 to 12 % progesterone in a silicone elastomer. No difference in conception rates is observed between the two intravaginal therapy methods. Prostaglandin (PG) therapy depends on the presence of an active corpus luteum and therefore can be used only during the breeding season. Prostaglandin causes the corpus luteum to regress and thereby inhibits progesterone production. It is effective only between days 5 and 14 of the estrous cycle. Therefore, two injections of PG are required 10 to 14 days apart to be effective in synchronizing the entire breeding group. AI conception rates are lower when PG therapy is used than with the progesterone pessary method. PG can be used in combination with short periods of progesterone therapy and PMSG. This method requires a 7-day treatment period with a vaginal pessary, and on the sixth day a single injection of PG is administered. The PMSG is given at pessary removal.

## *Ram Effect*

Teaser rams can be used to synchronize ewes naturally, because pheromones produced by the ram stimulate the advancement of the breeding season by 2 to 3 weeks and

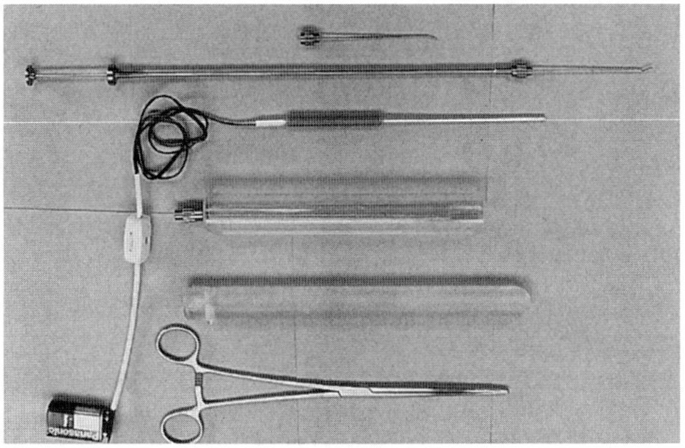

**FIGURE 26-19.** Transcervical AI equipment. Bozeman forceps, vaginoscope with light source, and 0.5 mL Cassou insemination gun with angled insemination tip.

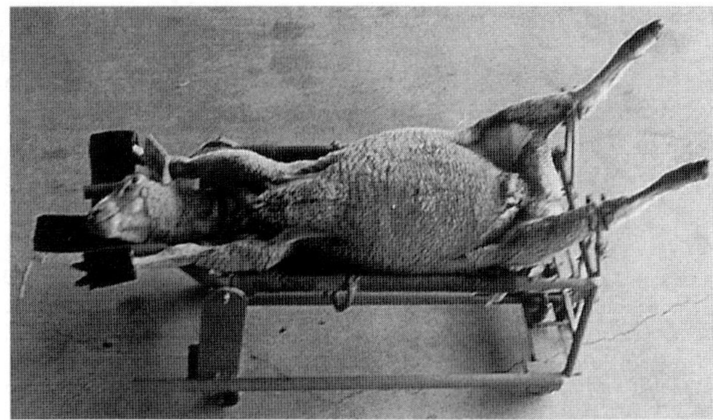

**FIGURE 26-20.** Ewe in laparoscopy cradle.

synchronize the ewes. Pheromones are specialized hormones released by the ram and smelled by the ewe. They are found in the wool and wax that accumulate around the ram's eyes. Visual or physical contact with the ram is not necessary to stimulate the ewe. Wool from a Dorset ram was rubbed on the muzzle of a group of ewes 3 times a day for 2 days. This treatment resulted in half of the ewes being stimulated. Different breeds of rams may differ in their ability to stimulate ewes. When Dorset rams were used as teasers, 67% of the ewes were bred during the first two weeks of their breeding season, compared to only 34% with Romney rams. No significant difference was found between Dorset and Suffolk teaser rams in their ability to stimulate onset of estrus during May. Within 10 min of the introduction of the ram or pheromones, ewes that are stimulated will start secreting gonadotrophins. The hormones cause the ewe to ovulate within three days.

Ewes must be completely isolated from rams for approximately two months before introduction of the teaser rams in order to have a stimulation effect from the ram pheromones. It is also suggested that rams be kept at least a half mile away from the ewes to prevent the ewes from picking up the scent of the rams' pheromones during this period. A ratio of one teaser ram per 100 ewes is normally required to assure a stimulating effect. Vasectomized, epididectomized, or intact rams can be used to stimulate ewes. However, if an intact ram is allowed to be in direct contact with the ewes, any ewe that has a behavioral estrus during the teasing period might be bred. Since direct contact with the ram is

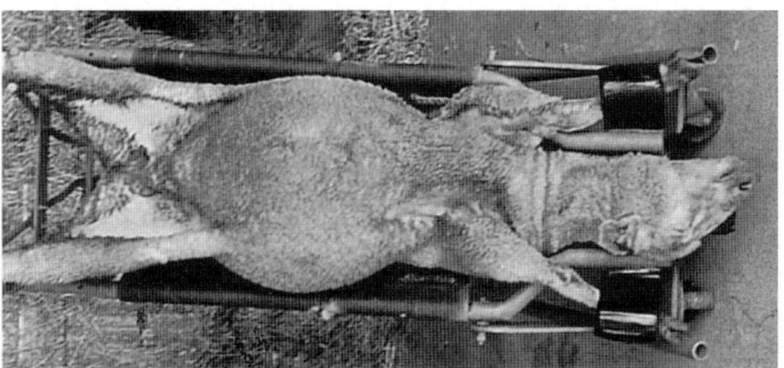

**FIGURE 26-21.** Laparoscopy cradle in surgical position, 40° angle.

FIGURE 26-22. Laparoscopy AI gun, 0.25 mL straw, and insemination glass pipette.

not required to stimulate the ewe, it is advisable when using intact rams to place them in an adjacent field. Long periods of teasing are not required; studies have shown that allowing ewes to be exposed to rams for 2 days is as effective as teasing for 17 days.

Wethers that have been treated with testosterone propionate (105 mg/injection 3 times a week for 2 to 3 weeks) are almost as effective at stimulating ewes as rams. Buck goats have also been found to have a stimulating effect on ewes.

### Insemination Methods

There are four methods of artificially inseminating the ewe: vaginal (VAI), cervical (CAI), transcervical (TAI), and laparoscopic (LAI) or intrauterine. Each method has its advantages and disadvantages. The first sheep was successfully artificially inseminated in 1936. Today sheep AI is widely used throughout the world. Insemination procedures have been previously published (19–21). Various insemination methods are summarized in Table 26-6 and Figures 26-19 to 26-22.

### Time of Insemination

When progesterone pessary and PMSG are used in combination, and VAI or CAI is performed, a single insemination should be conducted 54 to 56 h after the pessary is removed. If the ewes are to be inseminated twice, the first insemination should take place 48 h after pessary removal and the second 12 h later. Double insemination normally results in a 5 to 10% increase in conception rate and increases prolificacy as well. When ewe lambs are inseminated it is recommended that insemination take place 50 h after pessary removal, since ewe lambs come into estrus earlier than mature ewes.

When the TAI is performed, insemination should take place between 48 and 56 h following pessary removal. If the CIDR without PMSG is used to synchronize estrus, insemination is performed 48 to 57 h after removal. If the short term progesterone therapy combined with prostaglandin and PMSG is used, insemination is performed 48 to 60 h following pessary removal.

When LAI is performed and the progesterone and PMSG therapy is used, insemination should be conducted 56 to 62 h following pessary removal. If the ewes are superovulated, given higher levels of PMSG or FSH, insemination should take place earlier. When fresh semen is used the insemination is performed 36 to 48 h after withdrawing the pessary. Superovulation insemination should be conducted 44 to 48 h after pessary withdrawal when frozen-thawed semen is used. LAI is performed 48 to 52 h after CIDR is withdrawn.

## REFERENCES


1. Hunter RHF. Reproduction of Farm Animals. London: Longman, 1982.
2. Amann RP, Almquist JO. Bull management to maximize semen output. Proc 6th Tech Conf on AI and Reprod NAAB 1976;1–9.
3. Almquist JO. Effect of long term ejaculation at high frequency on output of sperm, sexual behavior, and fertility of holstein bulls; relation of reproductive capacity to high nutrient allowance. J Dairy Sci 1982;6:814–823.
4. Herman HA, Mitchell JR, Doak GA. Evaluation of semen—general considerations, appearance and viability. In: The Artificial Insemination and Embryo Transfer of Dairy and Beef Cattle. Danville, IL: Interstate Publishers, 1994;59–72.
5. Herman HA., Mitchell JR, Doak GA. Evaluation of semen: live-dead staining and morphology. In: The Artificial Insemination and Embryo Transfer of Dairy and Beef Cattle. Danville, IL: Interstate Publishers, 1994;81–92.
6. Walkes WL, Nebel RL, McGilliard ML. Time of ovulation relative to mounting activity in dairy cattle. J Dairy Sci 1996; 7:1551–1561.
7. Peters JL. Radiographic evaluation of bovine artificial insemination technique among professional A.I. technicians and herdsman-insemination using .5 and .25 ml french straws. Masters thesis. Pennsylvania State University Department of Dairy and Animal Science, 1984.
8. Hemsworth PH, Galloway DB. The effect of sexual stimulation on the sperm output of the domestic boar. Anim Reprod Sci 1979;2:387–394.
9. Gerritts RJ, Graham EF, Cole RJA. Effect of collection interval on the characterization of the ejaculate in the boar. J Anim Sci 1962;2:1002(abst #233).
10. Hughes PE, Varley MA. Artificial insemination. In: Hughes PE, Varley MA, eds. Reproduction in the Pig. Butterworths, 1980;187–195.

11. Weitze KF. Timing of AI and ovulation in breeding herds I. In: Rath D, Johnson LA, Weitze KF, eds. Reproduction in Domestic Animals. Blackwell Science, 1996; 31:1–342.
12. Reed HCB. Current use of frozen boar semen-Future needs of frozen boar semen. In: Johnson LA, Larsson K, eds. Deep Freezing of Boar Semen. Uppsala, Sweden: Swedish Univ Agric Sci, 1985;225–238.
13. Johnson LA. Fertility results using frozen boar spermatozoa: 1970 to 1985. In: Johnson LA, Larsson K, eds. Deep Freezing of Boar Semen. Uppsala, Sweden: Swedish Univ Agric Sci, 1985;199–224.
14. Johnson LA. Verified sex pre-selection in farm animals. In: Johnson LA, Rath D, eds. Boar Semen Preservation II. Berlin and Hamburg: Paul Parey Scientific Publishers, 1990;213–219.
15. Didion BA, Schoenbeck RA. Fertility of frozen boar semen used for AI in commercial settings. In: Rath D, Johnson LA, Weitze KF, eds. Reproduction in Domestic Animals. Blackwell Science, 1996;31:1–342.
16. Soede NM, Kemp B. Timing of AI and ovulation in sows. In: Rath D, Johnson LA, Weitze KF, eds. Reproduction in Domestic Animals. Blackwell Science, 1996;31:1–342.
17. Blanchard TL, Varner DD, eds. Stallion Management. Veterinary Clinics of North America—Equine Practice. Philadelphia: WB Saunders, 1992.
18. Varner DL, Schumacher J, Blanchard TL, Johnson L. Diseases and Management of Breeding Stallions. St. Louis: Mosby-Year Book, 1991.
19. Evans G, Maxwell WMC. Salmon's Artificial Insemination of Sheep and Goats. Buttersworths, 1987.
20. Sheep Production Handbook. American Sheep Industry Association Production Education and Research Council, 1988.
21. Chemineau P, Cagnie Y, Guerdon Y, Roger P, Valet JC. Training Manual on Artificial Insemination in Sheep and Goats. FAO Animal Production and Health Paper 83, 1991.

# Chapter 27

# *X and Y Chromosome-Bearing Spermatozoa*

E.S.E. Hafez and B. Hafez

Female animals have two similar sex chromosomes (X and X), whereas males have two different sex chromosomes (one X chromosome and one smaller Y chromsome). The gametes (egg and sperm) are haploid cells containing either the X or the Y chromosome. Diploid somatic cells of females (homogametic sex) contain a pair of X chromosomes, but somatic cells of males (heterogametic sex) have XY sex chromosomes. The genetic sex is determined in the oviduct at the time of fertilization, and the sex of the offspring is determined by the sex chromosome within the sperm.

Extensive investigations have been carried out for preselection and complete separation of X and Y sperm before artificial insemination (AI). Sex of the offspring can also be predetermined in embryos arising from diploid or haploid nuclear transplantation into recipient ova, parthenogenetic activation of ova, or fusion of two oocytes. Different cytogenetic and cytologic techniques are used to examine the diploid cells at an appropriate stage of fertilization to diagnose the genetic sex of the embryo. For example, fluorescence microscopy is used to detect the presence of a Y chromosome. Chromosome analysis is performed by culturing leukocytes or fetal cells to study the individual chromosomes using karyotyping procedures (1).

This chapter addresses four concepts:

1. morphologic, physiologic, biophysical, and immunologic differences between X and Y sperm
2. factors affecting primary and secondary sex ratio
3. techniques for separation of X and Y sperm based on valid statistical evaluation of the results
4. attempts to alter the sex ratio by the use of "sexed" sperm

## Biology of Sperm

When sperm are transported through the female reproductive tract, they undergo capacitation to acquire their fertilizing potential. Sperm release and/or acquire various micromolecules and macromolecules on their plasmalemma as they migrate through the vaginal secretions, cervical mucus, endometrial secretions, oviductal fluid, and peritoneal fluid.

The degree of maturation and age of sperm in an ejaculate can influence density. Packed cell volume of bovine sperm is markedly affected by the osmolality of the medium. Live bull sperm placed in a hypo-osmotic saline solution swell to three times their normal size. Dead sperm do not swell or react osmotically. Live sperm placed in hyperosmotic media shrank from a volume of about 25 $\mu m^3$ to 20 $\mu m^3$.

### *Cytogenetics of X and Y Sperm*

There are many potential differences between sperm containing an X or a Y chromosome (Table 27-1). Sex chromosomes are responsible for any differences in DNA content. The presence of an X or a Y chromosome (Fig. 27-1) could cause a difference in size and shape of sperm, weight, density, motility (type and velocity), surface charge, and surface biochemistry or internal biochemistry (2, 3). The degree of difference may also be affected by other factors such as age of semen, repeat breeding (possible differential embryo mortality), and use of bulls that had been born co-twin with heifers (and have circulating XX leukocytes).

There are species variations in the mass differential of the X and Y chromosomes. The presence of large X chromosomes could result in greater weight and density of the X-containing sperm if size and other constituents are the same.

### *Sperm Plasmelemma*

The external plasmalemma has different characteristics in different parts of the sperm. X and Y sperm have different surface characteristics at spermiation from the germinal epi-

TABLE 27-1. ***Some Differences Between X and Y Sperm***

| PARAMETER | DIFFERENCE | EVALUATION |
|---|---|---|
| DNA size | Less in Y sperm<br>X sperm is larger | Measurable and accepted<br>Y sperm measured may or may not be representative of random sperm population |
| Identify motility | Y chromosome fluoresces<br>Y sperm faster | Species specific<br>Evidence primarily dependent on accuracy of F-body staining technique |
| Surface charge | X sperm migrate to cathode | No charge difference between X and Y sperm |

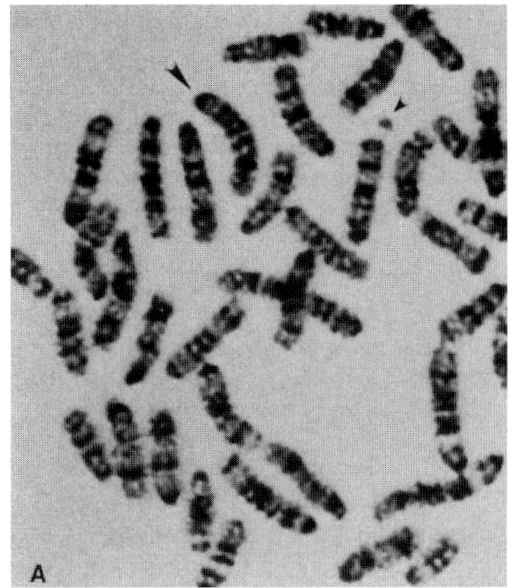


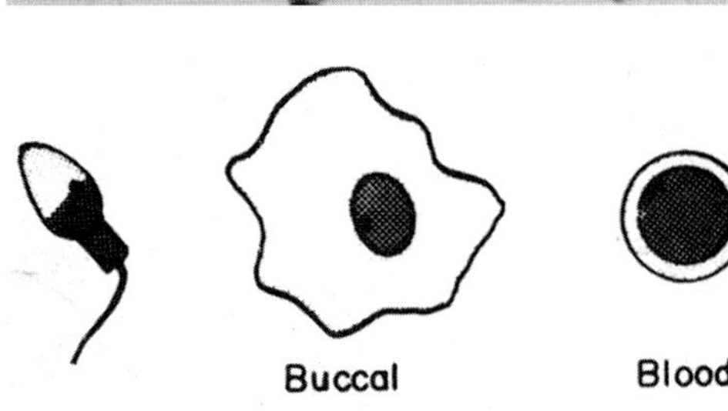


FIGURE 27-1. Mitotic metaphase chromosome spreads stained to reveal G-banding. (**A**) Chromosomes from a female $XY^x$. The *large arrowhead* designates the X and *small arrowhead* the $Y^x$ chromosome (From: Eicher EM. Primary sex determining genes in mice. In: Amann RP, Seidel GE Jr, eds. Prospects for Sexing Mammalian Sperm. Boulder: Colorado University Associated Press, 1982.) (**B**) Localization of Y body in these cell types. Buccal cells: Y body usually found anywhere within the nucleus. Blood cells: lymphocyte Y body usually found near periphery of nucleus, appears crescent shaped. Spermatozoon: Y body usually found equatorially within sperm head. (From: Lueck J, Zanaveld LJD. Cytogenetics of spermatozoa: Y-chromosome staining. In: Hafez ESE, ed. Techniques in Human Andrology. Amsterdam: Elsevier, 1977.)

thelium. If ejaculated sperm are examined, such differences would be masked by components absorbed from the seminal plasma.

### *Karyotyping of Sperm*

The distinction of X and Y sperm based on the fluorescence of the Y chromosome is facilitated by (a) quinacrine staining of sperm, which causes fluorescence of the long arm of the Y chromosome, and (b) a fluorescent spot (F body), which appears in 39 to 47% of the sperm in smears stained with quinacrine. Banding techniques are recommended: G-band and Q-band methods. Such procedures permit the accurate identification of individual chromosomes. The staining of chromosomes is carried out using a Giemsa dye mixture.

## TECHNIQUES OF SPERM SEPARATION

Techniques used to separate sperm are discussed in Table 27-2. Experimental attempts have been hampered by the lack of laboratory tests to evaluate the degree of sperm separation. The presence of the F-body appears to be associated with the Y chromosome (Fig. 27-1).

Most of the techniques employed for sperm separation are based on nonequilibrium sedimentation (based on velocity of fall) or an equilibrium sedimentation on a density gradient (sedimentation to the level where specific gravities of sperm and the medium are equal). These techniques use simple gravity or centrifugation and are based on Stoke's law of sedimentation of a rigid sphere through an incompressible, viscous fluid at a low Reynolds' number (nonturbulent conditions). Aggregation of cells in the buffer is evaluated, and a concentration chosen at which aggregation is negligible.

Only two laboratory methods for separation of animal and human X and Y sperm appear valid, reproducible, and clinically applicable: albumin separation, which yields 75 to 80% Y sperm, and Sephadex filtration, which yields 70

TABLE 27-2. ***Techniques Employed to Separate X and Y Chromosome-Bearing Sperm***

| TECHNIQUES | RESULTS |
|---|---|
| Sedimentation of immobilized sperm on media | Insemination with sperm that had sedimented the greatest distance produced 70% females. |
| Skim-milk powder, glycine, sodium citrate, glycerol | Increase in number of male offspring when sperm from the top layers was used. |
| Albumin column | Successful results with frozen bull sperm preselected on albumin column before cryopreservation. |
| Velocity sedimentation | Sedimentation rates depend on size, density, and shape of sperm.<br>Cell size difference is predominant factor in separation of types; shape is usually the least important factor.<br>Sperm heads have extremely aspherical shapes. |
| Centrifugation through density gradients | Sperm separated according to their sedimentation rates by centrifugation through density gradients, provided the density of the gradient material is less than that of the sperm. The advantage is that the time required for separation is much shorter. Shorter time does not improve theoretical resolution of separation, because diffusion is insignificant. |
| Motility and electrophoretic separation | Immotile sperm electrophoretically attracted to the anode at neutral pH. When electrophoretic separation is under conditions consistent with sperm motility, sperm migrate to the cathode. Sperm are oriented by electric field and swim in direction the head is facing. If negatively charged, sperm can be oriented so that the tail is facing the anode by virtue of its greater negative charge density and their intrinsic motility is greater than the electrophoretic mobility. |
| Isoelectric focusing | Separation performed in columns with the fluid stabilized using density gradients.<br>Sperm layered on, or suspended in, this solution migrate electrophoretically until reaching an isoelectric point. |
| H-Y antigens | Sperm treated with H-Y antisera. Insemination with mouse sperm treated with antisera to a Y-linked histocompatibility antigen produced 45% males compared with 53% for controls. |
| Flow sorting by DNA content | Y-sorting is 72–80% successful. Disadvantages: low sorting rate and lack of sperm viability after sorting. |
| Sephadex column | Some 70% of X sperm found in certain fractions of the filtrate when sperm was placed on top of a column of Sephadex.<br>65–85% X sperm were found in certain fractions of filtrate. |

Data from: Beernink FJ. Factors influencing the human sex ratio. Presented at the Annual Meeting of the American Fertility Society, New Orleans, 1984.
Bennet D, Boyce EA. Sex ratio in progeny of mice inseminated with sperm treated with H-Y antiserum. Nature 1973;246:308.
Bhattacharya BC, Bangham AD, Cro RJ, Keynes RD, Rowson L. An attempt to determine the sex of calves by artificial insemination with spermatozoa separated by sedimentation. Nature 1966;211:863.
Corson SL, Baatzer FR, Alexander NH, Shlaff S, Otis C. Sex selection by sperm separation and insemination. Fertil Steril 1984;42:756.
Ericsson RJ, Glass RH. Functional differences between sperm bearing the X- or Y-chromosome. In: Amann RP, Seidel GE Jr, eds. Prospects for Sexing Mammalian Sperm. Boulder: Colorado University Associated Press, 1982.
Hafs HD, Boyd LJ. Galvanic separation of X- and Y-chromosome-bearing sperm. In: Kiddy CA, Hafs HD, eds. Sex Ratio at Birth Prospects for Control. American Society for Animal Science, 1971.
James WH. Gonadotrophin and the human secondary sex ratio. Br Med J 1980;281:711.
Meistrich ML. Potential and limitations of physical methods for separation of sperm bearing an X- and Y-chromosome. In: Amann RP, Seidel GE Jr, eds. Prospects for Sexing Mammalian Sperm. Boulder: Colorado University Associated Press, 1982.
Moore HDM, Hibbitt KG. Isoelectric focusing of boar spermatozoa. J Reprod Fertil 1975;44:329–332.
Pinkel D, Gledhill BL. Sex preselection in mammals: separation of sperm bearing Y and "O" chromosomes in the vole *(Microtus oregoni)*, Science 1982;218:904.
Sherbet GV, Lakshmi MS, Rao KV. Characterization of ionogenic groups and estimation of the net negative electric charge on the surface of cells using natural pH gradients. Exp Cell Res 1972;70:113–123.

to 75% X sperm (4). The separation of X and Y sperm is based on the following:

1. Differences in the weight, density, or size of the X and Y chromosomes as a result of differences in the size of different components of the sperm.
2. Differences in haploid expression of X and Y chromosomes as a result of differences in the nature of sperm components: defective allocation (nondisjunction) of sex chromosomes, to either the gametes or, after fertilization, to early cleavage products, will result in individuals with somatic cells containing only a single X chromosome (XO; YO is lethal) or an extra X or Y chromosome (XXX, XXY, or XYY).

### *Layered Separation Over Albumin Columns*

When semen is layered over columns of serum albumin, increased numbers of Y sperm are recovered from the albumin layers. Semen aliquots of 0.5 ml (diluted 1 : 1 with Tyrode's solution) are layered for 1 h over a 7.5% solution of serum albumin in a glass column (8 × 75 mm). The initial sperm layer is then removed by pipette, the albumin centrifuged at 2800 to 3200 rpm for 10 min, and the sperm disc is resuspended in Tyrode's solution. The resuspended sperm is then layered over a two-layer serum albumin column. At 1 h, the sperm layer is removed, and after another 30 min, the 13% layer is removed. The 20% serum albumin is then centrifuged for 10 minutes, and the sperm disc is resuspended in 0.25 ml of Tyrode's solution, which is then inseminated into the uterus (5).

### *Flow Cytometry and Sorting*

With flow cytometry, high-speed measurements of components and properties of individual cells are made in a liquid suspension. Laser light is used for monochromatic illumination of cells stained with fluorescent dyes. Light detectors sample the fluorescence produced by the interaction of light with dye and produce electrical signals proportionate to the intensity of fluorescent light from each object. This technique is useful in the evaluation of the degree of separation needed to produce populations enriched in X or Y sperm (2, 3).

### *Practical Application*

Gender selection in farm animals is used for several purposes:

1. produce more female progeny from superior females, or from herd and flock replacements, and increased milk, meat, and pelt production
2. produce more males for meat production from culled females and cross-breeding schemes, e.g., dairy-beef crosses
3. ensure male progeny as herd sires from tom dam-sire crosses
4. ensure appropriate progeny when progeny testing young bulls
5. avoid intersexes in multiple births

Gender selection in horses will provide more progeny for sale or for brood mare replacements. Good fertility of sexed sperm is important for commercial purposes. The fertility level also must be considered when determining how many breedings are needed to produce the desired number of sexed progeny. The number of inseminations needed to obtain an accurate assessment of reproductive ability of cattle is not precisely known (6). Several thousand inseminations are required to evaluate true reproductive efficiency within a few percentage points.

## FUTURE RESEARCH

Additional research is needed in the following areas:

1. Sperm motility: Sperm isolate themselves based on different progressive motility.
2. Sperm dimensions or density: Cells sorted through a device sensitive enough to detect minute differences.
3. Sperm cytogenetics: Chemical or immunologic reaction capable of selecting on sex chromosome content.
4. Sperm environment: Hormone or chemical condition resulting in penetration of the egg by an X or Y sperm (7).
5. Search for Robersonian chromsome rearrangements that include a sex chromosome: the availability of such chromosomes could facilitate specific breeding schemes suitable for selection for or against a female or male.
6. Detection of a t-like system associated with a Robertsonian translocation.
7. Cytogenetic sexing of cells isolated from an embryo and transfer of the selected embryo after short *in vitro* culture.

## REFERENCES

1. Forsling ML. Pocket Examiner in Endocrinology. London: Pitman Publishing, 1984.
2. Foote RH. Functional differences between sperm bearing the X- or Y-chromosome. In: Amann RP, Seidel GE Jr, eds. Prospects for Sexing Mammalian Sperm. Boulder: Colorado University Associated Press, 1982.
3. Foote RH. Prospects for sexing: present status, future prospects and overall conclusions. In: Amann RP, Seidel GE Jr, eds. Prospects for Sexing Mammalian Sperm. Boulder: Colorado University Associated Press, 1982.
4. Beernink FJ. Techniques for separating X- and Y-spermatozoa.

In: Fredericks CM, et al, eds. Foundations of *In Vitro* Fertilization. New York: Hemisphere, 1986.
5. Beernink FJ, Ericsson RJ. Male sex preselection through sperm isolation. Fertil Steril 1982;38:493.
6. Foote RH, Oltenacu EAB. Increasing fertility in artificial insemination by culling bulls or ejaculates within bulls. Proc 8th Tech Conf Artif Insem Reprod NAAB, British Columbia, 1980;6–12.
7. Ericsson RJ, Glass RH. Functional differences between sperm bearing the X- or Y-chromosome. In: Amann RP, Seidel GE Jr, eds. Prospects for Sexing Mammalian Sperm. Boulder: Colorado University Associated Press, 1982.

# Chapter 28

# *Pregnancy Diagnosis*

M.R. Jainudeen and E.S.E. Hafez

An early diagnosis of pregnancy is essential for reproductive management as well as economic production. This chapter begins with the importance of pregnancy diagnosis. It is followed by the traditional practice of establishing pregnancy: suppression of the estrous cycle. Clinical and immunologic methods are described for the diagnosis of pregnancy (Fig. 28-1). The choice of method depends on the species, stage of gestation, cost, accuracy, and speed of diagnosis. Rectal palpation of the uterus, real-time ultrasonography, and on-farm tests for progesterone based on ELISA kits are covered in detail.

## Importance of Pregnancy Diagnosis

Knowing whether or not an animal is pregnant is of considerable economic value, as well as being an important tool in reproductive management. In general, an early diagnosis of pregnancy is required:

a) to identify nonpregnant animals soon after mating or insemination so that production time lost from infertility may be reduced by appropriate treatment or culling,
b) to certify animals for sale or insurance purposes,
c) to reduce waste in breeding programs using expensive hormonal techniques, and
d) to assist in the economic management of livestock.

### *Nonreturn to Estrus*

During pregnancy, the conceptus inhibits the regression of the corpus luteum (CL) and prevents the animal from returning to estrus. Therefore, an animal not returning to estrus after service is assumed to be pregnant.

Cattle and Buffalo. Absence of estrus after mating is widely used by farmers and artificial insemination (AI) centers as an indicator of pregnancy, but the reliability of the method depends on the accuracy of estrous detection in the herd. Both anestrus and the rare occurrence of estrus during pregnancy in cattle may affect the reliability of this method. Almost all artificial insemination centers worldwide use computerized monthly reports of the 60-to-90–day nonreturn rate (NR) from records of inseminations. Two months after each month when inseminations are performed (about 90 days after the beginning of that month), the records of all cows which were inseminated are checked to determine what proportion of them returned to estrus and were re-inseminated. In general, a 60-to-90–day NR of 70% on first service will correspond to about 60 to 65% pregnancy rate. In the buffalo, NR is unreliable due to difficulties of estrous detection.

Sheep and Goat. Estrus is difficult to detect in ewes. Therefore, a vasectomized ram with crayon or colored grease applied to the brisket or contained in special harness is used. The ram will mark ewes returning to estrus. By changing the color of the crayon at two-week intervals, it is possible to identify nonpregnant ewes during the mating season. The same technique is used in goats.

Pig. In most pig herds, sows are examined for signs of estrus 18 to 25 days after mating or insemination. Despite being laborious and failing to detect pregnant sows whose estrus is delayed due to embryonic mortality, it is still the most valuable and cheapest technique available for the pig herdsman. The technique of estrous detection is described in Chapter 13, Pigs.

Horse. Mares do not show homosexual behavior, but in the presence of a stallion or gelding will assume a stance characteristic of urination. The testing should commence at 16 days after the previous service.

## Clinical Methods of Pregnancy Diagnosis

Clinical methods depend on the detection of the conceptus—fetus, fetal membranes, and fetal fluids. The methods

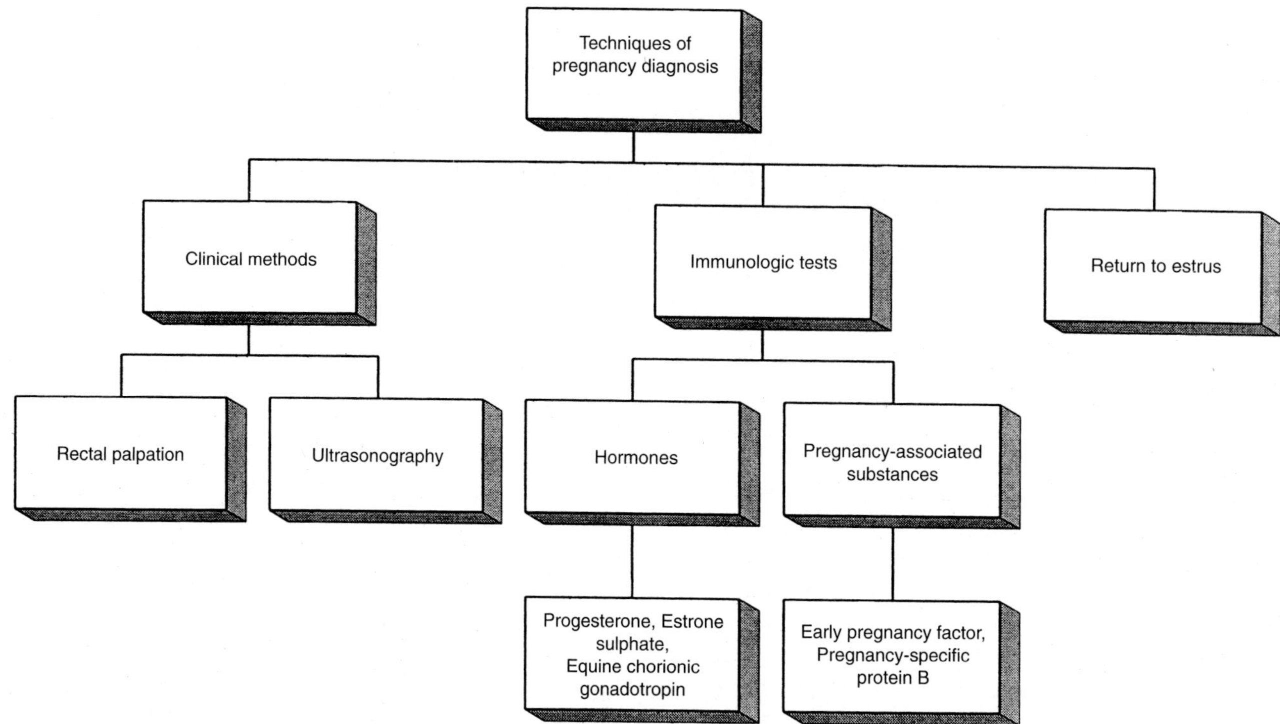


FIGURE 28-1. Pregnancy diagnosis techniques in farm animals.

TABLE 28-1. ***Diagnosis of Pregnancy in the Cow, Buffalo, and Mare by Rectal Palpation***

| ANIMAL | MONTH OF GESTATION | MAJOR FINDINGS |
|---|---|---|
| Cow | First | Quiescent uterus and a fully developed corpus luteum in one ovary. |
| Buffalo[a] | Second[b] | Enlargement and dorsal bulging of a pregnant horn due to fetal fluids; on application of digital pressure, gives a resilient sensation. "Fetal membrane slip" or palpation of allantochorion; amniotic vesicles represent anterior to the intercornual ligament. |
| | Third[b] | Descent of uterus commences; fetus is palpable. |
| | Fourth to seventh | Uterus on abdominal floor, fetus difficult to palpate; cotyledons, 2–5 cm in diameter, are palpated as circumscribed areas in uterine wall; middle uterine arteries hypertrophy and pulse changes to a distinct fremitus. |
| | Seventh to term | Cotyledons, fremitus, and fetal parts are palpable. |
| Mare | First | Contracted and firm cervix; turgid uterine horns. |
| | Second[b] | Chorioallantoic sac (size of an orange) bulges ventrally in lower third of uterine horn; uterine horns are turgid. |
| | Third | Chorioallantoic sac grows rapidly and descends into uterine body, changes from spherical to ovoid, and tenseness is gradually lost. Uterus begins to descend. |
| | Fourth | Dorsal surface of the uterus is felt as a distended dome between the stretched broad ligaments. Fetus and/or fetal parts palpable. |
| | Fifth to seventh | Uterus lies deep in abdominal cavity. Usually possible to palpate fetus, except in large pluriparous mares. |
| | Seventh to term | Fetus easier to palpate. Uterus begins to ascend. |

[a]Findings occur later than in cattle as a result of longer gestation length.
[b]Period when pregnancy can be accurately diagnosed.

include rectal examination and ultrasonic techniques. Radiography as method of pregnancy diagnosis in sheep, goats, and swine has now been abandoned because of the radiation hazards to the operator.

### *Rectal Examination*

Rectal examination is the accepted method of pregnancy diagnosis in the mare, buffalo, and cow. In this procedure, the uterus is palpated through the rectal wall to detect the uterine enlargement occurring during pregnancy, and the fetus or fetal membranes (Table 28-1). This technique, which can be performed at an early stage of gestation, is accurate, and the result is known immediately. For a detailed discussion the reader is referred to Arthur et al (1).

Because of the small pelvic cavity, the ewe, goat, and sow are unsuitable for rectal exploration of uterine contents. However, the middle uterine arteries in parous sows are readily accessible for palpation through the rectal wall. The detection of a fremitus in one or both uterine arteries is a rapid and simple test for pregnancy in the sow from 28 days onward.

### *Ultrasonography*

Ultrasound waves are inaudible to the human ear and operate at frequencies of 1 to 10 megahertz (MHz). Two types of ultrasound are employed in human and veterinary medicine: the Doppler phenomenon and the pulse-echo principle.

Doppler Phenomenon. In the Doppler phenomenon, sound waves striking a moving object are reflected to the transmitting source at a slightly altered frequency. The ultrasonic fetal pulse detector that is based on the Doppler phenomenon consists of a transducer and amplifier. The transducer (probe), when applied to the animal's abdominal wall or inserted into the rectum, emits a narrow beam of high-frequency waves (ultrasonic). Movements of the fetal heart or blood flow in the fetal (umbilical vessels) or maternal (uterine artery) circulation alter the frequency of these waves, which are reflected back to the probe, where they are converted into audible sound and amplified (earphones or speaker) or illuminated (oscilloscope).

Pulse-Echo Ultrasound. Pulses of ultrasound, generated by piezoelectric crystals in a transducer, on contacting tissues of varying acoustic impedance (resistance to the transmission), are reflected (echoed) to the transducer, then converted into electrical energy and displayed on a cathode ray oscilloscope in various ways. A-mode and B-mode are the basic forms currently in use. A-mode (amplitude) is a one-dimensional display of echo amplitude versus distance, whereas B-mode (brightness) produces an accurate two-dimensional image of soft tissue cross section. The brightness of the dots on the oscilloscope is projected in various shades of gray, comparable to a black and white succession; they will reveal any motion in the tissue being imaged. This is the basis of B-mode "real-time" scanning.

B-Mode Real-Time Ultrasound. The basic physical and diagnostic principles of ultrasonography have been reviewed elsewhere (2–5).

The major components of an ultrasound machine (Fig. 28-2) are:

a) an electrical pulse generator,
b) a transducer,
c) a scan converter, and
d) a video display.

A high-voltage electrical pulse of a few microseconds causes the piezoelectric transducer to vibrate and convert electrical to mechanical energy (ultrasound). The reflection of these

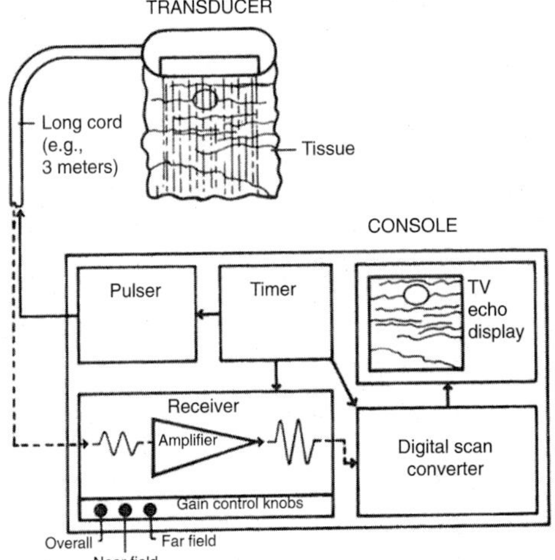


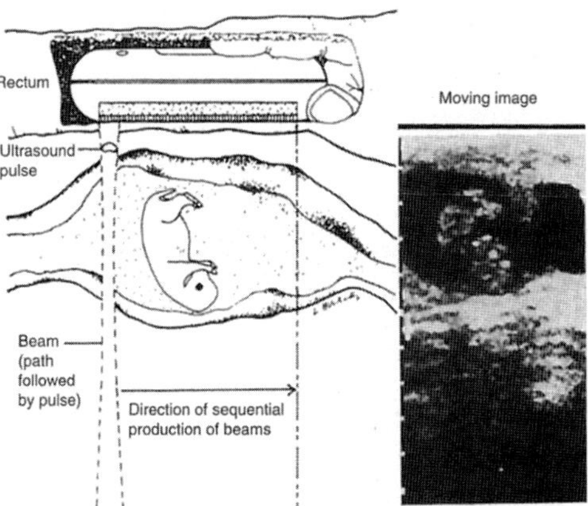


Figure 28-2. (**A**) Basic components of ultrasound scanner: a pulse generator, transducer, a scan converter, and a video display. (**B**) The development of a moving image of a 48-day bovine fetus by transrectal ultrasonography. (From Pierson RA, et al. Theriogenology 1988; 29:3–20.)

TABLE 28-2. *Ultrasound Techniques of Pregnancy Diagnosis in Farm Animals*

| Species | Technique | Placement of Transducer | Earliest Day After Mating | Diagnostic Criteria | Accuracy (%) |
|---|---|---|---|---|---|
| Horse | B-mode RT | Transrectal | 9 | Embryonic vesicle | 100 |
| Cattle | B-mode RT | Transrectal | 12 | Embryonic vesicle | 33 |
| | | | 20 | Embryo, heart beat | 100 |
| Buffalo | B-mode RT | Transrectal | 30 | Embryo, fetal fluids | ? |
| Sheep and goats | Doppler | Transabdominal | 60 | Fetal heart sounds | 90 |
| | A-mode | Transabdominal | | Fetal fluids | 70–90 |
| | B-mode RT | Transabdominal | 45–50 | Fetus(es), placentomes | 100 |
| | | Transrectal | 20–22 | Fetal fluids | <20 |
| Pig | Doppler | Transabdominal | 60 | Fetal heart sounds | 80 |
| | A-mode | Transabdominal | 60 | Fetal fluids | 70–90 |
| | B-mode RT | Transabdominal | 22 | Allantoic fluid | |

Adapted from literature cited in this chapter.
RT = real-time.
Transducer, 3.5 MHz (transabdominal); 5.0–7.5 MHz (transrectal).

waves (echoes) from tissue surfaces, on reaching the transducer, produces an electrical signal that is processed by a scan converter and displayed on a video monitor.

Depending on the display patterns they produce, transducers are of two types. A linear transducer produces a rectangular image, whereas the sector transducer produces a sector image similar to that of a "slice of a pie." The linear array type transducers are commonly used and have a frequency range of 3.5 to 7.5 MHz. Transducers with low frequencies (3.0 to 3.5 MHz) penetrate deeper and image deeper tissues than higher frequencies (5.0 to 7.5 MHz) that image closer to the surface. The images produced by low-frequency and high-frequency transducers are comparable to the view of a tissue as seen under a microscope at low and high magnifications, respectively.

For scanning the uterus, the transducer is placed on the ventrolateral abdominal wall (transabdominal) or in the rectum (transrectal) of the test animal. Contact between transducer and the skin or the rectal wall is made with coupling gel or vegetable oil.

The ultrasound techniques, placement of transducer and the earliest day after mating, the diagnostic criteria, and accuracy are summarized in Table 28-2. The 3.5 MHz transducer is used for the transabdominal approach (goat, sheep, pig) and the 5.0 to 7.5 MHz transducers for the transrectal route (horse, cattle, sheep). Images of tissues seen on the screen are either black (nonechogenic) or various shades of gray (echogenic). The urinary bladder, embryonic vesicle, and fetal fluids appear black; the fetal skeleton, white; and the fetal membranes and maternal tissues, various shades of grey. The ultrasonographs of pregnant uteri are shown in Figure 28-3. Some of the advantages of real-time ultrasonography in farm animals are listed in Table 28-3.

## IMMUNOLOGIC DIAGNOSIS

The immunologic techniques for diagnosis of pregnancy rely on detecting or measuring the level of substances originating in the conceptus, the uterus, or ovaries that enter the maternal blood, urine, or milk. Immunologic tests (Table 28-4) measure two types of substances.

1. Pregnancy specific, and appear in maternal blood (equine chorionic gonadotropin [eCG], early pregnancy factor [EPF]).
2. Pregnancy not specific, but their levels in maternal blood, urine, or milk change during pregnancy, e.g., progesterone, estrone sulphate.

### *Pregnancy-Associated Substances*

Several protein-like substances have been identified in maternal blood during pregnancy. Some of these substances are products originating in the conceptus, whereas others may be secreted at higher levels during gestation; thus, they can be used as indicators of pregnancy.

EARLY PREGNANCY FACTOR. An early pregnancy factor (EPF) was first reported in the circulation of pregnant

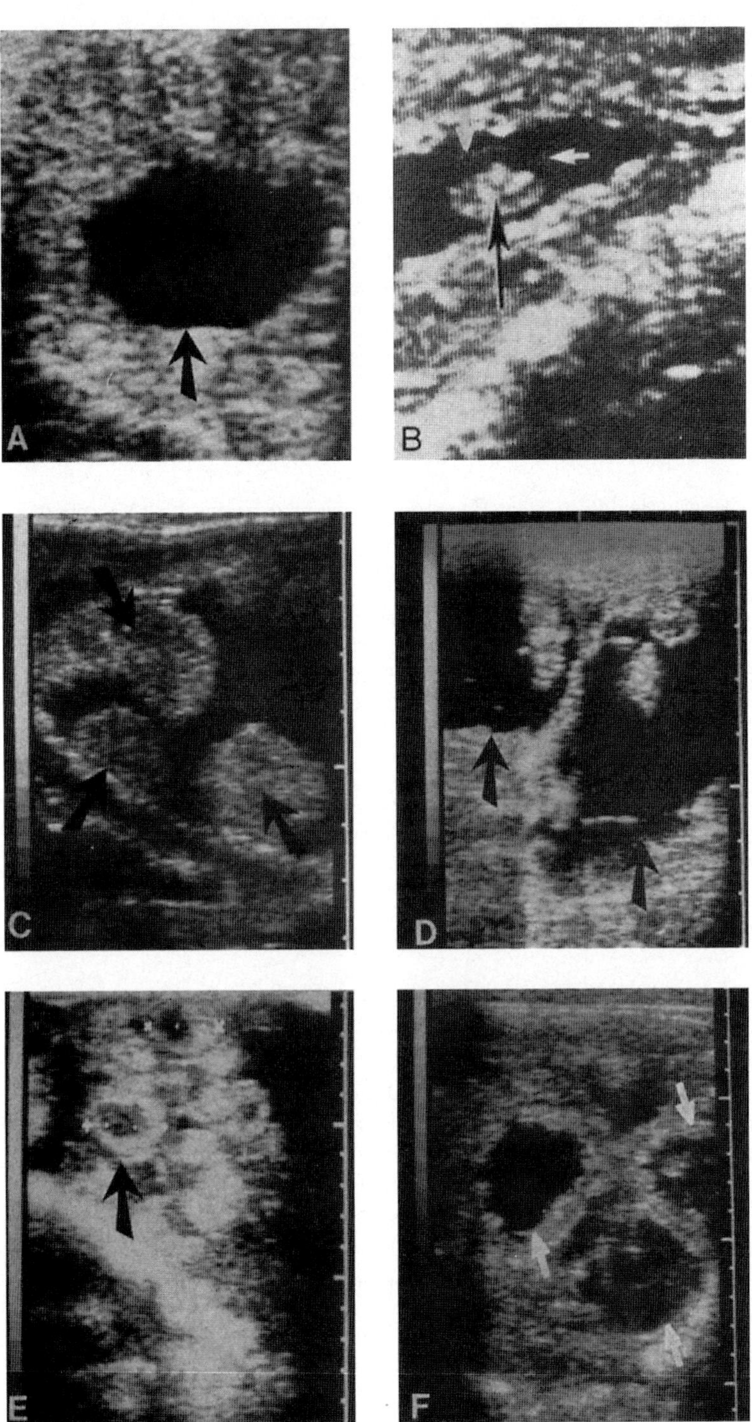


FIGURE 28-3. Ultrasonographs of pregnant uteri. (**A**) Mare day 17 conceptus (vesicle). (**B**) Cow, day 31, embryo (*black arrow*), amnion (*white arrow*) encircling the fetus. (**C**) Buffalo, day 50, placentomes. (**D**) Ewe day 37, twins (*arrows*). (**E**) Doe, day 45, uterus. (**A** from Squires et al. Theriogenology 1988;29:55–70; **B** from Kastellic et al. Theriogenology 1988;29:39–54.)

women (preimplantation stage) and subsequently in the sow, ewe, and cow. EPF, which has immunosuppressive properties, can be detected in serum within a few days after conception in pig, sheep, and cattle. It is a bioassay based on the inhibition of rosette formation. Because the rosette-inhibition test is time-consuming, it has limited use in routine pregnancy testing in farm animals. Besides diagnosing conception, a potential application for the EPF test could be for the early detection of fertilization failure or early embryonic mortality.

PREGNANCY-ASSOCIATED ANTIGENS. Antigens specific to pregnancy have been reported in maternal tissues of various species including that of sheep, cattle, and horses. Most of these antigens are detected in maternal blood during

TABLE 28-3. *Some Advantages of Real-Time Ultrasonography in Farm Animals*

| SPECIES | ADVANTAGES |
|---|---|
| Horse | Detection of twins by day 10–15 compared with rectal palpation (day 17–21) enables termination of pregnancy without loss in breeding time.[a] |
| Cattle | Assessment of viability of embryo heart beat (day 20–25) can be a tool in the study of embryonic mortality.[b] |
| | Detection of genital tubercle (day 55) and scrotal swelling and mammary teats (day 90) enables gender selection in valuable herds.[c,d] |
| Sheep | Determining fetal numbers after day 40 allows twin-bearing ewes to be fed energy supplements towards the later stages of pregnancy and prevent pregnancy toxemia.[e] |
| | The only method of differentiating hydrometra (a fluid-filled uterus) from pregnancy; progesterone concentration will remain elevated as in pregnancy.[f] |
| Goat | Determining fetal numbers after day 35.[g] |
| | The only method of differentiating hydrometra (a fluid-filled uterus) from pregnancy; progesterone concentration will remain elevated as in pregnancy.[h] |
| Pig | Can diagnose pregnancy earlier (day 28) than with A-mode ultrasonography (day 60).[h] |

[a]Bowman T. Ultrasonic diagnosis and management of early twins in the mare. Proc Amer Assoc Equine Practitioners 1986;32:35–43.
[b]Boyd JS, Omran SN, Ayliffe TR. Evaluation of real time B-mode ultrasound scanning for detecting early pregnancy in cows. Vet Rec 1990;127:35–52.
[c]Curran S, Pierson RA, Ginther OJ. Ultrasonographic appearance of the bovine conceptus from days 10 through 20. JVMA 1986;189:1289–1294.
[d]Muller E, Wittkowski G. Visualization of male and female characteristics of bovine fetuses by real-time ultrasonics. Theriogenology 1986;25:571–574.
[e]Gearhart MA, Wingfield WE, Knight AP, et al. Real-time ultrasonography for determining pregnancy status and viable fetal numbers in ewes. Theriogenology 1988;30:323–338.
[f]Bretzlaff KN. Development of hydrometra in a ewe flock after ultrasonography for determination of pregnancy. J Am Vet Med Assoc 1993;203:122–125.
[g]Buckrell BC, Bonnett BN, Johnson WH. The use of real-time ultrasound rectally for early pregnancy diagnosis in sheep. Theriogenology 1986;25:665–673.
[h]Taverne MAM, Willemse AA, eds. Diagnostic ultrasound and animal reproduction. London: Kluwer Academic Publishers, 1989.

the latter half of pregnancy and are of limited value in pregnancy tests.

The bovine conceptus produces numerous signals during early pregnancy. Currently only one protein from placental tissue has been partially purified—pregnancy-specific protein B (bPSPB). bPSPB can be detected by radioimmunoassay (RIA) in pregnant cow serum from day 24 of pregnancy until parturition (6). This RIA is more accurate than the progesterone RIA in detecting pregnant and nonpregnant dairy cows 30 days after AI because bPSPB is pregnancy specific, whereas the progesterone assay (see next section) is not. Unlike the progesterone assay, the timing of bPSPB test is independent of the breeding date. The disadvantages are that it is not detectable in cow's milk or urine and also persists in the blood for several months after parturition, which could interfere with early diagnosis of the subsequent pregnancy.

Besides bPSPB, another pregnancy specific protein is pregnancy serum protein (PSP60) which can be detected by RIA at day 28 of pregnancy in cattle (7). It has the same

TABLE 28-4. *Immunologic Methods of Pregnancy Diagnosis in Farm Animals*

| PREGNANCY TEST | PRINCIPLE | STAGE OF PREGNANCY | SPECIES |
|---|---|---|---|
| Early pregnancy factor | Detects immunosuppressive factor resulting in fertilization | Preimplantation | Cattle, sheep, and pigs |
| Progesterone | Predicts luteal activity | Implantation | All species |
| Estrone sulfate | Determines fetoplacental function | Postimplantation | All species |
| Equine chorionic gonadotropin | Determines fetoplacental function | Postimplantation | Horse |
| Pregnancy associated substances | Identifies antigens specific to pregnancy | Postimplantation | Cattle |

Low P4 - Not pregnant

Test

P4

Day bred

Next estrus

High P4 - pregnant

Test

P4

Day bred

Next estrus

Figure 28-4. Principles of the progesterone (P4) assay for pregnancy diagnosis in farm animals. The test is conducted either in milk or blood one estrous cycle length from mating or insemination.

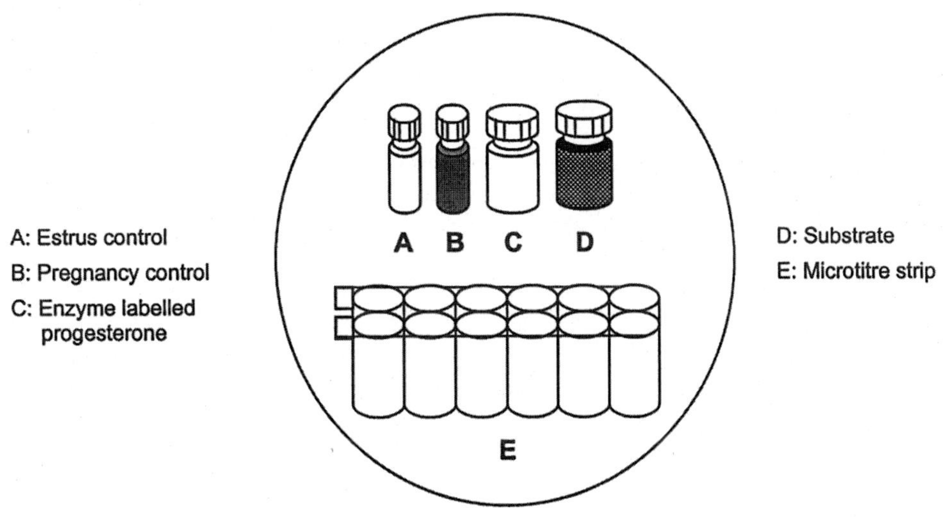


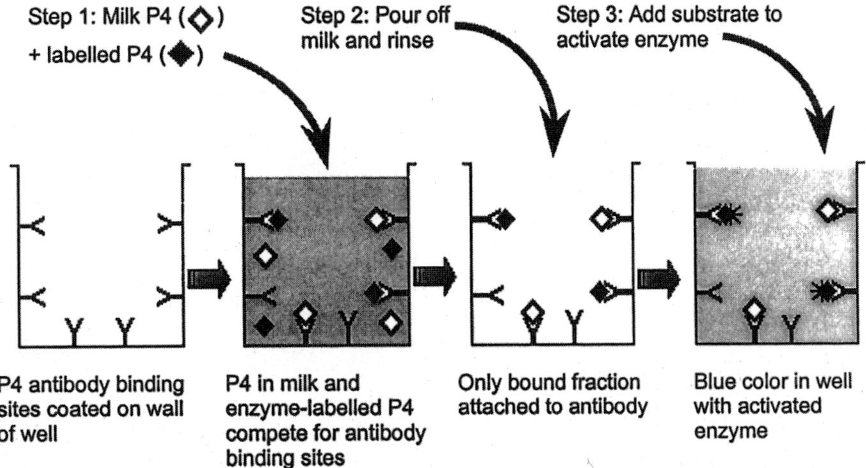


Figure 28-5. An ELISA Kit for "on farm" determination of milk progesterone in lactating dairy cows. The test relies on simple color changes and comparing with standards (Manufacturer Manuals).

accuracy as the P4 test, but more flexible and useful in naturally mated suckling herds where mating dates are not known.

### *Hormones*

Sensitive RIA and ELISA are available for the measurement of pregnancy-dependent hormones in body fluids. For example, pregnancy can be diagnosed in farm animals at a much earlier stage using the plasma or milk P4 than was possible using rectal palpation.

PROGESTERONE. The measurement of P4 has so far been the most widely used method of pregnancy detection in farm species. Although pregnancy nonspecific, progesterone can be used as a pregnancy test because the CL persists during early pregnancy in all farm animals. Progesterone levels are measured in biologic fluids such as blood and milk when progesterone is declining in nonpregnant animals. Normally, the sample is collected one estrous cycle length after an insemination or mating, e.g., 22 to 24 days in cattle and buffalo, 16 to 18 days in sheep, 18 to 21 days in goat, 16 to 22 days in horse, and 21 days in pigs. At this sampling time, the progesterone is low in a nonpregnant animal, whereas it is elevated in a pregnant animal (Fig. 28-4). However it is unreliable in the horse because prolonged diestrus (high P4) results in a false positive.

Milk is preferred to blood, particularly because of the higher progesterone levels in milk than in plasma. Also samples can be collected at milking time without inflicting much discomfort or pain on the animal.

Commercial pregnancy testing services based on milk progesterone are available for dairy herds in several countries. Milk samples are tested for progesterone using automated RIA. A sample of milk is collected between days 22 and 24 after insemination. The sampling technique will vary from one laboratory to another, but most prefer strippings from the afternoon milk. A preservative, e.g., potassium dichromate or mercuric chloride, is added to prevent spoilage of milk during transport to the laboratory. These methods are accurate but are relatively expensive, require laboratory facilities, and results are available only after several days.

A major disadvantage of the RIA is the rigid safety standards—safety of handlers, users, and disposal of radioactive material. Milk progesterone "kits" are commercially available for on-farm use and should overcome some of the problems inherent in RIA. The tests are either enzyme-linked immunosobant assay (ELISA) or latex agglutination assay. The steps in conducting the ELISA test are illustrated in Figure 28-5. On-farm tests are designed to determine the relative P4 concentration ("high" or "low") rather than obtaining a precise concentration. Evaluation of results is based on either a color or agglutination reaction with comparison to known standards. Correct interpretation of the test results depends upon accurate estrous detection and good recording.

A cow with high milk progesterone does not necessarily signify pregnancy, and a cow with low progesterone will not be pregnant. The accuracy of predicting pregnancy has ranged from 75 to 90%. On the contrary, the accuracy for nonpregnancy is 100%. The reasons for a cow to be incorrectly diagnosed as pregnant (false-positive) is listed in Table 28-5. Therefore, the milk progesterone test is more

TABLE 28-5. ***Interpretation of the "On-farm Milk Progesterone" Test for Pregnancy Diagnosis in Cattle***

| PROGESTERONE CONCENTRATION | INTERPRETATION | ACCURACY | ERRORS |
|---|---|---|---|
| High | Pregnant | 75% | 1. A cow incorrectly inseminated during the luteal phase (diestrus) will be in the luteal phase 3 weeks with elevated milk progesterone.<br>2. A cow with a longer than normal cycle length (e.g., 28 days).<br>3. A cow with a short interestrous interval (e.g., 17 days).<br>4. Embryonic mortality between sampling and confirmation of pregnancy by rectal palpation. |
| Low | Not pregnant | 100% | 1. Error in animal identification.<br>2. Human error in differentiating the color reaction in the ELISA test. |

reliable for diagnosing nonpregnancy than pregnancy and can identify nonpregnant animals at a much earlier time than is possible by rectal palpation.

The milk progesterone test has found limited application in other species. The ELISA assay for milk P4 on day 24 postinsemination was 100% accurate for nonpregnancy and 77% for pregnancy (8). Since sheep are not lactating at breeding time, the test has to be conducted on blood samples. In the goat, ELISA tests can be used for early diagnosis of pregnancy in milk samples collected 20 days after breeding (9), but it fails to differentiate pregnancy from hydrometra. In pig and horse, the accuracy of the test is low because of the persistence of CL (pseudopregnancy) in the nonpregnant animal.

**ESTRONE SULPHATE.** Estrone sulphate is the major estrogen produced by the conceptus and can be measured in maternal plasma, milk, or urine in all farm species. Estrone sulphate is detectable in the plasma earlier in the sow (day 20) and mare (day 40) than in the goat and sheep (day 40 to 50) or cow (day 72).

In the pig, estrone sulphate can be detected in maternal plasma as early as day 17 postmating, rising to a peak by day 26 to 29 and declining thereafter. It is more accurate earlier in gestation and is a better detector of nonpregnant sows than Doppler ultrasound. The main disadvantage of the procedure is the difficulty of collecting blood or urine, but this could be circumvented by measuring estrone sulphate in feces (10).

Both estrone sulphate and eCG levels (see the following section) may be used to diagnose pregnancy in the mare after day 40 of gestation. Because the developing fetus releases large quantities of estrone sulphate into the maternal circulation between days 75 to 100 of gestation, estrone sulphate has the advantage over eCG for determining the viability of the fetus.

**GONADOTROPIN.** Equine chorionic gonadotropin (eCG or PMSG) appears in the blood of mares as early as 40 days following conception, and its detection has been regarded as evidence of pregnancy. Immunologic diagnosis of pregnancy in mares is based on the principle that eCG, when present in the blood sample to be tested, prevents agglutination of sensitized sheep red cells by anti-eCG (hemagglutination-inhibition test, or HI). A kit containing all the reagents, containers, and pipettes needed is available that can be used on farms. Agglutination of red cells means a negative result (i.e., no pregnancy) and inhibition of agglutination, a positive result (Fig. 28-6). This test is most accurate between 50 and 100 days of gestation. If the fetus dies during this period, plasma eCG levels remain elevated. Therefore, if eCG is measured after fetal death, false-positive results will be obtained.

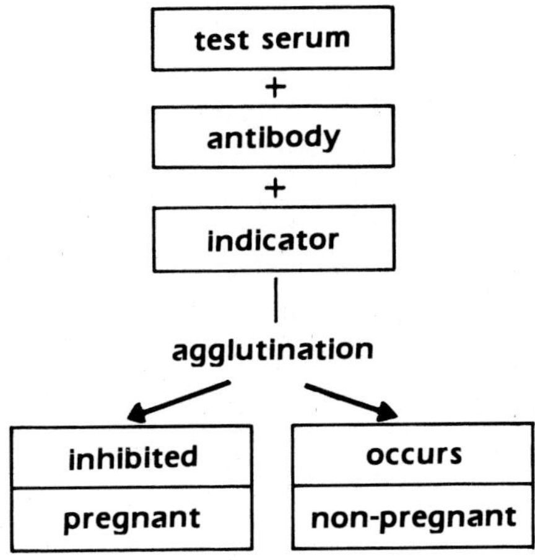


FIGURE 28-6. The principle of the hemagglutination test for the detection of equine chorionic gonadotropin (eCG, PMSG). The antibody is raised against eCG and the indicator system is sensitized sheep erythrocytes. Note the inhibition of hemagglutination is positive for pregnancy and occurrence of hemagglutination is negative for pregnancy.

**TABLE 28-6. *A Summary of the Techniques of Pregnancy Diagnosis in Farm Animals in Chronologic Order After Mating***

| SPECIES | DIAGNOSTIC TECHNIQUE | DAYS FROM MATING |
|---|---|---|
| Cattle and buffalo | EPF | First week |
| | Failure to return to estrus | 21–14 |
| | Progesterone | 22–24 |
| | Real-time ultrasonography | 24 |
| | bPSPB | 24–30 |
| | Rectal palpation | 35–40 |
| | Estrone sulfate | 72 |
| Sheep and goat | EPF (sheep) | Within 24 h |
| | Return to estrus | 16–21 |
| | Real-time ultrasonography | 35–40 |
| | P4 (goat) | 20 |
| | Estrone sulfate | 40–50 |
| Horse | Real-time ultrasonography | 9–16 |
| | Return to estrus | 16–21 |
| | P4 | 16–22 |
| | Rectal palpation | 17–25 |
| | eCG | 40–120 |
| | Estrone sulfate | 40–100 |
| Pig | Return to estrus | 18–25 |
| | P4 | 21 |
| | Real-time ultrasonography | 24 |
| | Estrone sulfate | 26 |
| | Fremitus in middle uterine artery | 28 |
| | A-mode ultrasonography | 30–90 |

Adapted from the literature cited in this chapter.

## CONCLUDING REMARKS

The various methods of diagnosing pregnancy in farm animals have been reviewed. Real-time ultrasonography is gaining popularity. It offers an array of information—pregnancy status, fetal numbers, and aging—but the ultrasound machines are expensive. Within each species, the methods that may be used are summarized in Table 28-6. Since all pregnancy tests early after insemination possess inherent errors, a follow-up examination might be indicated to confirm pregnancy in intensively managed herds or flocks with high prevalence of embryonic or fetal deaths.

## REFERENCES


1. Arthur GF, Noakes DE, Pierson H, Parkinson TM. Veterinary reproduction & obstetrics. London: WB Saunders, 1996.
2. Kahn W, Kenney R, Volkmann D. Veterinary Reproductive Ultrasonography. London: Mosby-Wolfe, 1994.
3. Pierson RA, Kastelic JP, Ginther OJ. Basic principles and techniques for transrectal ultrasonography in cattle and horses. Theriogenology 1988;29:3–20.
4. Powis RL. Ultrasound science for the veterinarian. Vet Clin North Am Equine Pract 1986;2:3–27.
5. Taverne MAM, Willemse AA, eds. Diagnostic ultrasound and animal reproduction. London: Kluwer Academic Publishers, 1989.
6. Sasser RG, Ruder CA, Ivani KA, Butler JE, Hamilton WC. Detection of pregnancy by radioimmunoassay of a novel pregnancy-specific protein in serum of cows and a profile of serum concentrations during gestation. Biol Reprod 1986;35:936–942.
7. Mialon MM, Renand G, Camous S, Martal J, Menissier F. Detection of pregnancy by radioimmunoassay of a pregnancy serum protein (PSP60) in cattle. Reprod Nutr Dev 1994;34:65–72.
8. Kaul V, Prakash BS. Accuracy of pregnancy/no pregnancy diagnosis in zebu and crossbred cattle and Murrah buffaloes by milk progesterone determination post insemination. Trop Anim Health Prod 1994;26:187–192.
9. Engeland IV, Ropstad E, Andresen O, Eik LO. Pregnancy diagnosis in dairy goats using progesterone assay. Anim Reprod Sci 1997;47:237–243.
10. Choi HS, Kiesenhofer E, Gantner H, Hois J, Bamberg E. Pregnancy diagnosis in sows by estimation of oestrogens in blood, urine or faeces. Anim Reprod Sci 1987;15:209–216.

# CHAPTER 29

# *Ovulation Induction, Embryo Production and Transfer*

M.R. JAINUDEEN, H. WAHID, AND E.S.E. HAFEZ

The expanding field of Embryo Transfer (ET) can be viewed as the female counterpart of artificial insemination. Females of superior genetic merit are superovulated with gonadotropic hormones, their eggs fertilized *in vivo* or oocytes fertilized *in vitro*, then the resultant embryos are transferred to recipients, genetically less distinguished surrogate mothers.

Synchronization of the estrous cycle is the first step in ET. It has progressed from prolonging or reducing the luteal phase, to modifying ovarian follicular waves with GnRH. A novel approach uses the protocol of GnRH-$PGF_{2\alpha}$-GnRH to improve synchrony of ovulation and timed insemination without the detection of estrus—the "dream" of the dairy farmer.

Techniques of collecting oocytes and embryos at slaughter or surgery of the donor have been superceded by the noninvasive techniques of ultrasonography, laparoscopy, and the transcervical approach.

Alternative approaches are available to overcome the problems associated with the induction of superovulation. Transvaginal ultrasound-guided oocyte aspiration has enabled the repeated collection of oocytes from adults whereas laparoscopy has significantly contributed to harvesting oocytes from juvenile donors, which can be fertilized *in vitro*. These advances have significantly contributed to the *in vitro* production of embryos in all farm animals, which hitherto depended upon the use of slaughterhouse ovaries of unknown genetic merit.

Cryopreservation technology is gradually replacing the age-old method of slow cooling and freezing of embryos in expensive freezers, to the simple method of vitrification. The ability to freeze and thaw embryos with very little detrimental effect on their survival facilitates not only routine ET but also has led to an international trade in frozen embryos of cattle, sheep and goat. Besides, the zona pellucida's ability to prevent the entry of viruses into the embryo makes the export of embryos considerably safer and cheaper than exporting live animals or semen. However, strict quarantine measures must be adopted to prevent contamination of embryos and reduce the risk of disease transmission.

Remarkable progress has been made during the past decade in the refinement of procedures for induction of ovulation, synchronization of estrus, *in vivo* and *in vitro* production and cryopreservation of embryos. The noninvasive techniques of ultrasonography for oocyte aspiration from adult and prepuberal animals, and the nonsurgical techniques and laparoscopy for routine embryo transfer (ET) have accelerated the growth of embryo transfer technology in farm animals.

This chapter will deal with the induction of ovulation, synchronization of the estrous cycle, and embryo transfer in farm animals.

## INDUCTION OF OVULATION

Methods of inducing ovulation are needed for treatment of anestrus and synchronization of the estrous cycle for timed artificial insemination (TAI). All farm species ovulate spontaneously during estrus. However, lactational anestrus in all species particularly during periods of undernutrition, postpubertal animals, and sheep and goats early in the breeding season may require hormonal therapy.

Hormonal preparations and methods of hormonal induction of ovulation in the different farm animals are summarized in Table 29-1. Mention has already been made to hormones directly related to reproduction (Chapter 3), their uses in different species (Chapters 10 through 16) and in reproductive failure (Chapters 17 and 18).

TABLE 29-1. ***Hormones Used for Induction of Estrus and Ovulation***

| TYPE OF HORMONE | METHOD OF ADMINISTRATION | BIOLOGIC ACTIVITY |
|---|---|---|
| GONADOTROPINS | | |
| eCG or PMSG | Single injection | Mimics FSH and stimulates follicular growth; long half-life |
| FSH | Single/multiple injections | Stimulates follicular growth; short half-life |
| hCG | Single injection | Mimics LH and induces ovulation |
| GONADOTROPIN RELEASING HORMONE AGONIST | | |
| aGnRH-buselerin | Single injection | Induces release of LH and FSH from the anterior pituitary; recruitment and selection of new dominant follicle |
| PROGESTOGENS | | |
| Progesterone | Multiple injections | Inhibits ovulation by suppressing LH secretion; mimics action of CL |
| Synthetic progestogens[a] | Oral, subcutaneous implant, intravaginal pessary/device | Inhibits ovulation by suppressing LH secretion; mimics action of CL |
| ESTROGENS | | |
| Estradiol conjugates[b] | Injection, implant | Induces premature regression of CL and enhances response to progestogens |
| Prostaglandins | | |
| $PGF_{2\alpha}$ or synthetic analogs | Single intramuscular injection | Induces regression of CL during responsive phases |

[a]Examples: oral preparations include Norgestomet, medroxyacetate progesterone (MAP), melengestrol acetate (MGA), fluorogestone acetate (FGA, Cronolone), and Altrenogest; intravaginal devices include Progesterone Releasing Intravaginal Device (PRID), Controlled Internal Drug Releasing Device (CIDR); intravaginal sponges include MAP and FGA

[b]Examples include estradiol valerate, estradiol benzoate, estradiol cypionate

A natural luteinizing hormone (LH) surge occurs as a result of a positive feedback of estrogen secretion by the developing follicle. Therefore, it may be appropriate to stimulate a surge of LH by the administration of gonadotropin-releasing hormone (GnRH), or induce an artificial LH-like surge by administration of human chorionic gonadotropin (hCG).

The growth of ovarian follicles in anestrous (acyclic) females can be stimulated with follicle stimulating hormone (FSH) of pituitary origin or equine chorionic gonadotropin (eCG) previously known as pregnant mare serum gonadotropin (PMSG) (Table 29-2).

FSH and LH have shorter biologic half-lives than the placental gonadotropins (eCG and hCG). Thus, multiple injections of FSH and LH are necessary to stimulate the same amount of follicular growth and ovulation that would result from a single injection of eCG. A single subcutaneous injection of porcine FSH (pFSH) dissolved in polyvinylpyrrolidine (PVP), a macromolecule, is as effective as multiple injections of pFSH for superovulating cattle (1).

Besides FSH, one large dose of GnRH causes a mature follicle to ovulate through release of endogenous LH and FSH. It should also be noted that cattle and sheep exhibit estrus in response to gonadotropin injection only after previous exposure to elevated progesterone or synthetic progestogen.

## SYNCHRONIZATION OF ESTROUS CYCLES

In a group of randomly cycling females, the time of estrus cannot be predicted with certainty for an individual animal. Detection of estrus is time consuming, laborious, and subject to human error.

Synchronization of estrus and ovulation in a group of females allows one to predict the time of estrus with reasonable accuracy. This reduces the time required for detection of estrus, or in some cases makes it possible for timed AI (TAI) without detection of estrus. TAI is considered effective when females are synchronized within a period of about 24 h, but this is seldom achieved.

### *Methods of Synchronization*

There are two basic methods of synchronization of the estrous cycles in farm species. These methods depend on either

TABLE 29-2. ***Protocols for Inducing Estrus and Ovulation in Acyclic Farm Animals***

| SPECIES | TREATMENT | END OF TREATMENT TO ESTRUS |
|---|---|---|
| CATTLE AND BUFFALO | | |
| Prepubertal or postpartum suckled cows | Estrogen on day 1 followed by 7–12 days of progestogen, eCG given on last day (optional) | Within 5 days |
| Postpartum milked cows | aGnRH on day 14 postpartum | 1 day |
| | aGnRH (day 0) and PGF (day 6)[a] | 2–4 days |
| SHEEP AND GOATS | | |
| Prepubertal or seasonal anestrus | Progestogen for 12–21 days with eCG given near the end of progestogen treatment | 2–4 days; eCG required for good response |
| SWINE | | |
| Prepubertal or postpartum anestrus | eCG alone | 3–5 days |
| | eCG on day 1 with hCG given 48–96 h later | 3–5 days |
| | eCG + hCG given on day 1 | 3–5 days |
| HORSES | | |
| Seasonal anestrus | Lengthen photoperiod by 4 h per day | 4–6 weeks earlier than normal |
| Late anestrus | Progestogen for 15 days | Within 1 week |

[a]Twagiramungu H, Guilbault LA, Dufour JJ. Synchronization of ovarian follicular waves with a gonadotropin-releasing hormone agonist to increase the precision of estrus in cattle: a review. J Anim Sci 1995;73:3143.

inhibiting LH secretion, or shortening the life span of the corpus luteum (CL) and the subsequent onset of estrus and ovulation.

EXTENDING THE LUTEAL PHASE. The first method involves long-term administration of a progestogen so that the CL regresses naturally during the period when progestogen is being administered (Table 29-1). With this approach, the exogenous progestogen continues to exert a negative feedback on LH secretion after regression of the CL. On progestogen withdrawal, follicular growth, estrus, and ovulation occur within 2 to 8 days. The interval from withdrawal of progestogen to the onset of estrus varies among species and among methods of progestogen treatment within species. Generally, long-term progestogen treatment lasts for 14 to 21 days depending on the species.

Several methods of administering progestogens are commercially available (Fig. 29-1). These include orally active progestogens, pessaries, ear implants, and intravaginal devices.

SHORTENING THE LUTEAL PHASE. The second method induces the premature regression of a cyclic CL (luteolysis) (Table 29-1). The two primary luteolytic agents are estrogen and prostaglandin $F_{2\alpha}$ ($PGF_{2\alpha}$), or its analogue (Cloprostenol). Estrogen is luteolytic in ruminants but not in horse or pig whereas $PGF_{2\alpha}$ is luteolytic in all species, at least during certain phases of CL development.

A single injection of $PGF_{2\alpha}$ will regress the CL usually within 24 to 72 h, and estrus and ovulation occur within 2 to 3 days. In all species, the CL is responsive to luteolytic agents only during certain stages of its development. Luteolytic agents will not cause regression of the CL during the first 4 to 6 days of the cycle in ruminants and horses, and during the first 12 or 13 days of the cycle in the pig.

Estrus and ovulation can also be synchronized in cyclic animals through a combination of progestogen and a luteolytic agent. This approach uses a luteolytic agent to regress the CL and the progestogen to mimic the action of progesterone and prevent estrus until its withdrawal.

### *Synchronization Protocols*

Methods for synchronizing estrus in farm animals are summarized in Table 29-3.

CATTLE. $PGF_{2\alpha}$ and its analogs are the most effective method for estrous cycle control in dairy cattle. Long-term progestogen treatment of cattle is unsatisfactory because of reduced fertility, even though estrus is well-synchronized. The following treatment protocols are available for cycling cattle and buffalo.

1. *Two $PGF_{2\alpha}$ injections 11 or 12 days apart.* After the second injection, animals may be bred/AI at detected

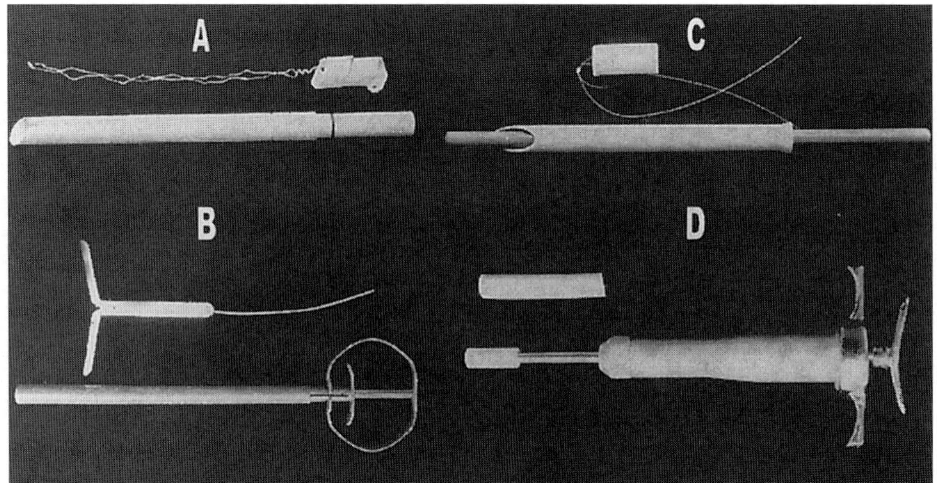


FIGURE 29-1. Methods of progesterone administration in cattle, buffalo, sheep, and goat. (**A**) Progesterone Intravaginal Device (PRID), a stainless spiral coil covered with an inert silicone rubber matrix, coated with progesterone, and an applicator for insertion into the vagina of a cow or buffalo; (**B**) Controlled Internal Drug Release (CIDR), a T-shaped silicon elastomer device containing progesterone, and applicator for insertion into the vagina of a cow or buffalo; (**C**) Progestogen-impregnated intravaginal sponge with speculum and introducer; (**D**) Progestogen-ear implant and an implanting device. (Adapted from the literature; catalogue of various IUD manufacturers.)

estrus or inseminated at 72 and 96 h without reference to estrus.

2. *Progestogen and* $PGF_{2\alpha}$. A progestogen (CIDR, PRID) is administered as a vaginal pessary for 7 days with $PGF_{2\alpha}$ injected on the sixth day (Table 29-3). Cows are inseminated based estrus or at about 84 h after $PGF_{2\alpha}$.
3. *Progestogen and Estrogen.* An estrogen (5-mg estradiol valerate) and progestogen (3 mg Norgestomet) are injected on the first day of treatment. Then a progestogen

TABLE 29-3. ***Techniques for Synchronizing Estrus in Cyclic Farm Animals***

| SPECIES | METHOD | TREATMENT REGIMEN | END OF TREATMENT TO ESTRUS |
|---|---|---|---|
| Cattle and buffalo | PGF | Two injections (11–12 days apart) | 3–5 days: AIDE/TAI |
| Cattle | aGnRH + PGF | Inject aGnRH (day 0), PGF (day 6) | 2–4 days: TAI |
| | aGnRH + PGF + aGnRH | Inject aGnRH (day 0), PGF (day 7), aGnRH (day 8 or 9) | 2–4 days: TAI |
| | Progestogen + estrogen | Estrogen injection (day 1), CIDR (days 1–9) | 3–5 days: AIDE/TAI |
| | Progestogen + PGF | Progestogen (days 1–7), PGF (day 6) | 2–3 days: AIDE/TAI |
| Sheep | Progestogen (pessary) + eCG | Progestogen (12–14 days), eCG (day of pessary removal) | 2 days; AIDE or double AI |
| | PGF | Two injections (9 days apart) | 2–3 days; breed or AIDE |
| Goat | Progestogen (pessary) + eCG | Progestogen (18–21 days), eCG (day of pessary removal) | 2–3 days; breed or AIDE |
| | PGF | Two injections (11–12 days apart) | 2–3 days; breed at estrus or double AI |
| Swine | Progestogen in feed | Altrenogest (14–18 days) | 4–7 days; breed at estrus |
| Horse | Progestogen in feed | Altrenogest (15 days) | 4–7 days; breed at estrus |
| | PGF | One dose to mares in diestrus | 3–5 days; breed at estrus |
| | PGF + hCG | PGF (day 1), hCG (day 7–8), PGF (day 15), hCG (day 21–22) | 2–4 days |

(Norgestomet) is implanted for 9 days beginning on Day 1 (Table 29-3). Cows are inseminated based on estrus (AIDE) or at a fixed time (TAI) (54 hours) after implant removal.

4. *GnRH agonist.* This novel protocol controls follicular development and the life span of the CL. On Day 0 (Fig. 29-2), a GnRH agonist (aGnRH) is injected and on Day 6, $PGF_{2\alpha}$ is injected (2). This regimen synchronizes the estrous cycles of 70 to 80% of cyclic cows to within a 4-day interval without affecting the fertility rate (65 to 85%). The precision of estrus and high fertility rates are due to the aGnRH luteinizing or ovulating the mature follicle, and initiating recruitment and selection of a new dominant follicle. The injection of $PGF_{2\alpha}$ causes regression of the spontaneous CL or a potential CL induced by GnRH, or both. An advantage of this regimen is that it can be used at any stage of the cycle and eliminates the use of progestogen. Besides, it promotes the resumption of ovarian activity in acyclic postpartum cows and heifers. For TAI without the need for estrus detection, a protocol of aGnRH (Day 0)-$PGF_{2\alpha}$ (Day 7)-GnRH (Day 8) and AI at predetermined time may be used (3).

**SHEEP AND GOATS.** Progestogen and $PGF_{2\alpha}$ are effective for synchronizing estrus in both species, but duration of progestogen treatment varies because of differences in the length of the normal estrous cycle between ewes (16 days) and does (21 days)

1. *Progestogen pessary.* A progestogen pessary or implant is given for 12 to 14 days in sheep, or for 18 to 21 days in goats (Table 29-3). In both species, eCG (400 to 800 IU) is given at the time of progestogen withdrawal. For TAI, ewes should be inseminated at 48 and 60 h after progestogen withdrawal, and does at about 30 and 48 h.
2. *$PGF_{2\alpha}$.* $PGF_{2\alpha}$ can be used to synchronize ewes or does, but $PGF_{2\alpha}$ offers no real advantage over the combination of progestogen and eCG; the latter will work effectively in both anestrous and cyclic females. In ewes, 2 injections of prostaglandin are given 9 days apart, and the ewes bred at estrus or given a double AI (Table 29-3). In does, the 2 doses of prostaglandin are injected 11 to 12 days apart. Natural mating or double AI can be used at the synchronized estrus. Since $PGF_{2\alpha}$ will cause abortion, pregnancy should be eliminated before the $PGF_{2\alpha}$ injection.

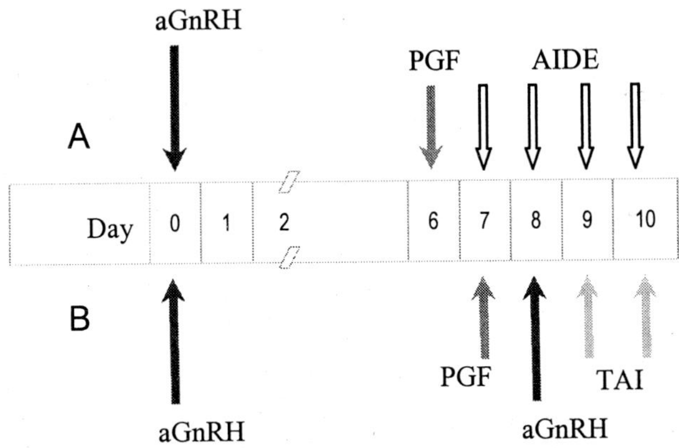


FIGURE 29-2. Protocols for synchronization of estrus. (**A**) Using a GnRH agonist (Twagiramungu H, Guilbault LA, Dufour JJ. Synchronization of ovarian follicular waves with a gonadotropin-releasing hormone agonist to increase the precision of estrus in cattle: a review. J Anim Sci 1995;73:3143); (**B**) using ovulation (Britt JS, Gaska J. Comparison of two estrus synchronization programs in a large, confinement-housed dairy herd. J Am Vet Med Assoc 1998;212:210). *AIDE* = artificial insemination at detected estrus; *TAI* = timed artificial insemination; *aGnRH* = GnRH agonist-buserilin.

**SWINE.** Progestogen (Altrenogest) fed for 14 to 18 days is effective in synchronizing estrus in cyclic gilts and sows (Table 29-3). Normally estrus begins on the fourth or fifth day after progestogen withdrawal, and most animals are in estrus during a 2 to 4 day period. In individually fed animals, fertility is acceptable from two fixed-time inseminations given on Days 6 and 7 after progestogen withdrawal.

$PGF_{2\alpha}$ is not useful for synchronizing estrus in cyclic swine because the CL do not respond to $PGF_{2\alpha}$ during the first 12 or 13 days of the estrous cycle. Estrogen or hCG on day 12 of an estrous cycle prolongs the life span of CL in pigs. Thus, one potential way of synchronizing estrus in swine is to inject 500 to 1000 IU of hCG to each female on day 12 of an estrous cycle, then inject $PGF_{2\alpha}$ about 3 weeks later. At that time all females in a group would have prolonged CL maintenance.

**HORSES.** Mares can be synchronized with either progestogen (Altrenogest) or $PGF_{2\alpha}$.

1. *Altrenogest.* Feeding mares Altrenogest for 15 days induces estrus about 3 days after progestogen withdrawal. Fertility in synchronized mares is similar to that for controls, and satisfactory fertility can be obtained by mating on alternate days during estrus.
2. *Prostaglandin.* Diestrous mares will respond to a single injection of prostaglandin by exhibiting estrus within 3 to 5 days. If a group of mares are in diestrus at the same time, their cycles can be synchronized and fertility is normal. In a group of randomly cycling mares, estrus can be synchronized by a regime that involves two doses of $PGF_{2\alpha}$ and two doses of hCG. The treatment protocol is as follows: Inject $PGF_{2\alpha}$ (Day 1), hCG (Day 7 or 8), $PGF_{2\alpha}$ (Day 15), and hCG (Day 21 or 22). Estrus is synchronized within a 2 to 4 day period and fertility is normal.

## EMBRYO TRANSFER

The history of embryo transfer dates back to 1891 when Heape performed the first successful embryo transfer in rabbits. Since then successful embryo transfers have been reported in all farm animals (Table 29-4). Commercialization of the embryo transfer technology began in North America in the 1970s.

A female farm animal (donor) can increase the number of offspring produced in her lifetime by repeatedly conceiving, recovering embryos in early pregnancy, and transferring them to the reproductive tracts of other females (recipients) to complete gestation (Fig. 29-3). This procedure will depend entirely upon the availability of a source of good quality embryos and the proper uterine environment in the recipient at the time of transfer (synchrony).

During the past decade, ET has continued to make major strides, particularly *in vitro* production of embryos and embryo manipulation techniques. However, progress in developing embryo transfer techniques to a practical scale comparable to artificial insemination has been rather slow.

There were several limitations in the induction of superovulation for the production of embryos on a large scale, and a simple nonsurgical technique for collecting and transferring embryos. Some of these problems have been resolved, and embryo transfer, just as artificial insemination, could play a significant role in animal reproduction.

Cryopreservation of embryos has enabled an international trade in cattle embryos. Commercial companies for embryo transfer in farm animals have been established in Australia, Argentina, Canada, New Zealand, the United States, and several countries in Europe.

The history of ET in farm animals has been reviewed elsewhere (4–6) and summarized (Table 29-4). A training manual for embryo transfer in cattle is also available (7). This section describes the basic concepts of producing embryos by both superovulation and *in vitro* fertilization (IVF) and the cryopreservation of embryos and embryo transfer in farm animals. Manipulation of embryos is discussed in Chapter 31.

The basic requirements for an ET program are:

1. a source of embryos,
2. a reliable method of transferring the embryos, and
3. suitably synchronized recipients.

Embryos may be harvested from a donor treated with a dose of FSH or by *in vitro* maturation (IVM)/*in vitro* fertilization (IVF) and *in vitro* culture (IVC).

### *In Vivo Production of Embryos*

The mammalian ovary contains thousands of oocytes, but domestic ruminants shed only one or two eggs per estrous cycle.

TABLE 29-4. ***Milestones in Mammalian Embryo Transfer and Related Techniques***

| YEAR | SPECIES | EVENT | RESEARCHER(S) |
|---|---|---|---|
| 1890 | Rabbit | Birth of an offspring born from embryo transfer | Heape |
| 1933 | Rat | Birth of an offspring born from embryo transfer | Nicholas |
| 1949 | Sheep and goat | Birth of a lamb and kid from embryo transfer | Warwick and Berry |
| 1951 | Pig | Birth of piglets from embryo transfer | Kvansnickii |
| 1951 | Cattle | Birth of calf from embryo transfer | Willett et al. |
| 1952 | Rabbit | First intercontinental shipment of embryos stored at 10°C | Marden and Chang |
| 1971 | Cattle | First commercial embryo transfer company formed for farm animals | Alberta Livestock Transplants Ltd. |
| 1972 | Mouse | Birth of an offspring from long-term frozen embryos | Whittingham et al. |
| 1973 | Cattle | Birth of a calf produced from frozen embryos | Wilmut and Rowson |
| 1974 | Horse | Birth of a pony after egg transfer | Oguri and Tsutsumi |
| 1978 | Human | Birth of a girl after IVF | Steptoe and Edwards |
| 1982 | Cattle | Birth of calf after IVF | Brackett et al. |
| 1983 | Asian buffalo | Birth of buffalo calf from embryo transfer | Drost et al. |
| 1986 | Sheep | Birth of cloned lamb derived from 8-cell to 16-cell sheep embryo | Willadsen |
| 1987 | Cattle | Birth of cloned calf derived from 9-cell to 15-cell morulae | Prather et al. |
| 1996 | Sheep | Birth of lamb cloned from adult somatic cells | Wilmut et al. |

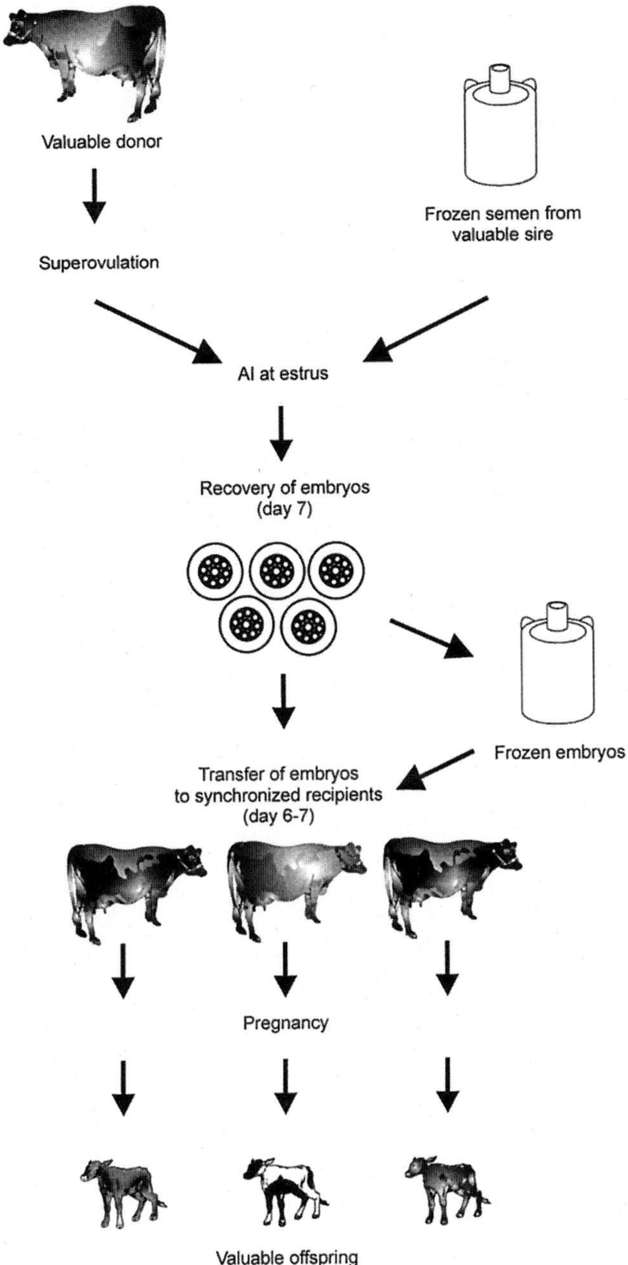


FIGURE 29-3. Diagrammatic representation of the steps associated with embryo production *in vivo* and subsequent transfer to synchronized recipients in cattle. (From the literature.)

Since FSH has a shorter biologic half-life than eCG, it is usually necessary to divide the total dose and inject at 12 hour intervals over 3 to 4 days to stimulate the same amount of follicular growth that would result from a single injection of eCG. Despite the superiority of FSH, eCG continues to be used alone or in combination with antisera, which was believed to bind any excess eCG in the circulation after the onset of estrus. However, anti-eCG serum had no significant effect on the numbers of corpora lutea or the numbers of embryos (8).

During the past decade Prostaglandin $F_{2\alpha}$ and its analogue cloprostenol have made a major contribution to superovulation in cattle. Not only does $PGF_{2\alpha}$ increase the flexibility of timing superovulation, but it is also an excellent treatment for producing large numbers of normal embryos. The superovulatory treatment can be initiated anytime between day 6 of the estrous cycle and natural CL regression. The optimal time for treatment, however, is between days 8 and 12 of the cycle in cattle. Most donors are in estrus 2 to 3 days after prostaglandin injection. Methods of superovulation are summarized in Table 29-5.

A novel protocol for superovulating cattle has been reported (9). The GnRH agonist (desloren)-LH protocol controls the timing of ovulation after hyperstimulation with FSH. The GnRH agonist (desloren implant) blocks the preovulatory LH surge, then injecting exogenous LH induces ovulation. In this protocol, the donor is inseminated concurrently with the LH injection and does not require detection of estrus (Fig. 29-6). Besides cattle, sheep can also be superovulated by chronic treatment with a GnRH agonist (buserilin) and pFSH for the production of viable embryos (10).

Both intrinsic and extrinsic factors influence the variability in the superovulatory response in cattle (11). Among the physiologic factors, the dominant functional follicle may exert a deleterious effect on the superovulatory response and decrease the number of embryos recovered. Of the extrinsic factors, undernutrition and lactation can exert a harmful effect on pulsatile LH secretion and follicular development.

With current collection procedures, superovulation increases the yield of normal embryos about five-fold in the cow, buffalo, goat, and sheep, but only slightly in pigs and horses.

**METHODS OF SUPEROVULATION.** As previously mentioned, exogenous FSH (eCG or FSH) injections are widely used in multiple ovulation/embryo transfer (MOET) programs to increase the supply of embryos from animals of superior genetic merit. Usually, subcutaneous or intramuscular injections of eCG or FSH will stimulate additional growth of the follicles, which will ovulate spontaneously without the need for exogenous LH or hCG in adult cattle, buffalo (Fig. 29-4), sheep, and goats (Fig. 29-5).

**REPEATED SUPEROVULATION.** Generally, donors respond similarly to first, second, and third superovulatory treatments. The response to subsequent treatments, however, is less in some individuals, probably due to the production of antibodies against gonadotropins, which are protein hormones. This may be avoided to some extent by increasing the interval between hormone treatments and using gonadotropins derived from the same species as the one being treated.

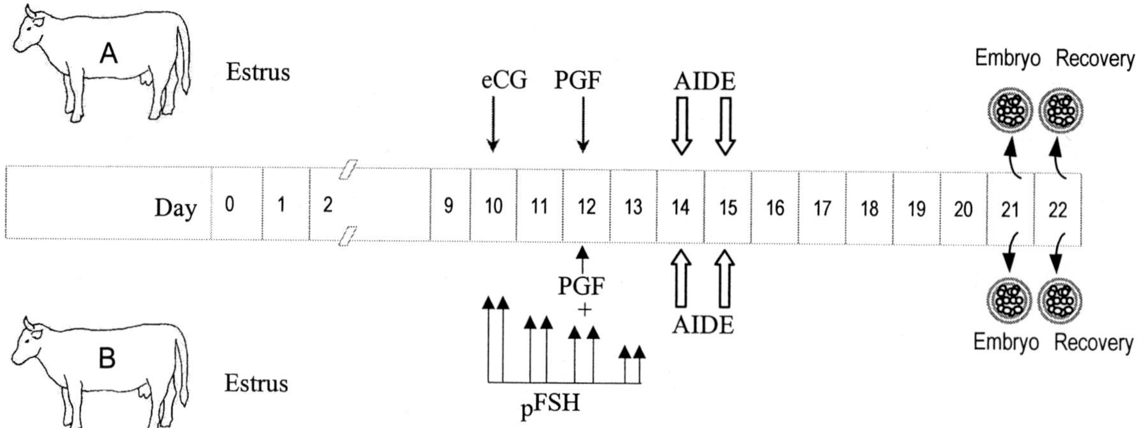


FIGURE 29-4. Protocols for superovulation for cattle and buffalo based on a gonadotropins. (A) eCG + $PGF_{2\alpha}$; (B) pFSH + $PGF_{2\alpha}$. eCG = equine chorionic gonadotropin; *pFSH* = porcine Follicle Stimulating Hormone; *PGF* = prostaglandin $F_{2\alpha}$; *AIDE* = artificial insemination at detected estrus.

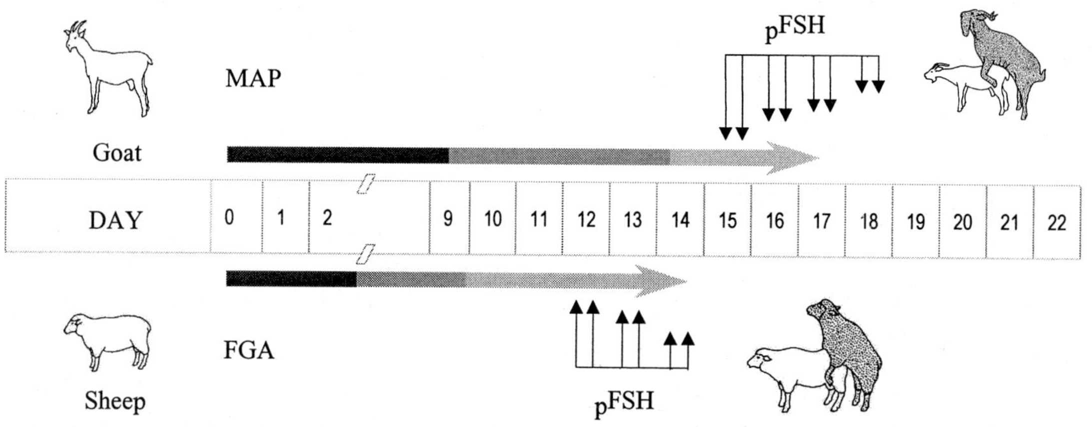


FIGURE 29-5. Protocols for superovulation of sheep and goat based on a progestogen pessary (MAP/FGA) and multiple injections of porcine FSH.

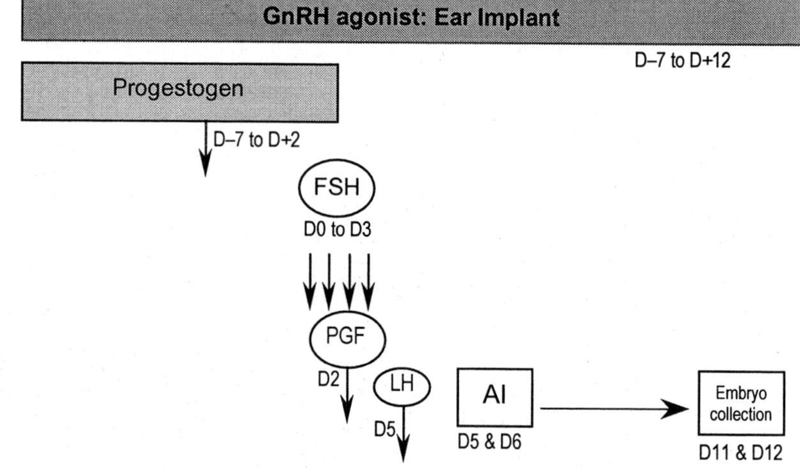


FIGURE 29-6. A novel protocol for superovulation in cattle using GnRH agonist + FSH + $PGF_{2\alpha}$ + LH (adapted from D'Occio MJ, Sudha G, Jillella D, et al. Use of a GnRH agonist to prevent endogenous LH surge and injection of exogenous LH to induce ovulation in heifers stimulated with FSH: A new model for superovulation. Theriogenology 1997; 47:601.). The GnRH agonist bioimplant, placed subcutaneously in the ear, releases about 20 $\mu$g deslorein/24 h. Day 0 = Day of first FSH. Treated cows are inseminated at time of the LH injection.

TABLE 29-5. ***Protocols for Superovulation in Farm Animals***

| SPECIES | PRETREATMENT | GONADOTROPIN[a] | PGF | LH |
|---|---|---|---|---|
| Goat | Fit a progestogen pessary for 17 days | Inject 20 mg pFSH one day before pessary removal | Inject 125–250 $\mu$g cloprostenol | None |
| Sheep | Fit a progestogen pessary for 12 days | Inject 20 mg pFSH one day before pessary removal | | None |
| Cattle and buffalo | Progestogen for 7–8 days | Inject 20–30 mg pFSH | Inject 1000 $\mu$g cloprostenol | |
| Cattle[b] | Day-7 progestogen + aGnRH implant[c] | Inject 80 mg FSH (day 0–4) | Inject 25 mg PGF (Lutelase) (day 2) | Inject (IM) 25 mg porcine LH (day 5) |
| Pig | Feed altrenogest for 15 days | Inject 1500 IU eCG one day before end of feeding period | None | None |

[a]The FSH total dose is divided into four decreasing twice daily doses.
[b]Cattle data from D'Occhio MJ, Sudha G, Jillella D, et al. Use of a GnRH agonist to prevent endogenous LH surge and injection of exogenous LH to induce ovulation in heifers stimulated with FSH: A new model for superovulation. Theriogenology 1997;47:601.
[c]Pessary: MAP or FGA; intravaginal device CIDR/PRID

TABLE 29-6. ***Current Methods of Collection and Transfer of Embryos in Farm Animals***

| SPECIES | COLLECTION TECHNIQUE | DAYS FROM ESTRUS | TRANSFER TECHNIQUE |
|---|---|---|---|
| Cattle | Transcervical using a 2-way or 3-way Foley catheter | 7 | Transcervical with Cassou AI gun and either 0.5 or 0.25 mL French straws |
| Buffalo | Transcervical using a 2-way or 3-way Foley catheter | 5–6 | Transcervical with Cassou AI gun and either 0.5 or 0.25 mL French straws |
| Horse | Transcervical using a 2-way or 3-way Foley catheter | 6–9 | Flank laparotomy/transcervical |
| Sheep | Midventral laparotomy | 3–6 | Midventral laparotomy uterine transfer |
| | Transcervical[a] | 5–6 | Transcervical |
| | Laparoscopy[b] | 5–6 | Laparoscopy, uterine transfer[b] |
| Goat | Laparotomy | 3–4 | Midventral laparotomy |
| | Transcervical[c] | | Transcervical |
| | Laparoscopy | | Laparoscopy |
| Pig | Midventral laparotomy, fluid flushed into the uterus from the fimbriated end of the oviduct | 4–6 | Midventral laparotomy, deposited into uterine horn or through the oviduct; about 14 embryos are transferred to each recipient |
| | Transcervical[d] | 4–6 | Transcervical[d] |
| | Laparoscopy[e] | 3 | Laparoscopy[e] |

[a]Data from Mylne MJA, McKelvey WAC, Fernie, K, Mathews K. Use of a transcervical technique for embryo recovery in sheep. Vet Rec 1992;130:450.
[b]Data from McKelvey WAC, Robinson JJ, Aitken RP, Robertson IS. Repeated recoveries of embryos from ewes by laparoscopy. Theriogenology 1986;25:855.
[c]Data from Pereira RJ, Sohnrey, B, Holtz W. Nonsurgical embryo collection in goats treated with prostaglandin F2$\alpha$ and oxytocin. J Anim Sci 1998;76:360.
[d]Data from Li J, Rieke A, Day BN, Prather RS. Technical Note: Porcine non-surgical embryo transfer. J Anim Sci 1996;74:2263.
[e]Data from Besenfelder U, Modl J, Muller M, Brem G. Endoscopic embryo collection and embryo transfer into the oviduct and the uterus of pigs. Theriogenology 1997;47:1051.

**Insemination.** Superovulated donors are usually inseminated more often and with more sperm per insemination. Yet, fertilization rates of eggs from superovulated donors are usually considerably below those from untreated donors. This may be due partly to suboptimum sperm transport, ovulation over a period of time, defective oocytes, or other causes.

**Collection of Embryos.** Historically, embryos were collected from the oviducts or uteri of donors after slaughter or at surgery. Since 1976, the transcervical recovery (nonsurgical) of embryos from the cow, buffalo, and mare is routinely practiced (Table 29-6). Similarly, embryos from sheep, goat, and pigs were routinely collected by laparotomy, but from the early 1990s, laparoscopic and transcervical techniques are increasingly being used.

*Surgical Methods.* The surgical method most often used in sheep, goats, and pigs consists of exposing the reproductive tract by a midventral incision under general anesthesia. Various methods and catheters are used to collect embryos (Fig. 29-7). Embryos may be recovered from the uterine horns after they have left the oviducts, usually 5 days after estrus or later. The basic component of the flushing medium is phosphate buffered saline (PBS). It is introduced into the base of the uterine horn and flushed toward the utero-tubal junction (UTJ), where the medium is collected through a blunt syringe needle or a small glass tube inserted into the uterine lumen. The procedure may also be carried out in the reverse direction. Fewer embryos are recovered with these procedures than by flushing the oviducts. A volume of 2 to 20 mL is used to flush the oviducts, whereas 10 mL is used to flush the uterus depending on its size.

*Nonsurgical Methods.* For many applications, nonsurgical techniques for collection of embryos are desirable because all surgical techniques invariably lead to the formation of adhesions, and there is less risk to the life and health of the donor with nonsurgical methods.

***The Transcervical Method.*** In this approach, a 3-way Foley catheter is used for collecting embryos in cattle, buffalo, and mare (Fig. 29-8). In cattle and buffalo, the Foley catheter with the stilette in place is guided through the cervix by rectal manipulation. The catheter can be positioned either in the uterine body or in one horn. Most prefer to flush each horn separately. After the catheter is positioned in one horn, the balloon is inflated. The uterine horn is filled with 30 to 60 mL of warm PBS medium, which is then allowed to flow into the collection vessel while the uterus is gently massaged through the rectum. This is repeated until 300 to 800 mL of medium have been used. The Foley catheter is then inserted into the other uterine horn and the process repeated. The same technique is used to recover embryos from mares, except that the balloon is inflated in the cervix and both horns are flushed simultaneously.

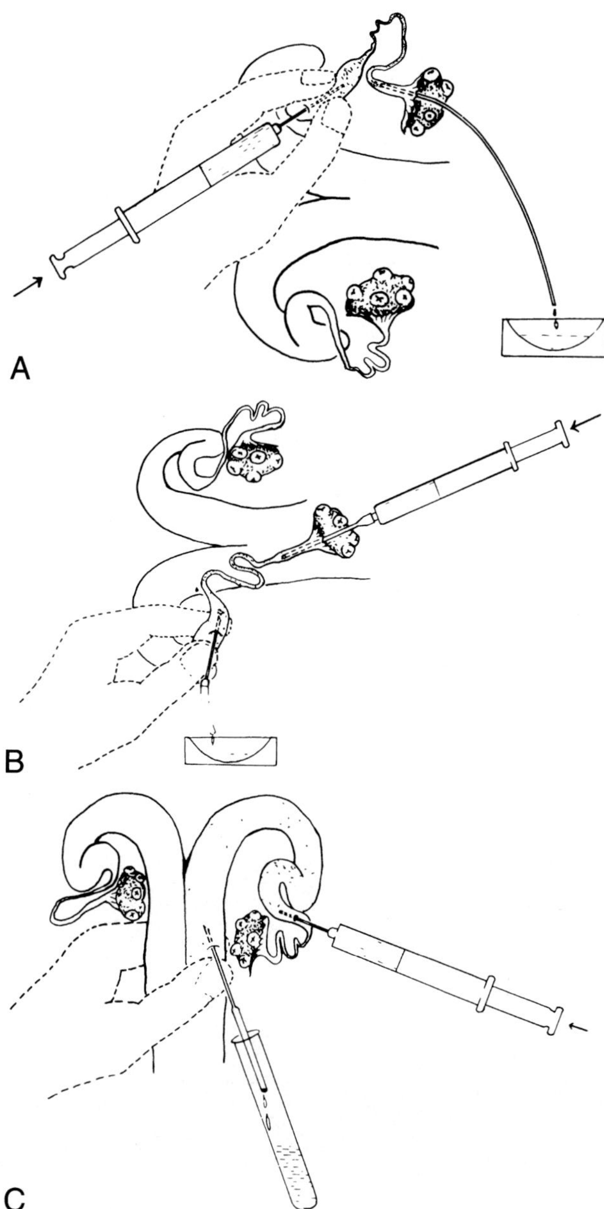


**Figure 29-7.** Surgical techniques of embryo recovery from superovulated sheep and goat. (**A**) Flushing oviduct toward fimbriae. (**B**) Flushing oviduct toward uterotubal junction. (**C**) Flushing uterus toward base of the uterine horn.

The transcervical route has been successful for embryo collection in sheep (12) and goat. Injections of $PGF_{2\alpha}$ and oxytocin facilitate the introduction of the catheter in the goat (13).

***Laparoscopy.*** McKelvey et al (14) first reported the use of laparoscopy under general anesthesia for collection of embryos from the uterus of sheep. Subsequently, this approach has been used in goat and pig (15). The basic difference between surgical technique and laparoscopy is that instruments for flushing are inserted through stab wounds rather than by a midventral incision.

A laparoscope is inserted through one stab wound in

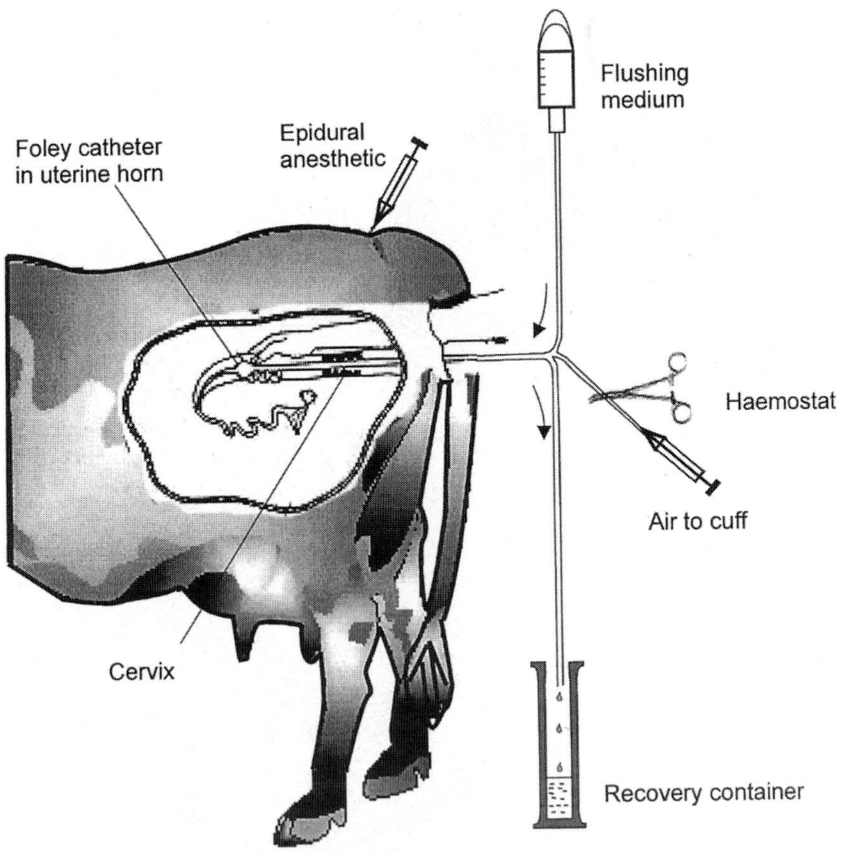


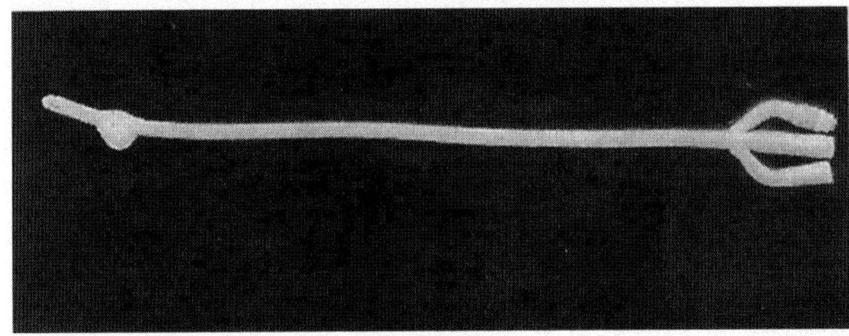

FIGURE 29-8. Transcervical recovery of embryos from the uterus of a cow on Day 6–8 after estrus. A 3-way Foley catheter is passed through the cervix and directed to one uterine horn and the cuff inflated to prevent leakage of fluid. The flushing medium is allowed to flow continuously by gravity and the uterine flushings collected in a graduated cylinder.

the skin. While visualizing the uterus, a 2-way Foley catheter is inserted through another stab wound and guided into one uterine horn before inflating the balloon. Next an intravenous catheter is inserted into the uterine lumen close to the uterotubal junction (Fig. 29-9). About 40 to 50 mL of fluid are injected through the intravenous catheter and the flushings collected via the Foley catheter. The other horn is similarly flushed.

**SELECTION OF EMBRYOS FOR TRANSFER.** The detailed procedure for isolating embryos from uterine flushings from the cattle and buffalo are described elsewhere (7). The flushings in sheep, goat, and pig are examined directly under a stereomicroscope. The embryos should be kept in a container that prevents evaporation of the culture medium. Paraffin oil may be used frequently to cover the medium to prevent evaporation and contamination with micro-organisms. Usually, only morphologically normal embryos are transferred; however, a few that appear morphologically abnormal may also develop into normal young.

Stages of embryonic development normally found at various times after ovulation are presented in Table 29-7 and Fig. 29-10. Eggs at any stage, from one cell to the hatched blastocyst, can develop to term following transfer to a suitable recipient, but success rates may be lower with very early and very late stages. Under most conditions, embryos between the eight-cell (four-cell in pigs) and blastocyst stage result in the highest pregnancy rates. Older embryos may tolerate *in vitro* handling better than younger embryos.

Most bovine embryos are collected from the uterus from the morula to the expanded blastocyst stage (Fig. 29-11). The grading of pre-attachment embryos is shown in Table 29-8.

In general, only excellent and good embryos are considered as "*transferable embryos*" in cattle. Defective embryos

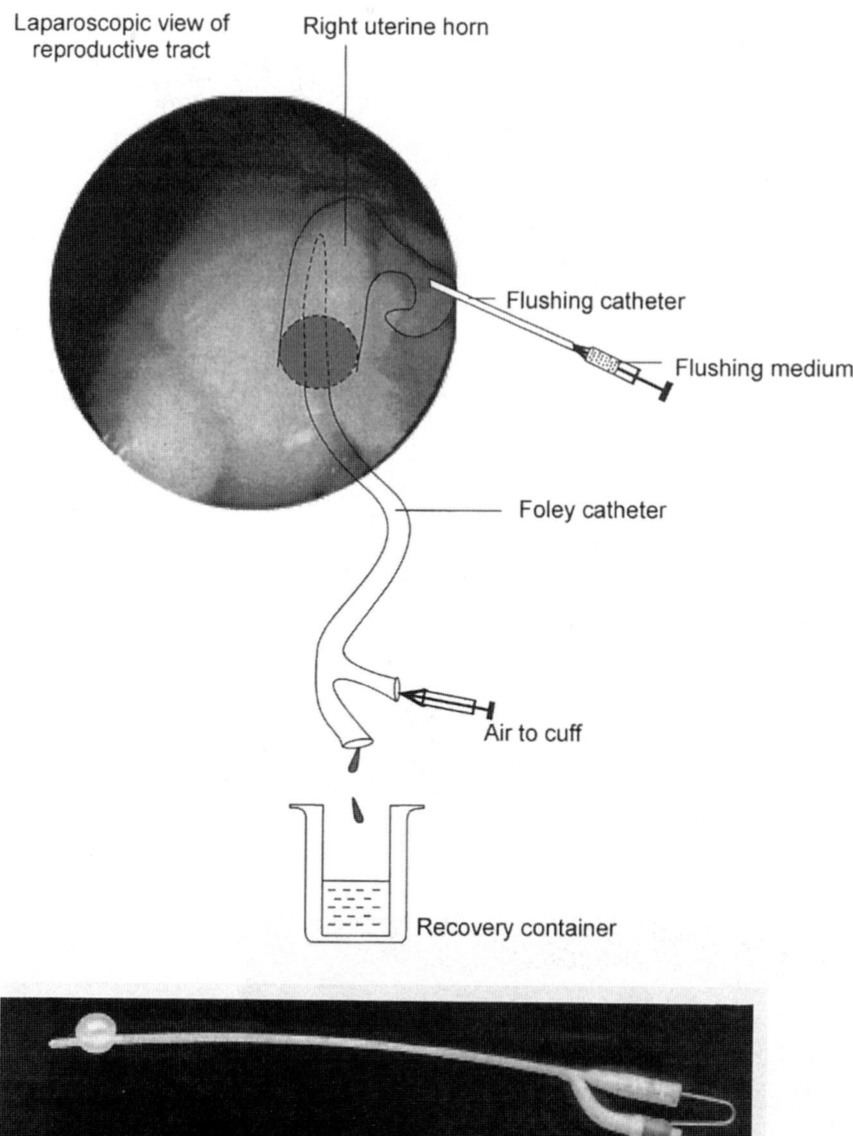

FIGURE 29-9. A laparoscopic view of the uterus in a ewe showing a Foley catheter placed within the right uterine horn, with the cuff inflated to recover embryos by infusing medium through a catheter inserted close to the tip of the horn.

showing any of the following morphologic anomalies must be discarded

1. blastomeres of variable, nonuniform size,
2. cellular debris in the morula,
3. collapse of the degenerated blastocyst within an oblong-shaped zona pellucida,
4. disintegrating mitotic figure,
5. indistinct foamy blastomeres,
6. fragmentation of cytoplasmic and nuclear material,
7. abnormal shape of morula or blastocyst (Fig. 29-12).

## *In Vitro* Embryo Production (IVEP)

The procedure involves collection of oocytes from ovarian follicles, then completing three biologic steps: *in vitro* maturation of oocytes (IVM); *in vitro* fertilization (IVF); and *in vitro* culture (IVC) (Fig. 29-13). Some examples of IVEP in farm species are presented in Table 29-9.

CAPACITATION OF SPERM. Spermatozoa do not attain their full capacity for fertilization until after they are transported in the female reproductive tract. Sperm have to undergo further physiologic changes (sperm capacitation) before they can penetrate the zona pellucida and fuse with the vitellus of the eggs. Most early experiments with IVF were unsuccessful because the sperm were not capacitated—a term that refers to a modification of ejaculated sperm in the female reproductive tract, making them capable of fertilizing eggs. Capacitation allows sperm to undergo a normal acrosome reaction before fertilization.

In early studies, capacitated sperm were often obtained

TABLE 29-7. ***Location and Stages of Embryonic Development at Various Times After Ovulation in Farm Species***

| Location | Stage of Embryonic Development | Days After Ovulation | | | |
|---|---|---|---|---|---|
| | | *Cow and Buffalo* | *Mare* | *Ewe and Doe* | *Pig* |
| Oviduct | 1-Cell | 0–1 | 0–1 | 0–1 | 0–1 |
| | 2-Cell | 0–2 | 0–2 | 0–1 | 0–1 |
| | 4-Cell | 1–2 | 1–2 | 1–2 | 2–3 |
| | 8-Cell | 2–4 | 2–3 | 2–3 | 3–4 |
| | Early morula | 3–5 | 2–4 | 2–4 | 3–4 |
| Uterus | Compacted morula | 4–6 | 4–5 | 4–5 | 3–5 |
| | Early blastocyst | 6–7 | 5–6 | 5–6 | 4–5 |
| | Blastocyst | 6–8 | 6–7 | 6–7 | 5–6 |
| | Expanded blastocyst | 7–9 | 7–8 | 7–8 | 5–7 |
| | Hatching blastocyst | 8–10 | 8–9 | 8–9 | 6–8 |

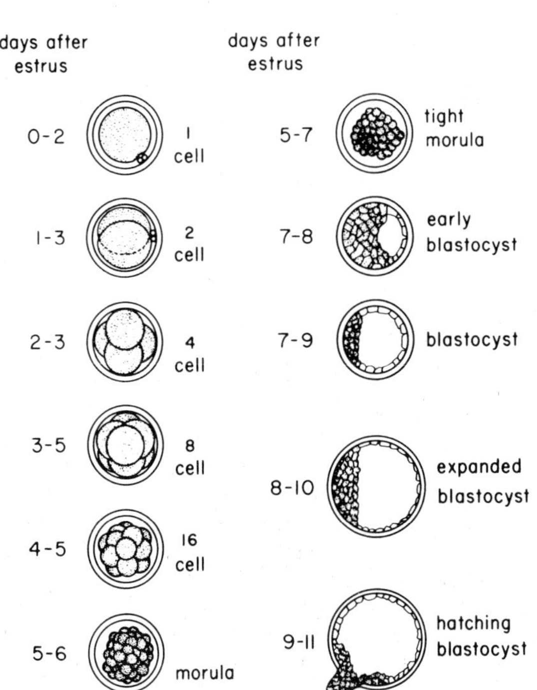


FIGURE 29-10. Diagram to illustrate the different stages of development of pre-attachment bovine embryos based on days after estrus.

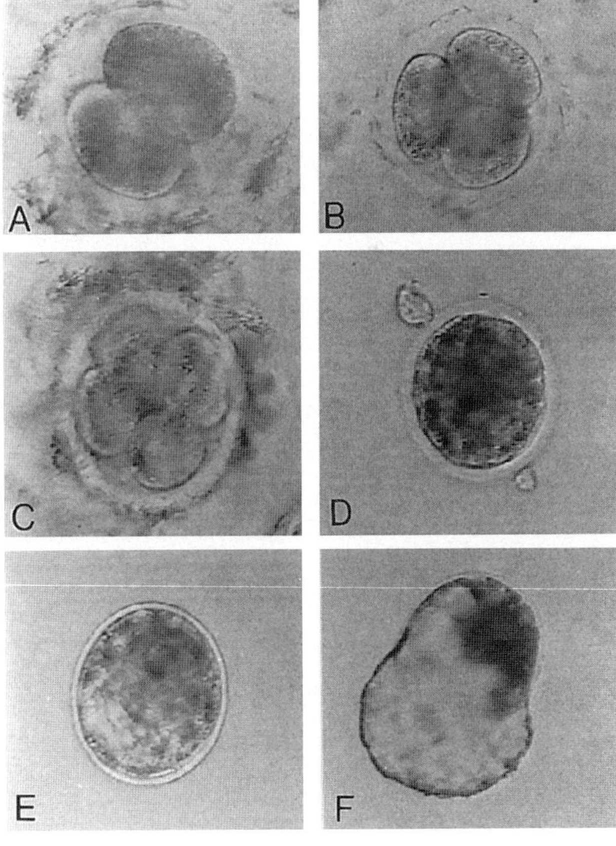


FIGURE 29-11. Photographs of pre-attachment bovine embryos at different stages of development. **(A–C)** *In vitro* fertilized 2-cell, 4-cell, and 8-cell embryos, respectively. **(D–F)** Compact morula, expanded blastocyst, and hatching blastocyst, respectively, obtained by superovulation and recovered from uterine flushing on Days 6–9.

TABLE 29-8. ***Characteristics of Bovine Follicle, Cumulus-Oocyte-Complex, Grades, and Development of Preattachment Embryos***

| CATEGORY | TYPE | FEATURES |
|---|---|---|
| Ovarian follicles | Healthy nonatretic | · Uniformly bright<br>· Translucent<br>· Extensive vascularization<br>· Normal granulosa layer<br>· Absence of floating particles in the follicular fluid<br>· At least 75% of expected number of granulosa cells for a given follicle size<br>· Theca interna pink to red |
| | Slightly atretic (Intermediate) | · Slight loss of translucency<br>· Slightly grayish<br>· White theca interna<br>· Few very small floating particles in follicle cavity |
| | Atretic | · Dull gray, poorly vascularized<br>· Blood vessels empty or irregularly filled with clotted blood<br>· Detached granulosa membrane<br>· Free particles in antral cavity |
| Cumulus-oocyte-complex | A | · Greater than 5 layers of cumulus cells |
| | B | · Between 3–5 layers of cumulus cells |
| | C | · Between 1–3 layers of cumulus cells |
| | D | · Denuded oocytes |
| | E | · Oocytes with expanded cumulus or atretic |
| Grading of preattachment embryos | Excellent | · Embryo evenly granulated and perfectly symmetrical embryo with distinct outline<br>· Blastomere extrusion absent<br>· Embryo at expected stage of development for its age |
| | Good | · Embryo evenly granulated and with distinct outline<br>· Some blastomere extrusion or degeneration<br>· Shape somewhat asymmetric |
| | Fair | · Intact embryo with hazy outline<br>· Extruded cells<br>· Vesiculation or degenerate blastomeres |
| | Poor | · Embryo with uneven granulation or hazy outline<br>· Some blastomere extrusion or degeneration<br>· Abnormal shape |
| | Degenerate | · Development stage difficult to determine |
| Embryonic development | Morula | · Individual blastomeres not distinct<br>· Perivitelline space mostly occupied by embryo |
| | Compact morula | · Individual blastomeres come together, forming a compact embryo mass occupying two-thirds of the perivitelline space |
| | Early blastocyst | · Embryo with a fluid filled cavity or blastocele (signet ring)<br>· Embryo occupied three-quarters of the perivitelline space<br>· Trophoblast and inner cell mass can be differentiated |
| | Mid blastocyst | · Outer trophoblast differentiation pronounced<br>· Inner cell mass compact and darker<br>· Blastocyst very prominent and embryo occupies almost all of the perivitelline space |
| | Expanded blastocyst | · Embryo markedly increased in size<br>· Thinning of zona pellucida |
| | Hatched blastocyst | · Embryo in the process of hatching<br>· Zona pellucida shed |
| | Hatched expanded blastocyst | · Re-expanded embryo with a large blastocyst<br>· Circular, very fragile, and in later stages elongated |

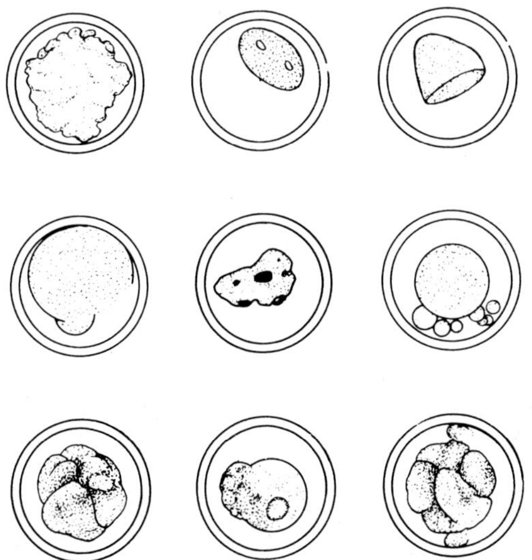

FIGURE 29-12. Degenerating one-cell ova and embryos, which should not be used for routine embryo transfer.

by flushing the uterus or oviducts of a mated female. Capacitation may be accomplished *in vitro,* although the mechanism as well as the duration of the process may differ from the *in vivo* phenomenon. *In vitro* fertilization has been accomplished with sperm capacitated by high ionic strength medium, $Ca^{2+}$ ionophore, caffeine, long incubation (18 to 24 h), high pH, and washing through percoll gradient, but results were not repeatable.

The discovery that glyocosaminoglycan heparin capacitates bull sperm (16) has significantly advanced IVF technology in farm animals. Both embryo development and birth of offspring have resulted from *in vitro* fertilization with heparin-capacitated sperm in cattle and other farm species.

The first step in sperm capacitation is to obtain a sample of ejaculated semen with a high percentage of sperm showing progressive motility. If frozen semen is used, sperm motility can be enhanced (hypermotility) by either physical methods (swim-up technique, percoll density gradient) or chemical agents (caffeine, theophylline). The swim-up technique is illustrated in Figure 29-14.

To capacitate bovine sperm, the required number of sperm is diluted in bicarbonate buffered medium containing 10 $\mu$g/mL of heparin (16). Medium containing sperm is dispensed in microdroplets under paraffin oil, or in wells without oil, and incubated for 4 h.

IN VITRO MATURATION OF OOCYTES (IVM). Unlike sperm, the oocyte requires no exposure to the reproductive tract following release from the gonad to be fertile. In the past, oocytes for IVEP were obtained mostly by aspirating follicles from slaughterhouse ovaries (17). Oocytes are collected by dissecting, slicing, or aspirating. The dissection technique allows the isolation of individual follicles. Slicing of ovarian tissues gives the highest number of oocytes, while aspiration is the most efficient technique in terms of the time to obtain oocytes. The features of ovarian follicles are summarized in Table 29-8. Only healthy follicles are selected for oocyte aspiration.

Since the early 1990s, ovum pick up (OPU) by puncture of ovarian follicles in the live donor (*in vivo*) by laparoscopy (18) or ultrasonography (19) is gaining acceptance. Transvaginal ultrasound guided OPU (Fig. 29-15) can be performed in live donors at weekly intervals from adult and prepuberal cattle, sheep, and goat (20). OPU can provide four to eight oocytes per collection and may be an alternative to superovulation in the future.

In most laboratories, bovine oocytes are matured in TCM199 medium with 10% fetal calf serum and gonadotropins (FSH, LH). Oocytes are transferred into a dish containing this maturation medium. After rupturing follicles to release the cumulus oocyte complexes (COC), four to five or a group of COC are placed in microdroplets of the same medium under paraffin oil in Petri dishes and incubated at 39°C in 5% $CO_2$ and 95% air with high humidity for 24 h.

IN VITRO FERTILIZATION (IVF). During coincubation of an IVM oocyte with capacitated sperm, one sperm penetrates the oocyte, triggering a series of events leading to fertilization (Fig. 29-16). The IVF procedure involves preparing microdroplets of 25 $\mu$l of sperm suspension and 25 $\mu$l of medium containing 10 $\mu$g/mL heparin. Next four to five COC are placed in a droplet of the fertilization medium (final volume 50 $\mu$l) under paraffin oil and incubated in 5% $CO_2$ and 95% air with high humidity at 39°C for 24 h.

In aged oocytes, the incidence of polyspermy is high and if the oocyte is too old, embryonic development is abnormal or fertilization may not take place at all.

Modified, balanced salt solutions, such as Krebs-Ringer bicarbonate, support *in vitro* fertilization. The acrosome reaction seems to occur much more readily in media containing serum albumin in the form of either heat-treated serum or bovine serum albumin. It is also critical to provide an energy source, usually glucose or pyruvate, to support spermatozoal motility and the metabolism of the oocytes.

Fertilization rate can be assessed by microscopic examination for cleavage but for more accurate analysis, some oocytes, 18 to 22 h after insemination, should be fixed, stained, and examined under phase contrast microscopy. High fertilization rates in IVF depend upon optimal number of fertilizable sperm with vigorous motility, and a fertilizable ovum with a first polar body.

Some criteria (Table 29-10) used as evidence for fertilization are

a) penetration of sperm into the ooplasm,
b) swelling of the sperm head, pronuclear formation,
c) morphologically normal cleavage, blastocyst formation,

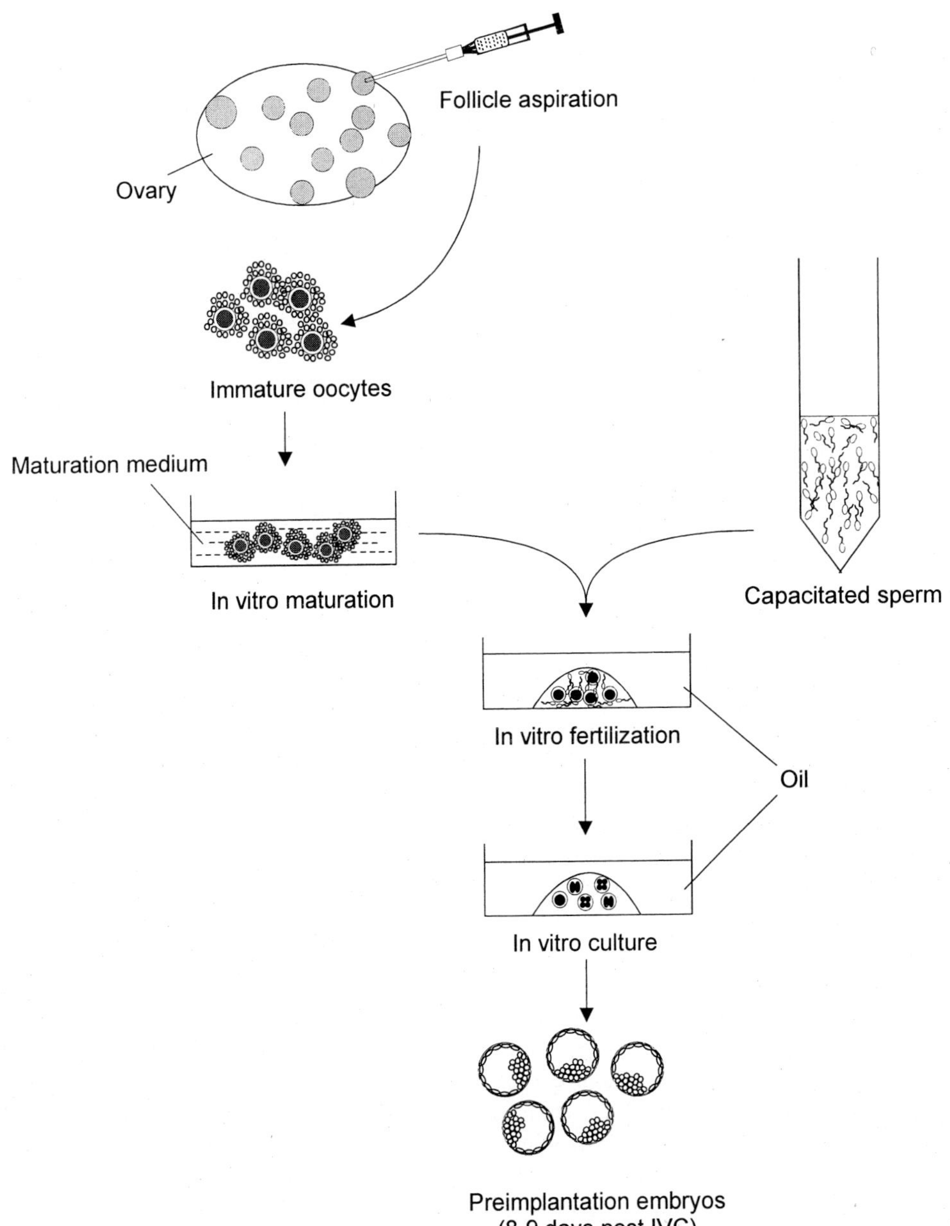


FIGURE 29-13. Basic steps in the *in vitro* production of embryos in cattle. Oocytes are aspirated from ovarian follicles and matured (*in vitro maturation*), fertilized with capacitated sperm (*in vitro fertilization*), and zygotes cultured (*in vitro culture*) for 8 to 9 days to obtain blastocysts for transfer to the uterus.

d) breakdown of cortical granules, and
e) evidence of a sperm tail in the ooplasm.

None of these alone is sufficient proof of normal fertilization; for example parthenogenetic embryos also exhibit some of these traits.

IN VITRO CULTURE (IVC). Following IVF, the zygotes must be cultured for further development before they are transferred into the uterus or cryopreserved. There are three systems of IVC of embryos

a) Transferring to the ligated oviduct of a temporary recipient, e.g., sheep or rabbit, and four or five days later, embryos are recovered, graded, and frozen or transferred.
b) Zygotes cocultured *in vitro* with somatic cells (oviductal epithelial cells, granulosa cells) in medium TCM199.
c) Simple medium without somatic cell support such as synthetic oviductal fluid (SOF) (21).

The mammalian oviduct has the ability to support the development of embryos across many species, indicat-

TABLE 29-9. ***Some Examples of*** *In Vitro* **Production of Embryos**

| Species | Sperm Capacitation | IVM | IVC | Results |
|---|---|---|---|---|
| Cattle[a] | Heparin | 20–30 h | Sheep oviduct (4–6 days) | 60–70% pregnancy rate |
| Buffalo[b] | Heparin | TCM199 + buffalo estrus serum + gonadotropin | Oviductal epithelial cells | Birth of 5 IVF buffalo calves |
| Sheep[c] | Heparin | 24–26 h | Oviductal epithelial cells | 31.5% embryos |
| Goat[d] | Heparin | Caprine follicular fluid + FSH + TCM199 (5% $CO_2$ at 39°C) | SOF supplemented with amino acids and serum, and incubated (5% $CO_2$ at 39°C) | 61% blastocysts resulted in kids |
| Pig[e] | None | Cumulus-oocyte-complexes were cultured in NCSU 23 medium with hormonal supplements for 20–22 h. Cultured for an additional 20–22 h without hormone. Then cumulus-free oocytes were coincubated with frozen-thawed spermatozoa for 5–6 h. | Putative zygotes were transferred to NCSU 23 medium containing 0.4% BSA and cultured for 144 h. | Pregnancies in 5 of 9 recipients with the birth of 18 live piglets |

[a]Data from Galli C, Lazzari G. Practical aspects of IVM/IVF in cattle. Anim Reprod Sci 1996;42:371.

[b]Data from Madan ML, Das SK, Palta P. Application of reproductive technology to buffaloes. Anim Reprod Sci 1996;42:299.

[c]Data from Wahid H, Gordon I, Sharif H, Lonergan P, Monaghan P, Gallagher M. Development of ovine blastocysts following maturation, fertilization and culture of oocytes *in vitro*. Proc 7th European Embryo Transfer Assoc. Cambridge 1991;214.

[d]Data from Poulin N, Guler A, Pignon P, Cognie Y. *In vitro* production of goat embryos: heparin in IVF medium affects development ability. In: Proc Int Conf On Goats, Vol 2. Beijing, China, 1996;838.

[e]Data from Abeydeera LR, Wang WH, Cantley TC, Rieke A, Day BN. Coculture with follicular shell pieces can enhance the developmental competence of pig oocytes after *in vitro* fertilization: relevance to intracellular glutathione. Biol Reprod 1998;58:213.

ing that many of the beneficial effects of the oviduct environment may actually be nonspecific concerning species. Pig early embryos (1-cell to 8-cell stage) cultured in "organ coculture" in mouse excised oviducts, can develop to the morula and blastocyst stage (22). Similarly, bovine embryos can develop *in vivo* sheep and rabbit oviduct coculture (23).

**CULTURE CONDITIONS, MEDIA, AND SUPPLEMENTS.** Embryo development occurs in several culture conditions, media and supplements, and gaseous atmospheres.

*CULTURE CONDITIONS.* Culture in sealed tubes yields results equal to those noted for microdrops of media under paraffin oil. A reduced oxygen atmosphere of 5% $CO_2$, 5% $O_2$, and 90% $N_2$ is at least equal to, and in some species superior to, 5% $CO_2$ in air in promoting embryo development.

*CULTURE AND COCULTURE MEDIA.* Several culture and coculture media have been used for *in vitro* physiologic maturation and subsequent cleavage at various stages of development. Some of the commonly used media are modified Krebs-Ringer's bicarbonate, modified Dulbecco's, TCM199, modified Ham's F-10, Whitten medium, Eagle's basal medium with Hank's salts, and modified minimum essential medium (MEM) with Earl's salts.

*MACROMOLECULAR SUPPLEMENTS.* Media supplemented with a large protein molecule decreases surface tension, thereby reducing embryos tendencies to float or adhere to plastic or glass surfaces. Media may contain either bovine serum albumin (BSA) or blood serum (often from fetal calves) that has been inactivated by being held at 56°C for 30 min. BSA is usually added at 0.3 to 1%, but concentrations from 0.1% to 50% have been used.

Several biologic culture media have been used for the manipulation of embryos (see Appendix). Usually, 50 mg of streptomycin sulfate and 100,000 IU of potassium penicillin G are added per liter, but other concentrations and other antibiotics and antifungal agents are frequently used as well. Media should be forced through a filter of 0.45 $\mu$m or smaller to remove bacteria.

All media except modified phosphate-buffered saline are bicarbonate-buffered and therefore require an atmosphere of 5% $CO_2$ to maintain proper pH. This is accomplished with a mixture of 5% $CO_2$ in air, or better, 5% $CO_2$,

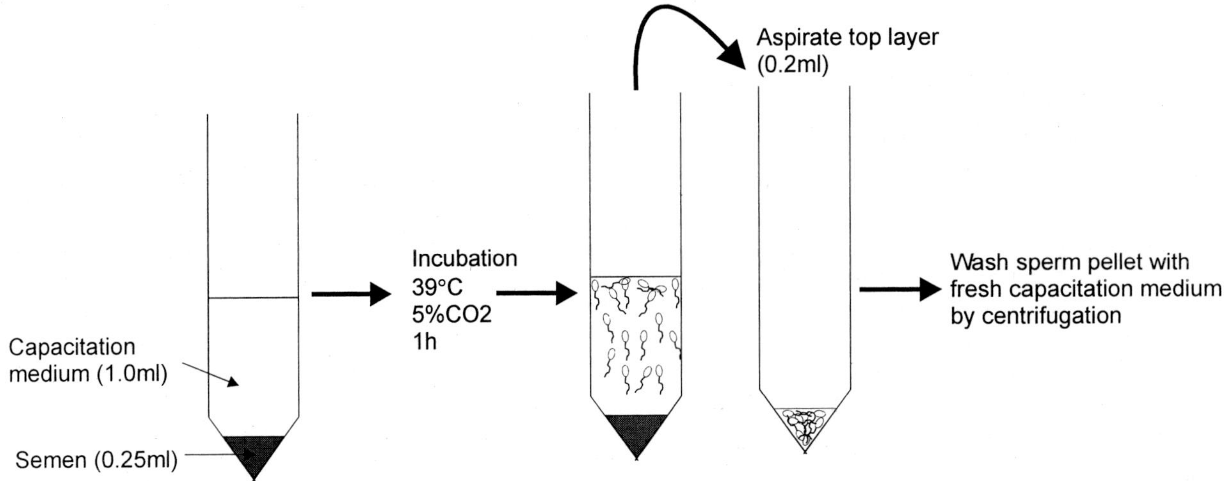


FIGURE 29-14. Diagram illustrating the "swim up" technique for the production of hypermotile sperm for *in vitro* fertilization.

5% $O_2$, and 90% $N_2$. A $CO_2$ incubator or small, gassed, and airtight containers may be used. When media must be kept in an air environment (without $CO_2$) for long periods, 25 mL HEPES buffer is usually added and the NaCl decreased to maintain proper osmolality.

The pH of media may range from 7 to 8, but best results are obtained between 7.2 and 7.6. Osmolalities between 270 and 300 mOsm/kg are most commonly used for embryos. Water is the principal ingredient, and purity is important. Double distillation or glass distillation of deionized water is usually adequate. The media are passed through a 0.2 $\mu$m membrane filter and stored in bottle sterilized in an autoclave.

QUALITY CONTROL. Table 29-10 summarizes the procedures and physiologic parameters of gametes, IVF, and embryos for transfer, and Table 29-11, the laboratory equipment and facilities required for an ET program.

### *Cryopreservation of Embryos*

The efficacy of embryo transfer depends on maintaining the viability of embryos from the time of collection to the time of transfer. The successful freezing of bull sperm at −195°C led immediately to attempts at freezing mammalian embryos, but nearly 25 years elapsed before cattle embryos were successfully frozen. To date, successful results based on pregnancy rates have been obtained with cryopreserved embryos of cattle, sheep, goat, and horse, but few successes have been reported in pig. Post-thaw embryo survival has been shown to be dependent on the initial embryo quality, developmental stage, species, time from collection to freezing, type of cryoprotectant, and cooling protocol.

Cryopreservation of embryos is covered in greater detail in Chapter 30. There are two methods of cryopreservation of embryos.

CONVENTIONAL OR "EQUILIBRIUM" CRYOPRESERVATION. This is the freezing technique that is most frequently used in research and by commercial companies. In this technique, the embryos are placed in a concentrated glycerol solution (1.4 M in PBS supplemented with BSA) at room temperature and the embryo is allowed to equilibrate for a 20-min period. One embryo is loaded into a 0.25 or 0.5 mL French straw. During the cooling process the straws are seeded (−4 to −7°C) and cooling is continued at a rate of 0.3 to 0.5°C/min to −30°C, when bovine embryos are plunged into $LN_2$.

The principles of freezing embryos in other farm species are essentially similar to those for bovine embryos. Sheep embryos are successfully frozen with ethylene glycol (1.5 M) or DMSO (1.5 M) rather than with glycerol. Horse embryos have been frozen in 0.5 mL straws rather than 0.25 mL straws, but with cooling rates and seeding and plunging temperatures similar to those used with bovine embryos.

Swine embryos are highly sensitive to temperature and cryoprotectants, which may be due to their high lipid content. Cooling to 15 or 10°C causes a dramatic increase in the percentage of degenerated embryos.

"NONEQUILIBRIUM" CRYOPRESERVATION OR VITRIFICATION. During the past decade, embryos have also been frozen by a "nonequilibrium" method. This rapid freezing (vitrification) consists of dehydration of the embryo at room temperature by a very highly concentrated vitrification media and a very rapid freeze that avoids the formation of ice crystals, allowing the solution to change from a liquid to a glassy state (Fig. 29-17). A low toxicity vitrification solution (EFS 40) consists of three cryoprotective agents (24)

a) a rapidly permeating low toxic agent, e.g., 40% (v/v) ethylene glycol,

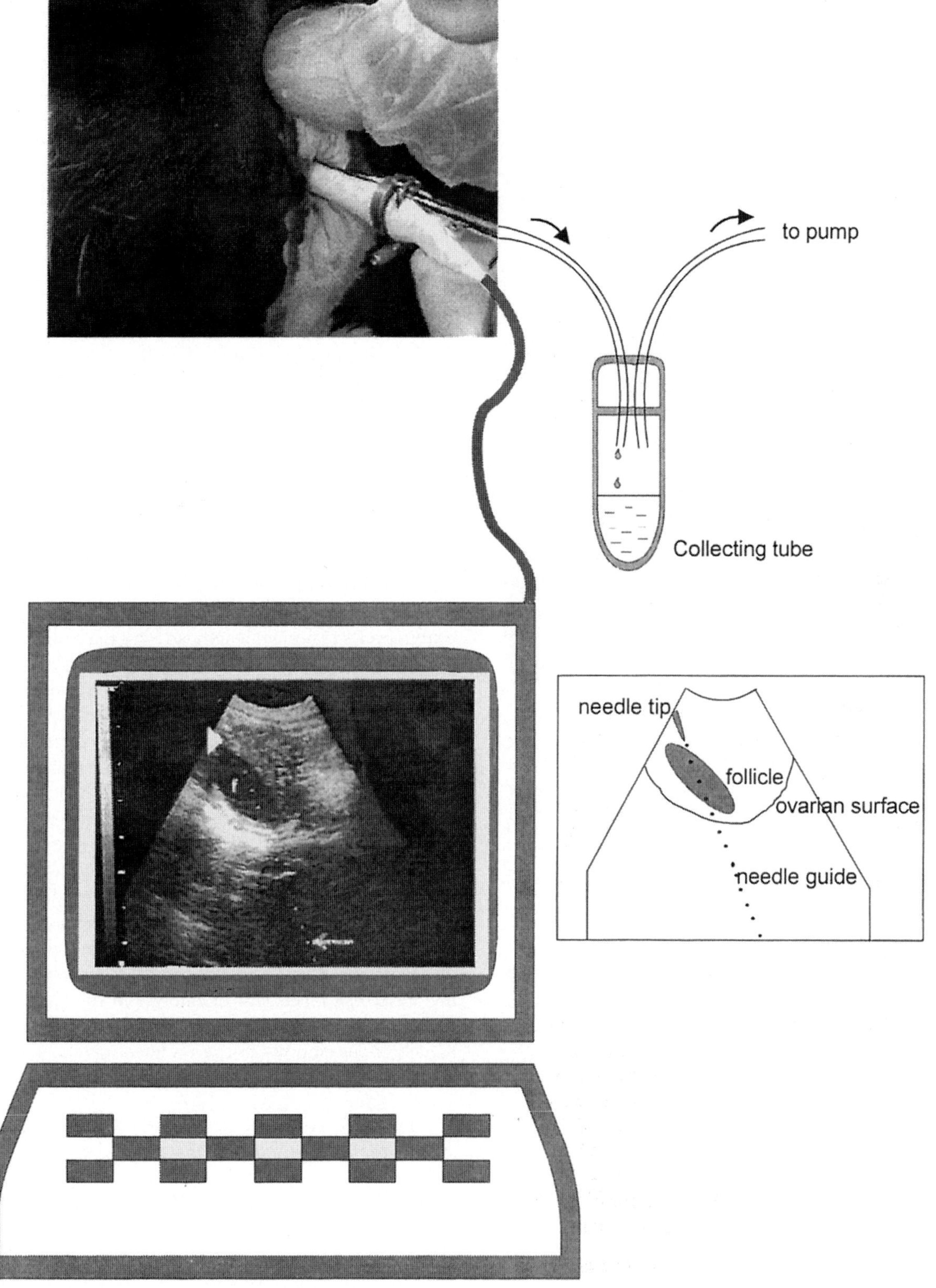


FIGURE 29-15. Transvaginal ultrasound guided oocyte aspiration in a cow. The transducer is inserted into the vagina and the ovary fixed by rectal palpation. When the ultrasonographic image of the follicle is aligned with the puncture line on the monitor, the aspiration cannula is advanced through the vaginal wall into the cavity of the ovarian follicle to aspirate the contents.

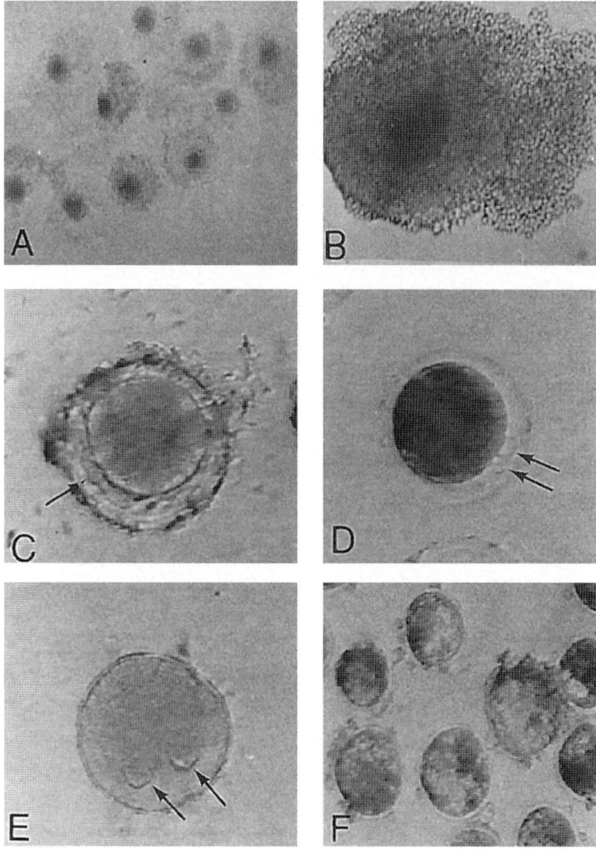


FIGURE 29-16. *In vitro* embryo production from slaughterhouse ovaries in cattle. (**A**) A group of oocyte-cumulus-complexes (COC) after IVM. Note expanded cumulus cell. (**B**) A COC with 4 to 5 layers of cumulus cells before IVM. (**C**) A IVM oocytes surrounded by sperm. Note the extrusion of the first polar body (*arrow*). (**D**) *In vitro* fertilized egg. Note the extrusion of the second polar body (*arrows*). (**E**) Formation of pronuclei. (**F**) A group of IVC blastocysts.

b) a macromolecule, e.g., 18% (w/v) Ficoll, and
c) a disaccharide, e.g., 0.3 M sucrose.

The above solution is efficient for vitrifying several mammalian embryos. Brief exposure at room temperature to the solution of blastocysts of cattle (1 min), sheep (0.5 min), and horse (2 min), is done before plunging into $LN_2$. In cattle, 74% of the blastocysts survived the freezing and thawing, and 60% of the recipients delivered a calf.

Vitrification has considerable promise in providing a successful method for the cryopreservation of bovine embryos. Some advantages are listed below:

a) Eliminates the need for expensive freezing machines.
b) Reduces the time required for equilibration and cooling.
c) Provides for simple and rapid one-step dilution of cryoprotectant after thawing.
d) Enables more embryos to be thawed and transferred per unit time.
e) Provides direct transfer of the embryo into the recipient upon thawing.

ADVANTAGES OF CRYOPRESERVED EMBRYOS. Some advantages of cryopreserved embryos are as follows:

a) Offers a practical solution for long-term storage.
b) Facilitates greater use of embryo transfer.
c) Eliminates synchronization of estrus in recipients; transfer can be done when the recipient is in the appropriate stage of the cycle.
d) Collect and transfer embryos at any time or place.
e) Distribute germplasm worldwide.
f) Conserve endangered species and exotic breeds.

## *Embryo Transfer Techniques*

SYNCHRONIZATION OF ESTRUS OF DONOR AND RECIPIENT. Pregnancy rate after embryo transfer is greatly influenced by the conditions and preparation of the recipients. An animal that is not fit for natural service cannot be used for embryo transfer. Females selected to be recipients must be good breeders with an infection-free genital tract and estrous cycles of normal length, and in good body condition.

Synchronization between the stage of embryo and the reproductive tract of the recipient is a prerequisite. This is usually accomplished by selecting recipients that were in estrus at the same time as the donor, either naturally or as a result of estrus synchronization. For optimum results, the recipient should be in estrus within 12 h of the donor. Pregnancy rates decline drastically if the difference is greater than 24 h in cows and 48 h in sheep and goats.

Recipients for frozen embryos should be selected to be in physiologic synchrony with the stage of development of the embryo. Thus, 7-day old frozen embryos should be transferred to recipients that were in estrus 7 days earlier.

Pregnancy losses from asynchronous transfers are probably due to the placement of embryos in the horn opposite to that of the side containing the CL, or to an inability of asynchronous embryos to exert a luteotropic action on the CL of the recipient.

THAWING OF EMBRYOS. In cattle, embryos in 0.5 mL straws are thawed in air for 20 s followed by 20 s in water (37°C), while those in 0.25 mL straws are thawed for 15 s in air and 20 s in water (37°C). The exposure to air reduces damage to the zona pellucida.

Several procedures are available for the removal of the cryoprotectant (e.g., glycerol). In the conventional method, glycerol is diluted with PBS in six or four steps, each step takes about 6 min. In transferring embryos between steps, a microscope is needed and the procedure is conducted under laboratory conditions.

TABLE 29-10. ***Procedures and Physiologic Parameters of Gametes and Fertilization***

| STAGES AND PROCEDURES | PHYSIOLOGIC PARAMETERS AND REGULATORY MECHANISM |
|---|---|
| Oocyte aspiration | Size of follicle |
| | Oocyte maturation, techniques, and timing |
| | Follicular fluid |
| | Biochemistry |
| | Hormones |
| | Cumulus mass |
| | Superovulation |
| Spermatozoa | Sperm maturity, motility, and concentration in media |
| | Sperm capacitation |
| | Acrosome reaction, changes in sperm surface |
| | Ion concentration and enzyme activity in milieu |
| *In vitro* fertilization | Quantity and quality of sperm in culture |
| | Sperm capacitation |
| | Basic culture medium |
| | Additives |
| | Energy source |
| | Sperm stimulants |
| | Hormones |
| | pH |
| | Gas phase ($O_2$ tension) |
| | Absence of seminal plasma |
| | Microscopic characteristics of fertilized ova |
| Criteria of *in vitro* fertilization | Penetration of spermatozoa within the vitellus |
| | Presence of sperm tail in the vitellus |
| | Presence of male and female pronuclei in the egg |
| | Presence of two polar bodies in the perivitelline space |
| | Cleavage and formation of two blastomeres with equal size, shape, and no fragmentation |
| Embryo transfer | State of embryo |
| | Cleavage rate and regularity of blastomeres |
| | Development stage of endometrium |
| | Transfer technique |

To overcome the step-wise dilution of the cryoprotectant, Leibo (25) described a method of diluting the glycerol within the straw by incorporating sucrose (rehydrating solution) between two air bubbles before freezing. After thawing, the cryoprotectant and the sucrose solution are mixed by shaking the straw (Fig. 29-18). It avoids the need to unload the embryos for rehydration and reloading embryos in a new straw, making a microscope, an embryologist, and laboratory equipment superfluous.

However, Leibo's method has not been widely adopted by the ET industry because the pregnancy rates are lower than with the conventional thawing procedures. Meanwhile, several laboratories are engaged in developing a one-step thawing procedure using other cryoprotectants, e.g., ethylene glycol for direct transfers. Once an ideal one-step thawing of embryos is found, thawing embryos will be as simple as thawing frozen semen.

**TRANSFER TECHNIQUES. CATTLE AND BUFFALO.** In the early days of ET, embryos were transferred by laparotomy under general or local anesthesia. Since 1978, the surgical technique has been discarded in favor of the transcervical route (26).

In the transcervical approach, the recipient is rectally palpated to determine the ovary containing the corpus luteum. Next, posterior epidural anesthesia is induced to prevent straining during the procedure. The dose of local anesthetic is adjusted to ensure that the animal remains standing throughout the transfer.

TABLE 29-11. ***Equipment and Laboratory Supplies for Embryo Transfer***

| | | |
|---|---|---|
| Glassware | Petri dishes, pipettes, embryo dishes, thermos flask for short-term storage of embryos, and assorted laboratory glassware/polyware | |
| Instruments and equipment | Instrument kits for recipients<br>Refrigerator<br>Deep freeze<br>Laundry bin<br>Water baths<br>Microscope and spare bulbs<br>Thermometers<br>Hot air oven<br>$CO_2$ incubator | Washing machine and dryer<br>Autoclave<br>Dry-heat sterilizer<br>Distillation units to produce distilled ultrafiltered water<br>Small gas sterilizer and refills<br>Liquid nitrogen container with mobile base<br>Instrument trolley<br>Operating lamp |
| Biologic safety cabinet | Ventilated cabinets (fume hoods) for personnel protection, with uncirculated inward flow of air away from the operator<br>Ventilated cabinet for personnel and product protection with open front with inward airflow for personnel protection, HEPA-filtered mass recirculated airflow for product protection; exhaust air is filtered<br>Closed-front ventilated cabinet (glove box), filtered with rubber gloves, with negative pressure of gastight construction | |
| Sterilizing and cleaning | Sterilization bags<br>Sterile market indicator tape<br>Laboratory coats, caps, and masks | Surgical gowns, caps parturition gloves, and masks<br>Hair clippers and spare blades<br>Scrub brushes, scrub fluid dispensers |

Under aseptic conditions, the embryo, loaded in a 0.25 mL straw, is fitted into the Cassou transfer gun and covered by a sterile sheath. The gun is inserted into the vagina and passed through the cervix by rectal manipulation and guided into the uterine horn ipsilateral to the corpus luteum. The contents of the straw are deposited in the uterine horn.

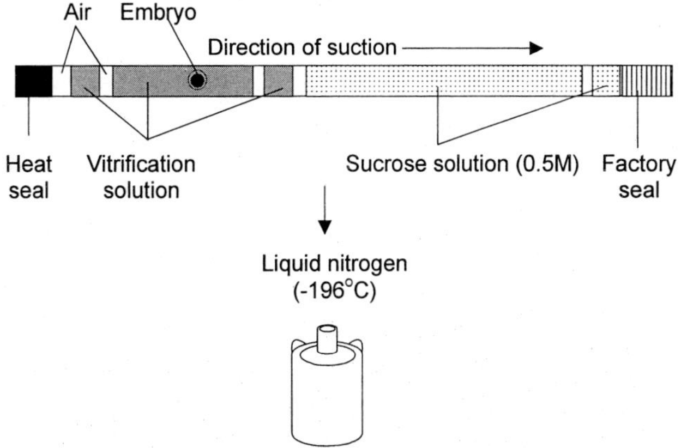


FIGURE 29-17. Steps in the vitrification of a bovine embryo. Loading a French straw (0.25 mL) by applying suction → sucrose solution → air → vitrification solution + embryo → air → heat seal; Plunging straw into liquid nitrogen for Vitrification.

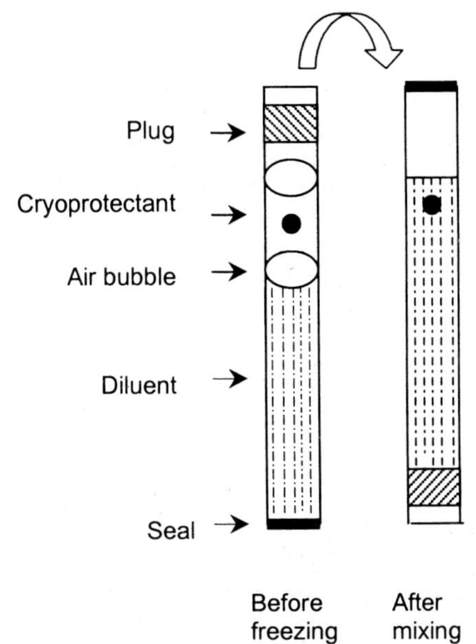


FIGURE 29-18. One-step thawing of an embryo within a straw (Leibo SP. A one-step method for direct non-surgical transfer of frozen-thawed bovine embryos. Theriogenology 1984;21:767.). Embryo in cryoprotectant (glycerol) is separated from the rehydrant (sucrose) by an air bubble (*Before freezing*). On thawing, fluid columns are mixed by inverting the straw and shaking it towards the seal end (*After mixing*).

Sheep and Goats. Most transfers are conducted by midventral laparotomy under general or local anesthetic with the animal restrained in a laparotomy cradle. Through a midventral incision, embryos are transferred with one or two drops of medium into the oviduct or the uterine horn. For transfer into the oviduct, the tip of a capillary pipette containing the embryos is inserted through the infundibulum to deposit embryos into the ampulla. When transfer is made to the uterus, the wall of the uterine horn is punctured with a blunt needle, and the embryos are expelled from the tip of the capillary pipette inserted into the uterine lumen. The transfer of embryos into the uterus can be performed by laparoscopy.

Maintenance of Pregnancy After Embryo Transfer. Pregnancy rates (the percentage of recipients becoming pregnant) should not be confused with the percentage of embryos surviving. Pregnancy and embryo survival rates that have been determined in early pregnancy will usually be only slightly inflated relative to term pregnancy rates. Under certain ideal conditions, up to 80% of the embryos survive to term following transfer to a synchronous recipient. The highest pregnancy rates in sheep, cattle, and goats are obtained with the transfer of one embryo into each uterine horn of the recipient. This frequently results in twins. In pigs, six to ten embryos should be transferred into each side to obtain a normal-sized litter because only about one-half of the embryos transferred are represented by viable young at birth.

### *Current Status of ET Technology in Farm Species*

Cattle. In MOET schemes, when all treated donors are considered, the average number of calves produced per superovulation is between three and four, even with the best technology. The median is two. Occasionally, litters of more than 20 calves are produced, but this occurs less than once in 100 attempts. The major contribution to this variability is the unpredictable response to superovulation and many unfertilized or abnormal eggs. Because cows can be superovulated four or five times a year, more than 10 calves can be obtained per cow per year on the average.

IVEP in cattle can be obtained from oocytes of slaughtered donors or from live donors by ultrasound guided aspiration. Among the factors influencing the efficiency of IVEP are the status of the donor, and techniques of IVC from the zygote to the blastocyst stage (27).

Oocytes can be collected *in vivo* from calves by laparoscopy or laparotomy by follicular aspiration, but transvaginal aspiration under ultrasonographic guidance has not been effective with calves less than 6-months old because of the small size of the vagina and the difficulty of rectal manipulation (20). Fresh IVF embryos per oocyte collection from 10-week to 12-week old calves may be expected to result in 8 to 10 pregnancies. Thus juvenile donors not only offer an alternative source of embryos but also reduce the generation interval. Both conventional cryopreservation and vitrification are successful for *in vivo* and *in vitro* produced bovine embryos from adult and juvenile donors.

Buffalo. Progress in the field application of ET in the buffalo has been slow. Since the birth of a buffalo calf by surgical transfer (28), most investigators prefer the nonsurgical transfer technique because less sophisticated handling facilities are required.

The ovulatory response at the same dose levels of gonadotropin is much lower in buffalo than in cattle. A disadvantage of PMSG is the high incidence of unovulated follicles (larger than 20 mm), which are larger than normal follicles.

Apparently, the rate of development through the morula and blastocyst stages occurs faster in buffalo than in cattle, such that the blastocyst emerges from the zona pellucida by day 6 or 7 in buffalo compared with day 9 in cattle. Since identification of hatched blastocysts in the flushing media is difficult, this species difference should be recognized in timing embryo recovery in the buffalo.

In Bulgaria and India, where most embryo transfers in buffalo have been conducted, the success rates have been less than 10%, as compared with pregnancy rates of 50 to 70% in dairy cattle. Some laboratories have achieved *in vitro* fertilization and embryonic development up to the morula stage in both the river and swamp type buffalo, and a few calves have been born in the river type (29). Some of the problems associated with ET in buffalo are summarized in Figure 29-19.

Sheep. In general, use of ET technology for genetic improvement in sheep is limited. This is because the conventional supply of embryos by superovulation and AI followed by surgical collection is both time consuming and expensive. While the level of performance is sufficient for producing lambs from barren ewes, further improvements are needed for MOET. An alternative approach is to aspirate follicles from slaughterhouse ovaries and followed by IVM and IVF procedures. About 60% of the original oocytes can develop into blastocysts (21). Apart from slaughterhouse ovaries, laparoscopic aspiration can yield more than 180 mature oocytes, which can yield about 25 offspring from a single collection (30).

In Australia, efforts are progressing to improve quality and production of wool by recombinant DNA techniques and transgenesis. IVEP can supply the one-cell zygotes needed for microinjection and the ET technology to transfer the manipulated embryos to surrogate mothers for the production of offspring. Thus, ET is expected to play a crucial role in Australia's transgenesis program.

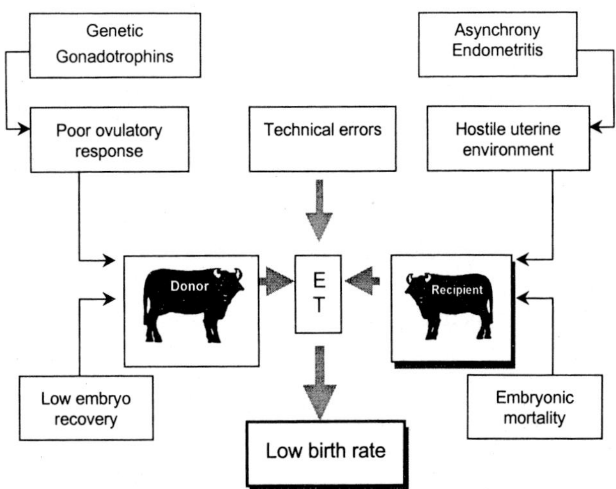


FIGURE 29-19. Factors associated with low birth rates to embryo transfer in buffalo (*Bubalus bubalis*).

GOAT. The recovery and transfer of embryos, the transvaginal ultrasound-guided oocyte aspiration from adult and prepuberal goats, and IVEP could contribute to the production of meat, milk, and other products. In a recent study, about 60% of *in vitro* produced blastocysts resulted in live kids, which was similar to the rates of those developed *in vivo*.

PIG. In pig breeding, embryo transfer is of limited value. The transfer of supersized litters to unmated females or of additional embryos to previously bred recipients does not appreciably increase litter size. One important use of embryo transfer in swine, however, is the introduction of new genetic material into specific pathogen free herds.

The failure to form a male pronucleus and the high incidence of polyspermy are serious problems in efforts to produce embryos efficiently *in vitro* from pig oocytes. Several studies have been conducted to reduce polyspermy. *In vitro*-matured and *in vivo*-matured pig oocytes possess equal ability to release cortical granules on sperm penetration (31). Unknown changes in the extracellular matrix and/or cytoplasm of the oocytes while in the oviduct may play an important role(s) in the establishment of a functional block to polyspermy in pig oocytes. By coculturing spermatozoa with oviductal cells, it is possible to reduce the number of spermatozoa confronting the eggs at fertilization, thereby decreasing the incidence of polyspermy and increasing the incidence of male pronuclei (32).

Despite the successful cryopreservation of embryos in most farm species, development of this technology in swine is rather slow (33). Normal piglets have been obtained after cryopreservation of pig blastocysts hatched *in vitro*, whereas efforts to freeze embryos with intact zona pellucida have been unsuccessful.

Pig embryos are sensitive to hypothermic conditions, limiting their ability to withstand conventional cryopreservation methods. The damage to the embryonic cytoskeleton may be overcome by using cytoskeleton stabilizers, and such embryos cryopreserved by conventional freezing and vitrification have resulted in pregnancies and live offspring.

HORSE. The application of embryo transfer in the horse is very limited. Superovulation is not very effective in the horse. A single embryo, however, can usually be recovered nonsurgically during each estrous cycle 6 or 7 days after ovulation. Furthermore, foals have been born by nonsurgical transfer (34). The scarcity of embryos has restricted cryopreservation of embryos.

IVEP, as an alternative source of equine embryos, has been successful and the birth of the first foal reported in 1991. Bruck et al (35) reported an ultrasound-guided transvaginal technique for repeated aspiration of oocytes from cyclic and FSH-treated mares. Thus embryo transfer may be especially useful for obtaining additional progeny from old, infertile brood mares.

## *Applications and Limitations of Embryo Transfer*

Successful embryo transfer depends on various factors including superovulation, estrus detection in the donor and recipients, insemination of the donor, recovery of embryos, short-term storage of embryos *in vitro*, embryo transfer, proper management of the recipient through parturition, and keeping the progeny healthy until useable or saleable. If even one of these steps is done poorly, the entire process may fail.

APPLICATIONS. Embryo transfer can be used to rapidly increase rare bloodlines, to obtain more offspring from valuable females, and to accelerate genetic progress by facilitating progeny testing of females and thus reducing the generation interval.

Embryo transfer is a useful technique that permits critical experimental approaches to problems in genetics, cytology, animal breeding, immunology, evolution, and the physiology and biochemistry of reproduction. For example, the technique can be used to evaluate the relative contributions of the aging oocyte and the aging reproductive tract to decreased reproduction in older animals.

The transport of frozen embryos over long distances can be an inexpensive means of exporting livestock. Frozen bovine embryos were first transported successfully from New Zealand to Australia in 1977. Since then an international trade in frozen embryos of cattle, sheep, and goats has emerged.

For the production of twins in cattle, transferring either a single embryo into each uterine horn of an unmated cow or a second embryo to the contralateral horn of a recipient cow that conceived a few days earlier is more effective than mild superovulation.

ET can play an important role in biotechnology, e.g., production of chimeras and other techniques of micromanipulation of gametes and embryos (see Chapter 31).

Limitations. Embryo transfer methods, however, are not nearly as effective as AI for making genetic progress. One problem is that reproductive rates of donors are increased at the expense of decreased reproductive rates of the recipients because the females in the recipient pool frequently remain nonpregnant for prolonged periods until the embryo is transferred to them.

Risk of Disease Transmission. The risk of disease transmission in the international trade of embryos is of major concern. The zona pellucida (ZP) forms an effective barrier preventing the entry of infectious agents into the embryo proper in cattle, sheep, and pigs. Thus transmission of infectious diseases through the embryo is less likely than live animals or semen. However, some agents adhere firmly to the outer surface of the ZP, especially onto those of the pig (36). The accidental rupture of the zona pellucida during freeze-thaw process might pose problems in the international trade of embryos.

Infection of the embryo may occur at fertilization through infected gametes, or during development within the uterus of the surrogate mother. As stated above, the ZP prevents not only the entry of viruses but also bacteria. For the latter, the uterine flushing media contain antibiotics that are bacteriostatic as well as bactericidal. Thus of major concern is the transmission of viral rather than bacterial diseases.

The chances of disease transmission is greater with frozen than fresh embryos. This is because cracks in the zona pellucida during the freeze-thaw process and the movement of water during thawing could expose the embryo to infectious agents.

Bovine diseases that are of negligible risk of transmission with embryos include leucosis, foot and mouth disease, brucellosis, and blue tongue. All embryos do not require treatment with trypsin to remove viruses sticking to the ZP. On the contrary, infectious bovine rhinotracheitis and pseudorabies must be subjected to trypsin treatment.

Strict governmental control by veterinary certification of health of embryos is still vital. Guidelines for the safe international movement of livestock embryos are provided in the International Animal Health Code of the Office International des Epizooties, and are given in the Manual of the International Embryo Transfer Society. The essence of the recommendations is the washing of embryos ten times in sterile culture medium and, where necessary, trypsin to remove viruses adhering to the ZP.

Sutmoller and Wrathall (37) divided the risk scenario into three phases.

1. The first phase deals with the potential for embryo contamination, which depends on the disease situation in the exporting region, the health status of donor herds and donor cows, and on the pathogenic properties of the disease agent.
2. The second phase covers risk mitigation by use of the internationally accepted standards for embryo processing.
3. The third phase considers the risk reductions resulting from post-collection surveillance of donors and donor herds, and also from testing of embryo-collection (flushing) fluids for the disease agent.

## References


1. Suzuki T, Yamamoto M, Oe M, Takagi M. Superovulation of beef cows and heifers with a single injection of FSH diluted in polyvinylpyrrolidone. Vet Rec 1994;135:41.
2. Twagiramungu H, Guilbault LA, Dufour JJ. Synchronization of ovarian follicular waves with a gonadotropin-releasing hormone agonist to increase the precision of estrus in cattle: a review. J Anim Sci 1995;73:3143.
3. Britt JS, Gaska J. Comparison of two estrus synchronization programs in a large, confinement-housed dairy herd. J Am Vet Med Assoc 1998;212:210.
4. Betteridge KJ. Embryo transfer. In: King GJ, ed. Reproduction in Domesticated Animals. Amsterdam: Elsevier Science Pub, 1993.
5. Gordon I. Controlled Reproduction in cattle and buffaloes. Oxon Cab International, 1996.
6. Gordon I. Controlled Reproduction in sheep and goats. Oxon Cab International, 1996.
7. Seidel GE, Seidel. Training Manual for Embryo Transfer in Cattle. FAO animal production and health paper No. 77, Rome, 1991;164.
8. Bevers MM, Dieleman SJ, Gielen JT, et al. Yield of embryos in PMSG-superovulated cows treated with anti-PMSG six or 18 hours after the peak of luteinizing hormone. Vet Rec 1993;132:186.
9. D'Occhio MJ, Sudha G, Jillella D, et al. Use of a GnRH agonist to prevent endogenous LH surge and injection of exogenous LH to induce ovulation in heifers stimulated with FSH: A new model for superovulation. Theriogenology 1997; 47:601.
10. Evans G, Brooks J, Struthers W, McNeilly AS. Superovulation and embryo recovery in ewes treated with gonadotropin-releasing hormone agonist and purified follicle stimulating hormone. Reprod Fertil Dev 1994;6:247.
11. Kafi M, McGowan MR. Factors associated with variation in the superovulatory response of cattle. Anim Reprod Sci 1997;48:137.

12. Mylne MJA, McKelvey WAC, Fernie K, Mathews K. Use of a transcervical technique for embryo recovery in sheep. Vet Rec 1992;130:450.
13. Pereira RJ, Sohnrey B, Holtz W. Nonsurgical embryo collection in goats treated with prostaglandin F2alpha and oxytocin. J Anim Sci 1998;76:360.
14. McKelvey WAC, Robinson JJ, Aitken RP, Robertson IS. Repeated recoveries of embryos from ewes by laparoscopy. Theriogenology 1986;25:855.
15. Besenfelder U, Modl J, Muller M, Brem G. Endoscopic embryo collection and embryo transfer into the oviduct and the uterus of pigs. Theriogenology 1997;47:1051.
16. Parrish JJ, Susko-Parrish JL, Leibfried-Rutledge ML, Crister ES, Eyestone WE, First NL. Bovine *in vitro* fertilization with frozen-thawed semen. Theriogenology 1986;25:591.
17. Xu KP, Greve T, Greve T, Callesen H, Hyttel P. Pregnancy resulting from cattle oocytes matured and fertilized *in vitro*. J Reprod Fertil 1987;81:501.
18. Reichenbach HD, Wiebke NH, Modl J, Zhu J, Brem G. Laparoscopy through the vaginal fornix of cows for the repeated aspiration of follicular oocytes. Vet Rec 1994;135:353.
19. Kruip TA, Pieterse MC, van Beneden TH, Vos PL, Wurth YA, Taverne MA. A new method for bovine embryo production: a potential alternative to superovulation. Vet Rec 1991; 128:208.
20. Armstrong DT, Kotaras PJ, Earl CR. Advances in production of embryos *in vitro* from juvenile and prepubertal oocytes from the calf and lamb. Reprod Fertil Dev 1997;9:333.
21. Walker SK, Hill JL, Bee CA, Warner DM. Improving the rate of production of sheep embryos using *in vitro* maturation and fertilization. Theriogenology 1994;41:330.
22. Krisher RL, Petters RM, Johnson BH. Effect of oviductal condition on the development of one-cell embryos in mouse or rat oviducts maintained in organ culture. Theriogenology 1989;32:885.
23. Westhusin ME, Slapak JR, Fuller DT, Kraemer DC. Culture of agar-embedded one and two cell bovine embryos and embryos produced by nuclear transfer in the sheep and rabbit oviduct. Theriogenology 1989;31:271.
24. Kassai M. Simple and efficient methods for vitrification of mammalian embryos. Anim Reprod Sci 1996;42:67.
25. Leibo SP. A one-step method for direct non-surgical transfer of frozen-thawed bovine embryos. Theriogenology 1984; 21:767.
26. Sreenan JM. Non-surgical embryo transfer in the cow. Theriogenology 1978;9:69.
27. Galli C, Lazzari G. Practical aspects of IVM/IVF in cattle. Anim Reprod Sci 1996;42:371.
28. Drost M, Wright JM Jr, Cripe WS, Richter AR. Embryo transfer in water buffalo (Bubalus bubalis). Theriogenology 1983;20:579.
29. Madan ML, Das SK, Palta P. Application of reproductive technology to buffaloes. Anim Reprod Sci 1996;42:299.
30. Tervit HR. Laparoscopy/laparotomy oocyte recovery and juvenile breeding. Anim Reprod Sci 1996;42:227.
31. Wang WH, Abeydeera LR, Prather RS, Day BN. Morphologic comparison of ovulated and *in vitro*-matured porcine oocytes, with particular reference to polyspermy after *in vitro* fertilization. Mol Reprod Dev 1998;49:308.
32. Dubuc A, Sirard MA. Effect of coculturing spermatozoa with oviductal cells on the incidence of polyspermy in pig *in vitro* fertilization. Mol Reprod Dev 1995;41:360.
33. Dobrinsky JR. Cryopreservation of pig embryos. J Reprod Fertil 1997;52(Suppl):301.
34. Oguri N, Tsutsumi Y. Non-surgical egg transfer in mares. J Reprod Fertil 1974;42:313.
35. Bruck I, Synnestvedt B, Greve T. Repeated transvaginal oocyte aspiration in unstimulated and FSH-treated mares. Theriogenology 1997;47:1157.
36. Chen SS, Wrathall AE. The importance of the zona pellucida for disease control in livestock by embryo transfer. Brit Vet J 1989;14:129.
37. Sutmoller P, Wrathall AE. The risks of disease transmission by embryo transfer in cattle. Rev Sci Tech 1997;16:226.

## SUGGESTED READING

Dieleman SJ, Bevers MM, Wurth YA, Gielen JT, Willemse AH. Improved embryo yield and condition of donor ovaries in cows after PMSG superovulation with monoclonal antisera administered shortly after the preovulatory LH peak. Theriogenology 1989;9:17.

Totey SM, Singh G, Taneja M, Pawshe CH, Talwar GP. *In vitro* maturation fertilization and development of follicular oocytes from buffalo (Bubalus bubalis). J Reprod Fertil 1992;95:597.

CHAPTER 30

# Preservation and Cryopreservation of Gametes and Embryos

E.S.E. HAFEZ

The main advantage of cryopreservation of embryos instead of just the sperm or oocyte is that the embryo contains the complete genome, i.e., the quota of chromosomes for the individual, and it can be transferred to a foster mother of known or unknown genetic background without the risk of genetic change. Embryo cryopreservation enables animal breeding centers to carry a wider range of stocks and to store stocks not in immediate use, thereby saving space and money as well as affording protection against loss through fire, disease, and other hazards. Inbred strains, mutations, and special genetic combinations can be preserved; this is a valuable asset for advanced research in animal genetics. In addition, genetic pedigree standards can be established and checked for genetic drift in subsequent generations.

Since the pioneering efforts of Audrey Smith in 1952 concerning the effect of low temperature on further development of mammalian ova, much progress in embryo cryopreservation has occurred (Table 30-1). Cryopreservation of embryos of different mammalian species was tried with variable degrees of success. These differences are due to the varied response of certain stages of embryonic development to different biophysical and physiochemical parameters such as cooling media, the nature and concentration protocol of the cryoprotectant used, the type of programmable freezer, the thawing rate, and the dilution protocol of the concentration of the cryoprotectant after thawing. The transport of frozen embryos over long distances is an inexpensive way to export farm animals. The successful transport of frozen bovine embryos from New Zealand to Australia is one example (1, 2).

## PRINCIPLES OF CRYOBIOLOGY

The biophysical principles that apply to cryopreservation of living cells and tissues also apply to cryopreservation of embryos. Embryos may be damaged during cryopreservation and/or thawing either by the formation of large intracellular ice crystals or by the increased intracellular concentration of solutes and accompanying changes that result from the dehydration of cells during cryopreservation (solution effects). Whereas fast freezing minimizes damage from solution effects, it leads to the formation of large ice crystals that cause severe mechanical damage. On the other hand, while slow freezing prevents large ice crystal formation, it leads to increased damage from solution effects. Therefore the optimal freezing rate for a given tissue depends on its relative tolerance to damage from ice crystals and toxicity from solution effects.

When a cell suspension is cooled below 0°C, extracellular ice crystals form, resulting in a concentration of the solutes in the remaining liquid water. The cell membrane acts as a barrier to prevent the spread of ice crystals into the intracellular compartments. Adding cryoprotectants such as glycerol or dimethyl sulfoxide to the freezing medium results in freezing at lower temperatures. This probably retards dehydration of cells and the resultant harmful solution effects; thus, embryos may be cooled slowly enough to prevent the formation of large ice crystals.

The critical ranges of temperature of which low rates are necessary for optimal survival are from −4°C to −60°C during cooling, and from −70°C to −20°C during rewarming.

Mammalian embryos can be preserved for prolonged periods in a state of suspended animation if they are able to withstand cryopreservation to temperatures at which no further biologic activity occurs. Liquid nitrogen at −196°C satisfies this condition. The embryos of cattle, sheep, and mice can survive rapid thawing provided that slow cooling is terminated between −30°C and −50°C by direct transfer to liquid nitrogen at −196°C.

TABLE 30-1. *First Successful Cryopreservation of Mammalian Embryos*

| SPECIES | AUTHORS | YEAR |
|---|---|---|
| Mouse | Whittingham et al. | 1972 |
| | Whittingham et al. | 1979 |
| | Kassai et al. | 1980 |
| | Wood and Farrant | 1980 |
| Rat | Whittingham et al. | 1975 |
| Rabbit | Bank and Maurer | 1974 |
| Cattle | Wilmut and Rowson | 1973 |
| | Willadsen et al. | 1978 |
| Sheep | Willadsen et al. | 1976 |
| | Willadsen | 1977 |
| Goat | Bilton and Moore | 1976 |
| | Bilton and Moore | 1979 |
| Human | Trounson et al. | 1982 |

## CRYOPRESERVATION OF EMBRYOS

Various techniques have been used for cryopreservation and thawing of cattle, sheep, swine, and horses (Table 30-2). Embryos selected for cryopreservation should be of the highest quality and at the correct stage of cleavage. They are handled with sterile techniques using a dissecting microscope. Embryos are transferred to sterile, freshly prepared culture media for microscopic classification and storage until use. If embryos are stored longer than 2 h before transfer, they are transferred into fresh medium every 2 h. The embryos are aspirated into micropipettes with a small volume of medium (less than 0.2 mL) to prevent contamination of the fresh medium. The morphologic classifications of embryos are summarized in Table 30-3.

The embryos are handled gently to avoid any physical damage. Manipulation and evaluation are accomplished as quickly as possible to return the embryos to a stable culture environment. To gain experience with handling embryos, operators are trained to use commercially available micropipettes to pick up sephadix particles with a diameter similar to mammalian eggs. Pieces of debris, unfertilized ova, or degenerating ova can also be used for practice.

### *Embryo Containers*

Embryos are stored in containers that are transparent, sealable, inert, convenient, and of small volume (less than 5 mL). Small, stoppered test tubes can be used, although they must be emptied into another container to locate the embryos under the stereoscope. The medium may be covered with a thin layer of paraffin oil to prevent evaporation, reduce bacterial contamination, and retard the rate of gas exchange between the medium and the atmosphere.

### *Culture and Storage Between 0 and 37°C*

For experimental manipulations and storage between recovery and transfer, embryos are kept in culture medium at 37°C. The development of embryos *in vitro* is slowed to two-thirds of the normal *in vivo* rate. Embryos frequently continue to develop for 2 to 3 days or more, although pregnancy rates are usually reduced if they are transferred after more than 24 h *in vitro* (3).

Embryos can be held in culture for several hours to a day between collection and transfer at ambient temperature (15 to 25°C). If they are cooled to 0 to 10°C or transferred to the ligated oviduct of a rabbit, they can be stored for several days with little reduction in viability. Porcine embryos are an exception and do not survive cooling below 15°C.

Tissue culture medium (TCM 199) or Dulbecco's phosphate-buffered saline (PBS) (which does not require 5% atmosphere) are suitable media and easy to use. TCM 199 with Hanks salts (without phenol red to facilitate locating the embryos) is used to flush out the embryos. Media for embryo storage contains: 25 mM HEPES buffer, and 10 to 20% calf or steer serum which has been Millipore-filtered and heat inactivated for 30 min at 56°C; these macromolecules prevent embryos from sticking to glass or plastic.

### *Embryo Cryopreservation Procedures*

The medium used for cryopreservation is modified Dulbecco's PBS supplemented with bovine serum albumin or serum, with various modifications (4–6). Cryoprotectant is added in steps either at 0° or 20°C. Embryos are cooled rapidly to 0°C and at a rate of 1°C/min to −7°C, at which point freezing is initiated by adding a small crystal of ice to the medium (seeding). Seeding minimizes temperature fluctuations resulting from the heat of fusion. Various types of glassware and computerized freezers are commercially used for cryopreservation and storage of semen and embryos (Figs. 30-1 through 30-4).

### *International Sales of Frozen Bovine Embryos*

Frozen embryos of various cattle breeds and production standards are available. In dairy cattle, for example, Brown Swiss, Holstein, and Jersey embryos have 50,000 to 70,000 production and up to 350-day lactation. Frozen embryos are also available for various beef cattle breeds. Prices of frozen embryos are based on production records and pedigrees.

**Table 30-2. *Summary of Precooling, Cooling, Seeding, Plunging, Storage, and Thawing of Embryos***

| Process | Techniques Employed |
|---|---|
| Collection of embryos | Selection and superovulation of donor, insemination during estrus<br>Collection of embryos from female reproductive tract or ovaries (surgical, nonsurgical, or postmortem)<br>Washing of embryos in sterile culture media<br>Microscopic evaluation and classification of embryos |
| Cryoprotectant solutions | Gradual step-wise concentration of cryoprotectant (DMSO, glycerol, or ready-made cryoprotectant available commercially)<br>Small volume is freshly prepared<br>Solutions to which serum is added are not stored more than 3–5 days, because protein denaturation occurs even under optimal temperatures<br>Solutions are kept refrigerated or frozen until use |
| Precooling preparation | Embryos transferred in serial concentrations of cryoprotectant<br>Straws attached to syringe using rubber adapter to aspirate medium/air bubbles and embryo<br>Straws and cane labeled for future identification<br>Straws heated or filled with phosphate-buffered saline<br>Straws dipped in blue or red PVS at both ends |
| Cooling procedures | Slow cooling rate ranges from 0.5–1.6°C/min<br>Rapid cooling rate ranges from 17–30°C/min<br>Cooling rate 1°C/min from ambient temperature to −7°C<br>Cooling rate 0.3°C/min to −35°C<br>Cooling rate 0.1°C/min to −38°C |
| Freezing, seeding, and plunging | Straws placed in freezer at −6°C and maintained for 10 min<br>Forceps cooled in liquid nitrogen<br>Straws grasped near embryos with cooled forceps until ice crystals form<br>Seeded straw placed into programmable freezer and cooling regimen applied<br>Thermos flask filled with liquid nitrogen<br>Cane containing frozen embryos removed from freezer and plunged into liquid nitrogen<br>Straws loaded in aluminum canes and stored in liquid nitrogen container at −196°C |
| Thawing | Thawing ranges from 20°C/min in slow warming to 360–500°C/min for the rapid thawing; optimal temperature for cryopreservant thawing ranges between 20–37°C<br>Temperature of water bath adjusted to 37°C<br>Color-marked canes identified and straws removed from cane to small canister containing liquid nitrogen; labels are checked before removing from liquid nitrogen<br>Straws are held by neck, placed in 37°C water bath, and removed when ice melts<br>Embryos remain on bottom of vial and are observed under a microscope, counted, and removed with a micropipette to avoid the occasional loss of embryos experienced by washing embryos out of the straw<br>Straws are thawed for 4 s in 37°C water bath and removed when ice melts<br>Water is wiped from straws |
| Cryoprotectant removal | Heat seal or PVC plug cut from tips of straws<br>Embryos washed through drops of serial dilutions of cryoprotectant mixture in sterile petri dish (35 mm diameter)<br>Embryos examined using a stereoscope to evaluate their quality |

Other breeds are available by custom order. Frozen embryos are sold with pedigree, health records, embryo certificates, and required breed registration forms.

The selection of embryo donor and sire matings has been governed by the parents' ability to significantly increase herd averages in the next generation. The use of embryos in developing nations can replace 25 to 30 years of breeding in one generation. Freezing facilitates handling and transporting embryos for transfer, making it superior to animal shipments between countries. Prospective buyers can

TABLE 30-3. ***Morphologic Classification of Embryos Before and After Cryopreservation and Thawing***

| PARAMETERS | CLASSIFICATION | | |
|---|---|---|---|
| Stage of embryonic development | Unfertilized (UFO)<br>2–12 cell<br>Early morula<br>Morula<br>Early blastocyst | | Blastocyst<br>Expanded blastocyst<br>Hatched blastocyst<br>Expanding hatched blastocyst |
| Criteria for classification of embryos | Compactness of blastomeres<br>Regularity in shape of embryo<br>Variation in cell size<br>Color and texture of the cytoplasm<br>Presence of vesicles | | Presence of extruded cells<br>Diameter<br>Regularity of the zona pellucida<br>Presence of cellular debris |
| Quality of embryo | Excellent | Perfect embryo for its stage. Blastomeres are of similar size with even color and texture; they are neither very light nor very dark. Cytoplasm is not granular or unevenly distributed and contains some moderate-sized vesicles. Perivitelline space empty and of regular diameter; zona pellucida even and neither wrinkled nor collapsed | |
| | Good | Trivial imperfections such as an oval zona, a few small excluded blastomeres, and slight asymmetry | |
| | Fair | Definite but not severe problems such as moderate numbers of excluded blastomeres, small size, and small amounts of degeneration | |
| | Poor | Partly degenerate, vesiculated cells, greatly varying cell size, very small, and/or similar problems | |
| | Very Poor | Severely degenerate, probably not worth transferring, unfertilized, zona only, ghostlike, 3 cell, debris, bacteriologic contamination | |
| Artifacts | Air bubble, debris, empty zona pellucida, denuded oviductal epithelium | | |

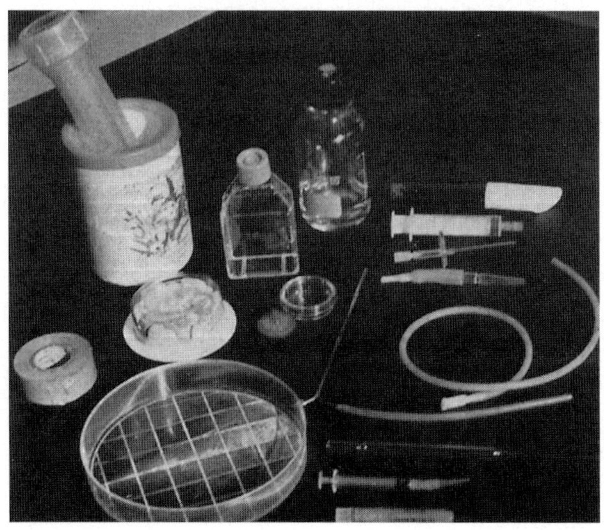

FIGURE 30-1. Glassware used for cryopreservation of embryos.

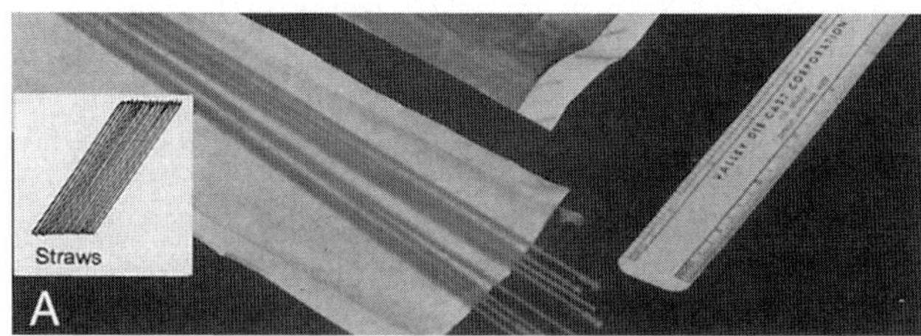


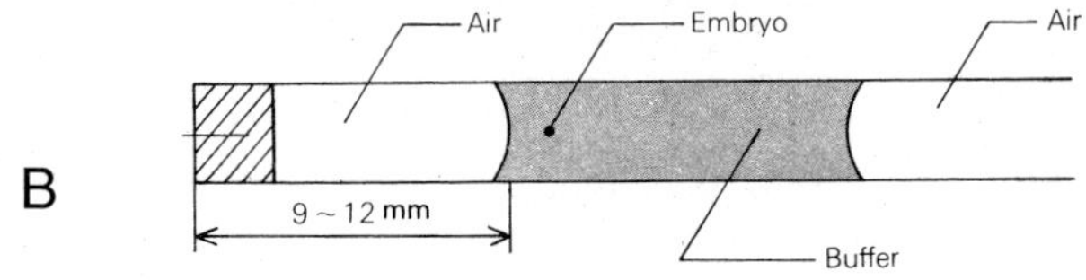


FIGURE 30-2. Various types of straws and ampules used for cryopreservation (A) and the methods used to transfer embryos to straws (B).

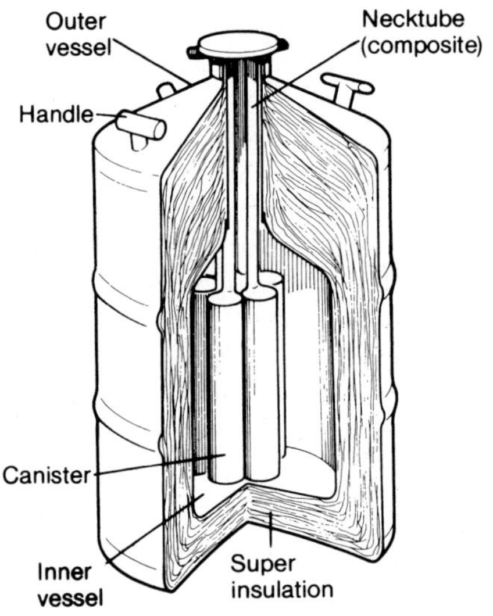


Figure 30-3. Liquid nitrogen containers showing inner construction and including storage area, absorbent, and vacuum and insulation. High-strength aluminum shell is durable and lightweight.

obtain listings of embryos available from any country of origin throughout the world.

## *Equipment, Glassware, and Accessories for Cryopreservation*

The necessary equipment, glassware, and accessories for cryopreservation include the following:

- Programmable freezer for cryopreservation of embryo
- Refrigerator for media, solutions, and hormones
- Liquid nitrogen tank with aluminum canes
- Microscope and stereoscope
- Laminar flow hood
- Quantitative pipettes for preparation of cryoprotectant solutions
- Catheters and pipettes for manipulation of embryos
- Culture dishes of various sizes
- Straws and ampules (Fig. 30-2) and selective sealer to seal ampules

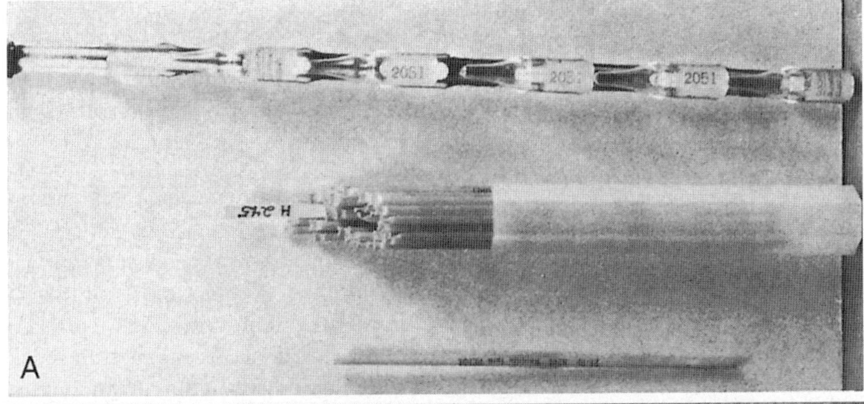


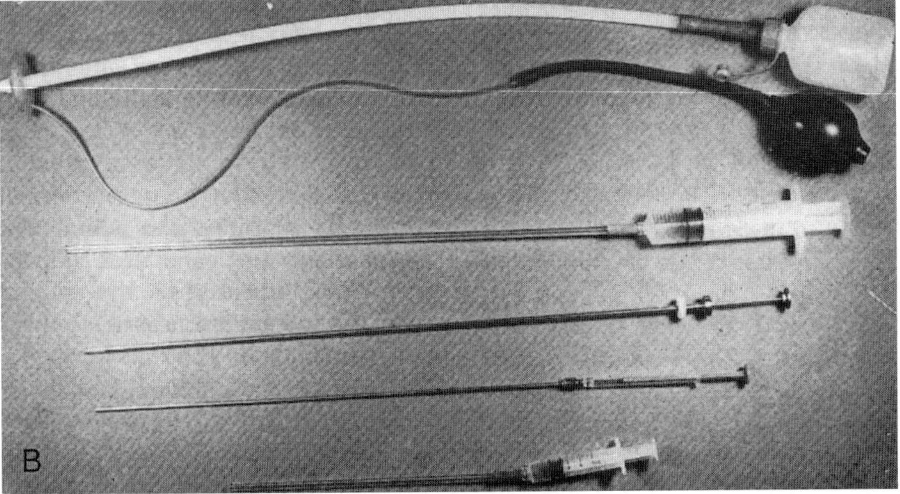


Figure 30-4. (*Top*) A 0.5-mL straw and goblet holding 36 straws in comparison with a 1.0-mL ampule on a six-ampule cane. (*Bottom*) Insemination equipment for sows, mares, cows, ewes, and bitches (top to bottom).

### *Programmable Freezers*

Electronically programmed machines are used to monitor the temperature over the critical phase of the cooling curve before the vials containing embryos are plunged into liquid nitrogen. Several types are completely self-contained and capable of obtaining controlled rates of cryopreservation with or without liquid nitrogen and without mechanical refrigeration devices or the use of conventional refrigerants. These are the three major systems:

a) Freezers with a cylindrical chamber with circulating air cooled by microprocessor controlled thermoelectric cells.
b) Freezers operated with liquid nitrogen.
c) Freezers operated with alcohol or other agents.

Important features of cryopreservation units include the following:

1. Portability (thermoelectric devices are air cooled, which precludes the use of liquid nitrogen or any other compressed gas).
2. Low maintenance without mechanical refrigeration devices.
3. Safety without danger of rapid gas volatilization or mechanical compressors.
4. Warming capabilities (may be warmed rather than cooled by activating a protected button).
5. Digital thermometer for reliable monitoring and subsequent control of the cryogenic program.

### *Thawing of Embryos*

At thawing, the straws containing cryopreserved embryos are transferred from the storage tank of liquid nitrogen to a small container with a wide top and filled with liquid nitrogen. The label is then checked before thawing the straw. Straws are held by the neck, quickly placed in a 37°C water bath, and gently agitated in the water until the ice has disappeared. If care is taken, embryos remain on the bottom of the vial and can be observed easily under a microscope, counted, and removed with a micropipette. This technique avoids the occasional loss of embryos experienced when they are washed out of the vial. Straws can also be directly thawed in a 37°C water bath.

The serial dilution is started with the cryoprotectant solution; allow 10 min for each step. Then the embryos are placed in PBS + 20% fetal calf serum (FCS) for 30 min, and the surviving embryos are transferred. Embryos in straws are ejected and treated as mentioned or diluted in one or two steps within the straw. The various concentrations of cryoprotectants are separated by air bubbles. The embryo can be transferred from one solution to the next one by tapping the straw.

The optimum rate of thawing depends on the cryopreservation technique. A precise thawing curve must also be followed and the embryos rehydrated by bathing in progressively weaker solutions of the cryoprotectant. Using this technique, pregnancy rates of more than 50% can be obtained when freezing the best ova, with poorer quality ova being transferred fresh.

Rapid warming limits the amount of growth of ice crystals in the frozen samples and often results in survival. If the samples have been frozen at a rate slow enough so that the cells are in osmotic equilibrium with the surrounding medium, the rate of warming need not be rapid. Embryos are sensitive to rapid warming, presumably as a result of the large transient osmotic stress that occurs during warming. This stress occurs as the ice is converted into free water, resulting in the transient exposure to a solution which is hypertonic with respect to the inside of cells. Embryos must absorb water from their environment to remain in osmotic equilibrium and to return to their normal isotonic volume. Because most metabolic reactions are arrested or drastically slowed down during cryopreservation, they are especially susceptible to warming or dilution shock at this stage.

### *Procedures to Test Embryo Survival*

The main parameters used to evaluate embryo survival are based on the following:

a) morphologic characteristics before and after freeze/thawing,
b) post-thaw embryo survival,
c) percentage of embryos remaining viable in culture, and
d) treatment × time interaction of (b) and (c).

A scoring system is recommended to grade the embryos after cryopreservation.

Several effective methods are used to evaluate survival after freezing, namely, morphologic appearance on thawing and development in culture; these are closely correlated with the ultimate survival of the frozen embryos. In species where morphologic examination and culture techniques are unreliable, other indirect methods are of value, i.e., transfer to interspecific oviducts and histologic examination. The development of a fluorescent dye test for the examination of these latter embryos would make assessment of viability much simpler. The main procedures to be used for embryos of farm animals is as follows:

1. Embryo viability after thawing is first assessed by testing the ability of the embryo to develop under conditions *in vitro* to the expanded blastocyst stage.
2. A second step includes the assessment of the frozen-thawed embryos' ability to develop into viable fetuses when blastocyst-stage embryos are transferred into pseudopregnant recipients.
3. Nonfrozen embryos are cultured to the blastocyst stage and then transferred to pseudopregnant recipients.

4. The survival of frozen-thawed embryos is compared to the survival of nonfrozen controls from the same animal.

### *Factors Affecting Post-Thaw Embryo Survival*

A number of maternal, technical, and operational factors influence the survival rate of embryos:

a) Physiologic and biophysical characteristics and developmental stage of embryos.
b) Time interval and *in vitro* treatment from embryo collection to initiation of cryopreservation.
c) Type of computerized freezers and program of cryopreservation.
d) Osmotic shock during various stages of cryopreservation.
e) Number of embryos in each straw and percentage of serum albumin in Dulbecco's PBS.
f) Exposure of embryos to excessive light during microscopic examination.
g) Osmotic and colloid osmotic pressures of fluids, prepared media, and cryoprotectants.
h) Nature and extent of "seeding" and "plunging."
i) Microbiologic contaminants in glassware, freezer, and storage.
j) Liquid nitrogen tank.
k) Faults of the freezer, computer, or operator.
l) Synchrony and nature of the recipient on embryo replacements (7).

### *Future Research*

Future research is needed to improve pregnancy rates from the cryopreserved embryos of farm animals. Physiologic and cytologic techniques can be employed to evaluate post-thaw survival of embryos with emphasis on the rate of cryopreservation and thawing, the application of programmable freezers, the maturation of ova transferred into surrogate animal follicles, the optimum number of stepwise concentrations and of dilution of cryoprotectants, the criteria to evaluate the rate of embryo survival, and the possible effects of the culture of embryos before the cryopreservation effects of relative concentration of serum, culture media, and cryoprotectants.

## CRYOPRESERVATION OF SEMEN

The agents that comprise good extending media have the following functions:

a) provide nutrients as a source of energy,
b) protect against the harmful effect of rapid cooling,
c) provide a buffer to prevent harmful shifts in pH as lactic acid is formed,
d) maintain the proper osmotic pressure and electrolyte balance,
e) inhibit bacterial growth,
f) increase the volume of the semen so that it can be used for multiple inseminations, and
g) protect the sperm cells during freezing (8–10).

### *Semen Extenders*

Pure substances and clean equipment should be used to exclude toxic materials from the sperm environment. Extenders should be prepared aseptically and stored for less than a week unless frozen. A simple carbohydrate, such as glucose, usually is added as a source of energy for the sperm. Both egg yolk and milk are used to protect against cold shock of the sperm cells as they are cooled from body temperature to 5°C. These substances also contain nutrients used by sperm. A variety of buffers may be used to maintain a nearly neutral pH and an osmotic pressure of approximately 300 mMol, which is equivalent to that of semen, blood plasma, and milk. To inhibit the growth of microorganisms in semen, penicillin, streptomycin, polymyxin B, or other combinations of antibiotics are added.

Bovine semen is usually diluted with egg yolk-citrate solution, homogenized whole milk, fresh and dried skim milk, coconut milk, or lactose solution. Semen has been successfully preserved in diluents based on the organic buffer, Tris(hydroxymethyl)aminomethane.

Buffer solutions such as phosphate or a 3.2% 2,9-trisodium citrate dihydrate adjusted to pH 6.9 by the addition to citric acid have been commonly used in combination with egg yolk. The addition of citric acid is unnecessary because the egg yolk component (20% by volume) has sufficient buffering capacity to return the pH to neutral.

The ultimate goal of semen preservation is to obtain pregnancies after artificial insemination as effectively as after natural mating. This depends on several factors apart from semen quality. Semen of farm animals was successfully cryopreserved more than 30 years ago; however, the techniques have been continually modified and improved. Semen cryopreservation, formerly in solid carbon dioxide (dry ice at −79°C), has been replaced with liquid nitrogen (−196°C) with the advantage of a more stable condition of the cryopreserved semen. The application of cryopreservation procedures has been more successful in cattle than in other species of farm animals. The freezability (post-thaw survival of cryopreserved semen) varies between species and among individual males of the same species. These species and individual variations are related to the biophysical and biochemical characteristics of sperm membranes. The functional integrity of cryopreserved-thawed semen is evaluated by its capacity to fertilize the ovum and to sustain embryogenesis.

The survival of ejaculated sperm in seminal plasma alone is limited to a few hours. To maintain sperm for longer periods and to cool or cryopreserve semen, dilution with a protective solution is necessary. Different solutions have been used as diluents or extenders for semen, most of which are variations of a few principal formulas.

Kallikrein and caffeine seem to stimulate sperm motility when added to semen after thawing. The action of caffeine is probably brought about by its stimulation of cyclic adenosine monophosphate (cAMP) levels in the sperm. Such additives are of doubtful value because they would be removed during sperm transport through the female reproductive tract.

Glycerol usually is added to protect sperm against the otherwise lethal effects of freezing. Dimethysulfoxide (DMSO) and sugars such as lactose and raffinose also may be beneficial, as they serve as dehydrating agents.

Practically all extenders for liquid or frozen semen have either egg yolk or heated milk or a combination of the two as basic ingredients. Egg yolk, simply combined with sodium citrate or organic buffers and heated milk or skim milk, has been used widely for bull semen, and with modifications for ram, buck, boar, and stallion semen.

For many years, the emphasis in artificial insemination (AI) programs was on the use of unfrozen semen. Numerous extender formulations were recommended (11). The ones used most widely were egg yolk buffered with sodium citrate or tris, or heated milk extenders for bull semen. These were adapted for use with other species. With the remarkable discovery by Polge and coworkers of the protective effect of glycerol during freezing, the emphasis shifted to the use of frozen semen. Even with the best freezing techniques, more sperm must be put into each breeding unit than with liquid (unfrozen) semen, because of the loss of some viable cells during freezing.

In areas where little refrigeration is available, semen may be stored at ambient temperatures. A carbonated egg-yolk extender called Illinois Variable Temperature extender (IVT) and coconut milk have given satisfactory fertility when semen was stored for up to a few days at moderate ambient temperatures. Most cattle are inseminated with frozen semen. This offers the user a wide variety or choice. It permits semen to be collected at one time and place and to be used anywhere, even after long periods of storage, provided that it is stored continuously at −196°C with a good supply of liquid nitrogen.

Pelleting extended bull semen and freezing it on solid carbon dioxide (dry ice) is practiced in a few countries. A sugar such as raffinose or 11% lactose may be used. Pellets offer an inexpensive way of preserving sperm, but they are difficult to properly identify when large numbers of bulls are involved. However, in some species in which successful freezing of sperm is difficult, the pellet method has been the most successful. Goat semen can be frozen in skim milk with about 9 g of glucose per liter and 7% glycerol by volume (12). Glycerol is detrimental to boar fertility (13), and 2% by volume or less is included in the extended semen during freezing. Some frozen boar semen is available commercially.

Stallion semen also can be pelleted or frozen in straws. Egg yolk-tris cream-gelatin extenders also have been used (14). Glycerol depresses the fertility of stallion semen; semen from some stallions freezes poorly, so the methods of freezing stallion semen are less than optimal (15). Nevertheless, commercial AI with frozen stallion semen has been successful. Vegetable dyes may be included in the extender at sufficient concentrations to distinctly color it. This will not harm the sperm and facilitates identification of semen from different males or breeds.

## *Semen Processing*

The processing of semen through cooling it to 5°C is similar whether it is to be used frozen or unfrozen. Semen is collected at body temperature. Following collection, it is kept warm (30°C) before extension to avoid cold shock. This is done by placing semen and extender in a water bath kept at 30°C. An aliquot of semen is removed for sample evaluation, and the remainder can be mixed with three to four parts of extender at 30°C. It is recommended that semen be held for 30 min at 30°C to increase the antibiotic action of the extender. The mixture is cooled gradually to 5°C for all species, except unfrozen boar semen, which usually is held at 15°C. Buck semen frequently is centrifuged first to prevent possible coagulation (12). Cooling should be slow, taking at least 1 h to cool the mixture from 30 to 5°C. Cooling usually is done with a surrounding water jacket to prevent cold shock.

EXTENSION OF SEMEN. Semen is extended at specific rates so that the volume of semen inseminated will contain sufficient sperm to give high fertility without wasting many cells.

Extension rates are higher with unfrozen semen than with frozen semen. Unfrozen bull semen can be extended 200 to 300 times with fewer than 5 million motile cells per insemination required for high fertility. Processing liquid semen after cooling to 5°C (or 15°C for boar semen) is simple. Tubes of extended semen should be nearly full to avoid excess air and agitation in shipment. They should be packaged in a manner that maintains the temperature constant and avoids exposure to light. With unfrozen bull, buck, ram, boar, and especially stallion semen, fertility declines within a few days of collection. It is recommended that semen be used the day of collection or the next day.

GLYCEROL ADDITION FOR FREEZING BULL SEMEN. Glycerol is used almost universally as the cryoprotective agent for freezing semen. The amounts and methods of adding glycerol vary, depending on the extenders, freezing methods, and species.

Glycerol usually is added to semen after cooling to 5°C; however, it affords just as much protection when added just before freezing. The final amount varies from less than 5% in some yolk-sugar media to 10% in milk. Some add glycerol slowly by dripping or by adding small amounts over a period of 1 h; others recommend a one-step addition. Extended semen normally is held for several hours at 5°C before freezing. Tris buffers and the sugar buffers used with pellet freezing offer the advantage that glycerol can be included in the initial media used for cooling sperm.

The semen-extender mixture is held for several hours before freezing to allow sperm cells to equilibrate with the extender (usually 5°C). About 4 to 6 h are optimal, depending on the medium used.

Bull sperm are packaged in three ways:

a) polyvinyl chloride straws containing 0.25 to 0.5 mL of extended semen;
b) glass ampules containing 0.5 to 1 mL;
c) pellets containing approximately 0.1 to 0.2 mL.

When the smaller volumes are frozen as a unit, the sperm concentration per milliliter is increased correspondingly, so that the total sperm per insemination dose is maintained. For example, semen frozen in 0.1-mL packages should have ten times as many sperm per unit volume as semen frozen 1.0-mL packages in order to contain the same total number of sperm.

Ampules provide a sterile container that can be automatically labeled, filled, and sealed. The latter prevents any cross-contamination. Each ampule contains sufficient sperm for a single insemination. Six to eight ampules are attached to a metal cane (Fig. 30-2), which also carries the bull's identification.

Pelleted semen is prepared by pipetting about 0.1-mL drops of extended semen into hemispheric depressions made in a block of dry ice. Sperm survival is good following freezing. Pellets take little space when they are stored in bulk; they offer the cheapest storage method. The main disadvantage is the difficulty of placing bull identification on each pellet, although this has been done by incorporating a small printed paper disc during freezing.

**FREEZING BULL SEMEN.** Mechanical freezers and freezers using dry ice, liquid air, liquid $O_2$, and liquid $N_2$ have all been tried successfully. Liquid $N_2$ has increased in popularity because it is also the refrigerant of choice for low-temperature, long-time storage of semen. Extended semen frozen as pellets, in straws, or in ampules is held at about 5°C before freezing. Straws usually are frozen in nitrogen vapor and stored at −196°C. Because of the large surface area of the straw and its thin wall, heat transfer is rapid and semen freezes rapidly, usually within a few minutes. Ampules often are frozen at about 3°C per minute to −15°C. At this point, the rate of freezing is increased until −150°C is reached. The ampules on canes then are transferred to liquid $N_2$ at −196°C. Freezing too rapidly may cause thermal shock and internal ice formation. Slow freezing causes salt concentrations to increase as water freezes out. This increase in osmotic pressure over a prolonged period of slow freezing may damage the proteins and lipoproteins of the sperm and the acrosome.

A variety of efficient vacuum-sealed liquid $N_2$ refrigerators is available for storing frozen semen. These range in size from central units with a storage capacity of several hundred thousand 0.25-mL "ministraws" or 0.5-mL "midistraws" with an $N_2$ reserve that lasts about 6 months, to the common field units that hold up to several thousand straws and an $N_2$ reservoir that lasts for up to 6 weeks. Ampules require more space; pellets stored in bulk occupy the least space. The large central storage units can hold up to 750,000 0.1-mL pellets and possibly provide economic banking of semen from young bulls in sampling programs. In some countries, after a large number of "breeding units" is frozen, the bulls are slaughtered, thereby decreasing total costs.

It is extremely important to check the liquid nitrogen refrigerator periodically to see that the nitrogen level is maintained. Loss of all liquid nitrogen, permitting the temperature to rise considerably, can result in killing the sperm, even when the semen still appears to be frozen.

**THAWING BULL SEMEN.** Frozen semen should be held continuously at low temperatures until used. After thawing, frozen sperm do not survive as long as unfrozen sperm, and they refreeze poorly. Therefore, one must be certain that the semen will be used soon once it has been thawed. Straws have been successfully thawed at temperatures ranging from that of ice water to 65°C or higher. Thaw time must be controlled carefully to avoid killing the cells by overheating. It is recommended that under field conditions ampules be thawed in ice water; this takes about 8 min. Higher temperatures (37°C) may be superior for straws but may depend on the extender. Pellets are best thawed in a liquid medium at 40°C, but under practical field conditions, an ice-water thawing bath is easier to maintain and is satisfactory.

**FROZEN SEMEN OF OTHER FARM ANIMALS.** The same general principles described for cattle semen appear to apply to handling frozen semen of other species. However, AI with frozen semen has not been developed extensively on a commercial scale for these species. Either the semen has been more difficult to freeze, resulting in lower fertility, or problems with the management of the females, including detection of estrus, have not made AI programs with frozen semen attractive or economic on an extensive basis.

Ram semen can be pelleted or frozen in straws with a milk, yolk-lactose, or yolk-tris extender. Semen collected during the normal breeding season freezes well. In the pellet method, the semen is cooled to 5°C, glycerol added as necessary, and the semen held for about 2 h before freezing as 0.1-mL to 0.4-mL pellets on dry ice. Storage is in liquid nitrogen at −196°C. Pellets are thawed in a solution similar to the freezing extender but with glycerol and egg yolk omitted. Sperm should be concentrated by centrifugation and a small volume containing the desired number of sperm cells (Table 30-4) inseminated, if possible, through the cervix. Fertility is considerably higher, and fewer sperm are required with intrauterine insemination (Fig. 30-4).

Buck (goat) sperm also can be frozen with good survival when semen is collected during the breeding season. The semen is pre-extended, centrifuged, and resuspended in heated milk (12) or yolk-tris media (16). The centrifugation removes seminal plasma, which contains an enzyme that can cause coagulation. Following cooling, the semen is frozen in straws and stored at −196°C. Thawing should be done quickly, and intrauterine insemination is highly desirable, if possible.

Boar semen has been difficult to freeze, but there are several successful methods (17, 18). Sperm survival is improved by holding the raw semen for 2 h to expose sperm cells to the seminal plasma. Then the cell concentration is increased by centrifugation, extender is added, and the extended semen is cooled to 5°C (Table 30-5). About 2% by volume of glycerol is added, and the semen pelleted as described previously. Following storage at −196°C, enough pellets are rapidly thawed in a solution such as that given in Table 30-6 to provide the necessary sperm for insemination.

The success with which stallion semen can be frozen varies greatly. The Nagase type of yolk-lactose-glycerol or yolk-raffinose-glycerol extender, or a more complex extender (19), can be used for straws as well. Only the sperm-rich fraction is collected, or much of the seminal plasma is removed by centrifugation. Semen is extended and cooled to 5°C. Stallion sperm are sensitive to glycerol and this compound may be added just before freezing. Storage is at −196°C. The fertility of stallion semen is decreased by freezing.

### *Evaluation of Sperm Motility*

Sperm motility is evaluated before cryopreservation and again after thawing. To evaluate sperm motility before cryopreservation, semen samples are diluted 1 : 20 in the same medium used for cryopreservation. The hemocytometer is filled then placed in a moist atmosphere for 3 min to stabilize before observation. The percentage of sperm with progressive forward motility, an important indicator of fertilizability, is evaluated. The number of sperm with forward

TABLE 30-4. *Extension, Storage, and Insemination Requirements with Frozen Semen (Based on Average Conditions)*

| | ALL FROZEN SEMEN | | | | |
|---|---|---|---|---|---|
| PARAMETERS | *Cattle* | *Sheep* | *Goat* | *Swine* | *Horse* |
| Extension rate of 1 mL semen (mL) | 10–75 | 5–10 | 10–25 | 4 | 2 |
| Inseminatin dose | | | | | |
| Volume (mL) | 0.2–1 | 0.05–0.2 | 0.5 | 50 | 20–50 |
| Motile sperm ($10^6$) | 15 | 200 | 200 | 5000 | 1500 |
| Best time to inseminate during estrus | 9 h after onset to end of estrus | 10–12 h after onset of estrus | 12–36 h after onset of estrus | 15–30 h after onset of estrus | Every second day, starting on day 2 of estrus |
| Site of semen deposition | Uterus and cervix | Uterus if possible | Uterus if possible | Cervix into uterus | Uterus |
| Number of breeding units per male | | | | | |
| Per ejaculate | 300 | 15 | 15 | 10 | 5 |
| Per week | 1000 | 150 | 150 | 30 | 15 |

**TABLE 30-5. *Cooling, Freezing, and Thawing Procedure of Bovine Embryos***

| | |
|---|---|
| Two step addition of glycerol | (5%, 10%) |
| ↓ | Place at −6°C |
| −6°C | Hold for 5–10 min |
| ↓ | Seed |
| −33°C | 0.3°C/min |
| Plunge into liquid nitrogen | |
| ↓ | |
| Thaw at 37°C | |
| ↓ | |
| Evaluate and record results | |
| ↓ | |
| Dilute out cryoprotectant in 4 steps | *or* 2 steps with sucrose |
| 7.5% glycerol in PBS with serum | |
| 5.0% glycerol in PBS with serum | |
| 2.5% glycerol in PBS with serum | *or* sucrose in PBS with serum |
| 0% glycerol in PBS with serum | PBS with serum |
| ↓ | |
| Wash 3 times in PBS | |
| Evaluate and record results | |

**TABLE 30-6. *Some Biophysical Characteristics of Some Cryoprotectants***

| PARAMETERS | DMSO | GLYCEROL | ETHYLENE GLYCOL |
|---|---|---|---|
| Chemical formula | $(CH_3)_2SO$ | $C_3H_5(OH)_3$ | $(CH_2OH)_2$ |
| Molecular weight | 78.13 | 92.10 | 62.07 |
| Specific gravity ($g/cm^3$ at 20°C) | 1.10 | 1.25 | 1.11 |
| Mass (g/L) | | | |
| 1.0 M | 78.13 | 92.10 | 62.07 |
| 3.0 M | 234.39 | 276.30 | 186.21 |
| Volume (mL/L) | | | |
| 1.0 M | 71.00 | 73.70 | 55.90 |
| 3.0 M | 213.10 | 221.10 | 167.70 |
| Grade | Laboratory Grade | Laboratory Grade | Laboratory Grade |
| Sigma Chemical Catalog No. | D-5879 | G-7757 | E-9129 |

· Specific gravity: the ratio of the weight of a given volume of a substance to the weight of the same volume of water at 0°C.

movement is divided by the total number of sperm (motile and nonmotile) and multiplied by 100.

When cryopreserved semen is thawed, it is transferred from the liquid nitrogen tank to a controlled water bath at 37°C for 3 to 5 min, or to an automatic thawing unit. Motility is estimated immediately after thawing and after 30 or 60 min of incubation at 37°C. Sperm motility is compared after cryopreservation with motility before cryopreservation to evaluate the effect of cryoprotectant on the cryosurvival:

$$\text{Recovery Rate} = (\text{Motility after freezing}) / (\text{Initial motility before freezing}) \times 100\%$$

## REFERENCES


1. Bilton RJ, Moore NW. *In vitro* culture, storage and transfer of goat embryos. Aust J Biol Sci 1976;29:125–129.
2. Bilton RJ, Moore NW. Proceedings: storage of cattle embryos. J Reprod Fertil 1976;46:537–538.
3. Davis DL, Day BN. Cleavage and blastocyst formation by pig eggs *in vitro*. J Anim Sci 1978;46:1043.
4. Hafez ESE. Reproduction in Farm Animals, 6th ed. Philadelphia: Lea & Febiger, 1993.
5. Bilton RJ, Moore NW. Factors affecting the viability of frozen stored cattle embryos. Aust J Biol Sci 1979;32:101–107.
6. Schneider U, Maurer RR. Factors affecting survival of frozen-thawed mouse embryos. Biol Reprod 1983;29:121.
7. Schneider J, Maurer RR. Factors affecting survival of frozen-thawed mouse embryos. Biol Reprod 1983;29:121.
8. Berndtson WE, Pickett BW. Techniques for the cryopreservation and field handling of bovine spermatozoa. In: The Integrity of Frozen Spermatozoa. Washington, DC: Conf Natl Acad Sci 1978;53–57.
9. Foote RW. Semen quality from the bull to the freezer: an assessment. Theriogenology 1975;3:219
10. Graham EF. Fundamentals of the preservation of spermatozoa. In: The Integrity of Frozen spermatozoa. Washington, DC: Proc Conf Natl Acad Sci 1978;4–44.
11. Salisbury GW, VanDemark NL, Lodge JR. Physiology of Reproduction and Artificial Insemination of Cattle, 2nd ed. San Francisco: WH Freeman, 1978.
12. Corteel JM. Production, storage and insemination of goat semen. Proceedings of the Symposium on Management of Reproduction in Sheep and Goats. Am Soc Anim Sci 1977;41–57.
13. Wilmut I, Polge C. The low temperature preservation of boar spermatozoa. (3) The fertilizing capacity of frozen and thawed semen. Cryobiology 1977;14:483.
14. Pickett BW, et al. Effect of seminal extenders on equine fertility. J Anim Sci 1975;40:1136.
15. Sullivan JJ. Characteristics and cryopreservation of stallion spermatozoa. Cryobiology 1978;15:355.

16. Fougner UA. Uterine insemination with frozen semen in goats. VIII Int Congr Anim Reprod Artif Insem Krakow. 1976;4:987.
17. Pursel VG, Johnson LA. Freezing of boar spermatozoa: fertilizing capacity with concentrated semen and new thawing procedure. J Anim Sci 1975;40:99.
18. Larsson K. Deep-freezing of boar semen. Cryobiology 1978; 15:352.
19. Nishikawa Y, Iritani A, Shinomiya S. Studies on the protective effects of egg yolk and glycerol on the freezability of horse spermatozoa. VII Int Congr Anim Reprod Artif Insem Munich 1972;1545.

## SUGGESTED READING

Bilton RJ, Moore NW. Factors affecting the viability of frozen stored cattle embryos. Aust J Biol Sci 1979;32: 101–107.

Pace MM, Sullivan JJ. A biological comparison of the .5 ml ampule and .5 ml French straw systems for packaging bovine spermatozoan. NAAB Proc 7th Tech Conf Artif Insem Reprod 1978;22–32.

Salamon S. Artificial Insemination of Sheep. Sidney, Australia: University of Sidney NSW, 1976.

CHAPTER 31

# Micromanipulation of Gametes and Embryos: In Vitro Fertilization and Embryo Transfer (IVF/ET)

B. HAFEZ AND E.S.E. HAFEZ

This chapter is an illustrative brief review dealing with recent advances in the following parameters:

a) Genetic engineering: emphasis on chromosome/genes; micromanipulation of gametes, embryos, and zona pellucida of cattle, sheep, and horses.
b) Gamete interaction: recognition between sperm receptors and oocyte receptors located on the zona pellucida, and cloning.
c) Intracytoplasmic injection (ICSI).
d) Molecular andrology: spermatid/Sertoli cell interaction, spermicidal activity.
e) Instrumentation, water/air filtration, culture/coculture/organ culture media and macromolecular supplementation.

## GENETIC ENGINEERING

Fertilization involves the union of the DNA of the nucleus in the sperm head with the DNA in the nucleus of the ovum. The egg undergoes complex maturational changes known as *meiosis* before it is ready for fertilization. These changes begin during fetal life and are completed only after ovulation and sperm penetration.

### Chromosomes and Genes

Chromosomal arrangements occur during mitosis/meiosis (Fig. 31-1). Normally the ovum (X) is fertilized by sperm X or sperm Y. In abnormal cases of nondisjunction of oogenesis or spermatogenesis, fertilization may occur between an abnormal sperm and/or an abnormal egg resulting in various chromosomal anomalies (Tables 31-1 and 31-2). Structural anomalies of the chromosomes include translocation, deletions, rings, and inversions of chromosomes during either mitosis or meiosis. Such anomalies effect individual autosomes or sex chromosomes.

The animal cell comprises a nucleus, protein-manufacturing units, and energy-production points. Spiraling double strands of atoms are the DNA, the master chemical of genes. The sequence or layout of these atoms contains all the instructions the cell needs to function. Recent advances in genetic engineering enable scientists to uncover, rearrange, and make copies, or clones of genes. For example, each human or animal cell contains some 100,000 genes. At least 22,000 of these genes have been isolated, and some of their specific functions have been identified.

## MICROMANIPULATION OF GAMETES, EMBRYOS, AND ZONA PELLUCIDA

Micromanipulation of embryos has shown that the embryos, in spite of a great reduction in their cell number, can develop through early cleavage (1) and to blastocyst formation (2). The simple bisection of fully compacted late morulae or early blastocysts allows the production of identical twins

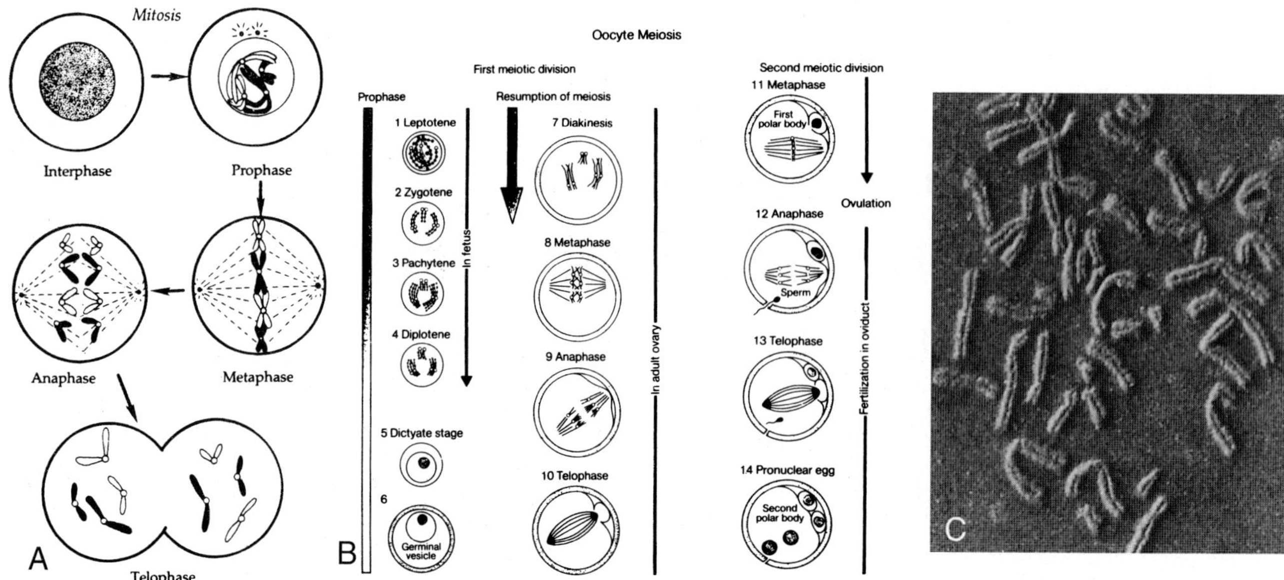


FIGURE 31-1. Chromosome arrangement during mitosis and meiosis. (**A**) Chromosome arrangement during mitosis. (Feingold M, Pashaya H. In: The Chromosome, Genetics and Birth Defects in Clinical Practice. Boston: Little Brown, 1983;2.) (**B**) Oocyte meiosis. For simplicity, only three pairs of chromosomes are depicted. Prophase stages (*1 to 4*) of the first meiotic division that occur in most mammals during fetal life. The meiotic process is arrested at the diplotene stage (first meiotic arrest), and the oocyte enters the dictyate stages (*5 to 16*). When meiosis is resumed, the first maturation division is completed (*7 to 11*). Ovulation occurs usually at the metaphase II stage (*11*), and the second meiotic division (*12 to 14*) takes place in the oviduct only following sperm penetration. (Tsafriri A, Bar-Ami S, Lindner HR. Control of the development of meiotic competence and of oocyte maturation in mammals. In: Fertilization of the Human Egg *In Vitro*. Berlin: Springer Verlag, 1983.). (**C**) Scanning electron micrograph of chromosomes.

in routine embryo transplantation procedures. Methods of producing identical twins, however, can only be fully explored in association with techniques of cryopreservation, which would permit transfer of each "half" of the same embryo at different times (Fig. 31-3). After the first irreversible cellular differentiation that occurs at the blastocyst stage, it is still possible to produce identical cattle twins by bisection of the day-8 blastocyst (3).

Embryo multiplication by nuclear transplantation has been successful in several domestic species: cattle, sheep, pigs, and rabbits. Several sets of clones are used as animal models for research on pathology or nutrition. Work con-

TABLE 31-1. *Types and Physiologic Mechanisms of Chromosome Anomalies*

| | | |
|---|---|---|
| Types of chromosome anomalies | Monosomy | Absence of one chromosome |
| | Trisomy: single | One additional chromosome |
| | Trisomy: double | Two additional chromosomes |
| | Polyploidy | One or two additional haploid sets |
| | Structural anomaly of chromosomes | Unbalanced chromosome constitution |
| Physiologic mechanisms of chromosome anomalies | Errors during oogenesis causing chromosomally abnormal ova | |
| | Errors during spermatogenesis causing chromosomally abnormal sperm | |
| | Errors during early stages of cleavage of zygote | |

TABLE 31-2. ***Normal and Abnormal Sex-Chromosome Constitutions Arising at Fertilization***

| SPERM | | OVA | | |
|---|---|---|---|---|
| | | Normal X | Nondisjunctive XX | O |
| Normal | X | XX (normal female) | XXX | XO |
| | Y | XY (normal male) | XXY | YO |
| Nondisjunctive | XY | XXY | | |
| | XX | XXX | | |
| | YY | XYY | | |
| | O | XO | | |

From McLaren A. Fertilization, cleavage and imaging plantation. In: Hafez ESE, ed. Reproduction in Farm Animals 4th ed. Philadelphia: Lea & Febiger, 1980. An O sperm or ovum is one that carries neither an X nor a Y chromosome. Nondisjunctive gametes arise through faulty sharing-out (nondisjunction) of the sex chromosomes. YO individuals probably are not viable; XXX individuals, in humans, are abnormal females.

cerns the biochemical characterization of the recipient cytoplasm at the time of introduction of foreign nucleus. Preactivation treatment of the cytoplasm induces an interphasic stage that matches the cell cycle stage of most donor nuclei. Chromatin reorganization after nuclear transfer as it affects normal development of nuclear transfer embryos is a key area for research (4–10).

## ZONA PELLUCIDA

The zona pellucida is an extracellular glycoprotein matrix. These glycoprotein deposits are assembled during the growth phase. The zona does not attain the full ability to be recognized and penetrated until the final stages of oocyte maturation. Throughout the maturation stage of the oocyte, the zona pellucida undergoes various ultrastructural changes.

During the period from germinal vesicle breakdown until metaphase I, the oocyte secretes proteoglycan-type molecules into the developing zona pellucida. During subsequent phases of meiotic maturatin (between metaphases I and II) the zona becomes more penetrable by sperm, due to the presence of proteoglycan-filled pores that develop in its structure. The zona pellucida serves various important functions:

a) during the induction of sperm acrosome reaction which is stimulated upon exposure of sperm to intact or digested zonae,
b) species-specific fertilization,
c) during cleavage, and
d) hatching of the blastocyst.

Release (hatching) of the blastocyst from the zona pellucida occurs in the uterus 4 to 8 days postovulation according to the species.

In the rabbit, zona removal occurs through an enzymatic (termed blastomase) dissolution of the zona layer by cells of the underlying trophoblast. Zona layer removal by the mouse may involve rhythmic expansions and contractions of the blastocyst aided by production of zona lysin from the estrogen-sensitized uterine epithelium. Changes in zona integrity that are due to enzymatic factors produced by the uterus or embryo have been implicated in hatching of pig blastocysts (11).

Exposure to the estrogen-stimulated uterine environment may cause a softening of the zona pellucida. The blastocyst appears to play the major role in hatching as zona becomes torn by distension of the blastocyst to squeeze between the two edges of the opening. Expansion of the blastocyst involves both cellular hyperplasia and fluid accumulation in the blastocoele. Fluid accumulation within the blastocoele appears to assist the hatching process since prostaglandin antagonists prevent both blastocyst expansion and hatching.

Extensive investigations have been carried out on surface properties of the zona pellucida (12), on the specificity of sperm-egg interactions (13), and on the mechanics of fertilization (13). The transfer of pronuclei between eggs has been employed to assess changes induced in the development of embryos following an unusual pronuclear history. Eggs with two female pronuclei can result from various forms of parthenogenetic activation, or from the use of micromanipulation to remove and insert specific pronuclei into the oocytes. Gynogenetic embryos, those containing two female pronuclei, develop abnormally; this is especially evident in their extraembryonic tissues. Micromanipulation is also used to establish mammalian eggs containing two male pronuclei.

Several techniques of embryo micromanipulation have been used to produce identical twins in cattle, sheep, and pigs (1, 14–16). The success of the technique depends on the use of agar gel to seal incisions made in the zona pellucida

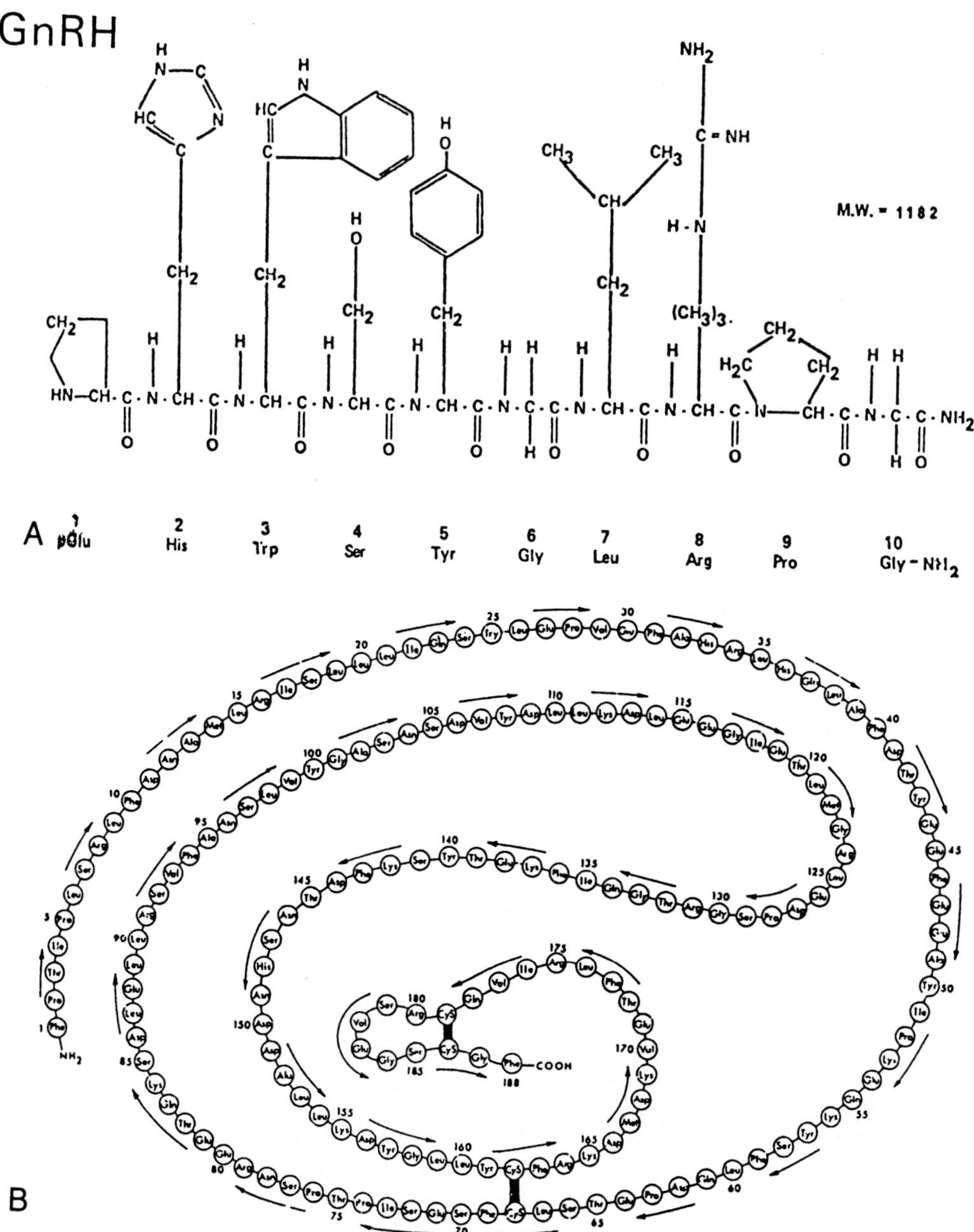


FIGURE 31-2. (A) Amino acid sequence of gonadotropin-releasing hormone (GnRH). (From Capen CC, Martin SL. The pituitary gland. In: McDonald LE, Pineda MH, eds. Veterinary Endocrinology and Reproduction. Philadelphia: Lea & Febiger, 1989.) (B) Amino acid sequence of the human somatotropin hormone (STH) molecule (Adapted from Lich, 1969).

during micromanipulation. The agar protects the blastomeres from damage by uterine secretions and leukocytes until the embryo has developed sufficiently to survive *in utero* without a zona (Figs. 31-3 through 31-5).

## *Protocol*

a) Eggs are obtained by superovulation denuded of cumulus cells with 0.1% hyaluronidase.
b) Zona pellucidae are then isolated when eggs are drawn into a micropipette with an inner diameter of about 60 $\mu$m and the contents are expelled.
c) The zonae are separated from the vitelli and washed several times (17).
d) The blastomeres of two-cell to eight-cell horse embryos recovered surgically 1 to 3 days after ovulation from pony mares were mechanically separated and inserted, in various combinations, into evacuated pig zona pellucidae to make "half" (demi) and "quarter" micromanipulated embryos.
e) The embryos are then embedded in agar and cultured *in vivo* in ligated oviducts of ewes for 3 1/2 to 5 days to allow development to the late morula-early blastocyst stage.

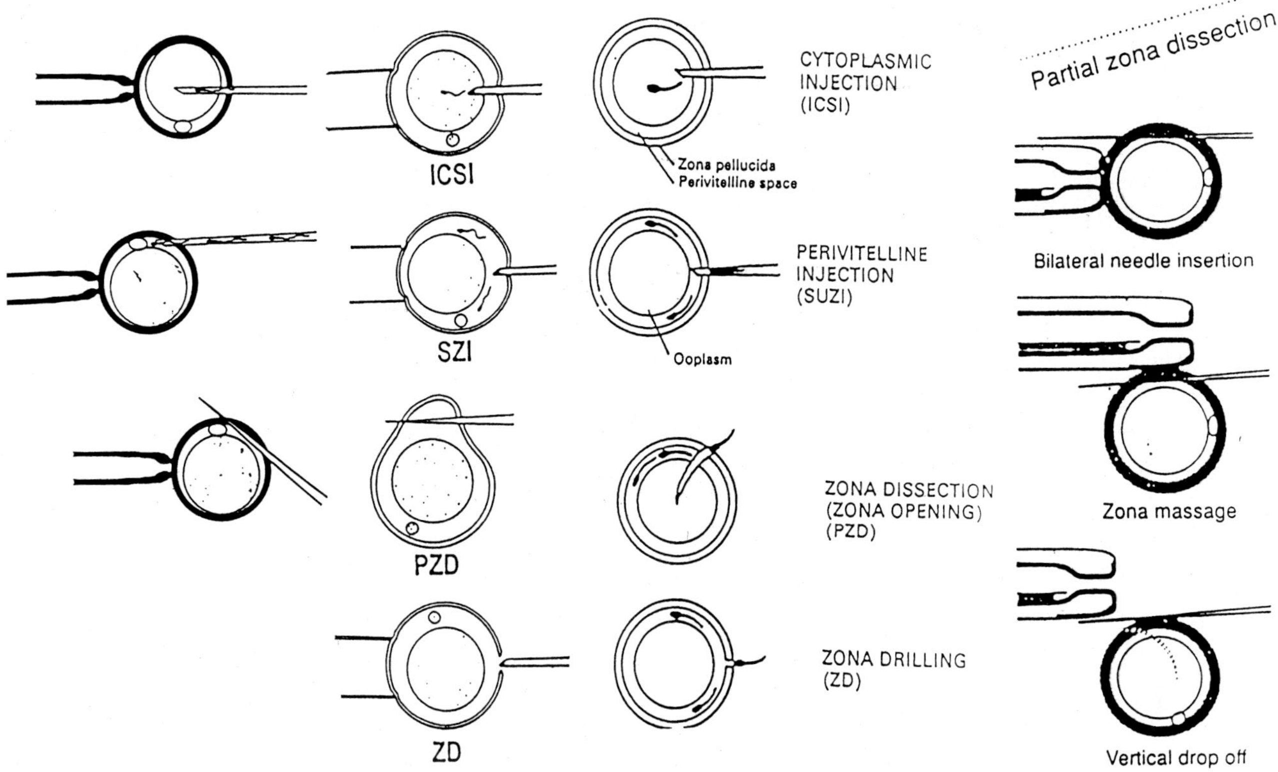


FIGURE 31-3. Patterns of micromanipulation of oocytes and assisted reproductive technology. (From the literature [see page 488]. Adapted from data by Ozil, 1983; Catt, 1996; Wassarman, 1988; Yanagimachi, 1981.)

TABLE 31-3. ***Embryo Sexing, Nuclear Transfer, Maturation Media, and Cloning in Mammals***

| | |
|---|---|
| Embryo sexing techniques | Separation on basis of sexual dimorphism<br>Detection of the sex chromatin mass<br>Fluorescent *in situ* hybridization<br>Detection of the H-Y antigen<br>Use of Y-specific DNA probes<br>Chromosome analysis |
| Factors involved in nuclear transfer | Use of particle gun<br>Sperm-mediated gene transfer<br>Injection of the pronuclei<br>Retroviral-mediated gene transfer<br>Injection of the oocyte cytoplasma<br>Germinal vesicle gene injection |
| Methods of gene transfer (cloning) | Quality of the cytoplast<br>Quantity of cytoplasm in the recipient oocyte<br>Age of cytoplast<br>Source of donor blastomeres<br>Cell stage of the cytoplast<br>Cell stage of donor blastomeres |
| Types of bovine serum for maturation media | Fetal calf serum<br>Pro-estrous serum<br>Steer serum<br>Estrous cow serum<br>Serum substitutes<br>Superovulated cow serum |

f) Subsequent surgical or nonsurgical transfer of "half" and "quarters" embryos to mares resulted in pregnancies, including monozygotic pairs (18).

## GAMETE INTERACTION

Recognition occurs between a sperm receptor located in plasma membrane, and an oocyte receptor located in zona pellucida (ZP3). ZP3 induces acrosome reaction. Closer interaction occurs between ZP2 and an inner acrosomal membrane receptor. Gamete interactions occur in round-headed sperm at the functional level where fertility is impaired. Round headed sperm were obtained from two infertile men whose semen analysis revealed this particular morphologic condition in over 90% of their sperm (Figs. 31-7 and 31-8).

Triple staining shows 100% of acrosomeless sperm have a complete absence of acrosome and various degrees of abnormalities in chromatin condensation.

Immunochemical studies with monoclonal antibodies to acrosin exhibited an abnormal pattern of weak fluorescence in the post nuclear region. Human ZP and zona-free hamster oocytes are used to study gamete interaction. Normal semen samples show an average of 46 sperm bound per zona.

a) round-headed sperm shows no binding to ZP
b) certain acrosomal proteins are needed for this process
c) acrosome is necessary for the correct organization of plasma membrane proteins

TABLE 31-4. ***Assisted Reproductive Technology/Andrology (ARTA) and In Vitro Semen Manipulation***

| METHOD | TECHNIQUES |
|---|---|
| Assisted Reproductive Technology (ARTA) | IVF-ET *in vitro* fertilization/uterine embryo transfer<br>GIFT gamete intrafallopian transfer<br>PROST pronuclear-stage tubal transfer<br>ZIFT zygot intrafallopian transfer<br>TEST tubal embryo-stage transfer, (embryos in (TET) in premorula cleavage stages)<br>Embryo Bank cryopreservation of oocytes/morulae |
| Zona drilling | Mechanical or by local application of a zona solvent like acid Tyode's or alpha chymotrypsin solution using a microneedle. |
| Partial Zona drilling (PZD) | Zona is mechanically torn with a glass needle or cracked by piercing on a glass bolding pipette. |
| Subzonal injection (SUZI) | Injection of one or more sperm into perivitelline space. |
| Intra-cytoplasmic injection (ICSI) | Injection of immotile live sperm directly into vitellus. |
| Semen manipulation *in vitro* | a. swim up/swin down<br>b. use of semen additives<br>c. *in vitro* capacitation<br>d. *in vitro* hyperactivation<br>e. separation of X and Y sperm<br>f. cryopreservation/semen banks |

Catt JW. Intracytoplasmic sperm injection (ICSI) and related technology. Anim Reprod Sci 1996;4:239–250.
ICSI method is in its initial stages.
Pregnancies are achieved in severe case of male infertility.
Babies born after micromanipulation of Zona Pellucida were normal and without any chromosomal anomalies.

TABLE 31-5. ***Manipulation/Micromanipulation of Eggs/Morulae***

| | |
|---|---|
| Micromanipulation of zona pellucida/ related techniques | "Zona drilling" by mechanical force<br>"Puncture" with acid Tryod, pronase, or trypsin solution with micropipette<br>"Cracking" using two fine glass hooks controlled by micromanipulator<br>"PZD" partial opening using mechanical force only, followed by microinsemination |
| Transfer of early germ cells | Transfer of male germ cells in PVS, chromosomes of male/female gametes undergo characteristics of species |
| Nuclear, cell/ blastomere transfer | Transfer part of cell/especially nuclei or whole cell (fusion of cytoblast/karyoplasts with host cells is inhibited by electrofusion) |
| Blastocyst biopsy | One or two blastomeres are removed (for preimplantation diagnosis of sex or genetic anomalies) allowing remaining embryos to develop into individual animal |
| Cloning (nuclear substitution) | Nuclear transplant into enucleated egg, to enable continual propagation of particular gene/trait/species |
| Transgenic animals | Cloned genes introduced into somatic cells or embryos |

TABLE 31-6. *Assisted Fertilization and Assisted Blastocyst Hatching*

| | | |
|---|---|---|
| Indications for assisted fertilization by ICSI | · Duct obstruction<br>· Duct absence<br>· Unexplained failure of fertilization<br>· Extreme oligozoospermia<br>· Extreme asthenozoospermia<br>· Extreme mixed teratozoospermia | · Uniform teratozoospermia<br>· Necrozoospermia<br>· Aneuploidy<br>· Pronuclear/syngamy disorder<br>· Antibodies to sperm<br>· Female infertility |
| Indications for assisted blastocyst/ fragment removal | · Elevated zona thickness<br>· Unexplained failure of implantation<br>· Reduced embryonic development rate<br>· ICSI | · Elevated maternal age<br>· Elevated basal FSH level<br>· Fragmentation above 15% |
| Advantages of assisted hatching | · Technically simple<br>· Not labor intensive<br>· Normal rate of congenital malformation | · Elevates implantation<br>· Promotes earlier implantation |
| Disadvantages of assisted hatching | · Possible risk of conjoint turning<br>· Embryo loss high with standard embryo transfer<br>· Low success with standard transfer techniques | |

There is complete absence of fusion with zona-free hamster oocytes due to the inability of reorganization of plasma membrane proteins in the post acrosomal region as a result of the absence of acrosome reaction in round headed sperms. The acrosome is necessary for sorting and the correct organization of plasma membrane.

## INTRACYTOPLASMIC SPERM INJECTION (ICSI)

Recently, various methods of assisted reproductive technology have been applied for different types of male and female infertility (Tables 31-4 through 31-8). The most popular method was intracytoplasmic sperm injection (ICSI) (Tables 31-4 and 31-6). The micromanipulation techniques used to enhance fertilization in both animals and humans are reviewed. Using knowledge derived from the human research direct sperm injection into the oocytes of domestic species was reinvestigated. Exogenous oocyte activation was not mandatory for fertilization. The birth of a lamb indicates that normal development can occur subsequent to sperm injection. The lamb was produced from sperm that had been sorted on a flow cytometer and was of the predicted sex. There are several potential uses of sperm injection for domestic and exotic species (19).

TABLE 31-7. *Time Required for Capacitation in Different Species*

| SPECIES | TIME REQUIRED FOR CAPACITATION | DURATION OF SPERM MOTILITY (h) | DURATION OF SPERM FERTILITY (h) | FERTILIZABLE LIFE OF OOCYTES (h) |
|---|---|---|---|---|
| Mouse | <1 | 13 | 6 | 15 |
| Sheep | 1–5 | 48 | 30–48 | 12–15 |
| Rat | 2–3 | 17 | 14 | 12 |
| Hamster | 2–4 | — | — | 9–12 |
| Pig | 3–6 | 50 | 24–48 | 10 |
| Rabbit | 5 | 43–50 | 28–36 | 6–8 |
| Rhesus monkey | 5–6 | — | — | 23 |
| Human | 5–6 | 48–60 | 24–48 | 6–24 |
| Dog | — | 268 | 134 | 24 |

From: Dale B, Elder K. *In Vitro* Fertilization, Cambridge, UK, Cambridge University Press, 1997.

TABLE 31-8. *The Zona Pellucida in Relative to Assisted Reproduction: Effect of Sperm Oocyte Interaction on the Binding to and Penetration of Sperm to the Zona Pellucida*

| PARAMETERS | |
|---|---|
| Sperm Binding/ Penetration[a] | 1. Oocyte maturity affects number of sperm bound to the zona.<br>2. Number of sperm bound to mature oocyte = 51 ± 50<br>Number of sperm bound to immature oocyte = 7 ± 12<br>Number of sperm bound to atretic oocyte = 10 ± 18<br>3. Fertilized mature oocytes have higher number of sperm bound to the zonae compared to unfertilized oocytes 81 ± 53 compared to 42 ± 47.<br>4. Sperm motility/the number of motile sperm used to inseminate oocytes correlated with number of sperm bound to the zona, whereas sperm morphology/sperm concentration do not correlate. |
| Second Insemination[b] | 5. Second insemination is performed if fertilization does not occur 18 h after first insemination.<br>6. The oocyte does not fertilize either due to a) its own maturity or b) due to sperm difficulty to penetrate the zona pellucida.<br>7. Secondary insemination leads to fertilization since blastomeres are seen 18 h after this secondary insemination.<br>8. This activity in the oocyte is delayed following the first insemination and not related to the second one.<br>9. Secondary insemination yields 5–7% of fertilization. Similar to that of immature oocytes.<br>10. Secondary insemination is performed only in cases of unfertilized oocytes which were immature when first insemination was performed. |
| Polyspermy[c] | 11. Despite the exposure of eggs to supernumerary sperm, the incidence of polypoid fertilization is 2–10%. This incidence may be related to the functional ability of the polyspermic block of the oocyte rather than to the high number of sperm in the dish.<br>12. Polypronuclear fertilization is more frequent in cycles with high fertilization/improved pregnancy rates.<br>13. This emphasizes the important role of the oocyte in polyspermy. |

[a]Mahadevan et al, 1987
[b]Ron-El et al, 1993
[c]Golan et al, 1992b
Adapted from the literature and Phillips/Shalgi, 1980; Ozil, 1983; Yanagimachi, 1977; Hartmann, 1983, Acosta AA, Kruger TF, 1996. Human Sperm in Assisted Reproduction, Parthenan Publishing, New York, NY.

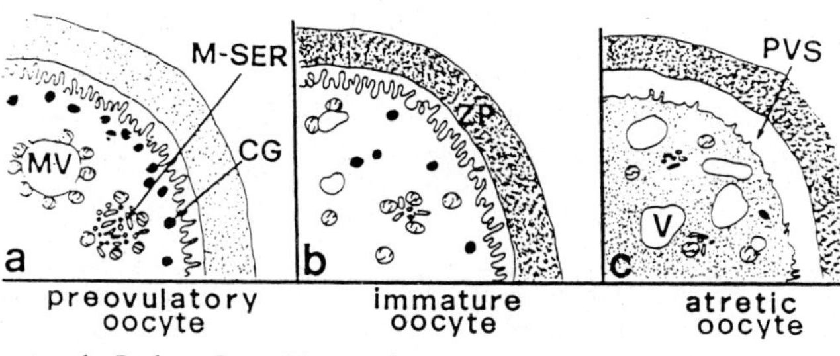


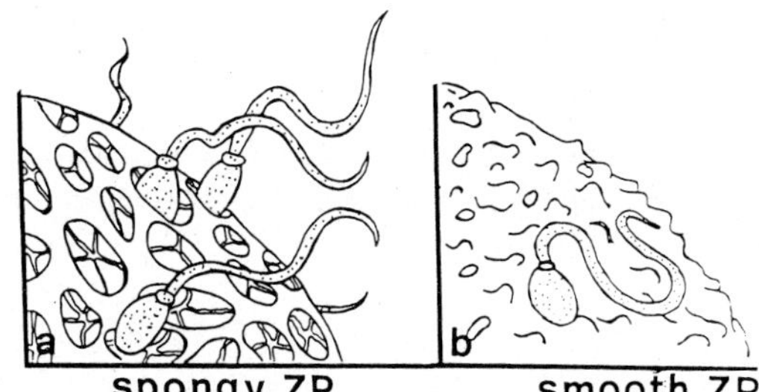


Drawings by Professor Pietro Motta and associates, Rome, Italy

# MOLECULAR ANDROLOGY

Several techniques have been applied to sperm/acrosome morphology acrosome assessment with PSA, computer sperm morphology assessment (28), and computer motility assessment (Fig. 31-6, top). Extensive investigations were conducted on the ultrastructural characteristics of neurosecretory material of the hypothalamus in relation to gamete physiology (Fig. 31-6, bottom).

## *Spermatid/Sertoli Cell Interaction*

When the nucleus, covered by the acrosome, moves toward the cell surface of the spermatids during midspermiogenesis, ectoplasmic specializations (ES) appear in the cytoplasm of Sertoli cells in apposition to the plasma membrane covering the acrosome. The ES is probably involved in attachment of the spermatids to the Sertoli cell, allowing for proper head-tail orientation of the spermatids, and remains apposed to the spermatid heads until spermiation (20, 21).

SPERMICIDAL ACTIVITY. D'Cruz et al (22) have applied computer-assisted sperm analysis (CASA) to evaluate the spermicidal activity of 8 metallocene dihalides (vanadocene dichloride [VDC], titanocene dichloride [TDC], zirconocene dichloride [ZDC], molybdocene dichloride [MDC], hafnocene dichloride [HDC], vanadocene dibromide [VDB], bis[methylcyclopentadienyl]vanadium dichloride

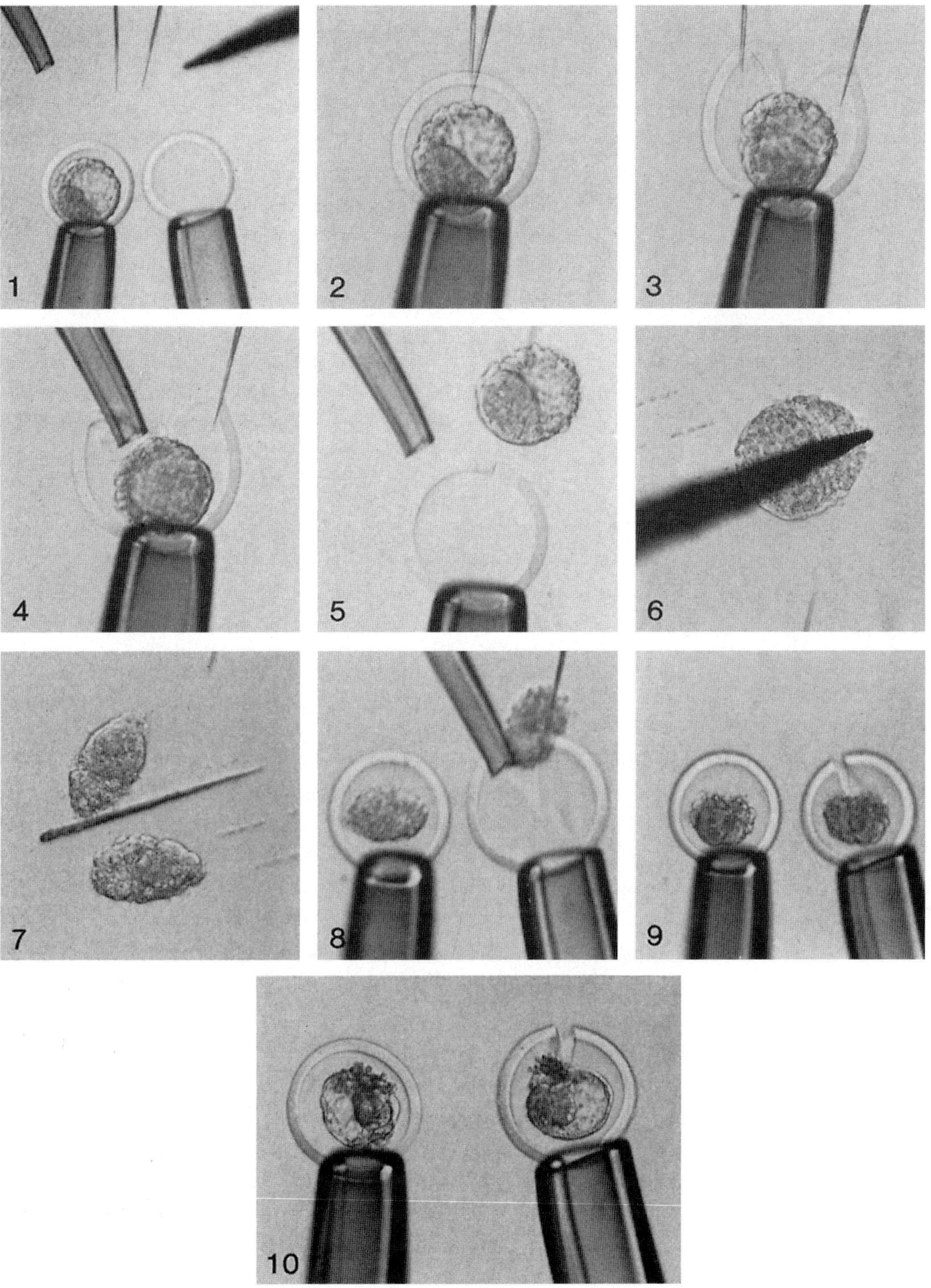

Figure 31-4. Method of bisection of cow blastocysts by micromanipulation. (**1**) Six microinstruments are placed in the optical field of an inverted microscope. Two micropipettes controlled by type-B micromanipulators hold the blastocyst and the empty zona pellucida by negative pressure. (**2**) Instruments with a sharp tip in front of the blastocyst are controlled by a type-A micromanipulator. The micropipette on the left and the microscalpel on the right are controlled by a type-B micromanipulator. This equipment allows the bisection of 6 to 8 blastocysts per hour. (From Willadsen SM. Micromanipulation of embryos of the large domestic species. In: Adams CE, ed. Mammalian Egg Transfer. Boca Raton, Florida: CRC Press, 1982.) (**2 and 3**) The two sharp microneedles cut the zona pellucida over as short a distance as possible along the middle. The blastocyst is subsequently rotated through 90° with the two microneedles to show the slit. (**4 and 5**) The micropipette is introduced through the slit inside the zona while a small volume of medium is injected to expel the embryo. (**6 and 7**) Bisection of the blastocyst is achieved using the microscalpel along the sagittal plane. (**8 and 9**) Using the suction of the micropipette, each "half" embryo is put back into an empty zona pellucida. (**10**) "Half" (demi) embryos are then incubated at 37°C for 2 hours. They reconstitute their blastocele, and it is possible to distinguish again the inner cell mass in each "half" blastocyst. The cells destroyed during the bisection adhere to the outer surface of the "half" blastocyst. (From Ozil JP. Production of identical twins by bisection of blastocysts in the cow. Repro Fertil 1983;69:463.)

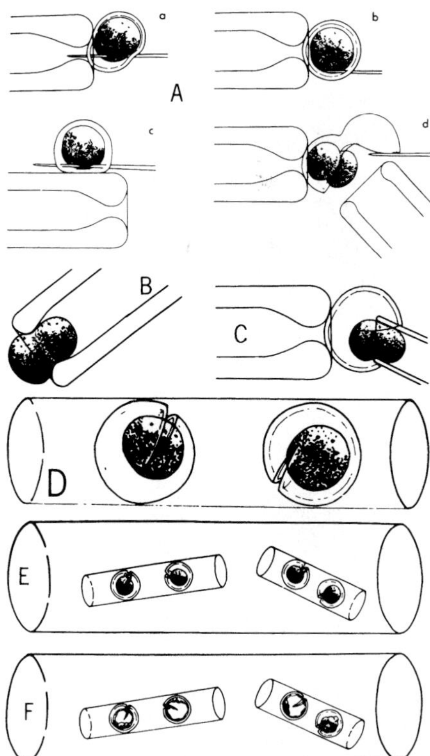


FIGURE 31-5. Micromanipulation of gametes and embryos. (**A**) Removal of the zona pellucida. (**B**) Separation of blastomeres. (**C**) Insertion of single blastomeres into evacuated zona pellucida. (**D**) First agar embedding. (**E**) Agar chip before transfer to the sheep oviduct after recovery from the sheep. The position of the individual embryo within the chip allows it to be readily identified after culture. (Willadsen SM. Micromanipulation of embryos of the large domestic species. In: Adams CE, ed. Mammalian Egg Transfer. Boca Raton, Florida: CRC Press, 1982.)

[VMDC], and vanadocene diiodide [VDI]; and 5 vanadocene di-pseudohalides (vanadocene diazide [VDA]). The sperm immobilizing activity of the vanadocene complexes was rapid and irreversible, since the treated sperm underwent apoptosis as determined by the flow cytometric annexin V binding assay, DNA nick end-labeling, and confocal laser scanning microscope. Thus metallocene complexes containing vanadium(IV), especially VDSeCN, may be ueful as contraceptive agents.

### *Dynamics of Sperm Motility*

Mammalian sperm exhibit different patterns of motility such as straight line velocity (VSL), curvilinear velocity (VCL), average path velocity (VAP), heat cross frequency (AHL), and angle of deviation (0) (Fig. 31-10). Sperm hyperactivation is of major physiological significance in binding to and penetration through the zona pellucida of the egg (Fig. 31-11).

## INSTRUMENTATION, WATER AND AIR FILTRATION, CULTURE MEDIA

### *Instrumentation and Supplies*

Equipment and laboratory supplies for embryo transfer, IVF, and embryo manipulation are listed in Table 31-9 and Figures 31-4 through 31-19.

### *Ultrapure Water*

Distilled and bottled water leach new organics as little as one hour after storage. Unfortunately, storage problems are just one of the drawbacks to using distilled or bottled water. There are also the problems of higher operating and maintenance costs and contaminant carryover. Laboratory water purification has undergone dramatic changes in the 1980s. Chemists, life scientists, and medical technicians are now routinely concerned with impurity levels that were impossible to measure 10 years ago. Today, deionization, reverse osmosis, carbon absorption, and membrane microfiltration are in some respects superior to distillation. Various systems of water ultrafiltration are now available commercially. These systems cost less than distilled or bottled water, and there is no contaminant carryover. Unlike stills, which require regular acid cleaning, ultrafiltration cartridges can be replaced in minutes.

### *Air Filtration*

Laminar airflow is airflow in which the entire body of air within a designated space moves with uniform velocity in a single direction along parallel flow lines. Laminar-flow biologic safety cabinets (hoods) are devices designed to minimize biohazards inherent in work with low- and moderate-risk biologic agents. Vertical lamina-flow containment hoods provide not only product protection by using a filtered down-flow of air but also provide operator protection through a negative pressure air barrier created along the front opening. With proper aseptic conditions and good laboratory procedures, risk levels are substantially reduced.

### *Culture, Coculture, and Organ Culture*

OVIDUCTAL SECRETIONS. The epithelial cells of the ovine and bovine oviduct secrete two classes of proteins.

a) The first class is uniformly secreted throughout the estrous cycle and represents a small proportion of the total protein output.
b) The second class displays cyclic pattern of secretion and is composed mainly of polypeptides. These two latter

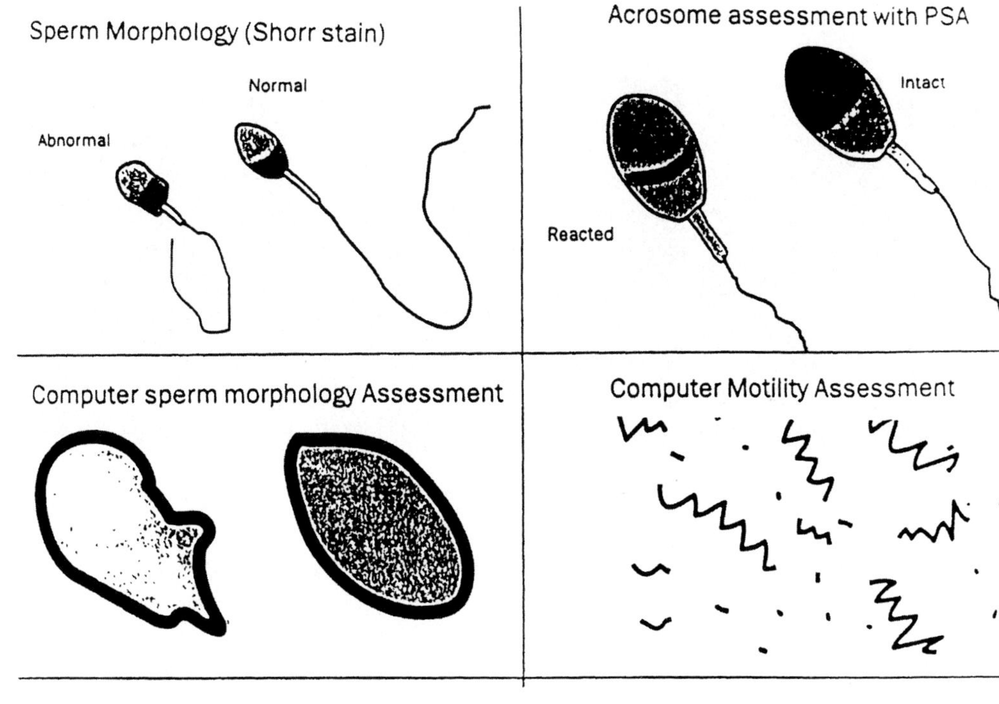


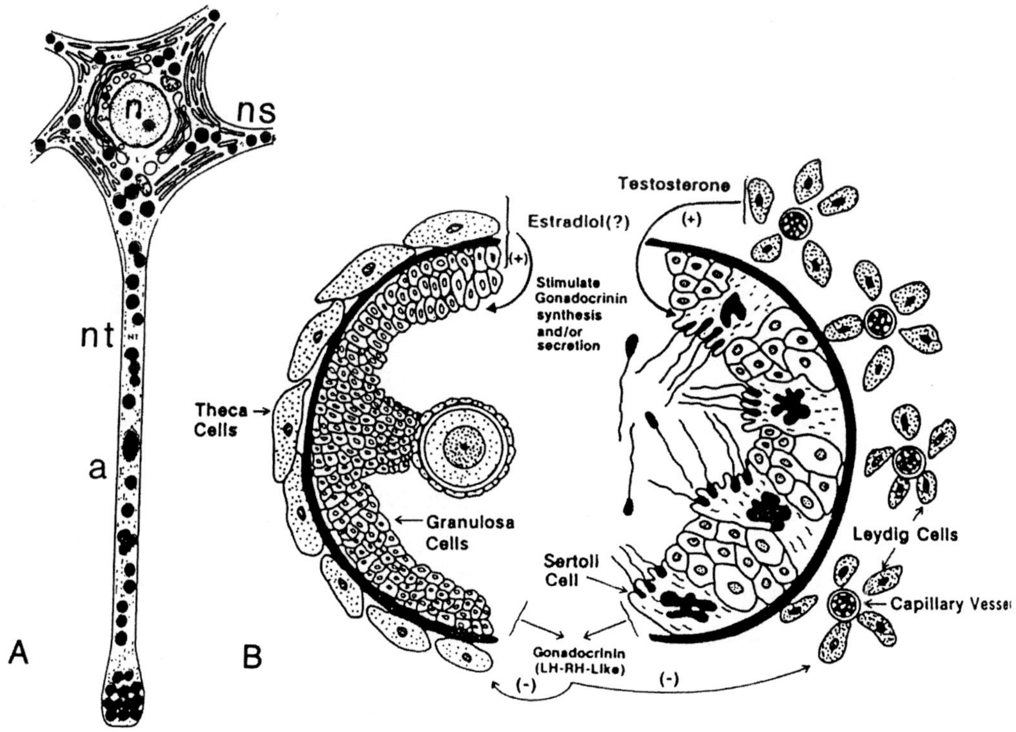


FIGURE 31-6. (*Top*) Techniques used to assess sperm/acrosome morphology. Computer assisted sperm motility. (Adapted from data in the literature.) (*Bottom*) (**A**) Ultra-structural characteristics of a neurosecretory neuron in the hypothalamus. The nerve cell body (*n*, nucleus) has dendritic and axonal (*a*) processes with arrays of rough endoplasmic reticulum, a prominent Golgi apparatus, and neurotubule (*nt*). Hormone-containing, membrane-limited neurosecretory granules (*ns*) are formed in the Golgi apparatus and transported along the axon to the site of release at the termination on capillaries. Neurosecretory neurons synthesize the releasing and release-inhibiting hormones of the adenohypophysis and the hormones of the neurohypophysis (oxytocin, antidiuretic hormone). The feedback to the theca cells and Leydig cells may inhibit steroidogenesis by decreasing the number of receptors; it also would interfere with the activation of the cAMP system (From Capen CC, Martin SL. The pituitary gland. In: McDonald LE, Pineda MH, eds. Veterinary Endocrinology and Reproduction. Philadelphia: Lea & Febiger, 1989.). (**B**) Postulated physiologic function of gonadotropins on the Sertoli and granulosa cells. (Adapted from different sources, including Sharp RM. Cellular aspects of the inhibitory actions of LH-RH on the ovary and testis. J Reprod Fertil 1982;64:517.)

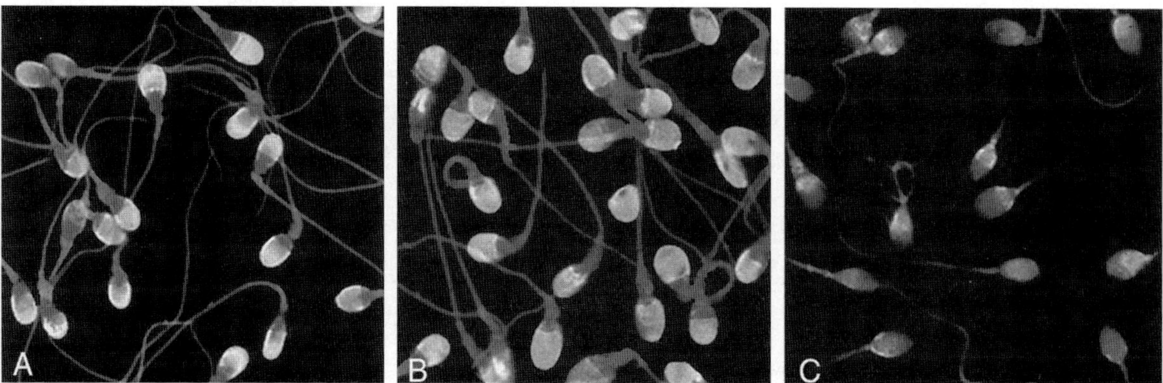


FIGURE 31-7. VCD lacks detergent-like membrane toxicity. Laser scanning confocal fluorescence image of sperm. All samples were triple labeled with FITC-Pisum sativum lectin for acrosome (green fluorescence), TOTO-3 for DNA (blue fluorescence), and Nile red for membrane lipid (red fluorescence). Triple labeling of sperm incubated for 3 h: (**A**) In the absence of VDC. (**B**) With of 100 $\mu$M VDC added. (**C**) With 100 $\mu$M nonoxynol-p. Original magnification 1200×. (From D'Cruz OJ, Ghosh A, Uckun FM. Spermicidal Activity of Metallocene Complexes Containing Vanadium(IV) in Humans. Reprod 1998;58:1515–1526.)

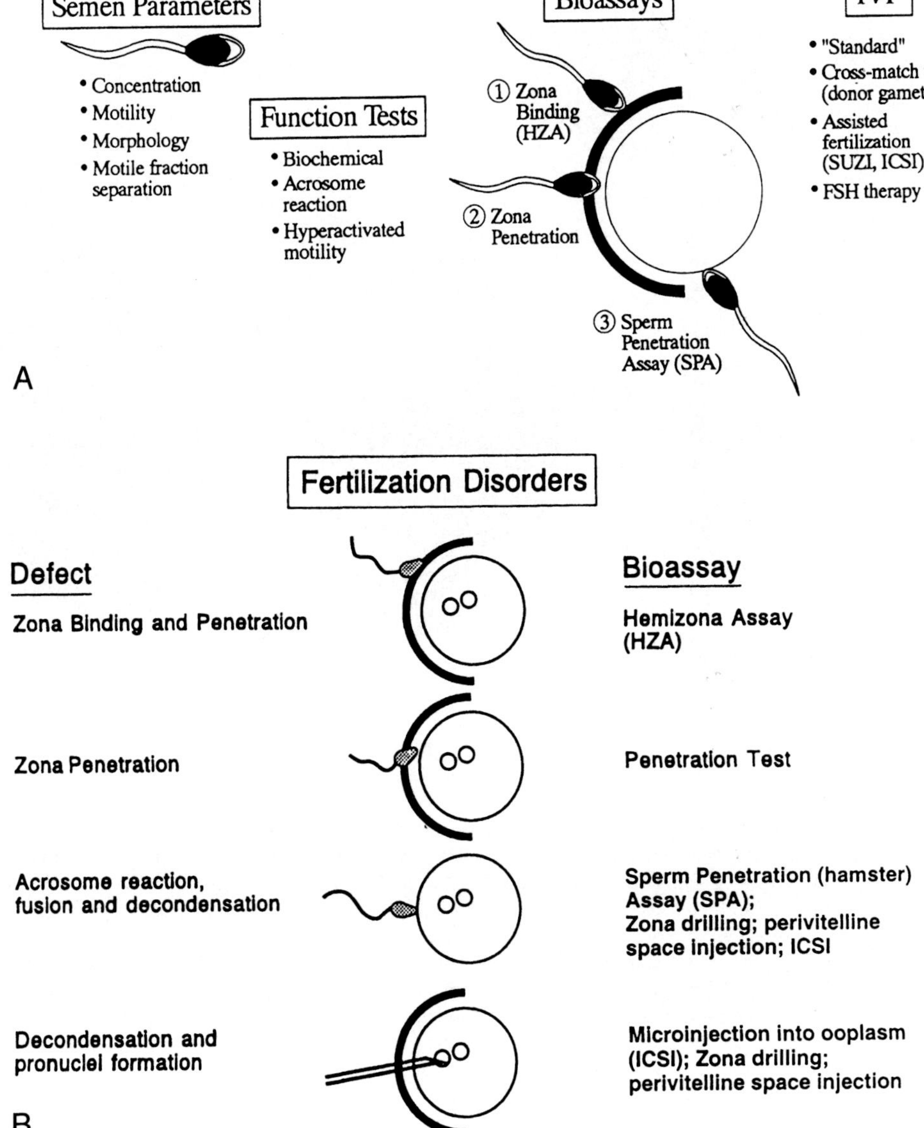


FIGURE 31-8. Diagnosis of failed IVF and sperm defects/fertilization failure. (**A**) Diagnostic scheme to establish a stepwise progressive diagnosis in cases of recurrent failed IVF. (**B**) Sequential analysis of specific sperm defects in cases of recurrent failed fertilization. (Reproduced with permission of Mosby-Year Book from Oehninger SC, Acosta AA, Veeck LL, Brzyski R, Kruger TF, Muasher SJ, Hodgen GC. Recurrent failure of *in vitro* fertilization: Role of the hemizona assay in the sequential diagnosis of specific sperm–oocyte defects. Am J Obstet Gynecol 1991;164:1210–1215.)

TABLE 31-9. ***Equipment, Supplies, Media, and Techniques for Sperm Preparation/IVF***

| | |
|---|---|
| Routine basic equipment for IVF | · Dissecting, inverted, and light microscopes<br>· Incubator with accurately regulated temperature and $CO_2$<br>· Centrifuge for sperm preparation<br>· Warmed stages or surfaces for culture manipulations<br>· Refrigerator/freezer<br>· Dry heat oven for drying and sterilizing |
| Disposable general supplies | · Nontoxic tissue culture<br>· Culture vessels<br>· Needles, catheters, oocyte aspiration/embryo<br>· Glass pipettes (soaked/rinsed in culture media) |
| Equipment for sperm preparation | · Semen sterile collection pot 60 mL<br>· Counting chamber (Makler, Sefi Medical Instruments, or Horwell hemocytometer)<br>· Centrifuge with swing-out rotor<br>· Microscope slides/coverslips<br>· Disposable test tubes: 4 mL, 10 mL<br>· Culture media: MediCult Percoll Medium, Sil-Select (MICROM)<br>· Glass Pasteur pipettes<br>· Disposable pipettes: 1 mL, 5 mL, 10 mL<br>· Spirit burner and methanol, or gas Bunsen burner<br>· Supply of liquid nitrogen/storage Dewar flasks |
| Sperm preparation techniques | 1. Overlay and swim-up, multiple overlay<br>2. Discontinuous buoyant density gradients<br>mini: 95/70/50%<br>two-step: 40/80%, 45/90%, 47.5/95%<br>one-step: 95%<br>3. High-speed centrifugation and washing<br>Sedimentation under oil<br>"fishing" with micromanipulator<br>Swim-out under oil |
| Manufacturing companies for IVF media | · Scandinavian: IVF Science AB, Mölndalsvägen 30A, PO Box 1410, Göthenburg, Sweden<br>· Menezo B2: Bio-Merieux, France<br>· Ham's F-10, EBSS: Flow Laboratories, UK<br>· HTF: Irvine Scientific, US<br>· Bio-Care International: San Diego, CA, US |

Adapted from Dale/Elder. (2,3,9; adapted from Adams CE, ed. Mammalian Egg Transfer. Boca Raton, Florida: CRC Press, 1983; Hunter RHF. Reproduction of Farm Animals. London: Longman, 1982; Daniel JC Jr, Methods in Mammalian Reproduction. New York: Academic Press, 1978.)

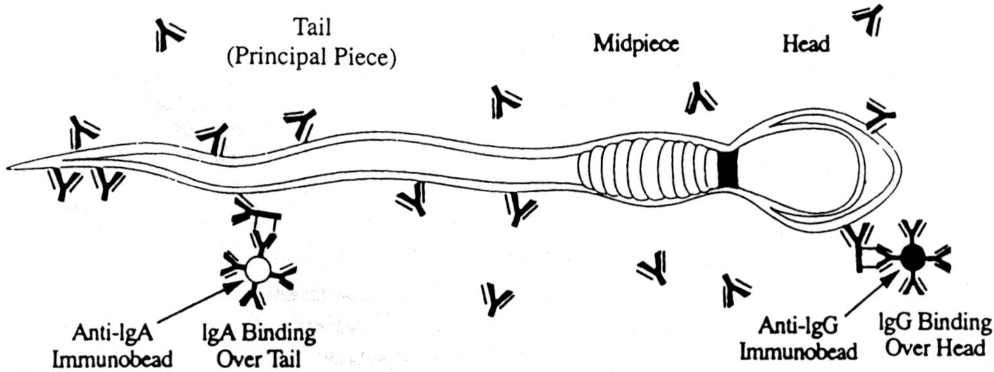


FIGURE 31-9. Schematic drawing of the immunobead test. Anti-IgA or anti-IgG covalently linked to polyacrylamide beads binds to IgA or IgG bound to the sperm surface. Quantification of antisperm antibody is by visualization of beads bound to the sperm surface. (Yeh W-R, Acosta AA, Van der Mereve JP. Antisperm antibodies 2: clinical aspects. In: Human Spermatozoa in Assisted Reproduction. Acosta AA, Kruger TF, eds. New York: Parthenon Publishing, 1996.).

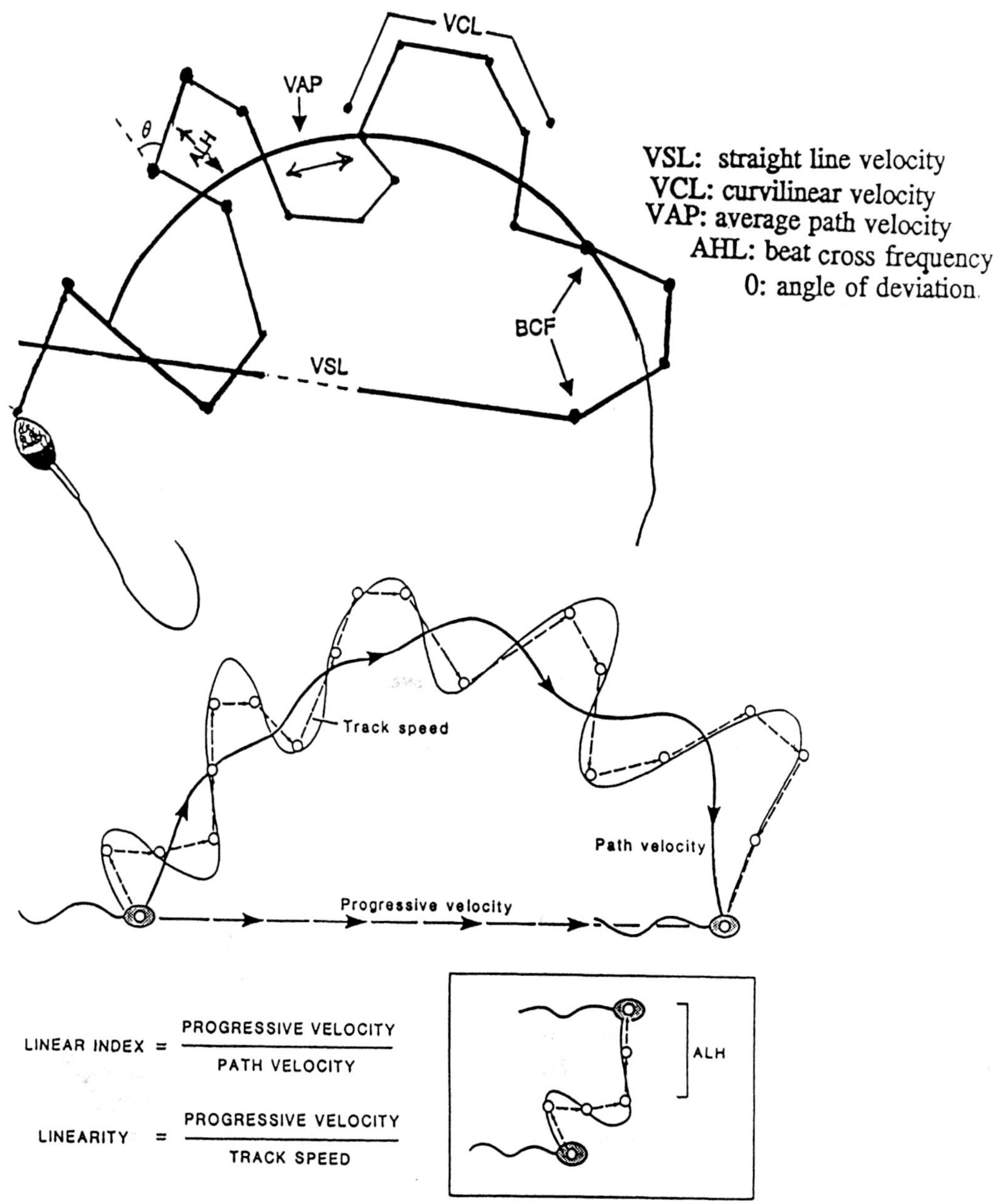


FIGURE 31-10. (*Top*) Different pattern of sperm motility. (*Bottom*) Measurements of "linear index" and "linearity" of sperm motility. (Adapted from literature; Kaskar K, Franken DR. Evaluation of Sperm Motility in Assisted Reproduction. Ch. 7 in Human Sperm in Assisted Reproduction. Acosta AA, Kruger TF, Parthenon, NY, 1996; Chan PJ, Tredway DR, Su BC, Corselli J, Davidson BJ, Sakugawa M. Sperm hyperactivation as quality control for sperm penetration assay. Urology 1992;39:63–66. Burkman LJ. Discrimination between nonhyperactivated and classical hyperactivated motility patterns in human spermatozoa using computerized analysis. Fertil Steril 1991;55:363–371. Mortimer D. Objective analysis of sperm motility and kinematics. In: Keel BA, Webster BW, eds. The CRC Handbook of Laboratory Diagnosis and Treatment of Infertility, Boca Raton, FL, CRC Press, 1990:97–133.)

proteins, detected soon after estrus, remain in the oviduct fluid for the same time frame as the ova (23). Oviductal levels of *de nova* synthesized proteins are highest during estrus and decline thereafter. Some 30 to 40 polypeptides are secreted, some of which are secreted at a greater rate during estrus. After ovulation, in spite of the surrounding cumulus and corona·radiata cells, signifi- amounts of oviductal glycoprotein bind firmly to porcine zona; however, the glycoproteins do not form ucin coat, as seen with rabbit oviductal ova.

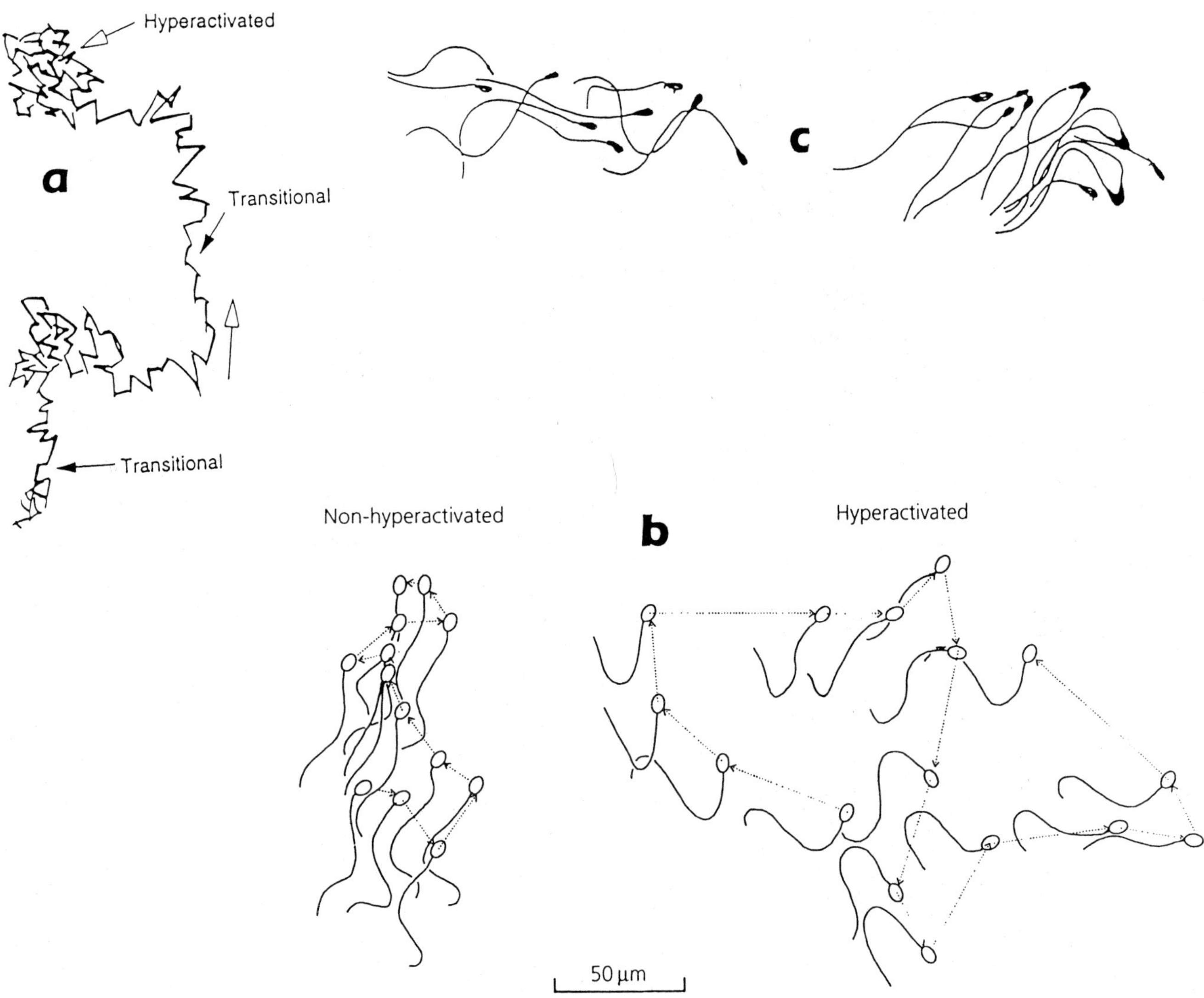


Figure 31-11. Sperm tail beating and head-centroid trajectory pattern for mammalian sperm. (a) Hyperactivated/transitional motility pattern. (b) Sperm motility before/after hyperactivation. (c) Various sperm motility *in vitro*. (Adapted from the literature and the following: Mortimer D. Objective analysis of sperm motility and kinematics. In: Keel BA, Webster BW, eds. Handbook of the Laboratory Diagnosis and Treatment of Infertility. Boca Raton: CRC Press, 1990:97–133; Mortimer ST. A critical review of the physiological importance and analysis of sperm movement in mammals. Hum Reprod Update 1997;3:403–439.)

The mammalian oviduct has the ability to support the development of embryos across many species, indicating that many of the beneficial effects of the oviduct environment may actually be nonspecific with regard to species. Extensive investigations were conducted using the oviduct *in vivo* or *in vitro* (cell or organ culture). Pig early embryos (one-cell to eight-cell stage) cultured in "organ coculture" in mouse excused oviducts, can develop to the morula and blastocyst stage (24). The rate of this embryonic development of pig embryos is enhanced when the oviduct is taken from mice mated to fertile or vasectomized males. Embryos may be transferred directly in the oviduct, or they can be placed in agar chips before placement in the oviduct. Bovine embryos can develop in *in vivo* sheep and rabbit oviduct coculture (25). Embryo viability was similar between both hosts; however, embryo recovery was slightly lower from the rabbit host as compared to the sheep.

Culture and Coculture. Several culture/coculture media are used for *in vitro* physiologic maturation and subsequent cleavage at various degrees: modified Krebs-Ringer's bicarbonate, modified Dulbecco's, TCM199, modified Ham's F-10, Whitten medium, Eagle's basal medium with

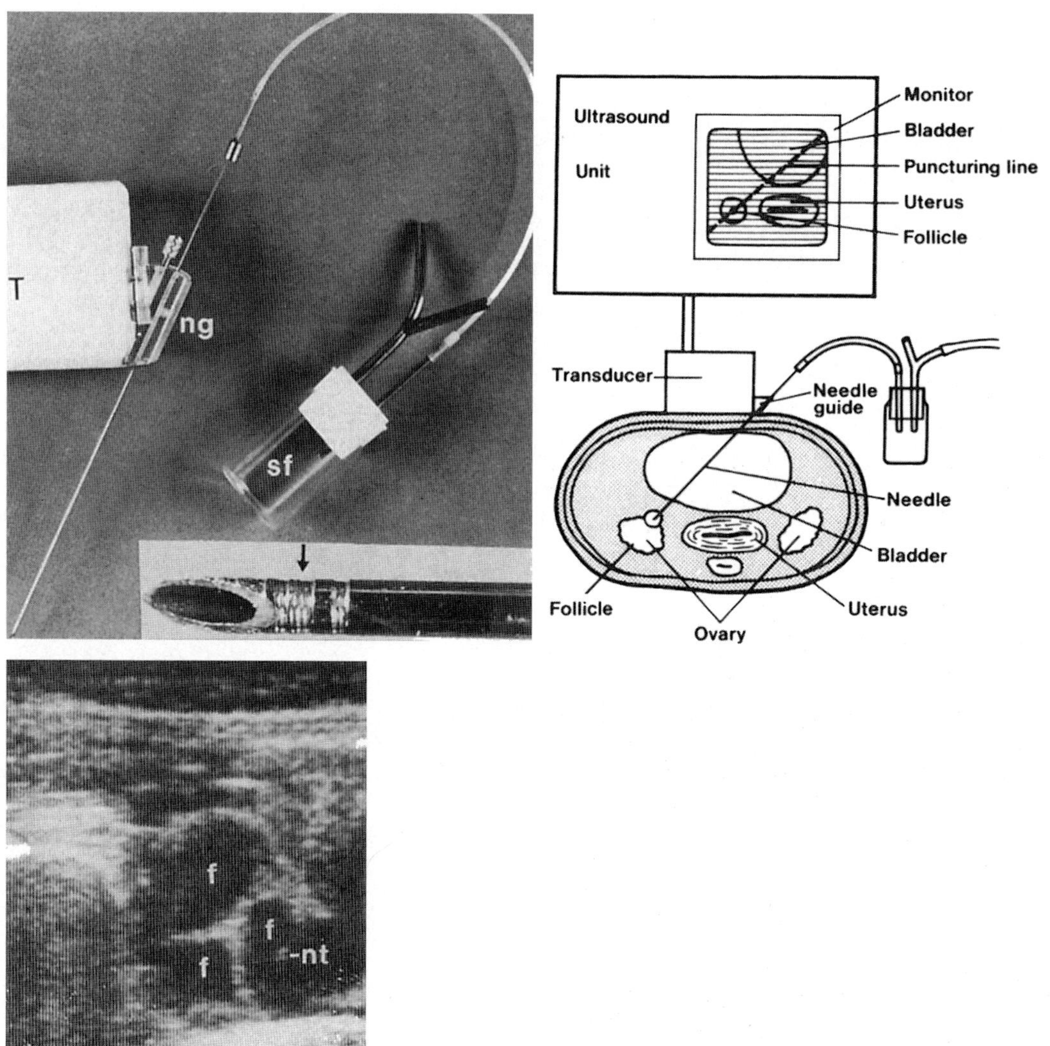


FIGURE 31-12. (*Left*) Aspiration equipment for ultrasonically guided percutaneous follicle puncture. *T*, transducer; *ng*, needle guide; *sf*, sampling flask. (*Inset, left*) Needle tip with the shallow tracks (*arrow*) in the needle tip. (*Right*) Schematic illustration of the ultrasonically guided puncture technique. (*Bottom*) Illustration of ultrasonically guided puncture of a human follicle. The white echo inside the follicle (f) represents the needle tip (nt). (Courtesy of R. Wikland.)

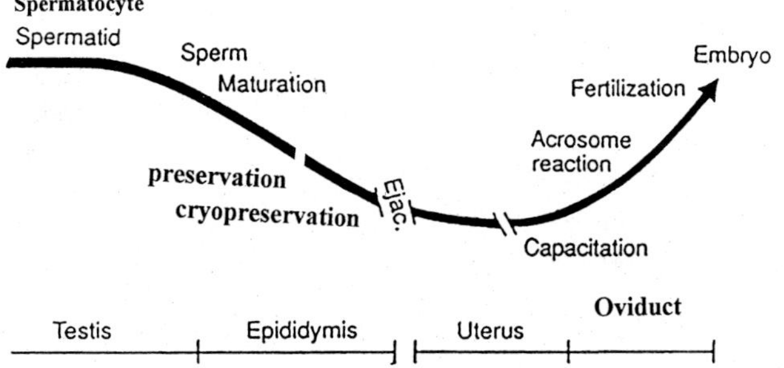


FIGURE 31-13. Physiology of sperm maturation-capacitation, acrosome reaction, fertilization, and implantation in the male and female reproductive organs.

Hank's salts, and modified minimum essential medium (MEM) with Earl's salts.

In human IVF centers, animal tissues are used in human coculture systems to evaluate pregnancy rates after embryo replacement. Fetal cattle uterine fibroblast monolayers are used to evaluate *in vitro* development in implantation of human embryos. Fetal uterine endometrial linings were obtained from healthy bovine fetuses and cells after several subcultures are used for coculture. Human embryos cocultured with cattle monolayers are transferred back to patients. The pregnancy rate is increased when human embryos cocultured *with* human ampullary cells are replaced back into patients.

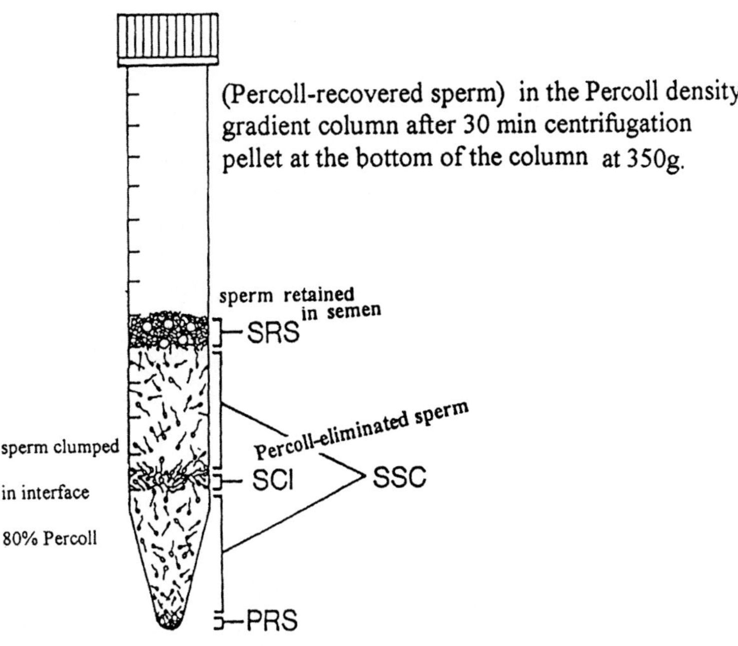


CALCULATION OF SPERM CELL CONCENTRATION:

Establish average sperm count from the two chambers.
Dimensions of the large central area of the Neubauer counting chamber are 1 mm (width) x 1 mm (height) x 0.1 mm (depth) for a volume of 0.1 mm³. Since sperm cell concentration is normally reported in sperm number per cubic centimeter (cc), the sperm count must be multiplied by a factor of 10,000.
Since the semen was diluted at a 1:100 ratio prior to the sperm count, the final sperm count must be multiplied by an additional factor of 100.

EXAMPLE: Sperm count of diluted semen in chamber 1 = 240
Sperm count of diluted semen in chamber 2 = 250
Average sperm count = 245
Sperm cell concentration =
$245 \times 10^4 \times 10^2$/cc or
$245 \times 10^6$/cc

B

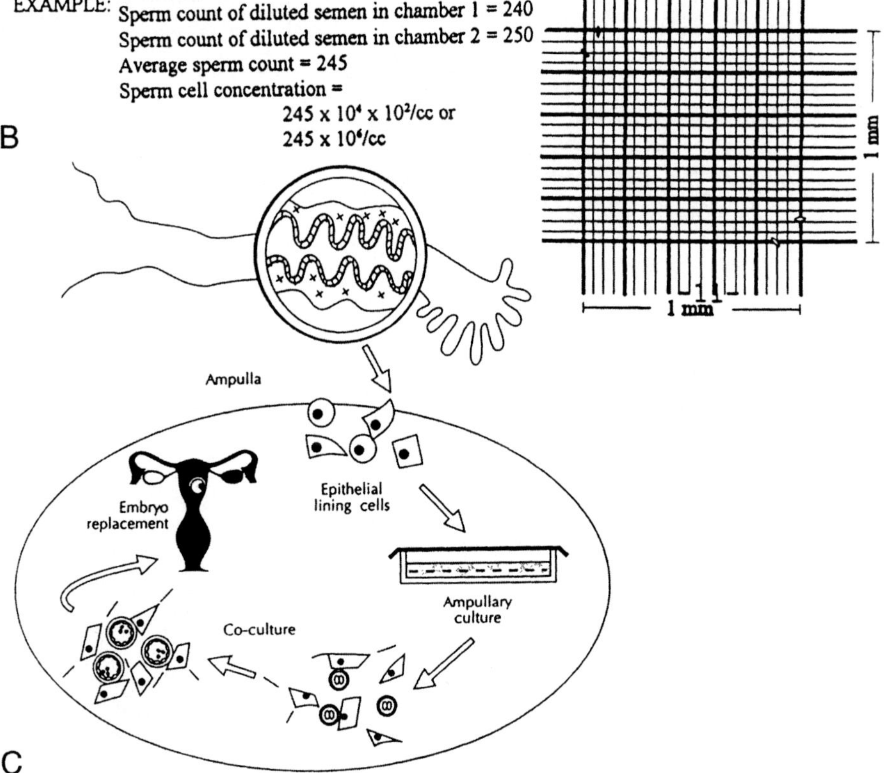


FIGURE 31-14. (A) Separation of sperm *in vitro* using "Percoll density gradient" and centrifugation. (B) Calculation of sperm concentration using "Neubauer counting chamber." (C) Organ culture/co-culture: epithelial lining of the ampullary portion of the oviduct *in vitro*, and co-cultured with fertilized egg used for embryo replacement. (Courtesy of Professor Bongso, University of Singapore, Singapore.)

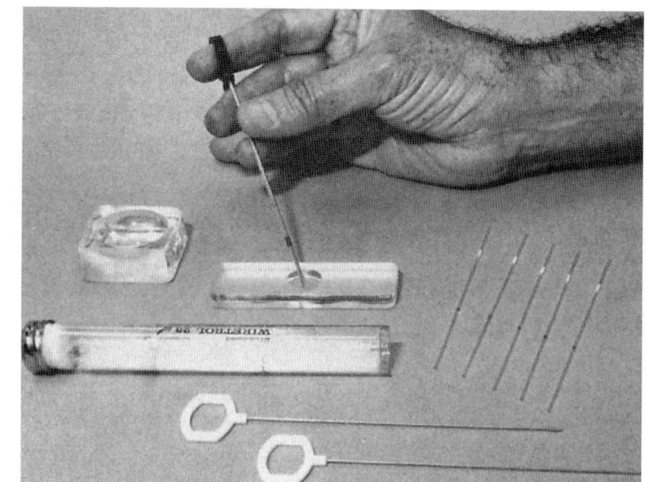

FIGURE 31-15. Wiretrol for micropipetting: color-coded permanent calibration line permits one-hand operation and eliminates mouth aspiration of micropipetting.

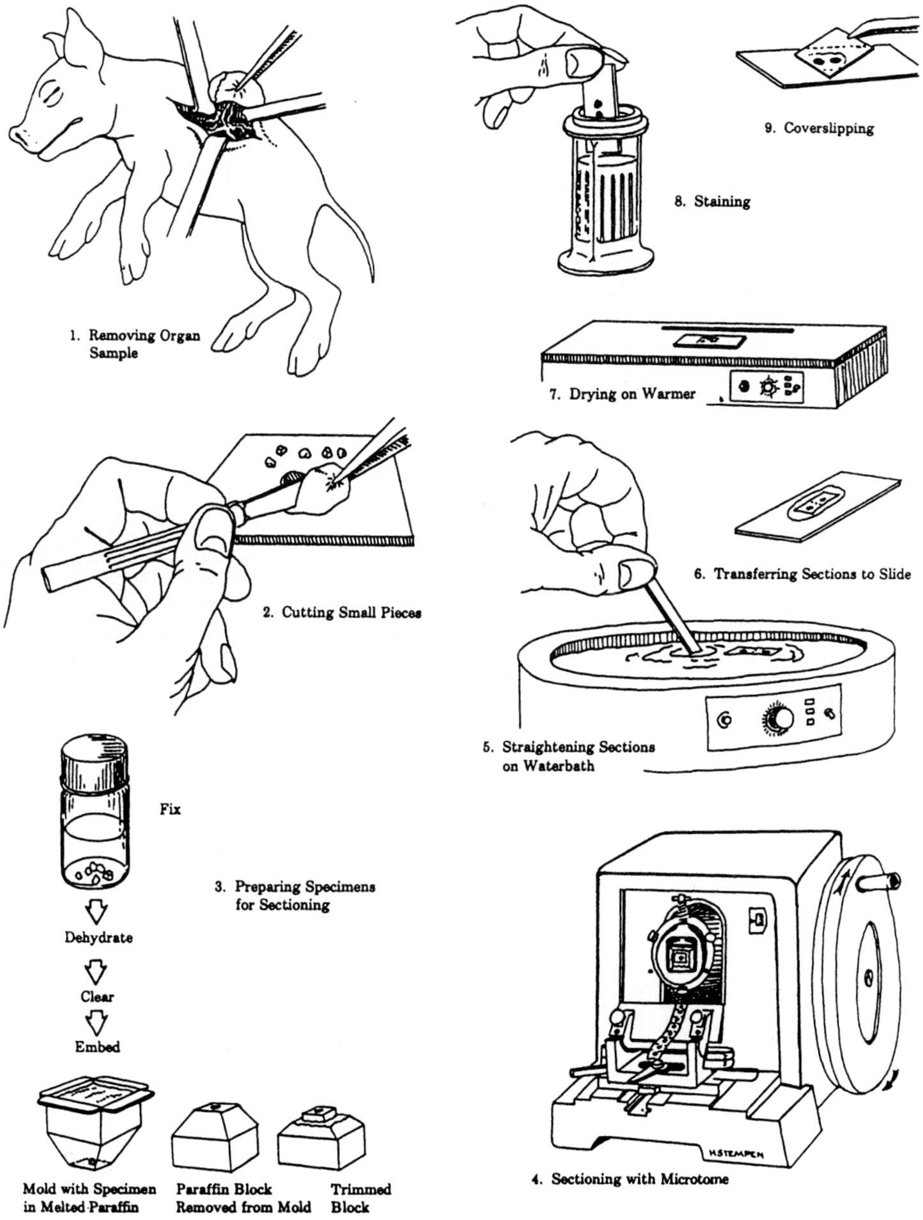

1. Removing Organ Sample

2. Cutting Small Pieces

Fix

3. Preparing Specimens for Sectioning

Dehydrate

Clear

Embed

Mold with Specimen in Melted Paraffin

Paraffin Block Removed from Mold

Trimmed Block

4. Sectioning with Microtome

5. Straightening Sections on Waterbath

6. Transferring Sections to Slide

7. Drying on Warmer

8. Staining

9. Coverslipping

FIGURE 31-16. Preparation of histological slides: fixation slicing, staining, and drying.

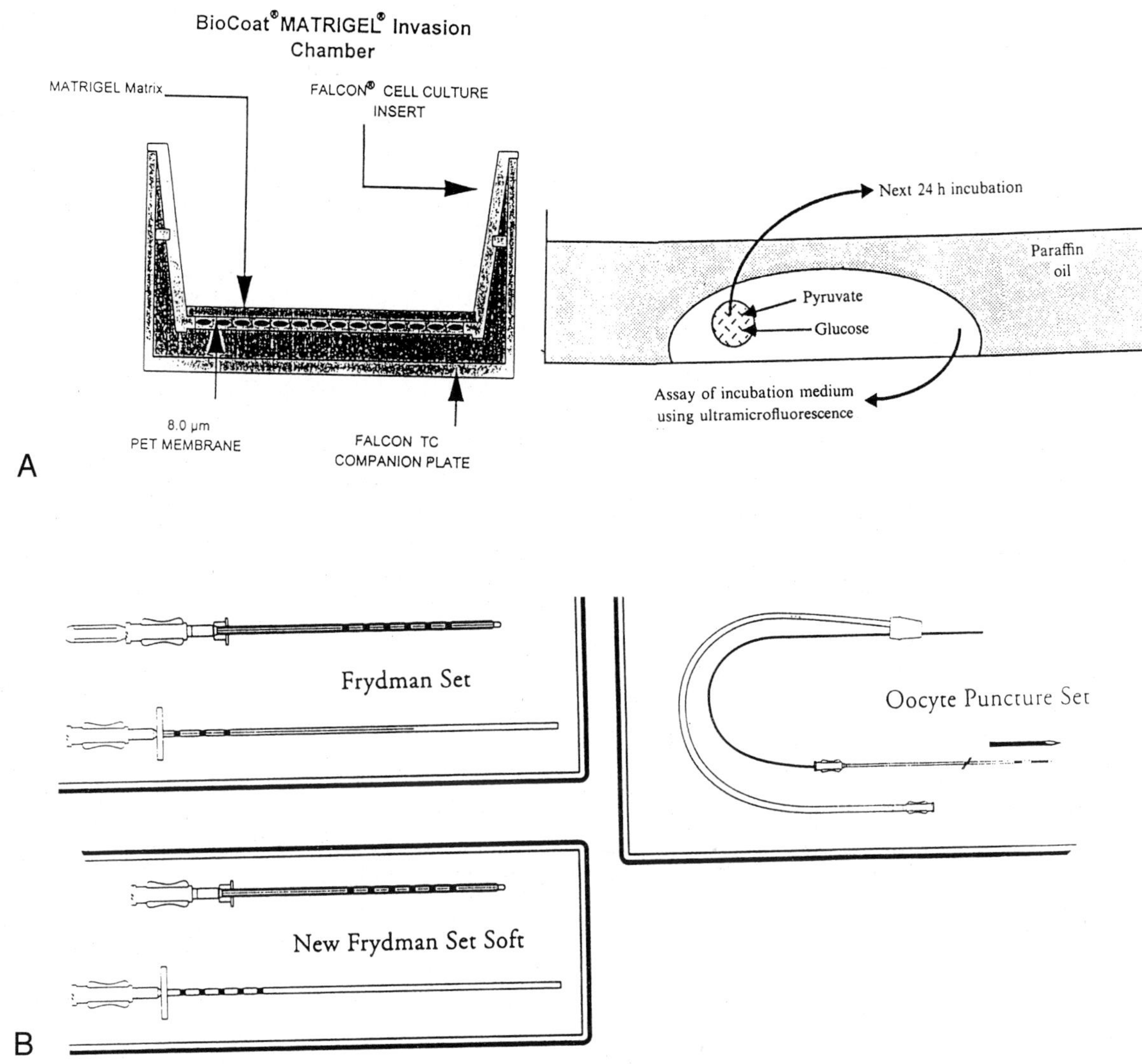


Figure 31-17. (**A**) BioCoat Matrigel Invasion Culture and assay of incubation media using ultramicrofluorescence. (**B**) Various types of micropipettes: Frydman set, New Frydman Set soft, and Oocyte puncture set.

## Macromolecular Supplementation

The preparation of serum added into maturation medium requires special attention. The serum obtained after coagulation of whole blood (delayed centrifuged [DC] serum) contains substances toxic to embryos. DC serum toxicity can be avoided completely by a serum preparation method that prevents the platelet-release reaction.

### *Culture Media*

Several biologic culture media have been used for the manipulation of embryos (see Appendix). Usually, 50 mg of streptomycin sulfate and 100,000 IU of potassium penicillin G are added per liter, but other concentrations and other antibiotics and antifungal agents are frequently used as well. Media should be forced through a filter of 0.45 $\mu$m or smaller to remove bacteria.

Media may contain either bovine serum albumin (BSA) or blood serum (often from fetal calves) that has been inactivated by being held at 56°C for 30 min. BSA is usually added at 0.3 to 1%, but concentrations from 0.1% to 50% have been used. All media except the modified phosphate-buffered saline are bicarbonate-buffered and therefore require an atmosphere of 5% $CO_2$ to maintain proper pH. This is accomplished with a mixture of 5% $CO_2$ in air, or better, 5% $CO_2$, 5% $O_2$, and 90% $N_2$. A $CO_2$ incubator or small, gassed, and airtight containers may be used. When media must be kept in an air environment (without $CO_2$) for long periods, 25 mL HEPES buffer is usually added and the NaCl decreased to maintain proper osmolality. Incubator or small, gassed, and airtight containers may be used when media must be kept in an air environment.

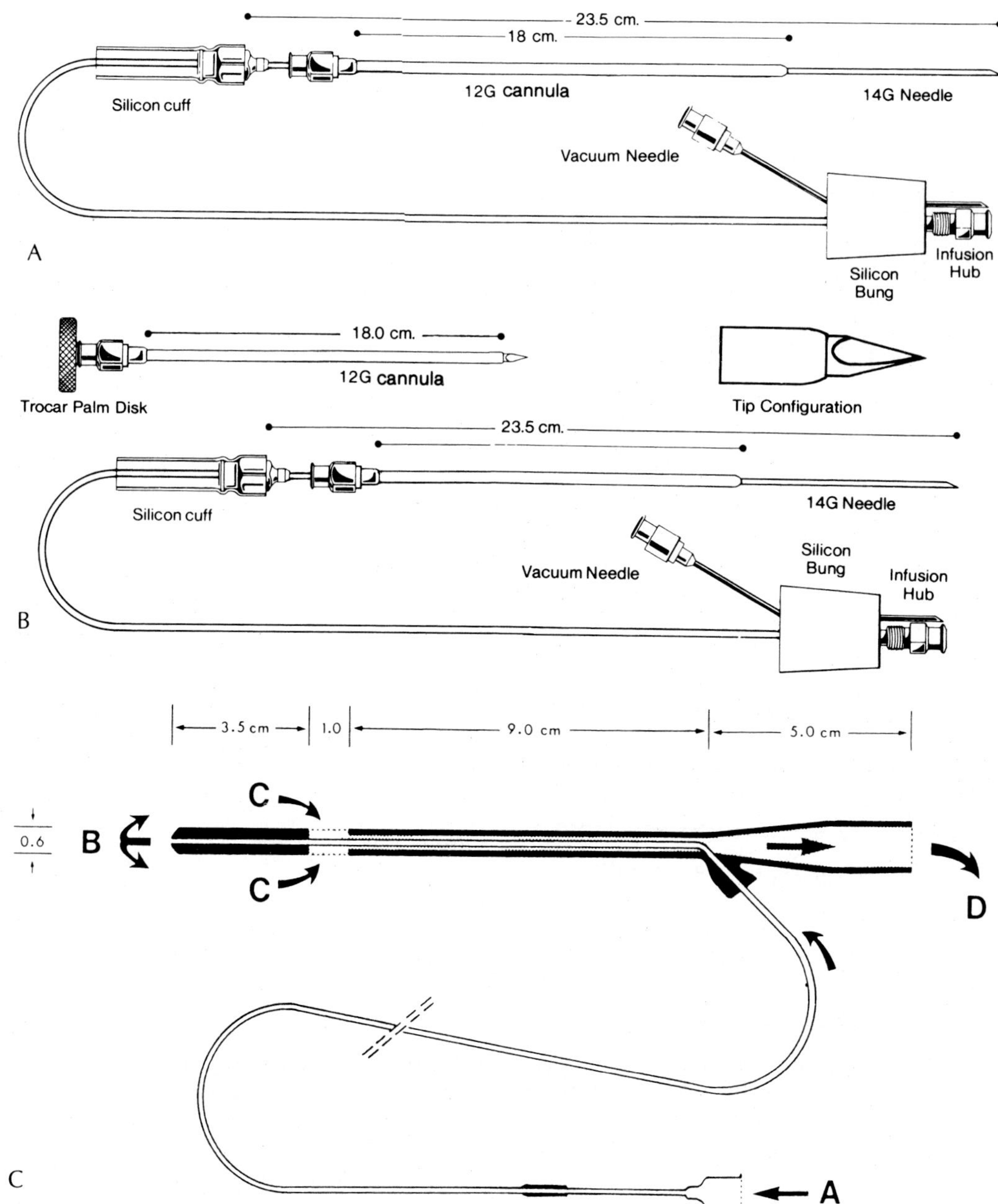


FIGURE 31-18. Different types of pipette and micropipette to recover eggs from donor cattle and transfer embryo non-surgically in recipient cattle.

Phenol red, 1 to 20 mg/L is often added as a pH indicator. The pH of media may range from 7 to 8, but best results are obtained between 7.2 and 7.6. The osmolality may be adjusted from 250 to 320 mOsm/kg by varying the NaCl concentration. Osmalalities between 270 and 300 mOsm/kg are most commonly used for embryos. Water is the principal ingredient, and purity is important. Double distillation or glass distillation of deionized water is usually adequate.

Modified, balanced salt solutions such as Krebs-Ringer bicarbonate support *in vitro* fertilization. The acrosome reaction seems to occur much more readily in media containing serum albumin in the form of either heat treated serum or bovine serum albumin (26). It is also critical to provide an energy source, usually glucose or pyruvate, to support sperm motility and the metabolism of the oocytes.

Development of early cleavage stage embryos is enhanced in the presence of oviductal epithelial cells, trophoblastic vesicles, uterine cells, or kidney cells. In some techniques, a whole chick embryo culture system is used. Embryos in agar chips are placed directly into the amniotic cavity of a developing chick embryo (27). Recovery of the agar chips is efficient, and embryonic development and viability are superior to that achieved *in vitro* for early cleavage stage goat and cattle embryos. In other

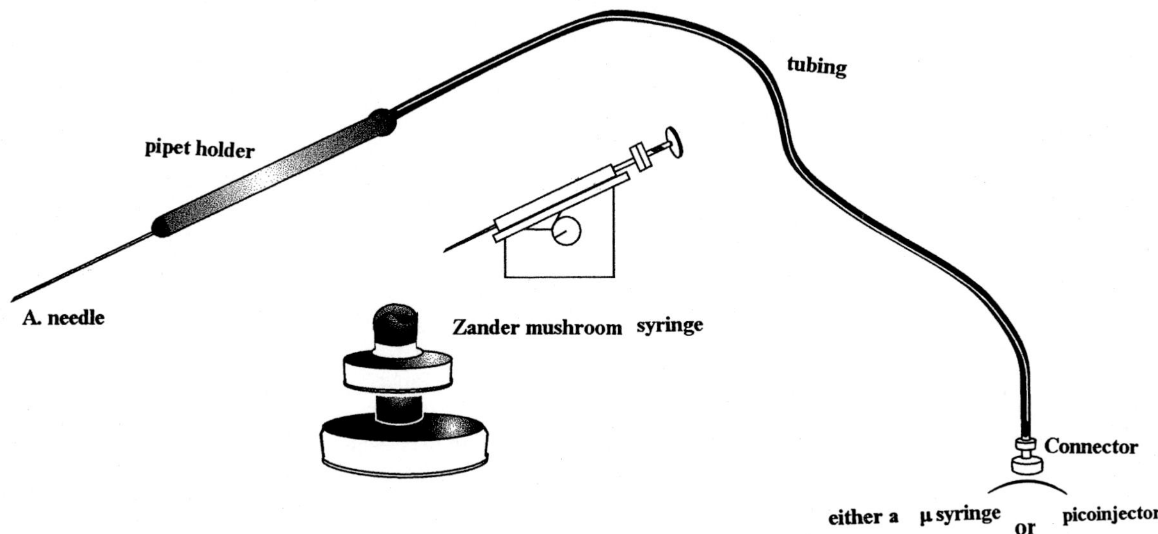


FIGURE 31-19. Zander mushroom syringe and attachments used to manipulate and select ova *in vitro* under the microscope or stereoscope.

techniques, bovine embryos (or blastomeres) are placed into hydrogel chambers, which are then placed into the peritoneal cavity of rodents.

## REFERENCES

1. Willadsen SM, Polge C. Attempts to produce monozygotic quadruplets in cattle by blastomere separation. Vet Rec 1981;108:211–213.
2. Ozil JP, Heyman Y, Renard JP. Production of monozygotic twins by micromanipulation and cervical transfer in the cow. Vet Rec 1982;110:126–127.
3. Ozil JP. Production of identical twins by bisection of blastocysts in the cow. Repro Fertil 1983;69:463.
4. Heyman Y, Renard JP. Cloning of domestic species. Anim Repro Sci, 1996;4:427–436.
5. Heyman Y, Chesne P, Renard JP. Reprogrammation complete de noyaux embryonnaires congeles apres transfert nucleaire chez le lapin. CR Acad Sci Paris (Ser III) 1990;31:321–326.
6. Heyman Y, Chesne P, Lebourhis D, Peynot N, Renard JP. Developmental ability of bovine embryos after nuclear transfer based on the nuclear source: in vivo versus in vitro. Theriogenology 1994;4:695–702.
7. Heyman Y, Chesne P, Thuard JM, Lebourhis D, Marchal J, Nibart M. Birth of cloned calves after nuclear transfer from sexed embryos. In: Proc 10th AETE Meeting. 1994:180.
8. Heyman Y, Camous S, Chesne P, Marchal J, Renard JP. Gestational profiles following transfer of cloned bovine blastocysts developed in vitro. Theriogenology 1995;4:234.
9. Heyman Y, Degrolard J, Adenot P, et al. Cellular evaluation of bovine nuclear transfer embryos developed in vitro. Reprod Nutr Dev 1996;3:713–723.
10. Kanka J, Hosak P, Heyman Y, et al. Transcriptional activity and nucleolar ultrastructure of rabbit nuclei after transplantation to enucleated oocytes. Mol Reprod Dev 1996;4:135–144.
11. Wassarman PM. The mammalian ovum. In: Knobil E, Neil JD, eds. The Physiology of Reproduction. New York: Raven Press, 1988;1.
12. Phillips DM, Shalgi RM. Surface properties of the zona pellucida. J Exp Zool 1980;213:1–8.
13. Yanagimachi R. Specificity of sperm-egg interaction. In: Edidin M, Jonson MH, eds. Immunobiology of Gametes. London and New York, Cambridge University Press, 1977.
14. Willadsen SM. The developmental capacity of blastomeres from 4 to 8-cell sheep embryos. J Embryol Exp Morp 1981;65:165–172.
15. Willadsen SM. Micromanipulation of embryos of the large domestic species. In: Adams CE, ed. Mammalian Egg Transfer. Boca Raton, Florida: CRC Press, 1982.
16. Yanagimachi R. In: Mastroianni IL Jr, Biffers JD, eds. Fertilization and Embryonic Development in Vitro. New York: Plenum Press, 1981;5.
17. Hartmann JF. Mammalian fertilization: gamete surface interactions in vitro. In: Mechanism and Control of Animal Fertilization. New York: Academic Press, 1983.
18. Allen WR, Pashen RL. Production of monozygotic (identical twins) by embryo-micromanipulation. J Reprod Fertil 1984; 71:607.
19. Catt JW. Intracytoplasmis sperm injection (ICSI) and related technology. Anim Reprod Sci 1996;4:239–250.
20. Russell LD. Morphological and functional evidence for Sertoli-germ cell relationships. In: Russell LD, Griswold MD, eds. The Sertoli Cell. Clearwater, Florida: Cache River Press, 1993:365–390.
21. Russell LD, Ettlin RA, Sinha Hikim AP, Clegg ED. Histological and Histopathological Evaluation of the Testis. Clearwater, Florida: Cache River Press, 1990.
22. D'Cruz OJH, Ghosh P, Uckun FM. Spermicidal activity of metallocene complexes containing vanadium(IV) in humans. Reprod 1998;5:1515–1526.
23. Gandolfi F, Brevini TAL, Richardson L, Brown CR, Moor RM. Characterization of proteins secreted by sheep oviduct epithelial cells and their function in embryonic development. Development 1989;106:303–312.

24. Krisher RL, Petters RM, Johnson BH. Effect of oviductal condition on the development in organ culture. Theriogenology 1989;32:885–892.
25. Westhusin ME, Slapak JR, Fuller DT, Kraemer DC. Culture of agar-embedded one and two cell bovine embryos and embryos produced by nuclear transfer in the sheep and rabbit oviduct. Theriogenology 1989;31:271.
26. Bavister B, Yanagimachi R. The effects of sperm extracts and energy sources on the mobility and acrosome reaction of hamster spermatozoa in vitro. Biol Reprod 1977;16:228.
27. Blackwood EG, Godke RA. A method using the chick embry amnion for mammalian embryo culture. J Tissue Culture Meth 1989;12:73–76.
28. Acosta AA, Kruger TF. Human Spermatozoa in Assisted Reproduction, 2nd ed., New York: Parthenon Publishing Co., 1996.


## SUGGESTED READING


Adams CE. Egg transfer in carnivores and rodents, between species, and to extopic sites. In: Mammalian Egg Transfer. Boca Raton, FL: CRC Press, 1983.

Adams CE. Egg transfer in the rabbit. In: Mammalian Egg Transfer. Boca Raton, FL: CRC Press, 1983.

Aitken RJ. Fertilization and early embryogenesis. In: Hillier SG, Kitchener HC, Heilson JP, eds. Scientific Essentials of Reproductive Medicine. London: WB Saunders, 1996.

Allen WR. Hormonal control of early pregnancy in the mare. Anim Reprod Sci 1984;7:284.

Anderson GB. Methods of producing twins in cattle. Theriogenology 1978;9:3.

Bacha WS Jr, Wood LM. Color atlas of veterinary histology. Philadelphia: Lea & Febiger, 1990.

Bavister BD. In vitro fertilization: principles, practice and potential. In: Hafez ESE, Semm K, eds. In Vitro Fertilization and Embryo Transfer. Lancaster, England: MTP Press, 1982.

Bjorkman NH. Fine structure of the fetal-maternal area of exchange in the epitheliochorial and endotheliochorial type of placentation. Acta Anat 1973;86(Suppl 1):1.

Britt JH. Induction and synchronization of ovulation. Reproduction in Farm Animals 4th ed. Philadelphia: Lea & Febiger, 1986.

Calhoun ML. The microscopic anatomy of the digestive tract of Gallus domesticus. Iowa State Coll J Sci 1933;7:251.

Church RB, Shea BF. The role of embryo transfer in cattle improvement programs. Can J Anim Sci 1977;57:33.

Daniel JD Jr. Methods in mammalian embryology. San Francisco: WH Freeman, 1971.

Dauzier L, Thibault C, Wintenberger S. La fecondation in vitro de l'oeuf de la lapine. CR Acad Sci Paris 1954;238:844–845.

Dukelow WR. Methods in mammalian reproduction. Daniel JC Jr, ed. New York: Academic Press, 1978.

Dukelow WR. Ovum recovery and embryo transfer in primates. In: Adams CE, ed. Mammalian Egg Transfer. Boca Raton, Florida: CRC Press, 1983.

Dziuk PJ. Obtaining eggs and embryos from sheep and pigs. In: Daniel JC Jr, ed. Methods in Mammalian Embryology. San Francisco: WH Freeman, 1971.

Elsden RP, Hasler JF, Seidel GE Jr. Nonsurgical recovery of bovine eggs. Theriogenology, 1976;6:523.

Fleming AD. Developmental capability of superovulated ova. In: Hafez ESE, Semm K, eds. In vitro Fertilization and Embryo Transfer. Lancaster, England: MTP Press, 1982.

Foote RH, Onuma H. Superovulation, ovum collection, culture and transfer: a review. J Dairy Sci, 1970;53:1681.

Franchi LL, Baker TG. Oogenesis and folicular growth. In: Hafez ESE, Evans TN, eds. Human Reproduction: Conception and Contraception. New York: Harper & Row, 1973.

Getty R. Sisson and Grossman's The Anatomy of the Domestic Animals, 5th ed. Philadelphia: WB Saunders, 1975.

Gould KG. Fertilization in vitro of nonhuman primate ova: present status and rationale for further development of the technique. Report to the Ethics Advisory Board, HEW. Washington, DC: US Government Printing Office, 1979.

Gould KG. Ovum recovery and in vitro fertilization in the chimpanzee. Fertil Steril 1983;40:387–388.

Hare WCD, Betteridge KJ. Relationship of embryo sexing to other methods of prenatal sex determination in farm animals: a review. Theriogenology, 1978;9:27.

Hendricks AG. Embryology of the Baboon. Chicago: University of Chicago Press, 1971.

Hoshiai H, Tsuiki A, Takahashi K, Suzuki M. Sperm-egg interactions by scanning electron microscopy. Arch Androl 1984;12:146.

Hunter RHF. Reproduction of Farm Animals. London: Longman, 1982.

Iritani A, Niwa K. Capacitation of bull spermatozoa and fertilization in vitro of cattle follicular oocytes matured in culture. J Reprod Fertil 1977;50:119.

Iritani A, Niwa K, Imai H. *In-vitro* fertilization of pig follicular oocytes matured in culture. Biol Reprod 1978;18(Suppl 1):14a.

Jeffcoat LG, Whitwell K. Twinning as a cause of foetal and neonatal loss in Thoroughbred mares. J Comp Pathol 1976;83: 91–96.

Jinno M, Iizuka BA, Sandow BA, Hodgen GD. In vitro maturation of oocytes assisted reproduction. Tech Androl (ARTA) 1990;1:54–68.

Kanagawa H, Inouse I, Ishikawa T. Ovulation rate in beef cattle after repeated treatments with gonadotropins and prostaglandin. In: Hafez ESE, Semm K, eds. In vitro fertilization and embryo transfer. Lancaster, England: MTP Press, 1982.

Katska L. Comparison of two methods for recovery of ovarian oocytes from slaughter cattle. Anim Reprod Sci 1984; 7:461–463.

Keuhl TJ, Dukelow WR. Maturation and in vitro fertilization of follicular oocytes of the squirrel monkey (*Saimiri sciureus*). Biol Reprod 1979;21:545.

Koos RD, Jaccarino FJ, Magaril RA, LeMaire WJ. Perfusion of the rat ovary in vitro: methodology, induction of ovulation and pattern of steroidogenesis. Biol Reprod 1984;31:1135–1141.

Kuzan FB, Wright RW Jr. Observations of the development of bovine morulae on various cellular and noncellular substrata. J Anim Sci 1982;5:811–816.

Kvansnickii AV. Interbreed ova transplantation. Sovetsk Zootech 1951;1:36.

Land RB. The genetics of breed improvement. In: Betteridge KJ, ed. Embryo Transfer in Farm Animals. Ottawa, Canada, Dept. Agric Monograph 16, 1977.

Lucas AM, Stettenheim PR. Avian Anatomy. Integument part I. Washington, DC: United States Department of Agriculture (USDA), 1972

Lucas AM, Stettenheim PR. Avian Anatomy. Integument part II. Washington, DC: United States Department of Agriculture (USDA), 1972

Marden WGR, Chang MC. Aerial transport of mammalian ova for transplantation. Science 1952;115:705.

Maurer RR, Foote RH. Maternal aging and embryonic mortality in the rabbit. (I) Repeated superovulation, embryo culture, and transfer. J Reprod Fertil 1971;25:329–341.

McGaughey RW, Polge C. Cytogenetic analysis of pig oocytes matured in vitro. J Exp Zool 1971;176:383.

Newcomb R, Rowson LEA. Conception rate after uterine transfer of cow eggs in relation to synchronization of estrus and age of eggs. J Reprod Fertil 1975;4:539.

Nicholas JS. Development of transplanted rat eggs. Proc Soc Exp Biol Med 1933;30:1111.

Nickel R, Schilnimer A, Seiferle E, eds. Anatomy of the Domestic Birds. Siller WG, Wight PAL, trans. New York: Springer-Verlag, 1977.

Niwa K, Hosoi Y, O'Hara K, Iritani A. Fertilization in vitro of rabbit eggs with or without follicular cells by epididymal spermatozoa capacitated in a chemically defined medium. Anim Reprod Sci 1983;6:143–149.

Oguri N, Tsutsumi Y. Non-surgical transfer of equine embryos. In: Hafez ESE, Semm K, eds. In Vitro Fertilization and Embryo Transfer. Lancaster, England: MTP Press, 1982.

Onuma H, Hahan J, Foote. Factors affecting superovulation, fertilization and recovery of superovulated ova in prepuberal cattle. J Reprod Fertil 1970;21:119.

Pincus GW, Enzmann EV. The comparative behavior of mammalian eggs in vivo and in vitro (I) The activation of ovarian eggs. J Med 1935;6:665.

Rich LJ. The morphology of canine and feline blood cells, including equine references. St Louis: Ralston, Purina, 1976.

Roche JF, Ireland J, Mawhinney S. Control and induction of ovulation in cattle. J Reprod Fertil Suppl 1981;30:211.

Rogers BJ. Mammalian sperm capacitation and fertilization in vitro; a critique of methodology. Gamete Res. 1978;1:165.

Ross MH, Romrell LJ. Histology. 2nd ed. Baltimore: Williams & Wilkins, 1989

Rowson LEA, Lawson RAS, Moor RM. Production of twins in cattle by egg transfer. J Reprod Fert 1971;25:261.

Seidel GE Jr, Bowen RA, Kane MT. In vitro fertilization, culture and transfer of rabbit ova. Fertil Steril 1976;27:861.

Seidel GE Jr, Larson LL, Spilman CH, Hahn J, Foote RH. Culture and transfer of calf ova. J Dairy Sci 1971;54:923.

Seitz HM, Brackett BG, Mastroanni L. Fertilization. In: Hafez ESE, Evans TN, eds. Human Reproduction: Conception and Contraception. New York: Harper & Row, 1973.

Shalgi R, Phillips DM. Mechanics of in vitro fertilization in the hamster. Biol Reproduction 1980;23:433–444.

Shea BF, Hines DJ, Lightfoot DE, Ollis GW, Olson SM. The transfer of bovine embryos. In: Rowson LEA, ed. Egg Transfer in Cattle. Commission of the European Communities. EUR 5491, Luxembourg. 1976:145–152.

Sreenan JM. Non-surgical embryo transfer in the cow. Theriogenology 1978;9:69.

Sreenan JM, Behan D, Mulvehill P. Egg transfer in the cow: factors affecting pregnancy and twinning rates following bilateral transfer. J Reprod Fertil 1975;44:77.

Sugie T. Successful transfer of a fertilized bovine egg by non-surgical techniques. J Reprod Fertil 1965;10:197.

Sugie T, Soma T, Tsunoda Y, Mizuochi K. Embryo transfer in goat and sheep. In: Hafez ESE, Semm K, eds. In vitro Fertilization and Embryo Transfer. Lancaster, England: MTP Press, 1982.

Sundstrom P. Interaction of human gametes in vitro by scanning electron microscopy. Arch Androl 1984;12:145.

Sundstrom P. Interaction between spermatozoa and ovum in vitro. In: Hafez ESE, Kenemans OP, eds. Atlas of Human Reproduction by Scanning Electron Microscopy. Lancaster, England, MTP Press, 1982;24

Thibault C, Dauzier L. Fertilisines et fecondation in vitro de l'oeuf de la lapine. CR Acad Sci (Paris) 1960;250:1358–1359.

Thibault C, Dauzier L. Analyse des conditions de la fecondation in vitro de l'oeuf de la lapine. Ann Biol Anim Biochim Biophys 1961;1:227–294.

Trounson AO, Willadsen SM, Moor RM. Reproductive function in prepubertal lambs: ovulation, embryo development and ovarian steroidogenesis. J Reprod Fertil 1977;49:69.

Trounson AO, Rowson LEA, Willadsen SM. Non-surgical transfer of bovine embryo. Vet Rec 1978a;102:74.

Trounson AO, Shea BF, Ollis GW, Jacobson ME. Frozen storage and transfer of bovine embryos. J Anim Sci 1978b;47:677.

Warwick BL, Berry RO. Inter-generic and intra-specific embryo transfer. J Hered 1949;40:287.

Wassarman PM. The mammalian ovum. In: Knobil E, Neil JD, eds. The Physiology of Reproduction. New York: Raven Press, 1988;1.

Wheater PR, Burkitt HG, Daniels VG. Functional Histology. A text and colour atlas. New York: Churchill Livingstone, 1979.

Wittingham DG, Leibo SP, Mazur P. Survival of mouse embryos frozen to −196°C and −259°C. Science 1972;178:411.

Willett EL, et al. Successful transplantation of a fertilized bovine ovum. Science 1951;113:247.

Wilmut I, Rowsen LEA. Experiments on the low-temperature preservation of cow embryos. Vet Rec 1973;92:686.

Wright RW Jr, et al. In vitro culture of embryos from adult and prepuberal ewes. J Anim Sci 1976;42:912.

Wright RW Jr, Bondioli KR. Aspects of in vitro fertilization and embryo culture in domestic animals. J Anim Sci 1981;53:701.

Xu KP, Greve T, Callesen H, Hyttel P. Pregnancy resulting from cattle oocytes matured and fertilized in vitro. J Reprod Fertil 1987;81:501–504.

Yanagimachi R. In: Mastroianni IL Jr, Biffers JD, eds. Fertilization and Embryonic Development in Vitro. New York, Plenum Press, 1981;5.

# GLOSSARY

**Abortion** The termination of pregnancy with the expulsion of a fetus of recognizable size before it is viable.

**Acentric** A chromosome without the centromere.

**Acrocentric** A type of chromosome whereby the centromere is located very near to one end.

**Acrosome** Sac-like organelle on the anterior portion of the sperm head that contains several enzymes used during the penetration of egg membranes by the sperm.

**Activin** Dimer of the $\beta$ subunits ($\beta A \beta B$) of inhibin originally isolated from follicular fluid on the basis of its ability to stimulate production of FSH by cultured pituitary gonadotropes.

**Adipose tissue** Fatty connective tissue, commonly the part of the body where fat is stored.

**Albumin** A protein in many animal and vegetable tissues, including human plasma, soluble in water and coagulable by heat; a principal constituent of egg white.

**Allantois** Diverticulum of the hindgut fuses with chorion to form the chorioallantoic placenta.

**Allele** An alternative or different form of the same gene or DNA sequence, which occurs on either one of two homologous chromosomes in a diploid organism.

**Amnion** Innermost of the fetal membranes forming the waterbag that surrounds and protects the embryo/fetus.

**Androgen** Male sex hormone secreted by the Leydig cells in the testis

**Androgen-binding protein** Androgen carrier protein involved in delivery of hormone to target tissues through interaction with its cell surface receptor.

**Anestrus** 1) Absence of estrus without ovulation. 2) The interval of sexual quiescence between two estrous cycles in mammals, or prolonged failure of estrus in a mature animal. 3) Absence of estrus. True anestrus is a state of complete sexual inactivity with no manifestations of estrus, which should be distinguished from nondetected estrus. In the latter, a functional corpus luteum is present.

**Aneuploidy** A cell which has an additional chromosome or a deletion of a chromosome from the expected balanced diploid number of chromosomes.

**Anovulatory estrus** 1) Ovulation without estrus. 2) The animal shows normal behavioral estrus and the ovarian follicle reaches preovulatory size but does not rupture.

**Antibody** Protein molecules produced by B lymphocytes that are produced in response to exposure to a specific antigen and towards which the antibody can react with high affinity and specificity. Antibodies are members of the immunoglobulin protein family. Antibodies cause opsonization of microbes to promote phagocytosis by neutrophils and macrophages and also allow NK cells to recognize targets.

**Antigen** A substance not normally present in an animal that, following entry into an animal, elicits immune responses specific for that antigen mediated by B lymphocytes (antibody production) and T lymphocytes (cytotoxicity, helper functions).

**Antigen presentation** The process by which antigens are processed by antigen-presenting cells (macrophages, dendritic cells, B cells, endothelial cells, and some epithelial cells) so that they are bound by proteins of the major histocompatibility complex and can be identified by T-cell receptors.

**Areolae** Specialized parts of chorion opposite endometrial glands that are involved in uptake of nutrients and other molecules from maternal system (singular areolus).

**Atresia** The closure or the failure of development of a normal opening or channel in the body.

**Autocrine** Process in which ligands (hormones, growth factors, and neurotrophins) produced by a cell in turn act upon the cell itself to modulate (amplify or attenuate) growth/differentiation.

**Autoimmune disease** Several diseases of unknown cause may reflect a strange inability of the body to "recognize" itself, so that mechanisms that normally create immunity to foreign invaders somehow establish a specific sensitivity to certain of the body's own tissues.

**Autosome** A chromosome other than the sex chromosomes, or not involved in sex determination.

**Azoospermia** Absence of sperm in the semen.

**Basophil** Granulated cells present in the circulation whose granules contain substances that promote vasodilation, increased vascular permeability, and smooth muscle contraction. Basophils are similar in function to mast cells in tissue.

**Biopsy** Removal of tissue from the living body for diagnosis. The tissue specimen may be subjected to biochemical tests; more often, it is set in a paraffin block, cut into thin slices, stained, and studied under a microscope.

**Buck** Adult male goat or rabbit.

**CD4** Cluster of differentiation antigen 4. This protein is expressed on the surface of T lymphocytes and participates in recognition of antigen that is processed by proteins of the major histocompatability complex class II. Used as a marker for helper lymphocytes.

**CD8** Cluster of differentiation antigen 8. This protein is expressed on the surface of T lymphocytes and participates in recognition of antigen that is processed by major histocompatability complex class I. Used as a marker for cytotoxic T lymphocytes.

**CL-dependent species** A species in which progesterone needed for the maintenance of pregnancy is dependent upon a functional corpus luteum.

**Centromere** The constricted portion of the chromosome to which the spindle fibers attach during a cell division (meiosis and mitosis).

**Chimera** An individual with cell populations of more than one genotype produced from two or more zygotes.

**Chorion** Outermost of the fetal membranes. The fetal part of the placenta develops from it.

**Chorionic girdle** A ring of tissue that forms on the horse placenta around day 25 to 36 of pregnancy. Subsequently, cells from the chorionic girdle invade the endometrium to form endometrial cups.

**Chromatid** Each of the two daughter strands of a duplicated chromosome joined at the centromere during meiosis and mitosis.

**Chromosome** 1) A single DNA molecule, carrying genetic inheritance that is condensed into a compact structure by complexing with accessory histones or histone-like proteins. Chromosomes exist as homologous pairs in higher eukaryotes. 2) Any abnormal change in the chromosome aberration number or structure. 3) Threadlike bodies in the nucleus of a cell containing the genes and DNA. The chromosomes separate during a stage of cell division. Stained and prepared specimens can be studied under a microscope. Each parent contributes a chromosome to the pair. One of the pairs contains the sex chromosomes. A dam contributes the X (female-determining) chromosome to the pair, and a sire contributes either an X or a Y chromosome.

**Chromosome loss** Failure of a chromosome to become incorporated into the nucleus of a daughter cell at cell division.

**Cilia** Minute hairlike processes of specialized cells that beat rhythmically and keep debris-laden fluids flowing in one direction, for example, out of the lungs. The word also means eyelashes.

**Codominance** A heterozygous individual showing phenotypic effects of both alleles equally.

**Conceptus** 1) The products of conception, i.e., the embryo or fetus and its associated placental membranes. 2) The products of conception (it can be fertilized egg, embryo, or the fetal membranes).

**Conception rate (fertility)** The proportion of ewes or does mated that conceive.

**Congenital defects** Abnormalities of structure or function which are present at birth.

**Corpus luteum** The "yellow body" that develops from a follicle of the ovary after a ripened egg has been discharged. It produces progesterone, a hormone that prepares the lining of the uterus to receive a fertilized egg. If fertilization occurs, the corpus luteum enlarges and continues to produce pregnancy-sustaining hormone for several months. If conception does not occur, the corpus luteum degenerates.

**Cranium** The skull, containing the brain.

**Cremaster** Muscles that retract the testis.

**Crossing-over** The exchange of DNA sequences between chromatids of homologous chromosomes during meiosis.

**Cryptorchidism** Failure of the testicles to descend into the scrotum during fetal development; the undescended testis remains in the abdominal cavity or groin.

**Cystadenoma** A cystic neoplasm lined with epithelial cells and filled with retained secretions.

**Cytogenetics** The cytologic approach to genetics, mainly involving microscopic studies of chromosomes.

**Cytokines** 1) Small proteins that contribute to the endometrial immune system. 2) Regulatory proteins secreted by cells of the immune system that can modulate function of other immune cells and certain non-immune cells.

**Cytology** Scientific study of the structure, elements, and functions of cells.

**Cytoplasm** The substance of a cell outside of its nucleus. Transformations of energy, synthesis of proteins, and uncountable chemical exchanges that keep us alive occur incessantly in the cytoplasm.

**Cytotoxicity** Killing of cells. Lymphocytes that cause cytotoxicity include cytotoxic T lymphocytes and natural killer cells (adjective: cytotoxic).

**Decalcification** The withdrawal of calcium from the bones where it had been deposited. It may be caused by an inadequate supply of calcium in the ration so that calcium has to be taken from the bones, or it may be caused by hormonal imbalances.

**Deficiency** The absence of part of the normal genome or chromosome set.

**Deletion** Loss of a DNA (chromosome) segment from a chromosome. Deletions are recognized genetically by: absence of reverse mutation, presence of a deletion loop at meiosis visualized cytologically, revealing of recessive lethals, and pseudodominance.

**Dendritic cell** An antigen presenting cell present in tissues such as skin and other sites including, probably, the reproductive tract. Dendritic cells are of bone marrow origin and have long processes that can, via phagocytosis or endocytosis, process antigen and present it to lymphocytes.

**Diploid** The condition when the genome of an organism consists of two copies of each chromosome.

**Dizygotic** Developed at the same time from two fertilized eggs (fraternal twins).

**Doe** Adult female goat or rabbit.

**Dominant** An allele that determines the phenotype or trait of an individual even when present as a heterozygous with a recessive allele. For example, if A is dominant over a, then AA and Aa have the same phenotype.

**Dominant follicle** A single large follicle that continues to grow while suppressing the growth of follicles larger than 4 mm in diameter.

**Ductless gland (endocrine gland)** Secretes a hormone(s) into the blood that acts at a distant target tissue. A more modern definition includes hormones not necessarily produced by a ductless gland and that can act via a paracrine or autocrine mechanisms (e.g., prostaglandins).

**Dysgerminoma** A rare malignant ovarian tumor composed of undifferentiated germinal epithelium; the counterpart of seminoma of the testis. Also called Ovarian seminoma.

**Dystrophy** Degeneration, wasting, and abnormal development.

**Ejaculation** Ejaculation involves complex motor activity which is completed in two phases: emission of sperm and ejaculation of semen. Emission of semen: sperm from the epididymis/vas deferens as well as secretions from the seminal vesicles and prostate are transported into the posterior portion of the urethra by active concentration of the musculature around the epididymis, vas deferens, and seminal vesicle. Emission is associated with contraction of the internal urethral sphincter and closure of the bladder neck to prevent the ejection of the sperm backward into the bladder. Ejaculation of semen: This phase is triggered by the transport of semen in the prostatic part of the urethra. Afferent impulses stimulate the sacral/lumbar nerves to stimulate spasmodic contraction of bulbocavernosus and perineal muscles. The external urethral sphincter relaxes and the semen is propelled via the urethra. Semen is ejaculated in several forceful thrusts.

**Electrophoresis** The movement of charged particles in an electric field toward either the anode or the cathode; used as a means of separating substances in a medium.

**Embryo** In this period, rapid growth and differentiation occur, during which the major tissues, organs, and systems are established and the major features of external body form are recognizable.

**Embryonic** 1) Of, or relating to, an embryo. 2) Undeveloped, rudimentary.

**Endocrinology** Study of the classic endocrine system.

**Endocytosis** Uptake of fluid or specific molecules into a cell through formation of vesicles on the cell surface (adjective: endocytic).

**Endometrial cup** Knob or cup like structures on the endometrium of the pregnant mare that are formed from invading placental cells from the chorionic girdle. Cells of the endometrial cups, which produce equine chorionic gonadotropin, first form about day 36 to 38 of pregnancy and are destroyed by day 100 to 140 of pregnancy.

**Endometrial cups** Discrete, raised areas arranged in a circular fashion at the caudal portion of the gravid uterine horn in the horse. These cups are formed by the invasion of the endometrium by a band of specialized trophoblastic cells (chorionic girdle) that peel off the fetal membranes by day 38. The endometrial cups are the source of the eCG present in high concentrations in the blood of mares between 40 and 130 days of gestation.

**Endometritis** Infection of the endometrium; release of endometrial fragments outside the uterus.

**Eosinophil** A granulated cell which can release cytotoxic and vasoactive substances when activated.

**Epithelia** Cells that form the outer layer of the skin, i.e., those that line all the portions of the body that have contact with external air (eyes, ears, nose, throat, lungs), and tissues specialized for secretion such as the urogenital tract.

**Equine chorionic gonadotrophin** Gonadotrophin (eCG) of fetal origin that appears in maternal blood between 40 and 130 days of pregnancy in the horse. It is a rich source of FSH.

**Esterase** Any enzyme that promotes the hydrolysis of an ester.

**Estrogen** A hormone produced in the ovaries to stimulate growth of the inner lining of the uterus.

**Estrus** Period at which a female animal shows sexual desire towards the male.

**Ewe** Adult female sheep.

**Fecundity** The number of live offspring produced by an organism.

**Feedback loop** Mechanism of communication between the ovaries and hypothalamo-pituitary axist.

**Fertilization** Penetration of the ovum by the spermatozoan and completed by the fusion of the female and male chromosomes with subsequent formation of male and female pronuclei and expulsion of the second polar body, syngamy leading to cleavage to two blastomeres.

**Fetal maceration** In cases of incomplete abortion, bacteria enter through a partially dilated cervix to autolyze fetal soft tissues leaving fetal bones floating within the uterine lumen. This condition is referred to as *fetal maceration*, which is a septic process unlike mummification.

**Fetal membranes** Closely related to extra-embryonic or fetal membranes that are differentiated into the yolk sac, amnion, allantois, and chorion.

**Fetus** Growth and changes in the form of the fetus characterize this period.

**Fimbria** A fringelike structure, especially, fimbriae of the opening of the oviducts, close to the ovary. The fringelike projections are covered with cilia. The conversion of an unfrozen solution into the solid form.

**Flehmen** After sniffing the urine or vulva of a cow, the bull curls his upper lip in a characteristic manner.

**Flushing** Increasing the level of nutrition before mating; commonly practiced in sheep to increase ovulation rate.

**Follicle** 1) A somewhat spherical mass of cells usually containing a cavity. 2) A smalll crypt, such as the depression in the skin from which the hair emerges.

**Follicle stimulating hormone (FSH)** Protein made by the anterior pituitary, binds to cells with FSH receptors and promotes estradiol biosynthesis/follicle development/initiation of spermatogenesis.

**Follicular phase** First phase of the estrous cycle, at a time when a new cohort of follicles is recruited, from which the Graafian follicle will be selected.

**Follistatin** FSH-suppressing protein originally isolated from ovarian follicular fluid and having an important role as an activin-binding protein.

**Freemartin** A heifer born co-twin to a bull. About 95% are sterile.

**Frenulum** A small fold of mucous membrane that extends from a fixed to a movable part and limits the motion of the movable part.

**Fundamental number** The number of chromosome arms in a somatic cell of a particular species.

**Gamete** A haploid sex cell (egg or sperm) which contains a single copy of each chromosome.

**Gene** A unit of heredity or a segment of DNA on a chromosome that encodes a specific protein or several related proteins.

**Genotype** 1) The genetic constitution of an organism. 2) The structure of DNA or the genetic makeup of an organism which determines the expression of a trait (phenotype).

**Gestation** 1) The period from implantation of the blastocyst in the endometrium until the termination of pregnancy. 2) The period in which animals complete their embryonic and fetal development within the uterus. Length of gestation is calculated as the interval from fertile mating to parturition.

**Glycolosis** The energy-producing process in the body, especially in muscles, in which sugar is broken down into lactic acid; since oxygen is not consumed, it is frequently termed anaerobic glycolysis.

**Gonad** Primary sex glands, ovaries, or testes.

**Gonadal peptides** Peptides made in the ovary or testes that have paracrine roles in gametogenesis/endocrine roles to regulate FSH production. Inhibins, activins, and follistatin.

**Gonadotrophs** Cells within the anterior pituitary gland that, in response to stimulation by GNRH and modulation by circulating gonadal products, synthesize/secrete LH and FSH.

**Gonadotropin-releasing hormone (GnRH)** Decapeptide hypothalamic-releasing hormone controls pituitary gonadotropin synthesis/secretion and ultimately, reproductive competence. The peptide, secreted by hypothalamic neurons into the hypophyseal portal circulation, that induces pituitary (LH)/(FSH) secretion.

**Gonadotropin** A hormone or a substance that stimulates either the ovaries or the testes.

**Gonadotropins** LH and FSH are two pituitary hormones secreted in a pulsatile fashion to direct steroidogenesis/gametogenesis at level of gonad.

**Gonocyte** A primitive reproductive cell.

**Graafian follicle** Dominant follicle, completing its growth process.

**Gram-positive, Gram-negative** Classification of bacteria according to whether they do or do not accept a stain named for Hans Gram, a Danish bacteriologist. Different life processes and vulnerabilities of germs are reflected by their Gram-positive or Gram-negative characteristics.

**Growth factors** Small peptides that act by autocrine and paracrine pathways. Peptides which stimulate or inhibit the cell from which they are synthesized (autocrine) or of the adjacent cell (paracrine).

**Growth hormone (GH)** Polypeptide hormone secreted by anterior lobe of the pituitary gland, stimulates growth in various tissues indirectly by inducing insulin-like growth factor 1 generation. Direct growth-promoting and anti-insulin actions mediated by GH receptor.

**Haploid** 1) Each chromosome is present as one complete set of the genetic endowment of a eukaryotic organism. 2) Referring to the reduced number of chromosomes in the gametes relative to that in the zygotes or in the body cells (diploid); the haploid number is half the diploid number.

**Helper T cell** T cells which produce cytokines that promote activation and differentiation of other cells of the immune system. Most helper cells are CD4 T cells.

**Hematoma** A localized mass of blood outside of the blood vessels, usually found in a partly clotted state.

**Heredity** The biological similarity of offspring and parents.

**Hermaphrodite** An individual having both male and female genitalia.

**Heterogametic** An individual having two heteromorphic sex (differently shaped) chromosomes, for example, X and Y chromosomes.

**Heterozygote** A diploid cell with different paternal and maternal alleles.

**Histology** Microarchitecture of body tissues.

**Homogametic** An individual having similar shaped sex chromosomes (e.g., XX), producing only one kind of gamete.

**Homologous** A member of a pair of identical chromosomes which synapse during meiosis. Chromosomes that pair with each other at meiosis or chromosomes in different species that have retained most of the same genes during their evolution from a common ancestor.

**Homozygous** An individual having identical alleles at a locus.

**Hormone** Special chemicals made by the body that cause changes in the body.

**Hyaluronidase** An enzyme, found in sperm, snake and bee venom, and pathogenic bacteria; it causes the breakdown of hyaluronic acid in the tissue spaces, thus enabling the invading agent to enter cells and tissues. Also called Spreading factor.

**Hybrid** The progeny differing in at least one genetic characteristic (trait) from its parents.

**Hydrometra** An accumulation of fluid within the uterus associated with a persistent corpus luteum in goat.

**Hyperplasia** Overgrowth of an organ or tissue from increased numbers of cells that are in normal patterns.

**Hypertrophy** Increase in the size of an organ because of overgrowth of cells without an increase in the number of cells. The overgrowth of cells is in response to increased activity or functional demands.

**Hypophysis** The pituitary gland.

**Hypothalamic-pituitary-gonadal axis** GnRH controls the production of gonadotropin subunits ($\alpha$, FSH P, and LH P), which regulate gametogenesis/steroidogenesis. Sex steroids and gonadal peptides feed back at the hypothalamus and/or pituitary to ensure reproductive competence.

**Hypothalamus** Endocrine glands at the base of the brain, controls a variety of functions: body temperature, appetite, procreation, and regulates the secretion of hormones by the pituitary gland.

**Idiogram** A diagram of the chromosomes arranged in an orderly manner.

**Immune response** The coordinated response of the immune system to a foreign agent.

**Immune system** The collection of molecules, cells, and tissues that participate in development of immunity and which can also play roles in tissue repair, removal of tumors, and other functions.

**Immunity** Reactions to foreign substances, especially those that are of microbial origin, to protect the organism from the harmful effects of these substances. The immune system can also eliminate tumors from the body and generate reactions which are themselves harmful to the organism. Immunity is often divided into specific or adaptive immunity, which involves responses to specific antigens, and innate immunity, which involves reactions that are not specific to particular antigens, for example phagocytosis by neutrophils. Another distinction is made between humoral immunity, mediated by antibodies, and cell-mediated immunity, mediated by actions of T lymphocytes.

**Immunoglobulin** The family of proteins to which antibodies belong. The name is derived from the fact that antibodies are in the globulin fraction of blood serum. Several classes of immunoglobulin exist called IgG, IgM, IgA, IgE, and IgD.

**Implantation** The blastocyst adheres to, penetrates, and establishes nutritional support from maternal tissues, normally the endometrium.

**In vitro** In glass; pertaining to studies done in test tubes or laboratory hardware, outside of the living body.

**Infertility** A temporary inability to produce viable young within a stipulated time characteristic for each species.

**Inhibin** Glycoprotein hormone made up of two disulfide-linked and dissimilar subunits termed $\alpha$ and $\beta$ ($\beta$A or $\beta$B) involved in suppression of pituitary FSH.

**Insemination** Introduction of semen into the vagina by natural means or by artificial insemination.

**Insulin-like growth factor I (IGF-1)** Synthesized in the liver, IGF-1 is under **GH** control and is expressed in multiple extrahepatic tissues. It acts as a potent stimulator of cell growth and its major somatic growth factor.

**Interferons (IFNs)** Interferons (IFNs) are a group of proteins, which were initially identified by their ability to protect cells against viral infections. There are at least three classes: $\alpha$, $\beta$, and $\gamma$. Both $\alpha$ and $\beta$ IFNs are synthesized in response to viral infection whereas a IFN-$\gamma$ is produced in T lymphocytes following mitogenic or antigenic stimulation.

**Intersex** An individual having external genitalia with attributes of both sexes.

**Inversion** A chromosomal aberration/mutation whereby a segment of the chromosome is rotated through 180 degrees and is reinserted in the same location, resulting in a reverse gene sequence.

**Isochromosome** A chromosome with morphologically and genetically identical arms.

**Isoelectric** Having an equal number of positive and negative charges; electrically neutral; said of certain molecules.

**Isthmus** 1) A narrow section of tissue connecting two larger sections. 2) A narrow passage connecting two larger cavities or tubular structures.

**Karyotype** An individual's chromosomes arranged based on certain physical characteristics such as size, length, and morphology of the chromosomes.

**Karyotyping** Analysis of chromosomes.

**Kinetochore** The chromosomal attachment point for the spindle fibers located within the centromere.

**Klinefelter syndrome** An abnormal male individual having an extra X chromosome (XXY).

**Labia** Lips or liplike organs. Labia majora: folds of skin on either side of the entrance of the vulva. Labia minora: folds of tissue covered with mucous membrane within the labia majora.

**Lactation** The production of milk.

**Lambing percentage** The number of lambs born per 100 ewes exposed.

**Lambing rate (fecundity)** The number of lambs born of ewes lambing.

**Laparoscopy** The technique of viewing the internal organs using an optical instrument.

**Lesion** Alteration of tissue or function due to injury or disease, e.g., pimple, fracture, abscess, scratch, or wart.

**Leukocyte** White blood cells; cells of bone marrow origin that circulate in blood and function in immune responses. Leukocytes include lymphocytes, monocytes, eosinophils, basophils, and neutrophils. The term leukocyte is also sometimes used more broadly to include macrophages and mast cells.

**Leukocytosis** Abnormal increase in numbers of white blood cells. The cell count normally increases slightly after eating and in pregnancy, but the word implies an abnormal increase, often associated with bodily defenses against infection and inflammation.

**Leydig cell** 1) Terminally differentiated somatic cell in testis steroidogenesis. 2) Interstitial cells of the testes that produce testosterone, the male hormone (and small amounts of female hormone). The cells are separate structures from those that produce sperm. Thus, infertile males whose production of sperm is impaired may produce adequate amounts of male hormone and be entirely potent.

**Ligament** A band of tough, flexible fibrous tissue that connects bones or supports organs.

**Locus** A specific site on a chromosome.

**Luteal phase** Second phase of the estrous cycle, characterized by the presence of the corpus luteum when implantation occurs.

**Luteinizing hormone (LH)** Hormone released by pituitary serves dual purposes of causing a dominant follicle to release its egg and stimulating the corpus luteum to secrete progesterone. Gonadotropin is produced mostly to promote ovarian steroid secretion to induce ovulation.

**Luteolysin** An agent that causes regression of the corpus luteum.

**Luteolysis** Process of regression of the corpus luteum.

**Lymphocyte** 1) A type of white blood cell which plays a role in the immune response. 2) Cell of the immune system that generally mounts responses against specific antigens. The major effector actions of lymphocytes include antibody production (B cells), secretion of cytokines to regulate other immune cells (helper T cells) and cytotoxicity (cytotoxic T cells and natural killer cells).

**Lysis** The rupture or breakdown of a cell.

**Macrophage** Mononuclear cell located in tissues that participates in phagocytosis and antigen presentation. Called monocyte when in blood and various other names in specific tissues.

**Major histocompatibility complex (MHC)** Major proteins responsible for tissue rejection responses against tissue grafts. The role of MHC proteins is to bind antigen in a way that allows T cells to recognize the antigen and become activated. MHC class I proteins stimulate T cells expression CD8 and MHC class II proteins stimulate T cells expressing CD4.

**Male effect** The sudden introduction of a male in seasonally anestrus females leading to the induction of estrus.

**Mast cell** Granulated cells present in tissues whose granules contain substances that promote vasodilation, increased vascular permeability, and smooth muscle contraction. Mast cells are similar in function to basophils in the circulation.

**Maternal recognition of pregnancy** Before attaching to the endometrium, the blastocyst secretes substances which prolong the life span of the cyclic corpus luteum beyond the period of the estrous cycle. The time at which it occurs is known as maternal recognition of pregnancy (MRP).

**Meiosis** The reduction division process to produce haploid gametes, comprising of a single duplication of the genetic material.

**Melatonin** The hormone secreted by the pineal gland.

**Mesenchyme** Embryonic connective tissue consisting of an aggregation of cells in contact with one another by means of long processes, thus forming a loose network; the space between the cells is filled with a ground substance; the mesenchymal cell is multipotential, i.e., it can develop into many kinds of connective tissue.

**Metacentric** A chromosome with the centromere located in the middle.

**Metestrous bleeding** The presence of blood in the vulval discharge 48 to 72 hours after end of estrus. It is due to petechial hemorrhages in the endometrium. It is only an indication that a cow has been in estrus and not related to conception.

**Mitosis** The replication of a cell to form two daughter cells with identical sets of chromosomes.

**Modulation** The changes that take place in response to changes in the environment, such as the temporary change of osteoblasts into osteocytes and back to osteoblasts in response to altered conditions in the environment.

**Monozygotic** Developed from a single fertilized egg, as identical twins.

**Morphologic** Relating to the structure or form of organisms.

**Mosaic** An individual with cell populations or more than one genotype produced from one zygote.

**Mucosa** The inner lining of a cavity as the lining of the oral cavity.

**Mummification** It is characterized by fetal mortality but the fetus is not aborted. Instead, resorption of placental fluids, dehydration of the fetus and its membranes lead to a uterus which is tightly wrapped around the fetus. The corpus luteum is retained and the mummified fetus(es) parturition may not occur (cattle).

**Mutagen** A physical or a chemical agent which causes mutation.

**Mutation** An alteration of a gene sequence or in a DNA structure.

**Myoid** Resembling muscle.

**Myometrium** Muscular wall of the uterus.

**Natural killer (NK) cell** A lymphocyte that lacks typical B-cell and T-cell markers and which can recognize certain cell types (for example, those that do not display major histocompatibility complex class I on their cell surfaces) and kill those cells. Unlike cytotoxic T cells, natural killer cells do not require previous exposure to antigens on the target cell to initiate cytotoxicity.

**Negative feedback loop** Process whereby a hormone secreted by a target organ (e.g., the ovary) signals to the hypothalamic-pituitary axis to secrete stimulatory hormones (e.g., LH and FSH) to be readjusted to steady state.

**Neoplasm** The abnormal multiplication of cells with the formation of a mass or new growth of tissue; it may be localized (benign) or spreading and invasive (malignant). Also called Tumor. Cf. Hyperplasia; hypertrophy.

**Neuroendocrine** Denoting a relationship between the nervous system and the endocrine gland.

**Neuromuscular** Relating to nerve and muscle, such as the nerve endings in a muscle, or the interaction of nerve and muscle.

**Neutrophil** Polymorphonuclear leukocyte that participates in phagocytosis. Neutrophils, which are also called polymorphonuclear leukocytes (PMN), are one of the first cells to migrate to a site of inflammation.

**Nymphomania** Exaggerated sexual desire (mounting) in a female.

**Ocular** 1) Pertaining to the eye 2) The eyepiece of a microscope.

**Oocyte** A cell in the ovary derived from an oogonium that, upon undergoing meiosis, produces an ovum; a primitive egg in the ovary.

**Opsonization** Process by which particles are coated with antibody or complement to increase the affinity of phagocytes which have antibody or complement receptors for the particle.

**Orchitis** Inflammation of the testis. Also called Testitis.

**Ovariectomy** Removal of ovaries.

**Oviduct** Tubes through which the egg is transported to the uterus and in which fertilization usually occurs.

**Ovulatory surge** Abundant release of GnRH and gonadotropin in response to the estradiol positive feedback to induce ovulation.

**Paracellular transport** Transepithelial movement of fluid and solutes through the intercellular spaces.

**Paracrine** Produced by one cell act on adjacent cells to modify or modulate proliferation development.

**Parturition** Physiologic process by which the pregnant uterus delivers the fetus and placenta from the maternal organism (labor).

**Pedigree** A family tree drawn with standard genetic symbols, showing inheritance patterns for specific phenotypic characters. A representation of the ancestry of an individual or family; a family tree.

**Phagocyte** Cell capable of phagocytosis. Among the phagocytes are neutrophils and macrophages.

**Phagocyte** A white blood cell with properties of engulfing and digesting invading bacteria or other foreign particles.

**Phagocytosis** The process whereby cells engulf and digest microbes or other particles.

**Phenotype** The expression of gene alleles (genotype) that is detectable as a physical or biochemical trait.

**Phimosis** Elongation and tightening of the foreskin of the penis, preventing retraction of the head of the organ.

**Photoperiodism** The physiologic response of living organisms to varying periods of exposure to light (photoperiod).

**Photoreceptor** A nerve end-organ capable of being stimulated by light, as the rods and cones of the retina. Also called Photoceptor.

**Phytoestrogens** Plants that contain compounds with estrogenic activity.

**Pineal gland** Endocrine gland located at the base of the brain that secretes the hormone melatonin.

**Placenta** Apposition or fusion of the fetal membranes to the endometrium to permit physiologic exchange between fetus and mother. It originates as a result of various degrees of fetal-maternal interactions and is connected to the embryo by a cord of blood vessels.

**Placentome** In ruminants, the fetal cotyledons fuse with caruncles or specialized projections of the uterine mucosa to form placentomes or functional units.

**Plasma cell** An activated B cell that synthesizes large amounts of antibody.

**Plasmalemma** Cell membrane; see under Membrane.

**Polyspermy** Immediately following fertilization, the egg surface (zona pellucida) changes to prevent fusion of additional sperm. When this fails, one or more sperm enter the egg to form polyploid embryos.

**Prepartum** Prior to parturition/labor.

**Primiparous** Animal that is pregnant for the first time.

**Primordial** 1) Relating to the embryonic group of cells that develops into an organ or structure 2) Formed during the early stage of development.

**Progesterone** 1) Main ovarian steroid produced by the corpus luteum, secreted by follicle at the time of gonadotropin surge. 2) Sex steroid secreted by luteal tissue and the placenta. It acts as the "hormone of pregnancy" and suppresses myometrial activity during pregnancy.

**Prolonged gestation** The normal duration of gestation is extended beyond the length characteristic of the species.

**Prostaglandin** Chemical made by the body that causes the muscle of the uterus to contract.

**Prostaglandins** Prostaglandins are group of 20 carbon unsaturated hydroxy fatty acids with a cyclopentene ring. Most closely associated with reproduction are $PGF_{2\alpha}$, which plays a role in luteolysis and parturition, and prostaglandin $E_2$.

**Protamine** Any of a group of simple, highly basic proteins, rich in arginine and soluble in water; they neutralize the anticoagulant action of heparin.

**Pseudopregnancy** "False" pregnancy due to the prolongation of luteal activity (persistence of the corpus luteum, prolonged diestrus). The persistence of the corpus luteum beyond its normal cyclical lifespan (horse) or is associated with the accumulation of fluid in the uterus (goat).

**Puberty** The physical and biochemical changes, associated with activation of the hypothalamic-pituitary-gonadal axis, that lead to adult reproductive function.

**Puberty** The age at which the reproductive organs become functionally active.

**Puerperium** Postpartum period, is broadly defined as the period extending from delivery until the maternal organism has returned to its normal nonpregnant state.

**Purulent** Containing, exuding, or producing pus.

**Pyometra** Accumulation of pus within the lumen of the uterus associated with infection.

**Pyrexia** Elongation of body temperature above normal. Also called Fever.

**Ram** Adult male sheep.

**Receptor** Protein present on cell membranes that binds to a cognate hormone and mediates its effect on cell morphology and/or activity.

**Recessive** An allele that is expressed only in the homozygous condition.

**Resorption** Absorption of tissue debris or fluid by the body.

**Seasonally polyestrous** Commencing estrous cycle during specific breeding season.

**Seminiferous tubules** Convoluted tubes found in the testes, which contain cells that produce sperms.

**Sephadex** Proprietary name for gel particles composed of cross-linked dextrans; used as molecular sieves in gel filtration; used for research on egg transport.

**Sex steroid** Steroid hormones derived primarily from the gonads, are responsible for the development of the sex organs.

**Sex steroid-binding globulin** Carrier protein that transports testosterone/estradiol in blood.

**Silent estrus** Ovulation without estrus.

**Smear** Secretions or blood spread on a glass slide for examination under a microscope. Smears are often stained with various dyes to contrast details.

**Somatic cell** Any non-germ cell that makes up the body of an organism.

**Species** A group of related organisms belonging to the same biological species which can freely interbreed to produce fertile progenies.

**Spermatocytes** Immature sperm cells.

**Spermatogenesis** The formation and development of sperm.

**Stenosis** Abnormal constriction of a channel or orifice.

**Sterility** A permanent factor preventing procreation.

**Steroid** Natural hormones or synthetic drugs whose molecules share a common skeleton of four rings of carbon atoms (the steroid nucleus) but which have different actions according to the attachment of other atoms.

**Stroma** The supporting tissue of an organ, as opposed to its active "producing" tissue.

**Synapse** Close pairing of homologous chromosomes at meiosis.

**T-cell receptor** A molecule present on the surface of T cells that binds specifically to a particular antigen when that antigen is placed with a major histocompatibility complex protein present on an antigen-presenting cell. The T-cell receptor, which is a dimeric protein formed with either an

$\alpha$ and $\beta$ subunit or an $\gamma$ and $\delta$ subunit, confers specificity towards T cells so they only recognize one or a few antigens. Under appropriate conditions, binding of T-cell receptor to its antigen leads to activation of the T cell.

**Tendon** A band of tough white fibrous tissue that connects a muscle to a bone. Muscle fibers merge into one end of a tendon, the other end of which is attached to a bone.

**Testis** One of the two egg-shaped glands which produce spermatozoa, normally situated in the scrotum. Also called Testicle.

**Testosterone** A steroid hormone produced by cells of the testis independent from cells that produce spermatozoa. A primary circulating androgen.

**Theca** A sheath, such as the one covering a tendon or a vesicular ovarian follicle.

**Thoracolumbar** Relating to the thoracic and lumbar regions of the spine.

**Thyroxine** An active iodine-containing hormone, produced normally in the thyroid gland, that aids in regulating metabolism; produced synthetically or extracted from the thyroid gland in crystalline form for treatment of thyroid disorders such as hypothyroidism, cretinism, and myxedema. Also called Tetraiodothyronine.

**Tissue culture** The growing of cells in a suitable nutrient in flasks or test tubes outside of the body.

**Transrectal ultrasonography** Ultrasonic examination through the rectum.

**Transuterine migration** Migration of embryos from one uterine horn to the other for spacing within the uterus is common in swine to equally distribute them in the two horns.

**Trophoblast** In early development, the outer layer of the blastocyst which gives rise to the extra-embryonic membranes. Later in development, the term refers to epithelial cells of the chorion.

**Tunica** A coat or enveloping layer of tissue.

**Umbilical cord** It acts as the vascular link between mother and fetus.

**Vesicular** 1) Of, or relating to, vesicles. 2) Containing vesicles.

**Viviparity** Birth of live young, as compared to ovoviviparity (egg laying).

**X Chromosome** The female sex-determining chromosome; females have two of them, males only one. See Chromosome. The X chromosome is larger than the Y chromosome and contains some genes for which there are no complements on the Y chromosome.

**Y Chromosome** The male sex-determining chromosome. See Chromosome.

## GLOSSARY OF COMMON ABBREVIATIONS

| | |
|---|---|
| **ACTH** | Adenocorticotropic hormone |
| **ADH** | Antidiuretic hormone |
| **AFP** | $\alpha$-Fetoprotein |
| **AI** | Artificial insemination |
| **AIDS** | Acquired immune deficiency syndrome (HIV) |
| **AMH** | anti-Müllerian hormone |
| **AMP** | Adenosine monophosphate |
| **ARC** | AIDS-related complex |
| **ATP** | Adenosine triphosphate |
| **BBB** | Blood-brain barrier |
| **BBT** | Basal body temperature |
| **bFGF** | Basic fibroblast growth factor |
| **BP** | Blood pressure |
| **BSA** | Bovine serum albumin |
| **cAMP** | Cyclic AMP |
| **cDNA** | DNA complementary to RNA |
| **CDP** | Cytidine 5′-phosphate |
| **CIC** | Circulating immune complexes |
| **CL** | Corpus luteum (singular) |
| **CRH** | Corticotropin-releasing hormone |
| **CSF** | Colony-stimulating factor |
| **CT** | Computed tomography |
| **D&C** | Dilation and cutterage of uterus |
| **D&E** | Dilation and evacuation of uterus |
| **DES** | Diethylstilbestrol |
| **DHEA** | Dihydroepiandrosterone |
| **DHT** | Dihydrotestosterone |
| **DMB** | Diazobenzyloxymethyl |
| **DMSO** | Dimethyl sulfoxide ($Me_2SO$) |
| **DNA** | Deoxyribonucleic acid |
| **EF** | Elongation factor |
| **EGF** | Epidermal growth factor |
| **ELISA** | Enzyme-linked immunosorbant assay |
| **FCS** | Fetal calf serum |
| **FGF** | Fibroblast growth factor |

| | |
|---|---|
| **FHR** | Fetal heart rate |
| **FRP** | Follicular regulating protein |
| **FSH** | Follicle-stimulating hormone |
| **FSH-RH** | Follicle-stimulating hormone–releasing hormone |
| **GnRH** | Gonadotropin-releasing hormone |
| **GH-RH** | Growth hormone-releasing hormone |
| **GLC** | Gas-liquid chromatography |
| **GM-CSF** | Granulocyte-macrophage colony stimulating factor |
| **GTT** | Glucose tolerance test |
| **hCB** | Human cord blood |
| **hCG** | Human chorionic gonadotropin |
| **hMG** | Human menopausal gonadotropin |
| **hMT** | Human mammary tumor |
| **HPLC** | High-pressure liquid chromatography |
| **HSV** | Herpes simplex virus |
| **ICM** | Inner cell mass of blastocyst |
| **IF** | Immunofluorescence techniques |
| **IFN** | Interferon |
| **IFN-g** | Interferon-g |
| **Ig** | Immunoglobulin |
| **IGFS** | Insulin-like growth factor serum |
| **IL-1** | Interleukin-1 |
| **IL-6** | Interleukin-6 |
| **IM** | Intramuscular |
| **IUGR** | Intrauterine growth retardation |
| **IUGR-LBW** | Intrauterine growth retardation low birth weight |
| **IV** | Intravenous |
| **IVF** | In vitro fertilization |
| **kDa** | Kilodalton |
| **LBW** | Low birth weight |
| **LH** | Luteinizing hormone |
| **LH-RH** | Luteinizing hormone-releasing hormone |
| **LH-RF** | Luteinizing hormone-releasing factor |
| **LI** | Luteinizing inhibitor |
| **LPS** | Lipopolysaccharide |
| **MI** | Macrophages |
| **MIS** | Müllerian-inhibiting substance |
| **MRI** | Magnetic resonance imaging |
| **MT** | Mitochondria |
| **NA** | Neutralizing antibody |
| **NGF** | Nerve-growth factor |
| **NK** | Natural killer cell |
| **PAF** | Platelet-activating factor |
| **PAGE** | Polyacrylamide-gel electrophoresis |
| **PBL** | Peripheral blood lymphocytes |
| **PBS** | Phosphate-buffered saline |
| **PDGF** | Platelet-derived growth factor |
| **PG** | Prostaglandins |
| **$PGE_2$** | Prostaglandin $E_2$ |
| **$PGF_2$** | Prostaglandin $F_2$ |
| **PIF** | Prolactin-inhibiting factor |
| **PMSG** | Pregnant mare serum gonadotropin |
| **PVS** | Perivitelline space |
| **RNA** | Ribonucleic acid |
| **RRA** | Radioreceptor assay |
| **rRNA** | Ribosomal RNA |
| **SMC** | Somatomedin-c |
| **STH** | Somatotropic hormone |
| **TBG** | Thyroxine-binding globulin |
| **TDF** | Testis-determining factor |
| **TGF** | Transforming growth factor |
| **TGF-a** | Transforming growth factor-a |
| **TGF-b** | Transforming growth factor-b |
| **TNF** | Tumor necrosis factor |
| **VIP** | Vasoactive intestinal peptide |

## UNITS OF MEASURE

mg milligram ($10^{-3}$ g)
$\mu$g microgram ($10^{-6}$ g)
ng nanogram ($10^{-9}$ g)
pg picogram ($10^{-12}$ g)
IU International Unit

# Appendices

## Appendix I
## *Chromosome Numbers of Bovinae, Equinae, and Caprinae Species*

| Common Name | Scientific Name | Chromosome Number (2N) | Fundamental Number |
|---|---|---|---|
| Domestic cattle | *Bos taurus* | 60 | 62 |
| Banteng | *Bos banteng* | 60 | 62 |
| Zebu | *Bos indicus* | 60 | 62 |
| Yak | *Bos grunniens* | 60 | 62 |
| European bison | *Bison bonasus* | 60 | 62 |
| American bison | *Bison bison* | 60 | 62 |
| Gaur | *Bos gaurus* | 58 | 62 |
| Nyala | *Tragelaphus angasi* | 55 | 58 |
| Congo buffalo | *Syncerus caffer nanus* | 54 | 60 |
| African buffalo | *Syncerus caffer caffer* | 52 | 60 |
| Asiatic buffalo | *Bubalus bubalis* | 48 | 58 |
| Anoa | *Anoa depressicornis* | 48 | 60 |
| Nilgai | *Boselaphus tragocamelus* | 46 | 60 |
| Four-horned antelope | *Tetracerus quadricornis* | 38 | 38 |
| Sitatunga | *Tragelaphus spekei* | 30 | 58 |
| Mongolian wild horse | *Equus przewalskii* | 66 | 94 |
| Domestic horse | *Equus caballus* | 64 | 94 |
| Donkey | *Equus asinus* | 62 | 104 |
| Nubian ass | *Equus asinus africans* | 62 | 104 |
| Mongolian wild ass | *Equus hemionus* | 56 | 104 |
| Tibetan wild ass | *Equus kiang* | 56 | 104 |
| Persian wild ass | *Equus onager* | 56 | 104 |
| Grevy zebra | *Equus grevyi* | 46 | 78 |
| African zebra | *Equus burchelli* | 44 | 82 |
| Grant zebra | *Equus burchelli boehmi* | 44 | 82 |
| Mountain zebra | *Equus zebra* | 34(?) | 60 |
| Domestic goat | *Capra hircus* | 60 | 60 |
| Ibex | *Capra ibex* | 60 | 60 |
| Markhor | *Capra falconeri* | 60 | 60 |
| Saiga antelope | *Saiga tatarica* | 60 | 60 |
| Aoudad | *Ammotragus lervia* | 58 | 60 |
| Afghanistan sheep | *Ovis ammon cycloceros* | 58 | 60 |
| Kara-Tau sheep | *Ovis ammon nigimontana* | 56 | 60 |
| Domestic sheep | *Ovis aries* | 54 | 60 |
| Mouflon | *Ovis musimon* | 54 | 60 |
| Red sheep | *Ovis orientalis* | 54 | 60(?) |
| Bighorn sheep | *Ovis canadensis* | 54 | 60 |
| Laristan sheep | *Ovis ammon laristanica* | 54 | 60 |
| Musk ox | *Ovibos moschatus* | 48 | 60 |
| Himalayan tahr | *Hemitragus jemlahias* | 48 | 60 |
| Rocky Mountain goat | *Oreamnos americanus* | 42 | 60 |

# Appendix II
## *Chromosome Numbers and Reproductive Ability in Equine, Bovine, and Caprine Hybrids*

| Species and Chromosome Number (2N) | | Hybrids | |
|---|---|---|---|
| Sire | Dam | Chromosome Number (2n) | Reproductive Ability |
| Mongolian wild horse, 66 (*E. przewalskii*) | Domestic horse, 64 (*E. caballus*) | 65 | Fertility (?) |
| Donkey, 62 (*E. asinus*) | Domestic horse, 64 (*E. caballus*) | 63 (Mule) | Sterile |
| Domestic horse, 64 (*E. caballus*) | Donkey, 62 (*E. asinus*) | 63 (Hinny) | Males are sterile, females are fertile, only in very exceptional cases |
| Nubian ass, 62 (*E. asinus africanus*) | Donkey, 62 (*E. asinus*) | 62 | Fertile |
| Mongolian wild ass, 56 (*E. hemionus*) | Donkey, 62 (*E. asinus*) | 59 | Fertile (?) |
| Grevy zebra, 46 (*E. grevyi*) | Domestic horse, 64 (*E. caballus*) | 55 (Zebroid) | Sterile |
| African zebra, 44 (*E. burchelli*) | Donkey, 62 (*E. asinus*) | 53 (Zebronkey) | Sterile |
| Donkey, 62 (*E. asinus*) | Mountain zebra, 34(?) (*E. zebra*) | 48 | Sterile |
| American bison, 60 (*Bison bison*) | Zebu, 60 (*Bos indicus*) | 60 | Females are fertile |
| American bison, 60 (*Bison bison*) | Domestic cattle, 60 (*Bos taurus*) | 60 (Cattalo) | Male $F_1$ are sterile |
| Domestic cattle, 60 (*Bos taurus*) | American bison, 60 (*Bison bison*) | 60 (Cattalo) | Male $F_1$ are sterile |
| Domestic goat, 60 (*Capra hircus*) | Barbary sheep, 58 (*Ammotragus lorvia*) | 59 (?) | Full-term fetuses, but no live hybrid |
| Domestic goat, 60 (*Capra hircus*) | Domestic sheep, 54 (*Ovis aries*) | 57 | Embryos are resorbed or aborted at 6 weeks pregnancy |
| Domestic sheep, 54 (*Ovis aries*) | Mouflon, 54 (*Ovis musimon*) | 54 | Fertile in both sexes |
| Bighorn sheep, 54 (*Ovis canadensis*) | Domestic sheep, 54 (*Ovis aries*) | 54 | Reduced fertility |

# APPENDIX III
# *Preparation of Physiologic Solutions*

| DULBECCO'S PHOSPHATE-BUFFERED SALINE (PBS) | | |
|---|---|---|
| To make 10 L: | | |
| $CaCl_2 \cdot 2H_2O$ | 1.32 g | a |
| $MgSO_4 \cdot 7H_2O$ | 1.21 g | a |
| NaCl | 80 g | b |
| KCl | 2 g | b |
| $Na_2HPO_4$ | 11.5 g | b |
| $KH_2PO_4$ | 2 g | b |
| Glucose | 10 g | b |
| Streptomycin sulfate | 0.5 g | b |
| Na pyruvate | 0.36 g | b |
| Na penicillin G | 1,000,000 units | b |

a May be weighed in advance and stored indefinitely in a sterile bottle under refrigeration.
b May be weighed in advance and stored in sterile bottle under refrigeration for 1 month. Do not mix with $CaCl_2$ and $MgSO_4$ until just before use.

Before use:
1. Dissolve NaCl, KCl, $Na_2HPO_4$, $KH_2PO_4$, glucose, streptomycin, Na pyruvate, and penicillin in 8 L of deionized, distilled water.
2. Dissolve $CaCl_2$ and $MgSO_4 \cdot 7H_2O$ in 2 L of deionized, distilled water.
3. Add 2 L to 8 L with constant stirring. (Other methods of dissolving these ingredients often lead to formation of a precipitate.)
4. Add heat-treated bovine serum (1%) immediately prior to use for recovery of embryos and add 10% serum for storage of embryos.

### *Preparation of Stock Solutions*

Two stock solutions are made:

| | |
|---|---|
| 1. Modified phosphate buffered saline | 40 mL |
| Fetal calf serum (FCS) | 10 mL |
| PBS + 20% FCS | 50 mL |
| 2. PBS + 20% FCS | 45 mL |
| Glycerol | 5 mL |
| Cooling medium (10% glycerol, v/v) | ~50 mL |

## COMPOSITION OF SOME COMMON BUFFERS AND SOLUTIONS

Baker's solution:

| | |
|---|---|
| Glucose | 3 g |
| $Na_2HPO_4$ | 0.6 g |
| $KH_2PO_4$ | 0.01 g |
| NaCl | 0.2 g |
| Add distilled water to 100mL | |

Joel's solution:
80 mL of 5.42% destrose in distilled water
20 mL of 0.125 $N_2MgCl_2$in distilled water

Locke's solution:

| | |
|---|---|
| $CaCl_2$ | 0.24 g |
| KCl | 0.42 g |
| $NaHCO_3$ | 0.1 g |
| NaCl | 9.0 g |
| Add distilled water to 100 mL | |

Physiologic saline:

| | |
|---|---|
| NaCl | 0.85 g |
| Add distilled water to 100 mL | |

Modified Ringer's buffer solution:

| | |
|---|---|
| NaCl | 120 mM |
| KCl | 5 mM |
| $KH_2PO_4$ | 10 mM |
| $MgSO_4 \cdot 7H_2O$ | 5 mM |
| Tris HCl | 1 mM |

Ringer-Locke's solution:

| | |
|---|---|
| NaCl | 9.5 g |
| KCl | 0.075 g |
| $CaCl_2$ | 0.1–0.2 g |
| $NaHCO_3$ | 0.1–0.2 g |
| Glucose (optional) | 1.0 g |
| Water | 1000.0 g |

Ringer-Tyrodes' solution:

| | |
|---|---|
| NaCl | 8.0 g |
| KCl | 0.2 g |
| $CaCl_2$ | 0.2 g |
| $MgSO_4$ | 0.1–0.2 g |
| $NaHCO_3$ | 0.5–1.0 g |
| Glucose (optional) | 1.0 g |
| Water | 1000.0 ml |

Scott's solution:

| | |
|---|---|
| Sodium bicarbonate | 3.5 g |
| Magnesium sulphate | 20.0 g |
| Distilled water | 1000 mL |

The Scott's solution is to be used only when the ordinary tap water is "hard" and should be changed frequently, e.g., after rinsing 20 to 25 slides.

Hanks' BSS without bicarbonate (previously sterilized by autoclaving):

| | |
|---|---|
| Penicillin | 250 units/mL |
| Streptomycin | 250 μg/mL |
| Kanamycin | 100 μg/mL |
| or gentamycin | 50 μg/mL |
| Amphotericin B | 2.5 μg/mL |

(All preparations sterile, store at −20°C.)

Dexamethasone 1 mg/ml (100×):

This comes already sterile in glass vials. To dissolve, add 5 mL of water by syringe to vial, remove, and dilute to give a concentration of 1 mg/mL. Aliquot and store at −20°C. Betamethasone and methylprednisolone may be prepared in the same way.

Penicillin (e.g., crystapen benzylpenicillin sodium):

1,000,000 units per vial

Use 4 vials and 400 mL Hanks' BBS

Prepare as for kanamycin; final concentration 10,000 units/mL

Phosphate Buffered Saline (PBS) (Dulbecco "A"):

Oxoid tablets, Code BR14a, 1 tablet per 100 mL distilled water

Dispense and then autoclave

Store at room temperature, pH 7.3, osmolality 280 mOsm/LKg

PBSB contains the calcium and magnesium and should be prepared and sterilized separately. Mix with PBSA, if required, immediately before use.

# Appendix IV
# *Technique for Determining Spermatozoal Concentration Using a Hemacytometer*

## Recommended Equipment

**Platelet/WBC Unopette® Microcollection system (Becton-Dickinson, Rutherford, New Jersey)**

—Plastic reservoirs containing 1.98 mL of 1% buffered ammonium oxalate

—20 μL glass capillary pipettes with plastic shields

**Counting Chamber (Hemacytometer) with Neubauer Ruling and Coverslips**

**Lab Counter with One Counting Unit (0–999 range)**

## Technique

1. Mix semen thoroughly to evenly distribute sperm cells.
2. Mix semen with an appropriate diluent (such as 1% buffered ammonium oxalate) at a dilution ratio of 1:100 (e.g., 20 μL semen to 1.98 mL diluent).
3. Place a clean hemacytometer (with Neubauer ruling) on a flat surface and fit with an appropriate coverslip.
4. Thoroughly mix the diluted semen, then immediately fill the two chambers of the hemacytometer with the diluted semen. Do not overfill the chambers.
5. Wait 5 min for sperm to settle before starting sperm count. The hemacytometer can be placed in a covered humidified Petri dish to prevent dehydration during this waiting period.
6. The Neubauer ruling consists of 9 large squares. Using 200× magnification phase contrast microscopy, count all sperm heads within the large center square. This square is subdivided into 25 smaller squares. Sperm heads that overlie lines of each of these squares should only be included in the count if they touch the upper or left borders. Sperm heads touching the right or lower borders of each square are not counted.
7. Sperm counts are performed separately for each of the hemacytometer chambers. If the sperm count of the two chambers varies by more than 10%, disregard the results and prepare additional hemacytometer chambers for recounts.
8. Be certain to finish the counting process by focusing just underneath the coverslip because some sperm will adhere to the underside of the coverslip.

## Calculation of Sperm Cell Concentration

1. Establish average sperm count from the two chambers.
2. Dimensions of the large central area of the Neubauer counting chamber are 1 mm (width) × 1 mm (height) × 0.1 mm (depth) for a volume of 0.1 $mm^3$. Since sperm cell concentration is normally reported in sperm number per cubic centimeter (cc), the sperm count must be multiplied by a factor of 10,000.
3. Since the semen was diluted at a 1:100 ratio prior to the sperm count, the final sperm count must be multiplied by an additional factor of 100.
4. EXAMPLE:
   Sperm count of diluted semen in chamber 1 = 240
   Sperm count of diluted semen in chamber 2 = 250
   Average sperm count = 245
   Sperm cell concentration =
   $245 \times 10^4 \times 10^2$/cc or
   $245 \times 10^6$/cc

# APPENDIX V
## *Preparation of Sperm Stains*

### PAPANICOLAOU STAINING

The Papanicolaou stain clearly distinguishes between basophilic and acidophilic cell components and allows a detailed examination of the nuclear chromatin pattern. This method, therefore, has been commonly used for routine diagnostic cytology. The Papanicolaou staining technique has also proved useful in the analysis of sperm morphology and in the examination of immature germinal cells.

**1. Preparation of Specimen.** The smear should be slightly air dried and then fixed in equal parts of ethanol (95%) and ether for 5 to 15 min.

**2. Staining Procedure.** Fixed smears should be stained according to the following procedure:

| | |
|---|---|
| Ethanol 80%[1] | 10 dips[2] |
| Ethanol 70% | 10 dips |
| Ethanol 50% | 10 dips |
| distilled water | 10 dips |
| Harris' or Mayer's hematoxylin | 3 min exactly |
| Running water | 3 to 5 min |
| Acid ethanol | 2 dips |
| Running water | 3 to 5 min |
| Scott's solution[3] | 4 min |
| Distilled water | 1 dip |
| Ethanol 50% | 10 dips |
| Ethanol 70% | 10 dips |
| Ethanol 80% | 10 dips |
| Ethanol 95% | 10 dips |
| Orange G 6 | 2 min |
| Ethanol 95% | 10 dips |
| Ethanol 95% | 10 dips |
| EA-50[4] | 5 min |
| Ethanol 95% | 5 dips |
| Ethanol 95% | 5 dips |
| Ethanol 95% | 5 dips |
| Ethanol 99.5% | 2 min |
| Xylol (3 staining jars) | Approximately 1 min in each |

Change xylol if it turns milky. Mount at once with Depex or any mounting medium.

[1]Check the acidity of water before preparing the different grades of ethanol. The pH should be 7.0.

[2]One dip corresponds to approximately 1 sec.

[3]Scott's solution is used when the ordinary tap water is "hard."

[4]The prepared Papanicolaou stain (EA50 and OG 6) may be obtained commercially. The same companies usually manufacture the hematoxylin preparation. The commercially available stains are usually satisfactory, but the stains may be prepared in the laboratory at a substantial saving. The stains can be prepared as follows:

| | |
|---|---|
| Eosin Y | 10 g |
| Bismarck brown Y | 10 g |
| Light-green SF, yellowish | 10 g |
| Distilled water | 300 mL |
| Ethanol 95% | 2000 mL |
| Phosphotungstic acid | 4 g |
| Saturated lithium carbonate solution (in distilled water) | 0.5 mL |

### STOCK SOLUTIONS

Prepare separate 10% solutions of each of the stains as follows:

Eosin Y 10 g in 100 mL distilled water
Bismarck brown Y 10 g in 100 mL distilled water

Light-green SF 10 g in 100 mL distilled water

To prepare 200 ml of stain, mix the preceding stock solution as follows:

| | |
|---|---|
| Eosin Y | 50 mL |
| Bismarck brown Y | 10 mL |
| Light-green SF | 12.5 mL |

Make up to 2000 mL with 95% ethanol; add 4 g phosphotungstic acid and 0.5 mL saturated lithium carbonate solution. Mix well and store solution at room temperature in dark-brown tightly capped bottles. The solution is stable for 2 to 3 months. Filter before using.

Constituents of OG6:

| | |
|---|---|
| Orange G crystals | 10 g |
| Distilled water | 100 mL |
| Ethanol 95% | 1000 mL |
| Phosphotungstic acid | 0.15 g |

Stock solution number I:

Prepare 10% aqueous solution as follows: Orange G crystal 10 g in 100 mL distilled water. Shake well and allow to stand in a dark-brown bottle at room temperature for 1 week before using.

Belsey MA, Elliasson R, Gallegos AJ, Moghissi KS, Paulsen CA, Prasad MRN. Laboratory Manual for the Examination of Human Semen and Semen–Cervical Mucus Interaction, WHO Special Programme of Research, Development and Research Training in Human Reproduction. Singapore: Press Concern, 1980.

Stock solution number II (Orange G, 0.5% solution):

Stock solution number 1 — 50 mL

Prepare with 95% ethanol to 1000 mL

To prepare final solution of 1000 mL of the stain, add 0.15 g phosphotungstic acid to 1000 mL stock solution number II; mix well and store in dark-brown stoppered bottles at room temperature. Filter before using. The solution is stable for 2 to 3 months.

Harris hematoxylin without acetic acid:

| | |
|---|---|
| Hematoxylin (dark crystals) | 8 g |
| Ethanol 95% | 80 mL |
| Aluminum ammonium sulphate | 160 g |
| Distilled water | 1600 mL |
| Mercuric oxide | 6 g |

To prepare the staining mixture, dissolve aluminum ammonium sulfate in distilled water by heating. Dissolve hematoxylin crystal in 95% ethanol. Add hematoxylin solution to ammonium sulfate solution. Heat the mixture to 95°C. Remove from flame, and while stirring, slowly add the mercuric oxide. Solution will be dark purple in color. Immediately plunge the container in a cold-water bath and filter when the solution is cold. Store in dark-brown bottles at room temperature and let stand for 48 hours. Dilute the required amount with an equal part of distilled water and filter again.

Giemsa stain:

Layer undiluted methyl alcohol on the slide

Let stand for 10 min

Drain and let air dry

Cover the slide with Giemsa stain (17 drops of the stock Giemsa solution in enough distilled water to make the final volume 5 ml)

Let stand for 20 min

Rinse with distilled water

Meyer's hematoxylin stain:

Layer 10% formaldehyde on the slide

Let stand for 1 min

Rinse with distilled water

Stain for 2 min in Meyer's hematoxylin

Rinse in distilled water

Crystal violet-rose bengal stain:

Layer Chlorazene (chloramine-T)

(5% in distilled water) on the slide

Let stand for 5 min

Rinse with 95% alcohol

Immerse in crystal violet (25% in distilled water)

Let stand for 8 min

Rinse with 95% alcohol

Immerse in rose bengal (1% in distilled water) for 8 sec

Rinse with distilled water

Bryan's sperm stain, Graham and Leishman's blood stain:[5]

Fix the slide in formalin (10% for 3 min, and subsequently in 95% ethanol for 3 min and in 70% ethanol for 3 min; change every third time)

Rinse with distilled water for 3 min and submerge in alphanaphthol for 4.5 min

Rinse with tap water for 15 min and add pyronine B for 2 min

Immerse 3 times in tap water

Add modified Bryan's stain for 15 min (description follows)

Immerse 3 times in 1% acetic acid

Wash with tap water for 1 min and add Leishman's blood stain for 5 minutes

Immerse 3 times in tap water and air dry

Modified Bryan's sperm stain:

| | |
|---|---|
| Acetic acid 1% | 1500 mL |
| Eosin yellow | 0.5 g |
| Fast green | 0.5 g |
| Naphthol yellow S | 0.5 g |

Mix thoroughly and store in stoppered bottle, the stain is filtered before use.

Leishman's Blood Stain (Stock Solution):

Combine 0.5 g of eosinated methylene blue and 300 mL of absolute methyl alcohol (MeOH).

Mix thoroughly and allow to age in the dark at room temperature for 7 days.

Place the stain in an incubator (35 to 37°C) for 2 days.

The stock solution is now ready for use and should be stored in a tightly-stoppered dark bottle, away from heat and light.

Alternative blood stain stock solutions commercially available are Jenner's blood stain or Wright's blood stain. The timing involved with these stains must be varied at the "Leishman's" step in the procedure to achieve comparable results.

Buffer Solution: Combine 2 buffer tablets, pH 6.8, with 200 mL of distilled water. (If not used at once, recheck pH before use.)

Leishman's Blood Stain (Working Solution): Combine 10 mL formaldehyde solution with 90 mL of 95% E10H. (0.1 g of calcium acetate may be added per 200 mL of solution to ensure neutral pH of 7.0.)

[5]Ulstein M, Capell P, Holmes K, Paulsen CA. Nonsymptomatic genital tract infection and male infertility. *In* Human Semen and Fertility Regulation in Men. St. Louis: Mosby, 1976.

Alcoholic Formalin: Combine 10 mL formaldehyde solution with 90 mL of 95% EtOH; 0.1 g of calcium acetate may be added per 200 mL of solution to ensure neutral pH of 7.0.

Alphanaphthol: Dissolve 1 g alphanaphthol in 100 mL of 40% ethyl alcohol (EtOH). Immediately before initial use, add 0.2 mL of 3% hydrogen peroxide solution.

Pyronine Y: Combine 1 g of pyronine, 4 mL aniline, and 96 mL of 40% EtOH.

Sodium citrate buffer: Mix 7 g sodium citrate with 1 L of 0.9 NaCl and adjust pH to 7.5.

### *Bryan/Leishman Stain for Seminal Fluid Morphology Smears*

*Note:* Use freshly made, air-dried smears from fresh samples on clean slides.

| | | |
|---|---|---|
| Alcohol formalin 10% | 1 min | Fresh each time |
| Ethyl alcohol (EtOH) 80% | 5 min | Change every third time[a] |
| EtOH 70% | 5 min | Change every third time |
| EtOH 50% | 5 min | Change every third time |
| Alphanaphthol | 4 min | Change every 3 days |

Add 0.4 ml of 3% hydrogen peroxide to 200 mL of alphanaphthol just before initial use; the solution is active for 3 days at room temperature.

| | | |
|---|---|---|
| Running tap water | 15 min | Running slowly |
| Pyronine Y | 4 min | Fresh each week |
| Running tap water | 3 dips[b] | Running slowly |
| Sodium citrate buffer | 3 min | pH 7.5; fresh each time |
| Distilled water | 1 min | Fresh each time |
| Modified Bryan's stain | 15 min | Fresh every other time |
| Acetic acid 1% | 2 dips | Fresh each time |
| Running tap water | 1 min | Running slowly |
| Buffer and Leishman's stain | 30 min | Fresh each time |

Filter Leishman's stock 50 mL, add pH 6.8 buffer 150 mL filter again immediately before use.

| | | |
|---|---|---|
| Running tap water | 1 to 2 dips | Running slowly |
| Air dry (do not blot) | | |

[a]Change after every 30 slides if a staining jar holding 10 slides is being used.
[b]Each dip should be approximately of 1 second duration.

## SPECIAL CONSIDERATIONS

1. Pyronine Y, modified Bryan's and Leishman's stains should be filtered before initial use. In addition, the buffer and Leishman's working stain should be filtered before use to remove precipitated stain.
2. The final stain intensity can be increased by staining for a longer time in the buffered Leishman's stain or can be decreased by repeated washing. Check for the desired intensity with a microscope before mounting the slide.
3. Hydrogen peroxide deteriorates rapidly in the presence of light; thus, the stock 3% solution should be stored in an amber bottle in the dark.
4. The stock Leishman's stain should be aged before use by storing for 7 days at room temperature in the dark followed by incubation at 35 to 37°C for 2 days in the dark. The aged solution is stable for a month if kept in a sealed container in the dark.

# APPENDIX VI
## *Preparation of Trypsin for Zona-Free Hamster Ova*

| Trypsin diluent-buffered | |
|---|---|
| Sodium chloride | 6.0 g |
| Trisodium citrate | 2.9 g |
| Tricine [N-Tris(hydroxy-methyl)methyl glycine] | 1.79 g |
| Phenol red | 0.005 g |
| Distilled water to | 1000 mL |

Stir ingredients until dissolved, adjust pH to 7.8
Filter through Whatman No. 1 filter paper
Dispense and autoclave
Osmolality = 290 nOsm/kg

Trypsin Stock (2.5% in 0.85% (0.14 M) NaCl)

Trypsin solutions can be bought commercially. Alternatively, to make up a 2.5% solution in 0.85% NaCl, stir for 1 hour at room temperature or 10 hours at 4°C. If trypsin does not dissolve completely, clarify by filtration through Whatman No. 1 filter paper.

Sterilize by filtration, aliquot, and store at −20°C.

*Note:* Trypsin is available as crude (e.g., Difco 1:250) or purified (e.g., Sigma [3×] recrystallized) preparations. Crude preparations contain several other proteases that may be important in cell dissociation but may also be harmful to more sensitive cells. The usual practice is to use crude trypsin unless cell damage reduces viability or reduced growth is observed, then purified trypsin may be used. Pure trypsin has a higher specific activity and should therefore be used at a proportionally lower concentration, e.g., 0.05 or 0.01%.

| Trypsin Verene Phosphate (TVP) | |
|---|---|
| Trypsin (Difco 1:250) | 25 mg (or 1 mL Flow or Gibco 2.5%) |
| Phosphate buffered saline (PBS) | 98 mL |
| Disodium EDTA ($2H_2O$) | 37 mg |
| Chick serum (Flow) | 1 mL |

Mix PBS and EDTA and autoclave, then add chick serum and trypsin.

If using powdered trypsin, sterilize by filtration before adding chick serum. Aliquot and store at −20°C.

# APPENDIX VII
## *Evaluation of Chromosomes of Ova*

Morulae or blastocysts are incubated for 2 h at 37°C in tissue culture (TC) medium 199 to which Colcemid (0.5 g/mL) has been added. They are then placed in 0.9% sodium citrate in siliconized centrifuge tubes for 10 min and dissociated gently by aspiration with a siliconized Pasteur pipette. After further incubation for 10 min, the test tube is centrifuged at 800 rpm for 5 min, and the supernatant is removed and replaced with alcohol acetic fixative.

The preparations are stored overnight at 4°C, and after removal of the fixative by centrifugation, 45% aqueous acetic acid is added. The dissociated cells are resuspended following a second change of acetic acid, and small drops of the suspension are placed on a glass slide warmed to 56°C on a hot plate. The slides are then stained with carbol fuchsin.

# Appendix VIII
## *Book/IVF Companies*

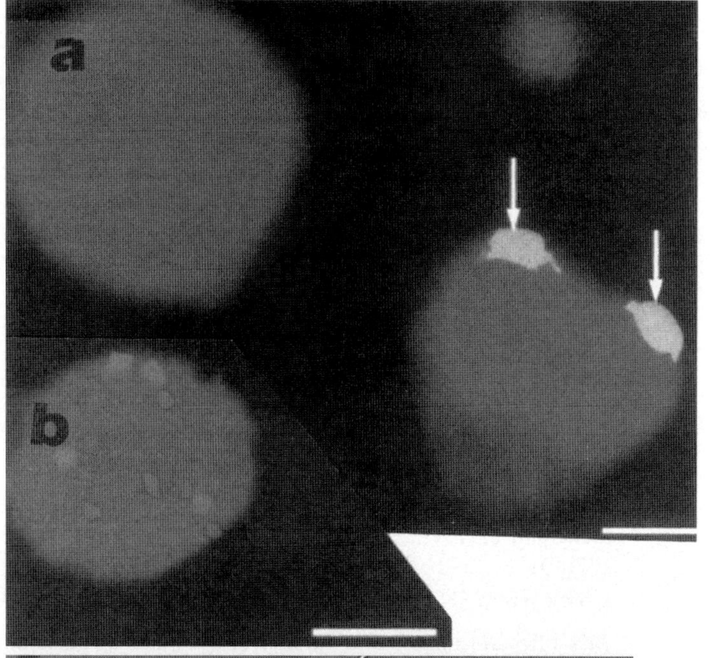


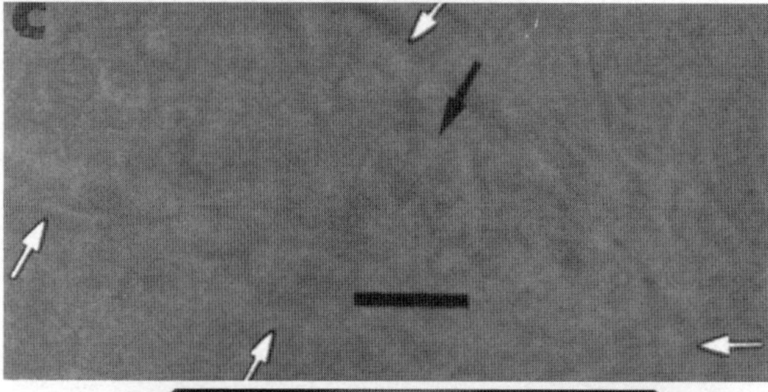


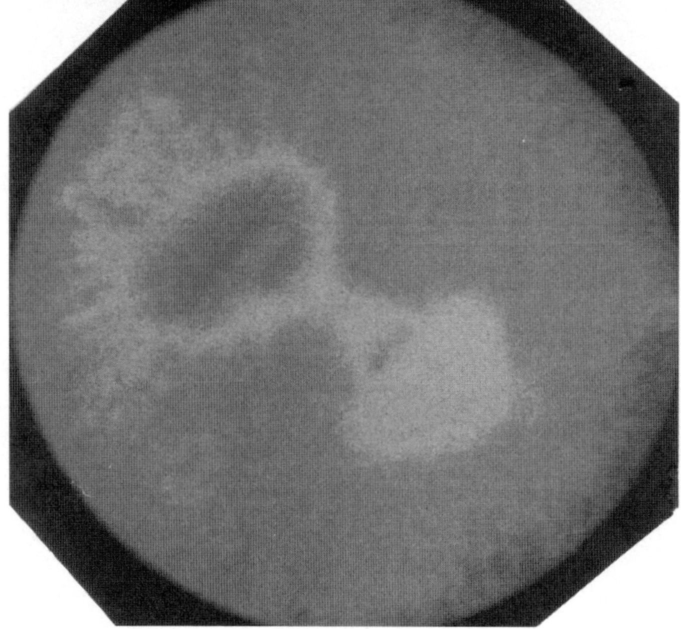

Zygote: The Biology of Gametes and Early Embryos

The biology of gametes/early embryos covers

- gametogenesis
- sperm-egg interaction
- sperm-egg interaction
- activation of gametes
- polarity in oocytes and zygotes
- cell-cycle control
- cell-cell interactions
- generation of early cell lineages

The basic architecture of an embryo is established soon after fertilization and usually within several cleavage divisions. This journal is centered on spatial/temporal regulation of cellular components within the oocyte/zygote, ranges from the programming of developmental information during oogenesis, through its modification at fertilization, to the integration of the maternal early embryonic genomes.

**a.** Human spermatogenic cells immunolabelled for proacrosin with 4D4 mAb (yellow fluorescence) and counter-stained with ethidium bromide (red fluorescence). Binucleate cell, probably a giant round spermatid, showing proacrosin immunoreactivity in two noncommunicating areas adjacent to each nucleus (arrows). The larger adjacent cell of monocyte nuclear (upper left) does not show any proacrosin immunoreactivity. Scale represents 5$\mu$m.
**b.** Evaluation of the meiotic maturity of human spermatozogenic cells using double color FISH with D15Z1 (light blue fluorescence spots) probes. Nuclei are counter-stained with DAPI (dark blue fluorescence). Primary spermatocyte in the first meiotic prophase showing four copies of both of the visualized DNA sequences, corresponding to two bivalents each consisting of two chromatids.
**c.** Egg cells and other cells derived from ovular tissue of Brassica napus. Bars = 10 $\mu$m. *In situ* egg cell (black arrow) in an embryo sac (white arrow) after cleaning treatment.
Cambridge University Press, North American Branch, 40 West 20th Street, New York, NY 10011-4211, USA.

*In Vitro* Fertilization

BRIAN DALE
*Director of Research Stazione Zoologia, Naples*
and
KAY ELDER
*Director of Training, Bourn Hall Clinic, Cambridge*

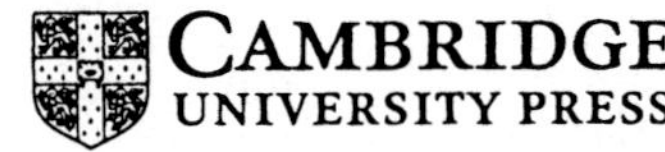


1. Microinsemination techniques include subzonal injection (SZI), intracytoplastic sperm injection (ICSI), zona drilling (ZD), and partial zona dissection (PZD).

2. Variations of fertilization after ICSI

   PN: pronuclei; PB: polar body
   a. two pronuclei, 2 polar bodies
   b. three pronuclei, one polar body
   c. one pronucleus, two polar bodies
   d. no pronuclei, one polar body
   e. early cleavage

3. Variations in egg maturity found after hyalase treatment and corona dissection.
   a. germinal vesicle
   b. metaphase I
   c. metaphase ii

4. Boyant density gradients
   (a–b) two-step gradients before and after centrifugation
   c. mini-gradient

5. The ARIC test: a population of spermatozoa are exposed to the calcium ionophore A23187 and then labelled with fluorescent lectins for specific surface sugars. The white area indicates fluorescence.
   I. acrosome intact
   II. incomplete acrosome reaction
   III. complete acrosome reaction
   IV. dead sperm
   V. abnormal sperm

6. Loading embryos into a cryostraw before freezing

7. Single sperm inside microinjection needle prior to injection

8. Injection and holding pipettes

References

Dale B (1996) In: Greger R, Windhorst U (eds). Comprehensive Human Physiology. Springer Verlag, Berlin.
Johnson M, Everitt B (1990) Essential Reproduction. Blackwell Scientific Publications, Oxford.
Sagata N (1996) Meiotic metaphase arrest in animal oocytes: its mechanisms and biological significance. Trends in Cell Biology 6:22–28.
Yanagimachi R (1994) Mammalian Fertilization. In: Knobil E and Neill J (eds). The Physiology of Reproduction. Raven Press, New York, pp 189–317.

(*see illustration on next page*)

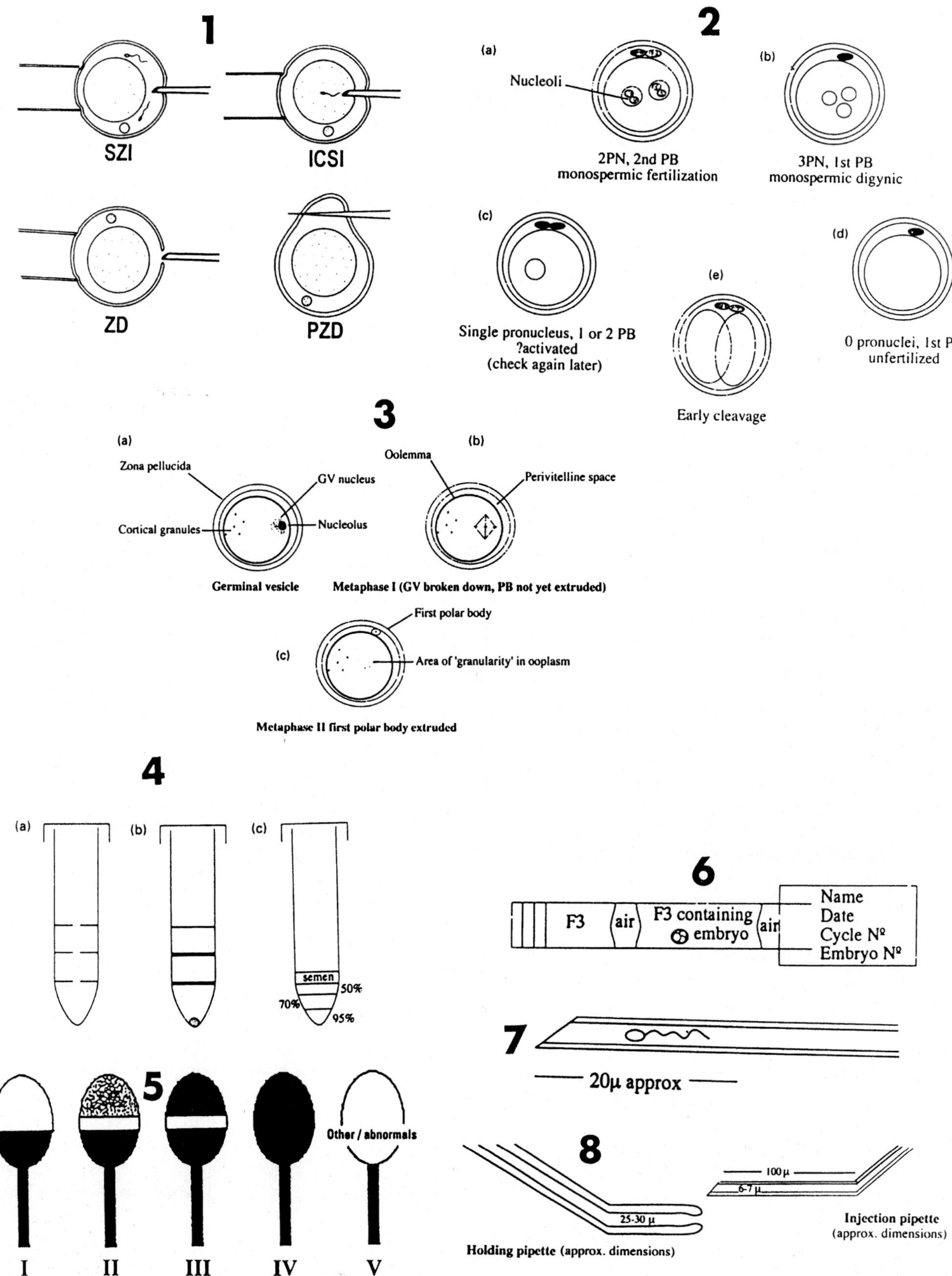
1
SZI
ICSI
ZD
PZD
2
(a)
Nucleoli
2PN, 2nd PB
monospermic fertilization
(b)
3PN, 1st PB
monospermic digynic
(c)
Single pronucleus, 1 or 2 PB
?activated
(check again later)
(d)
0 pronuclei, 1st PB
unfertilized
(e)
Early cleavage
3
(a)
Zona pellucida
GV nucleus
Cortical granules
Nucleolus
Germinal vesicle
(b)
Oolemma
Perivitelline space
Metaphase I (GV broken down, PB not yet extruded)
(c)
First polar body
Area of 'granularity' in ooplasm
Metaphase II first polar body extruded
4
(a)
(b)
(c)
semen
50%
70%
95%
5
Other / abnormals
I
II
III
IV
V
6
F3
air
F3 containing
embryo
air
Name
Date
Cycle Nº
Embryo Nº
7
20μ approx
8
25-30 μ
Holding pipette (approx. dimensions)
100 μ
6-7 μ
Injection pipette
(approx. dimensions)

# Appendix IX
## *In Vitro Fertilization by Microinjection*

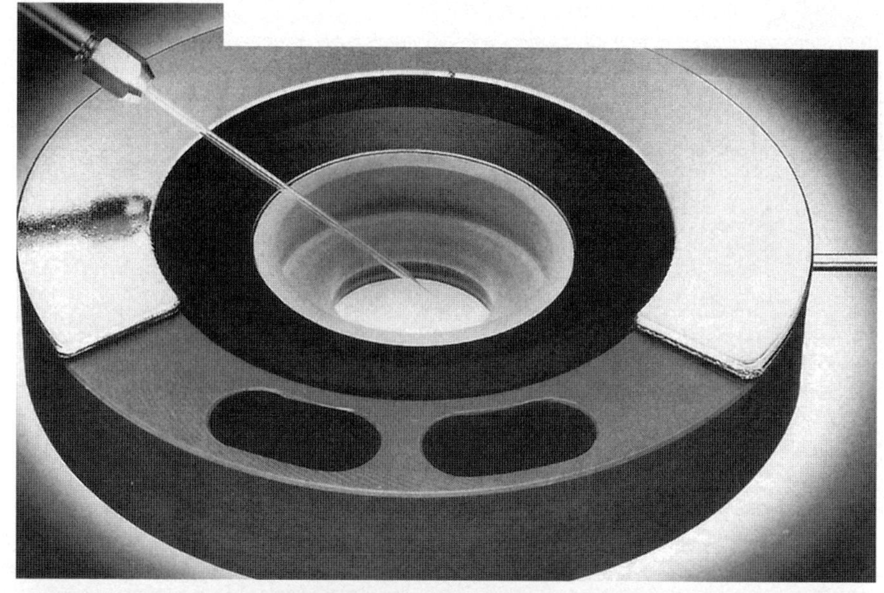

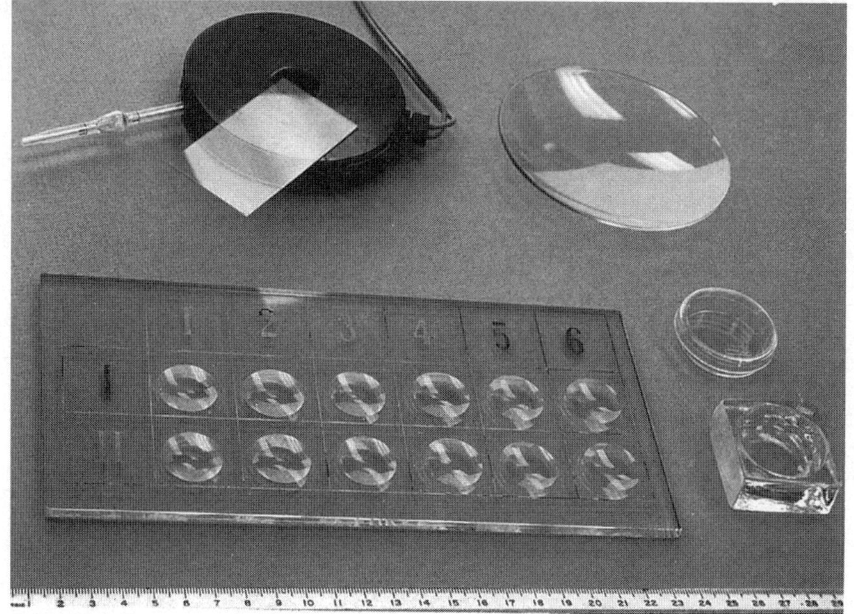


In vitro fertilization by microinjection

## REAL-TIME SPERM SEPARATION WANG TUBES
F.N. WANG

This system encompasses the application of newly designed separation tubes and innovative methods. Several biological and biophysical phenomena and basic and theoretical principles have been applied in the real-time sperm separation system:

- Nonpathological spermatozoa do not transfer microorganisms.
- The motility pattern and swim-up capacity of infected sperm or pathological sperm are limited or disturbed.
- The faster the sperm migrate and the greater distance they cover, the more normal the sperm are.
- Spermatozoa that are different from that expected for their stage of development and sperm with morphological or physiological disorders can be identified by characteristics such as different migration velocities and different distances of migration.
- Highly motile sperm can be easily separated from other live cells such as leukocytes, red blood cells, lymphocytes, and cellular debris.
- Tissue culture medium has a low viscosity, which does not favor the adhesion of the microorganisms to the highly motile sperm.
- The specific gravity of a sperm pellet is greater than that of the tissue culture medium so that the pellet will fall steadily to the bottom of a Wang tube, allowing the motile sperm to migrate.
- The velocity and direction of sperm migration are quite different from the random active or passive movement of microorganisms.
- The Wang tube system is a multidirectional challenge/migration (MCM) technique. It is not just a simple swim-up technique. The spermatozoa are allowed to migrate along multiple directions and pass through carefully designed, computerized curvatures of critical angles. The challenge effected facilitates the selection of high-quality sperm.
- These formulae have been based on the theories of Bernoulli's equation and application of hydrodynamics.

F.N. WANG
REAL-TIME SPERM SEPARATION
A REVIEW OF WANG TUBES
AND RELATED TECHNOLOGIES
ARCHIVES OF ANDROLOGY 34:13–32 (1995)

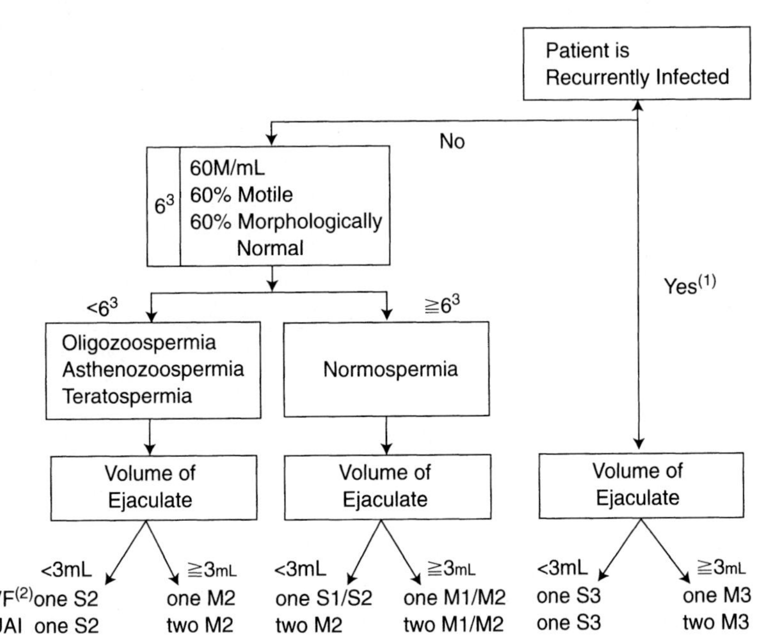


**Selection of the right Wang tube.**

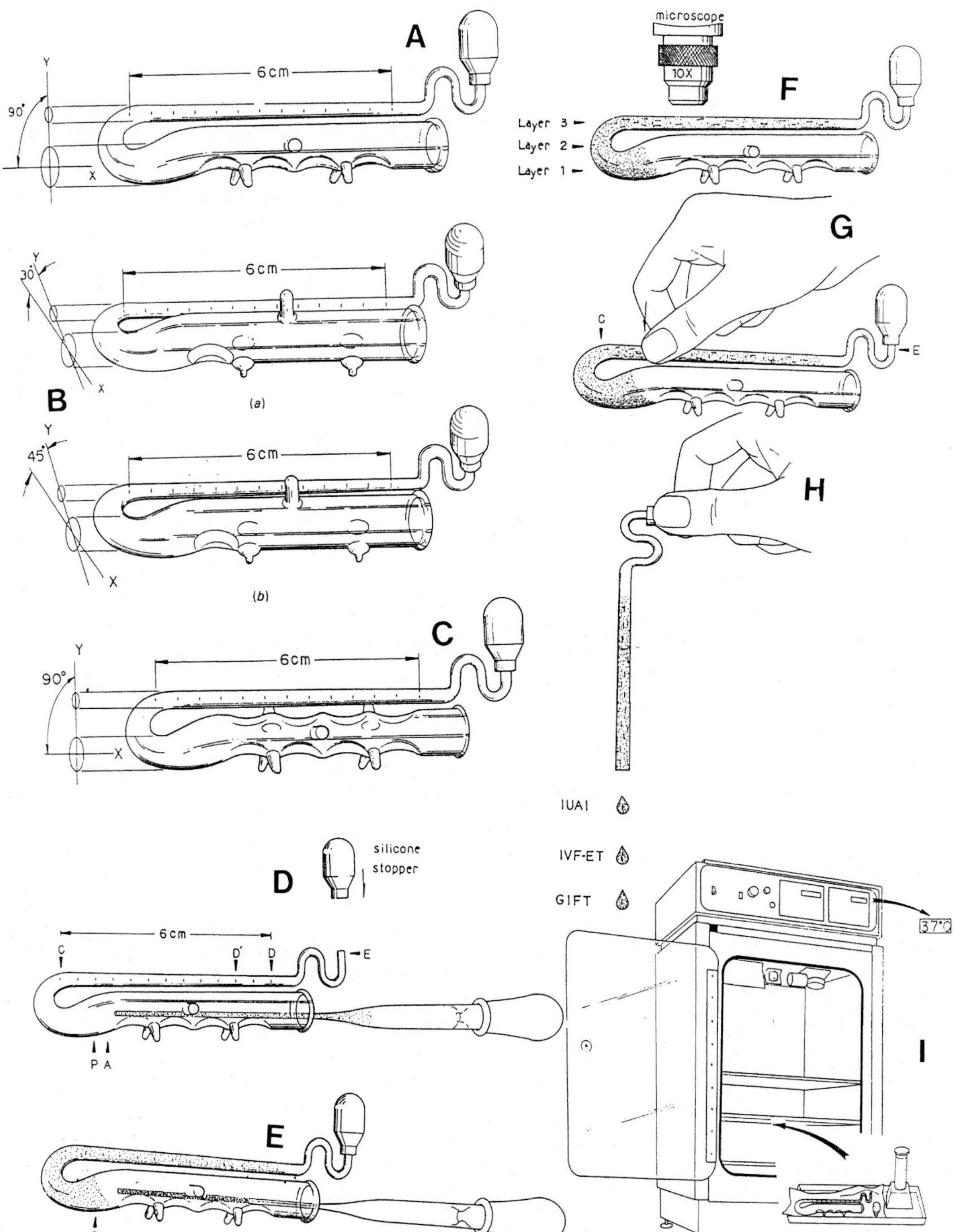


**A:** The Wang tube, standard type (frontal view). Upward standing position with a side arm at 6 cm length and 90° inclination.

**B:** The Wang tube, oblique type (fronto-ventral view): (*a*) with a side arm at 30° inclination; (*b*) at 45° inclination.

**C:** The Wang tube complex (frontal view). Supward standing position with four convex lenses symmetrical to those on the bottom wall, and two additional racks attached to the anterior wall of the low component of the tube.

**D:** Tissue culture medium is placed in a Wang tube with a long Pasteur pipette.

**E:** The sperm-pellet suspension is injected into the Wang tube.

**F:** Following incubation, the tissue culture medium inside the Wang tube is in three distinct layers: layer 1 is markedly turbid, layer 2 is turbid, while layer 3 is clear and contains high-quality sperm. The image of migrating sperm and the sperm parameters can be directly checked via microscopy before collection.

**G:** High-quality sperm is collected from a Wang tube. Pressing the side arm cuts off the Wang tube.

**H:** High-quality sperm is released from the side arm of the Wang tube by squeezing the silicone stopper with the right thumb and index finger.

**I:** The Wang tube, silicone stopper, and tissue culture medium are placed in an incubator before the tubes are filled with the tissue culture medium.

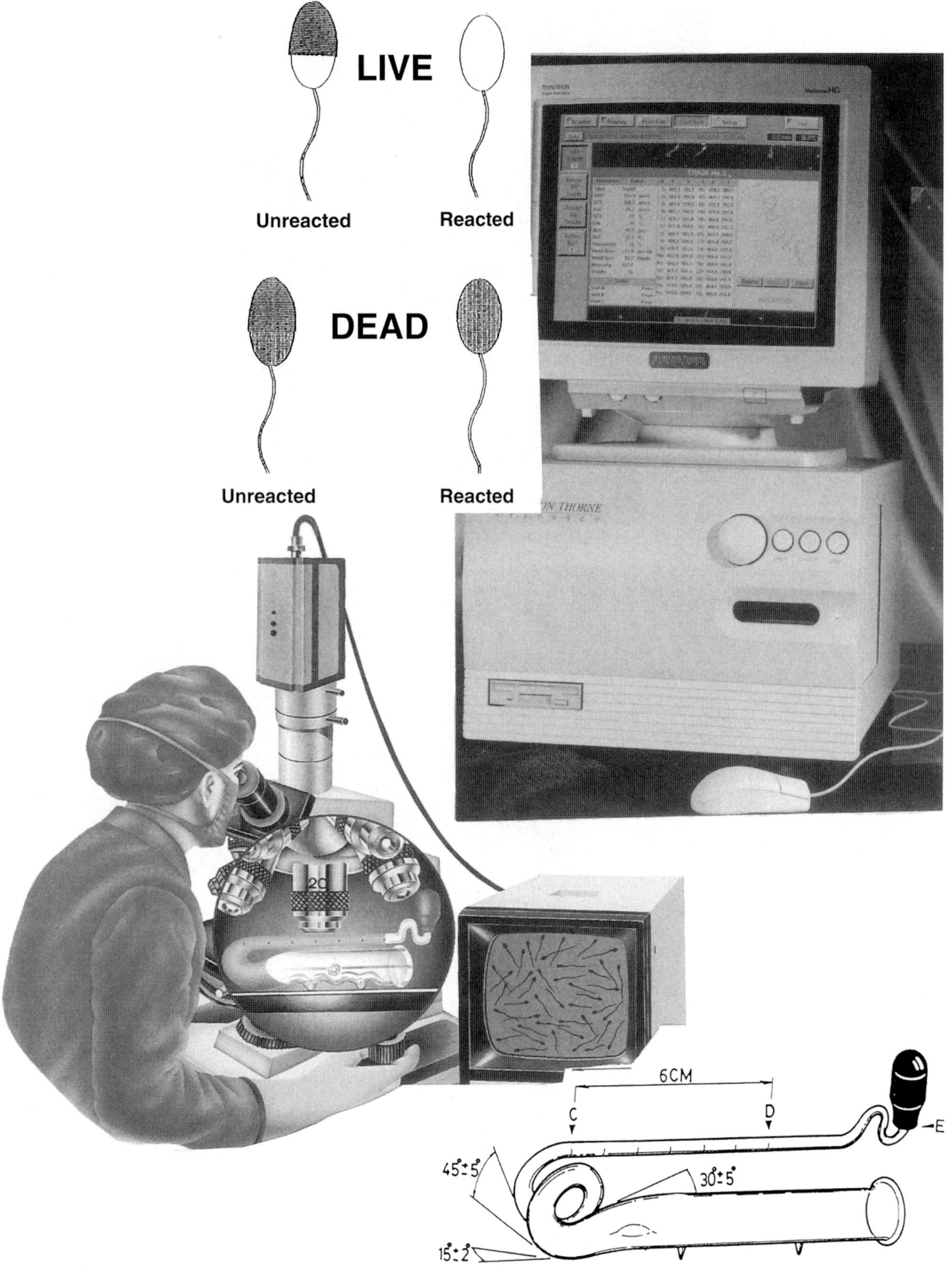


(*Top*) Hamilton-Thorn Computer-assisted sperm analysis (CASA) is applied to differentiate reacted and non-reacted live and dead sperm. (*Bottom*) Wang's Tube System for separation of sperm for IVF.

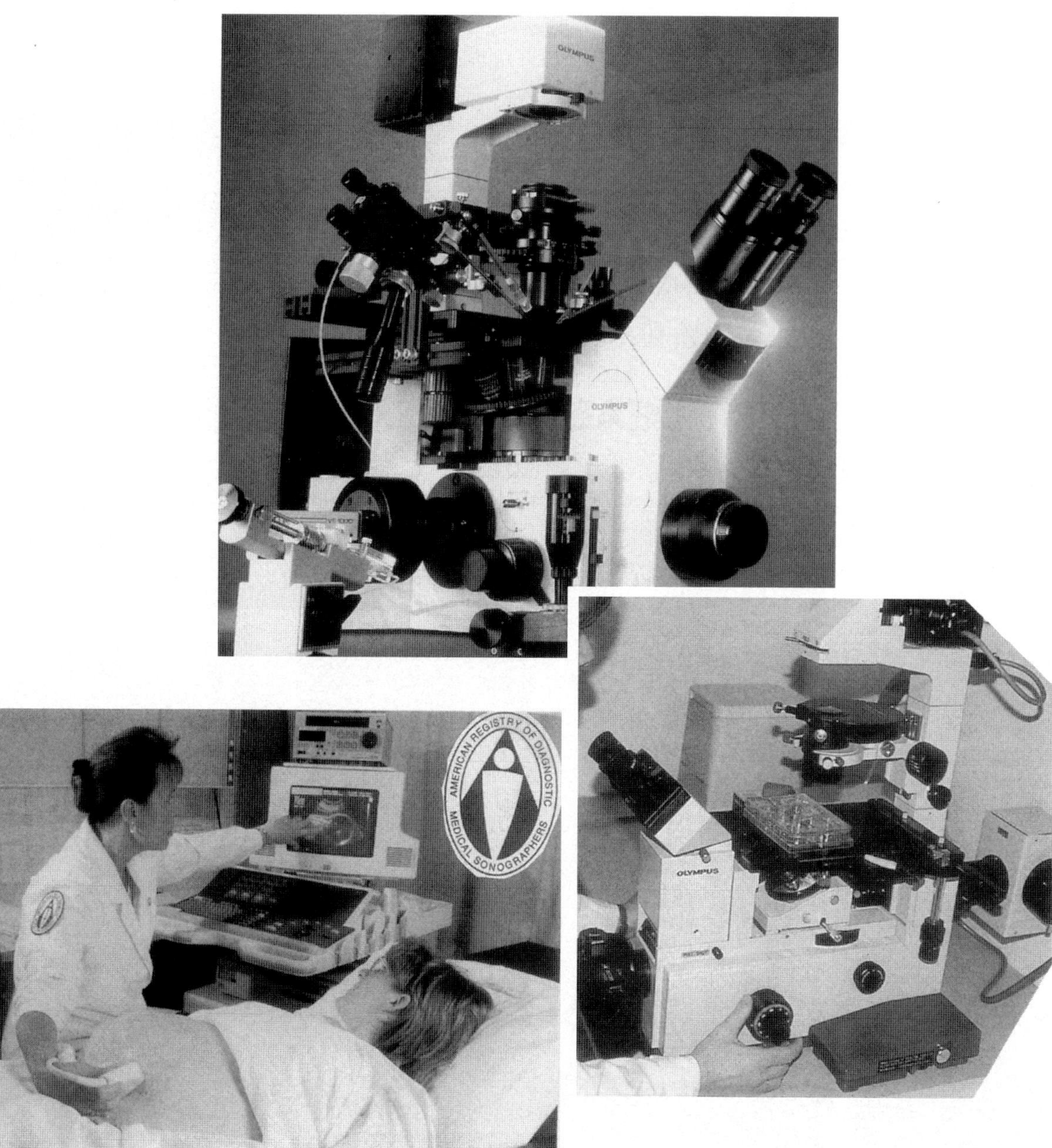


Evaluation of cell culture experiments using fluorescence technique.

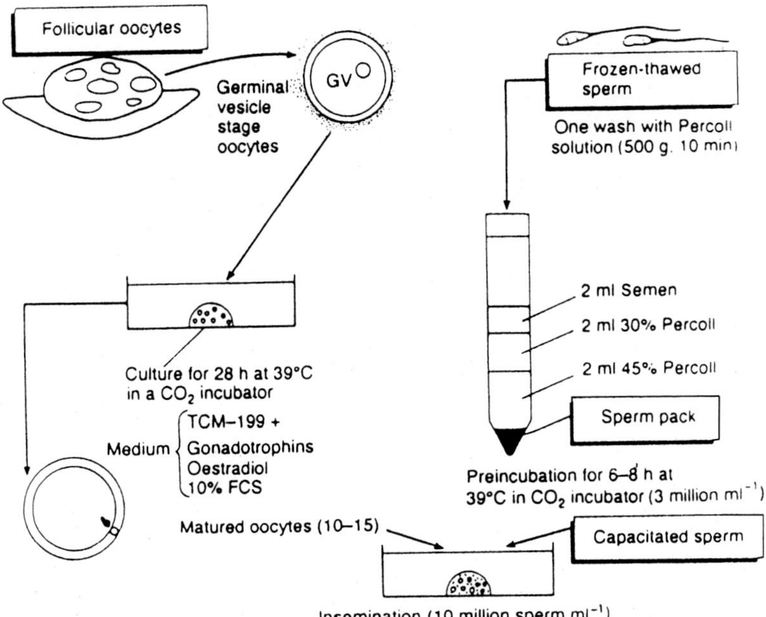


*In vitro* fertilization system (Kyoto University) for cattle (Iritani and associates). (Courtesy of Professor Iritani.)

# INDEX

Page numbers in *italics* indicate figures; those followed by a t indicate tables